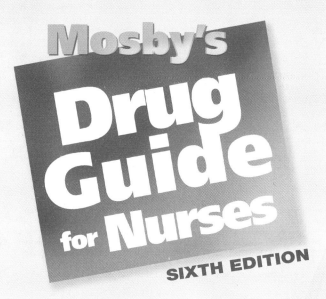

Mosby's Drug Guide for Nurses

SIXTH EDITION

Linda Skidmore-Roth, RN, MSN, NP
Consultant
Littleton, Colorado
Formerly, Nursing Faculty

New Mexico State University
Las Cruces, New Mexico;
El Paso Community College,
El Paso, Texas

*Mosby's DrugSmart CD-ROM to
accompany Mosby's Drug Guide
for Nurses*

with 190 *illustrations and* 2 *color inserts*

ELSEVIER
MOSBY

ELSEVIER
MOSBY

11830 Westline Industrial Drive
St. Louis, Missouri 63146

Mosby's Drug Guide for Nurses, SIXTH EDITION   **ISBN: 0-323-03450-0**
Copyright © 2005 Mosby Inc. All rights reserved.

No refund without mini CD-ROM.

NOTICE

Pharmacology is an ever-changing field. Standard safety precautions must be followed, but as new research and clinical experience broaden our knowledge, changes in treatment and drug therapy may become necessary or appropriate. Readers are advised to check the most current product information provided by the manufacturer of each drug to be administered to verify the recommended dose, the method and duration of administration, and contraindications. It is the responsibility of the appropriately licensed treating health care provider, relying on experience and knowledge of the patient, to determine dosages and the best treatment for each individual patient. Neither the publisher nor the author assumes any liability for any injury and/or damage to persons or property arising from this publication.

Previous editions copyrighted 1996, 1997, 1999, 2001, 2003

International Standard Book Number: 0-323-03450-0

Executive Publisher, Nursing: Darlene Como
Developmental Editor: Laura Selkirk
Publishing Services Manager: Melissa Lastarria
Design Manager: Teresa McBryan

Printed in the United States of America

Last digit is the print number: 9   8   7   6   5   4   3   2   1

The Latest *Evolution* in Learning.

Evolve provides online access to free resources designed specifically for you. The resources will provide you with information that is in addition to material covered in the drug cards and much more.

Visit the Web address listed below to start your learning evolution today!

▶ **LOGIN:** http://evolve.elsevier.com/nursingdrugupdates/Skidmore/NDG

- **Drug Monographs**
  Includes full monographs for drugs new to this edition, less common drugs not found in this text, and individual penicillins.
- **FDA Alerts**
  Provides updates on drug and lot recalls, labeling changes, new interactions, and safety warnings.
- **Recently Approved Drugs**
  Offers a table of drugs approved by the FDA after publication of the book, including links to approved product inserts.
- **Drug Dosage Calculators**
  Includes drug dosage calculators to help determine body surface area, pediatric drug dosages, IV rates, capsule and tablet doses, and more.
- **Drug Name Safety Information**
  Links to organizations and resources involved in reducing medication errors caused by drug name confusion.
- **WebLinks**
  Links to websites covering FDA drug information, Canadian Drugs, Herbs and Botanicals, and Related Pharmacology.

Think outside the book... **evolve.**

Consultants

Jean Krajicek Bartek, PhD, APRN
Nurse Practitioner
University of Nebraska Medical Center
College of Nursing
Courtesy Faculty
College of Medicine (Pharmacology)
Omaha, Nebraska

Doris M. Bates, RN
Oncology/OB Staff Nurse
Penobscot Valley Hospital
Lincoln, Maine

Rita Hanover Berdan, MS, RN, C
Nursing Faculty
St. Joseph's Hospital Health Center School
  of Nursing
Syracuse, New York

Barbara L. Cary, MSN, RN
Adjunct Faculty
University of Maine
Augusta, Maine

Tamara Conroy, RMA, CPT, SPN
Pittston, Pennsylvania

Linda M. DeLamar-Gallos, CRNA, MSN, MS
Capital Health Systems
Mercer Campus
Trenton, New Jersey

Jennifer L. DiGiacinto, Pharm D
Clinical Pharmacologist
Office of Clinical Pharmacology
  and Biopharmaceutics
US Food and Drug Administration
Rockville, Maryland

Henry B. Geiter, Jr, RN, C, CCRN
Vencor Hospital
St. Petersburg Junior College
St. Petersburg, Florida

F. James Grogan, PharmD
Executive Director
Grogan Communications
Swansea, Illinois

Jennifer L. Gudeman, PharmD
Product Surveillance Specialist
Corporate Product Monitoring
Mallinckrodt / Tyco Healthcare
St. Louis, Missouri

Scott Harrington, PharmD, RPh
Harrington Health Informatics
Tucson, Arizona

Phyllis Howard, RN, BSN
Associate Professor of Practical Nursing
Ashland Technical College
Ashland, Kentucky

Peter Huynh, PharmD
Pharmacotherapy Fellow
Washington State University
Spokane, Washington

Joan Ann Leach, RNC, MS, ME
Professor of Nursing
Capital Community College
Hartford, Connecticut

Mary Jo Mattocks, PhD, MN, BSN
Assistant Professor
Montana State University
Northern Great Falls Campus
Great Falls, Montana

Jennifer L. McQuade, PharmD
Medical Information Consultant
St. Louis, Missouri

Michelle M. Montpas, RN, MSN, OCN
CS Mott Community College
Flint, Michigan

Janet Rentfro, RN, ADN, ACLS
Medical Supervisor
Ascension Island
South Atlantic Ocean

Becky A. Ridenhour, PharmD
St. Louis College of Pharmacy
St. Louis, Missouri

Roberta J. Secrest, PhD, PharmD, RPh
Eli Lilly and Company
Indianapolis, Indiana

Patricia R. Teasley, APRN, BC
Professor
Nursing Department
Central Texas Collge
Killeen, Texas

Brenda L. Thompson, PharmD
Assistant Professor
Pharmacy Practice Division
St. Louis College of Pharmacy
St. Louis, Missouri

Joyce S. Willens, PhD, RN
Assistant Professor
College of Nursing
Villanova University
Villanova, Pennsylvania

Preface

Mosby's Drug Guide for Nurses, 6th edition, is the most in-depth handbook available for nursing students and practicing nurses! Since its first publication in 1996, more than 100 U.S. and Canadian pharmacists and consultants have reviewed the book's content closely. Today, *Mosby's Drug Guide for Nurses* is more up to date than ever—with features that make it easy to find critical information fast!

NEW FACTS

This edition features more than 2,000 new drug facts, including:
- new drugs and new dosage information
- newly researched side effects and adverse reactions
- the latest precautions, interactions, and contraindications, including highlighted pediatric and geriatric considerations
- IV therapy updates
- revised nursing considerations
- updated patient/family teaching guidelines

NEW FEATURES
- "Tall Man" lettering (required by the FDA for drug manufacturers) uses capitalization of distinguishing letters in 35 look-alike generic drug names to avoid medication errors.
- Error-prone abbreviations (μg, IU, U, MgSO4, MS, MSO4) no longer used as recommended by JCAHO.
- Monographs for 112 "high-alert" medications are highlighted with a blue background in the A-to-Z section to remind you to use extra care in administering these drugs. Appendix C provides a complete list of "high-alert" drugs most capable of causing significant harm to patients.
- Appendix A, "Selected new drugs," provides detailed monographs for 17 drugs recently approved by the FDA. (See Table of Contents for complete list.) Included are monographs for:
  - fosamprenavir (Lexiva) for treatment of HIV infection
  - memantine (Namenda) for treatment of Alzheimer disease
  - rosuvastatin (Crestor) for treatment of hypercholesterolemia
  - vardenafil (Levitra) for treatment of erectile dysfunction
- Appendix B, "Recent FDA drug approvals," lists generic/trade names and uses for 8 of the most recently approved drugs.
- *DrugSmart* CD-ROM offers monographs on 40 commonly used herbs, a drug interactions tool, drug dosage calculators and other clinically useful calculators, patient teaching guides in English and Spanish for commonly used drugs, and extra monographs for less frequently used drugs not included in the book

ORGANIZATION

This handbook is organized into three main sections:
- Individual drug monographs (in alphabetical order by generic name)
- Drug categories
- Appendixes (identified by the wide blue thumb tabs on the edge)

and three smaller sections that provide additional valuable information for nursing students:

- Disorders Index (follows the Appendixes)
- Drug Identification Guide (full-color center insert)
- Photo Atlas of Drug Administration (full-color center insert)

The guiding principle behind this book is to provide fast, easy access to drug information and nursing considerations. Every detail—from the cover, binding, and paper to the typeface, two-color design, eye-catching icons, and appendixes—has been carefully chosen with the user in mind. Here's what you'll find in each section of the handbook:

Individual Drug Monographs

This book includes monographs for more than 4,000 generic and trade name medications—those most commonly administered by students. Common trade names are given for all drugs regularly used in the United States and Canada, with drugs available only in Canada identified by a maple leaf icon (✤).

Each monograph provides the following information, whenever possible, for safe, effective administration of each drug:

High-alert status: Identifies drugs with the most potential to cause harm to patients, screened in light blue for easy identification.

Key drug status: Identifies drugs of special prominence within their functional class, often encountered by students during clinicals; denoted with a special icon (⚷).

Pronunciation: Helps the nurse master complex generic names.

Rx/OTC: Identifies prescription or over-the-counter drugs.

Functional and chemical classifications: Helps the nurse recognize similarities and differences among drugs in the same functional but different chemical classes.

Pregnancy category: FDA pregnancy categories A, B, C, D, or X are noted at the beginning of the monograph, as well as under Precautions or Contraindications depending on FDA category. Appendix J provides a detailed explanation of each category.

Controlled substance schedule: Includes schedules for the United States (I, II, III, IV, V) and Canada (F, G)

Action: Describes pharmacologic properties concisely.

Therapeutic outcome: Details all possible results of medication use, denoted with a special icon (➡).

Uses: Lists the conditions the drug is used to treat.

Investigational uses: Describes drug uses that may be encountered in practice but are not yet FDA-approved.

Dosage and routes: Lists all available and approved dosages and routes for adult, pediatric, and elderly patients.

"Pediatric" and "Geriatric" icons: Special icons (P and G) in the margins of the Dosage and routes, Contraindications, and Precautions sections that denote lifespan content.

Available forms: Includes tablets, capsules, extended-release, injectables (**IV**, IM, SC), solutions, creams, ointments, lotions, gels, shampoos, elixirs, suspensions, suppositories, sprays, aerosols, and lozenges.

Adverse effects: Groups potential reactions by body system, with common side effects *italicized* and life-threatening reactions in **bold type** for emphasis.

Contraindications: Lists conditions under which the drug absolutely should not be given, including FDA pregnancy safety categories D or X.

Precautions: Lists conditions that require special consideration when the drug is prescribed, including FDA pregnancy safety categories, A, B, and C.

"Do not confuse" icon (▨): Denotes drug names that might easily be confused, within each appropriate monograph.

Pharmacokinetics/pharmacodynamics: Features a quick-reference chart of concise facts on pharmacokinetics (absorption, distribution, metabolism, excretion, half-life) and pharmacodynamics (onset, peak, duration).

Interactions: Lists confirmed drug, food, and herbal interactions, grouped by effect.

"Herb-Drug Interaction" icon (▱): Highlights more than 400 potential interactions between herbal products and prescription or OTC drugs.

Lab test interferences: Identifies how the drug may affect lab test results.

Nursing considerations: Identifies key nursing considerations for each step of the nursing process: Assessment, Nursing Diagnoses (denoted with a special icon ☑), Implementation, Patient/Family Education, and Evaluation, including positive therapeutic outcomes. Instructions for giving drugs by various routes (e.g., **IV**, IM, SC, PO, topically, rectally) appear under Implementation, with route subheadings in bold.

Compatibilities: Lists syringe, Y-site, and additive compatibilities and incompatibilities. If no compatibilities are listed for a drug, the necessary compatibility testing has not been done and that compatibility information is unknown. To ensure safety, assume that the drug may not be mixed with other drugs unless specifically stated.

"Nursing Alert" icon (◆): Highlights situations in which the patient potentially could be at risk.

"Do Not Crush" icon (▧): Denotes drugs that may not be administered in crushed form.

Treatment of overdose: Lists drugs and treatments for overdoses where appropriate.

Drug Categories

The Drug Categories section, following the individual drug monographs, provides general information about the various functional classes to promote learning about the similarities and differences among drugs in the same functional class. It summarizes action, uses, adverse effects, contraindications, precautions, pharmacokinetics, interactions, and nursing considerations for each functional class.

Appendixes

Selected new drugs: Includes comprehensive information on 17 key drugs approved by the FDA during the last 12 months.

Recent FDA drug approvals: Summarizes basic information, such as generic name, trade name and uses, for drugs so recently approved by the FDA that complete information was not yet available when this book went to press.

High-alert drugs: Lists the 112 drugs in *Mosby's Drug Guide for Nurses* that are considered high-alert because of their potential to cause significant harm to patients.

Ophthalmic, otic, nasal, and topical products: Provides monographs for more than 150 ophthalmic, otic, nasal, and topical products commonly used today, grouped by chemical drug class.

Combination products: Provides details on the forms and uses of more than 700 combination products.

Rarely used drugs: Provides concise monographs for 125 infrequently used drugs, including dosage and routes, uses, and contraindications.

Less frequently used antihistamines: Includes names, uses, doses, forms, interactions, and contraindications.

Vaccines and toxoids: Features an easy-to-use table with generic and trade names, uses, dosages and routes, and contraindications for 32 key vaccines and toxoids.

Herbal products: Features basic usage information on more than 70 common herbs and natural supplements.

FDA pregnancy categories: Explains the 5 FDA pregnancy categories.

Controlled substance chart: Covers both United States and Canadian drug schedules, with examples.

Commonly used abbreviations: Lists abbreviations alphabetically with their meanings.

IV drug/solution compatibility chart: Lists compatibilities for 52 **IV** drugs and solutions.

Nomogram for calculation of body surface area: Provides a quick, handy chart for calculating body surface area for patient drug calculations.

Disorders Index

This book includes both a general index and a disorders index, both of which are updated and expanded in this edition. Dovetailing with the content nursing students encounter in medical-surgical courses, the disorders index lists major disorders and major drugs used in their management. The page number for each drug listed follows.

Drug Identification Guide

The Drug Identification Guide includes 160 full-color photos showing the top 60 prescribed drugs as tabulated in *Mosby's Drug Consult*. Photos are arranged alphabetically by generic name, with dosage strengths listed.

Photo Atlas of Drug Administration

This practical resource for students and practitioners lists standard precautions and provides 30 full-color illustrations depicting the physical landmarks and administration techniques used for **IV**, IM, SC, and ID drug delivery.

The following sources were consulted in the preparation of this edition:

Blumenthal M: *The complete German Commission E monographs: therapeutic guide to herbal medicines,* Austin, 2002, American Botanical Council.

Drug information: Bethesda, American Hospital Formulary Service.

Facts and comparisons: St Louis, updated monthly.

Gahart BL: *Intravenous medications,* ed 18, St Louis, 2004, Mosby.

Goodman A and others: *Goodman and Gilman's the pharmacological basis of therapeutics,* ed 11, New York, 2002, Pergamon Press.

McKenry LM, Salerno E: *Mosby's pharmacology in nursing,* ed 21, St Louis, 2003, Mosby.

Mediphor Editorial Group: *Drug interaction facts,* Philadelphia, updated quarterly, JB Lippincott.

Review of natural products: Philadelphia, updated monthly, *Facts and Comparisons.*

Acknowledgments

I am indebted to the nursing and pharmacology consultants who reviewed the manuscript and galley pages and thank them for their criticism and encouragement. I would also like to thank Darlene Como, Laura Selkirk, and Brian Dennison, my editors, whose active encouragement and enthusiasm have made this book better than it might otherwise have been. I am likewise grateful to Melissa Lastarria and Graphic World, Inc., for the coordination of the production process and assistance with the development of the new edition.

Linda Skidmore-Roth

Contents

Drug Monographs New to This Edition

abacavir (Rx)

(aba-ka'veer)

Ziagen

Func. class.: Antiretroviral

Chem. class.: Nucleoside reverse transcriptase inhibitor (NRTI)

Pregnancy category C

Action: A synthetic, nucleoside analog with inhibitory action against HIV. Inhibits replication of HIV by incorporating into cellular DNA by viral reverse transcriptase, thereby terminating the cellular DNA chain

→ **Therapeutic Outcome:** Decreased symptoms of HIV

Uses: In combination with other antiretroviral agents for HIV-1 infection

Dosage and routes

Adult: PO 300 mg bid with other antiretrovirals

Adolescents and children ≥3 mo: PO 8 mg/kg bid, max 300 mg bid with other antiretrovirals

Available forms: Tabs 300 mg; oral sol 20 mg/ml

Adverse effects

(*italic* = common; **bold** = life-threatening)

CNS: Fever, headache, malaise, insomnia, paresthesia

GI: Nausea, vomiting, diarrhea, anorexia, cramps, abdominal pain, ↑ *AST, ALT*

HEMA: **Granulocytopenia, anemia,** lymphopenia

INTEG: Rash, **fatal hypersensitivity reactions,** urticaria

META: **Lactic acidosis**

MISC: ↑ CPK

RESP: Dyspnea

Contraindications: Hypersensitivity

Precautions: Granulocyte count <1000/mm³ or Hgb <9.5 g/dl, pregnancy **C**, lactation, children, severe renal disease, severe hepatic function

Pharmacokinetics

Absorption	Well absorbed (PO)
Distribution	50% plasma protein binding
Metabolism	To inactive metabolite
Excretion	Kidneys, feces
Half-life	1½-2 hr

Pharmacodynamics

Unknown

Interactions

Individual drugs

Alcohol: ↑ abacavir levels; do not use with alcohol

Ribavirin: possible lactic acidosis

NURSING CONSIDERATIONS

Assessment

- Assess for lactic acidosis (elevated lactate levels, ↑ liver function tests) and severe hepatomegaly with steatosis; discontinue treatment
- Assess for fatal hypersensitivity reactions: fever, rash, nausea, vomiting, fatigue, cough, dyspnea, diarrhea, abdominal discomfort; treatment should be discontinued and not restarted
- Assess for pancreatitis: abdominal pain, nausea, vomiting, elevated liver enzymes; drug should be discontinued because condition can be fatal
- Monitor CBC, differential, platelet count qmo; withhold drug if WBC is <4000/mm³ or platelet count is <75,000/mm³; notify prescriber of results; monitor viral load and CD4 counts during treatment
- Monitor renal function studies; BUN, serum uric acid, urine CCr before, during therapy; these may be elevated throughout treatment
- Monitor temp q4h, may indicate beginning infection
- Monitor liver function tests before, during therapy (bilirubin, AST, ALT, amylase, alkaline phosphatase prn or qmo)

Nursing diagnoses

☑ Infection, risk for (uses)

☑ Injury, risk for physical injury (adverse reactions)

☑ Knowledge, deficient (teaching)

Implementation

PO route

- Give on empty stomach, q12h around the clock
- Give in combination with other antiretrovirals with or without food
- Store in cool environment; protect from light, do not freeze

Patient/family education

- Advise patient to report signs of infection: increased temp, sore throat, flu symptoms; to avoid crowds and those with known infections
- Instruct patient to report signs of anemia: fatigue, headache, faintness, shortness of breath, irritability
- Advise patient to report bleeding; avoid use of razors or commercial mouthwash

---

- Inform patient that drug is not a cure, but will control symptoms
- Inform patient that major toxicities may necessitate discontinuing drug
- Instruct patient to use contraception during treatment
- Caution patient to avoid OTC products or other medications without approval of prescriber
- Caution patient not to have any sexual contact without use of a condom, needles should not be shared, blood from infected individual should not come in contact with another's mucous membranes
- Give Medication Guide and Warning Card; discuss points on guide
- Advise patient to stop drug if skin rash, fever, cough, shortness of breath, GI symptoms occur, notify prescriber immediately; advise all health care providers that allergic reactions have occurred with this drug

Evaluation
Positive therapeutic outcome
- Decreased infection; symptoms of HIV

---

acarbose (Rx)
(a-kar'bose)
Prandese ✦, Precose
Func. class.: Oral antidiabetic
Chem. class.: α-Glucosidase inhibitor
Pregnancy category B

Action: Delays the digestion of ingested carbohydrates, results in a smaller rise in blood glucose after meals; does not increase insulin production

➡ Therapeutic Outcome: Decreased blood glucose levels in diabetes mellitus

Uses: Stable adult-onset diabetes mellitus (type 2), alone or in combination with a sulfonylurea

Dosage and routes
Initial dose
Adult: PO 25 mg tid with first bite of meal

Maintenance dose
Adult: PO may be increased to 50-100 mg tid; dosage adjustment at 4-8 wk intervals

Adult <60 kg: PO not to exceed 100 mg tid

Available forms: Tabs 25, 50, 100 mg

Adverse effects
(*italic* = common; **bold** = life-threatening)
GI: Abdominal pain, diarrhea, flatulence, increased serum transaminase level

Contraindications: Hypersensitivity, diabetic ketoacidosis, cirrhosis, inflammatory bowel disease, colonic ulceration, partial intestinal obstruction, chronic intestinal disease, serum creatinine >2 mg/dl

Precautions: Pregnancy **B**, renal disease, **P** lactation, children, hepatic disease

Pharmacokinetics	
Absorption	Unknown
Distribution	Unknown
Metabolism	GI tract
Excretion	Kidneys as intact drug
Half-life	Elimination 2 hr

Pharmacodynamics
Peak 1 hr

Interactions
Individual drugs
Digoxin: ↓ acarbose effect
Insulin, phenytoin: ↑ hypoglycemia
Isoniazid, nicotinic acid, thyroid: ↑ hyperglycemia
Drug classifications
Calcium channel blockers, corticosteroids, diuretics, estrogens, oral contraceptives, phenothiazines, progestins, sympathomimetics: ↑ hyperglycemia
Digestive enzymes, intestinal absorbents: ↓ effect of acarbose
Sulfonylureas: ↑ hypoglycemia
⊘ Herb/drug
Alfalfa, aloe, basil, bay, bilberry, bitter melon, black catechu, buchu, burdock, coriander, dandelion, eyebright (po), fenugreek, garlic, ginseng, glucomannan, glucosamine, goat's rue, gymnema, horehound, horse chestnut, jambul, myrrh, myrtle: ↑ antidiabetic effect
Bee pollen, blue cohosh, broom, chromium, elecampane, eucalyptus, gotu kola: ↓ antidiabetic effect
Lab test interferences
↑ AST, bilirubin
↓ Calcium, vit B_6

NURSING CONSIDERATIONS
Assessment
- Assess for hypoglycemia (weakness, hunger, dizziness, tremors, anxiety, tachycardia, sweating), hyperglycemia; even though this drug does not cause hypoglycemia, if on a sulfonylurea or insulin, hypoglycemia may be additive; if hypoglycemia occurs, treat with glucose or if severe, **IV** dextrose or IM glucagon
- Monitor 1 hr postprandial for establishing effectiveness, then glycosylated Hgb q3 mo

---

- Monitor AST, ALT q3 mo × 1 yr, and periodically thereafter, if elevated dose may need to be reduced or discontinued; obtain glycosylated Hgb periodically

Nursing diagnoses
☑ Nutrition: more than body requirements (uses), imbalanced
☑ Nutrition: less than body requirements (adverse reactions), imbalanced
☑ Knowledge, deficient (teaching)
☑ Noncompliance (teaching)

Implementation
PO route
- Give tid with first bite of each meal
- Provide storage in tight container in cool environment

Patient/family education
- Teach patient the symptoms of hypoglycemia, hyperglycemia and what to do about each
- Instruct that medication must be taken as prescribed; explain consequences of discontinuing the medication abruptly; that insulin may need to be used during stress such as trauma, surgery, fever
- Tell patient to avoid OTC medications, herbal products unless approved by prescriber
- Teach patient that diabetes is a life-long illness; drug will not cure condition
- Instruct patient to carry/wear emergency ID as diabetic
- Teach patient that diet and exercise regimen must be followed

Evaluation
Positive therapeutic outcome
- Improved signs, symptoms of diabetes mellitus (decreased polyuria, polydipsia, polyphagia; clear sensorium, absence of dizziness, stable gait)

---

acebutolol (Rx)
(a-se-byoo′ toe-lole)
Monitan ♣, Sectral
Func. class.: Antihypertensive
Chem. class.: Selective β_1-blocker; group II antidysrhythmic (II)

Pregnancy category B

Action: Competitively blocks stimulation of β-adrenergic receptors within vascular smooth muscle (decreases rate of SA node discharge, increases recovery time), slows conduction of AV node resulting in decreased heart rate (negative chronotropic effect), which decreases O_2 consumption in myocardium because of β_1-receptor antagonism, also decreases renin-aldosterone-angiotensin system at high doses, inhibits β_2-receptors in bronchial system (high doses)

⇒**Therapeutic Outcome:** Decreased B/P, heart rate, AV conduction, control of dysrhythmias

Uses: Mild to moderate hypertension, sinus tachycardia, persistent atrial extrasystoles, tachydysrhythmias, management of PVCs

Investigational uses: Prophylaxis of MI, treatment of angina pectoris, tremor, mitral valve prolapse, thyrotoxicosis, idiopathic hypertrophic subaortic stenosis

Dosage and routes
Hypertension
Adult: PO 400 mg qd or in 2 divided doses; may be increased to desired response; maintenance 200-1200 mg/qd in 2 divided doses

Ventricular dysrhythmia
Adult: PO 200 mg bid, may increase gradually; usual range 600-1200 mg daily; should be tapered over 2 wk before discontinuing

G *Elderly:* PO not to exceed 800 mg/qd

Renal dose
Adult: PO CCr 25-50 ml/min, reduce dose by 50%; if <25 ml/min reduce dose by 75%

Available forms: Caps 200, 400 mg; tabs 100, 200, 400 mg ♣

Adverse effects
(*italic* = common; **bold** = life-threatening)
CNS: *Insomnia, fatigue, dizziness, mental changes,* memory loss, hallucinations, depression, lethargy, drowsiness, strange dreams, catatonia
CV: **Profound hypotension, bradycardia, CHF, cold extremities, postural hypotension, 2nd- or 3rd-degree heart block**
EENT: Sore throat; dry, burning eyes
ENDO: Increased hypoglycemic response to insulin
GI: *Nausea, diarrhea,* vomiting, **mesenteric arterial thrombosis, ischemic colitis,** flatulence
GU: *Impotence,* decreased libido, dysuria, nocturia
HEMA: **Agranulocytosis, thrombocytopenia, purpura**
INTEG: Rash, flushing, pruritus, sweating, alopecia, dry skin
MS: Joint pain, cramping
RESP: **Bronchospasm,** dyspnea, wheezing, cough
MISC: Facial swelling, weight gain, decreased exercise tolerance

Contraindications: Hypersensitivity to β-blockers, cardiogenic shock, heart block (2nd or 3rd degree), sinus bradycardia, CHF, cardiac failure

Precautions: Major surgery, pregnancy **B**, lactation, diabetes mellitus, renal disease, thyroid disease, COPD, asthma, well-**P** compensated heart failure, hepatic disease, peripheral vascular disease, children

Pharmacokinetics

Absorption	Well absorbed
Distribution	Crosses placenta, minimal CNS; protein binding 26%
Metabolism	Liver to diacetolol
Excretion	Urine
Half-life	8-13 hr diacetolol, 3-4 hr acebutolol

Pharmacodynamics

	PO (ANTIHYPERTENSIVE)	PO (ANTIDYSRHYTHMICS)
Onset	1-1½ hr	1 hr
Peak	2-4 hr	4-6 hr
Duration	12-24 hr	10-12 hr

Interactions
Individual drugs
Alcohol (large amounts), cimetidine, diltiazem, hydrALAZINE, prazosin: ↑ hypotension
Cholestyramine, colestipol: ↓ antihypertensive effect
Cimetidine, diltiazem, hydrALAZINE, prazosin: bradycardia
Ergots: ↑ peripheral ischemia
Insulin: ↑ hypoglycemia
Thyroid: ↓ effectiveness
Verapamil: ↑ myocardial depression
Drug classifications
Antidiabetics, oral: ↑ hypoglycemic effect
Antihypertensives: ↑ hypertension
Calcium channel blockers, diuretics, nitrates: ↑ hypotension
Calcium channel blockers, cardiac glycosides, diuretics: bradycardia
NSAIDs: ↓ antihypertensive effect
Theophyllines: ↓ bronchodilatation
Herb/drug
Aconite: ↑ toxicity, death
Aloe, buckthorn bark/berry, cascara sagrada bark, rhubarb root, senna leaf/fruits: ↑ acebutolol effect
Astragalus, cola tree: ↑ or ↓ antihypertensive effect

Barberry, betony, black catechu, black cohosh, bloodroot, broom, burdock, cat's claw, dandelion, figwort, fumitory, goldenseal, Irish moss, Jamaican dogwood, kelp, khella, kudzu, licorice, mistletoe, parsley: ↑ antihypertensive effect
Coltsfoot, guarana, khat, licorice: ↓ antihypertensive effect
Horehound: ↑ serotonin effect
Lab test interferences
False positive: Antinuclear antibodies titer
↑ serum lipoprotein levels, BUN, potassium, triglyceride, uric acid, LDH, AST, ALT, blood glucose, alkaline phosphatase

NURSING CONSIDERATIONS
Assessment
• Monitor B/P during beginning treatment, periodically thereafter; pulse q4h; note rate, rhythm, quality; apical/radial pulse before administration; notify prescriber of any significant changes (pulse <50 bpm)
• Check for baselines in renal, liver function tests before therapy begins
• Assess for edema in feet, legs daily, monitor I&O, daily weight; check for jugular vein distention, rales bilaterally, dyspnea (CHF)
• Monitor skin turgor, dryness of mucous membranes for hydration status, especially elderly

Nursing diagnoses
✓ Cardiac output, decreased (side effects)
✓ Injury, risk for physical (side effects)
✓ Knowledge, deficient (teaching)
✓ Noncompliance (teaching)

Implementation
PO route
• Given ac, hs; tablet may be crushed or swallowed whole; give with food to prevent GI upset; reduced dosage in renal dysfunction; check pulse before giving, hold dose and notify prescriber if pulse is <60 bpm
• Store protected from light, moisture; place in cool environment

Patient/family education
• Teach patient not to discontinue drug abruptly, severe cardiac reactions may occur, taper over 2 wk; may cause precipitate angina if stopped abruptly
• Advise patient that drug may mask signs of hypoglycemia or alter blood glucose levels
• Teach patient not to use OTC products containing α-adrenergic stimulants (such as nasal decongestants, cold preparations); to

---

avoid alcohol, smoking; to limit sodium intake as prescribed
• Teach patient how to take pulse and B/P at home, advise when to notify prescriber
• Instruct patient to comply with weight control, dietary adjustments, modified exercise program
• Tell patient to carry/wear emergency ID to identify drug(s) that patient is taking, allergies; tell patient that drug controls symptoms but does not cure
• Caution patient to avoid hazardous activities if dizziness or drowsiness is present; that drug may cause sensitivity to cold
• Teach patient to report symptoms of CHF: difficult breathing, especially on exertion or when lying down, night cough, swelling of extremities or bradycardia, dizziness, confusion, depression, fever
• Teach patient to take drug as prescribed, not to double or skip doses; take any missed doses as soon as remembered if several hours until next dose
• Advise patient to continue with required lifestyle changes (exercise, diet, weight loss, stress reduction)

Evaluation
Positive therapeutic outcome
• Decreased B/P in hypertension (after 1-2 wk)
• Absence of dysrhythmias

Treatment of overdose: Lavage, **IV** atropine for bradycardia, **IV** theophylline for bronchospasm, digitalis, O₂, diuretic for cardiac failure, hemodialysis, **IV** glucose for hypoglycemia, **IV** diazepam (or phenytoin) for seizures

---

acetaminophen ⊕ₐ (OTC)
(a-seat-a-mee′noe-fen)
Abenol ✦, Acephen, Aceta, Actimol, Aminofen, Apacet, APAP, Apo-Acetaminophen ✦, Arthritis Foundation Pain Reliever Aspirin-Free, Aspirin-Free Anacin, Aspirin-Free Pain Relief, Atasol ✦, Banesin, Children's Feverall, Dapa, Dapacin, Datril, Exdol ✦, FemEtts, Genapap, Genebs, Halenol, Liquiprin, Mapap, Maranox, Meda, Neopap, Oraphen-PD, Panadol, Redutemp, Robigesic ✦, Rounax ✦, Silapap, Tapanol, Tempra, Tylenol
Func. class.: Nonopioid analgesic
Chem. class.: Nonsalicylate, paraaminophenol derivative

Pregnancy category B

Action: May block pain impulses peripherally that occur in response to inhibition of prostaglandin synthesis; does not possess antiinflammatory properties; antipyretic action results from inhibition of prostaglandins in the CNS (hypothalamic heat-regulating center)

⮕**Therapeutic Outcome:** Decreased pain, fever

Uses: Mild to moderate pain or fever

Dosage and routes
℗ *Adult and child >12 yr:* PO/REC 325-650 mg q4h prn, max 4 g/day
ℙ *Child:* PO 10-15 mg/kg q4h
ℙ *Child 6-12 yr:* REC 325 mg q4-6h, max 2-6 g/day
ℙ *Child 3-6 yr:* REC 125 mg q4-6h, max 720 mg/day
ℙ *Child 1-3 yr:* REC 80 mg q4h
ℙ *Child 3-11 mo:* REC 80 mg q6h

Available forms: REC supp 80, 120, 125, 325, 600, 650 mg; chewable tabs 80, 160 mg; caps 500 mg; elix 120, 160, 325 mg/5 ml; liq 120, 160 mg/5 ml, 500 mg/15 ml; sol 100 mg/1 ml, 120 mg/2.5 ml; tabs 160, 325, 500, 650 mg; granules 80 mg/pkg or cup

Adverse effects
(*italic* = common; **bold** = life-threatening)
CNS: Stimulation, drowsiness
GI: Nausea, vomiting, abdominal pain; **hepatotoxicity, hepatic seizure (overdose)**
GU: **Renal failure** (high, prolonged doses)
HEMA: **Leukopenia, neutropenia, hemolytic anemia (long-term use), thrombocytopenia, pancytopenia**

INTEG: Rash, urticaria
SYST: **Hypersensitivity**
TOXICITY: **Cyanosis, anemia, neutropenia, jaundice, pancytopenia, CNS stimulation, delirium followed by vascular collapse, convulsions, coma, death**

Contraindications: Hypersensitivity; intolerance to tartrazine (yellow dye #5), alcohol, table sugar, saccharin, depending on product

Precautions: Anemia, hepatic disease, renal disease, chronic alcoholism, pregnancy **G** B, elderly, lactation

Pharmacokinetics

Absorption	Well absorbed (PO), variable (REC)
Distribution	Widely distributed; crosses placenta in low concentrations
Metabolism	Liver 85%-95%; metabolites are toxic at high levels
Excretion	Kidneys—metabolites, breast milk
Half-life	3-4 hr

Pharmacodynamics

	PO	REC
Onset	½-1 hr	½-1 hr
Peak	1-3 hr	1-3 hr
Duration	3-4 hr	3-4 hr

Interactions
Individual drugs
Alcohol, carbamazepine, diflunisal, isoniazid, rifabutin, rifampin, sulfinpyrazone: ↑ hepatotoxicity, ↓ effect
Colestipol, cholestyramine: ↓ absorption of acetaminophen
Warfarin: Hypoprothrombinemia; long-term use, high doses of acetaminophen
Zidovudine: ↑ bone marrow suppression
Drug classifications
Barbiturates, hydantoins: ↓ effect, ↑ hepatotoxicity
NSAIDs, salicylates: ↑ renal adverse reactions
Lab test interferences
Interference: Chemstrip G, Dextrostix, Visidex II, 5-HIAA

NURSING CONSIDERATIONS
Assessment
• Monitor liver function studies: AST, ALT, bilirubin, creatinine before therapy if long-term therapy is anticipated; may cause hepatic toxicity at doses >4 g/day with chronic use
• Monitor renal function studies: BUN, urine creatinine, occult blood; albumin indicates nephritis

• Monitor blood studies: CBC, pro-time if patient is on long-term therapy
• Check I&O ratio; decreasing output may indicate renal failure (long-term therapy)
• Assess for fever and pain: type of pain, location, intensity, duration, temperature, diaphoresis
• Assess for chronic poisoning: rapid, weak pulse; dyspnea; cold, clammy extremities; report immediately to prescriber
• Assess hepatotoxicity: dark urine, clay-colored stools, yellowing of skin and sclera; itching, abdominal pain, fever, diarrhea if patient is on long-term therapy
• Assess allergic reactions: rash, urticaria; if these occur, drug may have to be discontinued

Nursing diagnoses
☑ Pain (uses)
☑ Mobility, impaired physical (uses)
☑ Injury, risk for (side effects)
☑ Knowledge, deficient (teaching)

Implementation
PO route
• Administer to patient crushed or whole; chewable tabs may be chewed
• Give with food or milk to decrease gastric symptoms; give 30 min before or 2 hr after meals; absorption may be slowed

Patient/family education
◆● Teach patient not to exceed recommended dosage; acute poisoning with liver damage may result; acute toxicity includes symptoms of nausea, vomiting, and abdominal pain; prescriber should be notified immediately
• Tell patient to read label on other OTC drugs; many contain acetaminophen and may cause toxicity if taken concurrently
• Teach patient to recognize signs of chronic overdose: bleeding, bruising, malaise, fever, sore throat
• Inform patient that urine may become dark brown as a result of phenacetin (metabolite of acetaminophen)
• Tell patient to notify prescriber for pain or fever lasting more than 3 days

Evaluation
Positive therapeutic outcome
• Decreased pain
• Decreased fever

Treatment of overdose: Drug level q4h, gastric lavage, activated charcoal; administer oral acetylcysteine to prevent hepatic damage (*see acetylcysteine monograph,* pp. 9-10)

☑ Herb/drug   ⊘ Do Not Crush   ◆ Alert   ◆☊ Key Drug   **G** Geriatric   **P** Pediatric

*acetaZOLAMIDE (Rx)
(a-set-a-zole'-a-mide)
Apo-Acetazolamide ♣, acetaZOLAMIDE, Diamox, Diamox Sequels, Hydrazol
Func. class.: Diuretic carbonic anhydrase inhibitor; antiglaucoma agent, antiepileptic
Chem. class.: Sulfonamide derivative

Pregnancy category C

Action: Decreases the aqueous humor in the eye, which lowers intraocular pressure by the inhibition of carbonic anhydrase; also inhibits carbonic anhydrase activity in proximal renal tubules to decrease reabsorption of water, sodium, potassium, bicarbonate; decreases carbonic anhydrase in CNS, increasing seizure threshold; prevents uric acid or cysteine buildup in the renal system by the decrease in pH causing alkaline urine

→ **Therapeutic Outcome:** Decreased intraocular pressure; control of seizures; prevention and treatment of acute mountain sickness; prevention of uric acid/cysteine renal stones; decreased edema in lung tissue and peripherally; decreased B/P

Uses: Open-angle glaucoma, narrow-angle glaucoma (preoperatively if surgery delayed), epilepsy (petit mal, grand mal, mixed), edema in CHF, drug-induced edema, acute mountain sickness

Investigational uses: Prevention of uric acid/cysteine renal stones, decrease CSF production in infants with hydrocephalus

Dosage and routes
Closed angle glaucoma
Adult: PO/IM/**IV** 250 mg q4h or 250 mg bid, to be used for short-term therapy or 500 mg ES bid

Open angle glaucoma
Adult: PO/IM/**IV** 250 mg-1 g/day in divided doses for amounts over 250 mg or 500 mg SR bid

Edema in CHF
Adult: IM/**IV** 250-375 mg/day in AM

P Child: IM/**IV** 5 mg/kg/day in AM

Seizures
Adult: PO/IM/**IV** 8-30 mg/kg/day in 1-4 divided doses, usual range 375-1000 mg/day in divided doses tid or qid, or 300-900 mg/m²/day, not to exceed 1.5 g/day

P Child: PO/IM/**IV** 8-30 mg/kg/day in divided doses tid or qid, or 300-900 mg/m²/day, not to exceed 1 g/day

Mountain sickness
Adult: PO 250 mg q8-12h

Renal stones
Adult: PO 250 mg hs

P Infants with hydrocephalus
Infant: **IV** 5 mg/kg/day q6h, may be increased up to 100 mg/kg/day if tolerated

Available forms: Tabs 125, 250 mg; caps ext rel 500 mg; inj 500 mg

Adverse effects
*(italic = common; **bold** = life-threatening)*
CNS: Drowsiness, paresthesia, anxiety, depression, headache, dizziness, confusion, stimulation, fatigue, **seizures,** sedation, nervousness
EENT: Myopia, tinnitus
ENDO: Hyperglycemia, hypokalemia, hypocalcemia, hypomagnesemia, hyponatremia, hyperchloremia
GI: Nausea, vomiting, anorexia, constipation, diarrhea, melena, weight loss, **hepatic insufficiency,** taste alterations
GU: Frequency, hypokalemia, polyuria, **uremia,** glucosuria, hematuria, dysuria, crystalluria, renal calculi
HEMA: Aplastic anemia, hemolytic anemia, leukopenia, agranulocytosis, thrombocytopenia, purpura, pancytopenia
INTEG: Rash, pruritus, urticaria, fever, **Stevens-Johnson syndrome,** photosensitivity

Contraindications: Hypersensitivity to sulfonamides, severe renal disease, severe hepatic disease, electrolyte imbalances (hyponatremia, hypokalemia), hyperchloremic acidosis, Addison's disease, long-term use in narrow-angle glaucoma

Precautions: Hypercalcemia, pregnancy C

⬛ Do Not Confuse:
acetaZOLAMIDE/acetoHEXAMIDE, Diamox/Dobutrex, Diamox/Trimox

Pharmacokinetics	
Absorption	GI tract—65% if fasting, 75% with food; **IV**—complete
Distribution	Crosses placenta; widely distributed
Metabolism	None
Excretion	Kidneys, unchanged (80% within 24 hr); breast milk
Half-life	2½-5½ hr

Pharmacodynamics			
	PO	**PO–EXT REL**	**IV**
Onset	1½ hr	2 hr	2 min
Peak	2-4 hr	3-6 hr	15 min
Duration	8-12 hr	18-24 hr	4-5 hr

Interactions
Individual drugs
Amphotericin B: ↑ hypokalemia
Aspirin: ↑ excretion of aspirin
Cyclosporine: ↑ toxicity
Diflunisal: ↑ side effects
Lithium: ↑ excretion of lithium
Methenamine: ↓ acetaZOLAMIDE effect
Primidone: ↓ primidone level
Drug classifications
Amphetamines: ↑ action
Anticholinergics: ↑ anticholinergic action
Salicylates: ↑ toxicity
Lab test interferences
False positive: Urinary protein, 17-hydroxysteroids
↓ Thyroid iodine uptake

NURSING CONSIDERATIONS
Assessment
• Assess patient for tinnitus, hearing loss, ear pain; periodic testing of hearing is needed when high doses of this drug are given by **IV** route
• Monitor manifestations of hypokalemia: *RENAL:* acidic urine, reduced urine osmolality, nocturia, polyuria, polydipsia; *CARDIAC:* hypotension, broad T wave, U wave, ectopy, tachycardia, weak pulse; *NEURO:* muscle weakness, altered LOC, drowsiness, apathy, lethargy, confusion, depression; *GI:* anorexia, nausea, cramps, constipation, distention, paralytic ileus; *RESP:* hypoventilation, respiratory muscle weakness
• Monitor for CNS, GI, cardiovascular, integumentary, neurologic manifestations of hypocalcemia: *CNS:* personality changes, anxiety, disturbances, depression, psychosis, nausea, vomiting; *GI:* constipation, abdominal pain from muscle spasm; *CV:* decreased contractility, decreased cardiac output, hypotension, lengthened ST segment, prolonged QT interval; *INTEG:* scaling eczema, alopecia, hyperpigmentation; *NEURO:* tetany, muscle twitching, cramping, grimacing, seizure, altered deep tendon reflexes, spasm
• Monitor for manifestations of hypomagnesemia: *CNS:* agitation; *NEURO:* muscle twitching, paresthesias, hyperactive reflexes, positive Babinski's reflex, dysphagia, nystagmus, seizures, tetany; *GI:* nausea, vomiting, diarrhea, anorexia, abdominal distention; *CARDIAC:* ectopy, tachycardia, broad, flat, or inverted T waves, depressed ST segment, prolonged QT, decreased cardiac output, hypotension
• Monitor for manifestations of hyponatremia: *CV:* increased B/P, cold, clammy skin, hypovolemia, or hypervolemia, vomiting, diarrhea, abdominal cramps; *NEURO:* lethargy, increased intracranial pressure, confusion, headache, seizures, coma, fatigue, tremors, hyperreflexia
• Monitor for manifestations of hyperchloremia: *NEURO:* weakness, lethargy, coma; *RESP:* deep, rapid breathing
• Assess fluid volume status: I&O ratio and record, count or weigh diapers as appropriate, distended neck veins, crackles in lung, color, quality and sp gr of urine, skin turgor, adequacy of pulses, moist mucous membranes, bilateral lung sounds, peripheral pitting edema; dehydration symptoms of decreasing output, thirst, hypotension, dry mouth, and mucous membranes should be reported
• Monitor electrolytes: potassium, sodium, calcium, magnesium; also include BUN, blood pH, ABGs, uric acid, CBC, blood glucose
• Assess B/P before and during therapy with patient lying, standing, and sitting as appropriate; orthostatic hypotension can occur rapidly
• Monitor blood, urine glucose in diabetic patients; glucose levels may be increased
• Assess for eye pain, change in vision when using drug for intraocular pressure
• Assess neurologic status when using drug for seizures
• Assess for decreased symptoms of acute mountain sickness: headache, nausea, vomiting, dizziness, fatigue, drowsiness, shortness of breath, insomnia
• Assess for cross-sensitivity between other sulfonamides and this drug

Nursing diagnoses
☑ Sensory perception, disturbed: visual (uses)
☑ Fluid volume, deficient (side effects)
☑ Fluid volume, excess (uses)
☑ Knowledge, deficient (teaching)

Implementation
• Give in AM to avoid interference with sleep
• Administer fluids 2-3 L/day to prevent renal calculi, unless contraindicated
• Potassium replacement if potassium level is <3.0 ml/dl
PO route
• Give with food, if nausea occurs, crush tabs and mix with sweet substance to counteract

 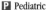

bitter taste; ES caps may be opened and sprinkled on food

🚫 • Do not crush or chew caps

Ⅳ **IV route**

• Do not use solution that is yellow or has a precipitate or crystals

IV: Dilute 500 mg of drug/5 ml or more sterile water for inj: use within 24 hr

Direct IV: Give over 1 min or more

Intermittent infusion: May be added to NS, D_5W, $D_{10}W$, 0.45% NaCl; give over 4-8 hr

Additive compatibilities: Cimetidine, ranitidine

Additive incompatibilities: Multivitamins

Patient/family education

• Teach patient to take the medication early in the day to prevent nocturia

• Instruct patient to take with food or milk if GI symptoms of nausea and anorexia occur

• Teach patient to maintain a record of weight on a weekly basis and notify prescriber of weight loss of >5 lb

• Caution patient that this drug causes a loss of potassium, so food rich in potassium should be added to the diet; refer to a dietician for assistance in planning

• Advise patient to wear protective clothing and sunscreen in the sun to prevent photosensitivity

• Teach patient not to use alcohol or any OTC medications without prescriber's approval; serious drug reactions may occur

• Emphasize the need to contact prescriber immediately if muscle cramps, weakness, nausea, dizziness, or numbness occurs

• Teach patient to take own B/P and pulse and record

• Teach patient to continue taking medication even if feeling better; this drug controls symptoms but does not cure the condition

• Teach patient to see ophthalmologist periodically; glaucoma is a slow process

• Advise patient to ↑ fluids to 2-3 L/day if not contraindicated

• Instruct patient to report nausea, vertigo, rapid weight gain, change in stools

Evaluation

Positive therapeutic outcome

• Decreased intraocular pressure

• Decreased edema

• Decreased seizures

• Prevention of mountain sickness

• Prevention of uric acid/cysteine stones

Treatment of overdose: Lavage if taken orally, monitor electrolytes, administer

dextrose in saline, monitor hydration, CV, renal status

---

acetylcysteine ⚷π (Rx)
(a-se-teel-sis'tay-een)
Mucomyst, Mucosil, Parvolex ✤
Func. class.: Mucolytic; antidote—acetaminophen
Chem. class.: Amino acid ʟ-cysteine
Pregnancy category B

Action: Decreases viscosity of secretions in respiratory tract by breaking disulfide links of mucoproteins; increases hepatic glutathione, which is necessary to inactivate toxic metabolites in acetaminophen overdose

➡ **Therapeutic Outcome:** Decreased hepatotoxicity from acetaminophen overdose (PO); decreased viscosity of mucus in respiratory disorders (inh)

Uses: Acetaminophen toxicity; bronchitis; pneumonia; cystic fibrosis; emphysema; atelectasis; tuberculosis; complications of thoracic surgery and cardiovascular surgery; diagnosis in bronchial lab tests

Investigational uses: Prevention of contrast media nephrotoxicity

Dosage and routes
Mucolytic
🅿 ***Adult and child:*** INH 2-20 ml (10% sol) q1-4h prn, or 1-10 ml (20% sol)

Acetaminophen toxicity
🅿 ***Adult and child:*** PO 140 mg/kg, then 70 mg/kg q4h × 17 doses to total 1330 mg/kg

Available forms: Sol 10%, 20%

Adverse effects
(*italic* = common; **bold** = life-threatening)
CNS: Dizziness, drowsiness, headache, fever, chills
CV: Hypotension
EENT: Rhinorrhea, tooth damage
GI: Nausea, stomatitis, constipation, vomiting, anorexia, **hepatotoxicity**
INTEG: Urticaria, rash, fever, clamminess
RESP: **Bronchospasm,** burning, **hemoptysis,** chest tightness

Contraindications: Hypersensitivity, increased intracranial pressure, status asthmaticus

Precautions: Hypothyroidism, Addison's disease, CNS depression, brain tumor, asthma, hepatic disease, renal disease, COPD, psychosis, alcoholism, seizure disorders, lactation, pregnancy **B**

Pharmacokinetics

Absorption	Extensive (PO), locally (inh)
Distribution	Unknown
Metabolism	Liver
Excretion	Kidneys
Half-life	Unknown

Pharmacodynamics

	PO	INH
Onset	Unknown	1 min
Peak	Unknown	Unknown
Duration	Up to 4 hr	5-10 min

Interactions
Individual drugs
Activated charcoal: ↓ absorption of acetylcysteine

Iron, copper, rubber: Do not use with acetylcysteine

NURSING CONSIDERATIONS
Assessment
Mucolytic use

• Assess cough: type, frequency, character, including sputum

• Assess characteristics, rate, rhythm of respirations, increased dyspnea, sputum; discontinue if bronchospasm occurs; ABGs for increased CO_2 retention in asthma patients

• Monitor VS, cardiac status including checking for dysrhythmias, increased rate, palpitations

Antidotal use

• Assess liver function tests, acetaminophen levels, pro-time, glucose, electrolytes; inform prescriber if dose is vomited or vomiting is persistent; provide adequate hydration; decrease dosage in hepatic encephalopathy

• Assess for nausea, vomiting, rash; notify prescriber if these occur

Nursing diagnoses
☑ Injury, risk for physical (uses) (antidote)
☑ Gas exchange, impaired (uses) (mucolytic)
☑ Airway clearance, ineffective (uses) (mucolytic)
☑ Poisoning, risk for (uses) (antidote)
☑ Knowledge, deficient (teaching)

Implementation
G • Give decreased dosage to elderly patients; their metabolism may be slowed; give gum, hard candy, frequent rinsing of mouth for dryness of oral cavity

• Use only if suction machine is available

PO route: *Antidotal use*

• Lavage, then give within 24 hr; give with cola or soft drink to disguise taste; can be given with H_2O through tubes; use within 1 hr

Inhalation route: *Mucolytic use*

• Use ac ½-1 hr for better absorption, to decrease nausea; only after patient clears airway by deep breathing, coughing

• Give by syringe 2-3 doses of 1-2 ml of 20% or 2-4 ml of 10% sol; 20% sol diluted with NS or water for injection; may give 10% sol undiluted

• Store in refrigerator: use within 96 hr of opening

• Provide assistance with inhaled dose: bronchodilator if bronchospasm occurs; wash face and rinse mouth after use to remove sticky feeling

• Use mechanical suction if cough insufficient to remove excess bronchial secretions

Patient/family education
Mucolytic use

• Tell patient to avoid driving or other hazardous activities until patient is stabilized on this medication; avoid alcohol, other CNS depressants; will enhance sedating properties of this drug

• Teach patient that unpleasant odor will decrease after repeated use; that discoloration of solution after bottle is opened does not impair its effectiveness; avoid smoking, smoke-filled rooms, perfume, dust, environmental pollutants, cleaners

Evaluation
Positive therapeutic outcome

• Absence of purulent secretions when coughing (mucolytic use)

• Clear lung sounds bilaterally (mucolytic use)

• Absence of hepatic damage (acetaminophen toxicity)

• Decreasing blood toxicology (acetaminophen toxicity)

---

activated charcoal (OTC)
Actidose, Actidose-Aqua, Charco-Aid 2000, CharcoCaps, Liqu-Char
Func. class.: Antiflatulent/antidote

Pregnancy category C

Action: Binds poisons, toxins, irritants; increases adsorption in GI tract; inactivates toxins and binds until excreted

---

 Herb/drug   Do Not Crush   Alert   Key Drug   **G** Geriatric   **P** Pediatric

A

⇒**Therapeutic Outcome:** Prevention of toxicity and death resulting from absorption of drugs

Uses: Poisoning

Dosage and routes
Poisoning

P Children should not get more than 1 dose of products with sorbitol

P *Adult and child:* PO 5-10 × weight of substance ingested; minimum dosage 30 g/250 ml of water; may give 20-40 g q6h for 1-2 days in severe poisoning

Available forms: Powder 15, 25, 30, 40, 120, 125, 240 g/container; oral susp 12.5 g/60 ml, 15 g/72 ml, 15 g/120 ml, 25 g/120 ml, 30 g/120 ml, 50 g/240 ml; ♣ 15 g/120 ml, 25 g/125 ml, 50 g/225 ml, 50 g/250 ml

Adverse effects
(*italic* = common; **bold** = life-threatening)
GI: Nausea, black stools, vomiting, constipation, diarrhea

Contraindications: Hypersensitivity to this drug, unconsciousness, semiconsciousness, poisoning of cyanide, mineral acids, alkalies

Precautions: Pregnancy C

Pharmacokinetics	
Absorption	None
Distribution	None
Metabolism	None
Excretion	Feces (unchanged)
Half-life	Unknown

Pharmacodynamics	
Onset	1 min
Peak	Unknown
Duration	4-12 hr

Interactions
Individual drugs
Acetylcysteine, ipecac: ↓ effectiveness of both drugs
Food/drug
Dairy products: ↓ effect of activated charcoal

NURSING CONSIDERATIONS
Assessment
• Assess neurologic status including LOC, pupil reactivity, cough reflex, gag reflex, and swallowing ability before administration; do not give if neurologic status is impaired; aspiration may occur unless a protected airway is present

• Assess toxin, poison ingested, time of ingestion, and amount
• Monitor respiration, pulse, B/P to determine charcoal effectiveness if taken for barbiturate/opioid poisoning

Nursing diagnoses
✓ Injury, risk for (uses)
✓ Poisoning, risk for (uses)
✓ Knowledge, deficient (teaching)

Implementation
• Give after inducing vomiting unless vomiting contraindicated (i.e., cyanide or alkalies); mix with 8 oz of water or fruit juice to form thick syrup; do not use dairy products to mix charcoal; repeat dose if vomiting occurs soon after dose
• Space at least 2 hr before or after other drugs, or absorption will be decreased; use a laxative to promote elimination; constipation occurs often
• Give alone; do not administer with ipecac; if patient unable to swallow, dilute to a less thick sol; keep container tightly closed to prevent absorption of gases
• Give through a nasogastric tube if patient unable to swallow

Patient/family education
• Tell patient stools will be black
• Teach patient about overdose/poison prevention and about keeping poison control chart available

Evaluation
Positive therapeutic outcome
• Alert, PERL (poisoning)
• Absence of distention
• Absence of odor in wounds

---

acyclovir ♣ (Rx)
(ay-sye′kloe-ver)
Avirax ♣, Zovirax
Func. class.: Antiviral
Chem. class.: Acylic purine nucleoside analog

Pregnancy category B

See Appendix D for topical products

Action: Interferes with DNA synthesis by conversion to acyclovir triphosphate, causing decreased viral replication, time of lesional healing

⇒**Therapeutic Outcome:** Decreased amount and time of healing of lesions

Uses: Mucocutaneous herpes simplex virus, herpes genitalis (HSV-1, HSV-2), herpes zoster;

simple mucocutaneous herpes simplex in immunocompromised clients with initial herpes genitalis; herpes simplex encephalitis, cytomegalovirus, HSV after transplant

Dosage and routes
Renal dose
P *Adult and child:* PO/**IV** CCr >50 ml/min dose q8h; CCr 25-50 ml/min dose q12h; CCr 10-25 ml/min dose q24h; CCr 0-10 ml/min 50% of dose q24h

Herpes simplex
P *Adult and child >12 yr:* **IV** inf 5 mg/kg over 1 hr q8h × 5 days

P *Child <12 yr:* **IV** inf 250 mg/m^2 or 30 mg/kg/day divided q8h over 1 hr × 5 days

Genital herpes
Adult: PO 200 mg q4h 5 times a day while awake × 5 days to 6 mo depending on whether initial, recurrent, or chronic

P *Adult and child:* TOP apply to all lesions q3h while awake, 6 times a day × 1 wk

Herpes simplex encephalitis
P *Child 3 mo-12 yr:* **IV** 20 mg/kg q8h × 10 days

Child birth-3 mo: **IV** 10 mg/kg q8h × 10 days

Herpes zoster
Adult: PO 800 mg q4h while awake × 7-10 days; **IV** 5 mg/kg q8h

Varicella-zoster
Adult: PO 1000 mg q6h × 5 days or 600-800 mg q4h (5×/day while awake); **IV** 500 mg/m^2 q8h or 10 mg/kg q8h × 7 days

Chickenpox
Adult/child: PO 20 mg/kg qid × 5 days, max 800 mg/dose

P *Child:* PO 10-20 mg/kg (max 800 mg) qid × 5 days; **IV** 500 mg/m^2 q8h, or 10 mg/kg q8h × 7 days

Available forms: Caps 200 mg; tabs 400, 800 mg; inj **IV** 500 mg; top ointment 5% (50 mg/g); oral susp

Adverse effects
(*italic* = common; **bold** = life-threatening)
CNS: Tremors, confusion, lethargy, hallucinations, **seizures,** *dizziness, headache,* encephalopathic changes
EENT: Gingival hyperplasia
GI: Nausea, vomiting, diarrhea, increased ALT, AST, abdominal pain, glossitis, colitis
GU: **Oliguria, proteinuria, hematuria,** vaginitis, moniliasis, **glomerulonephritis, acute renal failure,** changes in menses, polydipsia

INTEG: Rash, urticaria, pruritus, pain or phlebitis at **IV** site, unusual sweating, alopecia, stinging, burning, vulvitis
MS: Joint pain, leg pain, muscle cramps
HEMA: **Thrombotic thrombocytopenia purpura, hemolytic uremic syndrome** (immunocompromised patient)

Contraindications: Hypersensitivity

Precautions: Lactation, hepatic disease, renal disease, electrolyte imbalance, dehydration, pregnancy **B**

Pharmacokinetics
Absorption	Minimal (PO)
Distribution	Widely distributed, crosses placenta, CSF concentration 50% plasma
Metabolism	Liver, minimal
Excretion	Kidneys, 95% unchanged
Half-life	2.0-3.5 hr, increased in renal disease

Pharmacodynamics
	PO	IV	TOP
Onset	Unknown	Rapid	Unknown
Peak	1½-2½	Infusion's end	Unknown

Interactions
Individual drugs
Interferon: ↑ synergistic effect
Probenecid: ↑ neurotoxicity, nephrotoxicity
Zidovudine: ↑ CNS side effects

NURSING CONSIDERATIONS
Assessment
- Monitor for signs of infection, type of lesions, area of body covered, purulent drainage
- Check I&O ratio; report hematuria, oliguria, fatigue, weakness; may indicate nephrotoxicity; check for protein in urine during treatment
- Monitor any patient with compromised renal system, since drug is excreted slowly in poor renal system function; toxicity may occur rapidly
- Monitor liver studies: AST, ALT
- Monitor blood studies: WBC, RBC, Hct, Hgb, bleeding time; blood dyscrasias may occur; drug should be discontinued
- Monitor renal studies: urinalysis, protein, BUN, creatinine, CCr; increased BUN, creatinine indicates renal failure and nephrotoxicity
- Obtain C&S before drug therapy; drug may be taken as soon as culture is taken; repeat

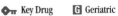

C&S after treatment; determine the presence of other sexually transmitted diseases
• Monitor bowel pattern before, during treatment; if severe abdominal pain with bleeding occurs, drug should be discontinued
• Assess allergies before treatment, reaction of each medication; place allergies on chart in bright red letters; allergic reaction: burning, stinging, swelling, redness, rash, vulvitis, pruritus

Nursing diagnoses
☑ Infection, risk for (uses)
☑ Knowledge, deficient (teaching)

Implementation
PO route
🚫• Do not break, crush, or chew caps
• Give with food to lessen GI symptoms; may give without regard to meals with 8 oz of water
• Store at room temperature in dry place
• Shake suspension before use
Topical route
• Use finger cot or rubber glove to prevent further infection
• Enough medication to cover lesions completely
• After cleansing with soap and water before each application, dry well
IV IV route
• Provide increased fluids to 3 L/day to decrease crystalluria
• Give by int inf after reconstituting with 10 ml sterile water for injection/500 mg of drug (50 mg/ml); shake; dilute in 0.9% NaCl, LR, D_5W, D_5/0.25% NaCl, D_5/0.45% NaCl, D_5/0.9% NaCl (7 mg/ml); give over at least 1 hr (constant rate) by infusion pump to prevent nephrotoxicity; do not reconstitute with sol containing benzyl alcohol or parabens; check infusion site for redness, pain, induration; rotate sites
• Lower dosage in acute or chronic renal failure
• Store at room temperature for up to 12 hr after reconstitution; if refrigerated, sol may show a precipitate that clears at room temperature, yellow discoloration does not affect potency

Y-site compatibilities: Allopurinol, amikacin, ampicillin, amphotericin B cholesteryl sulfate complex, cefamandole, cefazolin, cefonicid, cefoperazone, ceforanide, cefotaxime, cefoxitin, ceftazidime, ceftizoxime, ceftriaxone, cefuroxime, cephapirin, chloramphenicol, cimetidine, clindamycin, co-trimoxazole, dexamethasone sodium phosphate, dimenhyDRINATE, diphenhydrAMINE, doxycycline, DOXOrubicin, erythromycin, famotidine, filgrastim, fluconazole, gallium, gentamicin, granisetron, heparin, hydrocortisone sodium succinate, hydromorphone, imipenem/cilastatin, lorazepam, magnesium sulfate, melphalan, methylPREDNISolone sodium succinate, metoclopramide, metronidazole, multivitamin infusion, nafcillin, oxacillin, paclitaxel, penicillin G potassium, pentobarbital, perphenazine, piperacillin, potassium chloride, propofol, ranitidine, remifentanil, sodium bicarbonate, tacrolimus, teniposide, tetracycline, theophylline, thiotepa, ticarcillin, tobramycin, trimethoprim-sulfamethoxazole, vancomycin, zidovudine

Y-site incompatibilities: Dobutamine, DOPamine, ondansetron, verapamil

Additive compatibilities: Fluconazole

Additive incompatibilities: Blood products, protein-containing solutions, DOBUTamine, DOPamine

Patient/family education
Topical route
• Tell patient not to use in eyes; for use when there is no evidence of infection; apply with glove to prevent further infection
• Instruct patient to avoid use of OTC creams, ointments, lotions unless directed by prescriber; may cause reinfection, delayed healing
• Teach patient to use asepsis (hand washing) before, after each application and avoid contact with eyes; to adhere strictly to prescribed regimen to maximize successful treatment outcome
PO route
• Teach patient that drug may be taken orally before infection occurs; that drug should be taken when itching or pain occurs, usually before eruptions; that partners need to be told that patient has herpes; they can become infected, so condoms must be worn to prevent reinfections; that drug does not cure infection, just controls symptoms and does not prevent infection to others
⬥• Tell patient to report sore throat, fever, fatigue; may indicate superinfection; that drug must be taken in equal intervals around the clock to maintain blood levels for duration of therapy
• Tell patient to notify prescriber of side effects: bruising, bleeding, fatigue, malaise; may indicate blood dyscrasias
• Tell patient to seek dental care during treatment to prevent gingival hyperplasia

- Teach female patients with genital herpes to have regular Pap smears to prevent undetected cervical cancer
🚫 • Do not crush or chew caps

Evaluation
Positive therapeutic outcome
- Absence of itching, painful lesions
- Crusting and healed lesions

Treatment of overdose: Discontinue drug, hemodialysis, resuscitate if needed

---

adalimumab (Rx)
(add-a-lim'yu-mab)
Humira
Func. class.: Antirheumatic agent (disease modifying), immunomodulator

Pregnancy category B

Action: A form of human IgG1 monoclonal antibody specific for human tumor necrosis factor (TNF). Elevated levels of TNF are found in patients with rheumatoid arthritis

➡ **Therapeutic Outcome:** Decreased pain, inflammation in joints, better ROM

Uses: Reduction in signs and symptoms and inhibiting progression of structural damage in patients with moderate to severe active rheumatoid arthritis in patients ≥18 years of age who have not responded to other disease-modifying agents

Dosage and routes
Adult: SC 40 mg every other wk

Available forms: Inj 40 mg/0.8 ml

Adverse effects
(*italic* = common; **bold** = life-threatening)
CNS: Headache
EENT: Sinusitis
GI: Abdominal pain, nausea
INTEG: Rash, *inj site reaction*
MISC: Flulike symptoms, UTI, hypertension, back pain, lupuslike syndrome
RESP: *URI*

Contraindications: Hypersensitivity

P **Precautions:** Pregnancy (B), lactation,
G children, elderly, CNS demyelinating disease, lymphoma, latent TB

🚫 **Do Not Confuse:**
Humira/Humalin

Pharmacokinetics
Absorption	Unknown
Distribution	Unknown
Metabolism	Unknown
Excretion	Unknown
Half-life	Terminal 2 wk

Pharmacodynamics
Unknown

Interactions
Drug classification
Vaccines: Do not give concurrently; immunization should be brought up to date before treatment

NURSING CONSIDERATIONS
Assessment
- Assess for pain, stiffness, ROM, swelling of joints during treatment
- Check for inj site pain, swelling; usually occur after 2 inj (4-5 days)
◆ • Check for infections, stop treatment if present, some serious infections, including sepsis, may occur; patients with active infections should not be started on this drug

Nursing diagnoses
☑ Pain, chronic (uses)
☑ Mobility, impaired physical (uses)
☑ Activity intolerance (uses)
☑ Knowledge, deficient (teaching)

Implementation
SC route
- Do not admix with other sol or medications, do not use filter, protect from light

Patient/family education
- Teach patient about self-administration if appropriate: inj should be made in thigh, abdomen, upper arm; rotate sites at least 1 inch from old site; do not inject in areas that are bruised, red, hard
- Advise patient that if medication is not taken when due, inject next dose as soon as remembered and inject next dose as scheduled

Evaluation
Positive therapeutic outcome
- Decreased inflammation, pain in joints

---

adefovir dipivoxil (Rx)
(add-ee-foh'veer)

Hepsera
Func. class.: Antiviral

Pregnancy category C

Action: Inhibits hepatitis B virus DNA polymerase by competing with natural substrates and by causing DNA termination after its incorporation into viral DNA; causes viral DNA death

→**Therapeutic Outcome:** Improving liver function tests, lessening symptoms of chronic hepatitis B

Uses: Chronic hepatitis B

Dosage and routes
Adult: **PO** 10 mg qd, optimal duration unknown

Renal dose
Adult: **PO** CCr ≥50 ml/min 10 mg q24h; CCr 20-49 ml/min 10 mg q48h; CCr 10-19 ml/min 10 mg q72h; hemodialysis 10 mg q7 days following dialysis

Available forms: Tabs 10 mg

Adverse effects
(*italic* = common; **bold** = life-threatening)
CNS: Headache
GI: Dyspepsia, abdominal pain

Contraindications: Hypersensitivity

Precautions: Pregnancy (C), lactation, ▣children, severe renal disease, impaired ▣hepatic disease, elderly

Pharmacokinetics	
Absorption	Rapidly from GI tract
Distribution	Unknown
Metabolism	Unknown
Excretion	Kidneys 45%
Half-life	7.48 hr

Pharmacodynamics	
Onset	Unknown
Peak	1¾
Duration	Unknown

Interactions
Individual drugs
Acetaminophen, aspirin, indomethacin: ↑ granulocytopenia
Acetaminophen, acyclovir, adriamycin, amphotericin B, cimetidine, dapsone, DOXOrubicin, fluconazole, flucytosine, ganciclovir, indomethacin, interferon, morphine, pentamidine, phenytoin, probenecid, trimethoprim,

vinBLAStine, vinCRIStine: ↑ serum concentrations, toxicity
Drug Classifications
Benzodiazepines, nucleoside analogs (experimental), sulfonamides: ↑ serum concentrations, toxicity

NURSING CONSIDERATIONS
Assessment
• Assess for nephrotoxicity: increasing CCr, BUN
• Assess for HIV before beginning treatment, because HIV resistance may occur in chronic hepatitis B patients
• Assess for lactic acidosis, severe hepatomegaly with stenosis
▣• Assess elderly patients more carefully; may develop renal, cardiac symptoms more rapidly
• Assess for exacerbations of hepatitis after discontinuing treatment, monitor liver function tests

Nursing diagnoses
✓Infection, risk for (uses)
✓Knowledge, deficient (teaching)

Implementation
• Give by mouth without regard to food
• Store in cool environment; protect from light

Patient/family education
• Advise patient that optimal duration of treatment is unknown
• Advise patient to avoid use with other medications unless approved by prescriber
• Advise patient to notify prescriber of decreased urinary output

Evaluation
Positive therapeutic outcome
• Decreased symptoms of chronic hepatitis B, improving liver function tests

---

✦ HIGH ALERT

adenosine (Rx)
(ah-den'oh-seen)

Adenocard, Adenoscan
Func. class.: Antidysrhythmic—misc.
Chem. class.: Endogenous nucleoside

Pregnancy category C

Action: Slows conduction through AV node, can interrupt reentry pathways through AV node, and can restore normal sinus rhythm in patients with supraventricular tachycardia (SVT)

→**Therapeutic Outcome:** Normal sinus rhythm in patients diagnosed with SVT

Uses: SVT, as a diagnostic aid to assess myocardial perfusion defects in CAD

Dosage and routes
Antidysrhythmic
Adult: **IV** bol 6 mg; if conversion to normal sinus rhythm does not occur within 1-2 min, give 12 mg by rapid **IV** bol; may repeat 12 mg dose again in 1-2 min

P *Infants and children:* 0.05 mg/kg; if not effective, increase dose by 0.05 mg/kg q2 min to a max of 0.25 mg/kg or 12 mg

Diagnostic use
Adult: **IV** 140 mcg/kg/min × 6 min

Available forms: Inj 3 mg/ml (vial); 6 mg/2 ml (vial)

Adverse effects
*(italic = common; **bold** = life-threatening)*
CNS: Lightheadedness, dizziness, arm tingling, numbness, apprehension, blurred vision, headache
CV: Chest pain/pressure, **atrial tachydysrhythmias,** sweating, palpitations, hypotension, *facial flushing*
GI: Nausea, metallic taste, throat tightness, groin pressure
***RESP:** Dyspnea, chest pressure,* hyperventilation

Contraindications: Hypersensitivity, 2nd- or 3rd-degree heart block, AV block, sick sinus syndrome, atrial flutter, atrial fibrillation

P **Precautions:** Pregnancy **C,** lactation,
G children, asthma, elderly

◼ Do Not Confuse:
Adenocard/adenosine

Pharmacokinetics
Absorption	Complete bioavailability
Distribution	Erythrocytes, cardiovascular endothelium
Metabolism	Liver, converted to inosine and adenosine monophosphate
Excretion	Kidneys
Half-life	10 sec

Pharmacodynamics
Onset	Rapid
Peak	Unknown
Duration	1-2 min

Interactions
Individual drugs
Caffeine, theophylline: ↓ effects of adenosine
Carbamazepine: ↑ heart block

Digoxin: ↑ ventricular fibrillation
Dipyridamole: ↑ effects of adenosine
Smoking
↑ tachycardia
▨ *Herb/drug*
Aconite: ↑ toxicity, death
Aloe, broom, chronic buckthorn use, cascara sagrada (chronic use), Chinese rhubarb, figwort, fumitory, goldenseal, kudzu, licorice: ↑ effect
Coltsfoot: ↓ effect
Horehound: ↑ serotonin effect

NURSING CONSIDERATIONS
Assessment
- Monitor I&O ratio, electrolytes (potassium, sodium, chloride)
- Assess cardiopulmonary status: pulse, respiration, ECG intervals (PR, QRS, QT); check for transient dysrhythmias (PVCs, PACs, sinus tachycardia, AV block)
- Assess respiratory status: rate, rhythm, lung fields for rales, watch for respiratory depression; bilateral rales may occur in CHF patient; if increased respiration, increased pulse occurs, drug should be discontinued
- Assess CNS effects: dizziness, confusion, paresthesias; drug should be discontinued

Nursing diagnoses
✓ Cardiac output, decreased (uses)
✓ Gas exchange, impaired (adverse reactions)
✓ Knowledge, deficient (teaching)

Implementation
Ⅳ IV direct (bolus)
- Give **IV** bol undiluted; give 6 mg or less by rapid inj; if using an **IV** line, use port near insertion site, flush with 0.9% NaCl (50 ml); warm to room temperature before giving
Continuous infusion
- Give 30-ml vial undiluted via peripheral vein

Solution compatibilities: D_5LR, D_5W, LR, 0.9% NaCl
- Store at room temperature; sol should be clear; discard unused drug

Patient/family education
- Tell patient to report facial flushing, dizziness, sweating, palpitations, chest pain
- Instruct patient to rise from sitting or standing slowly to prevent orthostatic hypotension

Evaluation
Positive therapeutic outcome
- Normal sinus rhythm
- Diagnosis of perfusion defect

 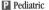

agalsidase beta
Fabrazyme
See Appendix A, Selected New Drugs

---

alatrofloxacin (Rx)
(ah-lat-troh-floks'ah-sin)
Trovan IV
trovafloxacin (Rx)
(troh-vah-floks'ah-sin)
Trovan (oral)
Func. class.: Antiinfective
Chem. class.: Fluoroquinolone
Pregnancy category C

Action: Interferes with conversion of intermediate DNA fragments into high molecular weight DNA in bacteria; DNA gyrase inhibitor

➡ **Therapeutic Outcome:** Bacterial action against the following: nosocomial pneumonia: *Escherichia coli, Pseudomonas aeruginosa, Haemophilus influenzae, Staphylococcus aureus;* community-acquired pneumonia: *Staphylococcus pneumoniae, Haemophilus influenzae, Staphylococcus aureus, Klebsiella pneumoniae, Mycoplasma pneumoniae, Mycoplasma catarrhalis, Legionella pneumophilia, Chlamydia pneumoniae*

Uses: Nosocomial pneumonia, community-acquired pneumonia, chronic bronchitis, acute sinusitis, complicated intraabdominal infections, gyn/pelvic infection, skin/skin structure infections, UTIs, chronic bacterial prostatitis, urethral gonorrhea in males, PID, cervicitis caused by susceptible organisms

Dosage and routes
Alatrofloxacin
Serious infections
Adult: **IV** 300 mg q24h

Other infections
Adult: **IV** 200 mg q24h

Perioperative prophylaxis
Adult: 200 mg ½-4 hr before surgery

Trovafloxacin
Gonorrhea
Adult: PO 100 mg as a single dose

Other infections
Adult: PO 100-200 mg q24h

Perioperative prophylaxis
Adult: PO 200 mg ½-4 hr before surgery

Available forms: Conc sol for inj 5 mg/ml (alatrofloxacin); tabs 100, 200 mg (trovafloxacin)

Adverse effects
(*italic* = common; **bold** = life-threatening)
CNS: Headache, *dizziness,* insomnia, anxiety, psychosis, **seizures**
GI: Nausea, flatulence, vomiting, diarrhea, abdominal pain, **pseudomembranous colitis**
GU: Vaginitis, crystalluria, ↑ BUN, creatinine
INTEG: Rash, pruritus, photosensitivity
HEMA: Anemia, **thrombocytopenia, leukopenia,** ↓ Hgb, Hct, ↑ platelets
MS: Arthralgia, myalgia
SYST: **Anaphylaxis, Stevens-Johnson syndrome**

Contraindications: Hypersensitivity to quinolones, seizure disorders, cerebral atherosclerosis, photosensitivity

Precautions: Pregnancy **C**, lactation,
P children

Pharmacokinetics
Absorption	Unknown
Distribution	Unknown
Metabolism	Liver
Excretion	Kidneys, unchanged
Half-life	Unknown

Pharmacodynamics
Onset	Unknown
Peak	Unknown
Duration	Unknown

Interactions
Individual drugs
Citric acid/sodium citrate, iron, sucralfate: ↓ absorption
Cyclosporine: ↑ nephrotoxicity
Morphine **IV**: ↓ absorption of trovafloxacin
Theophylline: ↑ theophylline level, ↑ toxicity
Warfarin: ↑ warfarin level
Drug classifications
Antacids with aluminum/magnesium: ↓ absorption

NURSING CONSIDERATIONS
Assessment
• Assess for previous sensitivity reaction to fluoroquinolones
• Monitor for signs and symptoms of infection: characteristics of sputum, WBC >10,000/mm^3, fever; obtain baseline information before and during treatment
• Obtain C&S before beginning drug therapy

---

to identify if correct treatment has been initiated

• Assess for allergic reactions: rash, urticaria, pruritus, chills, fever, joint pain; may occur a few days after therapy begins; epINEPHrine and resuscitation equipment should be available for anaphylactic reaction

• Assess bowel pattern qd; if severe diarrhea occurs, drug should be discontinued

• Assess for overgrowth of infection, perineal itching, fever, malaise, redness, pain, swelling, drainage, rash, diarrhea, change in cough, sputum

• Identify urine output; if decreasing, notify prescriber (may indicate nephrotoxicity); also check for increased BUN, creatinine

• Assess for CNS disorders; other fluoroquinolones cause seizures, stimulation

• Monitor blood studies: AST, ALT, CBC, Hct, bilirubin, LDH, alkaline phosphatase, Coombs' test monthly if patient is on long-term therapy

• Monitor electrolytes: potassium, sodium, chloride monthly if patient is on long-term therapy

• Assess for hepatotoxicity, use only for serious or life-threatening infection

Nursing diagnoses

☑ Infection, risk for (uses)
☑ Diarrhea (side effects)
☑ Injury, risk for (side effects)
☑ Knowledge, deficient (teaching)
☑ Noncompliance (teaching)

Implementation

IV Intermittent IV infusion

• Check for irritation, extravasation, phlebitis daily

• Dilute with compatible solution to a concentration of 1-2 mg/ml, run over 1 hr

Y-site compatibilities: Amikacin, cyclo-SPORINE, DOPamine, droperidol, fentanyl, gentamicin, ketorolac, lorazepam, midazolam, nitroglycerin, ondansetron, tobramycin, vancomycin

Incompatibilities: Do not use with magnesium in the same **IV** line

Solution compatibilities: D₅, ½% NaCl, D₅/0.2% NaCl, LR

Patient/family education

• Teach patient to report sore throat, bruising, bleeding, joint pain; may indicate blood dyscrasias (rare)

• Advise patient to avoid hazardous activities until response is known

• Advise patient to contact prescriber if vaginal itching, loose foul-smelling stools, furry tongue occur, may indicate

superinfection; report itching, rash, pruritus, urticaria

• Advise patient to rinse mouth frequently, use sugarless candy or gum for dry mouth

• Instruct patient to take all medication prescribed for the length of time ordered; drug must be taken around the clock to maintain blood levels; not to give medication to others; to avoid other medication unless approved by prescriber; not to use theophyllines, toxicity may occur

• Advise patient to notify prescriber of diarrhea with blood or pus, may indicate pseudomembranous colitis

• Advise patient to use sunscreen to prevent photosensitivity

• Teach patient that drug may be taken with or without food; separate sucralfate, antacids by ≥4 hr; to ↑ fluid intake to 2 L/day to prevent crystalluria

Evaluation

Positive therapeutic outcome

• Absence of signs/symptoms of infection (WBC <10,000/mm³, temp WNL)

• Reported improvement in symptoms of infection

---

albumin, human (Rx)
(al-byoo'min)

Albuminar 5%, Albutein 5%, Buminate 5%, Plasbumin 5%, Albuminar 25%, Albutein 25%, Buminate 25%, Plasbumin-25%

Func. class.: Blood derivative—volume expander

Chem. class.: Placental human plasma

Pregnancy category C

Action: Exerts colloidal oncotic pressure, which expands volume of circulating blood by pulling fluid from extravascular to intravascular spaces, and maintains cardiac output

⇒ **Therapeutic Outcome:** Restoration of plasma volume by extravascular to intravascular fluid shift

Uses: Restores plasma volume in burns, hyperbilirubinemia, shock, hypoproteinemia, prevention of cerebral edema, cardiopulmonary bypass procedures, ARDS, hemorrhage; also replacement in nephrotic syndrome, hepatic failure

---

Dosage and routes
Burns
Adult: **IV** dose to maintain plasma albumin at 30-50 g/L, use 5% sol initially, then 25% sol after 24 hr

Shock
Adult: **IV** 500 ml of 5% sol q30 min, as needed

P *Child:* 0.5-1 g/kg/dose

Hypoproteinemia
Adult: **IV** 1000-2000 ml of 5% sol qd, not to exceed 5-10 ml/min or 25-100 g of 25% sol qd, not to exceed 3 ml/min, titrated to patient response

Hyperbilirubinemia/erythroblastosis fetalis
P *Infant:* **IV** 1 g of 25% sol/kg before transfusion

Available forms: Inj 50, 250 mg/ml (5%, 25%)

Adverse effects
(*italic* = common; **bold** = life-threatening)
CNS: Fever, chills, flushing, headache
CV: **Fluid overload,** hypotension, erratic pulse, tachycardia
GI: Nausea, vomiting, increased salivation
INTEG: Rash, urticaria
RESP: Altered respirations, **pulmonary edema**

Contraindications: Hypersensitivity, CHF, severe anemia, renal insufficiency

Precautions: Decreased salt intake, decreased cardiac reserve, lack of albumin deficiency, hepatic disease, renal disease, pregnancy **C**

Pharmacokinetics
Absorption	Complete bioavailability
Distribution	Intravascular spaces
Metabolism	Liver
Excretion	Unknown
Half-life	Unknown

Pharmacodynamics
Onset	15-30 min
Peak	Unknown
Duration	Unknown

Interactions: None
Lab test interferences
↑ Alkaline phosphatase

NURSING CONSIDERATIONS
Assessment
- Monitor blood studies: Hct, Hgb; if serum protein declines, dyspnea, hypoxemia can result; check for decreasing B/P, erratic pulse, respiration
- Monitor CVP: pulmonary wedge pressure will increase if overload occurs; I&O ratio: urinary output may decrease; CVP reading: distended neck veins indicate circulatory overload; shortness of breath, anxiety, insomnia, expiratory rales, frothy blood-tinged sputum, cough, cyanosis indicate pulmonary overload
- Assess for allergy: fever, rash, itching, chills, flushing, urticaria, nausea, vomiting, hypotension; requires discontinuation of infusion, use of new lot if therapy reinstituted; premedicate with diphenhydrAMINE

Nursing diagnoses
☑ Fluid volume, deficit (uses)
☑ Injury, risk for physical (uses)
☑ Fluid volume, excess (adverse reactions)
☑ Knowledge, deficient (teaching)

Implementation
IV **IV route**
- Check type of albumin; some are stored at room temperature, some need to be refrigerated; use only amber-colored sol without precipitate; solution should be clear
- Give **IV** slowly to prevent fluid overload; 5% may be given undiluted; 25% may be given diluted (D$_5$W, 0.9% NaCl) or undiluted; give over 4 hr, use infusion pump
- Provide adequate hydration before, during administration; whole blood may need to be given to prevent anemia; monitor hydration during treatment

Y-site compatibilities: Diltiazem

Solution compatibilities: LR, NaCl, Ringer's, D$_5$W, D$_{10}$W, D$_{2\frac{1}{2}}$W, dextrose/saline, dextran$_6$ D$_5$, dextran$_6$ NaCl 0.9%, dextrose/Ringer's, dextrose/LR

Patient/family education
- Explain use, reason for albumin; provide information on what to report to prescriber (hypersensitivity, fluid overload)

Evaluation
Positive therapeutic outcome
- Increased B/P, decreased edema (shock, burns)
- Increased serum albumin levels
- Increased plasma protein (hypoproteinemia)

albuterol (Rx)
(al-byoo'ter-ole)
AccuNeb, Airet, albuterol, Gen-Salbutamol ✤, Novo-Salmol ✤, Proventil, Salbutamol, Ventodisk, Ventolin, Volmax

Func. class.: Bronchodilator
Chem. class.: Adrenergic β₂-agonist, sympathomimetic, bronchodilator

Pregnancy category C

Action: Causes bronchodilatation by action on β₂ (pulmonary) receptors by increasing levels of cyclic adenosine monophosphate (cAMP), which relaxes smooth muscle; produces bronchodilatation; CNS, cardiac stimulation, increased diuresis, and increased gastric acid secretion; longer acting than isoproterenol

➡ **Therapeutic Outcome:** Increased ability to breathe because of bronchodilatation

Uses: Prevention of exercise-induced asthma, acute bronchospasm, bronchitis, emphysema, bronchiectasis, reversible airway obstruction

Investigational uses: Hyperkalemia in dialysis patients

Dosage and routes
To prevent exercise-induced bronchospasm
Adult: INH (metered dose inhaler) 2 puffs 15 min before exercising
Other respiratory conditions
P *Adult and child ≥12 yr:* INH (metered dose inhaler) 2 puffs q4h; **PO** 2-4 mg tid-qid, not to exceed 8 mg; NEB/IPPB 2.5 mg tid-qid

G *Elderly:* PO 2 mg tid-qid, may increase gradually to 8 mg tid-qid

P *Child 2-12 yr:* INH (metered dose inhaler) 0.1 mg/kg tid (max 2.5 mg tid-qid); NEB/IPPB 0.1-0.15 mg/kg/dose tid-qid or 1.25 mg tid-qid for child 10-15 kg or 2.5 mg tid-qid >15 kg

P *Adult and child >4 yr:* INH CAP (Rotahaler inhalation) 200 mcg cap inhaled q4-6h; may use 15 min before exercise

Available forms: Aerosol 90, 100 mcg/actuation; tabs 2, 4 mg; oral sol 2 mg/5 ml, ✤ ext rel 4, 8 mg; inh sol 0.83, 0.5, 1, 2.5 mg/ml; powder for inh (Ventodisk) 200, 400 mcg; inh caps 200 mcg; oral sol 2 mg/5 ml; 100 mcg/spray, 80 inh/canister, 200 inh/canister

Adverse effects
(*italic* = common; **bold** = life-threatening)
CNS: *Tremors, anxiety,* insomnia, headache, dizziness, stimulation, *restlessness,* hallucinations, flushing, irritability
CV: *Palpitations, tachycardia, hypertension,* angina, hypotension, dysrhythmias
EENT: Dry nose, irritation of nose and throat
GI: *Heartburn, nausea, vomiting*
MISC: Flushing, sweating, anorexia, bad taste/smell changes
MS: Muscle cramps
RESP: Cough, wheezing, dyspnea, **bronchospasm,** dry throat

Contraindications: Hypersensitivity to sympathomimetics, tachydysrhythmias, severe cardiac disease, heart block

Precautions: Lactation, pregnancy C, cardiac disorders, hyperthyroidism, diabetes mellitus, hypertension, prostatic hypertrophy, narrow-angle glaucoma, seizures, exercise-induced bronchospasm (aero-sol) in children <12 yr **P**

🔲 **Do Not Confuse:**
Ventolin/Vantin, Proventil/ Prinivil, albuterol/atenolol

Pharmacokinetics	
Absorption	Well absorbed (PO)
Distribution	Unknown
Metabolism	Liver extensively, tissues
Excretion	Unknown, breast milk
Half-life	3-4 hr

Pharmacodynamics			
	PO	PO–EXT REL	INH
Onset	½ hr	½ hr	5-15 min
Peak	2½ hr	2-3 hr	1-1½ hr
Duration	4-6 hr	12 hr	4-6 hr

Interactions
Drug classifications
β-Adrenergic blockers: Block therapeutic effect
Antidepressants (tricyclic): ↑ chance of hypertension, do not use together
Bronchodilators (aerosol): ↑ action of bronchodilator
Diuretics (potassium-losing): ↑ ECG changes/hypokalemia
MAOIs: ↑ chance of hypertensive crisis, do not use together

Oxytocics: Severe hypotension, do not use together
Sympathomimetics: ↑ adrenergic side effects
Xanthines: ↑ toxicity
Food/drug
Caffeine products, chocolate: ↑ stimulation
☑ Herb/drug
Black tea, green tea, cola nut, guarana: ↑ stimulation

NURSING CONSIDERATIONS
Assessment
• Assess respiratory function: vital capacity, forced expiratory volume, ABGs, lung sounds; heart rate, rhythm; B/P, sputum (baseline and during therapy)
• Determine that patient has not received theophylline therapy before giving dose, to prevent additive effect; client's ability to self-medicate
• Monitor for evidence of allergic reactions; paradoxic bronchospasm; withhold dose; notify prescriber if bronchospasm occurs

Nursing diagnoses
☑ Airway clearance, ineffective (uses)
☑ Gas exchange, impaired (uses)
☑ Knowledge, deficient (teaching)

Implementation
PO route
• Give PO with meals to decrease gastric
🅟 irritation; oral sol for children (no alcohol, sugar)
🅖 • In elderly patients, a spacing device is advised
🚫 • Do not crush, break, or chew extended release tabs
Aerosol route
• Give after shaking metered dose inhaler; have patient exhale and place mouthpiece in mouth, inhale slowly while depressing inhaler, hold breath, remove inhaler, exhale slowly; allow at least 1 min between inhalations
• Store in light-resistant container; do not expose to temperatures over 86° F (30° C)

Nebulizer/IPPB
• Dilute 5 mg/ml sol/2.5 ml 0.9% NaCl for inhalation; other solutions do not require dilution for nebulizer O$_2$ flow or compressed air 6-10 L/min

Patient/family education
• Tell patient not to use OTC medications before consulting prescriber; excess stimulation may occur; instruct patient to use this medication before other medications and allow at least 5 min between each to prevent overstimulation; to limit caffeine products such as chocolate, coffee, tea, and cola

• Teach patient to use inhaler; review package insert with patient; to avoid getting aerosol in eyes or blurring may result; to wash inhaler in warm water and dry qd; to rinse mouth after using; to avoid smoking, smoke-filled rooms, persons with respiratory infections
◆ • Teach patient that if paradoxic bronchospasm occurs to stop drug immediately and notify prescriber
• Instruct patient on administration of dose, not to use more than prescribed; serious side effects may occur; if taking PO regularly and dose is missed, take when remembered; space other doses on new time schedule; do not double doses
🅖 • In elderly patients, a spacing device is advised

Evaluation
Positive therapeutic outcome
• Absence of dyspnea and wheezing after 1 hr
• Improved airway exchange
• Improved ABGs

Treatment of overdose: Administer a β$_1$-adrenergic blocker

❗ HIGH ALERT

aldesleukin (Rx)
(al-dess-loo′kin)
interleukin-2, IL-2, Proleukin
Func. class.: Miscellaneous antineoplastics
Chem. class.: Interleukin-2, human recombinant, cytotine

Pregnancy category C

Action: Enhancement of lymphocyte mitogenesis and stimulation of IL-2–dependent cell lines; enhancement of lymphocyte cytotoxicity; induction of killer cell activity; induction of interferon-γ production; results in activation of cellular immunity and cytokines and inhibition of tumor growth

➡ **Therapeutic Outcome:** Prevention of rapid growth of malignant cells

Uses: Metastatic renal cell carcinoma in adults, phase II for HIV in combination with zidovudine, melanoma

Investigational uses: Kaposi's sarcoma given with zidovudine, metastatic melanoma given with cyclophosphamide, non-Hodgkin's lymphoma given with lymphokine-activated killer cells, AIDS (phase I) given with zidovudine

---

Dosage and routes

Adult: **IV** inf 600,000 international units/kg (0.037 mg/kg) over 15 min q8h × 14 doses; off 9 days; repeat schedule for another 14 doses, for a maximum of 28 doses/course

Available forms: Powder for inj 2.2 million international units/vial

Adverse effects

(*italic* = common; **bold** = life-threatening)

CNS: Mental status changes, dizziness, sensory dysfunction, syncope, motor dysfunction, fever, chills, headache, impaired memory, depression, sleep disturbances, hallucinations, rigors

CV: Hypotension, sinus tachycardia, dysrhythmias, bradycardia, PVCs, PACs, myocardial ischemia, **myocardial infarction, cardiac arrest,** capillary leak syndrome, **CVA**

EENT: Reversible visual changes

GI: Nausea, vomiting, *diarrhea,* stomatitis, anorexia, GI bleeding, dyspepsia, constipation, **intestinal perforation/ileus,** jaundice, ascites

GU: **Oliguria/anuria, proteinuria, hematuria,** dysuria, **renal failure**

HEMA: *Anemia,* **thrombocytopenia, leukopenia, coagulation disorders, leukocytosis, eosinophilia**

INTEG: Pruritus, *erythema, rash,* dry skin, **exfoliative dermatitis,** purpura, petechiae, urticaria

MS: Arthralgia, myalgia

RESP: Pulmonary congestion, dyspnea, **pulmonary edema, respiratory failure,** tachypnea, pleural effusion, wheezing, **apnea**

SYST: Infection

Contraindications: Hypersensitivity, abnormal thallium stress test or pulmonary function tests, organ allografts

Precautions: CNS metastases, bacterial infections, renal/hepatic, cardiac/pulmonary disease, pregnancy **C,** lactation, children, anemia, thrombocytopenia

Do Not Confuse:
Proleukin/Prokine

Pharmacokinetics

Absorption	Complete bioavailability
Distribution	Rapid extracellular, intravascular
Metabolism	Kidneys (convoluted tubules)
Excretion	Kidneys
Half-life	85 min

Pharmacodynamics

Onset	4 wk
Duration	≤12 mo

Interactions

Individual drugs

Indomethacin, radiation: ↑ toxicity

Radiation: ↑ bone marrow suppression

Drug classifications

Aminoglycosides, antineoplastics: ↑ toxicity

Antihypertensives: ↑ hypotension

Antineoplastics: ↑ bone marrow suppression

Glucocorticosteroids: ↓ tumor effectiveness

Psychotropics: Unpredictable reactions

Lab test interferences

↑ Bilirubin, ↑ BUN, ↑ serum creatinine, ↑ transaminase, ↑ alkaline phosphatase, ↑ hypomagnesemia, ↑ acidosis hypocalcemia, ↑ hypophosphatemia, ↑ hypokalemia, ↑ hyperuricemia, ↑ hypoalbuminemia, ↑ hypoproteinemia, ↑ hyponatremia, ↑ hyperkalemia, ↑ alkalosis (toxic effect of drug)

NURSING CONSIDERATIONS
Assessment

• Monitor CBC, differential, platelet count weekly; withhold drug if WBC is <2000/mm³ or platelet count is <75,000/mm³; notify prescriber of these results; transfusion of RBCs, platelets may be required

◆• Identify capillary leak syndrome (CLS), including a drop in mean arterial pressure (2-12 hr after initiating therapy); hypotension and hypoperfusion will occur; if B/P <90 mm Hg, monitor ECG, CVP in cardiac patients

• Monitor renal function studies: BUN, serum uric acid, urine CCr, electrolytes before, during therapy; I&O ratio; report fall in urine output to <30 ml/hr

• Monitor temperature q4h; fever may indicate beginning infection

• Check liver function tests before, during therapy: bilirubin, AST, ALT, alkaline phosphatase, LDH as needed or monthly

• Monitor ECG; watch for ST-T wave changes, low QRS and T, possible dysrhythmias (sinus tachycardia, PVCs)

• Monitor baselines in pulmonary function; document FEV >2 L or ≥75% before therapy; check daily VS, pulse oximetry, dyspnea, rales, ABGs, watch for respiratory failure, intubate if necessary

• Obtain stress thallium study before therapy; document normal ejection fraction, unimpaired wall motion

• Assess for bleeding: hematuria, guaiac, bruising or petechiae, mucosa, or orifices q8h

• Assess for GI symptoms: frequency of stools, cramping

• Assess for acidosis, signs of dehydration: rapid respirations, poor skin turgor, decreased urine output, dry skin, restlessness, weakness

---

- Assess for cardiac status: B/P, pulse, character, rhythm, rate, ABGs, ECG
- Assess for infection: sore throat; antibiotics may be prescribed prophylactically

Nursing diagnoses
☑ Injury, risk for (adverse reactions)
☑ Body image, disturbed (adverse reactions)
☑ Infection, risk for (adverse reactions)
☑ Knowledge, deficient (teaching)

Implementation
Ⅳ **Intermittent IV infusion**
- Give by intermittent **IV** inf after diluting 22 million international units (1.3 mg)/1.2 ml sterile (1.1 mg/ml) H₂O for inj at side of vial and swirl, do not shake; dilute dose with 50 ml D₅W and give over 15 min; use plastic bag; do not use an in-line filter; give through Y-tube or 3-way stopcock
- Give DOPamine 1-5 kg/min before onset of hypotension; ↓ dose preserves kidney output
- Give hydrocortisone, dexamethasone, or sodium bicarbonate (1 mEq/1 ml) for extravasation, apply ice compresses
- Store in refrigerator any diluted drug; do not freeze; administer within 48 hr; bring to room temperature before infusing; discard unused portion

Y-site compatibilities: Amikacin, **IV** fat emulsion, gentamicin, morphine, piperacillin, potassium chloride, ticarcillin, tobramycin, TPN #145, amphotericin B, calcium gluconate, diphenhydrAMINE, DOPamine, fluconazole, foscarnet, heparin, magnesium sulfate, metoclopramide, ondansetron, ranitidine, trimethoprim/sulfamethoxazole

Patient/family education
- Teach patient to avoid use of products containing aspirin or ibuprofen, razors, commercial mouthwash because bleeding may occur; to report symptoms of bleeding, hematuria, tarry stools
- Tell patient to report signs of anemia: fatigue, headache, irritability, faintness, shortness of breath
- Tell patient to report any changes in breathing or coughing even several months after treatment
- Advise patient that contraception will be necessary during treatment; teratogenesis may occur
- Teach patient to report signs/symptoms of infection: fever, chills, sore throat; patient should avoid crowds or persons with known infections

- Advise patient to avoid alcohol, NSAIDs, salicylates; GI bleeding may occur
- Advise patient that visual problems may occur but are reversible

Evaluation
Positive therapeutic outcome
- Decreased spread of malignancy

---

alefacept
Amevine
See Appendix A, Selected New Drugs

---

alemtuzumab (Rx)
(al-em-tuz'uh-mab)
Campath
Func. class.: Antineoplastic—misc.
Chem. class.: Monoclonal antibody
Pregnancy category C

Action: Composed of recombinant DNA-derived humanized monoclonal antibody (campath-1H), binds to CD52 antigen that is present on surface of B and T lymphocytes, causes lysis of leukemic cells

⇨**Therapeutic Outcome:** Decrease in number of white blood cells

Uses: B-cell chronic lymphocytic leukemia that has been treated with alkylating agents

Dosage and routes
Adult: **IV** 3 mg over 2 hr daily; when tolerated, increase to 10 mg; when 10 mg tolerated, increase to 30 mg qd; maintenance is 30 mg/day 3×/wk on alternate days

Available forms: Sol for inj 30 mg/3 ml

Adverse effects
(*italic* = common; **bold** = life-threatening)
CNS: Dizziness, insomnia, depression, headache, tremor, somnolence, fatigue
CV: Hypotension, tachycardia, hypertension, edema, chest pain, supraventricular tachycardia
GI: Anorexia, diarrhea, constipation, *nausea, stomatitis, vomiting, abdominal pain, dyspepsia*
HEMA: **Anemia, neutropenia, thrombocytopenia, pancytopenia,** purpura, epistaxis
INTEG: Rash, local reaction, pruritus
META: Hypokalemia, hypomagnesemia
MISC: Rigors, fever
RESP: Cough, pneumonia, rhinitis, **bronchospasm,** dyspnea, pharyngitis

Contraindications: Hypersensitivity, active systemic infection, immunodeficiency

Precautions: Pregnancy **C**, lactation, children

Pharmacokinetics

Absorption	Unknown
Distribution	Unknown; steady state 6 wk
Metabolism	Unknown
Excretion	Unknown
Half-life	12 days

Pharmacodynamics

Onset	Unknown
Peak	Unknown
Duration	Unknown

Interactions
Drug classifications
Live virus vaccines: Do not administer

Lab test interferences
Diagnostic tests using antibodies

NURSING CONSIDERATIONS
Assessment
• Assess CBC, platelets qwk or more often if myelosuppression occurs; assess CD4⁺ after therapy until recovery of >200 cells µ/L
• Assess for symptoms of infection; chills, fever, headache, may be masked by drug fever; do not administer drug if infection is present
• Assess CNS reaction: LOC, mental status, dizziness, confusion
• Assess cardiac status: lung sounds; ECG before and during treatment, especially in those with cardiac disease
• Assess for bone marrow depression: bruising, bleeding, blood in stools, urine, sputum, emesis

Nursing diagnoses
☑ Infection, risk for (adverse reactions)
☑ Injury, risk for (adverse reactions)
☑ Nutrition: less than body requirements, imbalanced (side effects)
☑ Body image, disturbed (adverse reactions)
☑ Knowledge, deficient (teaching)

Implementation
Ⅳ **IV route**
• Do not give **IV** push or bolus
• Withdraw amount needed; do not shake ampule; use 5 µm filter prior to dilution, check for particulate matter and discoloration; inject into 100 ml sterile 0.9% NaCl or D₅W, invert to mix, do not add other drugs or infuse in same **IV** tubing

• Store reconstituted sol for ≤8 hr at room temp, do not freeze; protect from light

Patient/family education
• Instruct patient to take acetaminophen for fever
• Advise patient to avoid hazardous tasks, since confusion, dizziness may occur
• Instruct patient to report signs of infection: sore throat, fever, diarrhea, vomiting

Evaluation
Positive therapeutic outcome
• Decrease in production of malignant lymphocytes

---

alendronate (Rx)
(al-en′droe-nate)
Fosamax
Func. class.: Bone-resorption inhibitor
Chem. class.: Bisphosphonate
Pregnancy category C

Action: Absorbs calcium phosphate crystal in bone and may directly block dissolution of hydroxyapatite crystals of bone; inhibits normal and abnormal bone resorption

⇒**Therapeutic Outcome:** Decreased symptoms of osteoporosis, Paget's disease

Uses: Treatment and prevention of osteoporosis in postmenopausal women, Paget's disease, treatment of corticosteroid-induced osteoporosis in postmenopausal women not receiving estrogen, or in men who are continuing corticosteroid treatment with low bone mass

Dosage and routes
Osteoporosis in postmenopausal women
Ⓖ *Adult and elderly:* PO 10 mg qd or 70 mg qwk

Paget's disease
Ⓖ *Adult and elderly:* PO 40 mg qd × 6 mo, consider retreatment for relapse

Prevention of osteoporosis
Adult: PO 5 mg qd or 35 mg qwk

Corticosteroid-induced osteoporosis in postmenopausal women (not receiving estrogen)
Adult: PO 10 mg qd

Corticosteroid-induced osteoporosis in men or premenopausal women (not receiving estrogen)
Adult: PO 5 mg qd

A

Available forms: Tabs 5, 10, 35, 40, 70 mg

Adverse effects
(*italic* = common; **bold** = life-threatening)
CNS: Headache
GI: Abdominal pain, anorexia, constipation, nausea, vomiting, esophageal ulceration
META: Anemia, hypokalemia, hypomagnesemia, hypophosphatemia
MS: Bone pain

Contraindications: Hypersensitivity to bisphosphonates, delayed esophageal emptying, inability to sit or stand for 30 min

P Precautions: Children, lactation, pregnancy **C**, CCr <35 ml/min, esophageal disease, ulcers, gastritis

Pharmacokinetics	
Absorption	Unknown
Distribution	Mainly to bones
Metabolism	Unknown
Excretion	Via kidneys
Half-life	Unknown

Pharmacodynamics
Unknown

Interactions
Individual drugs
Ranitidine: ↑ alendronate effect
Drug classifications
Antacids, calcium supplements: ↓ absorption
NSAIDs, salicylates: ↑ GI reactions
Food/drug
Caffeine, food, orange juice: ↓ drug absorption

NURSING CONSIDERATIONS
Assessment
• For osteoporosis: bone density testing
• For Paget's disease: ↑ skull size, bone pain, headache
• Monitor renal studies and Ca, P, Mg, K
• Assess for hypercalcemia: paresthesia, twitching, laryngospasm, Chvostek's, Trousseau's signs
• Monitor alkaline phosphatase; level of 2× upper limit of normal is indicated for Paget's disease

Implementation
• Give PO for 6 mo to be effective in Paget's disease; take with 8 oz of water 30 min before 1st food, beverage, or medication of the day
• Store in cool environment out of direct sunlight

Patient/family education
• Teach patient to remain upright for 30 min after dose to prevent esophageal irritation; if dose is missed, skip dose, do not double doses or take later in day
• Teach patient to take in AM, only before food, other meds, to take with 6-8 oz of water (not mineral water)
• To take calcium, vit D if instructed by provider
• To use weight-bearing exercise to increase bone density
• Teach patient to let provider know if pregnancy is planned or suspected or if nursing

Evaluation
Positive therapeutic outcome
• Increased bone mass, absence of fractures

alfuzosin
Uroxatral
See Appendix A, Selected New Drugs

alitretinoin (Rx)
(al-ee-tret′i-noyn)
Panretin
Func. class.: Retinoid, 2nd generation
Pregnancy category D

Action: Controls cellular differentiation and proliferation of neoplastic and healthy cells by binding to retinoid receptors

⇒ Therapeutic Outcome: Decreased size and number of lesions

Uses: Kaposi's sarcoma cutaneous lesions

Dosage and routes
Adult: TOP apply enough gel to cover lesions with a generous coating, allow to dry for 3-5 min before covering with clothing, do not apply near mucosal areas, apply as long as benefit occurs

Available forms: Top gel 0.1%

Adverse effects
(*italic* = common; **bold** = life-threatening)
INTEG: Rash, stinging, pain, warmth, redness, erythema, blistering, crusting, peeling, dermatitis

Contraindications: Hypersensitivity to retinoids, pregnancy **D**

Precautions: Lactation, eczema, sunburn,
G elderly, cutaneous T-cell lymphoma

Pharmacokinetics

Absorption	Small amounts
Distribution	Unknown
Metabolism	Unknown
Excretion	Kidneys
Half-life	Unknown

Pharmacodynamics

Unknown

Interactions
Individual drugs
DEET: Do not use around DEET (an insect repellant)

NURSING CONSIDERATIONS
Assessment
- Assess part of body involved, including time involved, what helps or aggravates condition, cysts, dryness, itching
- Assess for dermal toxicity that may start as erythema, then edema; drug may need to be discontinued and restarted

Nursing diagnoses
☑ Skin integrity, impaired (uses)
☑ Body image, disturbed (uses)
☑ Knowledge, deficient (teaching)

Implementation
- Apply bid initially to lesions, can be increased to tid-qid according to tolerance, discontinue for a few days if severe reactions occur
- Store at room temp
- Wash hands after application

Patient/family education
- Instruct patient to avoid application on normal skin, and to avoid getting cream in eyes, nose, other mucous membranes
- Advise patient to avoid sunlight, sunlamps or to use protective clothing or sunscreen to prevent burns
- Advise patient that treatment may cause warmth, stinging; dryness; peeling will occur
- Caution patient that drug does not cure condition; only relieves symptoms; that therapeutic results may be seen in 2-3 wk but may not be optimal until after 6 wk

Evaluation
Positive therapeutic outcome
- Decrease in size and number of lesions

---

allopurinol (Rx)
(al-oh-pure′i-nole)
alloprim, allopurinol, Aloprim, Apo-Allopurinol ✚, Lopurin, Purinol ✚, Zyloprim
Func. class.: Antigout drug
Chem. class.: Xanthine enzyme inhibitor

Pregnancy category C

Action: Inhibits the enzyme xanthine oxidase, reducing uric acid synthesis

⮞Therapeutic Outcome: Decreasing serum uric acid levels, decreasing joint pain

Uses: Chronic gout, hyperuricemia associated with malignancies, recurrent calcium oxalate calculi, Chagas disease, cutaneous/visceral leishmaniasis

Investigational uses: Stomatitis (mouthwash)

Dosage and routes
Increased uric acid levels in malignancies
Adult: IV inf 200-400 mg/m^2/day, max 600 mg/day

🅿 *Child:* IV inf 200 mg/m^2/day, initially

Gout/hyperuricemia
Adult: PO 200-600 mg qd depending on severity, not to exceed 800 mg/day

🅿 *Child 6-10 yr:* 300 mg qd
🅿 *Child <6 yr:* 150 mg qd

Impaired renal function
Adult: PO CCr 30-40 ml/min: 200 mg qd
Adult: PO CCr <20 ml/min: 100 mg qd
Adult: IV CCr 10-20 ml/min: 200 mg/day; CCr 3-10 ml/min 100 mg/day; CCr <3 ml/min 100 mg/day at intervals

Recurrent calculi
Adult: PO 200-300 mg qd

Uric acid nephropathy prevention
🅿 *Adult and child >10 yr:* PO 600-800 mg qd × 2-3 days

Stomatitis
Adult: Mouthwash dose varies, do not swallow mouthwash

Available forms: Tabs, scored, 100, 300 mg; inj 500 mg/vial

Adverse effects
(*italic* = common; **bold** = life-threatening)
CNS: Headache, drowsiness, neuritis, paresthesia
EENT: Retinopathy, cataracts, epistaxis

 Herb/drug   Do Not Crush   Alert   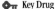 Key Drug   🅖 Geriatric   🅿 Pediatric

GI: Nausea, vomiting, anorexia, malaise, metallic taste, cramps, peptic ulcer, diarrhea, stomatitis
HEMA: **Agranulocytosis, thrombocytopenia, aplastic anemia, pancytopenia, leukopenia, bone marrow suppression, eosinophilia**
INTEG: Fever, chills, dermatitis, pruritus, purpura, erythema, ecchymosis, alopecia
MISC: Myopathy, arthralgia, hepatomegaly, **cholestatic jaundice, renal failure, exfoliative dermatitis**

Contraindications: Hypersensitivity

Precautions: Pregnancy **C,** lactation, renal disease, hepatic disease, children

Do Not Confuse:
allopurinol/apresoline, Lopurin/Lupron

Pharmacokinetics

Absorption	80%
Distribution	Widely distributed
Metabolism	Liver to oxypurinol
Excretion	Kidneys
Half-life	2-3 hr, terminal 18-30 hr

Pharmacodynamics

	PO	IV
Onset	Unknown	Unknown
Peak	2-4 hr	Unknown
Duration	Unknown	Unknown

Interactions
Individual drugs
Ammonium chloride potassium/sodium phosphate, vit C: ↑ kidney stone formation
Ampicillin, bacampicillin: ↑ risk of rash
Azathioprine: ↑ action of azathioprine
Chlorpropamide: ↑ action of chlorproPAMIDE
Cyclophosphamide, theophylline: ↑ action of allopurinol
Mercaptopurine: ↑ action of mercaptopurine
Drug classifications
ACE inhibitors: ↑ action of ACE inhibitors
Aluminum salts: ↓ effects of allopurinol
Anticoagulants (oral): ↑ action of oral anticoagulants
Antineoplastics: ↑ bone marrow suppression
Diuretics (thiazide): ↑ allopurinol toxicity

NURSING CONSIDERATIONS
Assessment
• Assess for pain including location, characteristics, onset/duration, frequency, quality, intensity or severity of pain, precipitating factors
• Monitor uric acid levels q2 wk; normal uric

acid levels are 6 mg/dl or less; check I&O ratio; increase fluids to 2 L/day to prevent stone formation, toxicity
• Monitor CBC, AST, BUN, creatinine before starting treatment, monthly; check blood glucose in diabetic patients receiving oral antidiabetic agents
• Monitor nutritional status: discourage organ meat, sardines, salmon, legumes, gravies (high-purine foods), alcohol

Nursing diagnoses
☑ Nutrition, more than body requirements (uses)
☑ Knowledge, deficient (teaching)

Implementation
PO route
• Give with meals to prevent GI symptoms; crush and mix with food or fluids for patients with swallowing difficulties
• Give a few days before antineoplastic therapy if using for hyperuricemia associated with malignancy
IV Infusion
• Reconstitute 30-ml vial with 25 ml of sterile water for inj; dilute to desired conc with 0.9% NaCl for inj or D₅ for inj, begin inf within 10 hr

Solution incompatibilities: Amikacin, amphotericin B, carmustine, cefotaxime, chlorproMAZINE, cilastatin, cimetidine, clindamycin, cytarabine, dacarbazine, DAUNOrubicin, diphenhydrAMINE, DOXOrubicin, doxycycline, droperidol, floxuridine, gentamicin, haloperidol, hydrOXYzine, idarubicin, imipenem, mechlorethamine, meperidine, metoclopramide, methylPREDNISolone, minocycline, nalbuphine, netilmicin, ondansetron, prochlorperazine, promethazine, sodium bicarbonate, streptozocin, tobramycin, vinorelbine

Patient/family education
• Tell patient to increase fluid intake to 2 L/day; to avoid taking large doses of vit C; kidney stone formation may occur; to maintain a diet enhancing urine alkalinity (e.g., milk, other dairy products); if taking for calcium oxalate stones, reduce dairy products, refined sugar, sodium, meat
• Tell patient to report skin rash, stomatitis, malaise, fever, aching; drug should be discontinued
• Advise patient to avoid hazardous activities if drowsiness or dizziness occurs; response may take several days to determine
• Tell patient to avoid alcohol, caffeine; these substances increase uric acid levels and decrease allopurinol levels

- Teach patient to report side effects and adverse reactions to prescriber, including rash, itching, nausea, vomiting

Evaluation
Positive therapeutic outcome
- Decreased pain in joints
- Decreased stone formation in kidney
- Decreased uric acid level to 6 mg/dl

---

almotriptan (Rx)
(al-moh-trip'tan)
Axert
Func. class.: Antimigraine agent
Chem. class.: 5-HT₁ receptor agonist

Pregnancy category C

Action: Binds selectively to the vascular 5-HT_1 receptor subtype, exerts antimigraine effect; causes vasoconstriction in cranial arteries

→ **Therapeutic Outcome:** Absence of migraines

Uses: Acute treatment of migraine with or without aura

Dosage and routes
Adult: PO may use 6.25 mg dose initially, but 12.5 mg is more effective; may repeat dose after 2 hr; do not give more than 2 doses/24 hr

Hepatic/renal dose
Adult: PO 6.25 mg initially, max 12.5 mg

Available forms: Tabs 6.25, 12.5 mg

Adverse effects
(*italic* = common; **bold** = life-threatening)
CV: Flushing, palpitations, tachycardia, **coronary artery vasospasm, MI, ventricular fibrillation, ventricular tachycardia**
EENT: Throat, mouth, nasal discomfort; vision changes
GI: Abdominal discomfort
INTEG: Sweating
MS: Weakness, neck stiffness, myalgia
NEURO: Tingling, hot sensation, burning, feeling of pressure, tightness, numbness, dizziness, sedation, headache, anxiety, fatigue, cold sensation
RESP: Chest tightness, pressure

Contraindications: Concurrent use of ergotamine-containing preparations, uncontrolled hypertension, hypersensitivity, basilar or hemiplegic migraine; concurrent MAOI therapy or within 2 wk

Precautions: Postmenopausal women, men >40 yr, risk factors for coronary artery disease, hypercholesterolemia, obesity, diabetes, **P** impaired hepatic or renal function, pregnancy **G** C, lactation, children, elderly

Pharmacokinetics

Absorption	Well absorbed (~70%)
Distribution	35% protein bound
Metabolism	Liver (metabolite); metabolized by MAO-A, CYP2D6, CYP3A4
Excretion	Urine, feces
Half-life	3-4 hr

Pharmacodynamics

Onset	Unknown
Peak	1-3 hr
Duration	3-4 hr

Interactions
Individual drugs
Ergot: ↑ vasospastic effects
Ketoconazole: ↑ plasma concentration of almotriptan
Drug classifications
5-HT_1 agonists, ergot derivatives: ↑ vasospastic effects
MAOIs: ↑ almotriptan effect
CYP2D6 inhibitors: ↑ almotriptan effect
Herb/drug
Butterbur: ↑ almotriptan effect

NURSING CONSIDERATIONS
Assessment
- Assess B/P, signs/symptoms of coronary vasospasms
- Assess for tingling, hot sensation, burning, feeling of pressure, numbness, flushing
- Assess for stress level, activity, recreation, coping mechanisms
- Assess neurologic status: LOC, blurring vision, nausea, vomiting, tingling in extremities preceding headache
- Assess for ingestion of tyramine-containing foods (pickled products, beer, wine, aged cheese), food additives, preservatives, colorings, artificial sweeteners, chocolate, caffeine, which may precipitate these types of headaches

Nursing diagnoses
☑ Pain, acute (uses)
☑ Knowledge, deficient (teaching)

Implementation
⊘• PO, swallow whole
- Provide quiet, calm environment with decreased stimulation from noise, bright light, excessive talking

---

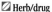

Patient/family education
- Instruct patient to use contraception while taking drug, notify prescriber if pregnancy is planned or suspected, avoid breastfeeding
- Advise patient to have dark, quiet environment available
- Inform patient that drug does not prevent or reduce number of migraine attacks
- Advise patient to report chest pain, drowsiness, dizziness, tingling, flushing, pressure

Evaluation
Positive therapeutic outcome
- Decrease in severity of migraine

Treatment of overdose: Gastric lavage followed by activated charcoal; clinical and ECG monitoring for ≥20 hr after overdose

---

alprazolam (Rx)
(al-pray′zoe-lam)
Apo-Alpraz ✦, Novo-Alprazol ✦, Nu-Alpraz ✦, Xanax
Func. class.: Antianxiety/sedative/hypnotic
Chem. class.: Benzodiazepine

Pregnancy category D
Controlled substance schedule IV

Action: Depresses subcortical levels of CNS, including limbic system, reticular formation; potentiates GABA (γ-aminobutyric acid)

➔ Therapeutic Outcome: Decreased anxiety

Uses: Anxiety, panic disorders, anxiety with depressive symptoms

Investigational uses: Depression, social phobia, premenstrual syndrome, dysphoric disorders

Dosage and routes
Anxiety disorder
Adult: PO 0.25-0.5 mg tid, not to exceed 4 mg/day in divided doses

G *Elderly:* PO 0.125-0.25 mg bid; increase by 0.125 mg as needed

Panic disorder
Adult: PO 0.5 mg tid, max 10 mg/day; may ↑ q 3-4 days by 1 mg/day or less

Premenstrual dysphoric disorders
Adult: PO 0.25 mg bid-qid, starting on day 16-18 of menses, taper over 2-3 days when menses occurs

Social phobia
Adult: PO 2-8 mg/day

Hepatic dose
Reduce dose by 50%

Available forms: Tabs 0.25, 0.5, 1, 2 mg; oral sol 0.1, 1 mg/ml

Adverse effects
(*italic* = common; **bold** = life-threatening)
CNS: Dizziness, drowsiness, confusion, headache, anxiety, tremors, stimulation, fatigue, depression, insomnia, hallucinations
CV: Orthostatic hypotension, **ECG changes, tachycardia,** hypotension
EENT: Blurred vision, tinnitus, mydriasis
GI: Constipation, dry mouth, nausea, vomiting, anorexia, diarrhea
INTEG: Rash, dermatitis, itching

Contraindications: Hypersensitivity to benzodiazepines, narrow-angle glaucoma, **P** psychosis, pregnancy **D**, child <18 yr

G Precautions: Elderly, debilitated, hepatic disease, renal disease

◼ Do Not Confuse:
alprazolam/lorazepam, Xanax/Lanoxin, Xanax/Tylox, Xanax/Zantac

Pharmacokinetics	
Absorption	Slow, complete
Distribution	Widely distributed; crosses placenta; crosses blood-brain barrier
Metabolism	Liver, to active metabolites
Excretion	Kidneys, breast milk
Half-life	12-15 hr

Pharmacodynamics	
Onset	1 hr
Peak	1-2 hr
Duration	4-6 hr, therapeutic response 2-3 days

Interactions
Individual drugs
Alcohol: ↑ CNS depression
Cimetidine, disulfiram, erythromycin, fluoxetine, isoniazid, ketoconazole, levodopa, metoprolol, propoxyphene, propranolol, valproic acid: ↑ action of alprazolam
Rifampin: ↓ action of alprazolam
Drug classifications
Anticonvulsants, antihistamines: ↑ CNS depression
Barbiturates: ↓ action of alprazolam
Contraceptives (oral): ↑ action of alprazolam
Sedative/hypnotics: ↑ CNS depression
Xanthines: ↑ sedation
Food/drug
Grapefruit juice: ↑ drug level

Cat's claw, chamomile, cowslip, goldenseal, hops, kava, licorice, Queen Anne's lace, Skullcap, St. John's wort, valerian, wild cherry: ↑ CNS depression

Lab test interferences
↑ ALT, ↑ AST, ↑ alkaline phosphatase; ↑ neutropenia

NURSING CONSIDERATIONS
Assessment
• Assess mental status: mood, sensorium, anxiety, affect, sleeping pattern, drowsiness, dizziness, especially elderly; physical dependency, withdrawal symptoms: anxiety, panic attacks, agitation, seizures, headache, nausea, vomiting, muscle pain, weakness; suicidal tendencies; indications of increasing tolerance and abuse; withdrawal seizures may occur after rapid decrease in dose or abrupt discontinuation; short duration of action **G** makes it the drug of choice in the elderly
• Monitor B/P (with patient lying, standing), pulse; if systolic B/P drops 20 mm Hg, hold drug, notify prescriber
• Monitor blood studies: CBC during long-term therapy; blood dycrasias have occurred rarely; decreased hematocrit, neutropenia may occur
• Monitor hepatic studies: AST, ALT, bilirubin, creatinine LDH, alkaline phosphatase, if on long-term treatment
• Monitor I&O; indicate renal dysfunction if on long-term treatment

Nursing diagnoses
☑ Anxiety (uses)
☑ Injury, risk for (adverse reactions)
☑ Knowledge, deficient (teaching)

Implementation
• Give with food or milk for GI symptoms; tab may be crushed, if patient is unable to swallow medication whole, and mixed with foods or fluids; may divide total daily dose into more times/day, if anxiety occurs between doses
• Give sugarless gum, hard candy, frequent sips of water for dry mouth

Patient/family education
• Tell patient that drug may be taken with food or fluids, and tabs may be crushed or swallowed whole
• Tell patient not to use for everyday stress or longer than 4 mo unless directed by prescriber; not to take more than prescribed amount; may be habit forming; not to double doses or skip doses; memory impairment is a sign of long-term use

• Tell patient to avoid OTC preparations unless approved by prescriber; alcohol and CNS depressants will increase CNS depression
• Tell patient to avoid driving, activities that require alertness, since drowsiness may occur; to avoid alcohol ingestion or other psychotropic medications; to rise slowly or fainting may **G** occur, especially elderly; that drowsiness may worsen at beginning of treatment
• Tell patient not to discontinue medication abruptly after long-term use; withdrawal symptoms include vomiting, cramping, tremors, seizures

Evaluation
Positive therapeutic outcome
• Decreased anxiety, restlessness, sleeplessness (short-term treatment only)

Treatment of overdose: Lavage, VS, supportive care, flumazenil

---

! HIGH ALERT

alteplase (Rx)
(al-ti-plaze')
Activase, Activase rt-PA ✦, Lysatec rt-PA ✦, Cathflo tissue plasminogin activator, t-PA
Func. class.: Thrombolytic enzyme
Chem. class.: Tissue plasminogen activator (TPA)

Pregnancy category C

Action: Produces fibrin conversion of plasminogen to plasmin; able to bind to fibrin, convert plasminogen in thrombus to plasmin, which leads to local fibrinolysis, limited systemic proteolysis

Therapeutic Outcome: Lysis of thrombi in MI, pulmonary emboli (life threatening)

Uses: Lysis of obstructing thrombi associated with acute MI; conditions requiring thrombolysis (e.g., PE, DVT, unclotting arteriovenous shunts, acute ischemic CVA)

Investigational uses: Unstable angina, occluded central venous catheters

Dosage and routes
Pulmonary embolism
Adult: **IV** 100 mg over 2 hr, then heparin

Acute ischemic stroke
Adult: **IV** 0.9 mg/kg, max 90 mg; give as inf over 1 hr, give 10% of dose

---

Myocardial Infarction (standard infusion)
Adult >65 kg: IV a total of 100 mg; 6-10 mg given **IV** bol over 1-2 min, 60 mg given over 1st hr, 20 mg given over 2nd hr, 20 mg given over 3rd hr; or 1.25 mg/kg given over 3 hr for <65 kg patient

Adult <65 kg: IV 0.75 mg over 1st hr, 0.075-0.125 mg/kg given **IV** bol over first 1-2 min, 0.25 mg/kg over 2nd hr, 0.25 mg/kg over 3rd hr to a total dose of 1.25 mg/kg, max 100 mg total

Myocardial Infarction (Accelerated infusion)
Adult: IV bol 15 mg; then 0.75 mg/kg over ½ hr; then 0.5 mg/kg over 1 hr

Occluded central venous catheters
Adult: 2 mg/2 ml infused in each port of dual lumen catheter; dwell time varies widely

Available forms: Powder for inj 50 mg (29 million international units/vial), 100 mg (58 million international units/vial)

Adverse effects
*(italic = common; **bold** = life-threatening)*
CV: **Sinus bradycardia, ventricular tachycardia, accelerated idioventricular rhythm, bradycardia**
INTEG: Urticaria, rash
SYST: **GI, GU, intracranial, retroperitoneal bleeding, surface bleeding, anaphylaxis**

Contraindications: Hypersensitivity, active internal bleeding, recent CVA, severe uncontrolled hypertension, intracranial/intraspinal surgery/trauma, aneurysm

P **Precautions:** Pregnancy **C**, lactation, G children, elderly, neurologic deficits

Pharmacokinetics
Absorption	Complete
Distribution	Unknown
Metabolism	>80% liver
Excretion	Kidneys
Half-life	35 min

Pharmacodynamics
Onset	Immediate
Peak	30-45 min
Duration	4 hr

Interactions
Individual drugs
Abciximab, aspirin, clopidrogrel, dipyridamole, eptifibatide, heparin, plicamycin, ticlopidine, tirofiban, valproic acid: ↑ bleeding

Drug classifications
Anticoagulants (oral), cephalosporins (some), NSAIDs: ↑ bleeding
Lab test interferences
↑ PT, ↑ APTT, ↑ TT
Herb/drug
Agrimony, alfalfa, angelica, anise, basil, bay, bilberry, black haw, bogbean, bromelain, buchu, chondroitin, cinchona bark, dong quai, fenugreek, feverfew, garlic, ginger, ginkgo, ginseng, horse chestnut, Irish moss, kelp, kelpware, khella, lovage, lungwort, meadowsweet, motherwort, mugwort, nettle, papaya, parsley (large amounts), pau d'arco, pineapple, poplar, prickly ash, safflower, saw palmetto, tonka bean, turmeric, wintergreen, yarrow: ↑ risk of bleeding
Chamomile, coenzyme Q10, flax, glucomannan, goldenseal, guar gum: ↓ anticoagulant effect

NURSING CONSIDERATIONS
Assessment
• Monitor VS q15 min, B/P, pulse, respirations (including peripheral), neurologic signs, temp at least q4h; temp >104° F (40° C) indicates internal bleeding; monitor rhythm closely; ventricular dysrhythmias may occur with hyperfusion; monitor heart, breath sounds, neurologic status, and peripheral pulses
◆• Assess for bleeding during 1st hr of treatment and 24 hr after procedure: hematuria, hematemesis, bleeding from mucous membranes, epistaxis, ecchymosis, puncture sites; guaiac all body fluids and stools; obtain blood studies (Hct, platelets, PTT, PT, TT, APTT) before starting therapy; PT or APTT must be less than 2 times control before starting therapy; TT or PT q3-4h during treatment; obtain CPK-MB to identify drug effectiveness
• Assess hypersensitivity: fever, rash, facial swelling, dyspnea, itching, chills; mild reaction may be treated with antihistamines; report to prescriber
• Monitor ECG; on monitor, watch for segment changes, changes in rhythm: sinus bradycardia, ventricular tachycardia, accelerated idioventricular rhythm may occur due to reperfusion; cardiac enzymes, radionuclide myocardial scanning/coronary angiography

Nursing diagnoses
☑ Pain, chronic (uses)
☑ Tissue perfusion, ineffective (uses)
☑ Injury, risk for (adverse reactions)

Implementation

IV Intermittent IV infusion
- Give after reconstituting with provided diluent; add appropriate amount of sterile water for injection (no preservatives); 20-mg vial/20 ml or 50-mg vial/50 ml (1 mg/ml); mix by slow inversion or dilute with 0.9% NaCl, D_5W to a concentration of 0.5 mg/ml further dilution; 1.5 to <0.5 mg/ml may result in precipitation of drug; use 18-G needle; flush line with NaCl after administration; use reconstituted IV sol within 8 hr or discard, within 6 hr of coronary occlusion for best results
- ◆ Do not use 150 mg or more total dose; intracranial bleeding may occur
- Give heparin therapy after thrombolytic therapy is discontinued and when TT, ACT, and APTT less than 2 times control (about 3-4 hr)
- Avoid invasive procedures, inj, rec temp; apply pressure for 30 sec to minor bleeding sites; 30 min to sites of atrial puncture, followed by pressure dressing; inform prescriber if this does not attain hemostasis; apply pressure dressing
- Store powder at room temperature or refrigerate; protect from excessive light

Y-site compatibilities: Lidocaine, metoprolol, propranolol

Y-site incompatibilities: DOBUTamine, DOPamine, heparin, nitroglycerin

Additive compatibilities: Lidocaine, morphine, nitroglycerin

Patient/family education
- Teach patient reason for alteplase, signs and symptoms of bleeding, allergic reactions, when to notify prescriber

Evaluation

Positive therapeutic outcome
- Lysis of pulmonary thrombi
- Adequate hemodynamic state
- Absence of congestive heart failure

---

aluminum hydroxide (OTC)
AlternaGEL, Alu-Cap, Alugel ✤, Aluminet, Aluminett, aluminum hydroxide, Alu-Tab, Amphojel, Basalgel, Basaljel, Dialume, Nephrox
Func. class.: Antacid, hypophosphatemic, antiulcer
Chem. class.: Aluminum product, phosphate binder

Pregnancy category C

Action: Neutralizes gastric acidity, binds phosphates in GI tract; these phosphates are excreted

Uses: Peptic, gastric, duodenal ulcers; hyperphosphatemia in chronic renal failure; reflux esophagitis, hyperacidity, heartburn, stress ulcer prevention in critically ill, GERD

Investigational uses: GI bleeding

→ **Therapeutic Outcome:** Decreased acidity, healing of ulcers; decreased phosphate levels in chronic renal failure

Dosage and routes
Adult: SUSP 5-10 ml 1 hr pc, hs; PO 600 mg 1 hr pc, hs, chewed with milk or water

GI bleeding
P *Infant:* PO 2-5 ml/dose q1-2h
P *Child:* PO 5-15 ml/dose q1-2h

Hyperphosphatemia in renal failure
Adult: SUSP 500 mg-2 g bid-qid

Available forms
Caps 475, 500 mg; tabs 300, 500, 600 mg; susp 320 mg/5 ml, 450 mg/5 ml, 600 mg/5 ml; 675 mg/5 ml

Adverse effects
(*italic* = common; **bold** = life-threatening)
GI: Constipation, anorexia, **obstruction,** fecal impaction
META: Hypophosphatemia, hypercalciuria

Contraindications: Hypersensitivity to this drug or aluminum products, abdominal pain of unknown origin

G **Precautions:** Elderly, fluid restriction, decreased GI motility, GI obstruction, dehydration, renal disease, sodium-restricted diets, pregnancy C

Pharmacokinetics	
Absorption	Not usually absorbed
Distribution	Widely distributed if absorbed; crosses placenta
Metabolism	Unknown
Excretion	Feces, kidneys (small amounts), breast milk
Half-life	Unknown

Pharmacodynamics	
Onset	20-40 min
Peak	½ hr
Duration	1-3 hr

Interactions
Individual drugs
Allopurinol: ↓ allopurinol effect
Amphetamine, mexiletine, quinidine: ↑ levels
Amprenavir: ↓ amprenavir effect
Chlorpromazine, isoniazid, tetracycline: ↓ absorption
Ciprofloxacin: ↓ effectiveness
Delavirdine: ↓ delavirdine effect
Diflunisal: ↓ diflunisal effect
Gabapentin: ↓ gabapentin effect
Gatifloxacin: ↓ gatifloxacin effect
Salicylate: ↓ levels
Ticlopidine: ↓ ticlopidine effect

Drug classifications
Cephalosporins: ↓ cephalosporin effect
Corticosteroids, H₂ antagonists: ↓ corticosteroid effect
Thyroid hormones: ↓ thyroid effect

▨ Herb/drug
• Buckthorn, cascara sagrada, castor, Chinese rhubarb: ↓ action of these herbs

NURSING CONSIDERATIONS
Assessment
• Assess pain symptoms: location, duration, intensity, alleviating precipitating factors
• Monitor phosphate levels, since drug is bound in GI system; urinary pH, calcium, electrolytes; hypophosphatemia: anorexia, weakness, fatigue, bone pain, hyperreflexia
• Monitor constipation; increase bulk in diet if needed

Nursing diagnoses
☑ Pain, chronic (uses)
☑ Constipation (adverse reactions)
☑ Knowledge, deficient (teaching)

Implementation
• 2 tsp (10 ml) will neutralize 20 mEq of acid; 2 tabs will neutralize 16 mEq of acid

PO route
• Give laxatives or stool softeners if constipa-
🄶 tion occurs, especially elderly
• Give after shaking liq; follow with water to facilitate passage
• Tab may be chewed if patient is unable to swallow; drink 8 oz of water after chewing; or by nasogastric tube if patient unable to swallow
• Give with 8 oz of water for hyperphosphate-mia unless contraindicated
• Give 1 hr before or after other medications to prevent poor absorption
• Give 15 ml 30 min pc and hs (esophagitis)
NG Tube
• May be given as prescribed q1-2h and given by gastric tube after diluting with water (peptic ulcer)

Patient/family education
• Instruct patient to increase fluids to 2000 ml/day unless contraindicated
• Instruct patient to avoid phosphate-containing foods (most dairy products, eggs, fruits, carbonated beverages) during drug therapy; to add cheese, corn, pasta, plums, prunes, lentils after drug (hypophosphatemia)
• Instruct patient not to use for prolonged periods if serum phosphate is low or if on a low-sodium diet; CHF patients should check for sodium content and use sodium-reduced products
• Instruct patient that stools may appear white or speckled; constipation may result; to report black tarry stools, which indicate gastric bleeding
• Instruct patient to check with prescriber after 2 wk of self-prescribed antacid use; may be used for 4-6 wk after symptoms subside or as prescribed
• Instruct patient to separate other medications by 2 hr

Evaluation
Positive therapeutic outcome
• Absence of pain, decreased acidity
• Increased pH of gastric secretions
• Decreased phosphate levels

amantadine (Rx)
(a-man'ta-deen)
amantadine HCl, Symadine, Symmetrel
Func. class.: Antiviral, antiparkinsonian agent
Chem. class.: Tricyclic amine

Pregnancy category C

Action: Prevents uncoating of nucleic acid in viral cell, preventing penetration of virus to host; causes release of dopamine from neurons

→ **Therapeutic Outcome:**
Resolution of infection, lessening of parkinsonism symptoms

Uses: Prophylaxis or treatment of influenza type A, extrapyramidal reactions, parkinsonism, respiratory tract infections

Investigational uses: Neuroleptic malignant syndrome, cocaine dependency, enuresis

Dosage and routes
Influenza type A
P **Adult and child >12 yr:** PO 200 mg/day in single dose or divided bid

P **Child 9-12 yr:** PO 100 mg bid

P **Child 1-9 yr:** PO 4.4-8.8 mg/kg/day divided bid-tid, not to exceed 200 mg/day

Extrapyramidal reaction/ parkinsonism
Adult: PO 100 mg bid, up to 400 mg/day in EPS; give for 1 wk, then 100 mg as needed up to 400 mg in parkinsonism; CCr 40-50 ml/min 100 mg/day; CCr 30 ml/min 200 mg 2×/wk; CCr 20 ml/min 100 mg 3×/wk; CCr 10 ml/min 100 mg alternating with 200 mg q7days

Available forms: Caps 100 mg; syr 50 mg/5 ml

Adverse effects
(*italic* = common; **bold** = life-threatening)
CNS: *Headache, dizziness,* drowsiness, fatigue, *anxiety,* psychosis, *depression, hallucinations,* tremors, **seizures,** confusion, *insomnia*
CV: *Orthostatic hypotension,* **CHF**
INTEG: Photosensitivity, dermatitis
EENT: Blurred vision
HEMA: Leukopenia
GI: *Nausea, vomiting,* constipation, dry mouth
GU: *Frequency, retention*

Contraindications: Hypersensitivity,
P lactation, child 1 yr, eczematous rash

Precautions: Epilepsy, CHF, orthostatic hypotension, psychiatric disorders, hepatic
G disease, renal disease, peripheral edema,
P elderly, pregnancy (C)

⚠ **Do Not Confuse:**
amantadine/ranitidine, amantadine/ rimantadine, Symmetrel/Synthroid

Pharmacokinetics
Absorption	Unknown
Distribution	Crosses placenta
Metabolism	Not metabolized
Excretion	Urine unchanged (90%), breast milk
Half-life	24 hr

Pharmacodynamics
Onset	48 hr
Peak	Unknown
Duration	Unknown

Interactions
Individual drugs
Atropine: ↑ anticholinergic response
Triamterene, hydrochlorothiazide: ↓ excretion of amantadine
Drug classifications
CNS stimulants: ↑ CNS stimulation
Anticholinergics (other): ↑ anticholinergic response
⚠ *Herb/drug*
Belladonna, henbane: ↑ anticholinergic response
Pheasant's eye, scopolia: ↑ action
Kava: ↓ action

NURSING CONSIDERATIONS
Assessment
- Monitor I&O ratio; report frequency, hesitancy
- Assess CHF, confusion, mottling of skin
- Assess bowel pattern before, during treatment
- Assess skin eruptions, photosensitivity after administration of drug
- Assess respiratory status: rate, character, wheezing, tightness in chest
- Assess allergies before initiation of treatment, reaction of each medication
- Assess signs of infection

Nursing diagnoses
✓ Infection, risk for (uses)
✓ Knowledge, deficient (teaching)

Implementation
- Give before exposure to influenza; continue for 10 days after contact

---

- Give at least 4 hr before hs to prevent insomnia
- Give after meals for better absorption, to decrease GI symptoms
- Give in divided doses to prevent CNS disturbances: headache, dizziness, fatigue, drowsiness
- Store in tight, dry container

Patient/family education
- Advise patient to change body position slowly to prevent orthostatic hypotension
- Teach about aspects of drug therapy: need to report dyspnea, weight gain, dizziness, poor concentration, dysuria, behavioral changes
- Advise patient to avoid hazardous activities if dizziness, blurred vision occurs
- Advise patient to take drug exactly as prescribed; parkinsonian crisis may occur if drug is discontinued abruptly; do not double dose; if a dose is missed, do not take within 4 hr of next dose; caps may be opened and mixed with food
- Teach to avoid alcohol

Evaluation
- Therapeutic response: absence of fever, malaise, cough, dyspnea in infection; tremors, shuffling gait in Parkinson's disease

Treatment of overdose: Withdraw drug, maintain airway, administer epiNEPHrine, aminophylline, O$_2$, IV corticosteroids, physostigmine

---

amifostine (Rx)
(a-mi-foss′teen)
Ethyol
Func. class.: Cytoprotective agent for cisplatin

Pregnancy category C

Action: Binds and detoxifies damaging metabolites of cisplatin by converting this drug by alkaline phosphatase in tissue to an active free thiol compound

➡ **Therapeutic Outcome:** Decreased toxic reaction from cisplatin

Uses: Used to reduce renal toxicity when cisplatin is given in ovarian cancer, reduces xerostomia in radiation therapy for head, neck cancer

Dosage and routes
Reduction of Renal Damage With Cisplatin
Adult: IV 910 mg/m^2 qd, within ½ hr before chemotherapy, may reduce dose to 740 mg/m^2 if higher dose is poorly tolerated

Xerostomia
Adult: IV 200 mg/m^2 qd over 3 min as inf 15-30 min before radiation therapy

Available forms: Powder for inj 500 mg/vial with 500 mg mannitol

Adverse effects
(*italic* = common; **bold** = life-threatening)
CNS: Dizziness, somnolence
CV: Hypotension
EENT: Sneezing
GI: Nausea, vomiting, hiccups
INTEG: Flushing, feeling of warmth
MISC: Hypocalcemia, rash, chills

Contraindications: Hypersensitivity to mannitol, aminothiol; hypotension, dehydration, lactation

Precautions: Elderly, CV disease, pregnancy **C,** children

Pharmacokinetics

Absorption	Complete
Distribution	Unknown
Metabolism	To free thiol compound
Excretion	Unknown
Half-life	5-8 min

Pharmacodynamics
Unknown

Interactions
Drug classfications
Antihypertensives: ↑ hypotension

NURSING CONSIDERATIONS
Assessment
- Assess for xerostomia: mouth lesion, dry mouth during therapy
- Assess fluid status before administration; administer antiemetic before administration to prevent severe nausea and vomiting; also, dexamethasone 20 mg **IV** and a serotonin antagonist such as ondansetron, dolasetron, or granisetron
- Monitor calcium levels before and during treatment; calcium supplements may be given for hypocalcemia
- Monitor blood pressure before and q5 min during infusion; if severe hypotension occurs, give **IV** 0.9% NaCl to expand fluid volume, place in Trendelenburg position

Nursing diagnoses
✓ Injury, risk for (uses)
✓ Knowledge, deficient (teaching)

Implementation
IV Intermittent IV Infusion
- Give by **IV** intermittent inf after reconstituting with 9.5 ml of sterile 0.9% NaCl, further dilute with 0.9% NaCl to a concentration of 5-40 mg/ml, give at a rate over 15 min within ½ hr of chemotherapy

Y-site compatibilities: Amikacin, aminophylline, ampicillin, ampicillin/sulbactam, aztreonam, bleomycin, bumetanide, buprenorphine, butorphanol, calcium gluconate, carboplatin, carmustine, cefazolin, cefonicid, cefotaxime, cefotetan, cefoxitin, ceftazidime, ceftizoxime, ceftriaxone, cefuroxime, cimetidine, ciprofloxacin, clindamycin, cyclophosphamide, cytarabine, dacarbazine, dactinomycin, DAUNOrubicin, dexamethasone, diphenhydrAMINE, dobutamine, DOPamine, DOXOrubicin, doxycycline, droperidol, enalaprilat, etoposide, famotidine, floxuridine, fluconazole, fludarabine, fluorouracil, furosemide, gallium, gentamicin, granisetron, haloperidol, heparin, hydrocortisone, hydromorphone, idarubicin, ifosfamide, imipenemcilastatin, leucovorin, lorazepam, magnesium sulfate, mannitol, mechlorethamine, meperidine, mesna, methotrexate, methylPREDNISolone, metoclopramide, metronidazole, mezlocillin, mitomycin, mitoxantrone, morphine, nalbuphine, netilmicin, ondansetron, piperacillin, plicamycin, potassium chloride, promethazine, ranitidine, sodium bicarbonate, streptozocin, teniposide, thiotepa, ticarcillin, ticarcillin/clavulanate, tobramycin, trimethoprim/sulfamethoxazole, trimetrexate, vancomycin, vinBLAStine, vinCRIStine, zidovudine

Additive incompatibilities: Do not mix with other drugs or solutions

Patient/family education
- Teach reason for medication and expected results, supine position during infusion
- Teach that side effects may cause severe nausea, vomiting, decreased B/P, chills, dizziness, somnolence, hiccups, sneezing

Evaluation
Positive therapeutic outcome
- Absence of renal damage

amikacin (Rx)
(am-i-kay'sin)
amikacin sulfate, Amikin
Func. class.: Antibiotic
Chem. class.: Aminoglycoside

Pregnancy category D

Action: Interferes with protein synthesis in bacterial cell by binding to ribosomal subunit, which causes misreading of genetic code; inaccurate peptide sequence forms in protein chain, causing bacterial death

➡ **Therapeutic Outcome:** Bactericidal effects for the following organisms: *Pseudomonas aeruginosa, Escherichia coli, Enterobacter, Acinetobacter, Providencia, Citrobacter, Staphylococcus, Serratia, Proteus*

Uses: Severe systemic infections of CNS, respiratory, GI, urinary tract, bone, skin, soft tissues

Investigational uses: *Mycobacterium avium* complex (intrathecal or intraventricular) in combination; aerosolization

Dosage and routes
Severe systemic infections
P *Adult and child:* **IV** inf 15 mg/kg/day in 2-3 divided doses q8-12h in 100-200 ml D₅W over 30-60 min, not to exceed 1.5 g; decreased dosages are needed in poor renal function as determined by blood levels, renal function studies; IM 15 mg/kg/day in divided doses q8-12h; qd or extended internal dosing as an alternative dosing regimen

P *Infants:* **IV**/IM 10 mg/kg initially, then 7.5 mg/kg q12h

P *Neonates:* IM/**IV** inf 10 mg/kg initially, then 7.5 mg/kg q12h in D₅W over 1-2 hr

P *Premature neonates:* **IV** 10 mg/kg initially, then 7.5 mg/kg q8-12h

Severe urinary tract infections
Adults: IM 250 mg bid

Renal dose
Adult: **IV**/IM 7.5 mg/kg initially, then increased as determined by blood levels, renal function studies

Available forms: Inj IM, **IV** 50, 250 mg/ml

Adverse effects
(*italic* = common; **bold** = life-threatening)
CNS: Confusion, depression, numbness, tremors, **seizures,** muscle twitching, **neurotoxicity,** dizziness, vertigo, tinnitus
CV: Hypotension or hypertension, palpitations

EENT: Ototoxicity, deafness, visual disturbances
GI: *Nausea, vomiting, anorexia,* increased ALT, AST, bilirubin, hepatomegaly, **hepatic necrosis,** splenomegaly
GU: **Oliguria, hematuria, renal damage, azotemia, renal failure, nephrotoxicity**
HEMA: **Agranulocytosis, thrombocytopenia, leukopenia, eosinophilia, anemia**
INTEG: *Rash,* burning, urticaria, dermatitis, alopecia

Contraindications: Mild to moderate infections, hypersensitivity to aminoglycosides, pregnancy **D**, sulfites

P *Precautions:* Neonates, mild renal disease, myasthenia gravis, lactation, hearing deficits, **G** parkinsonism, elderly

N **Do Not Confuse:**
Amikin/Amicar

Pharmacokinetics	
Absorption	Well absorbed (IM), completely absorbed (**IV**)
Distribution	Widely distributed in extracellular fluids, poor in CSF; crosses placenta
Metabolism	Minimal; liver
Excretion	Mostly unchanged (79%) in kidneys, removed by hemodialysis
Half-life	2-3 hr, prolonged up to 7 hr in infants; increased in renal disease
P	

Pharmacodynamics		
	IM	IV
Onset	Rapid	Rapid
Peak	15-30 min	1-2 hr

Interactions
Individual drugs
Dimenhydrinate, ethacrynic acid: ↑ masking of ototoxicity
Indomethacin: ↑ serum trough and peak
Drug classifications
Aminoglycosides, diuretics (loop): ↑ ototoxicity
Aminoglycosides: ↑ neurotoxicity, nephrotoxicity
Anesthetics, nondepolarizing neuromuscular blockers: ↑ neuromuscular blockade, respiratory depression
Cephalosporins, penicillins: Inactivation of amikacin
Z *Herb/drug*
Lysine (large amounts): ↑ toxicity
Acidophilus: Do not use with antiinfectives

Lab test interferences
↑ BUN, ↑ ALT, ↑ AST, ↑ bilirubin, ↑ LDH, ↑ alkaline phosphatase, ↑ creatinine, ↓ calcium, ↓ sodium, ↓ potassium, ↓ magnesium

NURSING CONSIDERATIONS
Assessment
• Assess patient for previous sensitivity reaction
• Assess patient for signs and symptoms of infection, including characteristics of wounds, sputum, urine, stool, WBC >10,000/mm³, earache, temp; obtain baseline information before and during treatment
• Obtain C&S tests before beginning drug therapy to identify if correct treatment has been initiated
• Assess for allergic reactions: rash, urticaria, pruritus
• Identify urine output; if decreasing, notify prescriber (may indicate nephrotoxicity); also notify prescriber of increased BUN and creatinine, urine CCr <80 ml/min; lower dosage should be given in renal impairment; urinalysis daily for protein, cells, casts, nephrotoxicity may be reversible if drug stopped at first sign
• Monitor blood studies: AST, ALT, CBC, Hct, bilirubin, LDH, alkaline phosphatase; Coombs' test monthly if patient is on long-term therapy
• Monitor electrolytes: potassium, sodium, chloride, magnesium monthly if patient is on long-term therapy
• Assess bowel pattern qd; if severe diarrhea occurs, drug should be discontinued
• Monitor for bleeding: ecchymosis, bleeding gums, hematuria, stool guaiac daily if on long-term therapy
• Assess for overgrowth of infection: perineal itching, fever, malaise, redness, pain, swelling, drainage, rash, diarrhea, change in cough, sputum
• Obtain weight before treatment; calculation of dosage is usually based on ideal body weight, but may be calculated on actual body weight
• Monitor VS during infusion, watch for hypotension, change in pulse
• Assess **IV** site for thrombophlebitis including pain, redness, swelling q30 min; change site if needed; apply warm compresses to discontinued site
• Obtain serum peak, drawn 30-60 min after **IV** infusion or 60 min after IM injection; trough level drawn just before next dose; 20-30 mcg/ml, trough 4-8 mcg/ml, blood level should be 2-4 times bacteriostatic level

- Urine pH if drug is used for UTI; urine should be kept alkaline
- Deafness by audiometric testing, ringing, roaring in ears, vertigo; assess hearing before, during, after treatment
- Dehydration: high sp gr, decrease in skin turgor, dry mucous membranes, dark urine
- Vestibular dysfunction: nausea, vomiting, dizziness, headache; drug should be discontinued if severe

Nursing diagnoses
☑ Infection, risk for (uses)
☑ Diarrhea (side effects)
☑ Knowledge, deficient (teaching)
☑ Injury, risk for (side effects)

Implementation
IM route
- Give deeply in large muscle mass, rotate inj sites

IV Intermittent IV infusion
- Dilute 500 mg of drug in 100-200 ml of **IV** D$_5$W, D$_5$NaCl, or 0.9% NaCl and give over ½-1 hr; flush after administration with D$_5$W or 0.9% NaCl

Syringe compatibilities: Clindamycin, doxapram

Y-site compatibilities: Acyclovir, amifostine, amiodarone, amsacrine, aztreonam, cisatracurium, cyclophosphamide, dexamethasone, diltiazem, enalamprilat, esmolol, filgrastim, fluconazole, fludarabine, foscarnet, furosemide, granisetron, idarubicin, IL-2, labetalol, lorazepam, magnesium sulfate, melphalan, midazolam, morphine, ondansetron, paclitaxel, perphenazine, remifentanil, sargramostim, teniposide, thiotepa, TPN #54, #61, #91, #203, #204, #212, vinorelbine, warfarin, zidovudine

Patient/family education
- Teach patient to report sore throat, bruising, bleeding, joint pain; may indicate blood dyscrasias (rare)
- Advise patient to contact prescriber if vaginal itching, loose foul-smelling stools, furry tongue occur; may indicate superinfection
- Advise patient to report hypersensitivity: rash, itching, trouble breathing, facial edema and notify prescriber

Evaluation
Positive therapeutic outcome
- Absence of signs/symptoms of infection: WBC <10,000/mm^3, temp WNL; absence of red draining wounds; absence of earache
- Reported improvement in symptoms of infection

Treatment of overdose: Withdraw drug; administer epINEPHrine, O$_2$, hemodialysis, exchange transfusion in the newborn; monitor serum levels of drug; may give ticarcillin or carbenicillin

---

amiloride (Rx)
(a-mill'oh-ride)
Amiloride HCl, Midamor
Func. class.: Potassium-sparing diuretic
Chem. class.: Pyrazine

Pregnancy category B

Action: Acts primarily on proximal distal tubule by inhibiting reabsorption of sodium and water and increasing potassium retention and conserving hydrogen ions

Therapeutic Outcome: Diuretic and antihypertensive effect while retaining potassium

Uses: Diuretic-induced hypokalemia; used with other agents to treat edema, hypertension

Dosage and routes
Adult: PO 5 mg qd; may be increased to 10-20 mg qd if needed

Available forms: Tabs 5 mg

Adverse effects
(*italic* = common; **bold** = life-threatening)
CNS: *Headache,* dizziness, fatigue, weakness, paresthesias, tremor, depression, anxiety
CV: Orthostatic hypotension, dysrhythmias, angina
EENT: Loss of hearing, tinnitus, blurred vision, nasal congestion, increased intraocular pressure
ELECT: **Hyperkalemia**
GI: *Nausea, diarrhea,* dry mouth, *vomiting, anorexia,* cramps, constipation, abdominal pain, jaundice, bleeding
GU: *Polyuria,* dysuria, frequency, impotence
HEMA: **Aplastic anemia, neutropenia (rare)**
INTEG: *Rash, pruritus,* alopecia, urticaria
RESP: Cough, dyspnea, shortness of breath

Contraindications: Anuria, hypersensitivity, hyperkalemia, impaired renal function

Precautions: Dehydration, pregnancy **B,** diabetes, acidosis, lactation, hepatic disease

---

Pharmacokinetics

Absorption	Variable (10%-15%)
Distribution	Widely distributed
Metabolism	Unchanged in urine (50%), in feces (40%)
Excretion	Renal; breast milk
Half-life	6-9 hr

Pharmacodynamics

Onset	2 hr
Peak	6-10 hr
Duration	24 hr

Interactions

Individual drugs

Lithium: ↑ Lithium toxicity

Drug classifications

ACE inhibitors, diuretics (potassium-sparing), potassium products, salt substitutes: ↑ hyperkalemia

Antihypertensives: ↑ action

NSAIDs: ↓ effectiveness of amiloride

Food/drug

Potassium foods: ↑ hyperkalemia

Herb/drug

Arginine: Fatal hypokalemia

Bearberry, gossypol: ↑ hypokalemia

Cucumber, dandelion, horsetail, licorice, nettle, pumpkin, Queen Anne's lace: ↑ amiloride effect

Khella: ↑ hypotension

St. John's wort: ↑ severe photosensitivity

Lab test interferences

Interference: GTT

NURSING CONSIDERATIONS

Assessment

- Monitor manifestations of hyperkalemia: *MS:* fatigue, muscle weakness; *CARDIAC:* dysrhythmias, hypotension; *NEURO:* paresthesias, confusion; *RESP:* dyspnea
- Monitor for manifestations of hyponatremia: *CV:* increased B/P, cold, clammy skin, hypovolemia or hypervolemia; *GI:* anorexia, nausea, vomiting, diarrhea, abdominal cramps; *NEURO:* lethargy, increased ICP, confusion, headache, seizures, coma, fatigue, tremors, hyperreflexia
- Monitor for manifestations of hyperchloremia: *NEURO:* weakness, lethargy, coma; *RESP:* deep rapid breathing
- Assess fluid volume status: I&O ratios and record, weight, distended red veins, crackles in lung, color, quality, and sp gr of urine, skin turgor, adequacy of pulses, moist mucous membranes, bilateral lung sounds, peripheral pitting edema; dehydration symptoms of decreasing output, thirst, hypotension, dry mouth and mucous membranes should be reported
- Monitor electrolytes: potassium, sodium, calcium, magnesium; also include BUN, ABGs, uric acid, CBC, blood glucose
- Assess B/P before and during therapy with patient lying, standing, and sitting as appropriate; orthostatic hypotension can occur rapidly

Nursing diagnoses

☑ Fluid volume, deficient (side effects)

☑ Fluid volume, excess (uses)

☑ Knowledge, deficient (teaching)

Implementation

- Give in AM to avoid interference with sleep
- With food; if nausea occurs, absorption may be increased

Patient/family education

- Teach patient to take medication early in the day to prevent nocturia
- Instruct patient to take with food or milk if GI symptoms of nausea and anorexia occur
- Teach patient to maintain a weekly record of weight and notify prescriber of weight loss >5 lb
- Caution patient that this drug causes an increase in potassium levels, so foods high in potassium should be avoided; refer to dietician for assistance, planning
- Caution patient not to exercise in hot weather or stand for prolonged periods since orthostatic hypotension will be enhanced
- Teach patient not to use alcohol or any OTC medications without prescriber's approval; serious drug reactions may occur
- Emphasize the need to contact prescriber immediately if muscle cramps, weakness, nausea, dizziness, or numbness occurs
- Teach patient to take own B/P and pulse and record
- Advise patient that dizziness and confusion may occur; avoid driving or other hazardous activities if alertness is decreased
- Teach patient to continue taking medication even if feeling better; this drug controls symptoms but does not cure the condition
- Advise patient with hypertension to continue other medical treatment (exercise, weight loss, relaxation techniques, cessation of smoking)

Evaluation

Positive therapeutic outcome

- Prevention of hypokalemia (diuretic use)
- Decreased edema
- Decreased B/P
- Increased diuresis

Treatment of overdose: Lavage if taken orally; monitor electrolytes; administer **IV** fluids; monitor hydration, CV, renal status

---

amino acid (Rx)
(a-mee′noe)

Injection: Aminess, Aminosyn, BranchAmin, NephrAmine, FreAmine HBC, HepatAmine
Solution:
Aminosyn, Aminosyn II, Aminosyn-PF, FreAmine III, Novamine, ProcalAmine, RenAmin, Travasol, Trophamine
Func. class.: Caloric agent
Chem. class.: Nitrogen product

Pregnancy category C

Action: Needed for anabolism to maintain structure; decreases catabolism, promotes healing

Therapeutic Outcome: Positive nitrogen balance, decreased catabolism

Uses: Hepatic encephalopathy, cirrhosis, hepatitis, nutritional support in cancer trauma, intestinal obstruction, short bowel syndrome, severe malabsorption

Dosage and routes
Amino acid injection
Adult: **IV** 80-120 g/day; 500 ml of amino acids/500 ml D_{50} given over 24 hr

Amino acid solution
Adult: **IV** 1-1.5 g/kg/day titrated to patient's needs

P *Child:* **IV** 2-3 g/kg/day titrated to patient's needs

Available forms: Inj **IV** 2.75%, 3.5%, 4.25%, 5%, 5.5%, 6%, 8.5%, 10%, 11.4%, 15% amino acids

Adverse effects
(*italic* = common; **bold** = life-threatening)
CNS: Dizziness, headache, confusion, **loss of consciousness**
CV: Hypertension, **CHF, pulmonary edema**
ENDO: Hyperglycemia, rebound hypoglycemia, electrolyte imbalances, hyperosmolar syndrome, hyperosmolar hyperglycemic nonketotic syndrome, alkalosis, acidosis, hypophosphatemia, hyperammonemia, dehydration, hypocalcemia
GI: Nausea, vomiting, liver fat deposits, abdominal pain
GU: Glycosuria, osmotic diuresis
INTEG: Chills, flushing, warm feeling, rash, urticaria, extravasation necrosis, phlebitis at inj site

Contraindications: Hypersensitivity, severe electrolyte imbalances, anuria, severe liver damage, maple syrup urine disease, PKU

Precautions: Renal disease, pregnancy **C**, **P** children, diabetes mellitus, CHF

Pharmacokinetics
Absorption	Complete bioavailability
Distribution	Widely distributed
Metabolism	Anabolism
Excretion	Kidney to urea nitrogen
Half-life	Unknown

Pharmacodynamics
Unknown

Interactions
Drug classifications
Diuretics, glucocorticoids, tetracyclines: ↑ negative nitrogen balance

NURSING CONSIDERATIONS
Assessment
• Monitor electrolytes (potassium, sodium, calcium, chloride, magnesium), blood glucose, ammonia, phosphate, ketones; renal, liver function studies: BUN, creatinine, ALT, AST, bilirubin; urine glucose q6h using Chemstrips, which are not affected by infusion substances; if BUN increases over 15%, therapy may need to be discontinued
• Check inj site for extravasation: redness along vein, edema at site, necrosis, pain; for a hard, tender area
• Monitor respiratory function q4h: auscultate lung fields bilaterally for crackles; monitor respirations for quality, rate, rhythm that indicates fluid overload
• Monitor temperature q4h for increased fever, indicating infection; if infection is suspected, infusion is discontinued and tubing, bottle, catheter tip cultured; blood catheter may be obtained
• Monitor for impending hepatic coma: asterixis, confusion, fetor, lethargy
• Hyperammonemia: nausea, vomiting, malaise, tremors, anorexia, convulsions; increased ammonia, ketone levels may occur

Nursing diagnoses
✓ Nutrition: less than body requirements (uses), imbalanced
✓ Injury, risk for physical (uses, adverse reactions)
✓ Infection, risk for (adverse reactions)
✓ Knowledge, deficient (teaching)

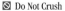 Herb/drug   Ⓢ Do Not Crush   ◆ Alert   ◆ Key Drug   **G** Geriatric   **P** Pediatric

Implementation

IV Continuous IV

- Give up to 40% protein and dextrose (up to 12.5%) via peripheral vein; stronger solutions require central **IV** administration; TPN only mixed with dextrose to promote protein synthesis
- Use immediately after mixing in pharmacy under strict aseptic technique using laminar flowhood; use infusion pump, in-line filter (0.22 µm) unless mixed with fat emulsion and dextrose (3 in 1)
- Use careful monitoring technique; do not speed up infusion; pulmonary edema, glucose overload will result
- Storage depends on type of solution; consult manufacturer
- Change dressing and **IV** tubing to prevent infection q24-48h or q5-7 days if transparent dressing is used

Y-site compatibilities: Amikacin, aminophylline, amoxicillin, ampicillin, ascorbic acid inj, atracurium, azlocillin, aztreonam, bumetanide, buprenorphine, calcium gluconate, carboplatin, cefamandole, cefazolin, cefonicid, cefoperazone, cefotaxime, cefotetan, cefoxtin, ceftazidime, ceftizoxime, ceftriaxone, cefuroxime, cephalothin, cephapirin, chloramphenicol, chlorproMAZINE, cimetidine, clindamycin, clonazepam, dexamethasone, diazepam, digoxin, diphenhydrAMINE, DOBUTamine, DOPamine, doxycycline, droperidol, enalaprilat, epINEPHrine, erythromycin lactobionate, famotidine, fentanyl, flucloxacillin, fluconazole, folic acid, foscarnet, gentamicin, granisetron, haloperidol, heparin, hydrocortisone, hydromorphone, hydrOXYzine, idarubicin, ifosfamide, IL-2, imipenem/cilastatin, insulin (regular), isoproterenol, kanamycin, leucovorin, levorphanol, lidocaine, lorazepam, magnesium sulfate, mannitol, meperidine, mesna, methicillin, metronidazole, mezlocillin, miconazole, morphine, moxalactam, multivitamins, nafcillin, netilmicin, nitroglycerin, norepINEPHrine, octreotide, ofloxacin, ondansetron, oxacillin, paclitaxel, penicillin G, penicillin G potassium, pentobarbital, phenobarbital, piperacillin, potassium chloride, prochlorperazine, ranitidine, salbutamol, sargramostim, tacrolimus, thiotepa, ticarcillin, ticarcillin/clavulanate, tobramycin, trimethoprim/sulfamethoxazole, urokinase, vancomycin, vecuronium, zidovudine

Y-site incompatibilities: Cephradine

Additive compatibilities: Amikacin, aminophylline, aztreonam, calcium gluconate, cefamandole, cefazolin, cefepime, cefotaxime, cefoxitin, cefsulodin, ceftazidime, ceftriaxone, cefuroxime, cimetidine, clindamycin, cyanocobalamin, cyclophosphamide, cycloSPORINE, cytarabine, DOPamine, epoetin, erythromycin, famotidine, folic acid, fosphenytoin, furosemide, heparin, insulin (regular), isoproterenol, lidocaine, meperidine, metaraminol, methicillin, methotrexate, methyldopate, methylPREDNISolone, metoclopramide, morphine, nafcillin, netilmicin, nizatidine, norepINEPHrine, ondansetron, oxacillin, penicillin G potassium, penicillin G sodium, phytonadione, polymyxin B, sodium bicarbonate, tacrolimus, tobramycin, vancomycin

Patient/family education

- Teach reason for use of amino acids as part of nutrition (TPN)
- Instruct patient to report at once to prescriber if chills, sweating are experienced

Evaluation

Positive therapeutic outcome

- Weight gain
- Decreased jaundice in liver disorders
- Increased LOC

---

aminophylline (Rx)
(am-in-off'i-lin)
Aminophyllin, Phyllocontin, Truphylline
Func. class.: Bronchodilator, spasmolytic
Chem. class.: Xanthine, ethylenediamine

Pregnancy category C

Action: Exact mechanism unknown; relaxes smooth muscle of respiratory system by blocking phosphodiesterase, which increases cyclic AMP; increased cyclic AMP alters intracellular calcium ion movements; produces bronchodilatation, increased pulmonary blood flow, relaxation of respiratory tract

Therapeutic Outcome: Increased ability to breathe

Uses: Bronchial asthma, bronchospasm associated with chronic bronchitis, emphysema, bradycardia

Investigational uses: Apnea in infancy for respiratory/myocardial stimulation, Cheyne-Stokes respirations as a respiratory stimulant

Dosage and routes

Adult: PO 6 mg/kg, then 3 mg/kg q6h × 2 doses, then 3 mg/kg q8h maintenance, max 900 mg/day or 13 mg/kg; PO in CHF 6 mg/kg, then 2 mg/kg q8h × 2 doses, then 1-2 mg/kg q12h maintenance; **IV** 4.7 mg/kg, then 0.55 mg/kg/hr × 12 hr, then 0.36 mg/kg/hr maintenance, **IV** in CHF 4.7 mg/kg, then 0.39 mg/kg/hr × 12 hr, then 0.08-0.16 mg/kg/hr maintenance

G *Elderly and in cor pulmonale:* PO 6 mg/kg, then 2 mg/kg q6h × 2 doses, then 2 mg/kg q8h maintenance; **IV** 4.7 mg/kg, then 0.47 mg/kg/hr × 12 hr, then 0.24 mg/kg/hr maintenance

P *Child 9-16 yr:* PO 6 mg/kg, then 3 mg/kg q4h × 3 doses, then 3 mg/kg q6h maintenance, max 18 mg/kg/day 12-16 yr, or 20 mg/kg/day 9-12 yr; **IV** 4.7 mg/kg, then 0.79 mg/kg/hr × 12 hr, then 0.63 mg/kg/hr maintenance

P *Child 6 mo-9 yr:* PO 4 mg/kg q4h × 3 doses, then 4 mg/kg q6h maintenance, max 24 mg/kg/day; **IV** 4.7 mg/kg, then 0.95 mg/kg/hr × 12 hr, then 0.79 mg/kg/hr maintenance

P *Infants 6-52 wk:* Dose (0.2 × age in wk) ÷ 5 × kg = 24 hr dose in mg

P *Premature <24 day postnatal:* 1 mg/kg q12h initially

P *>24 days postnatal:* 1.5 mg/kg q12hr

P *Neonates up to 40 wk premature postconception age:* PO/**IV** 1 mg/kg q12hr

P *Neonates at birth or 40 wk postconception age:* PO/**IV** >8 wk postnatal 1-3 mg/kg q6h; 4-8 wk postnatal 1-2 mg/kg q8h; up to 4 wk postnatal 1-2 mg/kg q12h

Hepatic disease
Adult: PO 6 mg/kg, then 2 mg/kg q8h × 2 doses, then 1-2 mg/kg q12h maintenance; **IV** 4.7 mg/kg, then 0.39 mg/kg/hr × 12 hr, then 0.08-0.16 mg/kg/hr maintenance

Available forms: Inj 250 mg/10 ml, 500 mg/21 ml, 100 mg/100 ml in 0.45% NaCl; rec supp 250 mg, 500 mg; oral liq 105 mg/5 ml; tabs 100, 200 mg; cont rel tabs 225, 350 mg

Adverse effects
(*italic* = common; **bold** = life-threatening)
CNS: Anxiety, restlessness, insomnia, *dizziness*, **seizures,** headache, lightheadedness, muscle twitching
CV: *Palpitations, sinus tachycardia,* hypotension, flushing, dysrhythmias
GI: *Nausea, vomiting,* diarrhea, dyspepsia, anal irritation (suppositories), epigastric pain
GU: Urinary frequency, SIADH

INTEG: Flushing, urticaria, *rec supp (irritation)*
RESP: Tachypnea, increased respiratory rate

Contraindications: Hypersensitivity to xanthines, tachydysrhythmias, active peptic ulcer disease

G **Precautions:** Elderly, CHF, cor pulmonale, hepatic disease, diabetes mellitus, hyperthyroidism, hypertension, seizure disorder, **P** irritation of the rectum or lower colon, children, pregnancy **C**, alcoholism

Pharmacokinetics

Absorption	Well absorbed (PO), slow (PO–ext rel), erratic (rec)
Distribution	Widely distributed; crosses placenta
Metabolism	Liver to caffeine
Excretion	Kidneys
Half-life	3-12 hr, increased in renal disease, CHF, geriatric patients, smokers

Pharmacodynamics

	PO	PO–EXT REL	IV
Onset	15-60 min	Unknown	Immediate
Peak	1-2 hr	4-7 hr	Infusion's end
Duration	6-8 hr	8-12 hr	6-8 hr

Interactions
Individual drugs
Adenosine, phenytoin, rifampin: ↓ aminophylline effect
Allopurinol, cimetidine, disulfiram, interferon: ↓ metabolism, ↑ toxicity of aminophylline
Carbamazepine, isoniazid: ↑ or ↓ aminophylline levels
Clarithromycin, fluvoxamine: ↑ aminophylline toxicity
Halothane: ↑ risk of dysrhythmias
Ketoconazole: ↓ effect of aminophylline
Lithium: ↓ effect of lithium
Methotrexate: ↑ effect of aminophylline
Mexiletine, thiabendazole: ↓ metabolism, ↑ toxicity
Phenytoin, rifampin: ↑ metabolism
Drug classifications
Antibiotics (macrolide), calcium channel blockers, diuretics (loop), oral contraceptives: ↑ aminophylline levels
Barbiturates, β-adrenergic blockers, diuretics (loop): ↓ effect of aminophylline
Corticosteroids, influenza vaccines: ↑ aminophylline toxicity

 Herb/drug   Do Not Crush   Alert   Key Drug   Geriatric   **P** Pediatric

Fluoroquinolones: ↓ metabolism, ↑ toxicity
Sympathomimetics: ↑ CNS, ↑ CV, adverse reactions

Smoking
↑ Metabolism, ↓ effect

Food/drug
Caffeinated foods (cola, coffee, tea, chocolate): ↑ CNS, CV, adverse reactions
Charcoal-smoked foods: ↓ effect

⊘ Herb/drug
Cola tree, ephedra, guarana, tea (black, green), yerba maté: ↑ effects
Ginseng, horsetail, Siberian ginseng, St. John's wort: ↓ effects

Lab test interferences
↑ Plasma free fatty acids

NURSING CONSIDERATIONS
Assessment
• Monitor theophylline blood levels (therapeutic level is 10-20 mcg/ml); toxicity may occur with small increase above 20 mcg/ml; especially elderly; determine whether theophylline was given recently (24 hr); check for toxicity: nausea, vomiting, anxiety, restlessness, insomnia, tachycardia, dysrhythmias, seizures; notify prescriber immediately
• Monitor I&O; diuresis will occur; dehydration may result in elderly or children in whom diuresis is great
• Monitor respiratory rate, rhythm, depth; auscultate lung fields bilaterally; notify prescriber of abnormalities; check ECG for tachycardia, PVCs, PACs in patients with cardiac problems
• Monitor allergic reactions: rash, urticaria; if these occur, drug should be discontinued, prescriber notified

Nursing diagnoses
✓ Airway clearance, ineffective (uses)
✓ Activity intolerance (uses)
✓ Injury, risk for (uses, adverse reactions)
✓ Knowledge, deficient (teaching)

Implementation
General
• Give around the clock to maintain blood (theophylline) levels
• If switching from **IV** to PO, give controlled-release dose at time of **IV** infusion discontinuation; if giving tab (immediate release), discontinue **IV** and wait >4 hr

PO route
• Avoid giving with food
⊘ • Do not crush or chew enteric-coated or controlled-release tabs

IV IV route
• May be diluted for **IV** inf in 100-200 ml in D_5W, $D_{10}W$, $D_{20}W$, 0.9% NaCl, 0.45% NaCl, LR
• Give loading dose over ½ hr, max rate of inf 25 mg/min, use infusion pump; after loading dose, give by cont inf
• Avoid IM inj; pain and tissue damage may occur
• Only clear sol; flush **IV** line before dose; store diluted sol for 24 hr if refrigerated

Syringe compatibilities: Heparin, metoclopramide, pentobarbital, thiopental

Y-site compatibilities: Allopurinol, amifostine, amphotericin B sulfate complex, amrinone, aztreonam, ceftazidime, cimetidine, cladribine, DOXOrubicin liposome, enalaprilat, esmolol, famotidine, filgrastim, fluconazole, fludarabine, foscarnet, gallium, granisetron, heparin sodium with hydrocortisone sodium succinate, labetalol, melphalan, meropenem, netilmicin, paclitaxel, pancuronium, piperacillin/tazobactam, potassium chloride, propofol, ranitidine, remifentanil, sargramostim, tacrolimus, teniposide, thiotepa, tolazoline, vecuronium

Y-site incompatibilities: DOBUTamine, hydrALAZINE, ondansetron

Additive compatibilities: Amobarbital, bretylium, calcium gluconate, chloramphenicol, cibenzoline, cimetidine, dexamethasone, diphenhydrAMINE, DOPamine, erythromycin lactobionate, esmolol, floxacillin, flumazenil, furosemide, heparin, hydrocortisone, lidocaine, mephentermine, meropenem, methyldopate, metronidazole/sodium bicarbonate, nitroglycerin, pentobarbital, phenobarbital, potassium chloride, ranitidine, secobarbital, sodium bicarbonate, terbutaline

Additive incompatibilities: Ascorbic acid, bleomycin, cephalothin, cefotaxime, chlorproMAZINE, cimetidine, clindamycin, codeine, dimenhyDRINATE, DOBUTamine, DOXOrubicin, doxycycline, epINEPHrine, erythromycin glucepate, hydrALAZINE, hydrOXYzine, insulin, isoproterenol, meperidine, methicillin, morphine, nafcillin, nitroprusside, norepinephrine, oxytetracycline, papaverine, penicillin G, pentazocine, phenobarbital, phenytoin, prochlorperazine, promazine, promethazine, sulfiSOXAZOLE, tetracycline, vancomycin

Rectal route
• Rec dose if patient is unable to take PO; retain rec dose for ½ hour

Patient/family education
• Teach patient to take doses as prescribed, not to skip dose; to check OTC medications,

current prescription medications for epHEDrine, which will increase CNS stimulation; advise patient not to drink alcohol or caffeine products (tea, coffee, chocolate, colas), which will increase action

• Teach patient to avoid hazardous activities; dizziness may occur

• Teach patient if GI upset occurs, to take drug with 8 oz of water or food; absorption may be decreased

• Teach patient to remain in bed 15-20 min after rec supp is inserted to prevent removal

• Instruct patient to avoid smoking; decreases blood levels and terminal half-life

• Instruct patient that smoking increases metabolism; dosage may need to be increased

• Teach patient to obtain blood levels of drug every few months to prevent toxicity; not to change brands, since effect may not be the same

• Teach patient to increase fluids to 2 L/day to decrease viscosity of secretions

• Advise patient to report toxicity: nausea, vomiting, anxiety, insomnia, rapid pulse, seizures, flushing, headache, diarrhea

Evaluation
Positive therapeutic outcome
• Decreased dyspnea
P • Respiratory stimulation in infants
• Clear lung fields bilaterally

! HIGH ALERT

amiodarone (Rx)
(a-mee-oh'da-rone)
Cordarone, Pacerone
Func. class.: Antidysrhythmic (Class III)
Chem. class.: Iodinated benzofuran derivative

Pregnancy category D

Action: Prolongs action potential duration and effective refractory period, slows sinus rate with increasing PR and QT intervals, noncompetitive α- and β-adrenergic inhibition; increases PR and QT intervals, decreases sinus rate, decreases peripheral vascular resistance

➡ **Therapeutic Outcome:** Decreased amount and severity of ventricular dysrhythmias

Uses: Severe ventricular tachycardia, supraventricular tachycardia, ventricular fibrillation or atrial fibrillation not controlled by 1st-line agents

Dosage and routes
Ventricular dysrhythmias
Adult: PO loading dose 800-1600 mg/day for 1-3 wk; then 600-800 mg/day × 1 mo; maintenance 400 mg/day; **IV** loading dose (first rapid) 150 mg over the first 10 min then slow 360 mg over the next 6 hr; maintenance 540 mg given over the remaining 18 hr, decrease rate of the slow infusion to 0.5 mg/min

P **Child:** PO loading dose 10-15 mg/kg/day in 1-2 divided doses for 4-14 days then 5 mg/kg/day (not recommended in children)

P **Child/infant:** **IV**/Intraosseous 5 mg/kg as a bolus (PALS guidelines)

Perfusion tachycardia: **IV** 5 mg/kg loading dose given over 20-60 min

Supraventricular tachycardia
Adult: PO 600-800 mg/day × 7 days or until desired response, then 400 mg/day × 21 days, then 200-400 mg/day maintenance

P **Child:** PO 10 mg/kg/day (800 mg/1.72 m²/day) × 10 days or until desired response, then 5 mg/kg/day (400 mg/1.72 m²/day) × 21-28 days, then 2.5 mg/kg/day (200 mg/1.72 m²/day) (not recommended in children)

Available forms: Tabs 200, 400 mg; inj 50 mg/ml

Adverse effects
(*italic* = common; **bold** = life-threatening)
CNS: *Headache, dizziness,* involuntary movement, tremors, peripheral neuropathy, malaise, fatigue, ataxia, paresthesias, insomnia
CV: *Hypotension,* **bradycardia, sinus arrest, CHF, dysrhythmias, SA node dysfunction**
EENT: Blurred vision, halos, photophobia, **corneal microdeposits,** dry eyes
ENDO: Hyperthyroidism or hypothyroidism
GI: Nausea, vomiting, diarrhea, abdominal pain, anorexia, constipation, **hepatotoxicity**
INTEG: Rash, photosensitivity, blue-gray skin discoloration, alopecia, spontaneous ecchymosis, **toxic epidermal necrolysis**
MISC: Flushing, abnormal taste or smell, edema, abnormal salivation, coagulation abnormalities
MS: Weakness, pain in extremities
RESP: **Pulmonary fibrosis,** pulmonary inflammation, **adult respiratory distress**
P **syndrome, gasping syndrome in neonates**

Contraindications: Sinus node dysfunction; 2nd- or 3rd-degree AV block;
P pregnancy **D**, neonates, infants, bradycardia, lactation

▨ Herb/drug   ⊠ Do Not Crush   ◈ Alert   ☞ Key Drug   G Geriatric   P Pediatric

Precautions: Goiter, Hashimoto's thyroiditis, electrolyte imbalances, CHF, severe hepatic, respiratory disease, children

Do Not Confuse:
Cordarone/Inocor

Pharmacokinetics

Absorption	Slow, variable (PO) up to 65%
Distribution	Body tissues; crosses placenta
Metabolism	Liver
Excretion	Bile, kidney (minimal)
Half-life	15-100 days

Pharmacodynamics

	PO
Onset	1-3 wk
Peak	Unknown
Duration	Up to months

Interactions
Individual drugs
Digoxin, disopyramide, flecainide, mexiletine, procainamide, quinidine, warfarin: ↑ blood levels, ↑ toxicity
Phenytoin: ↑ blood levels
Theophylline: ↑ levels
Warfarin: ↑ bleeding
Drug classifications
β-Adrenergic blockers, calcium channel blockers: ↑ dysrhythmias, cardiac arrest
Herb/drug
Aconite: ↑ toxicity, death
Aloe, broom, buckthorn (chronic use), cascara sagrada (chronic use), Chinese rhubarb, figwort, fumitory, goldenseal, kudzu, licorice: ↑ effect
Coltsfoot: ↓ effect
Horehound: ↑ serotonin effect

Lab test interference
↑ T_4

NURSING CONSIDERATIONS
Assessment
• Monitor I&O ratio; monitor electrolytes: potassium, sodium, chloride
• Monitor chest x-ray, thyroid function tests
• Monitor liver function studies: AST, ALT, bilirubin, alkaline phosphatase
• Monitor ECG continuously to determine drug effectiveness; measure PR, QRS, QT intervals; check for PVCs, other dysrhythmias; monitor B/P continuously for hypotension, hypertension; check for rebound hypertension after 1-2 hr
• Monitor for dehydration or hypovolemia
• Assess for CNS symptoms: confusion, psychosis, numbness, depression, involuntary

movements; if these occur, drug should be discontinued
• Assess for hypothyroidism: lethargy, dizziness, constipation, enlarged thyroid gland, edema of extremities, cool, pale skin
• Monitor hyperthyroidism: restlessness, tachycardia, eyelid puffiness, weight loss, frequent urination, menstrual irregularities, dyspnea, warm, moist skin
• Assess for pulmonary toxicity including ARDS, pulmonary fibrosis: dyspnea, fatigue, cough, fever, chest pain; drug should be discontinued if these occur
• Monitor cardiac rate, respiration: rate, rhythm, character, chest pain, ventricular tachycardia, supraventricular tachycardia or fibrillation
• Assess sight and vision before treatment and throughout therapy; microdeposits on the cornea may cause blurred vision, halos, and photophobia

Nursing diagnoses
☑ Cardiac output, decreased (uses)
☑ Gas exchange, impaired (adverse reactions)
☑ Knowledge, deficient (teaching)

Implementation
Start with patient hospitalized and monitored
PO route
• Give reduced dosage slowly with ECG monitoring only
• Loading dose with food to decrease nausea
Intermittent IV infusion
• 1000 mg/24 hr during loading/maintenance
• Initial loading: add 3 ml (150 mg) 100 ml D_5W (1.5 mg/ml) give over 10 min
• Loading inf: add 18 ml (900 mg) 500 ml D_5W (1.8 mg/ml) give over next 6 hr
• Maintenance inf: Give remainder of loading inf 540 mg over 18 hr (0.5 mg/min)
Continuous inf:
• After 24 hr, give 1-6 mg/ml at 0.5 mg/ml, max 30 mg/min

Y-site compatibilities: Amikacin, bretylium, clindamycin, DOBUTamine, DOPamine, doxycycline, erythromycin, esmolol, gentamicin, insulin (regular), isoproterenol, labetalol, lidocaine, metaraminol, metronidazole, midazolam, morphine, nitroglycerin, norepinephrine, penicillin G potassium, phentolamine, phenylephrine, potassium chloride, procainamide, tobramycin, vancomycin

Additive compatibilities: DOBUTamine, lidocaine, potassium chloride, procainamide, verapamil

Solution compatibilities: D_5W, 0.9% NaCl

Patient/family education

- Instruct patient to report side effects immediately to prescriber
- Instruct patient that skin discoloration is usually reversible, but skin may turn bluish on neck, face, arms when used for long periods
- Advise patient that dark glasses may be needed for photophobia
- Instruct patient to use sunscreen and protective clothing to prevent burning associated with photosensitivity
- Instruct patient to take medication as prescribed, not to double doses
- Instruct patient to complete follow-up appointment with health care provider including pulmonary function studies, chest x-ray, ophthalmic examinations

Treatment of overdose: Administer O₂, artificial ventilation, ECG, DOPamine for circulatory depression, diazepam or thiopental for seizures, isoproterenol

---

amitriptyline (Rx)
(a-mee-trip'ti-leen)

amitriptyline HCl, Apo-Amitriptyline ✦, Elavil, Endep, Levate ✦, Novotriptyn ✦
Func. class.: Antidepressant—tricyclic
Chem. class.: Tertiary amine

Pregnancy category C

Action: Blocks reuptake of norepinephrine, serotonin into nerve endings that increase action of norepinephrine, serotonin in nerve cells

Uses: Major depression

Investigational uses: Chronic pain management, prevention of cluster/migraine headaches, fibromyalgia

➔Therapeutic Outcome: Decreased symptoms of depression after 2-3 wk

Dosage and routes
Depression
Adult: PO 75 mg/day in divided doses; may increase to 150 mg qd, not to exceed 300 mg/day; IM 20-30 mg qid, or 80-120 mg hs

P *Elderly/Adolescent:* PO 30 mg/day in
G divided doses; may be increased to 100 mg/day

Cluster/migraine headaches
Adult: PO 50-150 mg/day

Chronic pain
Adult: PO 75-150 mg/day

Fibromyalgia
Adult: PO 10-50 mg qhs

Available forms: Tabs 10, 25, 50, 75, 100, 150 mg; inj IM 10 mg/ml; syr 10 mg/5 ml

Adverse effects
(*italic* = common; **bold** = life-threatening)
CNS: Dizziness, drowsiness, confusion, headache, anxiety, tremors, stimulation, weakness, insomnia, nightmares, EPS
G (elderly), increased psychiatric symptoms, **hyperthermia**
CV: Orthostatic hypotension, **ECG changes, tachycardia, hypertension,** palpitations, dysrhythmias
EENT: Blurred vision, tinnitus, mydriasis, ophthalmoplegia
GI: Constipation, dry mouth, weight gain, nausea, vomiting, **paralytic ileus,** increased appetite, cramps, epigastric distress, jaundice, **hepatitis,** stomatitis
GU: Urinary retention
HEMA: **Agranulocytosis, thrombocytopenia, eosinophilia, leukopenia**
INTEG: Rash, urticaria, sweating, pruritus, photosensitivity

Contraindications: Hypersensitivity to tricyclic antidepressants, recovery phase of myocardial infarction, narrow-angle glaucoma

Precautions: Suicidal patients, seizure disorders, prostatic hypertrophy, schizophrenia, psychosis, severe depression, increased intraocular pressure, narrow angle glaucoma, urinary retention, cardiac disease, hepatic/renal disease, hyperthyroidism, electroshock
P therapy, elective surgery, child <12 yr, preg-
G nancy **C**, elderly

⊠ Do Not Confuse:
amitriptyline/nortriptyline, Elavil/Mellaril, Elavil/Oruvail

Pharmacokinetics

Absorption	Well absorbed
Distribution	Widely distributed; crosses placenta
Metabolism	Liver, extensively
Excretion	Kidneys, breast milk
Half-life	10-46 hr

Pharmacodynamics

	PO/IM
Onset	45 min
Peak	2-12 hr
Duration	Unknown

 Herb/drug   Do Not Crush   Alert   Key Drug   Geriatric   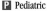 Pediatric

Interactions
Individual drugs
Alcohol: ↑ CNS depression
Carbamazepine: ↑ amitriptyline levels
Cimetidine, fluoxetine: ↑ levels, ↑ toxicity
Clonidine: ↑ hypertension; avoid use
Guanethidine: ↓ effects
Drug classifications
Antidepressants, antidysrhythmics IC: ↑ amitriptyline levels
Antihypertensives: Blocked response to antihypertensives
Antithyroid agents: ↑ risk of agranulocytosis
Barbiturates, benzodiazepines, CNS depressants: ↑ CNS effects
MAOIs: Hypertensive crisis, seizures
Oral contraceptives: ↑ effects, toxicity
Phenothiazines: ↑ amitriptyline levels, toxicity
Sympathomimetics (indirect acting): ↓ effects
Smoking
↑ Metabolism, ↓ effects
⊘ Herb/drug
Belladonna, henbane, jimsonweed, scopolia: ↑ anticholinergic effect
Chamomile, hops, kava, lavender, skullcap, valerian: ↑ CNS depression
SAM-e, St. John's wort: serotonin syndrome
Scopolia: ↑ amitriptyline action
Yohimbe: ↑ hypertension
Lab test interferences
↑ Blood glucose, ↑ alkaline phosphatase

NURSING CONSIDERATIONS
Assessment
• Monitor B/P (with patient lying, standing), pulse q4h; if systolic B/P drops 20 mm Hg, hold drug, notify prescriber; take VS q4h in patients with cardiovascular disease
• Monitor blood studies: CBC, leukocytes, differential, cardiac enzymes if patient is receiving long-term therapy
• Monitor hepatic studies: AST, ALT, bilirubin
• Check weight weekly; appetite may increase with drug
• Assess ECG for flattening of T wave, bundle branch block, AV block, prolongation of QTc interval, dysrhythmias in cardiac patients
G • Assess for EPS primarily in elderly: rigidity, dystonia, akathisia
• Assess mental status: mood, sensorium, affect, suicidal tendencies; increase in psychiatric symptoms: depression, panic
• Monitor urinary retention, constipation;
P constipation is more likely to occur in children
G or elderly
• Assess for withdrawal symptoms: headache, nausea, vomiting, muscle pain, weakness; do

not usually occur unless drug was discontinued abruptly
• Identify alcohol consumption; if alcohol is consumed, hold dose until morning
Nursing diagnoses
☑ Coping, ineffective (uses)
☑ Injury, risk for (side effects)
☑ Knowledge, deficient (teaching)
☑ Noncompliance (teaching)
Implementation
PO route
• Give with food or milk for GI symptoms
• Crush if patient is unable to swallow medication whole
• Give dosage hs if oversedation occurs
G during day; may take entire dose hs; elderly may not tolerate once/day dosing
• Store at room temp; do not freeze
Patient/family education
• Teach patient that therapeutic effects may take 2-3 wk
• Instruct patient to use caution in driving or other activities requiring alertness because of drowsiness, dizziness, blurred vision; to avoid rising quickly from sitting to standing, espe-
G cially elderly
• Advise patient to avoid alcohol ingestion, other CNS depressants; overheating
• Teach patient not to discontinue medication quickly after long-term use; may cause nausea, headache, malaise
• Advise patient to wear sunscreen or large hat, since photosensitivity occurs; hyperthermia can occur
• Teach patient to increase fluids, bulk in diet if constipation, urinary retention occur,
G especially elderly
• Teach patient to use gum, hard sugarless candy, or frequent sips of water for dry mouth
• Instruct patient to use contraception during treatment
Evaluation
Positive therapeutic outcome
• Decreased depression
• Absence of suicidal thoughts

Treatment of overdose: ECG monitoring, lavage, administer anticonvulsant, sodium bicarbonate

amlodipine (Rx)
(am-loe'di-peen)
Norvasc
Func. class.: Antianginal, calcium channel blocker, antihypertensive
Chem. class.: Dihydropyridine

Pregnancy category C

Action: Inhibits calcium ion influx across cell membrane during cardiac depolarization; produces relaxation of coronary vascular smooth muscle, peripheral vascular smooth muscle; dilates coronary vascular arteries; increases myocardial oxygen delivery in patients with vasospastic angina

➡ **Therapeutic Outcome:** Decreased angina pectoris, dysrhythmias, B/P

Uses: Chronic stable angina pectoris, hypertension, vasospastic angina (Prinzmetal's angina); may coadminister with other antihypertensives, antianginals

Dosage and routes
Angina
Adult: PO 5-10 mg qd

G *Elderly:* PO 2.5 mg qd

Hypertension
Adult: PO 5 mg qd initially, max 10 mg/day

Hepatic dose/Elderly
Adult: PO 25 mg/day, may ↑ to 10 mg/day (antihypertensive); 5 mg/day, may ↑ to 10 mg/day (antianginal)

Available forms: Tabs 2.5, 5, 10 mg

Adverse effects
(*italic* = common; **bold** = life-threatening)
CNS: Headache, fatigue, dizziness, asthenia, anxiety, depression, insomnia, paresthesia, somnolence
CV: Dysrhythmia, edema, bradycardia, hypotension, palpitations, syncope
GI: Nausea, vomiting, diarrhea, gastric upset, constipation, flatulence, anorexia, gingival hyperplasia, dyspepsia
GU: Nocturia, polyuria
INTEG: Rash, pruritus, urticaria, hair loss
MISC: Flushing, sexual difficulties, muscle cramps, cough, weight gain, tinnitus, epistaxis

Contraindications: Sick sinus syndrome, 2nd- or 3rd-degree heart block, hypersensitivity

P **Precautions:** CHF, hypotension, hepatic
G injury, pregnancy **C**, lactation, children, elderly

▶ Do Not Confuse:
Norvasc/Navane

Pharmacokinetics
Absorption	Well absorbed up to 90%
Distribution	Crosses placenta, protein binding 95%
Metabolism	Liver, extensively
Excretion	Kidneys to metabolites (90%)
Half-life	30-50 hr; ↑ in elderly, hepatic disease

Pharmacodynamics
Onset	Unknown
Peak	6-10 hr
Duration	24 hr

Interactions
Individual drugs
Alcohol: ↑ hypotension
Lithium: ↑ neurotoxicity
Drug classifications
Antihypertensives, nitrates: ↑ hypotension
NSAIDs: ↓ antihypertensive effect
Food/drug
Grapefruit juice: ↑ hypotension
▨ *Herb/drug*
Barberry, betel palm, burdock, goldenseal, khat, khella, lily of the valley, plantain: ↑ effect
Yohimbe: ↓ effect

NURSING CONSIDERATIONS
Assessment
• Assess fluid volume status: I&O ratio and record, weight, distended red veins, crackles in lung, color, quality and sp gr of urine, skin turgor, adequacy of pulses, moist mucous membranes, bilateral lung sounds, peripheral pitting edema; dehydration symptoms of decreasing output, thirst, hypotension, dry mouth and mucous membranes should be reported
• Monitor B/P and pulse; if B/P drops, call prescriber
• Monitor ALT, AST, bilirubin daily; if these are elevated, hepatotoxicity is suspected
• Monitor if platelet count is <150,000/mm^3; drug is usually discontinued and another drug started
• Monitor cardiac status: B/P, pulse, respiration, ECG

Nursing diagnoses
✓ Cardiac output, decreased (uses)
✓ Knowledge, deficient (teaching)

Implementation
PO route
- Give once a day, without regard to meals

Patient/family education
- Advise patient to avoid hazardous activities until stabilized on drug, dizziness is no longer a problem
- Instruct patient to avoid alcohol and OTC drugs unless directed by prescriber
- Advise patient to comply in all areas of medical regimen: diet, exercise, stress reduction, smoking cessation, drug therapy; to notify prescriber of irregular heartbeat, shortness of breath, swelling of feet and hands, severe dizziness, constipation, nausea, hypotension
- Teach patient to use as directed even if feeling better; may be taken with other cardiovascular drugs (nitrates, β-blockers)

Evaluation
Positive therapeutic outcome
- Decreased anginal pain
- Decreased B/P
- Increased exercise tolerance

Treatment of overdose: Defibrillation, β-agonists, **IV** calcium inotropic agents, diuretics, atropine for AV block, vasopressor for hypotension

---

amoxapine (Rx)
(a-mox′a-peen)
amoxapine, Asendin
Func. class.: Antidepressant
Chem. class.: Dibenzoxazepine derivative, secondary amine

Pregnancy category C

Action: Blocks reuptake of norepinephrine, serotonin into nerve endings, thereby increasing action of norepinephrine, serotonin in nerve cells

⊃ **Therapeutic Outcome:** Decreased symptoms of depression after 2-3 wk

Uses: Depression

Dosage and routes
Adult: PO 50 mg tid; may increase to 100 mg tid on 3rd day of therapy; not to exceed 300 mg/day unless lower doses have been given for at least 2 wk; may be given daily dose hs; not to exceed 600 mg/day in hospitalized patients

G *Elderly:* PO 25 mg hs, may increase by 25 mg/wk, up to 150 mg/day in divided doses

Available forms: Tabs 25, 50, 100, 150 mg

Adverse effects
(*italic* = common; **bold** = life-threatening)
CNS: *Dizziness, drowsiness,* confusion, headache, anxiety, tremors, stimulation, weakness, insomnia, nightmares, EPS **G** (elderly), increased psychiatric symptoms, paresthesia, impairment of sexual functioning, **neuroleptic malignant syndrome**
CV: *Orthostatic hypotension, ECG changes, tachycardia,* hypertension, palpitations
EENT: *Blurred vision,* tinnitus, mydriasis, ophthalmoplegia
GI: *Dry mouth, constipation,* nausea, vomiting, **paralytic ileus,** increased appetite, cramps, epigastric distress, jaundice, **hepatitis,** stomatitis, weight gain
GU: Urinary retention, **acute renal failure**
HEMA: **Agranulocytosis, thrombocytopenia, eosinophilia, leukopenia**
INTEG: Rash, urticaria, sweating, pruritus, photosensitivity
META: ↑ prolactin levels

Contraindications: Hypersensitivity to tricyclic antidepressants, recovery phase of myocardial infarction, seizure disorders, prostatic hypertrophy, narrow-angle glaucoma

Precautions: Suicidal patients, severe depression, increased intraocular pressure, urinary retention, cardiac disease, hepatic disease, hyperthyroidism, electroshock therapy, elective surgery, elderly, pregnancy **C**

N Do Not Confuse:
amoxapine/amoxicillin, amoxapine/Amoxil

Pharmacokinetics	
Absorption	Well absorbed
Distribution	Widely distributed; crosses placenta
Metabolism	Liver, extensively
Excretion	Kidneys, breast milk
Half-life	8 hr

Pharmacodynamics	
Onset	1-2 wk
Peak	2-6 wk
Duration	6-12 wk

Interactions
Individual drugs
Alcohol: ↑ CNS depression
Cimetidine, fluoxetine: ↑ amoxapine levels, ↑ toxicity of amoxapine
Clonidine: Severe hypotension; avoid use
Guanethidine: ↓ effects of amoxapine
Paroxetine, sertraline: ↑ amoxapine level, ↑ toxicity

Drug classifications
Barbiturates, benzodiazepines, CNS depressants: ↑ effects of amoxapine
Contraceptives (oral): ↑ effects, toxicity of amoxapine
◆ MAOIs: Hypertensive crisis, seizures
Sympathomimetics (indirect acting): ↓ effects of amoxapine
Smoking
↑ Metabolism, ↓ effects
⬛ *Herb/drug*
Chamomile, hops, kava, lavender, skullcap, St. John's wort, valerian: ↑ CNS depression
Belladonna, corkwood, henbane, jimsonweed: ↑ anticholinergic effect
Scopolia: ↑ amoxapine action
Lab test interferences
↑ Blood glucose, ↑ alkaline phosphatase, ↑ prolactin

NURSING CONSIDERATIONS
Assessment
• Monitor B/P (with patient lying, standing), pulse q4h; if systolic B/P drops 20 mm Hg hold drug, notify prescriber; take vital signs q4h in patients with cardiovascular disease
• Monitor blood studies: CBC, leukocytes, differential, cardiac enzymes if patient is receiving long-term therapy
• Monitor blood level: therapeutic 20-100 ng/ml
• Monitor hepatic studies: AST, ALT, bilirubin
• Check weight weekly; appetite may increase with drug
• Assess ECG for flattening of T wave, bundle branch block, AV block, dysrhythmias in cardiac patients
🅖 • Assess for EPS primarily in elderly: rigidity, dystonia, akathisia
• Assess mental status: mood, sensorium, affect, suicidal tendencies; increase in psychiatric symptoms: depression, panic; confusion
🅖 (elderly)
• Monitor urinary retention, constipation;
🅟 constipation is more likely to occur in children
🅖 and elderly
• Assess for withdrawal symptoms: headache, nausea, vomiting, muscle pain, weakness; do not usually occur unless drug was discontinued abruptly
• Identify alcohol consumption; if alcohol is consumed, hold dose until morning

Nursing diagnoses
✓ Coping, ineffective (uses)
✓ Injury, risk for (side effects)
✓ Knowledge, deficient (teaching)
✓ Noncompliance (teaching)

Implementation
• Give with food or milk for GI symptoms
• Crush if patient is unable to swallow medication whole
• Store at room temp; do not freeze

Patient/family education
• Teach patient that therapeutic effects may take 2-3 wk
• Instruct patient to use caution in driving or other activities requiring alertness because of drowsiness, dizziness, blurred vision; to avoid rising quickly from sitting to standing,
🅖 especially elderly
• Teach patient to avoid alcohol ingestion, other CNS depressants
• Teach patient not to discontinue medication quickly after long-term use: may cause nausea, headache, malaise
• Teach patient to wear sunscreen or large hat, since photosensitivity occurs
• Teach patient to increase fluids, bulk in diet if constipation, urinary retention occur,
🅖 especially elderly
• Advise patient to take gum, hard sugarless candy, or frequent sips of water for dry mouth

Evaluation
Positive therapeutic outcome
• Decreased depression
• Absence of suicidal thoughts

Treatment of overdose: ECG monitoring, induce emesis, lavage, activated charcoal, administer anticonvulsant

amoxicillin (Rx)
(a-mox-i-sill'in)
amoxicillin, Amoxil, Apo-Amoxi ✦, Novamoxin ✦, Nu-Amoxi ✦, Trimox, Wymox
Func. class.: Antiinfective, antiulcer
Chem. class.: Aminopenicillin
Pregnancy category B

Action: Interferes with cell wall replication of susceptible organisms by binding to the bacterial cell wall; the cell wall, rendered osmotically unstable, swells and bursts from osmotic pressure

➡ **Therapeutic Outcome:** Bactericidal effects for the following organisms: effective for gram-positive cocci (*Streptococcus pyogenes, Streptococcus faecalis, Streptococcus pneumoniae*), gram-negative cocci (*Neisseria gonorrhoeae, Neisseria meningitidis, Escherichia coli*), gram-negative bacilli (*Haemophilus influenzae, Proteus*

⬛ Herb/drug   🅢 Do Not Crush   ◆ Alert   ☚ Key Drug   🅖 Geriatric   🅟 Pediatric *mirabilis, Salmonella),* in combination for *Helicobacter pylori*

Uses: Infections of respiratory tract, skin, skin structures, genitourinary tract, otitis media, meningitis, septicemia, sinusitis, and bacterial endocarditis prophylaxis

Investigational uses: Lyme disease

Dosage and routes
Renal disease
Adult: PO CCr 10-50 ml/min dose q12h; CCr <10 ml/min dose q24h

Systemic infections
Adult: PO 750 mg-1.5 g qd in divided doses q8h

P *Child:* PO 20-50 mg/kg/day in divided doses q8h

Gonorrhea/urinary tract infections
Adult: PO 3 g given with 1 g probenecid as a single dose; followed by tetracycline or erythromycin

Chlamydia trachomatis
Adult: PO 500 mg/day × 1 wk

Bacterial endocarditis prophylaxis
P *Child:* PO 50 mg/kg/hr before and 25 mg/kg 6 hr after procedure

Helicobacter pylori
Adult: PO 1000 mg bid given with lansoprazole 30 mg bid, clarithromycin 500 mg bid × 2 wk; or 1000 mg bid given with omeprazole 20 mg bid, clarithromycin 500 mg bid × 2 wk; or 1000 mg tid given with lansoprazole 30 mg tid × 2 wk

Available forms: Caps 250, 500 mg; chewable tabs 125, 200, 250, 400, 500, 875; powder for oral susp 50 mg/ml, 125, 250 mg/5 ml; susp pedidrops 50 mg/ml; susp 125, 200, 250, 400 mg/5 ml

Adverse effects
(*italic* = common; **bold** = life-threatening)
CNS: Headache, fever, **seizures**
GI: *Nausea, vomiting, diarrhea,* increased AST, ALT, abdominal pain, glossitis, colitis, **pseudomembranous colitis**
HEMA: Anemia, increased bleeding time, **bone marrow depression, granulocytopenia**
INTEG: *Urticaria, rash*
SYST: **Anaphylaxis, respiratory distress, serum sickness**

Contraindications: Hypersensitivity to **P** penicillins; neonates

Precautions: Pregnancy **B,** hypersensitivity **P** to cephalosporins, neonates, renal disease

Do Not Confuse:
amoxicillin/amoxapine, Amoxil/amoxapine, Amoxil/amoxicillin, Trimox/Diamox, Trimox/Tylox, Wymox/Tylox

Pharmacokinetics

Absorption	Well absorbed (90%)
Distribution	Readily in body tissues, fluids, CSF; crosses placenta
Metabolism	Liver (30%)
Excretion	Breast milk, kidney, unchanged (70%)
Half-life	1-1.3 hr

Pharmacodynamics

Onset	½ hr
Peak	2 hr

Interactions
Individual drugs
Probenecid: ↑ amoxicillin levels, ↓ renal excretion
Warfarin: ↑ anticoagulant effects
Drug classifications
Anticoagulants (oral): ↑ anticoagulant effects
Contraceptives (oral): ↓ contraceptive effectiveness
Herb/drug
Acidophilus: Do not use with antiinfectives
Khat: ↓ absorption, separate by 2 hr
Lab test interferences
False positive: Urine glucose, urine protein, direct Coombs' test

NURSING CONSIDERATIONS
Assessment
• Assess patient for previous sensitivity reaction to penicillins or other cephalosporins; cross-sensitivity between penicillins and cephalosporins is common
• Assess patient for signs and symptoms of infection, including characteristics of wounds, sputum, urine, stool, WBC >10,000/mm³, earache, fever; obtain baseline information and monitor symptoms during treatment
• Obtain C&S before beginning drug therapy to identify if correct treatment has been initiated
• Assess for allergic reactions during treatment: rash, urticaria, pruritus, chills, fever, joint pain; angioedema may occur a few days after therapy begins; epINEPHrine and resuscitation equipment should be available for anaphylactic reactions
• Identify urine output; if decreasing, notify prescriber (may indicate nephrotoxicity); also, increased BUN, creatinine, urinalysis, protein, blood

- Monitor blood studies: AST, ALT, CBC, Hct, bilirubin, LDH, alkaline phosphatase, Coombs' test monthly if patient is on long-term therapy
- Monitor electrolytes: potassium, sodium, chloride monthly if patient is on long-term therapy
- Assess bowel pattern qd; diarrhea, cramping, blood in stools; if severe diarrhea occurs, notify prescriber; drug should be discontinued; pseudomembranous colitis may occur
- Monitor for bleeding: ecchymosis, bleeding gums, hematuria, stool guaiac daily if on long-term therapy
- Assess for overgrowth of infection: perineal itching, fever, malaise, redness, pain, swelling, drainage, rash, diarrhea, change in cough, sputum

Nursing diagnoses
✓ Infection, risk for (uses)
✓ Diarrhea (side effects)
✓ Injury, risk for (side effects)
✓ Knowledge, deficient (teaching)
✓ Noncompliance (teaching)

Implementation
PO route
- Give in even doses around the clock; if GI upset occurs, give with food; drug must be given for 10-14 days to ensure organism death and prevent superinfection; store in tight container
- The caps may be opened and contents taken with fluids
- Shake susp well before each dose, may be used alone or mixed in drinks, use immediately; susp may be stored in refrigerator for 14 days

Patient/family education
◆• Teach patient to report sore throat, bruising, bleeding, joint pain; may indicate blood dyscrasias (rare)
- Advise patient to contact prescriber if vaginal itching, loose foul-smelling stools, diarrhea, sore throat, fever, fatigue, furry tongue occur; may indicate superinfection or agranulocytopenia
- Instruct patient to take all medication prescribed for the length of time ordered; not to double dose; chew form is available
- Advise patient to notify prescriber of diarrhea with blood or pus, which may indicate pseudomembranous colitis

Evaluation
Positive therapeutic outcome
- Absence of signs/symptoms of infection (WBC <10,000/mm^3, temp WNL, absence of red draining wounds or earache)

- Prevention of endocarditis
- Resolution of ulcer symptoms

Treatment of anaphylaxis: Withdraw drug, maintain airway, administer epINEPHrine, aminophylline, O_2, **IV** corticosteroids

---

amoxicillin/clavulanate (Rx)
(a-mox-i-sill'in)
Augmentin, Augmentin ES-600, Augmentin XR, Clavulin ♣
Func. class.: Broad-spectrum antiinfective (extended spectrum)
Chem. class.: Aminopenicillin-β-lactamase inhibitor

Pregnancy category B

Action: Interferes with cell wall replication of susceptible organisms; the cell wall, rendered osmotically unstable, swells and bursts from osmotic pressure; combination increases spectrum of activity, β-lactamase resistance

➔**Therapeutic Outcome:** Bactericidal effects for the following organisms: *Escherichia coli, Proteus mirabilis, Haemophilus influenzae, Streptococcus faecalis, Streptococcus pneumoniae;* and β-lactamase–producing organisms: *Neisseria gonorrhoeae, Neisseria meningitidis, Shigella, Salmonella, Enterococcus, Streptococcus*

Uses: Infections of respiratory tract, skin, skin structures, genitourinary tract; otitis media, meningitis, septicemia, sinusitis, and endocarditis prophylaxis

Dosage and routes
Adult: PO 250-500 mg q8h or 500-875 mg q12h depending on severity of infection
P *Child ≤40 kg:* PO 20-40 mg/kg/day in divided doses q8h or 25-45 mg/kg/day in divided doses q12h
Renal dose
Adult: PO CCr 10-30 ml/min dose q12h; CCr <10 ml/min dose q24h

Available forms: Tabs 250, 500, 875 mg/125 mg clavulanate; chewable tabs 125, 200, 250, 400 mg; powder for oral susp 125, 200, 250, 400 mg/5 ml; (XR) ext rel tabs 1000 mg amoxicillin/62.5 mg clavulanate; (ES) powder for oral susp 600 mg amoxicillin; 42.9 mg clavulanate 5 ml

Adverse effects
(*italic* = common; **bold** = life-threatening)
CNS: Headache, fever, **seizures**

GI: *Nausea, diarrhea, vomiting,* increased AST, ALT, abdominal pain, glossitis, colitis, black tongue, **pseudomembranous colitis**
GU: **Oliguria, proteinuria, hematuria,** *vaginitis, moniliasis,* **glomerulonephritis**
HEMA: Anemia, **bone marrow depression, granulocytopenia, leukopenia, eosino-philia, thrombocytopenic purpura**
INTEG: Rash, urticaria
META: Hyperkalemia, hypokalemia, alkalosis, hypernatremia
SYST: **Anaphylaxis, respiratory distress, serum sickness, superinfection**

Contraindications: Hypersensitivity to
P penicillins; neonates

Precautions: Pregnancy **B**, lactation,
P hypersensitivity to cephalosporins; neonates; renal disease

Pharmacokinetics

Absorption	Well absorbed (90%)
Distribution	Readily in body tissues, fluids, CSF; crosses placenta
Metabolism	Liver (30%)
Excretion	Breast milk; kidney, unchanged (70%), removed by hemodialysis
Half-life	1-1.3 hr

Pharmacodynamics

Onset	½ hr
Peak	2 hr

Interactions
Individual drugs
Allopurinol: amoxicillin-induced skin rash
Probenecid: ↑ amoxicillin levels, decreased renal excretion
Drug classifications
Anticoagulants (oral): ↑ anticoagulant effects
Contraceptives (oral): ↓ contraceptive effectiveness
Herb/drug
Acidophilus: Do not use with antiinfectives
Khat: ↓ absorption
Lab test interferences
False positive: Urine glucose, urine protein, direct Coombs' test

NURSING CONSIDERATIONS
Assessment
• Assess patient for previous sensitivity reaction to penicillins or other cephalosporins; cross-sensitivity between penicillins and cephalosporins is common
• Assess patient for signs and symptoms of infection, including characteristics of wounds, sputum, urine, stool, WBC >10,000/mm^3, earache, fever; obtain baseline information and during treatment
• Complete C&S before beginning drug therapy to identify if correct treatment has been initiated
• Assess for anaphylaxis: rash, urticaria, pruritus, chills, dyspnea, laryngeal edema, fever, joint pain; angioedema may occur a few days after therapy begins; epINEPHrine and resuscitation equipment should be available for anaphylactic reaction
• Identify urine output; if decreasing, notify prescriber (may indicate nephrotoxicity)
• Monitor renal studies: urinalysis, protein, blood, BUN, creatinine
• Monitor blood studies: AST, ALT, CBC, Hct, bilirubin, LDH, alkaline phosphatase, Coombs' test monthly if patient is on long-term therapy
• Monitor electrolytes: potassium, sodium, chloride monthly if patient is on long-term therapy
• Assess bowel pattern qd; diarrhea, cramping, blood in stools, report to prescriber; if severe diarrhea occurs, drug should be discontinued; may indicate pseudomembranous colitis
• Monitor for bleeding: ecchymosis, bleeding gums, hematuria, stool guaiac daily if on long-term therapy
• Assess for overgrowth of infection: perineal itching, fever, malaise, redness, pain, swelling, drainage, rash, diarrhea, change in cough, sputum

Nursing diagnoses
☑ Infection, risk for (uses)
☑ Injury, risk for (side effects)
☑ Diarrhea (side effects)
☑ Knowledge, deficient (teaching)
☑ Noncompliance (teaching)

Implementation
PO route
• Give in even doses around the clock; if GI upset occurs, give with food; drug must be taken for 10-14 days to ensure organism death and prevent superinfection; store in tight container; cap can be opened and mixed with food or liq; chewable tabs should be chewed
• Administer only as directed; 2 250-mg tabs not equivalent to 1 500-mg tab due to strength of clavulanate
• Shake susp well before each dose; may be used alone or mixed in drinks, use immediately; susp may be stored in refrigerator for 10 days

Patient/family education

◆▶• Teach patient to report sore throat, bruising, bleeding, joint pain; may indicate blood dyscrasias (rare)
• Advise patient to contact prescriber if vaginal itching, loose foul-smelling stools occur; may indicate superinfection
• Instruct patient to take all medication prescribed for the length of time prescribed
• Advise patient to notify prescriber of diarrhea with blood or pus, which may indicate pseudomembranous colitis
• Advise patient to use alternative contraceptive measures if using oral contraceptives

Evaluation

Positive therapeutic outcome
• Absence of signs/symptoms of infection (WBC <10,000/mm^3, temp WNL)
• Reported improvement in symptoms of infection

Treatment of anaphylaxis: Withdraw drug, maintain airway, administer epINEPHrine, aminophylline, O$_2$, **IV** corticosteroids

---

amphotericin B deoxycholate (Rx)
(am-foh-tehr'ih-sin de-ox-ee-kohl'ate)
Fungizone
amphotericin B cholesteryl (Rx)
Amphotec
amphotericin B lipid based (Rx)
Abelcet
amphotericin B liposome (Rx)
AmBisome
Func. class.: Antifungal
Chem. class.: Amphoteric polyene

Pregnancy category B

Action: Increases cell membrane permeability in susceptible organisms by binding sterols in fungal cell membrane; decreases potassium, sodium, and nutrients in cell

▶**Therapeutic Outcome:** Fungistatic against histoplasmosis, blastomycosis, coccidioidomycosis, cryptococcosis, aspergillosis, phycomycosis, candidiasis, sporotrichosis

Uses: Treatment of severe, possibly fatal fungal infections (**IV**); treatment of topical fungal infections (top)

Investigational uses: Candiduria (bladder irrigation)

Dosage and routes
Deoxycholate
Adult: **IV** Give test dose of 1 mg; then 0.5 mg/kg, increase qd slowly to 0.5 mg/kg, may give 1 mg/kg/day or 1.5 mg/kg qid, alternate day dosing may be used

P *Child:* **IV** 0.25 mg/kg infused initially, increase by 0.25 mg/kg qod to max of 1 mg/kg/day

P *Adult and child:* TOP apply 2-4 × daily

P *Adult and child:* 1 ml qid

(Amphotec)
P *Adult and child:* **IV** 3-4 mg/kg/day, max 6 mg/kg/day

(Abelcet)
P *Adult and child:* **IV** 5 mg/kg/day as a 1 mg/ml inf given 2.5 mg/kg/hr

(AmBisome)
P *Adult and child:* **IV** Fungal infections 3-5 mg/kg q24h

Visceral leishmaniasis: 3 mg/kg q24h days 1-5 and 14 and 21; give 4 mg/kg on day 1-5, 10, 17, 24, 31, and 38 to immunocompromised patients

Available forms: *Amphotericin deoxycholate* inj 50-mg vial, oral susp 100 mg/ml; cream, ointment, lotion 3%; *amphotericin B lipid based* susp for inj 100 mg/20-ml vial

Adverse effects
(*italic* = common; **bold** = life-threatening)
CNS: Headache, fever, chills, peripheral nerve pain, paresthesias, peripheral neuropathy, **seizures,** dizziness
EENT: Tinnitus, deafness, diplopia, blurred vision
GI: Nausea, vomiting, anorexia, diarrhea, cramps, **hemorrhagic gastroenteritis, acute liver failure**
GU: Hypokalemia, axotemia, hyposthenuria, **renal tubular acidosis,** nephrocalcinosis, **permanent renal impairment, anuria, oliguria**
HEMA: Normochromic and normocytic anemia, **thrombocytopenia, agranulocytosis, leukopenia, eosinophilia,** hypokalemia, hyponatremia, hypomagnesemia
INTEG: Burning, irritation, pain, necrosis at inj site with extravasation, flushing, dermatitis, skin rash (top route)
MS: Arthralgia, myalgia, generalized pain, weakness, weight loss

---

🗍 Herb/drug   🚫 Do Not Crush   ◆ Alert   ◆ℼ Key Drug   🄶 Geriatric   🄿 Pediatric

Contraindications: Hypersensitivity, severe bone marrow depression

Precautions: Renal disease, pregnancy **B**

Pharmacokinetics

Absorption	Complete bioavailability (**IV**), rapidly absorbed (top)
Distribution	Body tissues
Metabolism	Liver
Excretion	Kidneys, detectable for several weeks
Half-life	Initial 24-48 hr, terminal 15 days

Pharmacodynamics

	IV	TOP
Onset	Immediate	Unknown
Peak	1-2 hr	Unknown

Interactions
Individual drugs
Mezlocillin, piperacillin, ticarcillin: ↑ hypokalemia
Drug classifications
Diuretics, nephrotoxic drugs: ↑ nephrotoxicity
Glucocorticoids, thiazides, diuretics: ↑ hypokalemia
☑ *Herb/drug*
Acidophilus: Do not use with antiinfectives
Gossypol: ↑ risk of nephrotoxicity

NURSING CONSIDERATIONS
Assessment
• Monitor VS q15-30 min during first inf; note changes in pulse, B/P
• Monitor blood studies: Hgb, Hct, potassium, sodium, calcium, magnesium q2 wk; BUN, creatinine weekly; decreased Hgb, Hct, and magnesium are common with increased potassium
• Monitor weight weekly; if weight increases over 2 lb/wk, edema is present; renal damage should be considered
• Monitor for renal toxicity: increasing BUN, serum creatinine; if BUN is >40 mg/dl or if serum creatinine >3 mg/dl, drug may be discontinued or dosage reduced; I&O ratio: watch for decreasing urinary output, change in sp gr; discontinue drug to prevent permanent damage to renal tubules; provide hydration of 2-3 L/day
• Monitor for hepatotoxicity: increasing AST, ALT, alkaline phosphatase, bilirubin
• Monitor for allergic reaction: dermatitis, rash; drug should be discontinued, antihistamines (mild reaction) or epINEPHrine (severe reaction) administered; check inj site for thrombophlebitis
• Monitor for hypokalemia: anorexia, drowsiness, weakness, decreased reflexes, dizziness, increased urinary output, increased thirst, paresthesias; if these occur, drug should be decreased or discontinued and potassium administered
Topical route
• Monitor for allergic reaction: burning, stinging, swelling, redness

Nursing diagnoses
☑ Infection, risk for (uses)
☑ Injury, risk for (adverse reaction)
☑ Knowledge, deficient (teaching)

Implementation
Topical route
• Provide enough medication to cover lesions completely; do not cover with occlusive dressing; apply liberally and rub thoroughly into affected area; administer after cleansing with soap, water before each application, dry well (as ordered), wear gloves during application
• Store at room temp in dry place
IV Intermittent IV infusion
Deoxycholate
• Give after diluting 50 mg in 10 ml sterile water (no preservatives) (5 mg-1 ml); shake well, further dilute with 500 ml of D_5W to concentration of 0.1 mg/ml; do not use other diluents or sol; use large needle (20 G); change needle for each step; wear gloves
• Use test dosage of 1 mg/20 ml D_5W; give over 10-30 min; if no reaction, drug is administered as ordered
• Administer **IV** using in-line filter (mean pore diameter >1 μm) using distal veins; check for extravasation, necrosis q8h; use an infusion pump; administer over 6 hr; rapid inf may result in circulation collapse; may also be given through central line
• Give acetaminophen and diphenhydrAMINE 30 min before inf to reduce fever, chills, headache
• Give drug only after C&S confirm organism, drug needed to treat condition; make sure drug is used in life-threatening infections
• Store protected from moisture and light; diluted sol is stable for 24 hr at room temp, 1 wk refrigerated

Syringe compatibilities: Heparin

Y-site compatibilities: Aldesleukin, diltiazem, DOXOrubicin liposome, famotidine, remifentanil, tacrolimus, teniposide, thiotepa, zidovudine

Y-site incompatibilities: Enalaprilat, fludarabine, foscarnet, ondansetron

Additive compatibilities: Fluconazole, heparin, hydrocortisone, methylPREDNISolone, sodium bicarbonate

Solution compatibilities: D₅W

**Cholesteryl
Liposomal complex**
IV IV route
• Reconstitute with 12 ml sterile water/50 ml vial (4 mg/ml), shake, use 5 micron filter, dilute in D₅W (1-2 mg/ml), give over 2 hr

Lipid complex
IV IV route
• Shake vial until dissolved, withdraw dose using 18-G needle, replace needle from syringe with drug using 5 micron filter needle (use needle for 4 vials or less), empty contents in **IV** of D₅W (1 mg/ml), give at 2.5 mg/kg/hr, use infusion pump

Patient/family education
Topical route
• Teach patient that skin and clothing may become discolored; to use asepsis (hand washing) before, after each application to prevent further infection
• Instruct patient to apply with glove to prevent further infection; not to cover with occlusive dressing; to continue even if condition improves
• Teach patient to avoid use of OTC creams, ointments, lotions, unless directed by prescriber
• Instruct patient to report increased itching, burning, rash, redness; ointment may irritate most hairy areas; to report if condition worsens
IV IV route
• Advise patient that long-term therapy may be needed to clear infection (2 wk-3 mo depending on type of infection)
• Teach patient side effects and when to notify prescriber

Evaluation
Positive therapeutic outcome
• Decrease in size, number of lesions (top)
• Decreased fever, malaise, rash
• Negative C&S for infecting organism

---

ampicillin (Rx)
(am-pi-sill′in)
Ampicin ✸, Apo-Ampi ✸, D-Amp ✸, Nu-Ampi ✸, NovoAmpicillin ✸, Penbriten ✸, Polycillin, Principen, Totacillin
Func. class.: Broad-spectrum antiinfective
Chem. class.: Aminopenicillin
Pregnancy category B

Action: Interferes with cell wall replication of susceptible organisms; the cell wall, rendered osmotically unstable, swells, and bursts from osmotic pressure

➔**Therapeutic Outcome:** Bactericidal effects for the following organisms: effective for gram-positive cocci *(Streptococcus pyogenes, Streptococcus faecalis, Streptococcus pneumoniae),* gram-negative cocci *(Neisseria gonorrhoeae, Neisseria meningitidis),* gram-negative bacilli *(Haemophilus influenzae, Proteus mirabilis, Salmonella, Shigella, Listeria monocytogenes),* gram-positive bacilli

Uses: Infections of respiratory tract, skin, skin structures, genitourinary tract; otitis media, meningitis, septicemia, sinusitis, and endocarditis prophylaxis

Investigational uses: C-section patients that are high risk for developing infection

Dosage and routes
Renal dose
CCr 30-50 ml/min dose q6-8hr; CCr 10-30 ml/min dose q8-12h; <10 ml/min dose q12h

Systemic infections
P Adult and child ≥40 kg (88 lb): PO 250-500 mg q6h or 1-2 g qd in divided doses q6h; **IV**/IM 250-500 mg q6h, (up to 2 g q4h in severe infections) or 2-8 g qd in divided doses q4-6h

P Child <40 kg: PO 25-100 mg/kg/day in divided doses q6h; **IV**/IM 25-50 mg/kg/day in divided doses q8h for septicemia or bacterial meningitis

Bacterial Meningitis
Adult: **IV** 8-14 g/day in divided doses q3-4h × 3 days

P Child: **IV** 100-200 mg/kg/day in divided doses q3-4h × 3 days

Gonorrhea
P Adult and child ≥ 45 kg (99 lb): PO 3.5 g given with 1 g probenecid as a single dose or IM/**IV** 500 mg q6h (≥40 kg); IM/**IV** 50 mg/kg/day in divided doses q6-8h (<40 kg)

Available forms: Powder for inj 125, 250, 500 mg, 1, 2, 10 g; **IV** inf 500 mg, 1, 2 g; caps 250, 500 mg; powder for oral susp, 125, 250, 500 mg/5 ml

Adverse effects
(*italic* = common; **bold** = life-threatening)
CNS: Lethargy, hallucinations, anxiety, depression, twitching, **coma, seizures**
GI: Nausea, vomiting, diarrhea, **pseudomembranous colitis**
GU: Oliguria, proteinuria, hematuria, *vaginitis, moniliasis,* **glomerulonephritis**
HEMA: Anemia, increased bleeding time, **bone marrow depression, granulocytopenia**
INTEG: Rash, urticaria
SYST: **Anaphylaxis, serum sickness**

Contraindications: Hypersensitivity to penicillins

Precautions: Pregnancy **B**; hypersensitivity to cephalosporins; neonates; renal disease

🔃 **Do Not Confuse:**
Omnipen/imipenem

Pharmacokinetics

Absorption	Moderate, duodenum (35%-50%)
Distribution	Readily in body tissues, fluids, CSF; crosses placenta
Metabolism	Liver (30%)
Excretion	Breast milk; kidney unchanged (70%), removed by dialysis
Half-life	50-110 min

Pharmacodynamics

	PO	IM	IV
Onset	Rapid	Rapid	Rapid
Peak	2 hr	1 hr	Infusion's end

Interactions
Individual drugs
Allopurinol: ↑ ampicillin-induced skin rash
Disulfiram: ↑ ampicillin concentrations
Probenecid: ↑ ampicillin levels, ↓ renal excretion
Drug classifications
Contraceptives (oral): ↓ contraceptive effectiveness
☑ *Herb/drug*
Acidophilus: Do not use with antiinfectives
Khat: ↓ absorption, separate by 2 hr
Lab test interferences
↑ AST, ↑ ALT

↓ conjugated estrone in pregnancy, ↓ conjugated estriol
False positive: Urine glucose, urine protein, direct Coombs' test

NURSING CONSIDERATIONS
Assessment
• Assess patient for previous sensitivity reaction to penicillins or other cephalosporins; cross-sensitivity between penicillins and cephalosporins is common
• Assess patient for signs and symptoms of infection, including characteristics of wounds, sputum, urine, stool, WBC >10,000/mm³, earache, fever; obtain baseline information and during treatment
• Obtain C&S before beginning drug therapy to identify if correct treatment has been initiated
• Assess for allergic reactions: rash, urticaria, pruritus, chills, fever, joint pain; angioedema may occur a few days after therapy begins; epINEPHrine and resuscitation equipment should be on unit for anaphylactic reaction; also, check for ampicillin rash: pruritic, red, raised
◄▶• Identify urine output; if decreasing, notify prescriber (may indicate nephrotoxicity)
• Monitor renal studies: urinalysis, protein, blood, BUN, creatinine
• Monitor blood studies: AST, ALT, CBC, Hct, bilirubin, LDH, alkaline phosphatase, Coombs' test monthly if patient is on long-term therapy
• Monitor electrolytes: potassium, sodium, chloride monthly if patient is on long-term therapy
• Assess bowel pattern qd; if severe diarrhea occurs, drug should be discontinued; may indicate pseudomembranous colitis
• Monitor for bleeding: ecchymosis, bleeding gums, hematuria, stool guaiac daily if on long-term therapy
• Assess for overgrowth of infection: perineal itching, fever, malaise, redness, pain, swelling, drainage, rash, diarrhea, change in cough, sputum

Nursing diagnoses
☑ Infection, risk for (uses)
☑ Injury, risk for (side effects)
☑ Diarrhea (side effects)
☑ Knowledge, deficient (teaching)
☑ Noncompliance (teaching)

Implementation
PO route
• Give in even doses around the clock; drug must be taken for 10-14 days to ensure organ-

ism death and prevent superinfection; store caps in tight container
• Tabs may be crushed or caps opened and mixed with water
• Shake susp well before each dose; store in refrigerator for 2 wk or 1 wk at room temp
IM route
• Reconstitute with 125 mg/0.9-1.2 ml; 250 mg/0.9-1.9 ml; 500 mg/1.2-1.8 ml; 1 g/2.4-7.4 ml; 2 g/6.8 ml
• Give deep in large muscle mass
IV IV route
• Reconstitute with 125 mg/0.9-1.2 ml; 250 mg/0.9-1.9 ml; 500 mg/1.2-1.8 ml; 1 g/2.4-7.4 ml; 2 g/6.8 ml
• Give by direct **IV** over 3-5 min in lower dosages (125-500 mg) or over 15 min in higher dosages (1-2 g)
• Give by intermittent inf after diluting with 0.9% NaCl, LR, D₅W, D₅/0.45% NaCl; use 50 ml of sol and dilute to concentration of <30 mg/ml

Syringe compatibilities: Chloramphenicol

Syringe incompatibilities: Erythromycin, gentamicin, kanamycin, lincomycin, metoclopramide, oxytetracycline, streptomycin, tetracycline

Y-site compatibilities: Acyclovir, amifostine, allopurinol, aztreonam, cyclophosphamide, DOXOrubicin liposome, enalaprilat, esmolol, famotidine, filgrastim, fludarabine, foscarnet, granisetron, heparin, regular insulin, labetalol, magnesium sulfate, melphalan, meperidine, morphine, multivitamins, oflaxacin, perphenazine, phytonadione, potassium chloride, propofol, remifentanil, thiotepa, tolazoline, vit B with C

Y-site incompatibilities: Calcium gluconate, epINEPHrine, fluconazole, hetastarch, hydromorphone, hydrALAZINE, ondansetron, sargramostim, verapamil, vinorelbine

Additive incompatibilities: Amikacin, aztreonam, chlorproMAZINE, DOPamine, gentamicin, hydrALAZINE, hydrocortisone, prochlorperazine

Additive compatibilities: Cefotiam, clindamycin, erythromycin, floxacillin, furosemide, tacrolimus, teniposide, theophylline, verapamil

Patient/family education
◆• Teach patient to report sore throat, bruising, bleeding, joint pain; may indicate blood dyscrasias (rare)

• Advise patient to contact prescriber if vaginal itching, loose foul-smelling stools, furry tongue occur; may indicate superinfection
• Instruct patient to take all medication prescribed for the length of time ordered
• Advise patient to notify prescriber of diarrhea with blood or pus, which may indicate pseudomembranous colitis
• Tab may be crushed; cap may be opened and mixed with water

Evaluation
Positive therapeutic outcome
• Absence of signs/symptoms of infection (WBC <10,000, temp WNL)
• Reported improvement in symptoms of infection

Treatment of anaphylaxis: Withdraw drug, maintain airway, administer epINEPHrine, aminophylline, O₂, **IV** corticosteroids

---

ampicillin/sulbactam (Rx)
(am-pi-sill'in/sul-bak'tam)
Unasyn
Func. class.: Broad-spectrum antiinfective
Chem. class.: Aminopenicillin
Pregnancy category B
(ampicillin)

Action: Interferes with cell wall replication of susceptible organisms; the cell wall, rendered osmotically unstable, swells and bursts from osmotic pressure; this combination extends the spectrum of activity and inhibits β-lactamase that may inactivate ampicillin

→**Therapeutic Outcome:** Bactericidal against *Pneumococcus, Enterococcus, Streptococcus, Escherichia coli, Proteus mirabilis, Neisseria meningitidis, Neisseria gonorrhoeae, Shigella, Salmonella,* and *Haemophilus influenzae* organisms; use only with β-lactamase–producing strain of infection

Uses: Skin and structure infections, intraabdominal infections, gynecologic infections, soft tissue infections, otitis media, sinusitis, meningitis, septicemia

Dosage and routes
Adult and child >40 kg: **IV**/IM 1 g ampicillin and 0.5 g sulbactam or 2 g ampicillin, and 1 g sulbactam q6h, not to exceed 4 g/day sulbactam

---

🅿 Herb/drug   🆂 Do Not Crush   ◆ Alert   ◆☞ Key Drug   🅖 Geriatric   🅟 Pediatric

P *Child <40 kg:* **IV** 100-200 mg/kg/day (ampicillin component) divided q6h, max 8 g/day

Renal dose
Adult ≥40 kg: IM/**IV** CCr 15-29 ml/min dose q12h; CCr 5-14 ml/min dose q24h

Available forms: Powder for inj 1.5 g (1 g ampicillin, 0.5 g sulbactam), 3 g (2 g ampicillin, 1 g sulbactam)

Adverse effects
(*italic* = common; **bold** = life-threatening)
CNS: Lethargy, hallucinations, anxiety, depression, twitching, **coma, seizures**
GI: Nausea, vomiting, diarrhea, increased AST, ALT, abdominal pain, glossitis, colitis, **pseudomembranous colitis**
GU: Oliguria, proteinuria, hematuria, *vaginitis, moniliasis,* **glomerulonephritis**
HEMA: Anemia, increased bleeding time, **bone marrow depression, granulocytopenia**
SYST: **Anaphylaxis, serum sickness**

Contraindications: Hypersensitivity to penicillins, ampicillin, or sulbactam

Precautions: Pregnancy **B**, hypersensitivity
P to cephalosporins, neonates, renal disease

Pharmacokinetics	
Absorption	Well absorbed (IM)
Distribution	Readily in body tissues, fluids, CSF; crosses placenta
Metabolism	Liver (10%-50%)
Excretion	Breast milk; kidney unchanged (75%)
Half-life	50-110 min (ampicillin)

Pharmacodynamics		
	IM	IV
Onset	Rapid	Immediate
Peak	1 hr	Infusion's end

Interactions
Individual drugs
Allopurinol: ampicillin-induced skin rash
Probenecid: ↑ ampicillin levels, ↓ renal excretion
Drug classifications
Contraceptives (oral): ↓ contraceptive effectiveness
☑ *Herb/drug*
Acidophilus: Do not use with antiinfectives
Khat: ↓ absorption, separate by 2 hr

Lab test interferences
False positive: Urine glucose, urine protein

NURSING CONSIDERATIONS
Assessment
• Assess patient for previous sensitivity reaction to penicillins or cephalosporins; cross-sensitivity between penicillins and cephalosporins is common
• Assess patient for signs and symptoms of infection; including characteristics of wounds, sputum, urine, stool, WBC >10,000/mm³, earache, fever; obtain baseline information and during treatment
• Complete C&S before beginning drug therapy to identify if correct treatment has been initiated
• Assess for allergic reactions: rash, urticaria, pruritus, chills, fever, joint pain; angioedema may occur a few days after therapy begins; epINEPHrine and resuscitation equipment should be on unit for anaphylactic reaction
◆• Identify urine output; if decreasing, notify prescriber (may indicate nephrotoxicity)
• Assess renal studies: urinalysis, protein, BUN, creatinine
• Monitor blood studies: AST, ALT, CBC, Hct, bilirubin, LDH, alkaline phosphatase, Coombs' test monthly if patient is on long-term therapy
• Monitor electrolytes: potassium, sodium, chloride monthly if patient is on long-term therapy
• Assess bowel pattern qd; if severe diarrhea occurs, drug should be discontinued; may indicate pseudomembranous colitis
• Monitor for bleeding: ecchymosis, bleeding gums, hematuria, stool guaiac daily if on long-term therapy
• Assess for superinfection: perineal itching, fever, malaise, redness, pain, swelling, drainage, rash, diarrhea, change in cough, sputum

Nursing diagnoses
☑ Infection, risk for (uses)
☑ Diarrhea (adverse reactions)
☑ Injury, risk for (adverse reactions)
☑ Knowledge, deficient (teaching)
☑ Noncompliance (teaching)

Implementation
IM route
• Reconstitute by adding 3.2 ml/1.5 g or 6.4 ml/3 g; use sterile water, 0.5% or 2% lidocaine; give within 1 hr of preparation; give deep in large muscle mass
• Give after C&S completed; on empty stomach

IV IV route
- Give **IV** after diluting 1.5 g/3.2 ml sterile H_2O for inj; or 3 g/6.4 ml (250 mg ampicillin/ 125 mg sulbactam); allow to stand until foaming stops; give directly over 15-30 min; dilute further in 50 ml or more of D_5W, D_5/10.45% NaCl, 10% invert sugar in water, LR, 6% sodium lactate, isotonic NaCl; administer within 1 hr after reconstitution; give as an intermittent inf over 15-30 min

Y-site compatibilities: Amifostine, aztreonam, cefepime, enalaprilat, famotidine, filgrastim, fluconazole, fludarabine, granisetron, heparin, regular insulin, meperidine, morphine, paclitaxel, remifentanil, tacrolimus, teniposide, theophylline, thiotepa

Y-site incompatibilities: Idarubicin, ondansetron, sargramostim

Additive compatibilities: Aztreonam

Additive incompatibilities: Aminoglycosides

Patient/family education
- Teach patient to report sore throat, bruising, bleeding, joint pain, persistent diarrhea; may indicate blood dyscrasias (rare) or superinfection
- Advise patient to contact prescriber if vaginal itching, loose foul-smelling stools, furry tongue occur; may indicate superinfection
- Instruct patient to use another form of contraception other than oral contraceptives
- To report immediately pseudomembranous colitis: fever, diarrhea with pus, blood, or mucus; may occur up to 4 wk after treatment
- To wear or carry emergency ID if allergic to penicillin products

Evaluation
Positive therapeutic outcome
- Absence of signs/symptoms of infection (WBC <10,000/mm³, temp WNL, absence of red draining wounds, earache)
- Reported improvement in symptoms of infection

Treatment of overdose: Withdraw drug, maintain airway, administer epINEPHrine, aminophylline, O_2, **IV** corticosteroids for anaphylaxis

---

amprenavir (Rx)
(am-pren′-a-ver)
Agenerase
Func. class.: Antiretroviral
Chem. class.: Protease inhibitor

Pregnancy category C

Action: Inhibits HIV protease

Therapeutic Outcome: Prevents maturation of the infectious virus

Uses: HIV in combination with other antiretroviral agents

Dosage and routes
Caps and solution are not interchangeable

Adult: PO (cap) 1200 mg bid

P *Child 13-16 yr:* PO (cap) 1200 mg bid

P *Child 4-12 yr or wt <50 kg:* PO (cap) 20 mg/kg qd or 15 mg/kg tid, max 2400 mg; PO (oral sol) 22.5 mg/kg bid or 17 mg/kg tid qd, max 2800 mg

Amprenavir/Ritonavir Regimen
Adult: PO 600 mg amprenavir, 100 mg ritonavir bid or 1200 mg amprenavir, 200 mg ritonavir bid

Hepatic Dose
P *Child:* PO (Child-Pugh score 5-8) 450 mg bid (caps), 513 mg bid (sol) in combination; (Child-Pugh score 9-12) 300 mg bid (caps) 342 mg bid (sol) in combination

Available forms: Cap 50, 150 mg; oral sol 15 mg/ml

Adverse effects
(*italic* = common; **bold** = life-threatening)
CNS: Paresthesia
ENDO: New-onset diabetes, hyperglycemia, exacerbation of preexisting diabetes mellitus
GI: Diarrhea, abdominal pain, nausea, **hepatotoxicity**
HEMA: **Acute hemolytic anemia**
INTEG: Rash, **Stevens-Johnson syndrome**

Contraindications: Hypersensitivity; oral sol: renal failure

Precautions: Liver disease, pregnancy **C**,
P lactation, children, hemophilia, sulfonamide
G sensitivity, elderly

Pharmacokinetics	
Absorption	Rapidly
Distribution	90% Protein Binding
Metabolism	Unknown
Excretion	Unknown
Half-life	7-10½ hr

 Herb/drug   Do Not Crush   ◆ Alert   ◆▥ Key Drug   **G** Geriatric   **P** Pediatric

Pharmacodynamics
Unknown

Interactions
Individual drugs
Alprazolam, carbamazepine, clozapine, dapsone, diazepam, diltiazem, flurazepam: Toxicity may occur
Amiodarone, lidocaine, quinidine: Serious life-threatening reactions
Bepridil, loratadine, lovastatin, midazolam: Do not use together; toxicity may occur
Cimetidine, indinavir, ritonavir: ↑ amprenavir levels
Clarithromycin, erythromycin, itraconazole: ↑ amprenavir levels; toxicity may occur
Didanosine, efavirenz, nevirapine, phenobarbital, rifamycin: ↓ amprenavir levels
Methadone: ↓ methadone effect
Warfarin: ↑ serious life-threatening interactions
Drug classifications
Antacids: ↓ amprenavir levels
Antidepressants (tricyclics): ↑ serious life-threatening reactions
Contraceptives (oral): ↓ effects of oral contraceptives
Ergots: Do not use together; toxicity may occur
☑ Herb/drug
St. John's wort: ↓ amprenavir level
Lab test interferences
↑ glucose, ↑ cholesterol, ↑ triglycerides
Interference: CPK, glucose (low)

NURSING CONSIDERATIONS
Assessment
• Assess for renal/hepatic failure, pregnancy, or those receiving disulfiram, metronidazole; oral sol contains propylene glycol in greater quantities
• Assess signs of infection, anemia
• Monitor liver studies: ALT, AST; viral load, CD4 count throughout treatment
• Monitor C&S before drug therapy; drug may be taken as soon as culture is taken; repeat C&S after treatment; determine the presence of other sexually transmitted diseases
• Assess bowel pattern before, during treatment; if severe abdominal pain with bleeding occurs, drug should be discontinued; monitor hydration
• Assess skin eruptions, rash, urticaria, itching
• Assess allergies before treatment, reaction of each medication; place allergies on chart

Nursing diagnoses
☑ Infection, risk for (uses)
☑ Knowledge, deficient (teaching)
Implementation
• Caps and oral sol are not interchangeable on a mg/mg basis
Patient/family education
• Advise patient to take as prescribed with or without food, avoid high-fat foods; if dose is missed, take as soon as remembered up to 1 hr before next dose; do not double dose, do not share with others
• Advise patient that drug must be taken in equal intervals around the clock to maintain blood levels for duration of therapy
• Advise patient to use nonhormonal method of contraception during treatment, use condoms
• Advise patient to notify prescriber of diarrhea, nausea, vomiting, rash
• Teach patient that drug does not cure AIDS or prevent transmission to others, only controls symptoms
Evaluation
Positive therapeutic outcome
• Increasing CD4 counts
• Decreased viral load
• Resolution of HIV

anagrelide (Rx)
(a-na′gre-lide)
Agrylin
Func. class.: Antiplatelet
Chem. class.: Imidazoquinazolinone
Pregnancy cetegory C

Action: Reduces platelet count (mechanism not clear) and prevents early platelet shape changes in response to aggregating agents thus inhibiting platelet aggregation

➔ **Therapeutic Outcome:** Inhibition of platelet aggregation

Uses: Essential thrombocythemia

Dosage and routes
Adult: PO 0.5 mg qid or 1 mg bid, may be adjusted after 1 wk, max 10 mg/day or 2.5 mg single dose

Available forms: Caps 0.5, 1.0 mg

Adverse effects
(*italic* = common; **bold** = life-threatening)
CNS: Headache, dizziness, **seizures,** paresthesia, **CVA**

CV: Postural hypotension, tachycardia, palpitations, **CHF, MI,** cardiomyopathy, cardiomegaly, **complete heart block, atrial fibrillation, arrhythmia,** chest pain
GI: Diarrhea, abdominal pain, nausea, flatulence, vomiting, anorexia, constipation, pancreatitis
GU: Dysuria
HEMA: Anemia, **thrombocytopenia,** ecchymosis, lymphadenoma
INTEG: Rash
MS: Asthenia, back pain
RESP: Dyspnea

Contraindications: Hypersensitivity, hypotension

P Precautions: Pregnancy **C,** lactation, child <16 yr, cardiac, renal, hepatic disease

Pharmacokinetics	
Absorption	Unknown
Distribution	Unknown
Metabolism	Liver, extensively
Excretion	Feces/urine
Half-life	1.3 hr

Pharmacodynamics	
Onset	Unknown
Peak	1 hr
Duration	>24 hr

Interactions
Individual drugs
Sucralfate: ↓ absorption
Food/drug
↓ absorption

NURSING CONSIDERATIONS
Assessment
• Monitor B/P, pulse baseline and during treatment until stable; take B/P with patient lying, standing; orthostatic hypotension is common
• Assess cardiac status: chest pain, what aggravates or ameliorates condition
• Monitor platelet counts q2 days × 1 wk, and qwk thereafter, response should begin after 1-2 wk; Hgb, WBC

Nursing diagnoses
☑ Cardiac output, decreased (uses)
☑ Knowledge, deficient (teaching)

Implementation
• Give with 8 oz of water; to improve absorption give on an empty stomach
• Store at room temp

Patient/family education
• Teach patient that this medication is not a cure; that drug may have to be taken continuously in evenly spaced doses only as directed; if a dose is missed, take one when remembered up to 4 hr; do not double doses
• Inform patient that it is necessary to quit smoking to prevent excessive vasoconstriction
• Advise patient to rise slowly from sitting or lying down to prevent orthostatic hypotension
• Caution patient not to use alcohol or OTC medication unless approved by prescriber
• Caution patient to avoid hazardous activities until stabilized on medication; dizziness may occur
• Teach patient to report cardiac reactions, ↑ bruising/bleeding
• Advise patient to use contraception (female, child-bearing age)

Evaluation
Positive therapeutic outcome
• Absence of thrombocythemia

---

anakinra (Rx)
(an-ah-kin′rah)
Kineret
Func. class.: Antirheumatic agent (disease modifying), immunomodulator
Chem. class.: Recombinant form of human interleukin-1 receptor antagonist (IL-1Ra)
Pregnancy category B

Action: A form of human interleukin-1 receptor antagonist (IL-1Ra) produced by DNA technology; blocks activity of IL-1, resulting in decreased cartilage degradation and decreased bone resorption

⇨**Therapeutic Outcome:** Decreased pain, inflammation

Uses: Reduction in signs and symptoms of moderate to severe active rheumatoid arthritis in patients 18 years of age or older who have not responded to other disease-modifying agents

Dosage and routes
Adult: SC 100 mg qd

Available forms: Sol for inj, 100 mg/ml

Adverse effects
(*italic* = common; **bold** = life-threatening)
CNS: Headache
EENT: Sinusitis
HEMA: **Neutropenia**
GI: Abdominal pain, nausea, diarrhea
INTEG: Rash, *inj site reaction*
MISC: Flulike symptoms
RESP: URI

☑ Herb/drug   🚫 Do Not Crush   ✦ Alert   ✦ᴛ Key Drug   Ⓖ Geriatric   🅿 Pediatric

Contraindications: Hypersensitivity to *Escherichia coli*-derived proteins or this product, sepsis

P **Precautions:** Pregnancy **B,** lactation,
G children, renal impairment, elderly

Pharmacokinetics

Absorption	Well absorbed (SC)
Distribution	Unknown
Metabolism	Unknown
Excretion	Unknown
Half-life	4-6 hr

Pharmacodynamics

Onset	Unknown
Peak	3-7 hr
Duration	Unknown

Interactions
Drug classifications
Etanercept, TNF blocking agents: ↑ risk of severe infection
Vaccines: Do not coadminister; immunizations should be brought up to date before treatment
⊘ *Herb/drug*
Arginine: ↑ gastric irritation
Bilberry, saw palmetto: ↓ effect
Bogbean, dong quai, feverfew, ginger, ginkgo: ↑ effect

NURSING CONSIDERATIONS
Assessment
• Assess pain, stiffness, ROM, swelling of joints during treatment
• Assess for inj site pain, swelling; usually occur after 2 inj (4-5 days)
• Assess for infections, stop treatment if present

Nursing diagnoses
✓ Pain, chronic (uses)
✓ Mobility, impaired physical (uses)
✓ Injury, risk for (side effects)
✓ Knowledge, deficient (teaching)

Implementation
• Do not use if cloudy or discolored or if particulate is present, protect from light
• Do not admix with other sol or medications, do not use filter

Patient/family education
Teach patient about self-administration if appropriate: inj should be made in thigh, abdomen, upper arm; rotate sites at least 1 in from old site
• Advise patient to notify prescriber if pregnancy is planned or suspected, avoid breast-feeding

Evaluation
Positive therapeutic outcome
• Decreased inflammation, pain in joints

---

anastrozole (Rx)
(an-ass-stroh'zole)
Arimidex
Func. class.: Antineoplastic
Chem. class.: Aromatase inhibitor
Pregnancy category D

Action: Lowers serum estradiol concentrations; many breast cancers have strong estrogen receptors

➔ Therapeutic Outcome:
Prevention of rapidly growing malignant cells

Uses: Advanced breast carcinoma that has not responded to other therapy in estrogen-receptor-positive patients (usually postmenopausal)

Dosage and routes
Adult: PO 1 mg qd

Available forms: Tab 1 mg

Adverse effects
(*italic* = common; **bold** = life-threatening)
CNS: Hot flashes, headache, light-headedness, depression, dizziness, confusion, insomnia, anxiety
CV: Chest pain, hypertension, thrombophlebitis, edema
GI: Nausea, vomiting, altered taste leading to anorexia, diarrhea, constipation, abdominal pain, dry mouth
GU: Vaginal bleeding, pruritus vulvae, vaginal dryness, pelvic pain
HEMA: **Thrombocytopenia, leukopenia**
INTEG: Rash, alopecia
MS: Bone pain, myalgia, asthenia
RESP: Cough, sinusitis, dyspnea

Contraindications: Hypersensitivity, pregnancy **D**

P **Precautions:** Leukopenia, thrombocytopenia,
G lactation, cataracts, children, elderly, liver disease, renal disease

Pharmacokinetics

Absorption	Adequately absorbed
Distribution	Unknown
Metabolism	Liver
Excretion	Feces, urine
Half-life	50 hr

Pharmacodynamics	
Onset	Unknown
Peak	4-7 hr
Duration	Unknown

Interactions
Lab test interferences
↑ GGT, ↑ AST, ↑ ALT, ↑ alkaline phosphatase, ↑ cholesterol, ↑ LDL

NURSING CONSIDERATIONS
Assessment
• Monitor CBC, differential, platelet count weekly; withhold drug if WBC is <4000/mm³ or platelet count is <75,000/mm³; notify prescriber of results; monitor calcium levels (hypercalcemia is common)
• Assess for tumor flare: increase in bone, tumor pain during beginning treatment; give analgesics as ordered to decrease pain
• Assess for bleeding: hematuria, guaiac, bruising or petechiae, mucosa or orifices, q8h; no rec temp

Nursing diagnoses
☑ Injury, risk for (adverse reactions)
☑ Knowledge, deficient (teaching)

Implementation
🚫 • Give with food or fluids for GI upset; do not break, crush, or chew enteric products; repeat dose may be needed if vomiting occurs
Store in light-resistant container at room temp

Patient/family education
• Instruct patient to report any complaints, side effects to health care prescriber; if dose is missed, do not double next dose
• Advise patient that vaginal bleeding, pruritus, hot flashes, can occur, and are reversible after discontinuing treatment
• Inform patient about who should be told about tamoxifen therapy
• Advise patient to report vaginal bleeding immediately; that tumor flare—increase in size of tumor, increased bone pain—may occur and will subside rapidly; may take analgesics for pain
• Caution patient to use sunscreen and protective clothing to prevent burns because photosensitivity is common
• Teach patient that hair loss may occur during treatment; a wig or hairpiece may make patient feel better; new hair may be different in color, texture after completion of therapy
• Inform patient that rash or lesions are temporary and may become large during beginning therapy

Evaluation
Positive therapeutic outcome
• Decreased spread of malignant cells in breast cancer

⚠ HIGH ALERT

anistreplase (Rx)
(an-is-tre-plaze′)
APSAC, Eminase
Func. class.: Thrombolytic enzyme
Chem. class.: Plasminogen activator
Pregnancy category C

Action: Promotes thrombolysis by promoting conversion of plasminogen to plasmin; complex is a combination of plasminogen and streptokinase

➡ **Therapeutic Outcome:** Thrombolysis in coronary arteries

Uses: Management of acute MI; for lysis of coronary artery thrombi

Dosage and routes
Adult: **IV** inj 30 units over 4-5 min as soon as possible after onset of symptoms

Available forms: Powder, lyophilized 30 units/vial

Adverse effects
(*italic* = common; **bold** = life-threatening)
CNS: Headache, fever, sweating, agitation, dizziness, paresthesia, tremor, vertigo, **intracranial hemorrhage**
CV: Hypotension, **dysrhythmias,** conduction disorders
GI: Nausea, vomiting
HEMA: Decreased Hct, **GI, GU, intracranial, retroperitoneal,** surface bleeding; **thrombocytopenia**
INTEG: Rash, urticaria, phlebitis at site, itching, flushing
MS: Low back pain, arthralgia
RESP: Altered respirations, dyspnea, **bronchospasm, lung edema**
SYST: Anaphylaxis (rare)

Contraindications: Hypersensitivity, active internal bleeding, intraspinal or intracranial surgery, neoplasms of CNS, severe, uncontrolled hypertension, cerebral embolism, thrombosis, hemorrhage, hypersensitivity to this drug or streptokinase

Precautions: Arterial emboli from left side of heart, pregnancy C, ulcerative colitis/enteritis, renal disease, hepatic disease, hypocoagulation, COPD, subacute bacterial

---

endocarditis, rheumatic valvular disease, intraarterial diagnostic procedure or surgery (10 days), recent major surgery, recent trauma, history of CVA, elderly

Pharmacokinetics

Absorption	Complete bioavailability
Distribution	Unknown
Metabolism	Binds to plasmin
Excretion	Kidneys
Half-life	105 min

Pharmacodynamics

Onset	Unknown
Peak	45 min
Duration	Unknown

Interactions
Individual drugs

Abciximab, aspirin, clopidogrel, dipyridamole, eptifibatide, heparin, plicamycin, ticlopidine, tirofiban, valproic acid: ↑ bleeding risk
Aminocaproic acid, aprotinen, tranexamic acid: ↓ action of anistreplase

Drug classifications

Anticoagulants, antiplatelets, cephalosporins (some), NSAIDs: ↑ bleeding risk

Herb/drug

Agrimony, alfalfa, angelica, anise, basil, bay, bilberry, black haw, bogbean, bromelain, buchu, chondroitin, cinchona bark, dong quai, fenugreek, feverfew, garlic, ginger, ginkgo, ginseng, horse chestnut, Irish moss, kelp, kelpware, khella, lovage, lungwort, meadowsweet, motherwort, mugwort, nettle, papaya, parsley (large amounts), pau d'arco, pineapple, poplar, prickly ash, safflower, saw palmetto, tonka bean, turmeric, wintergreen, yarrow: ↑ risk of bleeding
Chamomile, coenzyme Q10, flax, glucomannan, goldenseal, guar gum: ↓ anticoagulant effect

Lab test interferences

↑ PT, ↑ APTT, ↑ TT
↓ Fibrinogen, ↓ plasminogen

NURSING CONSIDERATIONS
Assessment

• Monitor VS, B/P, pulse, respirations, neurologic signs, temp at least q4h, temp >104° F (40° C) or indicators of internal bleeding
• Assess for hypersensitivity: fever, rash, itching, chills; mild reaction may be treated with antihistamines; hypersensitivity reactions/dyspnea, wheezing, facial swelling should be treated with epINEPHrine

• Monitor bleeding during 1st hr of treatment (hematuria, hematemesis, bleeding from mucous membranes, epistaxis, ecchymosis), continue to monitor for 24 hr after treatment; blood studies (Hct, platelets, PTT, PT, TT, APTT) before starting therapy; PT or APTT must be less than 2 × control before starting therapy; TT or PT q3-4h during treatment
• Monitor ECG, treat bradycardia, ventricular changes; assess neurologic status, neurologic change may indicate intracranial bleeding; cardiac enzymes, radionuclide, myocardial scanning/coronary angiography

Nursing diagnoses
☑ Tissue perfusion, ineffective (uses)
☑ Injury, risk for (uses, adverse reactions)
☑ Knowledge, deficient (teaching)

Implementation
• Give heparin therapy after thrombolytic therapy is discontinued, TT or APTT less than 2 × control (about 3-4 hr)
• Avoid invasive procedures: inj, rec temp; about 10% of patients have high streptococcal antibody titers, requiring increased loading doses
• Treat fever with acetaminophen
• Provide pressure for 30 sec to minor bleeding sites, 30 min to sites of arterial puncture followed by dressing; inform prescriber if hemostasis not attained; apply pressure dressing

IV, direct route
• Give after reconstituting single-dose vial/5 ml sterile water for inj (not bacteriostatic water), and roll (not shake) to enhance reconstitution, try to minimize foaming; give over 2-5 min by direct IV, give within ½ hr of reconstitution or discard, do not add other meds to vial or syringe; give within 6 hr of thrombi identification for best results; cryoprecipitate or fresh frozen plasma if bleeding occurs; store powder in refrigerator; use within 30 min after reconstitution

Incompatibilities: Do not mix with other drugs in sol or syringe

Patient/family education
• Teach patient action of drug and expected outcome; alert patient to possible hypersensitivity reactions and symptoms to report
• Advise patient bed rest is needed during entire course of treatment; handle patient as little as possible during therapy

Evaluation
Positive therapeutic outcome
• Absence of thrombolysis in MI
• Improved ventricular function

! HIGH ALERT

antihemophilic factor VIII (AHF) (Rx)
(an-tee-hee-moe-fill'ik)

Alphanate, antihemophilic factor, Bioclate, Helixate FS, Hemofilm, Humate-P, Hyate:C, Koate-DVI, Kogenate, Kogenate FS, Monoclate-P, Recombinate, ReFacto
Func. class.: Hemostatic, blood factor
Chem. class.: Factor VIII

Pregnancy category C

Action: Necessary for clotting. Activates factor X in conjunction with activated factor IX; transforms prothrombin to thrombin

➡ **Therapeutic Outcome:** Control of hemorrhage or excessive bleeding in factor VIII deficiency

Uses: Hemophilia A, patients with acquired circulating factor VIII inhibitors, factor VIII deficiency

Dosage and routes
Depends on severity of deficiency and level of antihemophilic factor

Massive hemorrhage
P *Adult and child:* **IV** 40-50 units/kg, then 20-25 units/kg q8-12h

Bleeding (overt)
P *Adult and child:* **IV** 15-25 units/kg, then 8-15 units/kg q8-12h × 4 days

Hemorrhage near vital organs
P *Adult and child:* **IV** 15 units/kg, then 8 units/kg q8h × 2 days, then 4 units/kg q8h × 2 days

Minor hemorrhage
P *Adult and child:* **IV** 8-10 units/kg q24h × 2-3 days or 8 units/kg q12h × 2 days, then q24h × 2 days

Joint bleeding
P *Adult and child:* **IV** 5-10 units/kg q8-12h × 1-2 days

Available forms: Inj 250, 500, 1000, 1500 units/vial (number of units noted on label)

Adverse effects
(*italic* = common; **bold** = life-threatening)
CNS: Headache, *lethargy, chills, fever, flushing*
CV: Hypotension, tachycardia
GI: Nausea, vomiting, abdominal cramps, jaundice, **viral hepatitis**
HEMA: **Thrombosis, hemolysis, risk of hepatitis B, HIV**

INTEG: Rash, flushing, *urticaria,* stinging at inj site
RESP: **Bronchospasm,** rhinitis, dyspnea, nosebleeds

Contraindications: Hypersensitivity to mouse, hamster, bovine protein

P Precautions: Neonates/infants, hepatic disease, blood types A, B, AB, pregnancy **C,** factor VIII inhibitor

Pharmacokinetics
Absorption	Complete availability
Distribution	Plasma
Metabolism	Not metabolized
Excretion	No excretion
Half-life	Biphasic 4 hr, 15 hr

Pharmacodynamics
Onset	Immediate
Peak	Unknown
Duration	12 hr

Interactions
Drug classifications
NSAIDs, salicylates: ↑ bleeding

NURSING CONSIDERATIONS
Assessment
• Monitor blood studies (coagulation factors assay by % normal): 5% prevents spontaneous hemorrhage, 30%-50% for surgery, 80%-100% for severe hemorrhage; blood group of patient, donors (if applicable; most factor VIII not from specific blood group donors)
• Monitor I&O, urine color; notify prescriber if urine becomes orange, red; change in urine color signifying hemolytic reaction; patients other than blood type O are more at risk
• Monitor pulse: discontinue infusion if significant increase
• Obtain test for factor VIII inhibitors before starting treatment, may require concomitant antiinhibitor coagulant complex therapy; Hct, Coombs' test with blood types A, B, AB
• Assess for allergy: fever, rash, itching, jaundice, wheezing, tachycardia, nausea, vomiting; give diphenhydrAMINE (Benadryl); continue therapy if reaction is mild, discontinue if severe; notify prescriber
◆• Monitor bleeding at ankles, knees, elbows, other joints; check for rebleeding after 15-30 min

Nursing diagnoses
☑ Tissue perfusion, ineffective (uses)
☑ Injury, risk for (uses, adverse reactions)
☑ Knowledge, deficient (teaching)

Implementation
IV IV route
- Administer **IV** slowly; use plastic syringe to reconstitute and administer; do not use glass, drug adheres to glass; use another needle as a vent when reconstituting; rotate gently to mix
- Administer after dilution with warm NS, D₅W, LR; give within 3 hr

IV infusion route
- Administer by **IV** inf: give at ≤2 ml/min if concentration exceeds 34 units/ml; or over 3 min if concentration is less than 34 units/ml; filter before using
- Store in refrigerator; do not freeze; after reconstitution, do not refrigerate; give within 3 hr

Additive compatibilities: Do not mix with other drugs in sol or syringe

Patient/family education
- Advise patient to report any signs of bleeding: gums, under skin, urine, stools, emesis; review methods to prevent bleeding; to be checked q2-3mo for HIV screen
- Instruct patient to avoid salicylates/NSAIDs; increases bleeding tendencies, decreases clotting
- Instruct patient to prepare, administer factor VIII concentrates at first sign of danger
- Instruct patient to advise health professionals of treatment for hemophilia
- Advise patient that immunization for hepatitis B may be given first
- Instruct patient to report hives, urticaria, chest tightness, hypotension; may be monoclonal antibody–derived factor VII; signs of viral hepatitis, AIDS
- Advise patient to carry/wear emergency ID describing disease process, drugs used

Evaluation
Positive therapeutic outcome
- Absence of bleeding
- Prevention of rebleeding

---

aprepitant
Emend
See Appendix A, Selected New Drugs

⚠ HIGH ALERT   A

ardeparin (Rx)
(are-de-pear′in)
Normiflo
Func. class.: Anticoagulant
Chem. class.: Low molecular weight heparin

Pregnancy category C

Action: Prevents conversion of fibrinogen to fibrin and prothrombin to thrombin by enhancing inhibitory effects of antithrombin III

➡ **Therapeutic Outcome:** Absence of deep vein thrombosis

Uses: Prevention of deep vein thrombosis after knee replacement surgery

Dosage and routes
Adult: SC 50 antifactor Xa units/kg q12h beginning the evening of the day of knee replacement surgery or the following AM, continued until patient is fully ambulatory or 2 wk, whichever is first
- To be used SC only

Available forms: Inj 5000, 10,000 anti-Xa units/0.5 ml

Adverse effects
(*italic* = common; **bold** = life-threatening)
CNS: **Intracranial bleeding,** fever, dizziness, headache
CV: Chest pain
GI: Nausea, vomiting, constipation, **hepatotoxicity**
HEMA: **Thrombocytopenia,** anemia
INTEG: Pruritus, superficial wound infection, ecchymosis, rash, inj site reactions
RESP: Dyspnea
SYST: Hypersensitivity, **hemorrhage, anaphylaxis** possible

Contraindications: Hypersensitivity to this drug, pork products, heparin, or other anticoagulants; hemophilia, leukemia with bleeding, thrombocytopenic purpura, cerebrovascular hemorrhage, cerebral aneurysm, severe hypertension, other severe cardiac disease

G **Precautions:** Elderly, pregnancy **C,** hepatic disease, severe renal disease, blood dyscrasias, subacute bacterial endocarditis, acute nephritis, lactation, child, recent childbirth, peptic ulcer disease, pericarditis, pericardial effusion, recent lumbar puncture, vasculitis, other diseases where bleeding is possible

---

Pharmacokinetics

Absorption	Well absorbed
Distribution	Widely
Metabolism	Unknown
Half-life	Unknown

Pharmacodynamics

Unknown

Interactions

Drug classifications

Anticoagulants (oral), NSAIDs, platelet inhibitors, salicylates: ↑ risk of bleeding

 Herb/drug

Agrimony, alfalfa, angelica, anise, basil, bay, bilberry, black haw, bogbean, bromelain, buchu, chrondroitin, cinchona bark, dong quai, fenugreek, feverfew, garlic, ginger, ginkgo, ginseng, horse chestnut, Irish moss, kelp, kelpware, khella, lovage, lungwort, meadowsweet, motherwort, mugwort, nettle, papaya, parsley (large amounts), pau d'arco, pineapple, poplar, prickly ash, safflower, saw palmetto, tonka bean, turmeric, wintergreen, yarrow: ↑ risk of bleeding

Chamomile, coenzyme Q10, flax, glucomannan, goldenseal, guar gum: ↓ anticoagulant effect

NURSING CONSIDERATIONS

Assessment

- Assess for blood studies (Hct, occult blood in stools, CBC, platelets) during treatment since bleeding can occur
- Assess for bleeding gums, petechiae, ecchymosis, black tarry stools, hematuria, epistaxis, decrease in Hct, B/P; may indicate bleeding, possible hemorrhage; notify prescriber immediately, drug should be discontinued; protamine should be equal to dose of drug given; 1 mg protamine = 100 anti-Xa units of drug
- Monitor for hypersensitivity: fever, skin rash, urticaria; notify prescriber immediately

Implementation

- Give by SC only; have patient sit or lie down; SC inj may be around the navel in a U-shape, upper outer side of thigh or upper outer quadrangle of the buttocks; rotate inj sites
- Changing needles is not recommended

Evaluation

- Therapeutic response: absence of deep vein thrombosis

Patient/family education

- Teach patient to avoid OTC preparations that may cause serious drug interactions unless directed by prescriber; may contain aspirin; other anticoagulants, NSAIDs
- Teach patient to use soft-bristle toothbrush to avoid bleeding gums, avoid contact sports, use electric razor, avoid IM inj
- Advise patient to report any signs of bleeding: gums, under skin, urine, stools; unusual bruising, hematoma at inj site

Treatment of overdose: Protamine sulfate 1% given **IV**

! HIGH ALERT

argatroban (Rx)

(are-ga-troe′ban)

Acova

Func. class.: Anticoagulant

Chem. class.: Thrombin inhibitor

Pregnancy category B

Action: Direct inhibitor of thrombin that is derived from L-arginine; it reversibly binds to the thrombin active site

➡ **Therapeutic Outcome:** Absence or decrease of thrombosis

Uses: Thrombosis, prophylaxis or treatment; anticoagulation prevention/treatment of thrombosis in heparin-induced thrombocytopenia; percutaneous coronary intervention (PCI)

Dosage and routes

Adult: **IV** 2 mcg/kg/min (1 mg/ml) give at 6 ml/hr for 50 kg of weight, at 8 ml/hr for 70 kg of weight, at 11 ml/hr for 90 kg of weight, at 13 ml/hr for 110 kg of weight, at 16 ml/hr for 130 kg of weight

Heparin-induced thrombocytopenia or heparin-induced thrombocytopenia and thrombosis syndrome Percutaneous coronary intervention (PCI)

Adult: **IV** inf 25 mcg/kg/min and a bolus of 350 mcg/kg given over 3-5 min, check ACT 5-10 min after bolus is completed, proceed if ACT >300 sec

Hepatic dose

Adult: **Cont Inf** 0.5 mcg/kg/min, adjust rate based on APTT

Available forms: Inj 100 mg/ml

Adverse effects

(*italic* = common; **bold** = life-threatening)

CNS: Fever

CV: **Atrial fibrillation, ventricular tachycardia**

GI: Nausea, vomiting, abdominal pain, diarrhea, **GI bleeding**
GU: Hematuria, abnormal kidney function, UTI
HEMA: Hemorrhage, thrombocytopenia
RESP: Pneumonia, dyspnea
SYST: Sepsis

Contraindications: Hypersensitivity, overt major bleeding

Precautions: Intracranial bleeding, renal P function impairment, lactation, children, hepatic disease, pregnancy **B**

Pharmacokinetics

Absorption	Unknown
Distribution	To extracellular fluid, 54% plasma protein binding
Metabolism	Liver
Excretion	Feces
Half-life	39-51 min

Pharmacodynamics
Unknown

Interactions
Drug classifications
Anticoagulants: ↑ risk of bleeding
Thrombolytics: ↑ action of argatroban
Herb/drug
Agrimony, alfalfa, angelica, anise, basil, bay, bilberry, black haw, bogbean, bromelain, buchu, chondroitin, cinchona bark, dong quai, fenugreek, feverfew, garlic, ginger, ginkgo, ginseng, horse chestnut, Irish moss, kelp, kelpware, khella, lovage, lungwort, meadowsweet, motherwort, mugwort, nettle, papaya, parsley (large amounts), pau d'arco, pineapple, poplar, prickly ash, safflower, saw palmetto, tonka bean, turmeric, wintergreen, yarrow: ↑ risk of bleeding
Chamomile, coenzyme Q10, flax, glucomannan, goldenseal, guar gum: ↓ anticoagulant effect

NURSING CONSIDERATIONS
Assessment
• Obtain baseline APTT before treatment; do not start treatment if APTT ratio ≥ 2.5, then APTT 4 hr after initiation of treatment and at least qd thereafter; if APTT above target, stop inf for 2 hr, then restart at 50%, take APTT in 4 hr; if below target, increase inf rate by 20%, take APTT in 4 hr, do not exceed inf rate of 0.21 mg/kg/hr without checking for coagulation abnormalities

• Monitor APTT, which should be 1.5-3 × control
◄ Assess for bleeding gums, petechiae, ecchymosis, black tarry stools, hematuria/epistaxis, B/P, vaginal bleeding and possible hemorrhage
• Fever, skin rash, urticaria

Nursing diagnoses
☑ Cardiac output, decreased (uses)
☑ Diarrhea (adverse reactions)
☑ Knowledge, deficient (teaching)

Implementation
• Avoid all IM inj that may cause bleeding
IV IV infusion
• Dilute in 0.9% NaCl, D_5, LR to a final conc 1 mg/ml; dilute each 2.5-ml vial 100-fold by mixing with 250 ml of diluents, mix by repeated inversion of the diluent bag for 1 min; may be slightly hazy
• Dosage adjustment may be made after review of APTT, not to exceed 10 mcg/kg/min

Patient/family education
• Advise patient to use soft-bristle toothbrush to avoid bleeding gums, avoid contact sports, use electric razor, avoid IM inj
• Instruct patient to report any signs of bleeding: gums, under skin, urine, stools

Evaluation
Positive therapeutic outcome
• Absence or decrease of thrombosis

---

aripiprazole (Rx)
(a-rip-ip-pra'zol)
Abilify
Func. class.: Antipsychotic/neuroleptic

Pregnancy category C

Action: Exact mechanism unknown; may be mediated through both dopamine type 2 (D_2) and serotonin type 2 (5-HT_2) antagonism

➔ **Therapeutic Outcome:** Decreased excitement, hallucinations, delusions, paranoia, reorganization of patterns of thought, speech

Uses: Schizophrenia

Dosage and routes
Adult: **PO** 10-15 mg/day; if needed, dosage may be increased to 30 mg qd after 2 wk

Available forms: Tabs 10, 15, 20, 30 mg

Adverse effects
(*italic* = common; **bold** = life-threatening)
CNS: Drowsiness, insomnia, agitation, anxiety, headache, **seizures, neuroleptic malignant syndrome**

CV: Orthostatic hypotension, **tachycardia**
EENT: Blurred vision
GI: Nausea, vomiting, jaundice, weight gain

Contraindications: Hypersensitivity, lactation, seizure disorders

P **Precautions:** Children, renal disease, **G** pregnancy **C,** hepatic disease, elderly

Pharmacokinetics

Absorption	Unknown
Distribution	Protein binding, 90%
Metabolism	Liver, extensively to major active metabolism
Excretion	Unknown
Half-life	Unknown

Pharmacodynamics

Unknown

Interactions
Individual drugs
Alcohol: ↑ sedation
Carbamazepine, fluoxetine, ketoconazole: ↑ effects of aripiprazole
Lithium: ↑ extrapyramidal symptoms (EPS)
Drug classifications
Antipsychotics: ↑ extrapyramidal symptoms
CNS depressants: ↑ sedation
CYP3A4/CYP2D6 inhibitors, CYP3A4 inducers: ↑ effects of aripiprazole
Herb/drug
Betel palm, kava: ↑ EPS
Cola tree, hops, nettle, nutmeg: ↑ neuroleptic effect

NURSING CONSIDERATIONS
Assessment
• Assess mental status before initial administration
• Check for swallowing of PO medication; check for hoarding or giving of medication to other patients
• Monitor I&O ratio; palpate bladder if urinary output is low
• Monitor bilirubin, CBC, liver function tests qmo
• Assess affect, orientation, LOC, reflexes, gait, coordination, sleep pattern disturbances
• Monitor B/P standing and lying; also pulse, respirations; take q4h during initial treatment; establish baseline before starting treatment; report drops of 30 mm Hg; watch for ECG changes
• Assess for dizziness, faintness, palpitations, tachycardia on rising
• Assess for extrapyramidal symptoms,

including akathisia (inability to sit still, no pattern to movements), tardive dyskinesia (bizarre movements of the jaw, mouth, tongue, extremities), pseudoparkinsonism (rigidity, tremors, pill rolling, shuffling gait)
◆• Assess for neuroleptic malignant syndrome: hyperthermia, increased CPK, altered mental status, muscle rigidity
• Assess skin turgor qd
• Assess for constipation, urinary retention qd; if these occur, increase bulk and water in diet

Nursing diagnoses
☑ Thought processes, disturbed (uses)
☑ Sensory perception, disturbed (uses)
☑ Noncompliance (teaching)
☑ Knowledge, deficient (teaching)

Implementation
G • Administer reduced dose in elderly
• Decrease stimulus by dimming lights, avoiding loud noises
• Supervise ambulation until patient is stabilized on medication; do not involve in strenuous exercise program because fainting is possible; patient should not stand still for a long time
• Store in tight, light-resistant container

Patient/family education
• Advise patient that orthostatic hypotension may occur and to rise from sitting or lying position gradually
• Advise patient to avoid hot tubs, hot showers, tub baths; hypotension may occur
• Instruct patient to avoid abrupt withdrawal of this drug; extrapyramidal symptoms may result; drug should be withdrawn slowly
• Teach patient to avoid OTC preparations (cough, hayfever, cold) unless approved by prescriber, because serious drug interactions may occur; avoid use with alcohol, CNS depressants; increased drowsiness may occur
• Advise patient to avoid hazardous activities if drowsy or dizzy
• Explain importance of compliance with drug regimen
• Advise patient, family to report impaired vision, tremors, muscle twitching, urinary retention
• Instruct patient to take extra precautions to stay cool in hot weather, that heat stroke may occur

Evaluation
Positive therapeutic outcome
• Decrease in emotional excitement, hallucinations, delusions, paranoia; reorganization of patterns of thought, speech

---

Treatment of overdose: Lavage if orally ingested; provide airway; *do not induce vomiting*

⚠ HIGH ALERT

arsenic trioxide (Rx)

Trisenox
Func. class.: Antineoplastic-miscellaneous

Pregnancy category D

Action: Not understood, causes morphologic changes and DNA fragmentation

➡ **Therapeutic Outcome:** Decrease in malignant cells

Uses: Acute promyelocytic leukemia

Dosage and routes
Induction
Adult: IV 0.15 mg/kg/day until bone marrow remission, max 60 doses
Consolidation treatment
Wait 3-6 wk after completion of induction

Adult: IV 0.15 mg/kg/day × 25 doses over a period of up to 5 wk

Available forms: Inj 1 mg/ml

Adverse effects
(*italic* = common; **bold** = life-threatening)
CNS: Anxiety, confusion, insomnia, headache, paresthesia, depression, dizziness, tremor, **seizures,** agitation, **coma,** weakness
CV: Hypotension, hypertension, prolonged QT interval, other ECG changes, chest pain, *tachycardia,* torsades de pointes
GI: Abdominal pain, constipation, diarrhea, dyspepsia, fecal incontinence, **GI hemorrhage,** dry mouth, *nausea, vomiting, anorexia*
GU: Vaginal hemorrhage, **renal failure,** incontinence
HEMA: Leukocytosis, anemia, thrombocytopenia, neutropenia, DIC
META: Increased ALT/AST, hyperkalemia, hypokalemia, hypomagnesemia, hyperglycemia
MISC: Weight gain or decrease, fatigue, severe edema, rigors, herpes simplex/zoster
RESP: **Pleural effusion,** dyspnea, cough, epistaxis, hypoxia, sinusitis, wheezing, rales, tachypnea

Contraindications: Hypersensitivity, pregnancy **D**

G Precautions: Elderly, lactation,
P children

Pharmacokinetics
Absorption	Unknown
Distribution	Stored in liver, kidney, heart, lung, hair, nails
Metabolism	Liver
Excretion	Kidneys
Half-life	Unknown

Pharmacodynamics
Unknown

Interactions
None known

NURSING CONSIDERATIONS
Assessment
◆ Monitor for APL differentiation syndrome: fever, dyspnea, pulmonary infiltrates, pleural or pericardial effusions, weight gain; this condition can be fatal; give high-dose steroids
• Assess for ECG changes: QT interval prolongation, complete AV block; obtain baseline ECG prior to drug therapy
• Monitor electrolytes: potassium, calcium, magnesium, creatine

Nursing diagnoses
☑ Risk for infection (adverse reactions)
☑ Nutrition: less than body requirements, imbalanced (adverse reactions)
☑ Knowledge, deficient (teaching)

Implementation
IV IV route
• Dilute with 100-250 ml D₅ or 0.9% NaCl immediately after withdrawing from ampule, give over 1-2 hr; may give over 4 hr if reactions occur

Patient/family education
• Teach patient to report planned or suspected pregnancy
• Inform patient that fertility impairment has not been studied

Evaluation
Positive therapeutic outcome
• Decrease in malignant cells

Treatment of overdose: Dimercaprol 3 mg/kg IM q4h, then 250 mg penicillamine PO, max 4×/day (≤1 g/day)

---

ascorbic acid (vitamin C) (OTC, Rx)
(as-kor′bic)
Apo-C ❦, ascorbic acid, Ascorbicap, C-Span, Cebid, Cecon, Cecore 500, Cemill, Cenolate, Cetane, Cevalin, Cevi-Bid, Ce-Vi-Sol, C-Crystals, Flavorcee, Kamu-Jay ❦, Mega-C/A Plus, Ortho/CS, Sunkist
Func. class.: Vitamin C, water-soluble vitamin

Pregnancy category C

Action: Needed for wound healing, collagen synthesis, antioxidant, carbohydrate metabolism, protein, lipid synthesis, prevention of infection

⮞ **Therapeutic Outcome:** Replacement and supplementation of vit C

Uses: Vit C deficiency, scurvy, delayed wound and bone healing, chronic disease, urine acidification, before gastrectomy; increased need: lactation, pregnancy, hyperthyroidism, emotional stress, trauma, burns, acidification of urine, dietary supplement

Investigational uses: Common cold prevention

Dosage and routes
RDA
🅿 *Neonates and up to 6 mo:* 30 mg/day
🅿 *Infants 6 mo-1 yr:* 35 mg/day
🅿 *Child 1-3 yr:* 40 mg/day
🅿 *Child 4-10 yr:* 45 mg/day
🅿 *Child 11-14 yr:* 50 mg/day
🅿 *Adult and child ≥14 yr:* 50-200 mg/day
Pregnancy: 70 mg/day
Lactation: 90 mg/day
Scurvy
Adult: PO/SC/IM/**IV** 100 mg-500 mg qd × 2 wk, then 50 mg or more qd
🅿 *Child:* PO/SC/IM/**IV** 100-300 mg qd × 2 wk, then 35 mg or more qd
Wound healing/chronic disease/fracture
Adult: SC/IM/**IV**/PO 200-500 mg qd
🅿 *Child:* SC/IM/**IV**/PO 100-200 mg added doses
Urine acidification
Adult: 4-12 g qd in divided doses
🅿 *Child:* 500 mg q6-8h

Available forms: Tabs 25, 50, 100, 250, 500, 1000, 1500 mg; effervescent tabs 1000 mg; chewable tabs 100, 250, 500 mg; timed release tabs 500, 750, 1000, 1500 mg; timed release caps 500 mg; crystals 4 g/tsp; powder 4 g/tsp; liq 35 mg/0.6 ml; sol 100 mg/ml; syr 20 mg/ml, 500 mg/5 ml; inj SC, IM, **IV** 100, 250, 500 mg/ml

Adverse effects
(*italic* = common; **bold** = life-threatening)
CNS: Headache, insomnia, dizziness, fatigue, flushing
GI: Nausea, vomiting, diarrhea, anorexia, heartburn, cramps
GU: Polyuria, urine acidification, oxalate or urate renal stones, dysuria
***HEMA:* Hemolytic anemia in patients with G6PD**
INTEG: Inflammation at inj site

Contraindications: Tartrazine, sulfite sensitivity; G6PD deficiency

Precautions: Gout, pregnancy C, diabetes, renal calculi (large doses)

Pharmacokinetics	
Absorption	Readily absorbed (PO)
Distribution	Widely distributed; crosses placenta
Metabolism	Oxidation
Excretion	Kidneys, inactive; breast milk
Half-life	Unknown

Pharmacodynamics
Unknown

Interaction
Individual drugs
Deferoxamine: ↑ iron toxicity
Iron (oral): ↑ effect of oral iron
Mexiletine: ↑ excretion in acidic urine
Primadone: ↑ requirements for vit C
Drug classifications
Anticoagulants (oral): ↓ action of anticoagulants (large doses)
Antidepressants (tricyclic): ↑ excretion in acidic urine
Estrogens: ↑ effect of estrogen
Salicylates: ↑ requirements of vit C
Smoking
Smoking decreases vit C levels
Lab test interferences
↓ Bilirubin, ↓ urine oxalate, ↓ cysteine
False positive: Negatives in glucose tests (Clinitest, Tes-Tape)
False negative: Occult blood (large dose), urine bilirubin, leukocyte determination

NURSING CONSIDERATIONS
Assessment
- Assess nutritional status for inclusion of foods high in vit C: citrus fruits, cantaloupe, tomatoes
- Assess for vit C deficiency before, during, and after treatment; scurvy (gingivitis, bleeding gums, loose teeth); poor bone development
- Monitor I&O ratio, polyuria; in patients receiving large doses renal stones may occur
- Monitor ascorbic acid levels throughout treatment if continued deficiency is suspected
- Assess inj sites for inflammation, pain, redness

Nursing diagnoses
☑ Nutrition: less than body requirements, imbalanced (uses)
☑ Knowledge, deficient (teaching)

Implementation
IV IV direct
- Give undiluted by *direct* **IV** 100 mg over at least 1 min, rapid inf may cause fainting

Intermittent infusion
- Give by intermittent inf after diluting with D_5W, $D_{10}W$, 0.9% NaCl, 0.45% NaCl, LR, Ringer's sol, dextrose/saline, dextrose/Ringer's combinations; temperature will increase pressure in ampules; wrap with gauze before breaking

Syringe compatibilities: Metoclopramide, aminophylline, theophylline

Syringe incompatibilities: Cefazolin, doxapram

Additive compatibilities: Amikacin, calcium chloride, calcium gluceptate, calcium gluconate, cephalothin, chloramphenicol, chlorproMAZINE, colistimethate, cyanocobalamin, diphenhydrAMINE, heparin, kanamycin, methicillin, methyldopate, penicillin G potassium, polymyxin B, prednisoLONE, procaine, prochlorperazine, promethazine, verapamil

Additive incompatibilities: Bleomycin, cephapirin, nafcillin, sodium bicarbonate, warfarin

Y-site compatibilities: Warfarin
PO route
- Mix oral sol with foods or fluids; ext rel caps should be swallowed whole
🚫 • Do not crush, break, or chew ext rel tab/cap
IM route
- Not to be diluted; give deep in large muscle mass

Patient/family education
- Teach patient necessary foods to be included in diet that are rich in vit C: citrus fruits, cantaloupe, tomatoes, chili peppers (red)
- Teach patient that smoking decreases vit C levels; not to exceed prescribed dose; increases will be excreted in urine, except time release
- Teach patient not to exceed RDA recommended dose, urinary stones may occur
- Teach patient using ascorbic acid for acidification of urine to test urine pH periodically

Evaluation
Positive therapeutic outcome
- Absence of anorexia, irritability, pallor, joint pain, hyperkeratosis, petechiae, poor wound healing
- Reversal of scurvy: bleeding gums, gingivitis, loose teeth

---

alfuzosin
Uroxatral
See Appendix A, Selected New Drugs

---

aprepitant
Emend
See Appendix A, Selected New Drugs

❗ HIGH ALERT

asparaginase (Rx)
(a-spar'a-gin-ase)
Elspar, Kidrolase ♣
Func. class.: Antineoplastic
Chem. class.: Escherichia coli enzyme

Pregnancy category C

Action: Indirectly inhibits protein synthesis in tumor cells; without amino acids, DNA, RNA synthesis is halted; asparagine, protein synthesis is halted; G_1 phase of cell cycle specific; a nonvesicant

➔ **Therapeutic Outcome:** Prevention of rapidly growing malignant cells in leukemia

Uses: Acute lymphocytic leukemia in combination with other antineoplastics unresponsive to other agents

---

Dosage and routes
In combination

P *Adult/child:* **IV** 1000 international units/kg/day × 10 days given over 30 min; IM 6000 international units/m²/day

Sole induction

P *Adult/child:* **IV** 200 international units/kg/day × 28 days

Desensitization

P *Adult/child:* **IV**/ID test dose of 2 international units ID, then 1 international unit, then double dose q10 min, until total dose is administered or reaction occurs

Available forms: Inj 10,000 international units with mannitol

Adverse effects
(*italic* = common; **bold** = life-threatening)

CNS: Neuritis, dizziness, headache, **coma,** depression, fatigue, confusion, hallucinations, lethargy, drowsiness, agitation, parkinsonism-like syndrome, **seizures**

CV: Chest pain

ENDO: Hyperglycemia

GI: Nausea, vomiting, anorexia, cramps, stomatitis, diarrhea, weight loss, **hepatotoxicity, pancreatitis**

GU: Urinary retention, **renal failure,** glycosuria, polyuria, azotemia, proteinuria, uric acid neuropathy

HEMA: **Thrombocytopenia, leukopenia, myelosuppression, anemia, decreased clotting factors** (V, VII, VIII, IX), decreased fibrinogen

INTEG: Rash, urticaria, chills, fever, perspiration

RESP: **Fibrosis, pulmonary infiltrate**

SYST: **Anaphylaxis**

Contraindications: Hypersensitivity, **P** infants, lactation, pancreatitis

Precautions: Renal disease, hepatic disease, pregnancy **C**

Pharmacokinetics

Absorption	Complete bioavailability (**IV**)
Distribution	Intravascular spaces
Metabolism	Unknown
Excretion	Reticuloendothelial system
Half-life	8-30 hr (**IV**), 39-49 hr (IM)

Pharmacodynamics

	IV	IM
Onset	Immediate	Immediate
Peak	14-24 hr	Unknown
Duration	3-5 wk	3-5 wk

Interactions
Individual drugs

Methotrexate: Blocked action of methotrexate
Vincristine: ↑ neurotoxicity

Drug classifications

Glucocorticosteroids: ↑ hyperglycemia
Hepatotoxic agents: ↑ hepatotoxicity
Live virus vaccines: ↓ response of vaccines

Lab test interferences

↓ Thyroid function tests
↑ Uric acid

NURSING CONSIDERATIONS
Assessment

• Assess for signs and symptoms of pancreatitis (nausea, vomiting, severe abdominal pain), anaphylaxis (bronchospasm, dyspnea), cyanosis; monitor amylase, glucose; more toxic in adults than children

• Assess symptoms indicating severe allergic reaction: rash, pruritus, urticaria, purpuric skin lesions, itching, flushing; joint pain, bronchospasm, hypotension; epINEPHrine and emergency equipment should be nearby

• Monitor for frequency of stools, characteristics: cramping, acidosis; signs of dehydration: rapid respirations, poor skin turgor, decreased urine output, dry skin, restlessness, weakness

• Monitor CBC, differential, platelet count weekly; withhold drug if WBC is <4000/mm³ or platelet count is <100,000/mm³, notify prescriber of results; also monitor PT, PTT, and TT, which may be increased

• Monitor pulmonary function tests, chest x-ray studies before, during therapy; chest x-ray film should be obtained q2 wk during treatment

• Monitor renal function studies: BUN, serum uric acid, ammonia urine CCr, electrolytes before, during therapy

• Check I&O ratio; report fall in urine output of 30/ml/hr

• Monitor temp q4h; elevated temp may indicate beginning infection

• Obtain liver function tests before, during therapy (bilirubin, AST, ALT, LDH) as needed or monthly

• Monitor RBC, Hct, Hgb, since these may be decreased; serum, urine glucose levels

- Assess for bleeding: hematuria, guaiac, bruising or petechiae, mucosa, or orifices q8h
- Assess for dyspnea, rales, nonproductive cough, chest pain, tachypnea, fatigue, increased pulse, pallor, lethargy, or swelling around eyes or lips; anaphylaxis may occur
- Assess for yellowing of skin and sclera, dark urine, clay-colored stools, itchy skin, abdominal pain, fever, diarrhea

Nursing diagnoses
✓ Injury, risk for (uses, adverse reactions)
✓ Body image, disturbed (adverse reactions)

Implementation
- Give after intradermal skin testing and desensitization, give 0.1 ml (2 international units) intradermally after reconstituting with 5 ml sterile H_2O or 0.9% NaCl for inj; then add 0.1 ml of reconstituted drug to 9.9 ml diluent (20 international units/ml); observe for 1 hr, check for wheal
- Use allopurinol or sodium bicarbonate to reduce uric acid levels, alkalinization of urine

IM route
- Reconstitute with 2 ml 0.9% NaCl/10,000 international units/vial, refrigerate, use within 8 hr, discard sooner if sol becomes cloudy

IV route
- Give by **IV** inf using 21-, 23-, 25-gauge needle; administer by slow **IV** inf via Y-tube or 3-way stopcock of flowing D_5W or 0.9% NaCl inf over 30 min after diluting 10,000 international units/5 ml of sterile H_2O or 0.9% NaCl (no preservatives) (2000 international units/ml); use of filter may be necessary if fibers are present

Y-site compatibilities: Methotrexate, sodium bicarbonate

Patient/family education
- Teach patient to report any complaints or side effects to nurse or physician
- Teach patient to report any changes in breathing or coughing
- Advise patient not to receive vaccinations while taking this drug
- Advise patient to use contraception, since drug is teratogenic

Evaluation
Positive therapeutic response
- Decreased replication of leukemia cells

Treatment of anaphylaxis: Administer epINEPHrine, diphenhydrAMINE, **IV** corticosteroids, O_2

---

aspirin ⚷ (OTC)
(as'pir-in)
Acuprin, Artria S.R., A.S.A., Aspergum, Aspirin ♣, Aspir-Low, Aspirtab, Astrin ♣, Bayer Aspirin, Coryphen ♣, Easprin, Ecotrin, 8-Hour Bayer Timed Release, Empirin, Entrophen ♣, Halfprin, Norwich Extra-Strength, Novasen ♣, PMS-ASA ♣, Sloprin, St. Joseph Children's Supasa ♣, Therapy Bayer, ZORprin
Func. class.: Nonopioid analgesic
Chem. class.: Salicylate

Pregnancy category D (3rd trimester)

Action: Blocks pain impulses in CNS, reduces inflammation by inhibition of prostaglandin synthesis; antipyretic action results from vasodilatation of peripheral vessels; decreases platelet aggregation

→**Therapeutic Outcome:** Decreased pain, inflammation, fever; absence of MI, transient ischemic attacks, thrombosis

Uses: Mild to moderate pain or fever including rheumatoid arthritis, osteoarthritis, thromboembolic disorders, transient ischemic attacks in men, rheumatic fever, post-MI, prophylaxis of MI

Investigational uses: Prevention of cataracts (long-term use), prevention of pregnancy loss in women with clotting disorders

Dosage and routes
Arthritis
Adult: PO 2.6-5.2 g/day in divided doses q4-6h
P *Child:* PO 90-130 mg/kg/day in divided doses q4-6h

Kawasaki disease
P *Child:* PO 80-120 mg/kg/day in 4 divided doses, maintenance 3-8 mg/kg/day as a single dose × 8 wk

MI, stroke prophylaxis
Adult: PO 81-650 mg/day

Pain/fever
Adult: PO/REC 325-650 mg q4h prn, not to exceed 4 g/day
P *Child:* PO/REC 40-100 mg/kg/day in divided doses q4-6h prn

Acute rheumatic fever
Adult: PO 5-8 g/day initially
P *Child:* PO 100 mg/kg/day × 2 wk, then 75 mg/kg/day × 4-6 wk

Thromboembolic disorders
Adult: PO 325-650 mg/day or bid

Transient ischemic attacks
Adult: PO 650 mg bid or 350 mg qid

Available forms: Tabs 81, 162.5, 325, 500, 650, 975 mg; chewable tabs 80, 81 mg; supp 60, 120, 125, 130, 150, 160, 195, 200, 300, 320, 325, 600, 640, 650 mg, 1.2 g; cream; gum 227.5 mg; dispersible tabs 325, 500 mg; tabs delayed release, enteric coated 80, 165, 300, 325, 500, 600, 650, 975 mg; ext rel 325, 650, 800 mg; del rel caps 325, 500 mg

Adverse effects
(*italic* = common; **bold** = life-threatening)
CNS: Stimulation, drowsiness, dizziness, confusion, **seizures,** headache, flushing, hallucinations, **coma**
CV: Rapid pulse, pulmonary edema
EENT: Tinnitus, hearing loss
ENDO: Hypoglycemia, hyponatremia, hypokalemia
GI: Nausea, vomiting, **GI bleeding,** diarrhea, heartburn, anorexia, **hepatitis**
HEMA: **Thrombocytopenia, agranulocytosis, leukopenia, neutropenia, hemolytic anemia,** increased pro-time, PTT, bleeding time
INTEG: Rash, urticaria, bruising
RESP: Wheezing, hyperpnea
P *SYST:* **Reye's syndrome (children), anaphylaxis, laryngeal edema**

Contraindications: Hypersensitivity to salicylates, tartrazine (FDC yellow dye #5), GI
P bleeding, bleeding disorders, children <12 yr, children with flulike symptoms, pregnancy **D** (3rd trimester), lactation, vit K deficiency, peptic ulcer, NSAIDs

Precautions: Anemia, hepatic disease, renal disease, Hodgkin's disease, pre/postoperatively, gastritis, asthmatic patients with nasal polyps or aspirin sensitivity

Pharmacokinetics	
Absorption	Well absorbed, small intestine (PO); erratic (enteric); slow (rec)
Distribution	Rapidly, widely distributed; crosses placenta
Metabolism	Liver, extensively
Excretion	Inactive metabolites, kidney; breast milk
Half-life	15-20 min (low doses); 30 hr (high doses)

Pharmacodynamics		
	PO	REC
Onset	15-30 min	Slow
Peak	1-2 hr	4-5 hr
Duration	4-6 hr	6-7 hr

Interactions
Individual drugs
Alcohol, cefamandole, clopidogrel, eptifibatide, heparin, insulin, plicamycin, ticlopidine, tirofiban: ↑ risk of bleeding
Ammonium chloride, nizatidine: ↑ salicylate level
Insulin, methotrexate, phenytoin: ↑ effects of each specific drug
Nitroglycerin: ↑ hypotension
PABA: ↑ toxic effects
Probenecid: ↓ effects of probenecid
Spironolactone, sulfinpyrazone: ↓ effects
Drug classifications
ACE inhibitors: ↓ antihypertensive effect
Antacids, corticosteroids, steroids, urinary alkalizers: ↓ effects of aspirin
Anticoagulants, thrombolytics: ↑ risk of bleeding
Carbonic anhydrase inhibitors: ↑ toxic effects
Diuretics (loop), sulfonylamides: ↓ effect of each specific drug
NSAIDs, steroids: ↑ gastric ulcers
Penicillins: ↑ effects of penicillins
Salicylates: ↓ blood glucose levels
Urinary acidifiers: ↑ salicylate levels

Food/drug
Foods acidifying urine may ↑ aspirin levels
Herb/drug
Agrimony, alfalfa, angelica, anise, basil, bay, bilberry, black haw, bogbean, bromelain, buchu, chondroitin, cinchona bark, dong quai, fenugreek, feverfew, garlic, ginger, ginkgo, ginseng, horse chestnut, Irish moss, kelp, kelpware, khella, lovage, lungwort, meadowsweet, motherwort, mugwort, nettle, papaya, parsley (large amounts), pau d'arco, pineapple, poplar, prickly ash, safflower, saw palmetto, tonka bean, turmeric, wintergreen, yarrow: ↑ risk of bleeding
Chamomile, coenzyme Q10, flax, glucomannan, goldenseal, guar gum: ↓ anticoagulant effect
Lab test interferences
↑ Coagulation studies, ↑ liver function studies, ↑ serum uric acid, ↑ amylase, ↑CO_2, ↑ urinary protein
↓ Serum potassium, ↓ PBI, ↓ cholesterol

Interference: Urine catecholamines, pregnancy test, urine glucose tests (Clinistix, Tes-Tape)

NURSING CONSIDERATIONS
Assessment
• Assess for pain: character, location, intensity, ROM before and 1 hr after administration
• Monitor liver function studies: AST, ALT, bilirubin, creatinine if patient is on long-term therapy
• Monitor renal function studies: BUN, urine creatinine if patient is on long-term therapy
• Monitor blood studies: CBC, Hct, Hgb, Pro-time if patient is on long-term therapy
• Check I&O ratio; decreasing output may indicate renal failure (long-term therapy)
◆• Assess hepatotoxicity: dark urine, clay-colored stools, yellowing of the skin and sclera, itching, abdominal pain, fever, diarrhea if patient is on long-term therapy
• Assess for allergic reactions: rash, urticaria; if these occur, drug may have to be discontinued; patients with asthma, nasal polyps, allergies; severe allergic reactions may occur
• Assess for ototoxicity: tinnitus, ringing, roaring in ears; audiometric testing needed before, after long-term therapy
• Monitor salicylate level: therapeutic level 150-300 mcg/ml
• Assess for visual changes: blurring, halos; corneal, retinal damage
• Check edema in feet, ankles, legs
• Identify prior drug history; there are many drug interactions

Nursing diagnoses
✓ Pain (uses)
✓ Mobility, impaired physical (uses)
✓ Injury, risk for (side effects)
✓ Knowledge, deficient (teaching)

Implementation
PO route
• Administer to patient crushed or whole; chewable tab may be chewed
🚫• Do not crush enteric product
• Give with food or milk to decrease gastric symptoms; separate by 2 hr of enteric product; absorption may be slowed
• Give antacids 1-2 hr after enteric products

Patient/family education
• Teach patient to report any symptoms of hepatotoxicity, renal toxicity, visual changes, ototoxicity, allergic reactions, bleeding (long-term therapy)
• Instruct patient to take with 8 oz of water

and sit upright for 30 min after dose to facilitate drug passing into the stomach; to discard tabs if vinegar-like smell is present; to avoid if allergic to tartrazine
• Instruct patient not to exceed recommended dosage; acute poisoning may result
• Advise patient to read label on other OTC drugs; many contain aspirin
• Inform patient that the therapeutic response takes 2 wk (arthritis); give ½ hr before planned exercise
• Teach patient to report tinnitus, confusion, diarrhea, sweating, hyperventilation
• Advise patient to avoid alcohol ingestion; GI bleeding may occur
• Advise patient with allergies, nasal polyps, asthma, that allergic reactions may develop
• Instruct patient to read labels on other OTC drugs: may contain salicylates
🅿• Teach patient not to give to children or teens with flulike symptoms or chicken pox; Reye's syndrome may develop

Evaluation
Positive therapeutic outcome
• Decreased pain
• Decreased inflammation
• Decreased fever
• Absence of MI
• Absence of transient ischemic attacks, thrombosis

Treatment of overdose: Lavage, activated charcoal, monitor electrolytes, VS

---

atazanavir
Reyataz
See Appendix A, Selected New Drugs

---

atenolol (Rx)
(a-ten'oh-lole)
Apo-Atenolol ✤, atenolol, Novo-Atenol ✤, Tenormin
Func. class.: Antihypertensive
Chem. class.: β-Blocker; β₁-, β₂-blocker (high doses)

Pregnancy category D

Action: Competitively blocks stimulation of β-adrenergic receptor within vascular smooth muscle; produces negative chronotropic activity, positive inotropic activity (decreases rate of SA node discharge, increases recovery time), slows conduction of AV node, decreases heart rate, decreases O_2 consumption in myocardium; also decreases renin-aldosterone-angiotensin system at high doses, inhibits β_2-receptors in bronchial system at higher doses

→ **Therapeutic Outcome:** Decreased B/P, heart rate, prevention of angina pectoris, MI

Uses: Mild to moderate hypertension; prophylaxis of angina pectoris; suspected or known MI (**IV** use)

Investigational uses: Dysrhythmia, mitral valve prolapse, pheochromocytoma, hypertrophic cardiomyopathy, vascular headaches, thyrotoxicosis, tremors, alcohol withdrawal

Dosage and routes
Adult: **IV** 5 mg; repeat in 10 min if initial dose is well tolerated, then start PO dose 10 min after last **IV** dose

Adult: PO 50 mg qd, increasing q1-2 wk to 100 mg qd; may increase to 200 mg qd for angina or up to 100 mg for hypertension

G *Elderly:* PO 25 mg/day initially

Renal dose
Adult: PO CCr 15-35 ml/min, max 50 mg/day; CCr <15 ml/min max 25 mg/day; hemodialysis 25-50 mg after dialysis

MI-Renal dose
Adult: **IV** 5 mg, then 5 mg over 10 min, then after 10 min give PO dose

Available forms: Tabs 25, 50, 100 mg; 500 inj mcg/ml

Adverse effects
(*italic* = common; **bold** = life-threatening)
CNS: *Insomnia, fatigue, dizziness, mental changes,* memory loss, hallucinations, depression, lethargy, drowsiness, strange dreams, catatonia
CV: **Profound hypotension, bradycardia, CHF, cold extremities, postural hypotension, 2nd- or 3rd-degree heart block**
EENT: Sore throat, dry burning eyes
ENDO: Increased hypoglycemic response to insulin
GI: *Nausea, diarrhea,* vomiting, **mesenteric arterial thrombosis, ischemic colitis**
GU: Impotence
HEMA: **Agranulocytosis, thrombocytopenia, purpura**
INTEG: Rash, fever, alopecia
RESP: **Bronchospasm,** dyspnea, wheezing

Contraindications: Hypersensitivity to β-blockers, cardiogenic shock, 2nd- or 3rd-degree heart block, sinus bradycardia, CHF, cardiac failure, pregnancy **D**

Precautions: Major surgery, lactation, diabetes mellitus, renal disease, thyroid disease, COPD, asthma, well-compensated heart failure

Do Not Confuse:
atenolol/albuterol, Tenormin/thiamine

Pharmacokinetics	
Absorption	50%-60% (PO)
Distribution	Crosses placenta; protein binding (5%-15%)
Metabolism	Not metabolized
Excretion	Breast milk, kidneys (50%), feces (50%—unabsorbed drug)
Half-life	6-9 hr

Pharmacodynamics		
	PO	IV
Onset	1 hr	Unknown
Peak	2-4 hr	5 min
Duration	24 hr	Unknown

Interactions
Individual drugs
Alcohol: ↑ hypotension (large amounts)
Diltiazem, hydralazine, methyldopa, prazosin, reserpine: ↑ hypotension, bradycardia
Epinephrine: α-adrenergic stimulation
Indomethacin: ↓ antihypertensive effect
Thyroid: ↓ effectiveness of atenolol
Verapamil: ↑ myocardial depression
Drug classifications
Antihypertensives: ↑ hypertension
β_2-Agonist, theophyllines: ↓ bronchodilatation
Cardiac glycosides: ↑ bradycardia
Nitrates: ↑ hypotension
Herb/drug
Aconite: ↑ toxicity, death
Astragalus, cola tree: ↑ or ↓ antihypertensive effect
Barberry, betony, black catechu, black cohosh, bloodroot, broom, burdock, cat's claw, dandelion, goldenseal, Irish moss, Jamaican dogwood, kelp, khella, mistletoe, parsley: ↑ antihypertensive effect
Coltsfoot, guarana, khat, licorice: ↓ antihypertensive effect
Lab test interferences
↑ Uric acid, ↑ potassium, ↑ triglyceride, ↑ lipoproteins
↑ Blood glucose, ↑ BUN, ↑ ANA titer

NURSING CONSIDERATIONS
Assessment
- Monitor B/P during beginning treatment, periodically thereafter; pulse q4h; note rate, rhythm, quality: apical/radial pulse before administration; notify prescriber of any significant changes (pulse <50 bpm)
- Check for baselines in renal, liver function tests before therapy begins
- Assess for edema in feet, legs daily; monitor I&O, daily weight; check for jugular vein distention, rales bilaterally, dyspnea (CHF)

Nursing diagnoses
☑ Cardiac output, decreased (uses)
☑ Injury, risk for physical (side effects)
☑ Knowledge, deficient (teaching)
☑ Noncompliance (teaching)

Implementation
PO route
- Given ac, hs, tablet may be crushed or swallowed whole; give with food to prevent GI upset; reduced dosage in renal dysfunction
- Store protected from light, moisture; place in cool environment

IV IV route
- Give **IV** direct over 5 min or diluted in 10-50 ml D₅W, 0.9% NaCl, and give at prescribed rate

Y-site compatibilities: Meperidine, meropenem, morphine

Patient/family education
- Teach patient not to discontinue drug abruptly; taper over 2 wk; may cause precipitate angina if stopped abruptly
- Teach patient not to use OTC products containing α-adrenergic stimulants (such as nasal decongestants, OTC cold preparations); to limit alcohol, smoking; to limit sodium intake as prescribed
- Teach patient how to take pulse and B/P at home; advise when to notify prescriber
- Instruct patient to comply with weight control, dietary adjustments, modified exercise program
- Advise patient to carry/wear emergency ID for drugs, allergies, conditions being treated; tell patient drug controls symptoms but does not cure
- Caution patient to avoid hazardous activities if dizziness, drowsiness is present
- Teach patient to report symptoms of CHF: difficult breathing, especially on exertion or when lying down, night cough, swelling of extremities or bradycardia, dizziness, confusion, depression, fever
- Teach patient to take drug as prescribed,

not to double doses, skip doses; take any missed doses as remembered if at least 6 hr until next dose
- Advise patient that drug may mask symptoms of hypoglycemia in diabetic patients
- Advise patient to use contraception while taking this drug; pregnancy category **D**

Evaluation
Positive therapeutic outcome
- Decreased B/P in hypertension (after 1-2 wk)
- Absence of dysrhythmias
- Absence of MI
- Decreased angina

Treatment of overdose: Lavage, **IV** atropine for bradycardia, **IV** theophylline for bronchospasm, digitalis, O₂, diuretic for cardiac failure, hemodialysis, **IV** glucose for hyperglycemia, **IV** diazepam (or phenytoin) for seizures

---

atomoxetine (Rx)
(at-o-mox'eh-teen)
Strattera
Func. class.: Psychotherapeutic—misc.

Pregnancy category C

Action: A selective norepinephrine reuptake inhibitor. May inhibit the presynaptic norepinephrine transporter. Exact mechanism of action is unknown

➡ **Therapeutic Outcome:** Decreased hyperactivity, impulsivity, increased attention, organization, ability to complete tasks

Uses: Attention deficit hyperactivity disorder

Dosage and routes
P *Child ≤70 kg:* **PO** 0.5 mg/kg, increase after 3 days to a target daily dose of 1.2 mg/kg in AM or evenly divided doses AM, late afternoon; max 1.4 mg/kg/day or 100 mg qd, whichever is less

P *Adult/child >70 kg:* **PO** 40 mg qd, increase after 3 days to a target daily dose of 80 mg in AM or evenly divided doses AM, late afternoon; max 100 mg qd

Available forms: Caps 10, 18, 25, 40, 60 mg

Adverse effects
(*italic* = common; **bold** = life-threatening)
CNS: *Insomnia,* dizziness, headache, irritability, crying, mood swings, fatigue
CV: *Palpitations,* hot flushes
ENDO: Growth retardation
GI: Dyspepsia, nausea, anorexia, dry mouth,

weight loss, vomiting, diarrhea, constipation
GU: Urinary hesitancy, retention, dysmenorrhea, erectile disturbance, ejaculation failure, impotence, prostatitis, abnormal orgasm
INTEG: **Exfoliative dermatitis,** sweating
MISC: Cough, rhinorrhea, dermatitis, ear infection

Contraindications: Narrow-angle glaucoma

Precautions: Hypertension, pregnancy **C,** **P** lactation, children >6 yr; hepatic, cardiac, or cerebrovascular disease

Pharmacokinetics

Absorption	Unknown
Distribution	Protein binding, 98%
Metabolism	Liver
Excretion	Kidneys
Half-life	Unknown

Pharmacodynamics

Unknown

Interactions
Individual drug
Albuterol: ↑ cardiovascular effects
Drug classifications
CYP2D6 inhibitors: ↑ effects of atomoxetine
MAOIs, vasopressors: Hypertensive crisis

NURSING CONSIDERATIONS
Assessment
• Monitor VS, B/P; check patients with cardiac disease more often for increased B/P
• Monitor height, growth rate q3mo in children; growth rate may be decreased
• Assess mental status: mood, sensorium, affect, stimulation, insomnia, aggressiveness
• Assess appetite, sleep, speech patterns
• Assess for attention span, decreased hyperactivity in ADHD persons

Nursing diagnoses
✓ Thought processes, disturbed (uses)
✓ Coping, ineffective (uses)
✓ Family coping, impaired (uses)
✓ Knowledge, deficient (teaching)

Implementation
• Provide gum, hard candy, frequent sips of water for dry mouth

Patient/family education
• Advise patient to avoid OTC preparations unless approved by prescriber
• Advise patient to avoid alcohol ingestion
• Advise patient to avoid hazardous activities until stabilized on medication

• Advise patient to get needed rest; patients will feel more tired at end of day

Evaluation
Positive therapeutic outcome
• Decreased hyperactivity (ADHD)

---

atorvastatin (Rx)
(a-tore′va-stat-in)
Lipitor
Func. class.: Antilipidemic
Chem. class.: HMG-CoA reductase inhibitor
Pregnancy category X

Action: Inhibits HMG-CoA reductase enzyme, which reduces cholesterol synthesis

Therapeutic Outcome:
Decreased cholesterol levels and LDLs, increased HDLs

Uses: As an adjunct in primary hypercholesterolemia (types Ia, Ib), dysbetalipoproteinemia, elevated triglyceride levels

Dosage and routes
Adult: PO 10 mg qd, usual range 10-80, dosage adjustments may be made in 2-4 wk intervals, max 80 mg/day

Available forms: Tabs 10, 20, 40, 80 mg

Adverse effects
(*italic* = common; **bold** = life-threatening)
CNS: Headache, asthenia
EENT: Lens opacities
GI: Abdominal cramps, constipation, diarrhea, heartburn, nausea, ↑ AST, dyspepsia, *flatus,* **liver dysfunction,** pancreatitis
INTEG: Rash, pruritus, alopecia
MS: Myalgia, **rhabdomyolysis,** arthralgia
GU: Impotence
RESP: Pharyngitis, sinusitis
MISC: Hypersensitivity

Contraindications: Hypersensitivity, pregnancy **X,** lactation, active liver disease

Precautions: Past liver disease, alcoholism, severe acute infections, trauma, hypotension, uncontrolled seizure disorders, severe metabolic disorders, electrolyte imbalance

Pharmacokinetics

Absorption	Unknown
Distribution	Unknown
Metabolism	Liver
Excretion	Bile, feces, kidneys
Half-life	14 hr

 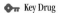

Pharmacodynamics
Unknown

Interactions
Individual drugs
Cholestyramine, colestipol: ↓ action of ator-vastatin

Clofibrate, cyclosporine, erythromycin, gemfibrozil, niacin: ↑ risk of rhabdomyolysis

Digoxin: ↑ action of digoxin

Warfarin: ↑ action of warfarin

Drug classifications
Antifungals (azole): Possible rhabdomyolysis

Contraceptives (oral): ↑ action

Food/drug
• Possible toxicity when used with grapefruit juice

• Food ↑ blood levels

Herb/drug
Glucomannan: ↑ effect

Gotu kola: ↓ effect

Lab test interferences
↑ bilirubin, ↑ alkaline phosphatase

Interference
Thyroid function tests

NURSING CONSIDERATIONS
Assessment
• Assess nutrition: fat, protein, carbohydrates; nutritional analysis should be completed by dietician before treatment

• Assess for muscle pain, tenderness, obtain CPK if these occur, drug may need to be discontinued

• Monitor bowel pattern daily; diarrhea may be a problem

• Monitor triglycerides, cholesterol at baseline and throughout treatment; LDL and VLDL should be watched closely; if increased, drug should be discontinued

• Monitor liver function studies q1-2 mo during the first 1½ yr of treatment; AST, ALT, liver function tests may be increased

• Monitor renal studies in patients with compromised renal system: BUN, I&O ratio, creatinine

• Assess eyes via ophthalmic exam 1 mo after treatment begins, annually

Nursing diagnoses
☑ Diarrhea (adverse reactions)

☑ Knowledge, deficient (teaching)

☑ Noncompliance (teaching)

Implementation
• Administer total daily dose at any time of day

• Store in cool environment in airtight, light-resistant container

Patient/family education
• Inform patient that compliance is needed for positive results to occur, not to double doses

• Teach patient that risk factors should be decreased: high-fat diet, smoking, alcohol consumption, absence of exercise

• Advise patient to notify prescriber if the GI symptoms of diarrhea, abdominal or epigastric pain, nausea, vomiting; chills, fever, sore throat; muscle pain, weakness occur

• Advise patient that treatment will take several years

• Advise patient that blood work and eye exam will be necessary during treatment

• Advise not to take if pregnant

• Advise patient to stay out of the sun, use protective clothing, or use sunscreen to prevent photosensitivity (rare)

Evaluation
Positive therapeutic outcome
• Decreased cholesterol levels, serum triglyceride

• Improved ratio of HDLs

atovaquone (Rx)
(a-toe'va-kwon)
Mepron
Func. class.: Antiprotozoal
Chem. class.: Aromatic diamide derivative; analog of ubiquinone

Pregnancy category C

Action: Interferes with DNA/RNA synthesis in protozoa, specifically ATP and nucleic acid synthesis

Therapeutic Outcome: Antiprotozoal for *Pneumocystis carinii* only

Uses: *Pneumocystis carinii* infections in patients intolerant of trimethoprim/sulfamethoxazole (co-trimoxazole)

Dosage and routes
Adult and adolescents 13-16 yr: PO 750 mg bid with food tid for 21 days

Available forms: 750 mg/5 ml

Adverse effects
(*italic* = common; **bold** = life-threatening)
CNS: Dizziness, headache, anxiety, insomnia
CV: Hypotension
GI: Nausea, vomiting, diarrhea, anorexia, increased AST and ALT, acute pancreatitis, constipation, abdominal pain
HEMA: Anemia, **leukopenia, neutropenia**
INTEG: Pruritus, urticaria, *rash,* oral monilia

META: Hyperkalemia, hypoglycemia, hyponatremia

Contraindications: Hypersensitivity or history of developing life-threatening allergic reactions to any component of the formulation

Precautions: Blood dyscrasias, hepatic **P** disease, diabetes mellitus, pregnancy **C**, **G** lactation, children, elderly

◤ Do Not Confuse:
Mepron (U.S.)/Mepron (meprobamate in Australia)

Pharmacokinetics

Absorption	Poor; increased when taken with fatty foods
Distribution	Unknown
Metabolism	Hepatic recycling
Excretion	Feces, unchanged (94%)
Half-life	2-3 days

Pharmacodynamics

Onset	Unknown
Peak	1-8 hr

Interactions
Individual drugs
Rifampin, rifabutin: ↓ effectiveness of atovaquone
Drug classifications
Use cautiously with highly protein-bound drugs
Food/drug
↑ absorption of drug, especially fatty foods

NURSING CONSIDERATIONS
Assessment
• Assess for *Pneumocystis carinii:* monitor WBC, bilateral lung sounds, sputum for C&S; these should be checked before, periodically during, and after treatment; after collection of 1st sputum, therapy may begin
• Monitor for symptoms of hyponatremia: *CV:* increased B/P, cold, clammy skin, hypovolemia or hypervolemia; *GI:* anorexia, nausea, vomiting, diarrhea, abdominal cramps; *NEURO:* lethargy, increased ICP, confusion, headache, seizures, coma, fatigue, tremors, hyperreflexia
• Monitor for symptoms of hypoglycemia/hyperglycemia in diabetic patients
• Monitor blood studies: blood glucose, CBC, platelets; I&O ratio; ECG for cardiac dysrhythmias, check B/P; liver studies: AST, ALT
• Monitor for signs of infection; anemia; monitor bowel pattern before, during treatment
• Monitor respiratory status: rate, character, wheezing, dyspnea

• Assess for dizziness, confusion, hallucination
• Assess for allergies before treatment, reaction of each medication; place allergies on chart; notify all people giving drugs

Nursing diagnoses
✓ Infection, risk for (uses)
✓ Diarrhea (adverse reactions)
✓ Knowledge, deficient (teaching)

Implementation
• Give with food (preferably fatty); increased absorption of the drug and higher plasma concentrations will occur; give tid × 3 wk

Patient/family education
• Instruct patient to take with food, preferably fatty foods, to increase plasma concentrations
• Advise patient to take drug exactly as prescribed

Evaluation
Positive therapeutic outcome
• Decreased temperature
• Ability to breathe
• Three negative sputum cultures

❗ HIGH ALERT

atropine ⊶ (Rx)
(a'troe-peen)
Atro-Pen
Methotrexate: ↑ blood levels, ↑ toxicity
Func. class.: Antidysrhythmic, anticholinergic parasympatholytic, mydriatic
Chem. class.: Belladonna alkaloid
Pregnancy category C

Action: Blocks acetylcholine at parasympathetic neuroeffector sites; increases cardiac output, heart rate by blocking vagal stimulation in heart; dries secretions, decreases sweating, salivation in low doses; mydriasis, increased heart rate and cycloplegia occur at moderate doses; motility of GI, GU systems at high dose

➲ Therapeutic Outcome: Drying of secretions, increased heart rate, cycloplegia, mydriasis

Uses: Bradycardia, bradydysrhythmia, reversal of anticholinesterase agents, insecticide poisoning, blocking cardiac vagal reflexes, decreasing secretions before surgery, antispasmodic with GU and biliary surgery, bronchodilator; ophthalmically for cycloplegia, mydriasis

---

Dosage and routes

Bradycardia/ bradydysrhythmias
Adult: **IV** bol 0.5-1 mg given q3-5 min, not to exceed 2 mg

P *Child:* **IV** bol 0.01-0.03 mg/kg up to 0.4 mg or 0.3 mg/m², may repeat q4-6h, min dose 0.1 mg to avoid paradoxical reaction

Organophosphate poisoning
P *Adult and child:* IM/**IV** 2 mg qh until muscarinic symptoms disappear; may need 6 mg qh

Presurgery
P *Adult and child >20 kg:* SC/IM/**IV** 0.4-0.6 mg before anesthesia

P *Child 12-16 kg:* SC/IM 0.3 mg 1 hr preop

Child 7-9 kg: SC/IM 0.2 mg 1 hr preop

Child 3 kg: SC/IM 0.1 mg 1 hr preop

Cycloplegic refraction
Adult: OPHTH ĩ-ĩĩ gtt of 1% sol 1 hr before exam

P *Child:* OPHTH ĩ-ĩĩ gtt of 0.5% sol bid-tid for up to 3 days before and 1 hr after exam

GI disorders
Adult: PO 0.3-1.2 mg q4-6h

Available forms: Inj 0.05, 0.1, 0.3, 0.4, 0.5, 0.8, 1 mg/ml; 2 mg/0.7 ml autoinjector; tabs 0.4 mg

Adverse effects
(*italic* = common; **bold** = life-threatening)
CNS: Headache, dizziness, involuntary movement, confusion, psychosis, anxiety, coma, flushing, drowsiness, insomnia, weakness,
G delirium (elderly)
CV: Hypotension, paradoxic bradycardia, angina, PVCs, hypertension, tachycardia, ectopic ventricular beats
EENT: Blurred vision, photophobia, glaucoma, eye pain, pupil dilatation, nasal congestion
GI: Dry mouth, nausea, vomiting, abdominal pain, anorexia, constipation, paralytic ileus, abdominal distention, altered taste
GU: Retention, hesitancy, impotence, dysuria
INTEG: Rash, urticaria, contact dermatitis, dry skin, flushing
MISC: Suppression of lactation, decreased sweating

Contraindications: Hypersensitivity to belladonna alkaloids, angle closure glaucoma, GI obstructions, myasthenia gravis, thyrotoxicosis, ulcerative colitis, prostatic hypertrophy, tachycardia/tachydysrhythmias, asthma, acute hemorrhage, hepatic disease, myocardial ischemia

Precautions: Pregnancy **C,** renal disease, lactation, CHF, tachydysrhythmias, hyperthy-
P roidism, COPD, hepatic disease, child <6 yr,
G hypertension, elderly, intraabdominal infections, Down syndrome, spastic paralysis, gastric ulcer

Pharmacokinetics

Absorption	Well absorbed (PO, SC, IM)
Distribution	Crosses blood-brain barrier, placenta
Metabolism	Liver
Excretion	Kidneys, unchanged (70%-90%); breast milk
Half-life	13-40 hr

Pharmacodynamics

	PO	IM/SC	IV	OPHTH
Onset	½ hr	15 min	2-4 min	½ hr
Peak	½-1 hr	30 min	2-4 min	30-60 min
Duration	4-6 hr	4-6 hr	4-6 hr	1-2 wk

Interactions
Individual drugs
Disopyramide: ↑ anticholinergic effect
Ketoconazole, levodopa: ↓ absorption
Potassium chloride (oral): ↑ GI lesions
Drug classifications
Antacids: ↓ absorption of atropine
Anticholinergics, antidepressants (tricyclic), antihistamines, antiparkinson agents: ↑ anticholinergic effect
⃠ Herb/drug
Aconite: ↑ toxicity, death
Aloe, broom, buckthorn (chronic use), cascara sagrada (chronic use), Chinese rhubarb, figwort, fumitory, goldenseal, kudzu, licorice: ↑ effect
Black root: Forms insoluble complex
Coltsfoot: ↓ effect
Horehound: ↑ serotonin effect
Jimsonweed, scopolia: ↑ atropine action

NURSING CONSIDERATIONS
Assessment
• Monitor I&O ratio; check for urinary
G retention and daily output in elderly or postoperative patients
• Monitor ECG for ectopic ventricular beats, PVC, tachycardia in cardiac patients
• Monitor for bowel sounds; check for constipation; abdominal distention and constipation may occur
• Monitor respiratory status: rate, rhythm, cyanosis, wheezing, dyspnea, engorged neck veins
• Monitor for increased intraocular pressure:

eye pain, nausea, vomiting, blurred vision, increased tearing; discontinue use if pain occurs (optic)
- Monitor cardiac rate: rhythm, character, B/P continuously
- Monitor allergic reaction: rash, urticaria

Nursing diagnoses
☑ Cardiac output, decreased (uses)
☑ Sensory perception, disturbed: visual (adverse reactions)
☑ Constipation (adverse reactions)
☑ Knowledge, deficient (teaching)

Implementation
IV IV route
- Give **IV** undiluted or diluted with 10 ml sterile H_2O; give at a rate of 0.6 mg/min; give through Y-tube or 3-way stopcock; do not add to **IV** sol; may cause paradoxic bradycardia lasting 2 min

Syringe compatibilities: Benzquinamide, butorphanol, chlorproMAZINE, cimetidine, dimenhyDRINATE, diphenhydrAMINE, droperidol, fentanyl, glycopyrrolate, heparin, hydromorphone, hydrOXYzine, meperidine, metoclopramide, midazolam, milrinone, morphine, nalbuphine, pentazocine, perphenazine, prochlorperazine, promazine, promethazine, propiomazine, ranitidine, scopolamine, sufentanil, vit B with C

Y-site compatibilities: Amrinone, etomidate, famotidine, heparin, hydrocortisone sodium succinate, meropenem, nafcillin, potassium chloride, sufentanil, vit B/C

Additive compatibilities: Dobutamine, furosemide, meropenem, netilmicin, sodium bicarbonate, verapamil
PO route
- PO 30 min ac
- Give increased bulk, water in diet if constipation occurs (anticholinergic effect)
IM route
- Expect atropine flush 15-20 min after inj; it
P may occur in children and is not harmful

Patient/family education
- Advise patient not to perform strenuous activity in high temperatures; heat stroke may result
- Instruct patient to take as prescribed; not to skip doses
- Instruct patient to report change in vision; blurring or loss of sight; trouble breathing; sweating; flushing, chest pain, allergic reactions, constipation, urinary retention
- Caution patient not to operate machinery if drowsiness occurs

- Advise patient not to take OTC products without approval of physician
Ophthalmic route
- Teach patient method of instillation: pressure on lacrimal sac for 1 min; do not touch dropper to eye
- Instruct patient that blurred vision will decrease with repeated use of drug; to omit next instillation if side effects are present
- Instruct patient not to perform hazardous tasks until able to see
- Advise patient to wait 5 min to use other drops; not to blink more than usual; use sunglasses to protect eyes

Evaluation
Positive therapeutic outcome
- Decreased dysrhythmias
- Increased heart rate
- Decreased secretions, GI, GU spasms
- Bronchodilatation
- Decrease in inflammation (iritis) or cycloplegic refraction (ophthalmic)

Treatment of overdose: O_2, artificial ventilation, ECG; administer DOPamine for circulatory depression; administer diazepam or thiopental for convulsion; assess need for antidysrhythmics

---

attapulgite (OTC)
(at-a-pull'gite)
Diar Aid, Diasorb, Fowler's Diarrhea Tablets ✤, Hydrated Magnesium Silicate, Kaopectate, Kaopectate Advanced Formula, Kaopectate Maximum Strength, Parepectolin, Rheaban, St. Joseph Antidiarrheal
Func. class.: Antidiarrheal
Chem. class.: Hydrous magnesium aluminum silicate

Pregnancy category C

Action: Decreases gastric motility, water content of stool; adsorbent, demulcent

→ **Therapeutic Outcome:** Decreased diarrhea

Uses: Diarrhea (cause undetermined), mild to moderate

Dosage and routes
Adult: PO 60-120 ml (45-90 ml conc) after each loose bowel movement

P *Child >12 yr:* PO 60 ml after each loose bowel movement

P *Child 6-12 yr:* PO 30-60 ml (30 ml conc) after each loose bowel movement

---

P *Child 3-6 yr:* PO 15-30 ml (15 ml conc) after each loose bowel movement

Available forms: Susp kaolin 0.87 g/5 ml, pectin 43 mg/5 ml; kaolin 0.98 g/5 ml, pectin 21.7 mg/5 ml

Adverse effects
(*italic* = common; **bold** = life-threatening)
GI: Constipation (chronic use)

Precautions: Pregnancy **C**

Pharmacokinetics	
Absorption	Not absorbed
Distribution	Unknown
Metabolism	Unknown
Excretion	Unknown
Half-life	Unknown

Pharmacodynamics
Unknown

Interactions
All drugs: ↓ action of all other drugs
🗹 *Herb/drug*
Nutmeg: ↑ effect

Nursing diagnoses
✔ Diarrhea (uses)
✔ Constipation (adverse reactions)
✔ Knowledge, deficient (teaching)

NURSING CONSIDERATIONS
Assessment
• Assess bowel pattern before, during, and after treatment; check for rebound constipation
P • Monitor for dehydration in children

Implementation
• For 48 hr only after each diarrhea stool

Patient/family education
• Advise patient not to exceed recommended dosage; notify prescriber if symptoms continue
• Instruct patient to shake well before administration

Evaluation
Positive therapeutic outcome
• Decreased diarrhea

---

azathioprine 🔑 **(Rx)**
(ay-za-thye'oh-preen)
Imuran
Func. class.: Immunosuppressant
Chem. class.: Purine antagonist

Pregnancy category D

Action: Produces immunosuppression by inhibiting purine synthesis, DNA, RNA in cells

➡ **Therapeutic Outcome:** Absence of graft rejection, slowing of rheumatoid arthritis

Uses: Renal transplants to prevent graft rejection, often used with corticosteroids, cytotoxics; refractory rheumatoid arthritis, refractory ITP, glomerulonephritis, nephrotic syndrome, bone marrow transplant

Investigational uses: Myasthenia gravis, chronic ulcerative colitis, Crohn's disease, Behçet's syndrome

Dosage and routes
Renal dose
CCr 10-50 ml/min 75% of dose; CCr <10 ml/min 50% of dose

Prevention of rejection
P *Adult and child:* PO, **IV** 3-5 mg/kg/day, then maintenance (PO) of at least 1-2 mg/kg/day

Refractory rheumatoid arthritis
Adult: PO 1/mg/kg/day; may increase dosage after 2 mo by 0.5 mg/kg/day; not to exceed 2.5 mg/kg/day

Available forms: Tabs 50 mg; inj **IV** 100 mg

Adverse effects
(*italic* = common; **bold** = life-threatening)
GI: Nausea, vomiting, stomatitis, esophagitis, **pancreatitis, hepatotoxicity, jaundice**
HEMA: Leukopenia, thrombocytopenia, **anemia, pancytopenia**
INTEG: Rash, alopeia
MS: Arthralgia, muscle wasting
MISC: Raynaud's symptoms, **serum sickness**

Contraindications: Hypersensitivity, pregnancy **D**

Precautions: Severe renal disease, severe
G hepatic disease, elderly

🗏 **Do Not Confuse:**
Imuran/Imferon

Pharmacokinetics

Absorption	Readily (PO)
Distribution	Crosses placenta
Metabolism	Liver to mercaptopurine
Excretion	Kidney, minimal
Half-life	3 hr

Pharmacodynamics

	PO	IV
Onset	Unknown	Unknown
Peak	4 hr	Unknown
Duration	Unknown	Unknown

Interactions
Individual drugs
Allopurinol: ↑ toxicity
Cyclosporine: ↑ myelosuppression
Warfarin: ↓ action of warfarin
Drug classifications
ACE inhibitors: ↑ leukopenia
Antineoplastics: ↑ myelosuppression
Vaccines: ↓ immune response
Herb/drug
Astragalus, echinacea, melatonin, safflower: ↑ immunosuppression
Ginseng, maitake, mistletoe, schisandra, St. John's wort, turmeric: ↓ effect
Lab test interferences
↓ Uric acid, ↑ liver function tests
Interference: CBC, diff count

NURSING CONSIDERATIONS
Assessment
• Assess symptoms of rheumatoid arthritis: pain in joints, stiffness, poor range of motion, inflammation before and during treatment
• Monitor blood studies: Hgb, WBC, platelets during treatment monthly; if leukocytes are <3000/mm³ or platelets <100,000/mm³, drug should be discontinued or reduced; decreased Hgb level may indicate bone marrow suppression
• Monitor liver function studies: alkaline phosphatase, AST, ALT, amylase, bilirubin; and for hepatotoxicity: dark urine, jaundice, itching, light-colored stools; drug should be discontinued
• Monitor I&O, weight qd, report decreasing urine output, toxicity may occur
• Assess for infection: increased temp, WBC; sputum, urine

Nursing diagnoses
☑ Mobility, impaired (uses)
☑ Infection, risk for (uses)
☑ Knowledge, deficient (teaching)

Implementation
PO route
• Give all medications PO if possible, avoiding IM inj, since bleeding may occur
• Give with meals to reduce GI upset; nausea is common
• For several days before transplant surgery, patients should be placed in protective isolation
IV **IV route**
• Prepare in biologic cabinet using gown, gloves, mask; give after diluting 100 mg/10 ml of sterile water for inj; rotate to dissolve; may further dilute with 50 ml or more saline or glucose in saline given over >30 min (intermittent inf)

Solution compatibilities: D₅W, NaCl 0.9%, NaCl 0.45%

Patient/family education
• Teach patient to take as prescribed, do not miss doses, if dose is missed on qd regimen, skip dose, if on multiple dosing/day, take as soon as remembered
• Teach patient that therapeutic response may take 3-4 mo in rheumatoid arthritis, to continue with prescribed exercise, rest, other medications; that drug is needed for life in renal transplant
• Instruct patient to report fever, rash, severe diarrhea, chills, sore throat, fatigue, since serious infections may occur; or clay-colored stools and cramping (hepatotoxicity)
• Advise patient to use contraceptive measures during treatment for 12 wk after ending therapy; drug is teratogenic
• Advise patient to avoid vaccinations
• Tell patient to avoid crowds and persons with known infections to reduce risk of infection
• Instruct patient not to use OTC medications without approval of prescriber
• Advise patient to use soft-bristled toothbrush to prevent bleeding

Evaluation
Positive therapeutic outcome
• Absence of graft rejection
• Immunosuppression in autoimmune disorders
• Increased joint mobility without pain in rheumatoid arthritis

---

azelastine (Rx)

(ay'ze-lass-teen)

Astelin

Func. class.: Leukotriene synthesis inhibitor
Chem. class.: Phthalazinone derivative

Pregnancy category C

Action: Inhibits the synthesis and release of leukotrienes; antagonizes action of acetylcholine, histamine, serotonin

➡ **Therapeutic Outcome:** Decreased nasal stuffiness, itching, swollen eyes

Uses: Seasonal allergic rhinitis

Dosage and routes

P *Adult and child ≥12 yr:* Nasal 2 sprays/nostril bid

Available forms: Spray 137 mcg/actuation

Adverse effects

(*italic* = common; **bold** = life-threatening)
CNS: Sedation (more common with increased dosages), drowsiness
MISC: Weight increase, myalgia

Contraindications: Hypersensitivity

Precautions: Pregnancy **C**

Pharmacokinetics	
Absorption	Unknown
Distribution	Unknown
Metabolism	Liver, extensively
Excretion	Feces
Half-life	25-42 hr

Pharmacodynamics	
Onset	Unknown
Peak	4-5 hr
Duration	Unknown

Interactions
Individual drugs
Alcohol: ↑ CNS depression

Drug classifications
CNS depressants, opioids, sedative/hypnotics: ↑ CNS depression

NURSING CONSIDERATIONS
Assessment

• Assess respiratory status: rate, rhythm, increase in bronchial secretions, wheezing, chest tightness; provide fluids to 2 L/day to decrease secretion thickness

Nursing diagnoses

✓ Airway clearance, ineffective (uses)
✓ Knowledge, deficient (teaching)
✓ Noncompliance (teaching, overuse)

Implementation

• Remove cap/safety clip from spray pump
• Prime pump if using for first time, push 4 times quickly, away from face, blow your nose, then place tip of pump into one nostril, while holding other nostril closed, tilt head forward, and spray into nostril
• Put cover/safety clip back on

Patient/family education

• Teach patient all aspects of drug uses; to notify prescriber if confusion, sedation occur; to avoid driving and other hazardous activity if drowsiness occurs; to avoid alcohol and other CNS depressants that may potentiate effect
• Caution patient not to exceed recommended dosage; dysrhythmias may occur

Evaluation
Positive therapeutic outcome

• Absence of runny or congested nose

azithromycin (Rx)

(ay-zi-thro-my'sin)

Zithromax

Func. class.: Antiinfective
Chem. class.: Macrolide (azalide)

Pregnancy category B

Action: Binds to 50S ribosomal subunits of susceptible bacteria and suppresses protein synthesis; much greater spectrum of activity than erythromycin

➡ **Therapeutic Outcome:** Bacteriostatic against the following susceptible organisms: *Moraxella catarrhalis, Streptococcus pneumoniae, Streptococcus pyogenes, Staphylococcus aureus, Haemophilus influenzae, Clostridium, Legionella pneumophila, Chlamydia trachomatis, Mycoplasma;* no effect on methicillin-resistant *S. aureus;* in

P children: acute otitis media *(H. influenzae, M. catarrhalis, S. pneumoniae)* PO, acute pharyngitis/tonsillitis (group A streptococcal) PO; acute skin/soft tissue infections (PO); community-acquired pneumonia *(C. pneumoniae, H. influenzae, M. pneumoniae, S. pneumoniae)* PO; pharyngitis/tonsillitis *(S. pyogenes)*

Uses: Mild to moderate infections of the upper respiratory tract, lower respiratory tract; uncomplicated skin and skin structure infections, nongonococcal urethritis, or cervicitis; prophylaxis of disseminated *Mycobacterium avium* complex (MAC)

Investigational uses: Bacterial endocarditis prevention, chlamydial infections, gonococcal infections, prophylaxis after sexual assault

Dosage and routes
Most infections
Adult: PO 500 mg on day 1, then 250 mg qd on days 2-5 for a total dose of 1.5 g
P *Child 2-15 yr:*
PO 10 mg/kg on day 1, then 5 mg/kg × 4 days

Pharyngitis/tonsillitis
Adult: PO 12 mg/kg qd × 5 days

Pelvic inflammatory disease
Adult: PO/**IV** 500 mg **IV** q24h × 2 doses, then 500 mg PO q24h × 7-10 days

Cervicitis, chlamydia, chancroid, nongonococcal urethritis
Adult: PO 1 g single dose

Gonorrhea
Adult: PO 2 g single dose

Endocarditis, prophylaxis
Adult: PO 500 mg 1 hr prior to procedure
P **Child:** PO 15 mg/kg 1 hr prior to procedure

Community acquired pneumonia
Adult: PO/**IV** 500 mg **IV** q24h × 2 doses, then 500 mg PO q24h × 7-10 days

Disseminated MAC infections
Adult: PO 600 mg/day in combination with ethambutol

Lower respiratory tract infections, acute skin/soft tissue infections, acute pharyngitis/tonsillitis
P **Child:** PO 3-day regimen, 10 mg/kg qd × 3 days

Acute otitis media
P **Child:** PO 30 mg/kg as a single dose or 10 mg/kg qd × 3 days or 10 mg/kg as a single dose on day 1, max 500 mg/day, then 5 mg/kg on days 2-5, max 250 mg/day

Prevention of acute otitis media
P **Child:** PO 10 mg/kg qwk × 6 mo

Available forms: Tabs 250, 600 mg; powder for inj 500 mg; powder for oral susp 1 g/packet; susp 100, 200 mg/5 ml

Adverse effects
(*italic* = common; **bold** = life-threatening)
CNS: Dizziness, headache, vertigo, somnolence
CV: Palpitations, chest pain
GI: *Nausea, vomiting, diarrhea,* **hepatotoxicity,** abdominal pain, stomatitis, heartburn, dyspepsia, flatulence, melena, **cholestatic jaundice, pseudomembranous colitis**
GU: Vaginitis, moniliasis, nephritis
INTEG: Rash, urticaria, pruritus, photosensitivity
SYST: **Angioedema**

Contraindications: Hypersensitivity to azithromycin, erythromycin, or any macrolide

Precautions: Pregnancy **B**, lactation, **G** hepatic/renal/cardiac disease, elderly, child <6 **P** mo for otitis media, child <2 yr for pharyngitis, tonsillitis

Do Not Confuse:
Zithromax/Zinacef

Pharmacokinetics
Absorption	Rapid, (PO) up to 50%
Distribution	Widely distributed
Metabolism	Unknown, minimal metabolism
Excretion	Unchanged (bile); kidneys, minimal
Half-life	11-70 hr

Pharmacodynamics
	PO	IV
Onset	Unknown	Unknown
Peak	2-4 hr	End of infusion
Duration	24 hr	24 hr

Interactions
Individual drugs
Carbamazepine, ergotamine, pimozide, theophylline: ↑ toxicity
Phenytoin: ↑ effects of oral anticoagulants
Pimozide: Fatal reaction
Tacrolimus: ↑ effects of tacrolimus
Triazolam: ↓ clearance of triazolam
Drug classifications
Aluminum antacids: ↓ peak serum
Anticoagulants (orals): ↑ effect of oral anticoagulants
Magnesium antacids: ↓ levels of azithromycin
Herb/drug
Acidophilus: Do not use with antiinfectives
Lab test interferences
↑ Bilirubin, ↑ LDH, ↑ alkaline phosphatase, ↑ CPK, ↑ K, ↑ Pro-time, ↑ BUN, ↑ creatinine, ↑ blood glucose, ↑ AST, ↑ ALT

NURSING CONSIDERATIONS
Assessment
• Assess for signs and symptoms of infection: drainage, fever, increased WBC >10,000/mm³, urine culture positive, sore throat, sputum culture positive

 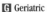

• Monitor respiratory status: rate, character, wheezing, tightness in chest; discontinue drug if these occur

• Monitor allergies before treatment, reaction of each medication; place allergies on chart, notify all people giving drugs; skin eruptions, itching

• Monitor I&O ratio, renal studies; report hematuria, oliguria in renal disease; check urinalysis, protein, blood

• Monitor liver studies: AST, ALT, bilirubin, LDH, alkaline phosphatase; CBC with differential

• Monitor C&S before drug therapy; drug may be taken as soon as culture is taken; C&S may be repeated after treatment

• Monitor bowel pattern before, during treatment

• Assess for superinfection: sore throat, mouth, tongue; fever, fatigue, diarrhea, anogenital pruritus

Nursing diagnoses
✓ Infection, risk for (uses)
✓ Diarrhea (adverse reactions)
✓ Knowledge, deficient (teaching)

Implementation
PO route
• Provide adequate intake of fluids (2 L) during diarrhea episodes

• Give with a full glass of water; give susp 1 hr before or 2 hr pc; tabs may be taken without regard to food; do not give with fruit juices

• Store at room temperature

• Reconstitute 1 g packet for susp with 60 ml water, mix, rinse glass with more water and have patient drink to consume all medication; packets not for pediatric use

IV route
• Reconstitute 500 mg drug/4.8 ml sterile water for inj (100 mg/ml), shake, dilute with ≥250 ml 0.9% NaCl, 0.45% NaCl, or LR to 1-2 mg/ml; diluted solution is stable for 24 hr or 7 days if refrigerated

• Give 500 mg or more/1 hr, never give IM or as a bol

Patient/family education
• Instruct patient to report sore throat, black furry tongue, fever, loose foul-smelling stool, vaginal itching, discharge, fatigue; may indicate superinfection

• Caution patient not to take aluminum/magnesium-containing antacids or food simultaneously with this drug; blood levels of azithromycin will be decreased

• Instruct patient to notify prescriber of diarrhea stools, dark urine, pale stools, yellow discoloration of eyes or skin, severe abdominal pain; cholestatic jaundice is a severe adverse reaction

• Teach patient complete dosage regimen; to notify prescriber if symptoms continue

• Teach patient that if pregnancy is suspected to notify prescriber

• Inform patient that sunburns may occur; wear protective clothing and sunscreen

Evaluation
Positive therapeutic outcome
• C&S negative for infection
• WBC within 5000-10,000/mm^3

---

balsalazide (Rx)
(ball-sal'a-zide)
Colazal
Func. class.: GI antiinflammatory
Chem. class.: Salicylate derivative

Pregnancy category B

Action: Delivered intact to the colon, bioconverted to 4-aminobenzoyl-β-alanine

➔ **Therapeutic Outcome:** Decreased inflammation in colon

Uses: Active, mild to moderate ulcerative colitis

Dosage and routes
Adult: PO 750 mg (3 tabs) tid × 8 wk, may take up to 12 wk

Available forms: Tabs 750 mg

Adverse effects
(*italic* = common; **bold** = life-threatening)
CNS: Headache, insomnia, fatigue, fever, dizziness
EENT: Dry mouth, dry eyes, rhinitis, sinusitis, watery eyes, blurred vision
GI: Nausea, vomiting, abdominal pain, diarrhea, rectal bleeding, flatulence, dyspepsia, dry mouth, constipation
MS: Arthralgia, back pain, myalgia
SYST: **Anaphylaxis**

Contraindications: Hypersensitivity to salicylates

Precautions: Pregnancy **B**, child <14 yr, lactation, pyloric stenosis

Pharmacokinetics
Absorption	Low, variable
Distribution	Plasma protein binding 99%
Metabolism	Unknown
Excretion	Kidneys, as metabolites
Half-life	Unknown

Pharmacodynamics
Unknown

Interactions
None known

Lab test interferences
↑ AST, ↑ ALT, ↑ GGT, ↑ LDH, ↑ bilirubin, ↑ alkaline phosphatase

False positive: Urinary glucose test

NURSING CONSIDERATIONS
Assessment
- Monitor kidney function studies: BUN, creatinine, urinalysis (long-term therapy)
- Assess for allergic reaction: rash, dermatitis, urticaria, pruritus, dyspnea, bronchospasm

Nursing diagnoses
☑ Injury, risk for (uses)
☑ Knowledge, deficient (teaching)

Implementation
- Give with food in evenly divided doses
- Use with resuscitative equipment available; severe allergic reactions may occur
- Give total daily dose evenly spaced to minimize GI intolerance
- Store in tight, light-resistant container at room temp

Patient/family education
- Advise patient to notify prescriber if symptoms do not improve, if rash, hives, or respiratory problems occur

Evaluation
Positive therapeutic outcome
- Absence of fever, mucus in stools, resolution of symptoms of ulcerative colitis

---

⚠ HIGH ALERT

basiliximab (Rx)
(bas-ih-liks'ih-mab)
Simulect
Func. class.: Immunosuppressant
Chem. class.: Murine/human monoclonal antibody (interleukin-2) receptor antagonist

Pregnancy category B

Action: Binds to and blocks the IL-2 receptor, which is selectively expressed on the surface of activated T-lymphocytes; impairs the immune system to antigenic challenges

➔ Therapeutic Outcome: Prevention of graft rejection

Uses: Acute allograft rejection in renal transplant patients when used with cycloSPORINE and corticosteroids

Dosage and routes
Adult: IV 20 mg × 2 doses; 1st dose within 2 hr before transplant surgery; 2nd dose given 4 days after transplantation

P *Child 2-15 yr:* **IV** 12 mg/m^2 × 2 doses; 1st dose within 2 hr before transplant surgery; 2nd dose given 4 days after transplantation

Available forms: Powder for inj 20 mg

Adverse effects
(*italic* = common; **bold** = life-threatening)
CNS: *Pyrexia, chills, tremors, headache, insomnia, weakness*
CV: *Chest pain,* angina, **cardiac failure,** hypotension, hypertension, edema
GI: *Vomiting, nausea, diarrhea,* constipation, abdominal pain, GI bleeding, gingival hyperplasia, stomatitis
INTEG: *Acne*
META: Acidosis, hypercholesterolemia, hyperuricemia, hyperkalemia, hypocalcemia, hypokalemia, hypophosphatemia
MISC: Infection, moniliasis, **anaphylaxis**
MS: Arthralgia, myalgia
RESP: *Dyspnea, wheezing, cough,* **pulmonary edema**

Contraindications: Hypersensitivity

P Precautions: Pregnancy **B**, infections,
G elderly, lactation, children

Pharmacokinetics	
Absorption	Unknown
Distribution	Unknown
Metabolism	Unknown
Excretion	Unknown
Half-life	7 days (adult)
	P 9½ days (child)

Pharmacodynamics	
Onset	Unknown
Peak	½ hr (adults)
Duration	Unknown

Interactions
Drug classifications
Immunosuppressants: ↑ immunosuppression
☑ **Herb/drug**
Astragalus, echinacea, melatonin, safflower: ↑ immunosuppression
Ginseng, maitake, mistletoe, schisandra, St. John's wort, turmeric: ↓ effect
Lab test interferences
↑ BUN, cholesterol, ↑ uric acid, ↑ creatinine,

 Herb/drug   Do Not Crush   Alert   Key Drug   Geriatric   **P** Pediatric

↑ potassium, ↑ calcium, ↑ blood glucose, ↑ Hgb, ↑ Hct

↓ Hgb, ↓ Hct, ↓ platelets, ↓ magnesium, ↓ phosphate

NURSING CONSIDERATIONS
Assessment
- Assess for infection, increased temp, WBC, sputum, urine
- Monitor blood studies: Hgb, WBC, platelets during treatment qmo; if leukocytes are <3000/mm^3, drug should be discontinued
- Monitor liver function studies: alkaline phosphatase, AST, ALT, bilirubin
- Assess hepatotoxicity: dark urine, jaundice, itching, light-colored stools; drug should be discontinued
- Assess for anaphylaxis, hypersensitivity: dyspnea, wheezing, rash, pruritus, hypotension, tachycardia; if severe hypersensitivity reactions occur, drug should not be used again

Nursing diagnoses
☑ Infection, risk for (adverse reactions)
☑ Knowledge, deficient (teaching)

Implementation
- Administer all medications PO if possible; avoid IM inj, since infection may occur

IV route
- After adding 5 ml sterile water for inj, shake gently to dissolve, reconstitute to a vol of 50 ml with 0.9% NaCl or D$_5$, gently invert bag, do not shake, do not admix

Patient/family education
- Instruct patient to report fever, chills, sore throat, fatigue, since serious infection may occur; avoid crowds, persons with known upper respiratory infections; use contraception during treatment

Evaluation
Positive therapeutic outcome
- Absence of graft rejection

---

beclomethasone (Rx)
(be-kloe-meth'a-sone)
Beclodisk ✢, Becloforte Inhaler ✢, Beclovent, QVAR, Vanceril, Vanceril Double Strength
Func. class.: Synthetic glucocorticoid (long acting)
Chem. class.: Beclomethasone diester

Pregnancy category C

Action: Antiinflammatory; vasoconstrictive properties; also immunosuppressive

→**Therapeutic Outcome:** Decreased inflammation and normal immunity

Uses: Seasonal, perennial allergic rhinitis, nasal polyps, chronic steroid-dependent asthma

Dosage and routes
P *Adult and child >12 yr:* INSTILL 1-2 sprays in each nostril bid-qid; INH 2-4 puffs tid-qid (42 mcg/actuations), max 20 inh/day; inh 2 puffs bid, max 10 inh/day (84 mcg/actuation)

P *Child 6-12 yrs:* INSTILL 1 spray in each nostril tid; INH 1-2 puffs tid-qid (42 mcg/actuation); 2 puffs bid, max 5 inh/day (84 mcg/actuation)

Available forms: Aero 42 mcg/spray (nasal); aero for nasal inh 42, 50, 84, 250 mcg/activation; aerosol for nasal inh 0.042%; inh cap 100, 200 mcg

Adverse effects
(*italic* = common; **bold** = life-threatening)
CNS: *Headache,* paresthesia
EENT: *Dryness, nasal irritation, burning, sneezing,* secretions with blood, nasal ulcerations, **perforation of nasal septum,** candidal infection, earache, *hoarseness*
ENDO: Adrenal suppression
GI: Dry mouth, dyspepsia
INTEG: Rash, urticaria, pruritus
MISC: **Angioedema adrenal insufficiency,** facial edema, Churg-Strauss syndrome
RESP: **Acute status asthmaticus,** wheezing, cough

Contraindications: Hypersensitivity, systemic corticosteroid therapy

P **Precautions:** Pregnancy **C,** children <12, nasal ulcers, recurrent epistaxis

Pharmacokinetics	
Absorption	Locally only
Distribution	Not distributed
Metabolism	Lungs, liver, GI system (by CYP3A)
Excretion	Feces, urine
Half-life	2.8 hr

Pharmacodynamics		
	INH	NASAL
Onset	10 min	10 min
Peak	Unknown	Unknown
Duration	Unknown	Unknown

✢ Canada Only   ◨ Do Not Confuse   * "Tall Man" lettering (See Preface)

NURSING CONSIDERATIONS
Assessment
- Assess adrenal suppression: 17-KS, plasma cortisol for decreased levels, adrenal function periodically for HPA axis suppression during prolonged therapy; monitor growth and development
- Assess blood studies, neutrophils, decreased platelets; WBC with diff baseline and q3 mo, if neutrophils <1000/mm^3, discontinue treatment
- Check nasal passages during long-term treatment for changes in mucus; check for burning, stinging; assess for glucocorticoid withdrawal: dizziness, hypotension, fatigue, muscle/joint pain; notify prescriber immediately
- Assess respiratory status: rest, rhythm, characteristics; auscultate lung bilaterally before and throughout treatment
- Assess for fungal infections in mucous membranes

Nursing diagnoses
☑ Airway clearance, ineffective (uses)
☑ Oral mucous membranes, impaired (adverse reactions)
☑ Knowledge, deficient (teaching)
☑ Noncompliance (teaching)

Implementation
- Give PO, using a spacer device for proper dose
- Use after cleaning aerosol top daily with warm water; dry thoroughly
- Store in cool environment; do not puncture or incinerate container

Patient/family education
- Teach patient to gargle/rinse mouth after each use to prevent oral fungal infections
- Teach patient that in times of stress, systemic corticosteroids may be needed to prevent adrenal insufficiency; do not discontinue oral drug abruptly, taper slowly
- Teach patient to continue using product even if mild nasal bleeding occurs; is usually transient
- Teach patient method of instillation after providing written instructions from manufacturer
- Teach patient to clear nasal passages before administration; use decongestant if needed; shake inhaler, invert, tilt head backward, insert nozzle into nostril, away from septum; hold other nostril closed and depress activator, inhale through nose, exhale through mouth

Evaluate
Positive therapeutic outcome
- Decrease in runny nose, improved symptoms of bronchial asthma

benazepril (Rx)
(ben-a′za-pril)
Lotensin
Func. class.: Antihypertensive
Chem. class.: ACE inhibitor

Pregnancy category
C (1st trimester)
D (2nd/3rd trimesters)

Action: Selectively suppresses renin-angiotensin-aldosterone system; inhibits ACE, preventing conversion of angiotensin I to angiotensin II

→**Therapeutic Outcome:** Decreased B/P in hypertension

Uses: Hypertension, alone or in combination with thiazide diuretics

Dosage and routes
Adult: PO 10 mg qd initially, then 20-40 mg/day divided bid or qd (without a diuretic); 5 mg PO qd (with a diuretic)

Renal dose
Adult: PO 5 mg qd with CCr <30 ml/min/ 1.73 m^2; increase as needed to maximum of 40 mg/day

G *Elderly:* PO 5-10 mg/day initially

Available forms: Tabs 5, 10, 20, 40 mg

Adverse effects
(*italic* = common; **bold** = life-threatening)
CNS: Anxiety, hypertonia, insomnia, paresthesia, headache, dizziness, fatigue
CV: Hypotension, postural hypotension, syncope, palpitations, angina
GI: Nausea, constipation, vomiting, gastritis, melena
GU: Increased BUN, creatinine, decreased libido, impotence, urinary tract infection
INTEG: Rash, flushing, sweating
MISC: **Angioedema**
META: Hyperkalemia, hyponatremia
MS: Arthralgia, arthritis, myalgia
RESP: Cough, asthma, bronchitis, dyspnea, sinusitis

Contraindications: Hypersensitivity to ACE inhibitors, pregnancy **D** (2nd/3rd trimesters), lactation, children P

Precautions: Impaired renal/liver function, dialysis patients, hypovolemia, blood dyscra-

 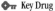

sias, CHF, COPD, asthma, elderly, bilateral renal artery stenosis; pregnancy **C** (1st trimester)

Do Not Confuse:
Lotensin/Lioresal, Lotensin/Loniten

Pharmacokinetics

Absorption	<40%
Distribution	Unknown; crosses placenta
Metabolism	Liver metabolites; protein binding 97%
Excretion	Kidney, breast milk (minimal)
Half-life	10-11 hr (metabolite); increased in renal disease

Pharmacodynamics

Onset	Unknown
Peak	½-1 hr
Duration	Unknown

Interactions
Individual drugs
Alcohol: ↑ hypotension (large amounts)
Lithium: ↑ serum levels
Drug classifications
Antihypertensives, diuretics: ↑ hypotension
Diuretics (potassium-sparing):
↑ hyperkalemia
Potassium supplements, sympathomimetics:
↑ toxicity
Herb/drug
Aconite: ↑ toxicity, death
Astragalus, cola tree: ↑ or ↓ antihypertensive effect
Barberry, betony, black catechu, black cohosh, bloodroot, broom, burdock, cat's claw, dandelion, goldenseal, Irish moss, Jamaican dogwood, kelp, khella, mistletoe, parsley: ↑ antihypertensive effect
Coltsfoot, guarana, khat, licorice, pineapple, yohimbe: ↓ antihypertensive effect
Lab test interferences
↑ BUN, ↑ creatinine, ↑ liver function tests, ↑ bilirubin, ↑ uric acid, ↑ blood glucose
Positive: ANA titer

NURSING CONSIDERATIONS
Assessment
• Monitor blood studies: neutrophils, decreased platelets
• Monitor B/P at peak/trough level of drug, check for orthostatic hypotension, syncope; if changes occur, dosage change may be required
• Monitor renal studies: protein, BUN, creatinine; watch for increased levels that may indicate nephrotic syndrome and renal failure;

monitor urine for protein; monitor renal symptoms: polyuria, oliguria, frequency, dysuria
• Establish baselines in renal, liver function tests before therapy begins
• Check potassium levels throughout treatment, although hyperkalemia rarely occurs
• Assess for allergic reactions: rash, fever, pruritus, urticaria; drug should be discontinued if antihistamines fail to help

Nursing diagnoses
✓ Cardiac output, decreased (uses)
✓ Injury, risk for (side effects)
✓ Knowledge, deficient (teaching)
✓ Noncompliance (teaching)

Implementation
PO route
• Store in air-tight container at 86° F (30° C) or less
• Severe hypotension may occur after 1st dose of this medication; decreased hypotension may be prevented by reducing or discontinuing diuretic therapy 3 days before beginning benazepril therapy

Patient/family education
• Instruct patient not to discontinue drug abruptly; advise patient to tell all persons associated with care
• Teach patient not to use OTC products (cough, cold, allergy) unless directed by prescriber; serious side effects can occur; xanthines such as coffee, tea, chocolate, cola can prevent action of drug
• Emphasize the importance of complying with dosage schedule, even if feeling better; to continue with medical regimen to decrease B/P: exercise, cessation of smoking, decreasing stress, diet modifications
• Emphasize the need to rise slowly to sitting or standing position to minimize orthostatic hypotension; not to exercise in hot weather because increased hypotension can occur
• Teach patient to notify prescriber of mouth sores, sore throat, fever, swelling of hands or feet, irregular heartbeat, chest pain, coughing, shortness of breath
• Caution patient to report excessive perspiration, dehydration, vomiting, diarrhea; may lead to fall in B/P
• Caution patient that drug may cause dizziness, fainting, light-headedness; may occur during 1st few days of therapy; to avoid activities that may be hazardous
• Teach patient how to take B/P; teach normal readings for age-group; ensure patient takes own B/P

- Advise patient to notify prescriber of pregnancy, drug will need to be discontinued

Evaluation
Positive therapeutic outcome
- Decreased B/P in hypertension

Treatment of overdose: 0.9% NaCl **IV** inf, hemodialysis

---

benztropine (Rx)
(benz'troe-peen)
Apo-Benztropin ✦, benztropine mesylate, Cogentin
Func. class.: Cholinergic blocker, antiparkinson agent
Chem. class.: Tertiary amine

Pregnancy category C

Action: Blockade of central acetylcholine receptors in the CNS, neurotransmitters are balanced

Therapeutic Outcome: Decreased involuntary movements

Uses: Parkinsonian symptoms, extrapyramidal symptoms (EPS) associated with neuroleptic drugs, acute dystonia

Dosage and routes
Drug-induced extrapyramidal symptoms
Adult: IM/**IV** 1-4 mg qd/bid; give PO dose as soon as possible; PO 1-2 mg bid/tid; increase by 0.5 mg q5-6 days

P *Child:* IM/**IV** 0.02-0.05 mg/kg/dose 1-2 × 1 day

G *Elderly:* PO 0.5 mg qd/bid, increase by 0.5 mg q5-6 days

Parkinsonian symptoms
Adult: PO 1-2 mg qd, in divided doses; increased 0.5 mg q5-6 days titrated to patient response

Acute dystonic reactions
Adult: IM/**IV** 1-2 mg, may increase to 1-2 mg bid (PO)

Available forms: Tabs 0.5, 1, 2 mg; inj IM, **IV** 1 mg/ml

Adverse effects
(*italic* = common; **bold** = life-threatening)
CNS: Confusion, anxiety, restlessness, irritability, delusions, hallucinations, headache, sedation, depression, incoherence, dizziness, **G** memory loss; delirium (elderly)
CV: Palpitations, tachycardia, hypotension, bradycardia

EENT: Blurred vision, photophobia, dilated pupils, difficulty swallowing, dry eyes, mydriasis, increased intraocular tension, angle closure glaucoma
GI: Dryness of mouth, constipation, nausea, vomiting, abdominal distress, **paralytic ileus,** epigastric distress
GU: Hesitancy, retention, dysuria
INTEG: Rash, urticaria, dermatoses
MISC: Increased temperature, flushing, decreased sweating, **hyperthermia, heat stroke,** numbness of fingers
MS: Muscular weakness, cramping

Contraindications: Hypersensitivity, narrow angle glaucoma, myasthenia gravis, **P** GI/GU obstruction, child <3 yr, peptic ulcer, megacolon, prostate hypertrophy

G Precautions: Pregnancy **C,** elderly, lactation, tachycardia, liver, kidney disease, drug abuse history, dysrhythmias, hypotension, **P** hypertension, psychiatric patients, children

Pharmacokinetics
Absorption	Well (PO, IM), completely (**IV**) absorbed
Distribution	Unknown
Metabolism	Unknown
Excretion	Unknown
Half-life	Unknown

Pharmacodynamics
	IM/IV	PO
Onset	15 min	1 hr
Peak	Unknown	Unknown
Duration	6-10 hr	6-10 hr

Interactions
Individual drugs
Disopyramide, quinidine: ↑ anticholinergic effects
Drug classifications
Antacids: ↓ absorption of benztropine
Antidepressants (tricyclic), antihistamines, phenothiazines: ↑ anticholinergic effects
Antidiarrheals: ↓ absorption
⊘ *Herb/drug*
Kava, jaborandi, pill-bearing spurge: ↓ benztropine effect
Butterbur, jimsonweed: ↑ benztropine effect
Black catechu: ↑ constipation

NURSING CONSIDERATIONS
Assessment
- Monitor I&O ratio; retention commonly causes decreased urinary output, distention, frequency, incontinence

---

- Assess for parkinsonism, EPS: shuffling gait, muscle rigidity, involuntary movements, loss of balance, pill rolling, muscle spasms, drooling before and during treatment
- Monitor for urinary hesitancy, retention; palpate bladder if retention occurs
- Monitor for constipation, cramping, pain in abdomen, abdominal distention; increase fluids, bulk, exercise if this occurs
- Assess for tolerance over long-term therapy; dosage may have to be increased or changed
- Assess for mental status: affect, mood, CNS depression, worsening of mental symptoms during early therapy
- Assess for benztropine "buzz" or "high," patients may imitate EPS

Nursing diagnoses
☑ Mobility, impaired (uses)
☑ Knowledge, deficient (teaching)
☑ Noncompliance (teaching)

Implementation
PO route
- Give with or after meals to prevent GI upset; may give with fluids other than water; hard candy, frequent drinks, gum to relieve dry mouth
- Give hs to avoid daytime drowsiness in patient with parkinsonism
- May be crushed and mixed with food
- Store at room temperature
IM route
- Give in large muscle mass for dystonic symptoms
IV **IV route**
- Give parenteral dose with patient recumbent to prevent postural hypotension; give undiluted 1 mg/1 min

Syringe compatibilities: Chlorpromazine, fluphenazine, metoclopramide, perphenazine, thiothixene

Y-site compatibilities: Fluconazole, tacrolimus

Patient/family education
- Teach patient to use caution in hot weather; drug may increase susceptibility to stroke since perspiration is decreased; patient should remain indoors
- Advise patient not to discontinue this drug abruptly; to taper off over 1 wk to prevent withdrawal symptoms (insomnia, involuntary movements, anxiety, tachycardias)
- Caution patient to avoid driving or other hazardous activities; drowsiness, dizziness may occur
- Teach patient to avoid OTC medication: cough, cold preparations with alcohol, antihistamines unless directed by prescriber; increased CNS depression may occur
- Advise patient to rise from sitting or recumbent position slowly to minimize orthostatic hypotension
- Teach patient to use gum, hard candy, frequent sips of water to decrease dry mouth; if dry mouth continues, saliva substitutes may be prescribed
- Instruct patient that doses should not be doubled, but missed dose may be taken up to 2 hr before next dose
- Advise patient to use good oral hygiene, use frequent sips of water, sugarless gum for dry mouth

Evaluation
Positive therapeutic outcome
- Absence of involuntary movements (pill rolling, tremors, muscle spasms)

---

bepridil (Rx)
(be'pri-dil)
Vascor
Func. class.: Calcium channel blocker, antianginal, antihypertensive
Pregnancy category C

Action: Inhibits calcium ion influx across cell membrane during cardiac depolarization; produces relaxation of coronary vascular smooth muscle, peripheral vascular smooth muscle; dilates coronary vascular arteries; increases myocardial oxygen delivery in patients with vasospastic angina, decreases SA/AV node conduction, inhibits fast sodium inward current

➡ **Therapeutic Outcome:** Decreased angina pectoris

Uses: Chronic stable angina, used alone or in combination with β-blockers, nitrates

Dosage and routes
Adult: PO 200 mg qd, after 10 days may increase dose if needed; max dose 400 mg/day

Available forms: Tabs, film-coated, 200, 300 mg

Adverse effects
(*italic* = common; **bold** = life-threatening)
CNS: Headache, fatigue, drowsiness, dizziness, anxiety, depression, weakness, insomnia, confusion, lightheadedness, nervousness
CV: **Dysrhythmias**, edema, **CHF**, bradycardia, hypotension, palpitations, **AV block, torsades de pointes**

GI: Nausea, vomiting, diarrhea, gastric upset, constipation, increased levels in liver function studies, gingival hyperplasia
GU: Nocturia, polyuria
HEMA: Agranulocytosis
MISC: Stevens-Johnson syndrome

Contraindications: Hypersensitivity, sick sinus syndrome, 2nd- or 3rd-degree heart block, Wolff-Parkinson-White syndrome, hypotension less than 90 mm Hg systolic, cardiogenic shock, history of serious ventricular dysrhythmias, uncompensated cardiac insufficiency

Precautions: CHF, hypotension, hepatic injury, pregnancy **C**, lactation, children, renal disease, IHSS, concomitant β-blocker therapy

Do Not Confuse:
bepridil/Prepidil

Pharmacokinetics	
Absorption	Well absorbed
Distribution	Plasma protein bound (99%), crosses placenta
Metabolism	Liver
Excretion	Urine, feces
Half-life	42 hr

Pharmacodynamics	
Onset	1 hr
Peak	2-3 hr
Duration	24 hr

Interactions
Individual drugs
Fentanyl: ↑ hypotension
Ritonavir: ↑ bepridil levels
Drug classifications
Antidepressants (tricyclic), antidysrhythmics, cardiac glycosides: ↑ prolongation of QT interval, depression of AV node
β-Adrenergic blockers: ↑ adverse reactions
Food/drug
Grapefruit: ↑ hypotension
Herb/drug
Barberry, betel palm, burdock, cat's claw, chicory, goldenseal, khat, khella, lily of the valley, plantain: ↑ antianginal effect
Yohimbe: ↓ effect
Lab test interferences
↑ Liver function tests, ↑ aminotransferase, ↑ CPK, ↑ LDH

NURSING CONSIDERATIONS
Assessment
• Assess fluid volume status: I&O ratio and record, weight, distended red veins, crackles in lung, color, quality, and sp gr of urine, skin turgor, adequacy of pulses, moist mucous membranes, bilateral lung sounds, peripheral pitting edema
• Assess cardiac status: B/P, pulse, respiration, ECG intervals (PR, QRS, QT), dysrhythmias; may prolong QT interval, alter T wave
• Obtain digoxin levels if cardiac glycosides are given with bepridil

Nursing diagnoses
✓ Cardiac output, decreased (uses)
✓ Knowledge, deficient (teaching)

Implementation
• Give once a day, with food for GI symptoms; adjust dose no more frequently than q10 days
• Do not break, chew, crush tabs

Patient/family education
• Instruct patient to avoid hazardous activities until stabilized on drug and dizziness is no longer a problem
• Instruct patient to limit caffeine consumption; to avoid alcohol and OTC drugs unless directed by prescriber
• Advise patient to comply in all areas of medical regimen: diet, exercise, stress reduction, drug therapy; to notify prescriber of irregular heartbeat, shortness of breath, swelling of feet and hands, pronounced dizziness, constipation, nausea, hypotension
• Teach patient to use as directed even if feeling better; may be taken with other cardiovascular drugs (nitrates, β-blockers)
• Teach patient to notify prescriber of swelling, weight gain, dyspnea, irregular heartbeat
• Advise patient to maintain good oral hygiene to prevent gingival hyperplasia

Evaluation
Positive therapeutic outcome
• Decreased anginal pain
• Increased activity tolerance

Treatment of overdose: Defibrillation, atropine for AV block, vasopressor for hypotension

betamethasone (Rx)
(bay-tah-meth′ah-sone)
Betnelan ✦, Betnesol ✦, Celestone, Cel-U-Jec, Selestoject ✦
Func. class.: Corticosteroid, synthetic; glucocorticoid, long acting

Pregnancy category C

Action: Decreases inflammation by suppression of migration of polymorphonuclear leukocytes, fibroblasts, reversal of increased

⬚ Herb/drug   Ⓢ Do Not Crush   ◆ Alert   ◆ₜₜ Key Drug   Ⓖ Geriatric   Ⓟ Pediatric capillary permeability and lysosomal stabilization

➡ **Therapeutic Outcome:** Decreased inflammation and normal immunity

Uses: Immunosuppression, severe inflammation, prevention of neonatal respiratory distress syndrome (by administration to mother), chronic asthma, rhinitis (inh); psoriasis, eczema, contact dermatitis, pruritus (top)

Dosage and routes
Adult: PO 0.6-7.2 mg qd; IM/**IV** 0.6-7.2 mg qd in joint or soft tissue (sodium phosphate)

P *Child:* PO 17.5 mcg/kg/day in 3 divided doses; IM 17.5 mcg/kg/day in 3 divided doses every 3rd day or 5.8-8.75 mcg/kg/day as a single dose (adrenal insufficiency)

P *Child:* PO 62.5-250 mcg/kg/day in 3 divided doses; IM 20.8-125 mcg/kg/day of the base q12-24h (other uses)

P *Adult and child:* TOP apply to affected area qid

Adult: INH 2-4 puffs tid-qid; not to exceed 20 inh/day

P *Child 6-12 yr:* INH 1-2 puffs tid-qid; not to exceed 10 inh/day

P *Adult and child >12 yr:* INSTILL 1-2 sprays in each nostril bid-qid

Available forms: Tabs 500, 600 mcg; tabs, effervescent 500 mcg ♣; syr 600 mcg/5 ml; ext rel tab 1 mg; sol for inj (phosphate) 3 mg/ml; susp for inj (phosphate/acetate) 6 mg/ml

Adverse effects
(*italic* = common; **bold** = life-threatening)
CNS: *Depression, flushing, sweating,* headache, ecchymosis, bruising, mood changes
CV: *Hypertension,* **circulatory collapse, thrombophlebitis, embolism,** tachycardia, **necrotizing angiitis, CHF**
EENT: Fungal infections, increased intraocular pressure, blurred vision
GI: *Diarrhea, nausea, abdominal distention,* **GI hemorrhage,** increased appetite, **pancreatitis**
HEMA: **Thrombocytopenia**
INTEG: *Acne, poor wound healing, ecchymosis, bruising,* petechiae
MS: Fractures, osteoporosis, weakness

Contraindications: Psychosis, hypersensitivity, idiopathic thrombocytopenia, acute glomerulonephritis, amebiasis, fungal infections, nonasthmatic bronchial disease, child <2 yr, AIDS, TB

Precautions: Pregnancy **C**, diabetes mellitus, glaucoma, osteoporosis, seizure disorders, ulcerative colitis, CHF, myasthenia gravis, renal disease, esophagitis, peptic ulcer

Pharmacokinetics

Absorption	Well absorbed (PO); systemic (top)
Distribution	Crosses placenta
Metabolism	Liver, extensively
Excretion	Kidney, breast milk
Half-life	3-5 hr, adrenal suppression 3-4 days

Pharmacodynamics

	PO	IM	IV	TOP
Onset	1-2 hr	Unknown	Rapid	Unknown
Peak	2 hr	4-8 hr	4-8 hr	Unknown
Duration	3 days	1-1½ days	1-1½ days	Unknown

Interactions
Individual drugs
Alcohol: ↑ GI bleeding
Amphotericin B, mezlocillin, ticarcillin: ↑ hypokalemia
Insulin: ↑ need for insulin
Phenytoin, rifampin: ↓ action, ↑ metabolism
Drug classifications
Barbiturates: ↓ action, ↑ metabolism
Diuretics: ↑ hypokalemia
Hypoglycemic agents: ↑ need for hypoglycemic agents
NSAIDs, salicylates: ↑ GI bleeding
Toxoids/vaccines: ↓ immune response
Food/drug
• Grapefruit juice should be avoided
⚠ *Herb/drug*
Aloe, goldenseal, hawthorn, hops, lemon balm, licorice, lily of the valley, mistletoe, perilla, pheasant's eye: ↑ corticosteroid effect
Buckthorn, cascara sagrada, Chinese rhubarb: ↑ hypokalemia
Lab test interferences
↑ Cholesterol, ↑ sodium, ↑ blood glucose, ↑ uric acid, ↑ calcium, ↑ urine glucose
↓ Calcium, ↓ potassium, ↓ T₄, ↓ T₃, ↓ thyroid ¹³¹I uptake test, ↓ urine 17-OHCS, ↓ 17-KS, ↓ PBI
False negative: Skin allergy tests

NURSING CONSIDERATIONS
Assessment
Systemic route
• Monitor potassium, blood glucose, urine glucose while on long-term therapy; hypokalemia and hyperglycemia; check weight daily; notify prescriber of weekly gain >5 lb
• Monitor B/P q4h, pulse; notify prescriber if chest pain occurs

- Monitor I&O ratio; be alert for decreasing urinary output and increasing edema
- Check plasma cortisol levels during long-term therapy (normal level: 138-635 nmol/L [SI units] when drawn at 8 AM); adrenal function periodically for HPA axis suppression
- Assess for symptoms of infection: increased temperature, WBC even after withdrawal of medication; drug masks infection symptoms
- Assess for symptoms of potassium depletion: paresthesias, fatigue, nausea, vomiting, depression, polyuria, dysrhythmias, weakness
- Monitor for edema, hypertension, cardiac symptoms
- Assess for mental status: affect, mood, behavioral changes, aggression

Topical route
- Check temperature; if fever develops, drug should be discontinued
- Assess for systemic absorption: increased temperature, inflammation, irritation

Nursing diagnoses
☑ Infection, risk for (adverse reactions)
☑ Knowledge, deficient (teaching)
☑ Noncompliance (teaching)

Implementation
PO route
- Give with food or milk to decrease GI symptoms

IM route
- Give IM inj deep in large mass, rotate sites, avoid deltoid, use 21-G needle; in one dose in AM to prevent adrenal suppression; avoid SC administration; may damage tissue

IV IV route
- Give **IV** (only sodium phosphate product); give over >1 min; may be given by **IV** inf in compatible sol after shaking susp (parenteral)
- Give titrated dose; use lowest effective dose

Y-site compatibilities: Heparin, hydrocortisone, potassium chloride, vit B/C

Inhalation route
- Give inh with water to decrease possibility of fungal infections; titrated dose; use lowest effective dose
- Use after cleaning aerosol top daily with warm water; dry thoroughly
- Store in cool environment; do not puncture or incinerate container

Topical route
- Apply only to affected areas; do not get in eyes; apply medication, then cover with occlusive dressing (only if prescribed), seal to normal skin, change q12h; systemic absorption may occur

- Apply only to dermatoses; do not use on weeping, denuded, or infected area
- Cleanse before applying drug; use treatment for a few days after area has cleared
- Store at room temperature

Patient/family education
Systemic route
- Advise patient that long-term therapy may be needed to clear infection (1-2 mo depending on type of infection); that emergency ID as steroid user should be carried or worn; dosage adjustment may be needed
◆• Instruct patient to notify prescriber if therapeutic response decreases; caution patient not to discontinue abruptly; adrenal crisis can result
- Instruct patient to avoid OTC products: salicylates, alcohol in cough products, cold preparations unless directed by prescriber
- Teach patient all aspects of drug usage including cushingoid symptoms
- Teach patient symptoms of adrenal insufficiency: nausea, anorexia, fatigue, dizziness, dyspnea, weakness, joint pain

Topical route
- Caution patient to avoid sunlight on affected area; burns may occur

Evaluation
Positive therapeutic outcome
- Ease of respirations, decreased inflammation (systemic)
- Absence of severe itching, patches on skin, flaking (top)

---

bethanechol ◆π (Rx)
(be-than′e-kol)
bethanechol chloride, Duvoid, Urebeth, Urecholine
Func. class.: Urinary tract stimulant, cholinergic
Chem. class.: Synthetic choline ester

Pregnancy category C

Action: Stimulates muscarinic acetylcholine receptors directly; mimics effects of parasympathetic nervous system stimulation; stimulates gastric motility, micturition; increases lower esophageal sphincter pressure

▶ **Therapeutic Outcome:** Absence of continued urinary retention

Uses: Urinary retention (postoperative, postpartum), neurogenic atony of bladder with retention

---

Dosage and routes
Adult: PO 25-50 mg bid-qid; SC 5-10 mg tid-qid prn

P *Child:* PO 0.6 mg/kg/day divided in 3-4 doses/day; SC 0.06 mg/kg tid or 0.15 mg/kg qid

Test dose
Adult: SC 2.5 mg repeated 15-30 min intervals × 4 doses to determine effective dose

Available forms: Tabs 5, 10, 25, 50 mg; inj SC 5 mg/ml

Adverse effects
(italic = common; bold = life-threatening)
CNS: Dizziness
CV: Hypotension, bradycardia, orthostatic hypotension, reflex tachycardia, **cardiac arrest, circulatory collapse**
EENT: Miosis, increased salivation, lacrimation, blurred vision
GI: Nausea, bloody diarrhea, belching, vomiting, cramps, fecal incontinence
GU: Urgency
INTEG: Rash, urticaria, flushing, increased sweating
***RESP:* Acute asthma, dyspnea, bronchoconstriction**

Contraindications: Hypersensitivity, severe bradycardia, asthma, severe hypotension, hyperthyroidism, peptic ulcer, parkinsonism, seizure disorders, CAD, COPD, coronary occlusion, mechanical obstruction, peritonitis, recent urinary or GI surgery

Precautions: Hypertension, pregnancy **C**, P lactation, child <8 yr, urinary retention

Pharmacokinetics	
Absorption	Poorly absorbed (PO); well absorbed (SC)
Distribution	Does not cross blood-brain barrier
Metabolism	Unknown
Excretion	Kidneys
Half-life	Unknown

Pharmacodynamics		
	PO	SC
Onset	30-90 min	5-15 min
Peak	1 hr	15-30 min
Duration	1-6 hr	2 hr

Interactions
Individual drugs
Donepezil: ↑ action of bethanechol
Procainamide, quinidine: ↓ action of bethanechol

Drug classifications
Cholinergic agonists: ↑ action, ↑ toxicity
Ganglionic blockers: ↑ severe hypotension

B

☑ Herb/drug
Jimsonweed, scopolia: ↓ effects
Jaborandi: ↑ cholinergic effect

Lab test interferences
↑ AST, ↑ lipase/amylase, ↑ bilirubin

NURSING CONSIDERATIONS
Assessment
• Monitor B/P, pulse, respirations; observe after parenteral dose for 1 hr
• Check I&O ratio; check for urinary retention or incontinence; if bladder emptying does not occur, notify prescriber; catheterization may be needed
• Assess for bradycardia, hypotension, bronchospasm, headache, dizziness, seizures, sweating, cramping, respiratory depression; drug should be discontinued if toxicity occurs; atropine administration

Nursing diagnoses
☑ Urinary elimination, impaired (uses)
☑ Injury, risk for (adverse reactions)
☑ Knowledge, deficient (teaching)

Implementation
SC route
◆• Give parenteral dose by SC route; use of IM, **IV** may result in cardiac arrest or cholinergic crisis (diarrhea with blood, cramping, hypotension, circulatory collapse)
◆• Administer only with atropine sulfate available for cholinergic crisis; give only after all other cholinergics have been discontinued
• Do not use sol with a precipitate, or if discolored
PO route
• Give increased doses if tolerance occurs as prescribed
• To avoid nausea and vomiting, take on an empty stomach; 1 hr ac or 2 hr pc
• Store at room temperature

Patient/family education
• Instruct patient to take drug exactly as prescribed; 1 hr ac or 2 hr pc; do not double doses; if dose is missed take within 1 hr of scheduled dose
• Caution patient to make position changes slowly; orthostatic hypotension may occur
• Instruct patient to report cramping, diarrhea with blood, flushing to prescriber

Evaluation
Positive therapeutic outcome
• Absence of urinary retention
• Absence of abdominal distention

Treatment of overdose: Administer atropine 0.6-1.2 mg **IV** or IM (adult)

bexarotene (Rx)
(bex-air'-oo-teen)
Targretin
Func. class.: Retinoid, 2nd generation
Pregnancy category X

Action: Selectively binds and activates retinoid X receptors (RXRs) that are partially responsible for cellular proliferation and differentiation; inhibits some tumor cells

Therapeutic Outcome: Decreased size and number of lesions

Uses: Cutaneous T-cell lymphoma

Investigational uses: Breast cancer

Dosage and routes
Adult: PO 300 mg/day/mm², may increase to 400 mg/day with proper monitoring

Available forms: Cap 75 mg

Adverse effects
(*italic* = common; **bold** = life-threatening)
CNS: Headache, fatigue, lethargy
GI: Nausea, abdominal pain, diarrhea,
acute pancreatitis
HEMA: **Leukopenia, neutropenia, anemia**
INTEG: Rash, asthenia, dry skin
SYST: Infection, hypothyroidism

Contraindications: Hypersensitivity to retinoids, pregnancy **X**

Precautions: Lactation, sunburn, hepatic, **P** renal disease, children

Pharmacokinetics	
Absorption	Unknown
Distribution	Unknown
Metabolism	Unknown
Excretion	Kidneys
Half-life	Unknown

Pharmacodynamics
Unknown

Interactions
Individual drugs
Phenytoin: ↓ bexarotene levels
Tamoxifen: ↓ action of tamoxifen
Vitamin A: limit intake to ≤15,000 international units/day
Drug classifications
Antidiabetics: ↑ action of antidiabetics
Azole antiinfectives: ↑ bexarotene levels
Barbiturates, rifampin: ↓ bexarotene levels
Oral contraceptives: ↓ action of oral contraceptives
Food/drug
Grapefruit juice: ↑ bexarotene levels

NURSING CONSIDERATIONS
Assessment
• Assess part of body involved, including time involved, what helps or aggravates condition, cysts, dryness, itching
• Assess cholesterol, HDL, triglycerides; these may be elevated
• Monitor CBC for leukopenia, neutropenia, anemia

Nursing diagnoses
✓ Skin integrity, impaired (uses)
✓ Body image, disturbed (uses)
✓ Knowledge, deficient (teaching)

Implementation
• Administer with food

Patient/family education
• Advise patient to avoid sunlight, sunlamps or to use protective clothing or sunscreen to prevent burns
• Instruct patient to avoid pregnancy while taking this drug and ≥1 mo after discontinuing therapy
• Teach patient to limit vit A to ≤15,000 international units/day to prevent toxicity
• Advise diabetic patients on insulin to watch for hypoglycemia

Evaluation
Positive therapeutic outcome
• Decrease in size and number of lesions

bicalutamide (Rx)
(bi-kal-yut'ah-mide)
Casodex
Func. class.: Antineoplastic hormone
Chem. class.: Nonsteroidal antiandrogen
Pregnancy category X

Action: Competitively inhibits the action to androgens by binding to cytosol androgen receptors in target tissue

Therapeutic Outcome: Prevention of growth of malignant cells

Uses: Prostate cancer in combination with luteinizing hormone-releasing hormone (LHRH) analog

Dosage and routes
Adult: PO 50 mg qd with LHRH

Available forms: Tab 50 mg

Adverse effects

(*italic* = common; **bold** = life-threatening)

CV: Hot flashes, hypertension, chest pain, **CHF**, edema

CNS: Dizziness, paresthesia, insomnia, anxiety, neuropathy, headache

GI: Diarrhea, constipation, nausea, vomiting, increased liver enzyme test, anorexia, dry mouth, abdominal pain

GU: Nocturia, **hematuria**, UTI, impotence, gynecomastia, urinary incontinence, frequency, dysuria, retention, urgency, breast tenderness, decreased libido, hot flashes

INTEG: Rash, sweating, dry skin, pruritus, alopecia

MISC: Infection, anemia, dyspnea, bone pain, headache, asthenia, *back pain,* flu-like symptoms

Contraindications: Hypersensitivity, pregnancy **X**

G **Precautions:** Renal, hepatic disease, elderly, lactation

Pharmacokinetics

Absorption	Well absorbed
Distribution	Unknown
Metabolism	Liver
Excretion	Urine, feces
Half-life	5.2 days

Pharmacodynamics

Onset	Unknown
Peak	31½ hr
Duration	Unknown

Interactions

Drug classifications

Anticoagulants: ↑ anticoagulation

Lab test interferences

↑ AST, ↑ ALT, ↑ bilirubin, ↑ BUN, ↑ creatinine
↓ Hgb, ↓ WBC

NURSING CONSIDERATIONS

Assessment

• Assess for diarrhea, constipation, nausea, vomiting

• Assess for hot flashes, gynecomastia; assure patient that these are common side effects

• Monitor PSA (prostate specific antigen), liver function studies

Nursing diagnoses

☑ Injury, risk for (uses, adverse reactions)

☑ Knowledge, deficient (teaching)

Implementation

• Give at same time each day (for both drugs) either AM or PM with or without food

• Give only with LHRH treatment

Patient/family education

• Teach patient to recognize and report signs of anemia, hepatotoxicity, renal toxicity

• Advise patient that hair may be lost, but is reversible after therapy is discontinued

• Advise patient not to use other products unless approved by prescriber

• Advise patient to use contraception

Evaluation

Positive therapeutic outcome

• Decreased tumor size, spread of malignancy

---

biperiden (Rx)

(bye-per′i-den)

Akineton

Func. class.: Antiparkinsonian agent, anticholinergic

Pregnancy category C

Action: Centrally acting competitive anticholinergic; blocks cholinergic responses in the CNS

➡ Therapeutic Outcome: Decreased involuntary movements

Uses: Parkinsonian symptoms, extrapyramidal symptoms (EPS) secondary to neuroleptic drug therapy

Dosage and routes

Extrapyramidal symptoms

Adult: PO 2 mg qd-tid; IM/**IV** 2 mg q30 min, if needed, not to exceed 8 mg/24 hr

P *Child:* IM 40 mcg/kg or 1.2 mg/m², may repeat q½h

Parkinsonian symptoms

Adult: PO 2 mg tid-qid; max 16 mg/24 hr

Available forms: Tabs 2 mg; inj IM/**IV** 5 mg/ml (lactate)

Adverse effects

(*italic* = common; **bold** = life-threatening)

CNS: Confusion, anxiety, restlessness, irritability, delusions, hallucinations, headache, sedation, depression, incoherence, dizziness, euphoria, tremors, memory loss

CV: Palpitations, tachycardia, postural hypotension, bradycardia

EENT: Blurred vision, photophobia, dilated pupils, difficulty swallowing, mydriasis, increased intraocular tension, angle closure glaucoma

GI: Dryness of mouth, constipation, nausea, vomiting, abdominal distress, **paralytic ileus**

GU: Hesitancy, retention, dysuria

INTEG: Rash, urticaria, dermatoses
MISC: Increased temperature, flushing, decreased sweating, **hyperthermia, heat stroke,** numbness of fingers
MS: Weakness, cramping

Contraindications: Hypersensitivity, narrow-angle glaucoma, myasthenia gravis, GI/GU obstruction, megacolon, stenosing peptic ulcers, prostatic hypertrophy

G Precautions: Pregnancy **C,** elderly, lactation, tachycardia, dysrhythmias, liver, kidney disease, drug abuse, hypotension, hyperten-
P sion, psychiatric patients, children

Pharmacokinetics

Absorption	Well absorbed (PO, IM)
Distribution	Unknown
Metabolism	Unknown
Excretion	Unknown
Half-life	18-24 hr

Pharmacodynamics

	IM/IV	PO
Onset	15 min	1 hr
Peak	Unknown	Unknown
Duration	6-10 hr	6-10 hr

Interactions
Individual drugs
Alcohol: ↑ sedation
Amantadine, quinidine: ↑ anticholinergic effects
Haloperidol: ↑ schizophrenic symptoms
Drug classifications
Antacids, antidiarrheals: ↓ biperiden absorption
Antidepressants (tricyclic), antihistamines, phenothiazines: ↑ anticholinergic effects
☑ *Herb/drug*
Black catechu: ↑ constipation
Kava, jaborandi, pill-bearing spurge: ↓ biperiden effect
Butterbur, jimsonweed: ↑ biperiden effect

NURSING CONSIDERATIONS
Assessment
• Monitor I&O ratio; retention commonly causes decreased urinary output, distention, frequency, incontinence
• Assess for parkinsonism, EPS: shuffling gait, muscle rigidity, involuntary movements, pill rolling, muscle spasms, drooling before and during treatment
• Assess patient response if anticholinergics are given
• Monitor for urinary hesitancy, retention; palpate bladder if retention occurs

• Monitor for constipation, cramping, pain in abdomen, abdominal distention; increase fluids, bulk, exercise if this occurs
• Assess for tolerance over long-term therapy; dosage may have to be increased or changed
• Assess for mental status: affect, mood, CNS depression, worsening of mental symptoms during early therapy

Nursing diagnoses
☑ Mobility, impaired (uses)
☑ Knowledge, deficient (teaching)

Implementation
PO route
• Give with food or pc to prevent GI upset; may give with fluids other than water; hard candy, frequent drinks, gum to relieve dry mouth
• Give hs to avoid daytime drowsiness in patients with parkinsonism
• Store at room temp
IV IV route
• Give parenteral dose with patient recumbent to prevent postural hypotension; give undiluted 2 mg or less over 1 min or more

Patient/family education
• Teach patient to use caution in hot weather; drug may increase susceptibility to heat stroke since perspiration is decreased; patient should remain indoors
• Teach patient not to discontinue this drug abruptly; to taper off over 1 wk to prevent withdrawal symptoms (insomnia, involuntary movements, anxiety, tachycardias)
• Teach patient to avoid driving or other hazardous activities; drowsiness, dizziness may occur
• Teach patient to avoid OTC medication: cough, cold preparations with alcohol, antihistamines unless directed by prescriber; increased CNS depression may occur
• Caution patient to rise from sitting or recumbent position slowly to minimize orthostatic hypotension
• Teach patient to use gum, hard candy, frequent sips of water to decrease dry mouth; if dry mouth continues, saliva substitutes may be prescribed
• Instruct patient that doses should not be doubled, but missed dose may be taken up to 2 hr before next dose

Evaluation
Positive therapeutic outcome
• Absence of involuntary movements (pill rolling, tremors, muscle spasms)

bisacodyl (OTC)

(bis-a-koe′dill)

Bisc-Evac ✤, Bisacolax ✤, Bisco-Lax ✤, Carter's Little Pills, Dacodyl, Deficol, Dulcagen, Dulcolax, Fleet Bisacodyl, Feen-a-Mint, Fleet Laxative, Modane, Reliable Gentle Laxative, Therelax

Func. class.: Laxative, stimulant
Chem. class.: Diphenylmethane

Pregnancy category C

Action: Acts directly on intestine by increasing motor activity; thought to irritate colonic intramural plexus; increases water in the colon

⮕ Therapeutic Outcome: Decreased constipation

Uses: Short-term treatment of constipation, bowel or rectal preparation for surgery, examination

Dosage and routes

P *Adult ≥12 yr:* PO 5-15 mg in PM or AM; may use up to 30 mg for bowel or rec preparation; REC 10 mg (single dose)

P *Child >3 yr:* PO 5-10 mg as a single dose; REC 10 mg as a single dose

P *Child <2 yr:* REC 5 mg as a single dose

Available forms: Enteric coated tabs 5 mg; supp 5, 10 mg; rec sol 10 mg/37 ml; enema 0.33 mg/ml, 10 mg/5 ml; powder for rec sol 1.5 mg bisacodyl/2.5 g tannic acid

Adverse effects

(*italic* = common; **bold** = life-threatening)
CNS: Muscle weakness
GI: Nausea, vomiting, anorexia, cramps, diarrhea, rectal burning (supp)
META: Protein-losing enteropathy, alkalosis, hypokalemia, **tetany,** electrolyte and fluid imbalances

Contraindications: Hypersensitivity, rectal fissures, abdominal pain, nausea, vomiting, appendicitis, acute surgical abdomen, ulcerated hemorrhoids, acute hepatitis, fecal impaction, intestinal/biliary tract obstruction

Precautions: Pregnancy **C**

Pharmacokinetics

Absorption	Poor
Distribution	Unknown
Metabolism	Liver, minimally
Excretion	Kidneys
Half-life	Unknown

Pharmacodynamics

	PO	RECT
Onset	6-10 hr	15-60 min
Peak	Unknown	Unknown
Duration	Unknown	Unknown

Interactions

Drug classifications
Antacids: ↓ of enteric coating of drugs
Gastric acid pump inhibitors: ↑ gastric irritation
H_2-blockers: ↑ gastric irritation

Herb/drug
Flax, lily of the valley, pheasant's eye, senna, squill: ↑ laxative action

NURSING CONSIDERATIONS
Assessment

• Monitor blood, urine electrolytes if used often by patient; check I&O ratio to identify fluid loss
• Assess cramping, rectal bleeding, nausea, vomiting; if these symptoms occur, drug should be discontinued; identify cause of constipation; identify whether fluids, bulk, or exercise missing from lifestyle

Nursing diagnoses

✓Constipation (uses)
✓Diarrhea (side effects)
✓Knowledge, deficient (teaching)
✓Noncompliance (teaching)

Implementation
PO route

• Give alone with water only for better absorption; do not take within 1 hr of antacids, milk
• Administer in AM or PM (oral dose)
🚫• Do not chew; swallow tabs whole
Rectal route
• Lubricate before insertion, patient should retain for ½ hr

Patient/family education

• Discuss with the patient that adequate fluid and bulk consumption is necessary
• Advise patient that normal bowel movements do not always occur daily
• Teach patient not to use in presence of abdominal pain, nausea, vomiting; tell patient to notify prescriber if constipation unrelieved or if symptoms of electrolyte imbalance occur: muscle cramps, pain, weakness, dizziness, excessive thirst

Evaluation
Positive therapeutic outcome

• Decreased constipation within 3 days

✤ Canada Only   ◪ Do Not Confuse   * "Tall Man" lettering (See Preface)

bismuth subsalicylate (OTC)
(bis'meth sub-sa-li'si-late)
Bismatrol, Bismatrol Extra Strength,
Bismed, Pepto-Bismol, Pepto-Bismol
Maximum Strength, Pink Bismuth,
PMS-Bismuth Subsalicylate
Func. class.: Antidiarrheal
Chem. class.: Salicylate

Pregnancy category C

Action: Inhibits prostaglandin synthesis responsible for GI hypermotility; stimulates absorption of fluid and electrolytes; antimicrobial, antisecretory effects

⇒**Therapeutic Outcome:** Absence of loose, watery stools

Uses: Diarrhea (cause undetermined); prevention of diarrhea when traveling; may be included to treat *Helicobacter pylori*

Dosage and routes
Antidiarrheal
Adult: PO 524 mg q½h or 1048 mg q1h, max 4.2 g/24 hr

P *Child 9-12 yr:* PO 15 ml; 262 mg q½-1h, max 2.1 g/24 hr

P *Child 6-9 yr:* PO 174.6 mg q½-1h, max 1.4 g/24 hr

P *Child 3-6 yr:* PO 88 mg q½-1h, max 704 mg/24 hr

Available forms: Chewable tabs 262 mg; susp 262, 300, 524 mg/15 ml

Adverse effects
(*italic* = common; **bold** = life-threatening)
CNS: Confusion, twitching
EENT: Hearing loss, tinnitus, metallic taste, blue gums
GI: Increased fecal impaction (high doses), dark stools, constipation
HEMA: Increased bleeding time

P **Contraindications:** Child <3 yr; impaction, children, teens with flulike symptoms, hypersensitivity (aspirin), history of GI bleeding, renal disease

Precautions: Anticoagulant therapy,
G pregnancy **C**, elderly, lactation, gout, diabetes mellitus, immobility

Pharmacokinetics

Absorption	Salicylate >90%
Distribution	None
Metabolism	None
Excretion	Feces (unchanged)
Half-life	Unknown

Pharmacodynamics

Onset	1 hr
Peak	2 hr
Duration	4 hr

Interactions
Individual drugs
Aminosalicylic acid: ↑ side effects, ↑ toxicity
Tetracycline: ↓ absorption
Drug classifications
Anticoagulants (oral): ↑ effect of anticoagulants
Antidiabetics (oral): ↑ effect of antidiabetics
Salicylates: ↑ risk of salicylate toxicity
⧄*Herb/drug*
Nutmeg: ↑ antidiarrheal effect
Sarsaparilla: ↑ bismuth absorption
Lab test interferences
Interference: Radiographic studies of GI system

NURSING CONSIDERATIONS
Assessment
• Monitor skin turgor; dehydration may occur in severe diarrhea; monitor electrolytes (potassium, sodium, chloride) if diarrhea is severe or continues long term
• Assess bowel pattern (frequency, consistency, shape, volume, color) before drug therapy, after treatment; check weight, bowel sounds; identify factors contributing to diarrhea (bacteria, diet, medications, tube feedings)

Nursing diagnoses
☑ Diarrhea (uses)
☑ Constipation (adverse reactions)
☑ Knowledge, deficient (teaching)

Implementation
• Shake susp before use; chewable tabs should not be swallowed whole

Patient/family education
• Teach patient to stop use if symptoms do not improve within 2 days or become worse, or if diarrhea is accompanied by high fever
• Teach patient to increase fluids for rehydration
• Tell patient to chew or dissolve chewable tabs in mouth; do not swallow whole; shake susp before using

---

⧄ Herb/drug   Ⓢ Do Not Crush   ◆ Alert   ◆ᴛᴛ Key Drug   G Geriatric   P Pediatric

- Tell patient to avoid other salicylates unless
P directed by prescriber; not to give to children
because of possibility of Reye's syndrome
- Tell patient that stools may turn gray; tongue
may darken; impaction may occur in debilitated patients

Evaluation
Positive therapeutic outcome
- Decreased diarrhea

---

bisoprolol (Rx)
(bis-oh'pro-lole)
Zebeta
Func. class.: Antihypertensive
Chem. class.: β_1-Blocker (selective)

Pregnancy category C

Action: Preferentially and competitively
blocks stimulation of β_1-adrenergic receptor
within cardiac muscle (decreases rate of SA
node discharge, increases recovery time),
slows conduction of AV node, decreases heart
rate, which decreases O_2 consumption in
myocardium; decreases renin-aldosterone-
angiotensin system; inhibits β_2-receptors in
bronchial and vascular smooth muscle at high
doses

→**Therapeutic Outcome:** Decreased B/P,
heart rate

Uses: Mild to moderate hypertension

Investigational uses: Stable angina
pectoris, stable CHF

Dosage and routes
Renal/hepatic dose
Adult: PO 2.5 mg, titrate upward

Hypertension
Adult: PO 5 mg qd; may increase if necessary
to 20 mg once daily; may need to reduce dose
in presence of renal or hepatic impairment

Available forms: Tabs 5, 10 mg

Adverse effects
(italic = common; **bold** = life-threatening)
CNS: Vertigo, headache, insomnia, fatigue,
dizziness, mental changes, memory loss,
hallucinations, depression, lethargy, drowsiness, strange dreams, catatonia, peripheral
neuropathy
CV: **Ventricular dysrhythmias, profound
hypotension, bradycardia, CHF,** cold
extremities, postural hypotension, 2nd- or
3rd-degree heart block
EENT: Sore throat, dry burning eyes

ENDO: Increased hypoglycemic response to
insulin
GI: Nausea, diarrhea, vomiting, **mesenteric
arterial thrombosis,** ischemic colitis,
flatulence, gastritis, gastric pain
GU: Impotence, decreased libido
HEMA: **Agranulocytosis, thrombocytopenia,** purpura, **eosinophilia**
INTEG: Rash, flushing, alopecia, pruritus,
sweating
MISC: Facial swelling, weight gain, decreased
exercise tolerance
MS: Joint pain, arthralgia
RESP: **Bronchospasm,** dyspnea, wheezing,
cough, nasal stuffiness

Contraindications: Hypersensitivity to
β-blockers, cardiogenic shock, heart block
(2nd or 3rd degree), sinus bradycardia, CHF,
cardiac failure

Precautions: Major surgery, pregnancy **C,**
P lactation, children, diabetes mellitus, renal or
hepatic disease, thyroid disease, COPD,
asthma, well-compensated heart failure, aortic
or mitral valve disease, peripheral vascular
disease, myasthenia gravis

Do Not Confuse:
Zebeta/Diabeta

Pharmacokinetics
Absorption	Well absorbed
Distribution	Unknown; protein binding (30%)
Metabolism	Liver, inactive metabolites
Excretion	Urine, unchanged (50%)
Half-life	9-12 hr

Pharmacodynamics
Onset	Unknown
Peak	2-4 hr
Duration	24 hr

Interactions
Individual drugs
Alcohol (large amounts), guanethidine,
reserpine: ↑ hypotension
Clonidine: Fatal reactions after discontinuing
clonidine
Epinephrine: ↑ hypertension, then bradycardia
Flecainide, haloperidol: ↑ effects of both drugs
Hydralazine, quinidine, prazosin: ↑ hypoten-
sion, bradycardia
Lidocaine: ↑ lidocaine toxicity
Theophylline: ↓ bronchodilatation
Drug classifications
Barbiturates, NSAIDs, penicillins, salicylates:
↓ antihypertensive effects

Calcium channel blockers, oral contraceptives: ↑ hypotension

Calcium channel blockers: ↑ myocardial depression

Diuretics (loop): ↑ CV effects

Ergots: ↑ peripheral ischemia

MAOIs: ↑ bradycardia

Sulfonylureas: ↓ hypoglycemic effect

☑ *Herb/drug*

Aconite: ↑ toxicity, death

Betel palm, butterbur, cola tree, figwort, fumitory, guarana, hawthorn, lily of the valley, motherwort, plantain: ↑ β-blocking effect

Coenzyme Q-10, ephedra, yohimbe: ↓ β-blocking effect

Lab test interferences

↑ AST, ↑ ALT, ↑ blood glucose, ↑ BUN, ↑ uric acid, ↑ potassium, ↑ lipoprotein, ↑ ANA titer

Interference: Glucose/insulin tolerance tests

NURSING CONSIDERATIONS
Assessment

• Monitor B/P during beginning treatment, periodically thereafter; pulse q4h: note rate, rhythm, quality; apical/radial pulse before administration; notify prescriber of any significant changes (pulse <50 bpm)

• Check for baselines in renal, liver function tests before therapy begins

• Assess for edema in feet, legs daily, monitor I&O, daily weight; check for jugular vein distention, rales bilaterally, dyspnea (CHF)

• Monitor skin turgor, dryness of mucous membranes for hydration status, especially 🅖 elderly

Nursing diagnoses

☑ Cardiac output, decreased (uses)

☑ Injury, risk for (side effects)

☑ Knowledge, deficient (teaching)

☑ Noncompliance (teaching)

Implementation

• Give qd; give with food to prevent GI upset; may be crushed

• Store protected from light, moisture; place in cool environment

Patient/family education

• Teach patient not to discontinue drug abruptly; may cause precipitate angina if stopped abruptly, evaluate noncompliance

• Teach patient not to use OTC products containing α-adrenergic stimulants (such as nasal decongestants, cold preparations); to avoid alcohol, smoking and to limit sodium intake as prescribed

• Teach patient how to take pulse and B/P at home; advise when to notify prescriber

• Instruct patient to comply with weight control, dietary adjustments, modified exercise program

• Tell patient to carry/wear emergency ID to identify drug being taken, allergies; tell patient drug controls symptoms but does not cure

• Caution patient to avoid hazardous activities if dizziness, drowsiness present

• Teach patient to take drug as prescribed, not to double doses, skip doses; take any missed doses as soon as remembered if at least 8 hr until next dose

• Advise patient to report bradycardia, dizziness, confusion, depression, fever, cold extremities

• Teach patient if diabetic, may mask signs of hypoglycemia, or alter blood glucose levels

Evaluation
Positive therapeutic outcome

• Decreased B/P in hypertension (after 1-2 wk)

Treatment of overdose: Lavage, **IV** atropine for bradycardia, **IV** theophylline for bronchospasm, digitalis, O_2, diuretic for cardiac failure, hemodialysis, **IV** glucose for hypoglycemia, **IV** diazepam (or phenytoin) for seizures

---

⚠ HIGH ALERT

bivalirudin (Rx)
(bye-val-i-rue'din)

Angiomax

Func. class.: Anticoagulant
Chem. class.: Thrombin inhibitor

Pregnancy category B

Action: Direct inhibitor of thrombin that is highly specific

➡ **Therapeutic Outcome:** Anticoagulation in percutaneous transluminal coronary angioplasty (PTCA)

Uses: Unstable angina in patients undergoing PTCA

Dosage and routes
Adult: **IV** bol 1 mg/kg, then **IV** inf 2.5 mg/kg/hr for 4 hr; another **IV** inf may be used at 0.2 mg/kg/hr for ≤20 hr; this drug is intended to be used with aspirin (325 mg qd) adjusted to body weight
Renal dose
Adult: **IV** GFR 30-59 ml/min, give 80% of dose; GFR 10-29 ml/min, give 40% of dose;

☑ Herb/drug   🚫 Do Not Crush   ◆ Alert   ◆🚋 Key Drug   🅖 Geriatric   🅟 Pediatric dialysis-dependent patients (not on dialysis) give 10% of dose

Available forms: Inj, lyophilized 250 mg vial

Adverse effects
(*italic* = common; **bold** = life-threatening)
CV: Hypo/hypertension, bradycardia
CNS: Headache, insomnia, anxiety, nervousness
GI: Nausea, vomiting, abdominal pain, dyspepsia
HEMA: Hemorrhage
MS: Back pain
MISC: Pain at inj site, pelvic pain, urinary retention, fever

Contraindications: Hypersensitivity, active bleeding

Precautions: Renal function impairment,
P lactation, children, hepatic disease, pregnancy
G B, elderly

Pharmacokinetics

Absorption	Unknown
Distribution	Unknown
Metabolism	Unknown
Excretion	Kidneys
Half-life	25 min

Pharmacodynamics
Unknown

Interactions
Drug classifications
Anticoagulants, thrombolytics: ↑ risk of bleeding
Herb/drug
Agrimony, alfalfa, angelica, anise, basil, bay, bilberry, black haw, bogbean, bromelain, buchu, chondroitin, cinchona bark, dong quai, fenugreek, feverfew, garlic, ginger, ginkgo, ginseng, horse chestnut, Irish moss, kelp, kelpware, khella, lovage, lungwort, meadowsweet, motherwort, mugwort, nettle, papaya, parsley (large amounts), pau d'arco, pineapple, poplar, prickly ash, safflower, saw palmetto, tonka bean, turmeric, wintergreen, yarrow: ↑ risk of bleeding
Chamomile, coenzyme Q10, flax, glucomannan, goldenseal, guar gum: ↓ anticoagulant effect

NURSING CONSIDERATIONS
Assessment
Assess for fall in B/P or Hct that may indicate hemorrhage
• Assess for fever, skin rash, urticaria

• Assess bleeding: check arterial and venous sites, IM inj sites, catheters; all punctures should be minimized

Nursing diagnoses
☑ Decreased cardiac output (uses)
☑ Knowledge, deficient (teaching)

Implementation
• Prior to PTCA, give with aspirin, 325 mg
IV **IV** direct 1 mg/kg as a bolus; then intermittent infusion
Intermittent infusion
• To each 250-mg vial add 5 ml of sterile water for inj, swirl until dissolved, further dilute reconstituted vial with 50 ml of D₅W or 0.9% NaCl (5 mg/ml); the dose is adjusted to body weight, run at 2.5 mg/kg/hr, do not admix before or during administration
• Give reduced dose in renal impairment

Patient/family education
• Explain reason for drug and expected results

Evaluation
Positive therapeutic outcome
• Anticoagulation in PTCA

⚠ HIGH ALERT

bleomycin ⚠ (Rx)
(blee-oh-mye'sin)
Blenoxane
Func. class.: Antineoplastic, antibiotic
Chem. class.: Glycopeptide
Pregnancy category D

Action: Inhibits synthesis of DNA, RNA, protein; derived from *Streptomyces verticillus;* replication is decreased by binding to DNA, which causes strand splitting; phase specific in the G₂ and M phases; a nonvesicant

Therapeutic Outcome: Prevention of rapidly growing malignant cells

Uses: Cancer of head, neck, penis, cervix, vulva of squamous cell origin, Hodgkin's disease, lymphosarcoma, reticulum cell sarcoma, testicular carcinoma, malignant pleural effusion

Dosage and routes
P *Adult and child:* SC/**IV**/IM 0.25-0.5 units/kg q1-2 wk or 10-20 units/m²; then 1 unit/day or 5 units/wk; may also be given intraarterially; do not exceed total dose, 400 units in lifetime

Available forms: Powder for inj 15 units/vial

Adverse effects
(*italic* = common; **bold** = life-threatening)
CNS: Fever, chills, pain at tumor site, headache, confusion
CV: Hypotension, peripheral vasoconstriction
GI: *Nausea, vomiting, anorexia, stomatitis, weight loss,* ulceration of mouth, lips
HEMA: Hypotension, peripheral vasoconstriction
IDIOSYNCRATIC REACTION: Hypotension, confusion, fever, chills, wheezing
INTEG: *Rash, hyperkeratosis, nail changes, alopecia,* fever and chills, pruritus, acne, striae, peeling
RESP: **Fibrosis,** pneumonitis, wheezing, **pulmonary toxicity**
SYST: **Anaphylaxis,** radiation recall, Raynaud's phenomenon

Contraindications: Hypersensitivity, pregnancy **D**

Precautions: Renal, hepatic, respiratory disease

Pharmacokinetics	
Absorption	Well absorbed (IM, SC, intrapleural, intraperitoneal)
Distribution	Widely distributed
Metabolism	Liver, 30%
Excretion	Kidneys, unchanged (50%)
Half-life	2 hr; ↑ in renal disease

Pharmacodynamics
Unknown

Interactions
Individual drugs
Phenytoin: ↓ phenytoin levels
Radiation: ↑ toxicity, bone marrow suppression
Drug classifications
Anesthetics (general), antineoplastics: ↑ toxicity
Antineoplastics: ↑ bone marrow suppression

NURSING CONSIDERATIONS
Assessment
• Assess buccal cavity q8h for dryness, sores or ulceration, white patches, oral pain, bleeding, dysphagia; obtain prescription for viscous lidocaine (Xylocaine)
◆• Assess symptoms indicating anaphylaxis: rash, pruritus, urticaria, purpuric skin lesions, itching, flushing, wheezing, hypotension; have emergency equipment available

• Monitor CBC, differential, platelet count weekly; withhold drug if WBC <4000/mm³ or platelet count <100,000/mm³; notify prescriber of results if WBC <20,000/mm³, platelets <150,000/mm³
• Monitor temp q4h (may indicate beginning of infection)
• Monitor liver function tests before and during therapy (bilirubin, AST, ALT, LDH) as needed or monthly
• Assess for bleeding: hematuria, stool guaiac, bruising or petechiae, mucosa or orifices q8h; inflammation of mucosa, breaks in skin
• Identify dyspnea, rales, unproductive cough, chest pain, tachypnea
• Identify effects of alopecia on body image; discuss feelings about body changes; if edema in feet, joint pain, stomach pain, shaking present, prescriber should be notified; identify inflammation of mucosa, breaks in skin

Nursing diagnoses
☑ Injury, risk for (adverse reactions)
☑ Body image, disturbed (adverse reactions)
☑ Infection, risk for (adverse reactions)
☑ Knowledge, deficient (teaching)

Implementation
• Avoid contact with skin, very irritating; wash completely to remove
• Give fluids **IV** or PO before chemotherapy to hydrate patient
• Give antacid before oral agent; give antiemetic 30-60 min before giving drug to prevent vomiting and prn and antibiotics for prophylaxis of infection
• Provide liq diet: carbonated beverages, gelatin may be added if patient is not nauseated or vomiting
• Rinsing of mouth tid-qid with water, club soda; brushing of teeth bid-qid with soft brush or cotton-tipped applicators for stomatitis; use unwaxed dental floss
SC/IM route
• IM test dose in lymphoma
• Reconstitute with 1-5 ml sterile water for inj; D₅W, 0.9% NaCl, rotate inj sites
IV **IV route**
• Drug should be prepared by experienced personnel using proper precautions
• Two test doses 2-5 units before initial dose in lymphoma; monitor for anaphylaxis
• Give by direct **IV** after reconstituting 15 units or less/5 ml or more of D₅W or 0.9% NaCl; give 15 units or less/10 min through Y-tube or 3-way stopcock initial dose; monitor for anaphylaxis

Intermittent infusion
• Administer after diluting 50-100 ml 0.9% NaCl, D_5W and giving at prescribed rate
Intrapleural route
• Give 60 units/50-100 ml of 0.9% NaCl, administered by physician through thoracotomy tube

Syringe compatibilities: Cisplatin, cyclophosphamide, DOXOrubicin, droperidol, fluorouracil, furosemide, heparin, leucovorin, methotrexate, metoclopramide, mitomycin, vinBLAStine, vinCRIStine

Y-site compatibilities: Allopurinol, amisostine, aztreonam, cisplatin, cyclophosphamide, DOXOrubicin, DOXOrubicin liposome, droperidol, filgrastim, fludarabine, fluorouracil, granisetron, heparin, leucovorin, melphalan, methotrexate, metoclopramide, mitomycin, ondansetron, paclitaxel, piperacillin/tazobactam, sargramostim, teniposide, thiotepa, vinBLAStine, vinCRIStine, vinorelbine

Additive compatibilities: Amikacin, cephapirin, dexamethasone, diphenhydrAMINE, fluorouracil, gentamicin, heparin, hydrocortisone, phenytoin, streptomycin, tobramycin, vinBLAStine, vinCRIStine

Additive incompatibilities: Aminophylline, ascorbic acid inj, carbenicillin, cefazolin, cephalothin, diazepam, hydrocortisone, methotrexate, mitomycin, nafcillin, penicillin G sodium, terbutaline

Solution compatibilities: 0.9% NaCl

Patient/family education
• Teach patient to avoid use of products containing aspirin or ibuprofen, razors, commercial mouthwash; bleeding may occur; to report symptoms of bleeding (hematuria, tarry stools)
• Instruct patient to report signs of anemia (fatigue, headache, irritability, faintness, shortness of breath)
• Instruct patient to report any changes in breathing or coughing even several months after treatment; to avoid crowds and persons with respiratory tract or other infections
• Inform patient that hair may be lost during treatment; a wig or hairpiece may make patient feel better; new hair may be different in color, texture
• Caution patient not to have any vaccinations without the advice of the prescriber; serious reactions can occur

• Advise patient contraception is needed during treatment and for several months after completion of therapy

Evaluation
Positive therapeutic outcome
• Prevention of rapid division of malignant cells

---

bortezomib
Velcade
See Appendix A, Selected New Drugs

---

bosentan (Rx)
(boh-sen-tan)
Tracleer
Func. class.: Vasodilator
Chem. class.: Endothelin receptor antagonist

Pregnancy category X

Action: Peripheral vasodilation occurs via antagonism of the effect of endothelin on endothelium and vascular smooth muscle

➔**Therapeutic Outcome:** Decreased pulmonary arterial hypertension

Uses: Pulmonary arterial hypertension with class III, IV symptoms

Investigational uses: Septic shock to improve microcirculatory blood flow

Dosage and routes
Adult >40 kg and >12 yr: PO 62.5 mg bid × 4 wk, then 125 mg bid

Adult <40 kg and >12 yr: PO 62.5 mg bid

Available forms: Tabs 62.5, 125 mg

Adverse effects
(*italic* = common; **bold** = life-threatening)
CNS: Headache, flushing, fatigue
CV: Hypotension, palpitations, edema of lower limbs
GI: Abnormal liver function, dyspepsia, **hepatotoxicity**
INTEG: Pruritus
MISC: Anemia

Contraindications: Pregnancy **X,** hypersensitivity, CVA, CAD

Precautions: Mitral stenosis, elderly, lactation, impaired hepatic function, children

Pharmacokinetics

Absorption	50% absorbed
Distribution	Protein binding >98%
Metabolism	Liver (metabolites); metabolized CYP2C9, CYP3A4, and possibly CYP2C19; steady state 3-5 days
Excretion	Biliary
Half-life	5 hr

Pharmacodynamics

Onset	Unknown
Peak	Unknown
Duration	Unknown

Interactions
Individual drugs
cycloSPORINE A, glyBURIDE: Do not coadminister
cycloSPORINE A, ketoconazole: ↑ bosetan level
cycloSPORINE: ↓ cycloSPORINE level
Glyburide: Glyburide level ↓ significantly, bosentan also ↓, ↑ liver function tests
Simvastatin: ↓ effects
Warfarin: ↓ anticoagulation
Drug classifications
Contraceptives (hormonal) statins: ↓ effects
Lab test interferences
↑ ALT, ↑ AST, ↓ Hgb, Hct

NURSING CONSIDERATIONS
Assessment
• Assess B/P, pulse during treatment until stable
• Assess hepatic tests: AST, ALT, bilirubin; liver enzymes may increase; if ALT/AST >3 and ≤5 × ULN, confirm lab value, decrease dose or interrupt treatment and monitor AST/ALT q2wk; if >8 × ULN, stop treatment
• Assess blood studies: Hct, Hgb may be decreased
• Assess hepatic involvement: vomiting, jaundice; drug should be discontinued

Nursing diagnoses
☑ Tissue perfusion, ineffective (uses)
☑ Knowledge, deficient (teaching)

Implementation
• Store at room temp

Patient/family education
• Instruct patient to report jaundice, dark urine, joint pain, fatigue, malaise, bruising, easy bleeding; may indicate blood dyscrasias
• Caution patient to avoid pregnancy; to use nonhormonal form of contraception

Evaluation
Positive therapeutic outcome
• Decrease in pulmonary hypertension

❗ HIGH ALERT

bretylium ⊙π (Rx)
(bre-til'ee-um)
Bretylate ✦, bretylium tosylate, Bretylol
Func. class.: Antidysrhythmic (Class III)
Chem. class.: Quaternary ammonium compound

Pregnancy category C

Action: After a transient release of norepinephrine, inhibits further release by postganglionic nerve endings; prolongs action potential, duration, and effective refractory period

➡ **Therapeutic Outcome:** Absence of dysrhythmias

Uses: Life-threatening ventricular tachycardia, cardioversion, ventricular fibrillation; for short-term use only

Dosage and routes
Renal dose
Adult: **IV** CCr 10-50 ml/min 25%-50% dose; CCr <10 ml/min avoid use

Severe ventricular fibrillation
Adult: **IV** bol 5 mg/kg; increase to 10 mg/kg repeated q15 min, up to 30 mg/kg; **IV** inf 1-2 mg/min or give 5-10 mg/kg over 10 min q6h (maintenance)

Ventricular tachycardia
Adult: **IV** inf 500 mg diluted in 50 ml D_5W or NS; infuse over 10-30 min; may repeat in 1 hr; maintain with 1-2 mg/min or 5-10 mg/kg over 10-30 min q6h; IM 5-10 mg/kg undiluted; repeat in 1-2 hr if needed; maintain with same dose q6-8h

🅿 *Child:* 2-5 mg/kg/dose

Available forms: Inj 50 mg/ml; 1, 2, 4 mg/ml prefilled syringes

Adverse effects
(*italic* = common; **bold** = life-threatening)
CNS: Syncope, dizziness, confusion, psychosis, anxiety
CV: Hypotension, postural hypotension, bradycardia, angina, PVCs, substernal pressure, transient hypertension, precipitation of angina
GI: Nausea, vomiting
RESP: Respiratory depression

Contraindications: Hypersensitivity, digitalis toxicity, aortic stenosis, pulmonary **P** hypertension, children

Precautions: Renal disease, pregnancy **C**, **P** lactation, children

Pharmacokinetics

Absorption	Complete bioavailability (**IV**)
Distribution	Unknown
Metabolism	Not metabolized
Excretion	Kidneys, unchanged
Half-life	4-17 hr

Pharmacodynamics

	IV	IM
Onset	5 min	½-2 hr
Peak	Infusion's end	Unknown
Duration	6-24 hr	6-24 hr

Interactions
Individual drugs
Caffeine: ↓ effects of adenosine
Carbamazepine: ↑ heart block
Dopamine, norepinephrine: ↑ pressor effects
Drug classifications
Cardiac glycosides: ↑ toxicity
Sympathomimetics: ↑ sympathomimetic effect
Herb/drug
Aconite: ↑ toxicity, death
Aloe, broom, buckthorn (chronic use), cascara sagrada (chronic use), Chinese rhubarb, figwort, fumitory, goldenseal, kudzu, licorice: ↑ effect
Coltsfoot: ↓ effect
Horehound: ↑ serotonin effect

NURSING CONSIDERATIONS
Assessment
• Monitor ECG continuously to determine drug effectiveness; measure PR, QRS, QT intervals; check for PVCs, other dysrhythmias; monitor B/P continuously for hypotension, hypertension; check for rebound hypertension after 1-2 hr

Nursing diagnoses
✓ Cardiac output, decreased (uses)
✓ Gas exchange, impaired (adverse reactions)
✓ Knowledge, deficient (teaching)

Implementation
IM route
• Give in large muscle mass, rotate sites to prevent necrosis
IV IV route
Direct
• Give **IV** bol undiluted; give 6 mg or less

over 1 min; if using an **IV** line, use port near insertion site, flush with normal saline (50 ml)
Intermittent infusion
• Give by intermittent inf after diluting 500 mg/50 ml or more with 0.9% NaCl, D₅W, D₅/0.45% NaCl, D₅/0.9% NaCl, LR, ⅙ mol/L sodium lactate; run over >8 min
Continuous infusion
• Give by cont inf diluted in sol; give 1-2 mg/min; use inf site
• Store at room temp; sol should be clear

Additive compatibilities: Aminophylline, atracurium, calcium chloride, calcium gluconate, digoxin, DOPamine, esmolol, regular insulin, lidocaine, potassium chloride, quinadine verapamil

Y-site compatibilities: Amiodarone, amrinone, cisatracurium, diltiazem, dobutamine, famotidine, isoproterenol, ranitidine, remifentanil

Additive incompatibilities: Phenytoin

Evaluation
Positive therapeutic outcome
• Decreased B/P, dysrhythmias, heart rate; normal sinus rhythm

---

bromocriptine (Rx)
(broe-moe-krip′teen)
Alti-Bromocriptine ♣, Apo-Bromocriptine ♣, Parlodel
Func. class.: Antiparkinsonian agent; DOPamine receptor agonist
Chem. class.: Ergot alkaloid derivative
Pregnancy category B

Action: Inhibits prolactin release by activating postsynaptic dopamine receptors; activation of striatal dopamine receptors may be reason for improvement in Parkinson's disease

Therapeutic Outcome: Decreased involuntary movements in Parkinson's disease; decreased lactation; decreased hormone levels in acromegaly; absence of amenorrhea in hyperprolactinemia

Uses: Adjunct with levodopa in Parkinson's disease, amenorrhea/galactorrhea caused by hyperprolactinemia, acromegaly

Investigational uses: Pituitary adenomas, neuroleptic malignant syndrome

Dosage and routes
Hyperprolactinemia
Adult: PO 1.25-2.5 mg with meals; may increase by 2.5 mg q3-7 days; usual dosage 5-7.5 mg

Acromegaly
Adult: PO 1.25-2.5 mg/day × 3 days hs; may increase by 1.25-2.5 mg q3-7 days; usual range 20-30 mg/day; max 100 mg/day

Parkinson's disease
Adult: PO 1.25 mg bid with meals; may increase q2-4 wk by 2.5 mg/day; not to exceed 100 mg/day

Pituitary adenoma
Adult: PO 1.25 mg bid-tid, may increase over several weeks

Neuroleptic malignant syndrome
Adult: PO 5 mg qd, max 20 mg/day

Available forms: Caps 5 mg; tabs 2.5 mg

Adverse effects
(*italic* = common; **bold** = life-threatening)
CNS: *Headache,* depression, restlessness, anxiety, nervousness, confusion, **seizures,** hallucinations, *dizziness,* fatigue, drowsiness, abnormal involuntary movements, psychosis
CV: *Orthostatic hypotension,* decreased B/P, palpitations, extrasystole, **shock,** dysrhythmias, bradycardia, **MI**
EENT: Blurred vision, diplopia, burning eyes, nasal congestion
GI: *Nausea, vomiting, anorexia,* cramps, constipation, diarrhea, dry mouth, GI hemorrhage
GU: Frequency, retention, incontinence, diuresis
INTEG: *Rash on face, arms,* alopecia, coolness, pallor of fingers, toes

Contraindications: Hypersensitivity to ergot, severe ischemic disease, severe peripheral vascular disease

Precautions: Lactation, hepatic disease, **P** renal disease, children, pituitary tumors, pregnancy **B**

Do Not Confuse:
Parlodel/pindolol

Pharmacokinetics

Absorption	Poorly absorbed
Distribution	Unknown
Metabolism	Liver, completely
Excretion	85%-98% feces
Half-life	4 hr (initial); 50 hr (terminal)

Pharmacodynamics

Onset	½-1½ hr
Peak	1-3 hr
Duration	8-12 hr

Interactions
Individual drugs
Alcohol: ↑ disulfiram-like reaction
Haloperidol, loxapine, methyldopa, metoclopramide, reserpine: ↓ levels of bromocriptine
Levodopa: ↑ neurologic effects
Drug classifications
Analgesics (opioid), antihistamines, sedative/hypnotics: ↑ CNS depression
Antidepressants (tricyclic), contraceptives (oral), estrogens, MAOIs, phenothiazines, progestins: ↓ levels of bromocriptine
Antihypertensives: ↑ hypotension
Herb/drug
Chaste tree fruit, kava: ↓ bromocriptine effect
Horehound: ↑ serotonin effect
Lab test interferences
↑ Growth hormone, ↑ AST, ↑ ALT, ↑ BUN, ↑ uric acid, ↑ alkaline phosphatase

NURSING CONSIDERATIONS
Assessment
• Assess symptoms of Parkinson's disease (extrapyramidal symptoms): shuffling gait, muscle rigidity, involuntary movements, pill rolling, muscle spasms, drooling before and during treatment
• Assess for resolution of symptoms of neuroleptic malignant syndrome: decreased temp, seizures, sweating, pulse
• Monitor for change in size of soft tissue volume in acromegaly
• Monitor B/P; establish baseline, compare with other readings; this drug decreases B/P; patient should remain recumbent for 2-4 hr after first dose; supervise ambulation

Nursing diagnoses
✓ Mobility, impaired (uses)
✓ Knowledge, deficient (teaching)

Implementation
• Give with meals or milk to prevent GI symptoms; crush tab if patient has swallowing difficulty
• Give hs so dizziness, orthostatic hypotension do not occur
• Store at room temp in air-tight container

Patient/family education
• Advise patient to change position slowly to prevent orthostatic hypotension

---

- Tabs may be crushed and mixed with food
- Caution patient to use contraceptives during treatment with this drug; pregnancy may occur; to use methods other than oral contraceptives
- Teach patient that therapeutic effect for Parkinson's disease may take 2 mo: galactorrhea, amenorrhea
- Caution patient to avoid hazardous activity if dizziness, drowsiness occurs during treatment start-up
- Advise patient to avoid alcohol and OTC medication unless approved by prescriber
- Teach patients with acromegaly to notify prescriber immediately if severe headache, nausea, vomiting, blurred vision occur; indicates change in enlargement of tumor
- Advise patient to report symptoms of MI immediately

Evaluation
Positive therapeutic outcome
- Parkinson's disease: decreased dyskinesia, decreased slow movements, decreased drooling
- Decreased breast engorgement with accompanied pain, tenderness
- Acromegly: decreased growth hormone levels

---

brompheniramine (OTC, Rx)
(brome-fen-eer'a-meen)
Bromfenac, brompheniramine, Chlorphed, Dehist, Diamine T.D., Dimetane, Dimetane Extentabs, Dimetapp Allergy Liqui-Gels, Nasahist-B
Func. class.: Antihistamine
Chem. class.: Alkylamine, H_1-receptor antagonist

Pregnancy category B

Action: Acts on blood vessels, GI, respiratory system by competing with histamine for H_1-receptor site; decreases allergic response by blocking histamine

➡ **Therapeutic Outcome:** Absence of allergy symptoms and rhinitis

Uses: Allergy symptoms, rhinitis, allergic dermatoses, nasal allergies, hypersensitivity reactions including blood transfusion reactions, anaphylaxis

Dosage and routes
P *Adult and child >12 yr:* PO 4-8 mg tid-qid, not to exceed 36 mg/day; TIME REL

8-12 mg bid-tid, not to exceed 36 mg/day; IM/**IV**/SC 5-20 mg q6-12h, not to exceed 40 mg/day
P *Child 6-12 yr:* PO 2 mg tid-qid, not to exceed 12 mg/day; IM/**IV**/SC 0.5 mg/kg/day divided tid or qid
P *Child 2-6 yr:* 1 mg q4-6h (not to exceed 6 mg/day)

Available forms: Tabs 4 mg; elix 2 mg/5 ml; inj 10 mg/ml; caps 4 mg

Adverse effects
(*italic* = common; **bold** = life-threatening)
CNS: Dizziness, drowsiness, poor coordination, fatigue, anxiety, euphoria, confusion, paresthesia, neuritis
CV: Hypotension, palpitations, tachycardia
EENT: Blurred vision, dilated pupils, tinnitus, nasal stuffiness, dry nose, throat, mouth
GI: Nausea, vomiting, anorexia, constipation, diarrhea
GU: Retention, dysuria, frequency, impotence
***HEMA:* Thrombocytopenia, agranulocytosis, hemolytic anemia**
INTEG: Photosensitivity
RESP: Increased thick secretions, wheezing, chest tightness

Contraindications: Hypersensitivity to H_1-receptor antagonists, acute asthma attack,
P lower respiratory tract disease, child <2 yr

Precautions: Increased intraocular pressure, renal disease, cardiac disease, hypertension, bronchial asthma, seizure disorder, stenosed peptic ulcers, hyperthyroidism, prostatic hypertrophy, bladder neck obstruction, pregnancy **B**

Pharmacokinetics

Absorption	Well absorbed (PO, IM)
Distribution	Widely distributed; crosses blood-brain barrier
Metabolism	Liver, extensively
Excretion	Kidneys, metabolite; breast milk (minimal)
Half-life	12-34 hr

Pharmacodynamics

	PO	SC/IM	IV
Onset	15-30 min	30 min	Immediate
Peak	2-5 hr	Unknown	Unknown
Duration	6-12 hr	8-12 hr	8-12 hr

Interactions
Individual drugs
Alcohol: ↑ CNS depression

Drug classifications
CNS depressants, opiates, sedative/hypnotics: ↑ CNS depression
MAOIs: ↑ anticholinergic effect

☑ *Herb/drug*
Corkwood, henbane leaf: ↑ anticholinergic effect
Hops, Jamaican dogwood, khat, senega: ↑ antihistamine effect
Kava: ↑ CNS depression

Lab test interferences
False negative: Skin allergy tests (discontinue antihistamines before testing)

NURSING CONSIDERATIONS
Assessment
• Assess respiratory status: rate, rhythm, increase in bronchial secretions, wheezing, chest tightness; provide fluids to 2 L/day to decrease secretion thickness
• Monitor I&O ratio: be alert for urinary retention, frequency, dysuria, especially in
G elderly; drug should be discontinued if these occur
• Monitor CBC during long-term therapy; blood dyscrasias may occur but are rare
• **IV** administration may result in rapid drop in B/P, sweating, dizziness, especially in
G elderly

Nursing diagnoses
✓ Airway clearance, ineffective (uses)
✓ Injury, risk for (side effects)
✓ Knowledge, deficient (teaching)
✓ Noncompliance (teaching, overuse)

Implementation
PO route
• May give with food to prevent GI upset; absorption is not altered by food
• Store in tight, light-resistant container

IV **IV route**
• Give undiluted or dilute 10 mg/ml using 0.9% NaCl at a rate of 1 min or more
• May be further diluted in 0.9% NaCl, D₅W; give as intermittent inf at prescribed rate

Patient/family education
• Teach patient all aspects of drug use; to notify prescriber if confusion, sedation, hypotension occur; to avoid driving or other hazardous activity if drowsiness occurs; to avoid alcohol or other CNS depressants that may potentiate effect
• Instruct patient not to exceed recommended dosage; dysrhythmias may occur
• Teach patient hard candy, gum, frequent rinsing of mouth may be used for dryness

Evaluation
Positive therapeutic outcome
• Absence of runny or congested nose, rashes

Treatment of overdose: Administer ipecac syrup or lavage, diazepam, vasopressors, barbiturates (short acting)

---

budesonide (Rx)
(byoo-des'oh-nide)
Entocort EC, Pulmicort, Rhinocort, Rhinocort Aqua
Func. class.: Glucocorticoid

Action: Prevents inflammation by depression of migration of polymorphonuclear leukocytes, fibroblasts, reversal of increased capillary permeability and lysosomal stabilization; does not suppress hypothalamus and pituitary function

Uses: Rhinitis; prophylaxis for asthma; Crohn's disease

Dosage and routes
Rhinitis (Rhinocort, Rhinocort Aqua)
P *Adult/child >6 yr:* SPRAY/INH 256 mcg qd (2 sprays in each nostril ᴀᴍ, ᴘᴍ or 4 sprays in each nostril, ᴀᴍ)

Asthma
P *Adult and child ≥6 yr:* INH 400-600 mcg/day

Crohn's disease
Adult: PO 9 mg qd ᴀᴍ × 8 wk

Available forms: Dry powder for INH 200 mcg/metered dose (turbuhaler); inh susp 0.25 mg/2 ml, 0.5 mg/2 ml; cap 3 mg; inhaler 32 mcg micronized/actuation (Rhinocort) 32 mcg/spray (Rhinocort Aqua)

Adverse effects
(*italic* = common; **bold** = life-threatening)
CNS: Headache, insomnia, hypertonia, syncope
EENT: Sinusitis, pharyngitis, rhinitis, oral candidiasis
GI: Dry mouth, dyspepsia, nausea, vomiting, abdominal pain, oral candidiasis
MISC: Ecchymosis, fever, *hypersensitivity,* flulike symptoms
MS: Back pain, myalgias, fractures
RESP: Nasal irritation, cough, nasal bleeding, *respiratory infections,* **bronchospasm**

Contraindications: Hypersensitivity, status asthmaticus

☑ Herb/drug   🚫 Do Not Crush   ◆ Alert   🔑 Key Drug   **G** Geriatric   **P** Pediatric

Precautions: Pregnancy **C,** inhaled form
(B); lactation, children, TB, fungal, bacterial,
systemic viral infections, ocular herpes simplex, nasal septal ulcers; hepatic disease
(caps)

Pharmacokinetics: Unknown

Interactions
• Ketoconazole: ↓ budesonide metabolism
• Avoid using with drugs metabolized by
CYP3A4 inhibition

NURSING CONSIDERATIONS
Assessment
• Assess respiratory status: rate, rhythm,
increase in bronchial secretions, wheezing,
chest tightness; provide fluids to 2 L/day to
decrease thickness of secretions; check for
oral candidiasis
• For bronchospasm, stop treatment and give
bronchodilator
• With viral infections, corticosteroid use can
mask infections
• For increased intraocular pressure, discontinue use if increase occurs

Implementation
INH route (asthma)
• Use scissors to open pouch
• Use Turbuhaler upright to load, prime when
using first time, turn grip to the right, then left
to click in place; to provide dose turn to right,
then to the left, click in place. Place mouthpiece between lips, inhale forcefully, do not
exhale through Turbuhaler, rinse after use
PO route (Crohn's disease)
• Caps: whole, do not chew, break
• May repeat 8-wk course if needed; may
taper to 6 mg/day for 2 wk before cessation

Perform/provide
• Storage at 59°-86° F (15°-30° C); keep
away from heat, open flame

Evaluate
• Therapeutic response: absence of asthma,
rhinitis

Patient/family education
• Teach patient to notify prescriber of pharyngitis, nasal bleeding
• Instruct patient not to exceed recommended
dose; adrenal suppression may occur
• Teach patient to carry/wear emergency ID
identifying steroid use
• Instruct patient to read and follow package
directions
• Instruct patient to prevent exposure to
infections, especially viral

bumetanide (Rx)
(byoo-met'a-nide)
Bumex
Func. class: Loop diuretic, antihypertensive
Chem. class.: Sulfonamide derivative
Pregnancy category C

B

Action: Acts on the ascending loop of Henle
in the kidney to inhibit the reabsorption of the
electrolytes sodium and chloride, causing
excretion of sodium, calcium, magnesium,
chloride, water, and some potassium; also
decreases reabsorption of sodium and chloride and increases the excretion of potassium
in the distal tubule of the kidney; responsible
for antihypertensive effect and peripheral
vasodilatation

Therapeutic Outcome: Decreased
edema in lung tissue and peripherally; decreased B/P

Uses: Edema in congestive heart failure,
nephrotic syndrome, ascites caused by hepatic
disease, hepatic cirrhosis

Investigational uses: May be used
alone or as adjunct with antihypertensives such
as spironolactone, triamterene

Dosage and routes
Adult: PO 0.5-2 mg qd; may give 2nd or 3rd
dose at 4-5 hr intervals; not to exceed 10
mg/day; may be given on alternate days or
intermittently; **IV**/IM 0.5-1 mg/day; may give
2nd or 3rd dose at 2-3 hr intervals; not to
exceed 10 mg/day

Child: PO/IM/**IV** 0.02-0.1 mg/kg q12h, max
10 mg/day

Available forms: Tabs 0.5, 1, 2 mg; inj
0.25 mg/ml

Adverse effects
(*italic* = common; **bold** = life-threatening)
CNS: Headache, fatigue, weakness, vertigo,
paresthesias
CV: Orthostatic hypotension, chest pain, ECG
changes, circulatory collapse
EENT: Ear pain, tinnitus, blurred vision
ELECT: Hypokalemia, hypochloremic alkalosis, hypomagnesia, hyperuricemia, hypocalcemia, hyponatremia, metabolic alkalosis
ENDO: Hyperglycemia
GI: Nausea, diarrhea, dry mouth, vomiting,
anorexia, cramps, oral and gastric irritations,
pancreatitis
GU: Polyuria, **renal failure,** *glycosuria*
HEMA: **Thrombocytopenia, leukopenia,
anemia**

INTEG: Rash, pruritus, purpura, urticaria
MS: Cramps, stiffness

Contraindications: Hypersensitivity to sulfonamides, anuria, electrolyte depletion

Precautions: Diabetes mellitus, dehydration, severe renal disease, pregnancy **C**, lactation

Do Not Confuse:
Bumex/Buprenex

Pharmacokinetics

	PO/IM
Absorption	Rapidly, completely absorbed
	PO/IM/IV
Distribution	Crosses placenta, protein binding >91%
Metabolism	Liver (30%-40%)
Excretion	Breast milk, urine (50% unchanged), feces (20%)
Half-life	1-1½ hr; 6-15 hr neonates

Pharmacodynamics

	PO	IM	IV
Onset	½-1 hr	40 min	5 min
Peak	1-2 hr	1-2 hr	½ hr
Duration	3-6 hr	4-6 hr	3-6 hr

Interactions
Individual drugs
Alcohol: ↑ orthostatic hypotension
Ethacrynic acid: Combination may cause ↑ chance of dysrhythmias (do not use together)
Indomethacin: ↓ diuretic and antihypertensive effects of bumetanide
Lithium: ↓ renal clearance causing ↑ toxicity
Metolazone: ↑ diuresis, electrolyte loss
Mezlocillin, piperacillin, ticarcillin: ↑ hypokalemia
Probenecid: ↓ effect of bumetanide
Drug classifications
Aminoglycosides: ↑ ototoxicity
Digitalis glycosides: ↑ potassium loss with relating dysrhythmias
Glucocorticoids, potassium-wasting drugs: ↑ hypokalemia
NSAIDs: ↓ diuretic effect
Herb/drug
Aloe, cucumber, dandelion, horsetail, pumpkin, Queen Anne's lace: ↑ diuretic effect
St. John's wort: Severe photosensitivity
Lab test interferences:
↑ Urinary phosphate

NURSING CONSIDERATIONS
Assessment
- Assess patient for tinnitus, hearing loss, ear

pain; periodic testing of hearing is needed when high doses of this drug are given by **IV** route
- Monitor for manifestations of hypokalemia: *RENAL:* acidic urine, reduced urine osmolality, nocturia, polyuria, polydipsia; *CV:* hypotension, broad T wave, U wave, ectopy, tachycardia, weak pulse; *NEURO:* muscle weakness, altered LOC, drowsiness, apathy, lethargy, confusion, depression; *GI:* anorexia, nausea, cramps, constipation, distention, paralytic ileus; *RESP:* hypoventilation, respiratory muscle weakness
- Monitor for manifestations of hypocalcemia: *CNS:* personality changes, anxiety, disturbances, depression, psychosis; *GI:* nausea, vomiting, constipation, abdominal pain from muscle spasm; *CV:* decreased contractility, decreased cardiac output, hypotension, lengthened ST segment, prolonged QT interval; *INTEG:* scaling eczema, alopecia, hyperpigmentation; *NEURO:* tetany, muscle twitching, cramping, grimacing, seizure, altered deep tendon reflexes, spasm
- Monitor for manifestations of hypomagnesemia: *CNS:* agitation; *NEURO:* muscle twitching, paresthesias, hyperactive reflexes, positive Babinski's reflex, dysphagia, nystagmus, seizures, tetany; *GI:* nausea, vomiting, diarrhea, anorexia, abdominal distention; *CV:* ectopy, tachycardia, broad, flat, or inverted T waves, depressed ST segment, prolonged QT, decreased cardiac output, hypotension
- Monitor for manifestations of hyponatremia: *CV:* increased B/P, cold, clammy skin, hypovolemia or hypervolemia; *GI:* anorexia, nausea, vomiting, diarrhea, abdominal cramps; *NEURO:* lethargy, increased ICP, confusion, headache, seizures, coma, fatigue, tremors, hyperreflexia
- Monitor for manifestations of hyperchloremia: *NEURO:* weakness, lethargy, coma; *RESP:* deep rapid breathing
- Assess fluid volume status: I&O ratio and record, distended red veins, crackles in lung, color, quality and sp gr of urine, skin turgor, adequacy of pulses, moist mucous membranes, bilateral lung sounds, peripheral pitting edema; dehydration symptoms of decreasing output, thirst, hypotension, dry mouth and mucous membranes should be reported; if urinary output decreases or azotemia occurs, drug should be discontinued
- Monitor electrolytes: potassium, sodium, calcium, magnesium; also include BUN, blood pH, ABGs, uric acid, CBC, blood glucose
- Assess B/P before and during therapy with patient lying, standing, and sitting as

 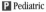

appropriate; orthostatic hypotension can occur rapidly

• Monitor for digoxin toxicity (anorexia, nausea, vomiting, confusion, paresthesia, muscle cramps) in patients taking digoxin; lithium toxicity in those taking lithium

Nursing diagnoses
✓ Urinary elimination, impaired (side effects)
✓ Fluid volume, deficient (side effects)
✓ Fluid volume excess (uses)
✓ Knowledge, deficient (teaching)

Implementation
• Give in AM to avoid interference with sleep
• Potassium replacement if potassium level is <3.0 mg/dl whole, or use oral solutions; drug may be crushed if patient is unable to swallow
PO route
• With food, if nausea occurs; absorption may be reduced; the safest dosage schedule is on alternate days
IV IV route
• Do not use solution that is yellow or has a precipitate or crystals
IV Direct IV
• Give undiluted through Y-tube or 3-way stopcock; give 20 mg or less/min
Intermittent infusion
• May be added to 0.9% NaCl, D_5W, $D_{10}W$, $D_{20}W$, invert sugar 10% in electrolyte #1, LR, sodium lactate ⅙ mol/L; use within 24 hr to ensure compatibility; give through Y-tube or 3-way stopcock; give at 4 mg/min or less; use infusion pump

Syringe compatibility: Doxapram

Y-site compatibilities: Allopurinol, amifostine, aztreonam, cefepime, cisatracurium, cladribine, diltiazem, filgrastim, granisetron, lorazepam, morphine, piperacillin/tazobactam, propofol, remifentanil, teniposide, thiotepa, vinorelbine

Additive compatibilities: Floxacillin, furosemide

Patient/family education
• Teach patient to take the medication early in the day to prevent nocturia
• Instruct the patient to take with food or milk if GI symptoms of nausea and anorexia occur
• Teach patient to maintain weekly record of weight and notify prescriber of weight loss of >5 lb
• Caution the patient that this drug causes a loss of potassium so food rich in potassium should be added to the diet; refer to a dietician for assistance in planning
• Caution the patient not to exercise in hot

weather or stand for prolonged periods since orthostatic hypotension will be enhanced

• Teach patient not to use alcohol or any OTC medications without prescriber's approval; serious drug reactions may occur
• Emphasize the need to contact prescriber immediately if muscle cramps, weakness, nausea, dizziness, or numbness occurs
• Teach patient to take own B/P and pulse and record
• Caution the patient that orthostatic hypotension may occur; patient should rise slowly from sitting or reclining positions and lie down if dizziness occurs
• Teach patient to continue taking medication even if feeling better; this drug controls symptoms but does not cure the condition
• Advise the patient with hypertension to continue other medical treatment (exercise, weight loss, relaxation techniques, cessation of smoking)

Evaluation
Positive therapeutic outcome
• Decreased edema
• Decreased B/P
• Increased diuresis

---

buprenorphine (Rx)
(byoo-pre-nor′feen)
Buprenex
Func. class.: Opioid analgesic
Chem. class.: Thebaine derivative

Pregnancy category C

Controlled substance schedule V

Action: Inhibits ascending pain pathways in limbic system, thalamus, midbrain, hypothalamus by binding to opiate receptor sites; this alters pain perception and response; generalized CNS depression

➔ **Therapeutic Outcome:** Relief of pain

Uses: Moderate to severe pain

Dosage and routes
Adult: IM/**IV** 0.3 mg q6h prn; may repeat
G dose after ½ hr; reduce dosage in elderly, may repeat after ½ hr; epidural 60-180 mcg over 48 hr

G *Elderly:* PO 0.15 mg q6h prn

Available forms: Inj 0.3 mg/ml (1-ml vials)

Adverse effects
(*italic* = common; **bold** = life-threatening)
CNS: *Drowsiness, dizziness, confusion, headache, sedation, euphoria,* **increased intracranial pressure,** amnesia
CV: Palpitations, bradycardia, change in B/P, tachycardia
EENT: Tinnitus, blurred vision, *miosis,* diplopia
GI: *Nausea,* vomiting, anorexia, constipation, cramps, dry mouth
GU: Increased urinary output, dysuria, urinary retention
INTEG: *Rash,* urticaria, bruising, flushing, diaphoresis, pruritus
RESP: **Respiratory depression,** dyspnea, hypo-/hyperventilation

Contraindications: Hypersensitivity, addiction (opioid)

Precautions: Addictive personality, pregnancy **C,** lactation, increased intracranial pressure, MI (acute), severe heart disease, respiratory depression, hepatic disease, renal disease, hypothyroidism, Addison's disease, addiction (opioid)

Do Not Confuse:
Buprenex/Bumex

Pharmacokinetics	
Absorption	Well absorbed (IM)
Distribution	Crosses placenta
Metabolism	Liver, extensively
Excretion	Kidneys, feces, breast milk
Half-life	2½-3½ hr

Pharmacodynamics		
	IM	IV
Onset	10-15 min	Immediate
Peak	1 hr	5 min
Duration	4 hr	2-5 hr

Interactions
Individual drugs
Alcohol: ↑ respiratory depression, hypotension, sedation
Drug classifications
Antihistamines, CNS depressants, sedative/hypotension: ↑ respiratory depression, hypotension
MAOIs: Do not use within 2 wk
Opioids: ↑ CNS depression
Herb/drug
Corkwood: ↑ anticholinergic effect
Kava, Jamaican dogwood, lavender, mistletoe, nettle, pokeweed, poppy, senega, valerian: ↑ CNS depression

NURSING CONSIDERATIONS
Assessment
• Assess pain characteristics: location, intensity, type, severity before medication administration and after treatment
• Monitor VS after parenteral route; note muscle rigidity, drug history, liver, kidney function tests, respiratory dysfunction: respiratory depression, character, rate, rhythm; notify prescriber if respirations are <10/min
• Monitor CNS changes: dizziness, drowsiness, hallucinations, euphoria, LOC, pupil reaction; withdrawal in opioid-dependent persons; if dependence occurs within 2 wk of discontinuing drug, withdrawal symptoms will occur
• Monitor allergic reactions: rash, urticaria

Nursing diagnoses
✓ Pain, acute (uses)
✓ Pain, chronic
✓ Sensory perception, disturbed: visual, auditory (adverse reactions)
✓ Breathing pattern, ineffective (adverse reactions)
✓ Knowledge, deficient (teaching)

Implementation
• Give by inj (IM, **IV**), only with resuscitative equipment available; give slowly to prevent rigidity
IM route
• Give deep in large muscle mass; rotate sites of inj
IV route
• Give **IV** direct undiluted over 3-5 min (0.3 mg/2 min); give slowly

Syringe compatibility: Midazolam

Y-site compatibilities: Allopurinol, amifostine, aztreonam, cefepime, cisatracurium, cladribine, filgrastim, granisetron, melphalan, piperacillin/tazobactam, propofol, remifentanil, teniposide, thiotepa, vinorelbine

Additive compatibilities: Atropine, bupivacaine, diphenhydrAMINE, droperidol, glycopyrrolate, haloperidol, hydrOXYzine, promethazine, scopolamine

Additive incompatibilities: Diazepam, floxacillin, furosemide, lorazepam

Patient/family education
• Instruct patient to report any symptoms of CNS changes, allergic reactions
• Caution patients to avoid CNS depressants: alcohol, sedative/hypnotics for at least 24 hr after taking this drug
• Discuss with patient that dizziness, drowsiness, and confusion are common; to avoid

 Herb/drug   Do Not Crush   Alert   Key Drug   Geriatric   **P** Pediatric

getting up without assistance, to avoid hazardous activities
- Discuss in detail all aspects of the drug
- Instruct patient to change position slowly to prevent orthostatic hypotension
- Teach patient to turn, cough, deep breathe after surgery to prevent atelectasis

Evaluation
Positive therapeutic outcome
- Relief of pain

---

*buPROPion (Rx)
(byoo-proe'pee-on)
buPROPion, Wellbutrin, Wellbutrin SR, Zyban
Func. class.: Antidepressant—misc., smoking deterrent
Chem. class.: Aminoketone

Pregnancy category B

Action: Inhibits reuptake of dopamine, serotonin, norepinephrine

▶ **Therapeutic Outcome:** Decreased symptoms of depression after 2-3 wk

Uses: Depression (Wellbutrin), smoking cessation (Zyban)

Dosage and routes
Depression
Adult: PO 100 mg bid initially, then increase after 3 days to 100 mg tid if needed; may increase after 1 mo to 150 mg tid; SR 150 mg bid, initially 150 mg AM, ↑ to 300 mg/day if initial dose is tolerated

G *Elderly:* PO 50-100 mg/day, may increase by 50-100 mg q3-4 days

Smoking cessation
Adult: PO 150 mg bid, begin with 150 mg qd × 3 days then 300 mg/day continue for 7-12 wk, not to exceed 300 mg/day

Available forms: Tabs 75, 100 mg; tabs, sus rel 50, 100, (Zyban) 150, 200 mg

Adverse effects
(*italic* = common; **bold** = life-threatening)
CNS: Headache, agitation, confusion, **seizures**, delusions, *insomnia, sedation, tremors,* dizziness, akinesia, bradykinesia
CV: **Dysrhythmias,** *hypertension,* palpitations, *tachycardia,* hypotension
EENT: Blurred vision, auditory disturbance
GI: Nausea, vomiting, dry mouth, anorexia, diarrhea, increased appetite, *constipation*
GU: Impotence, frequency, retention, *menstrual irregularities*
INTEG: Rash, pruritus, *sweating*
MISC: Weight loss or gain

Contraindications: Hypersensitivity, eating disorders, seizure disorder

Precautions: Renal and hepatic disease, recent MI, cranial trauma, pregnancy **B,** P lactation, children <18 yr, seizure disorders, G elderly

Do Not Confuse:
buPROPion/busPIRone

Pharmacokinetics	
Absorption	Well absorbed; bioavailability poor
Distribution	Unknown
Metabolism	Liver extensively
Excretion	Kidneys
Half-life	14 hr, steady state 1½-5 wk

Pharmacodynamics	
Onset	Up to 4 wk
Peak	Unknown
Duration	Unknown

Interactions
Individual drugs
Alcohol, levodopa, theophylline: ↑ risk of seizures
Carbamazepine: ↓ buPROPion effect
Cimetidine: ↑ levels
Cimetidine, phenytoin: ↑ toxicity
Ritonavir: ↑ buPROPion toxicity
Drug classifications
Antidepressants, benzodiazepines, MAOIs, steroids (systemic): ↑ risk of seizures
Antihistamines: ↑ CNS depression
Barbiturates, CYP450 drugs: ↓ buPROPion effects
CNS depressants: ↑ effects
MAOIs: Acute toxicity
Phenothiazines: ↑ toxicity, risk of seizures
🌿 *Herb/drug*
Belladonna, corkwood, jimsonweed: ↑ anticholinergic effect
Ephedra: Hypertensive crisis
Hops, kava, lavender: ↑ CNS depression
Lab test interferences
↑ Serum bilirubin, ↑ blood glucose, ↑ alkaline phosphatase
↓ VMA, ↓ 5-HIAA
False positive: Urinary catecholamines

NURSING CONSIDERATIONS
Assessment
- Monitor B/P (with patient lying, standing), pulse q4h; if systolic B/P drops 20 mm Hg

hold drug, notify prescriber; take vital signs q4h in patients with cardiovascular disease
• Assess smoking cessation progress after 7-12 wk, if progress has not been made, drug should be discontinued
• Assess for increased risk of seizures; if patient has used CNS depressant or CNS stimulants, dosage of buPROPion should not be exceeded
• Monitor blood studies: CBC, leukocytes, differential, cardiac enzymes if patient is receiving long-term therapy
• Monitor hepatic studies: AST, ALT, bilirubin if on long-term treatment
• Check weight weekly; appetite may increase with drug
• Assess ECG for flattening of T wave, bundle branch block, AV block, dysrhythmias in cardiac patients
G • Assess for EPS primarily in elderly: rigidity, dystonia, akathisia
• Assess mental status: mood, sensorium, affect, suicidal tendencies; increase in psychiatric symptoms: depression, panic
• Monitor urinary retention, constipation; **P** constipation is more likely to occur in children **G** or elderly
• Identify alcohol consumption; if alcohol was consumed, hold dose

Nursing diagnoses
☑ Coping, ineffective individual (uses)
☑ Injury, risk for (side effects)
☑ Knowledge, deficient (teaching)
☑ Noncompliance (teaching)

Implementation
• Give with food or milk for GI symptoms
• Give sugarless gum, hard candy, or frequent sips of water for dry mouth
• Store at room temp; do not freeze

Patient/family education
• Teach patient that therapeutic effects may take 2-3 wk; not to increase dose without prescriber's approval; that treatment for smoking cessation lasts 7-12 wk
• Teach patient to use caution in driving or other activities requiring alertness because of drowsiness, dizziness, blurred vision; to avoid rising quickly from sitting to standing, **G** especially elderly
• Teach patient to avoid alcohol ingestion, obtain approval for other drugs
• Teach patient to increase fluids, bulk in diet if constipation, urinary retention occur, **G** especially elderly; notify prescriber immediately if retention occurs
• Teach patient to take gum, hard sugarless candy, or frequent sips of water for dry mouth

• Advise patient not to use with nicotine patches unless directed by prescriber, may increase B/P
• Teach patient that risk of seizures increases when dose is exceeded, or if patient has seizure disorder
• Teach patient to notify prescriber if pregnancy is suspected or planned

Evaluation
Positive therapeutic outcome
• Decrease in depression
• Absence of suicidal thoughts
• Smoking cessation

Treatment of overdose: ECG monitoring, induce emesis, lavage, activated charcoal, administer anticonvulsant

---

*busPIRone (Rx)
(byoo-spye′rone)
BuSpar
Func. class.: Antianxiety, sedative
Chem. class.: Azaspirodecanedione

Pregnancy category B

Action: Acts by inhibiting the action of serotonin (5-HT) by binding to serotonin and dopamine receptors; also increases norepinephrine metabolism; has shown little potential for abuse

Therapeutic Outcome: Decreased anxiety

Uses: Management and short-term relief of anxiety disorders

Dosage and routes
Adult: PO 5 mg tid; may increase by 5 mg/day q2-3 days; not to exceed 60 mg/day

Available forms: Tabs 5, 10, 15, 30 mg

Adverse effects
(*italic* = common; **bold** = life-threatening)
CNS: Dizziness, headache, depression, stimulation, insomnia, nervousness, lightheadedness, numbness, paresthesia, incoordination, tremors, excitement, involuntary movements, confusion, akathisia, nightmares
CV: Tachycardia, palpitations, hypotension, hypertension, **CVA, CHF, MI**
EENT: Sore throat, tinnitus, blurred vision, nasal congestion, red, itching eyes, change in taste, smell
GI: Nausea, dry mouth, diarrhea, constipation, flatulence, increased appetite, rectal bleeding
GU: Frequency, hesitancy, menstrual irregularity, change in libido

---

INTEG: Rash, edema, pruritus, alopecia, dry skin
MISC: Sweating, fatigue, weight gain, fever
MS: Pain, weakness, muscle cramps, spasms
RESP: Hyperventilation, chest congestion, shortness of breath

Contraindications: Hypersensitivity, ■ child <18 yr

Precautions: Pregnancy **B,** lactation, ■ elderly, impaired hepatic/renal function

■ **Do Not Confuse:**
busPIRone/buPROPion

Pharmacokinetics

Absorption	Rapidly absorbed
Distribution	Unknown
Metabolism	Liver, extensively
Excretion	Feces
Half-life	2-3 hr

Pharmacodynamics
Unknown

Interactions
Individual drugs
Alcohol: ↑ CNS depression
Erythromycin, itraconazole: ↑ busPIRone levels
Rifampin: ↓ busPIRone effect
Drug classifications
MAOIs: ↑ B/P, do not use together
Psychotropics: ↑ CNS depression
CYP450 drugs: ↑ busPIRone levels
Food/drug
Grapefruit juice: ↑ busPIRone effect
◨ *Herb/drug*
Cowslip, kava, Queen Anne's lace, valerian: ↑ CNS depression

NURSING CONSIDERATIONS
Assessment
• Assess anxiety reaction: inability to sleep, apprehension, dread, foreboding, or uneasiness related to unidentified source of danger
• Assess for previous drug dependence or tolerance; if patient is drug dependent or tolerant, amount of medication should be restricted
• Monitor B/P (lying, standing), pulse; if systolic B/P drops 20 mm Hg, hold drug, notify prescriber; check I&O; may indicate renal dysfunction
• Monitor mental status: mood, sensorium, affect, sleeping patterns, drowsiness, dizziness, suicidal tendencies

• Assess for CNS reaction, some reactions may be unpredictable

Nursing diagnoses
☑ Anxiety (uses)
☑ Knowledge, deficient (teaching)
☑ Noncompliance (teaching)

Implementation
• Give with food or milk for GI symptoms; sugarless gum, hard candy, frequent sips of water for dry mouth
• May be crushed

Patient/family education
• Teach patient that drug may be taken with food; if dose is missed take as soon as remembered; do not double doses
• Caution patient to avoid OTC preparations unless approved by the prescriber; to avoid alcohol ingestion and other psychotropic medications unless prescribed; that 1-2 wk of therapy may be required before therapeutic effects occur
• Caution patient to avoid driving and activities requiring alertness since drowsiness may occur; until medication response is known, tell patient that drowsiness may worsen at beginning of treatment
• Instruct patient not to discontinue medication abruptly after long-term use; if dose is missed, do not double
• Advise patient to rise slowly or fainting may ■ occur, especially in elderly

Evaluation
Positive therapeutic outcome
• Increased well-being
• Decreased anxiety, restlessness, sleeplessness, dread

Treatment of overdose: Gastric lavage, VS, supportive care

! HIGH ALERT

busulfan (Rx)
(byoo-sul'fan)
Busulfex, Myleran
Func. class.: Antineoplastic alkylating agent
Chem. class.: Nitrosourea

Pregnancy category D

Action: Changes essential cellular ions to covalent bonding with resultant alkylation; this interferes with normal biologic function of DNA; activity is not phase specific; action is due to myelosuppression

⊅Therapeutic Outcome: Prevention of rapid growth of malignant cells in chronic myelocytic leukemia

Uses: Chronic myelocytic leukemia

Dosage and routes
Adult: PO 4-8 mg/day initially until WBC levels fall to 10,000/mm³; then drug is stopped until WBC levels rise over 50,000/mm³; then 1-3 mg/day; **IV** 0.8 mg/kg q6h × 4 days, given with cyclophosphamide

P *Child:* PO 0.06-0.12 mg/kg or 1.8-4.6 mg/m²/day; dosage is titrated to maintain WBC levels at 20,000/mm³

Available forms: Tabs 2 mg; sol for inj 6 mg/ml

Adverse effects
(*italic* = common; **bold** = life-threatening)
PO route
GI: Nausea, vomiting, *diarrhea, weight loss*
GU: Impotence, sterility, amenorrhea, gynecomastia, **renal toxicity**, hyperuremia, adrenal insufficiency–like syndrome
***HEMA:* Thrombocytopenia, leukopenia, pancytopenia, severe bone marrow depression**
INTEG: Dermatitis, hyperpigmentation, alopecia
***MISC:* Chromosomal aberrations**
***RESP:* Irreversible pulmonary fibrosis,** pneumonitis
CV: Hypotension, **thrombosis,** *chest pain,* **tachycardia, atrial fibrillation, heart block,** pericardial effusion, **cardiac tamponade** (high dose with cyclophosphamide)
IV **IV route**
***CNS:* Cerebral hemorrhage, coma, seizures,** *anxiety, depression, dizziness, headache,* encephalopathy, weakness, mental changes
CV: Hypotension, **thrombosis,** *chest pain,* **tachycardia, atrial fibrillation, heart block**
EENT: Pharyngitis, epistaxis
GI: Anorexia, constipation, diarrhea, dry mouth, nausea, vomiting
***RESP:* Alveolar hemorrhage, atelectasis,** cough, hemoptysis, hypoxia, pleural effusion, pneumonia, sinusitis

Contraindications: Radiation, chemotherapy, lactation, pregnancy **D** (3rd trimester), blastic phase of chronic myelocytic leukemia, hypersensitivity

Precautions: Child-bearing age men and women, leukopenia, thrombocytopenia, anemia, hepatotoxicity, renal toxicity

Pharmacokinetics
Absorption	Rapidly absorbed
Distribution	Unknown; crosses placenta
Metabolism	Liver, extensively
Excretion	Kidneys, breast milk
Half-life	2.5 hr

Pharmacodynamics
Unknown

Interactions
Individual drugs
Radiation: ↑ toxicity, bone marrow suppression
Drug classifications
Anticoagulants, salicylates: ↑ risk of bleeding
Antineoplastics: ↑ toxicity, bone marrow suppression
Live virus vaccines: ↓ antibody reaction
Lab test interferences
False positive: Breast, bladder, cervix, lung cytology tests

NURSING CONSIDERATIONS
Assessment
• Monitor CBC, differential, platelet count weekly; withhold drug if WBC <4000/mm³ or platelets <75,000/mm³; notify prescriber of results if WBC <15,000/mm³, platelets <150,000/mm³; institute thrombocytopenia precautions
• Monitor pulmonary function tests, chest x-ray films before, during therapy; chest film should be obtained q2 wk during treatment; check for dyspnea, rales, nonproductive cough, chest pain, tachypnea; pulmonary fibrosis may occur up to 10 yr after treatment with busulfan
• Assess for increased uric acid levels, swelling, joint pain primarily in extremities; patient should be well hydrated to prevent urate deposits
• Monitor renal function studies: BUN, serum uric acid, urine CCr before, during therapy; I&O ratio; report fall in urine output of 30 ml/hr; check for decreased hyperuricemia
• Monitor for cold, fever, sore throat (may indicate beginning infection); identify edema in feet, joint or stomach pain, shaking; prescriber should be notified
• Assess for bleeding: hematuria, guaiac, bruising or petechiae, mucosa or orifices q8h; no rectal temps

---

Nursing diagnoses
✓ Injury, risk for (adverse reactions)
✓ Body image, disturbed (adverse reactions)
✓ Infection, risk for (adverse reactions)
✓ Knowledge, deficient (teaching)

Implementation
• Give 1 hr before or 2 hr pc to lessen nausea and vomiting; give at same time qd
• Increase fluid intake to 2-3 L/day to prevent urate deposits, calculus formation
• Administer antibiotics for prophylaxis of infection; may be prescribed since infection potential is high
• Store in tight container

IV IV route
• Prepare in biologic cabinet using gloves, gown, mask; dilute with 10 times volume of drug using D₅W or 0.9% NaCl (0.5 mg/ml); when withdrawing drug, use needle with 5-micron filter provided, remove amount needed, remove filter, and inject drug into diluent; always add drug to diluent, not vice versa; stable for 8 hr at room temp using D₅W or 0.9% NaCl; give by central venous catheter over 2 hr q6h × 4 days, use infusion pump, do not admix
• Give antiemetic before **IV** route
• Give phenytoin before **IV** to prevent seizures in those with seizure disorders

Patient/family education
• Teach patient to avoid use of products containing aspirin or ibuprofen, razors, commercial mouthwash since bleeding may occur; to report symptoms of bleeding (hematuria, tarry stools)
• Instruct patient to report signs of anemia (fatigue, headache, irritability, faintness, shortness of breath)
• Instruct patient to report any changes in breathing or coughing even several months after treatment; to avoid crowds and persons with respiratory tract or other infections
• Teach patient that hair loss may occur; discuss the use of wigs or hair pieces
• Caution patient not to have any vaccinations without the advice of the prescriber; serious reactions can occur
• Advise patient that contraception is needed during treatment and for several months after the completion of therapy

Evaluation
Positive therapeutic outcome
• Decreased leukocytes to normal limits
• Absence of sweating at night
• Increased appetite, increased weight

---

butorphanol (Rx)
(byoo-tor'fa-nole)
Stadol, Stadol NS
Func. class.: Opiate analgesic
Chem class: Opioid antagonist, agonist

Pregnancy category C
Controlled substance schedule IV

Action: Inhibits ascending pain pathways in limbic system, thalamus, midbrain, hypothalamus by binding to opiate receptor sites; this alters pain perception and response

⟶ **Therapeutic Outcome:** Relief of pain

Uses: Moderate to severe pain, analgesia during labor, sedation preoperatively

Investigational uses: Migraine headache, pain

Dosage and routes
Adult: IM 1-4 mg q3-4h prn; **IV** 0.5-2 mg q3-4h prn; nasal spray in 1 nostril; may give another dose 1-1½ hr later; may repeat q3-4h

G *Elderly:* **IV** ½ adult dose at 2× the interval

Intranasal: May repeat q1-2h

Renal dose
Adult: **IV**/IM CCr 10-50 ml/min 75% dose; CCr <10 ml/min 50% dose

Severe Pain
Adult: Intranasal 1 spray in each nostril q3-4h

Available forms: Inj 1, 2 mg/ml; intranasal 10 mg/ml

Adverse effects
(*italic* = common; **bold** = life-threatening)
CNS: *Drowsiness, dizziness, confusion, headache, sedation, euphoria, weakness, hallucinations*
CV: Palpitations, bradycardia, hypotension
EENT: Tinnitus, blurred vision, miosis, diplopia, nasal congestion
GI: *Nausea, vomiting, anorexia, constipation, cramps*
GU: Increased urinary output, dysuria, urinary retention
INTEG: Rash, urticaria, bruising, flushing, diaphoresis, pruritus
RESP: **Respiratory depression,** pulmonary hypertension

Contraindications: Hypersensitivity to this drug or preservative, addiction (opioid), CHF, MI

Precautions: Addictive personality, pregnancy **C**, lactation, increased intracranial pressure, respiratory depression, hepatic disease, renal disease, child <18 yr

Do Not Confuse:
Stadol/Haldol

Pharmacokinetics

Absorption	Well absorbed (IM, nasal); complete (**IV**)
Distribution	Crosses placenta
Metabolism	Liver, extensively
Excretion	Feces (10%-15%); kidneys, unchanged (small amounts)
Half-life	3-4 hr

Pharmacodynamics

	IM	IV	NASAL
Onset	10-30 min	1 min	15 min
Peak	½ hr	5 min	1-2 hr
Duration	3-4 hr	2-4 hr	4-5 hr

Interactions
Individual drugs
Alcohol: ↑ respiratory depression, hypotension, sedation
Drug classifications
Antihistamines, CNS depressants, sedative/hypnotics: ↑ respiratory depression, hypotension
MAOIs: Do not use 2 wk before butorphanol, fatal reaction
Herb/drug
Chamomile, kava, Jamaican dogwood, lavender, mistletoe, nettle, pokeweed, poppy, senega, skullcap, valerian: ↑ CNS depression
Corkwood: ↑ anticholinergic effect

NURSING CONSIDERATIONS
Assessment
• Monitor VS after parenteral route; note muscle rigidity, drug history, liver, kidney function tests, respiratory dysfunction: respiratory depression, character, rate, rhythm; notify prescriber if respirations are <10/min
• Monitor CNS changes: dizziness, drowsiness, hallucinations, euphoria, LOC, pupil reaction
• Monitor allergic reactions: rash, urticaria

Nursing diagnoses
✓ Pain, acute (uses)
✓ Pain, chronic (uses)
✓ Sensory perception, disturbed: visual, auditory (adverse reactions)
✓ Injury, risk for (adverse reactions)
✓ Knowledge, deficient (teaching)

Implementation
• Store in light resistant container at room temp
IM route
• Give deeply in large muscle mass; rotate inj sites
Intranasal
• Give 1 spray in nostril
IV route
• Give **IV** undiluted at a rate of ≤2 mg/>3-5 min; titrate to patient response

Syringe compatibilities: Atropine, chlorproMAZINE, cimetidine, diphenhydrAMINE, droperidol, fentanyl, hydrOXYzine, meperidine, methotrimeprazine, metoclopramide, midazolam, morphine, pentazocine, perphenazine, prochlorperazine, promethazine, scopolamine, thiethylperazine

Syringe incompatibilities: Dimenhydrinate, pentobarbital

Y-site compatibilities: Allopurinol, amifostine, azetreonam, cefepime, cisatracurium, cladribine, DOXOrubicin liposome, enalaprilat, esmolol, filgrastim, fludarabine, granisetron, labetalol, melphalan, paclitaxel, piperacillin/tazobactam, propofol, remifentanil, sargramostim, teniposide, thiotepa, vinorelbine

Patient/family education
• Instruct patient to report any symptoms of CNS changes, allergic reactions; to avoid CNS depressants: alcohol, sedative/hypnotics for at least 24 hr after taking this drug
• Discuss with patient that dizziness, drowsiness, and confusion are common; to avoid getting up without assistance
• Discuss in detail all aspects of the drug
Nasal route
• Teach patient to blow nose to clear both nostrils before using; remove clip and cover, prime before using until spray appears; pump must be reprimed q48h; close nostril with finger and spray once quickly; have patient sniff
• Patient should replace clip and cover after use; caution patient not to shake medication

Evaluation
Positive therapeutic outcome
• Pain relief

Treatment of overdose: Narcan 0.2-0.8 **IV**, O_2, **IV** fluids, vasopressors

calcitonin (human) (Rx)
(kal-sih-toh'nin)
Cibacalcin
calcitonin (salmon) (Rx)
Calcimir, Miacalcin, Miacalin Nasal Spray,
Osteocalcin, Salmonine
Func. class.: Parathyroid agents (calcium
regulator)
Chem. class.: Polypeptide hormone

Pregnancy category C

Action: Decreases bone resorption, blood
calcium levels by direct action on bone, GI
system, and kidney; increases deposits of
calcium in bones; renal excretion of calcium
occurs; opposes parathyroid hormone

Therapeutic Outcome: Lowered
calcium level, decreasing symptoms of Paget's
disease

Uses: Paget's disease, postmenopausal
osteoporosis, hypercalcemia

Dosage and routes
Human
Paget's disease
Adult: SC 0.5 mg/day initially; may require
0.5 mg bid × 6 mo, then decrease until symp-
toms reappear

Salmon
Postmenopausal osteoporosis
Adult: SC/IM 100 international units/day;
nasal 200 international units (1 spray) alternating nostrils qd, activate pump before 1st
dose

Paget's disease
Adult: SC/IM 100 international units qd,
maintenance 50-100 international units qd or
qod

Hypercalcemia
Adult: SC/IM 4 international units/kg q12h,
increase to 8 international units/kg q6h if
response is unsatisfactory

Available forms: Human: Inj (SC) 500
mg/vial; **Salmon:** Inj 100 international units,
200 international units/ml, nasal spray 200
international units/actuation

Adverse effects
(*italic* = common; **bold** = life-threatening)
CNS: Headache, **tetany**, chills, weakness,
dizziness, fever
CV: Chest pressure
EENT: Nasal congestion, eye pain

GI: Nausea, diarrhea, vomiting, anorexia,
abdominal pain, salty taste, epigastric pain
GU: Diuresis, nocturia, urine sediment,
frequency
INTEG: Rash, flushing, pruritus of earlobes,
edema of feet, inj site reaction
MS: Swelling, tingling of hands
RESP: Dyspnea
SYST: **Anaphylaxis**

Contraindications: Hypersensitivity

Precautions: Renal disease, children,
lactation, osteogenic sarcoma, pregnancy **C**,
pernicious anemia

Pharmacokinetics
Absorption	Completely absorbed
Distribution	Unknown
Metabolism	Rapid; kidneys, tissue, blood
Excretion	Kidneys, inactive metabolite
Half-life	1 hr

Pharmacodynamics
	SC
Onset	15 min
Peak	4 hr
Duration	8-24 hr

Interactions: None

NURSING CONSIDERATIONS
Assessment
• Assess for GI symptoms, polyuria, flushing,
head swelling, tingling, headache; may indicate
hypercalcemia; nervousness, irritability,
twitching, seizures, spasm, paresthesia indicate
hypocalcemia during beginning of treatment
• Identify nutritional status; check diet for
sources of vit D (milk, some seafood), calcium
(dairy products, dark green vegetables),
phosphates
• Monitor BUN, creatinine, uric acid, chloride, electrolytes, urine pH, urinary calcium,
magnesium, phosphate, urinalysis (calcium
should be kept at 9-10 mg/dl; vit D 50-135
international units/dl), alkaline phosphatase
baseline and q3-6 mo; check urine sediment
for casts throughout treatment
• Assess for increased drug level, since toxic
reactions occur rapidly; have calcium chloride
or gluconate on hand if calcium level drops
too low; check for tetany

Nursing diagnoses
☑ Injury, risk for (adverse reactions)
☑ Pain, chronic (uses)
☑ Knowledge, deficient (teaching)

Implementation
- Store at <77° F (25° C); protect from light

SC route (human)
- Give by SC route only; rotate inj sites; use within 6 hr of reconstitution; give hs to minimize nausea, vomiting

IM route (salmon)
- After test dose of 10 international units/ml, 0.1 ml intradermally; watch 15 min; give only with epINEPHrine and emergency meds available
- IM inj in deep muscle mass slowly; rotate sites

Nasal route
- Use alternating nostrils for nasal spray

Patient/family education
- Teach method of inj if patient will be responsible for self-medication
- Instruct patient to notify prescriber for hypercalcemic relapse: renal calculi, nausea, vomiting, thirst, lethargy, deep bone or flank pain
- Teach patient that warmth and flushing occur and last 1 hr
- Provide a low-calcium diet as prescribed (Paget's disease, hypercalcemia)
- Advise patients with osteoporosis to increase calcium and vit D in diet and to continue with moderate exercise to prevent continued bone loss
- Advise patients to report difficulty swallowing or change in side effects to prescriber immediately

Evaluation
Positive therapeutic outcome
- Calcium levels 9-10 mg/dl
- Decreasing symptoms of Paget's disease, including pain
- Decreased bone loss in osteoporosis

---

calcitriol (Rx)
(kal-si-tree′ole)
Calcijex, Rocaltrol, (1,25-dihydroxy-cholecalciferol) Vitamin D₃
Func. class.: Parathyroid agent (calcium regulator)
Chem. class.: Vitamin D hormone

Pregnancy category C

Action: Increases intestinal absorption of calcium, provides calcium for bones, increases renal tubular resorption of phosphate

➡ Therapeutic Outcome: Calcium at normal level

Uses: Hypocalcemia in chronic renal disease, hyperparathyroidism, pseudohypoparathyroidism

Dosage and routes
Hypocalcemia
Adult: **IV** 0.5 mcg tid, initially; may increase by 0.25-0.5 mcg/dose q2-4 wk; 0.5-3 mcg tid maintenance

Predialysis
Adult: PO 0.25 mcg/day, max 0.5 mcg/day
P *Child:* PO 0.25 mcg/day, max 0.5 mcg/day
P *Child <3 yr: PO 1015 mcg/kg/day*

Hypocalcemia during chronic dialysis
Adult: PO 0.5-3 mcg/day
P *Child:* PO 0.25-2 mcg/day

Renal osteodystrophy
Adult: PO 0.25 mcg qod-3 mcg/day
P *Child:* PO 0.014-0.041 mcg/kg/day

Hypoparathyroidism
Adult: PO 0.25-2.7 mcg/day
P *Child:* PO 0.04-0.08 mcg/kg/day

Available forms: Caps 0.25, 0.5 mcg
Adverse effects
(*italic* = common; **bold** = life-threatening)
CNS: Drowsiness, headache, vertigo, fever, lethargy
CV: Palpitations
EENT: Blurred vision, photophobia
GI: Nausea, diarrhea, vomiting, jaundice, anorexia, dry mouth, constipation, cramps, metallic taste
GU: Polyuria, hypercalciuria, hyperphosphatemia, hematuria, thirst
MS: Myalgia, arthralgia, decreased bone development, weakness

Contraindications: Hypersensitivity, hyperphosphatemia, hypercalcemia, vit D toxicity

Precautions: Pregnancy **C**, renal calculi, lactation, CV disease

◩ Do Not Confuse:
calcitriol/Calciferol

Pharmacokinetics	
Absorption	Well absorbed
Distribution	To liver, crosses placenta
Metabolism	Liver
Excretion	Bile
Half-life	3-6 hr, undergoes hepatic recycling, excreted in bile

Pharmacodynamics	
Onset	2-6 hr
Peak	10-12 hr
Duration	Up to 5 days

Interactions
Individual Drugs
Cholestyramine, mineral oil: ↓ absorption of calcitriol
Phenytoin: ↑ vit D metabolism
Verapamil: ↑ dysrhythmias
Drug classifications
Antacids: ↑ hypermagnesemia
Diuretics (thiazide), calcium supplements: ↑ hypercalcemia
Cardiac glycosides: ↑ dysrhythmias
Vitamin D products: ↑ toxicity
Vitamins (fat-soluble): ↓ calcitriol absorption
Food/drug:
Large amounts of high-calcium foods may cause hypercalcemia
Lab test interferences
False: ↑ Cholesterol
Interference: Alkaline phosphatase, electrolytes

NURSING CONSIDERATIONS
Assessment
• Assess GI symptoms, polyuria, flushing, head swelling, tingling, headache; may indicate hypercalcemia
• Identify nutritional status; check diet for sources of vit D (milk, some seafood), calcium (dairy products, dark green vegetables), phosphates
• Monitor BUN, creatinine, uric acid, chloride, electrolytes, urine pH, urinary calcium, magnesium, phosphate, urinalysis (calcium should be kept at 9-10 mg/dl; vit D 50-135 international units/dl), alkaline phosphatase baseline and q3-6 mo
◆• Assess for increased drug level, since toxic reactions occur rapidly; have calcium chloride on hand if calcium level drops too low; check for tetany

Nursing diagnoses
☑ Injury, risk for (adverse reactions)
☑ Pain, chronic (uses)
☑ Knowledge, deficient (teaching)

Implementation
PO route
• Give with meals for GI symptoms
⊘• Do not crush or chew caps
Ⅳ IV route
• Give by direct **IV** over 1 min

Patient/family education
• Teach patient the symptoms of hypercalcemia and about foods rich in calcium
• Advise patient to avoid products with sodium: cured meats, dairy products, cold cuts, olives, beets, pickles, soups, meat tenderizers in chronic renal failure
• Advise patient to avoid products with potassium: oranges, bananas, dried fruit, peas, dark green leafy vegetables, milk, melons, beans in chronic renal failure
• Advise patient to avoid OTC products containing calcium, potassium, or sodium in chronic renal failure
• Instruct patient to avoid all preparations containing vit D
• Instruct patient to monitor weight weekly

Evaluation
Positive therapeutic outcome
• Calcium levels 9-10 mg/dl

---

calcium carbonate
(PO-OTC, IV-Rx)
Alka-Mints, Amitone, Apo-Cal ✤, BioCal, Calcarb, Calci-Chew, Calcilac, Calci-Mix, Calcite ✤, Calglycine ✤, Cal-Plus, Calsan ✤, Caltrate 600, Caltrate Jr., Chooz, Dicarbosil, Equilet, Gencalc, LIquid-Cal, Liquid-Cal-600, Maalox Antacid Caplets, Mallamint, Mylanta Lozenges ✤, Nephro-Calci, Nu-Cal ✤, Os-Cal 500, Oysco 500, Oystercal 500, Oyst-Cal 500, Rolaids Calcium Rich, Titralac, Tums, Tums E-X Extra Strength
Func. class.: Antacid, calcium supplement
Chem. class.: Calcium product

Pregnancy category C

Action: Neutralizes gastric acidity

▣**Therapeutic Outcome:** Neutralized gastric acidity; calcium at normal levels

Uses: Antacid, calcium supplement; not suitable for chronic therapy, hyperphosphatemia, hypertension in pregnancy, osteoporosis, prevention/treatment of hypocalcemia, hyperparathyroidism

Dosage and routes
Antacid
Adult: PO 0.5 mg-1.5 g or 2 pieces of gum 1 hr pc and hs

Hyperphosphatemia
Adult: PO 1 g or more in divided doses

Hypertension in pregnancy
Adult: PO 500 mg tid during 3rd trimester

Prevention of hypocalcemia, depletion, osteoporosis
Adult: PO 1-2 g qd

Available forms: Chewable tabs 350, 420, 450, 500, 750, 1000, 1250 mg; tabs 500, 600, 650, 1000, 1250 mg; gum 300, 450, 500 mg; susp 1250 mg/5 ml; lozenges 600 mg; caps 1250 mg; powder 6.5 g/packet

Adverse effects
(*italic* = common; **bold** = life-threatening)
GI: *Constipation,* anorexia, nausea, vomiting, flatulence, diarrhea, rebound hyperacidity, eructation

Contraindications: Hypersensitivity, hypercalcemia, hyperparathyroidism, bone tumors

G **Precautions:** Elderly, fluid restriction, decreased GI motility, GI obstruction, dehydration, renal disease, pregnancy **C**, lactation

Pharmacokinetics	
Absorption	⅓ absorbed by small intestine
Distribution	Unknown
Metabolism	Unknown
Excretion	Feces, urine, crosses placenta
Half-life	Unknown

Pharmacodynamics	
Onset	20 min
Peak	Unknown
Duration	20-180 min

Interactions
Individual Drugs
Quinidine: ↑ quinidine levels
Drug Classifications
Amphetamines: ↑ levels of amphetamines
Azole antiinfectives, calcium channel blockers, iron products, salicylates, tetracyclines: ↓ levels of each specific drug
Quinolone antiinfectives: ↓ levels of antiinfectives
⊘ *Herb/drug*
Lily of the valley, pheasant's eye, shark cartilage, squill: ↑ side effect, action
Lab test interferences
False increase: ↑ Chloride
False decrease: ↓ Magnesium, oxalate, lipase
False positive: benzodiazepines

NURSING CONSIDERATIONS
Assessment
• Monitor Ca⁺ (serum, urine), Ca⁺ should be

8.5-10.5 mg/dl, urine Ca⁺ should be 150 mg/day, monitor weekly
⬥• Assess for milk-alkali syndrome: nausea, vomiting, disorientation, headache
• Assess for constipation; increase bulk in the diet if needed
• Assess for hypercalcemia: headache, nausea, vomiting, confusion

Implementation
PO route
• Administer as antacid 1 hr pc and hs
• Administer as supplement 1½ hr pc and hs
• Administer only with regular tablets or capsules; do not give with enteric-coated tablets
• Administer laxatives or stool softeners if constipation occurs

Evaluation
• Therapeutic response: absence of pain, decreased acidity

Patient/family education
• Advise patient to increase fluids to 2 L unless contraindicated, to add bulk to diet for constipation; notify prescriber of constipation
• Advise patient not to switch antacids unless directed by prescriber, not to use as antacid for >2 wk without approval by prescriber
• Teach patient that therapeutic dose recommendations are figured as elemental calcium

calcium chloride
calcium gluceptate
calcium gluconate
calcium lactate
(PO-OTC, IV-Rx)
Func. class.: Electrolyte replacement—calcium product
Pregnancy category C

Action: Cation needed for maintenance of nervous, muscular, skeletal systems, enzyme reactions, normal cardiac contractility, coagulation of blood; affects secretory activity of endocrine, exocrine glands

➡ **Therapeutic Outcome:** Calcium at normal level, absence of increased magnesium, potassium

Uses: Prevention and treatment of hypocalcemia, hypermagnesemia, hypoparathyroidism, P neonatal tetany, cardiac toxicity caused by hyperkalemia, lead colic, hyperphosphatemia,

---

⊘ Herb/drug   Ⓢ Do Not Crush   ⬥ Alert   ☛ Key Drug   G Geriatric   P Pediatric vit D deficiency, osteoporosis prophylaxis, calcium antagonist toxicity (calcium channel blocker toxicity)

Dosage and routes
Calcium chloride
Adult: **IV** 500 mg-1 g q1-3 days as indicated by serum calcium levels; give at <1 ml/min; IAV 200-800 mg injected in ventricle of heart

P *Child:* **IV** 25 mg/kg over several min

Calcium gluceptate
Adult: **IV** 5-20 ml; IM 2-5 ml

P *Newborn:* 0.5 ml/100 ml of blood transfused

Calcium gluconate
Adult: PO 0.5-2 g bid-qid; **IV** 0.5-2 g at 0.5 ml/min (10% sol); max **IV** dose 3 g

P *Child:* PO/**IV** 500 mg/kg/day in divided doses

Calcium lactate
Adult: PO 325 mg-1.3 g tid with meals

P *Child:* PO 500 mg/kg/day in divided doses

Available forms: Many; check product listings

Adverse effects
(*italic* = common; **bold** = life-threatening)
CV: Shortened QT interval, heart block, hypotension, bradycardia, dysrhythmias; **cardiac arrest (IV)**
GI: Vomiting, nausea, constipation
HYPERCALCEMIA: Drowsiness, lethargy, muscle weakness, headache, constipation, **coma,** anorexia, nausea, vomiting, polyuria, thirst
INTEG: Pain, burning at **IV** site, severe venous thrombosis, necrosis, extravasation

Contraindications: Hypercalcemia, digitalis toxicity, ventricular fibrillation, renal calculi

Precautions: Pregnancy **C**, lactation, **P** children, renal disease, respiratory disease, cor pulmonale, digitalized patient, respiratory failure

Pharmacokinetics	
Absorption	Complete bioavailability (**IV**)
Distribution	Readily extracellular; crosses placenta
Metabolism	Liver
Excretion	Feces (80%), kidney (20%), breast milk
Half-life	Unknown

Pharmacodynamics		
	PO	IV
Onset	Unknown	Immediate
Peak	Unknown	Rapid
Duration	Unknown	½-1½ hr

C

Interactions
Individual drugs
Atenolol: ↓ effects of atenolol
Phenytoin: ↓ absorption of phenytoin when calcium is taken PO
Tetracycline: ↓ absorption of tetracycline (PO)
Verapamil: ↓ effects of verapamil, ↑ toxicity
Drug classifications
Antacids: Milk-alkali syndrome (renal disease)
Cardiac glycosides: ↑ toxicity
Diuretics (thiazide): ↑ hypercalcemia
Fluoroquinolones: ↓ absorption of fluoroquinolones when calcium is taken PO
Iron salts: ↓ absorption of iron when calcium is taken PO
Food/drug
Calcium (dairy products): ↑ hypercalcemia
Herb/drug
Lily of the valley, pheasant's eye, shark cartilage, squill: ↑ side effects, action
Lab test interferences
False: ↓ Magnesium, ↓ 17-OHCS, ↑ 11-OHCS

NURSING CONSIDERATIONS
Assessment
• Monitor ECG for decreased QT interval and T-wave inversion: in hypercalcemia, drug should be reduced or discontinued
• Monitor calcium levels during treatment (9-10 mg/dl is normal level)
• Assess cardiac status: rate, rhythm, CVP (PWP, PAWP if being monitored directly)

Nursing diagnoses
✓ Injury, risk for (uses, adverse reactions)
✓ Knowledge, deficient (teaching)

Implementation
IV **IV route**
• Administer **IV** undiluted or diluted with equal amounts of 0.9% NaCl for inj to a 5% sol; give 0.5-1 ml/min
• Give through small-bore needle into large vein; if extravasation occurs, necrosis will result (**IV**); IM inj may cause severe burning, necrosis, and tissue sloughing; warm sol to body temp before administering (only gluconate/gluceptate)
• Provide seizure precautions: padded side rails, decreased stimuli (noise, light); place airway suction equipment, padded mouth gag if calcium levels are low

Calcium chloride
Syringe compatibilities: Milrinone

Y-site compatibilities: Amrinone, DOBUTamine, epINEPHrine, esmolol, morphine, paclitaxel

Additive compatibilities: Amikacin, amphotericin B, ampicillin, ascorbic acid, bretylium, ceftriaxone, cephapirin, chloramphenicol, DOPamine, hydrocortisone, isoproterenol, lidocaine, methicillin, norepinephrine, penicillin G potassium, penicillin G sodium, pentobarbital, phenobarbital, verapamil, vit B/C

Calcium gluceptate
Additive compatibilities: Ascorbic acid inj, isoproterenol, lidocaine, norepinephrine, phytonadione, sodium bicarbonate

Calcium gluconate
Syringe compatibilities: Aldesleukin, allopurinol, amifostine, aztreonam, cefazolin, cefepime, ciprofloxacin, cladribine, DOBUTamine, enalaprilat, epINEPHrine, famotidine, filgrastim, granisetron, heparin/hydrocortisone, labetalol, melphalan, midazolam, netilmicin, piperacillin/tazobactam, potassium chloride, prochlorperazine, propofol, sargramostim, tacrolimus, teniposide, thiotepa, tolazoline, vinorelbine, vit B/C

Additive compatibilities: Amikacin, aminophylline, ascorbic acid inj, bretylium, cephapirin, chloramphenicol, corticotropin, dimenhyDRINATE, erythromycin, furosemide, heparin, hydrocortisone, lidocaine, magnesium sulfate, methicillin, norepinephrine, penicillin G potassium, penicillin G sodium, phenobarbital, potassium chloride, tobramycin, vancomycin, verapamil, vit B/C

PO route
• Give PO with or following meals to enhance absorption
• Store at room temp

Patient/family education
• Advise patient to remain recumbent 30 min after **IV** dose
• Caution patient to add food high in vit D content; to add calcium-rich foods to diet: dairy products, shellfish, dark green leafy vegetables; decrease oxalate-rich and zinc-rich foods: nuts, legumes, chocolate, spinach, soy
• Advise patient to prevent injuries, avoid immobilization

Evaluation
Positive therapeutic outcome
• Decreased twitching, paresthesias, muscle spasms
• Absence of tremors, convulsions, dysrhythmias, dyspnea, laryngospasm, negative Chvostek's sign, negative Trousseau's sign

calcium polycarbophil (OTC)
(pol-i-kar'boe-fil)
Equalactin, Fiberall, FiberCon, Fiber-Lax, Mitrolan
Func. class.: Laxative, bulk-forming
Pregnancy category C

Action: Attracts water, expands in intestine to increase peristalsis; also absorbs excess water in stool; decreases diarrhea

Therapeutic Outcome: Absence of constipation or diarrhea in irritable bowel syndrome

Uses: Constipation, irritable bowel syndrome (diarrhea), acute, nonspecific diarrhea

Dosage and routes
Adult: PO 1 g qd-qid prn, not to exceed 6 g/24 hr

Child 6-12 yr: PO 500 mg bid prn, not to exceed 3 g/24 hr

Child 3-6 yr: PO 500 mg bid prn, not to exceed 1.5 g/24 hr

Available forms: Chewable tabs 500, 1000 mg; tabs 500 mg

Adverse effects
(*italic* = common; **bold** = life-threatening)
GI: **Obstruction,** abdominal distention, flatus, laxative dependence

Contraindications: Hypersensitivity, GI obstruction

Precautions: Pregnancy C

Pharmacokinetics	
Absorption	None
Distribution	None
Metabolism	Unknown
Excretion	Feces
Half-life	Not known

Pharmacodynamics	
Onset	12-24 hr
Peak	1-3 days
Duration	Unknown

 Herb/drug   Do Not Crush   Alert   Key Drug   Geriatric   **P** Pediatric

Interactions
Individual drugs
Tetracycline: ↓ absorption of tetracycline
Herb/drug
Flax, lily of the valley, pheasant's eye, senna, squill: ↑ side effects, action

NURSING CONSIDERATIONS
Assessment
- Monitor blood, urine electrolytes if used often by patient; check I&O ratio to identify fluid loss
- Assess cramping, rectal bleeding, nausea, vomiting; if these symptoms occur, drug should be discontinued; identify cause of constipation; identify whether fluids, bulk, or exercise is missing from lifestyle
Nursing diagnoses
☑ Constipation (uses)
☑ Diarrhea (side effects)
☑ Knowledge, deficient (teaching)
☑ Noncompliance (teaching)
Implementation
- Give alone for better absorption; give after mixing with water immediately before use; administer with 6-8 oz of water or juice followed by another 8 oz of fluid
- Administer in AM or PM
Patient/family education
- Discuss with the patient that adequate fluid consumption is necessary; not to use laxatives long-term, laxative dependence will result
- Teach patient that normal bowel movements do not always occur daily
- Teach patient not to use in presence of abdominal pain, nausea, vomiting; tell patient to notify prescriber if constipation is unrelieved or if symptoms of electrolyte imbalance occur: muscle cramps, pain, weakness, dizziness, excessive thirst
Evaluation
Positive therapeutic outcome
- Decreased constipation within 3 days
- Decreased diarrhea in colitis within 1 wk

candesartan (Rx)
(can-deh-sar'tan)
Atacand
Func. class.: Antihypertensive
Chem. class.: Angiotensin II receptor (Type AT_1)

Pregnancy category C, 1st trimester; D, 2nd/3rd trimesters

Action: Blocks the vasoconstrictor and aldosterone-secreting effects of angiotensin II; selectively blocks the binding of angiotensin II to the AT_1 receptor found in tissues

→ **Therapeutic Outcome:** Decreased B/P

Uses: Hypertension, alone or in combination

Dosage and routes
Adult: PO (single agent) 16 mg qd initially in patients who are not volume depleted, range 8-32 mg/day; with diuretic or volume depletion 2-32 mg/day as a single dose or divided bid

Renal dose
Adult: PO Give lowest possible dose

Available forms: Tabs 4, 8, 16, 32 mg

Adverse effects
(*italic* = common; **bold** = life-threatening)
CNS: Dizziness, fatigue, headache
CV: Chest pain, peripheral edema
EENT: Sinusitis, rhinitis, pharyngitis
GI: Diarrhea, nausea, abdominal pain, vomiting
MS: Arthralgia, pain
GU: **Renal failure**
RESP: Cough, upper respiratory infection
SYST: **Angioedema**

Contraindications: Hypersensitivity; pregnancy **D** (2nd and 3rd trimesters)

Precautions: Hypersensitivity to ACE inhibitors; pregnancy C 1st trimester; lactation; children; elderly

Pharmacokinetics	
Absorption	Well absorbed
Distribution	Bound to plasma proteins
Metabolism	Extensive
Excretion	Feces, urine, breast milk
Half-life	9 hr

Pharmacodynamics	
Onset	Unknown
Peak	2 hr
Duration	24 hr

Interactions
Herb/drug

Aconite: ↑ toxicity, death

Astragalus, cola tree: ↑ or ↓ antihypertensive effect

Barberry, betony, black catechu, black cohosh, bloodroot, broom, burdock, cat's claw, dandelion, goldenseal, Irish moss, Jamaican dogwood, kelp, khella, mistletoe, parsley: ↑ antihypertensive effect

Coltsfoot, guarana, khat, licorice: ↓ antihypertensive effect

NURSING CONSIDERATIONS
Assessment

• Assess B/P, pulse q4h; note rate, rhythm, quality

• Monitor electrolytes: potassium, sodium, chloride; total CO_2

• Obtain baselines in renal, liver function tests before therapy begins

• Assess blood studies: BUN, creatinine, liver function tests before treatment

• Monitor for edema in feet, legs daily

• Assess for skin turgor, dryness of mucous membranes for hydration status; for angioedema: facial swelling, dyspnea

• Assess for pregnancy, this drug can cause fetal death when given in pregnancy

• Assess for adverse reactions, especially in renal disease

Nursing diagnoses

☑ Fluid volume, deficient (side effects)
☑ Noncompliance (teaching)
☑ Knowledge, deficient (teaching)

Implementation
PO route

• Administer without regard to meals

Patient/family education

• Teach patient not to take the drug if breastfeeding or pregnant, or have had an allergic reaction to this drug

• If a dose is missed, instruct patient to take as soon as possible, unless it is within an hour before next dose

• Advise patient to comply with dosage schedule, even if feeling better

• Teach patient to notify prescriber of fever, swelling of hands or feet, irregular heartbeat, chest pain

• Advise patient excessive perspiration, dehydration, diarrhea may lead to fall in blood pressure—consult prescriber if these occur

• Inform patient that drug may cause dizziness, fainting; lightheadedness may occur

• Caution patient to rise slowly to sitting or standing position to minimize orthostatic hypotension

• Advise patient to avoid all OTC medications unless approved by prescriber; to inform all health care providers of medication use

• Teach proper technique for obtaining B/P and acceptable parameters

Evaluation
Positive therapeutic outcome

• Decreased B/P

---

capecitabine (Rx)
(cap-eh-sit'ah-bean)
Xeloda
Func. class.: Antineoplastic, antimetabolite
Chem. class.: Fluoropyrimidine carbamate

Pregnancy category D

Action: Competes with physiologic substrate of DNA synthesis, thus interfering with cell replication in the S phase of cell cycle (before mitosis); drug is converted to 5-fluorouracil (5-FU)

Therapeutic Outcome: Decreasing symptoms of breast cancer

Uses: Metastatic breast, colorectal cancer

Dosage and routes:
Adult: PO 2500 mg/m²/day in 2 divided doses q12h at end of meal × 2 wk, then 1 wk rest period; given in 3 wk cycles; may be combined with Docetaxel, when capecitalane dose is lowered

Available forms: Tabs 150, 500 mg

Adverse effects
(*italic* = common; **bold** = life-threatening)
CNS: Dizziness, headache, *paresthesia, fatigue,* insomnia
GI: *Nausea, vomiting, anorexia, diarrhea, stomatitis, abdominal pain, constipation, dyspepsia,* **intestinal obstruction**
HEMA: **Neutropenia, lymphopenia, thrombocytopenia, myelosuppression,** anemia
INTEG: *Hand and foot syndrome,* dermatitis, nail disorder
MISC: Hyperbilirubinemia, eye irritation, pyrexia, edema, myalgia, limb pain, *pyrexia,* dehydration

P Contraindications: Hypersensitivity to 5-FU, infants, pregnancy **D**, severe renal impairment (CCr <30 ml/min)

P Precautions: Renal disease, hepatic
G disease, lactation, children, elderly

☑ Herb/drug   ⬢ Do Not Crush   ◆ Alert   ⬤π Key Drug   **G** Geriatric   **P** Pediatric

C

Xeloda/Xenical

Pharmacokinetics	
Absorption	Readily, food ↓
Distribution	Unknown
Metabolism	Liver, extensively
Excretion	Kidneys
Half-life	45 min

Pharmacodynamics	
Onset	Unknown
Peak	1½ hr
Duration	Unknown

Interactions
Individual drugs
Leucovorin: ↑ toxicity
Phenytoin: ↑ phenytoin level
Warfarin: ↑ risk of bleeding
Drug classifications
Antacids: ↑ capecitabine

NURSING CONSIDERATIONS
Assessment
• Assess buccal cavity q8h for dryness, sores or ulceration, white patches, pain, bleeding, dysphagia; obtain prescription for viscous lidocaine (Xylocaine)
• Assess symptoms indicating severe allergic reation: rash, pruritus, urticaria, purpuric skin lesions, itching, flushing; drug should be discontinued
• Monitor CBC, differential, platelet count weekly; withhold drug if WBC <4000/mm³ or platelet count is <100,000/mm³; notify prescriber of results if WBC <20,000/mm³, platelet count <150,000/mm³
• Monitor temp q4h (may indicate beginning of infection)
• Assess for hand/foot syndrome: paresthesia, tingling, painful/painless swelling, blistering, erythema with severe pain of hands/feet
• Assess for toxicity: severe diarrhea, nausea, vomiting, stomatitis
• Assess GI symptoms: frequency of stools, cramping; if severe diarrhea occurs, fluids/electrolytes may need to be given
• Monitor liver function tests before and during therapy (bilirubin, AST, ALT, LDH) as needed or monthly; note jaundice of skin or sclera, dark urine, clay-colored stools, itchy skin, abdominal pain, fever, diarrhea
• Assess for bleeding: hematuria, stool guaiac, bruising or petechiae, mucosa or orifices q8h; inflammation of mucosa, breaks in skin

Nursing diagnoses
☑ Injury, risk for (adverse reactions)
☑ Body image, disturbed (adverse reactions)
☑ Infection, risk for (adverse reactions)
☑ Knowledge, deficient (teaching)

Implementation
PO route
• Give antiemetic 30-60 min before giving drug to prevent vomiting and prn; give antibiotics for prophylaxis of infection
• Provide liq diet: carbonated beverages; gelatin may be added if patient is not nauseated or vomiting
• Help patient to rinse mouth tid-qid with water or club soda, brush teeth bid-qid with soft brush or cotton-tipped applicators for stomatitis, use unwaxed dental floss

Patient/family education
• Contraceptive measures are recommended during therapy; drug is teratogenic to fetus
• Advise patient to avoid use of products containing aspirin or ibuprofen, razors, commercial mouthwash, since bleeding may occur; to report symptoms of bleeding (hematuria, tarry stools)
• Instruct patient to report signs of anemia (fatigue, headache, irritability, faintness, shortness of breath)
• Advise patient not to become pregnant while taking this drug; to avoid using while lactating
• Advise patient not to double dose, if dose is missed
• Advise patient to report immediately severe diarrhea, vomiting, stomatitis, fever ≥100° F, hand/foot syndrome, anorexia

Evaluation
Positive therapeutic outcome
• Prevention of rapid division of malignant cells

---

captopril ⚷ (Rx)
(kap'toe-pril)
Capoten, Novo-Captopril ♦
Func. class.: Antihypertensive
Chem. class.: Angiotensin-converting enzyme (ACE) inhibitor

Pregnancy category C
(1st trimester); D (2nd/3rd trimesters)

Action: Selectively suppresses renin-angiotensin-aldosterone system; inhibits ACE; prevents conversion of angiotensin I to angiotensin II

➤ **Therapeutic Outcome:** Decreased B/P in hypertension; decreased preload, afterload in CHF

Uses: Hypertension, CHF, left ventricular dysfunction (LVD) after MI, diabetic nephropathy

Dosage and routes
Malignant hypertension
Adult: PO 25 mg increasing q2h until desired response; not to exceed 450 mg/day

Hypertension
Adult: Initial dose: PO 25 mg bid-tid; may increase to 50 mg bid-tid at 1-2 wk intervals; usual range 25-150 mg bid-tid; max 450 mg

P *Child:* PO 0.3-0.5 mg/kg/dose, titrate up to 6 mg/kg/day in 2-4 divided doses

P *Neonate:* PO 10 mcg (0.01 mg)/kg bid-tid, may increase as needed

CHF
Adult: PO 12.5 mg bid-tid; may increase to 50 mg bid-tid; after 14 days may increase to 150 mg tid if needed

LVD After MI
Adult: PO 50 mg tid, may begin treatment 3 days after MI; give 6.25 mg as a single dose, then 12.5 mg tid, increase to 25 mg tid for several days, then 50 mg tid

Diabetic nephropathy
Adult: PO 25 mg tid

Renal dose
Adult: PO 6.25-12.5 mg bid-tid

P *Child:* PO 150 mcg (0.15)/kg tid

Available forms: Tabs 12.5, 25, 50, 100 mg

Adverse effects
(italic = common; bold = life-threatening)
CNS: Fever, chills
CV: Hypotension, postural hypotension, *tachycardia,* angina
GI: Loss of taste, liver function tests
GU: Impotence, dysuria, nocturia, **proteinuria, nephrotic syndrome, acute reversible renal failure,** polyuria, oliguria, frequency
HEMA: **Neutropenia, agranulocytosis, pancytopenia, thrombocytopenia,** anemia
INTEG: Rash, **angioedema**
MISC: **Angioedema,** hyperkalemia
RESP: **Bronchospasm,** *dyspnea, cough*

Contraindications: Hypersensitivity,
P lactation, heart block, children, potassium-sparing diuretics, bilateral renal artery stenosis, pregnancy **D** (2nd/3rd trimesters)

Precautions: Dialysis patients, hypovolemia, leukemia, scleroderma, LE, blood dyscrasias, CHF, diabetes mellitus, pregnancy **C** (1st trimester), renal disease, thyroid disease, COPD, asthma

🚫 **Do Not Confuse:**
Captopril/Capitrol/Carvedilol

Pharmacokinetics	
Absorption	Well absorbed
Distribution	Widely distributed; crosses placenta, excreted in breast milk, small amounts
Metabolism	Liver (50%)
Excretion	Kidneys, unchanged (50%)
Half-life	2 hr increase in renal disease

Pharmacodynamics	
Onset	¼-1 hr
Peak	1 hr
Duration	6-12 hr

Interactions
Individual drugs
Alcohol (acute ingestion): ↑ hypotension (large amounts)
Digoxin, lithium: ↑ serum levels, toxicity
Insulin: ↑ hypoglycemia
Drug classifications
Antacids: ↓ absorption
Antidiabetics (oral): ↑ hypoglycemia
Antihypertensives, diuretics, nitrates, phenothiazines: ↑ hypotension
Diuretics (potassium-sparing), potassium supplements: ↑ toxicity, do not use
NSAIDs: ↓ captopril effect
Sympathomimetics: Do not use
🖉 *Herb/drug*
Aconite: ↑ toxicity, death
Astragalus, cola tree: ↑ or ↓ antihypertensive effect
Barberry, betony, black catechu, black cohosh, bloodroot, broom, burdock, cat's claw, dandelion, goldenseal, Irish moss, Jamaican dogwood, kelp, khella, mistletoe, parsley: ↑ antihypertensive effect
Coltsfoot, guarana, khat, licorice: ↓ antihypertensive effect
Lab test interferences
False positive: Urine acetone, ANA titer, ↑ AST, ↑ ALT, ↑ alkaline phosphatase, ↑ bilirubin, ↑ uric acid, ↑ glucose

NURSING CONSIDERATIONS
Assessment
• May be crushed and mixed with food
• Monitor blood studies: decreased platelets;

WBC with diff baseline and periodically q3 mo, if neutrophils <1000/mm³, discontinue treatment
• Monitor B/P, check for orthostatic hypotension, syncope; if changes occur, dosage change may be required
• Monitor renal studies: protein, BUN, creatinine; watch for increased levels that may indicate nephrotic syndrome and renal failure; monitor renal symptoms: polyuria, oliguria, frequency, dysuria
• Establish baselines in renal, liver function tests before therapy begins and check periodically; monitor for increased liver function studies; watch for increased uric acid, glucose
• Check potassium levels throughout treatment, although hyperkalemia rarely occurs
• Check for edema in feet, legs daily; monitor weight daily in CHF
• Assess for allergic reactions: rash, fever, pruritus, urticaria; drug should be discontinued if antihistamines fail to help

Nursing diagnoses
☑Cardiac output, decreased (uses)
☑Injury, risk for (side effects)
☑Knowledge, deficient (teaching)
☑Noncompliance (teaching)

Implementation
• Store in air-tight container at 86° F (30° C) or less
• Severe hypotension may occur after 1st dose of this medication; decreasing hypotension may be prevented by reducing or discontinuing diuretic therapy 3 days before beginning captopril therapy
• Administer 1 hr ac or 2 hr pc
• May crush tab and dissolve in water, give within ½ hr, make sure tab is completely dissolved

Patient/family education
• Caution patient not to discontinue drug abruptly; advise patient to tell all persons associated with care
• Teach patient not to use OTC products (cough, cold, allergy) unless directed by prescriber; serious side effects can occur; xanthines such as coffee, tea, chocolate, cola can prevent action of drug
• Teach patient importance of complying with dosage schedule, even if feeling better; to continue with medical regimen to decrease B/P: exercise, cessation of smoking, decreasing stress, diet modifications
• Emphasize the need to rise slowly to sitting or standing position to minimize orthostatic

hypotension; not to exercise in hot weather or increased hypotension can occur
• Teach patient to notify prescriber of mouth sores, sore throat, fever, swelling of hands or feet, irregular heartbeat, chest pain, coughing, shortness of breath
• Caution patient to report excessive perspiration, dehydration, vomiting, diarrhea; may lead to fall in B/P
• Caution patient that drug may cause dizziness, fainting, lightheadedness; may occur during 1st few days of therapy; to avoid activities that may be hazardous
• Teach patient how to take B/P, and teach normal readings for age-group; ensure patient takes regularly
• Advise patient to tell prescriber if pregnancy is suspected or planned

Evaluation
Positive therapeutic outcome
• Decreased B/P in hypertension

Treatment of overdose: 0.9% NaCl **IV** infusion, hemodialysis

carbamazepine (Rx)
(kar-ba-maz'e-peen)
Apo-Carbamazepine ♣, Atretol, Carbatrol, Epitol, Novo-Carbamaz ♣, Tegretol, Tegretol CR ♣, Tegretol-XR
Func. class.: Anticonvulsant
Chem. class.: Iminostilbene derivative
Pregnancy category D

Action: Exact mechanism unknown; appears to decrease polysynaptic responses and block posttetanic potentiation

Therapeutic Outcome: Absence of seizures; decreased trigeminal neuralgia pain

Uses: Tonic-clonic, complex-partial, mixed seizures; trigeminal neuralgia

Investigational uses: Diabetes insipidus, bipolar disorder, neurogenic pain, schizophrenia, psychotic behavior with dementia, rectal administration, diabetic neuropathy, restless leg syndrome

Dosage and routes
Seizures
Adult and child >12 yr: PO 200 mg bid; may be increased by 200 mg/day in divided doses q6-8h; maintenance 800-1200 mg/day; maximum 1600 mg/day (adult); max child 12-15 yr 1000 mg/day; max child >15 yr 1200 mg/day; adjustment is needed to minimum dose to control seizures; ext rel give bid; rec

administration of oral susp 200 mg/10 ml or 6 mg/kg as a single dose

P *Child 6-12 yr:* PO tabs 100 mg bid or susp 50 mg qid; may increase by <100 mg qwk, max 1000 mg/day; ext rel tabs qd-bid

P *Child <6 yr:* PO 10-20 mg/kg/day in 2-3 divided doses, may increase qwk

Trigeminal neuralgia
Adult: PO 100 mg/bid; may increase 100 mg q12h until pain subsides; not to exceed 1200 mg/day; maintenance is 200-400 mg bid

Available forms: Chewable tabs 100, 200 mg; tabs 200 mg; oral susp 100 mg/5 ml; ext rel 100, 200, 400 ✽ mg; ext rel caps 200, 300 mg

Adverse effects
(*italic* = common; **bold** = life-threatening)
CNS: Drowsiness, dizziness, confusion, fatigue, **paralysis,** headache, hallucinations, **worsening of seizures,** unsteadiness, speech disturbances
CV: **Hypertension, CHF,** hypotension, aggravation of CAD, dysrhythmias, **AV block**
EENT: Tinnitus, dry mouth, blurred vision, diplopia, nystagmus, conjunctivitis
ENDO: Syndrome of inappropriate antidi-
G uretic hormone (SIADH) (elderly)
GI: Nausea, constipation, diarrhea, anorexia, vomiting, abdominal pain, stomatitis, glossitis, increased liver enzymes, **hepatitis**
GU: Frequency, retention, albuminuria, glycosuria, impotence, ↑ BUN, **renal failure**
HEMA: **Thrombocytopenia, agranulocytosis, leukocytosis, leukopenia, aplastic anemia, eosinophilia,** increased pro-time
INTEG: Rash, **Stevens-Johnson syndrome,** urticaria, photosensitivity
RESP: Pulmonary hypersensitivity (fever, dyspnea, pneumonitis)

Contraindications: Hypersensitivity to carbamazepine or tricyclic antidepressants, bone marrow depression, concomitant use of MAOIs, pregnancy **D**

Precautions: Glaucoma, hepatic disease, renal disease, cardiac disease, psychosis,
P lactation, child <6 yr

◪ Do Not Confuse:
Tegretol/Toradol

Pharmacokinetics

Absorption	Slow; completely absorbed
Distribution	Widely distributed; protein binding 76%
Metabolism	Extensively, liver
Excretion	Urine, feces, breast milk
Half-life	14-16 hr or more

Pharmacodynamics

Onset	2-4 day
Peak	4-8 hr
Duration	Unknown

Interactions
Individual drugs
Benzodiazepines: ↓ effect of benzodiazepine, verapamil
Cisplatin, danazol, DOXOrubicin, felbamate, primidone, rifampin: ↓ carbamazepine levels
Clarithromycin, verapamil: ↑ toxicity
Contraceptives (oral): ↓ effect of oral contraceptives
Doxycycline: ↓ half-life
Felbamate, fluoxetine, fluroxamine: ↑ carbamazepine effect
Haloperidol: ↓ serum levels, ↓ therapeutic efficacy
Lithium: ↑ CNS toxicity
Phenobarbital: ↑ effect
Phenytoin: ↑ and ↓ plasma levels, ↓ carbamazepine plasma levels
Theophylline: ↓ effect of carbamazepine
Thyroid hormones: ↓ effect of thyroid hormones
Valproic acid: ↓ plasma levels, ↑ half-life of carbamazepine
Warfarin: ↓ effect of warfarin
Drug classifications
Barbiturates: ↓ serum levels of carbamazepine
◆MAOIs: Fatal reaction; do not use together
Food/drug
Grapefruit juice: ↓ carbamazepine level
◪ *Herb/drug*
Ginkgo, quinine: ↑ anticonvulsant action
Ginseng, santonica: ↓ anticonvulsant action

NURSING CONSIDERATIONS
Assessment
• Assess for seizures: character, location, duration, intensity, frequency, presence of aura
• Assess for trigeminal neuralgia: facial pain including location, duration, intensity, character, activity that stimulates pain
• Monitor liver function tests (AST, ALT) and urine function tests, BUN, urine protein periodically during treatments

- Check blood levels during treatment or when changing dose; therapeutic level 4-12 mcg/ml
- Assess for blood dyscrasias: fever, sore throat, bruising, rash, jaundice, epistaxis (long-term treatment only)
- Assess seizure activity including type, aura, location, duration, and character; provide seizure precaution

Nursing diagnoses
☑ Injury, risk for (side effects)
☑ Knowledge, deficient (teaching)

Implementation
- Give with food for GI symptoms
🚫 • Chew tab: tell patient to chew, not swallow whole, do not crush, break, chew ext rel product; ext rel cap may be opened and mixed with food
- Shake oral susp before use
- Mix an equal amount of water, D_5W, 0.9% NaCl when giving by NG tube, flush tube with 100 ml of above sol

Patient/family education
- Teach patient to carry/wear emergency ID stating patient's name, drugs taken, condition, prescriber's name, phone number
- Caution patient to avoid driving, other activities that require alertness until stabilized on medication
- Teach patient not to discontinue medication quickly after long-term use
- Teach patient to use a nonhormonal type of contraception to prevent harm to the fetus
- Advise patient to use sunscreen to prevent burns
- Teach patient to take exactly as prescribed, 🚫 do not double or omit doses, not to crush, break, or chew ext rel products
- Teach patient to report immediately chills, rash, light-colored stools, dark urine, yellowing of skin/eyes, abdominal pain, sore throat, mouth, ulcers, bruising, blurred vision, dizziness

Evaluation
Positive therapeutic outcome
- Decreased seizure activity

Treatment of overdose: Lavage, VS

carbidopa-levodopa (Rx)
(kar-bi-doe′pa lee-voe-doe′pa)
carbidopa/levodopa, Sinemet, Sinemet CR
Func. class.: Antiparkinsonism agent
Chem. class.: Catecholamine

Pregnancy category C

Action: Decarboxylation of levodopa to periphery is inhibited by carbidopa; more levodopa is made available for transport to brain and conversion to dopamine in the brain

Therapeutic Outcome: Absence of involuntary movements

Uses: Parkinsonism, restless legs syndrome, chronic manganese intoxication, cerebral arteriosclerosis

Dosage and routes
Beginning therapy for those not taking levodopa
Adult: PO 10 mg carbidopa/100 mg levodopa tid-qid or 25 mg carbidopa/100 mg levodopa tid, may increase qd to desired response

For those not taking levodopa ER
Adult: PO 50 mg carbidopa/200 mg levodopa bid

For those taking levodopa ER
Adult: Begin treatment with 10% more levodopa/day given PO q4-8h, may increase or decrease dose q3 days

For those taking levodopa <1.5 g/day
Adult: PO 25 mg carbidopa/100 mg levodopa tid-qid, may increase qd to desired response

For those taking levodopa >1.5 g/day
Adult: PO 25 mg carbidopa/250 mg levodopa tid-qid, may increase qd to desired response

Available forms: Tabs 10/100, 25/100, 25 mg carbidopa/250 mg levodopa; ext rel tab: 25 mg/100 mg, 50 mg/200 mg carbidopa/levodopa (Sinemet CR)

Adverse effects
(*italic* = common; **bold** = life-threatening)
CNS: *Involuntary choreiform movements, hand tremors, fatigue, headache, anxiety, twitching, numbness, weakness, confusion, agitation, insomnia, nightmares,* psychosis, hallucination, hypomania, severe depression, dizziness

CV: Orthostatic hypotension, tachycardia, hypertension, palpitation

EENT: Blurred vision, diplopia, dilated pupils

GI: Nausea, vomiting, anorexia, abdominal distress, dry mouth, flatulence, dysphagia, bitter taste, diarrhea, constipation

HEMA: Hemolytic anemia, leukopenia, agranulocytosis

INTEG: Rash, sweating, alopecia

MISC: Urinary retention, incontinence, weight change, dark urine

Contraindications: Hypersensitivity, narrow-angle glaucoma, malignant melanoma, history of malignant melanoma, or undiagnosed skin lesions resembling melanoma

Precautions: Renal disease, cardiac disease, hepatic disease, respiratory disease, MI with dysrhythmias, wide angle glaucoma, convulsions, peptic ulcer, pregnancy **C**

Pharmacokinetics

Absorption	Well absorbed (PO); ER dose slow
Distribution	Widely distributed
Metabolism	Liver, extensively
Excretion	Kidneys, metabolites
Half-life	Levodopa (1 hr); carbidopa (1-2 hr)

Pharmacodynamics

	PO	PO-ER
Onset	Unknown	Unknown
Peak	1 hr	2½ hr
Duration	6-24 hr	Unknown

Interactions
Individual drugs

Metoclopramide: ↑ effects of levodopa

Papaverine, pyridoxine: ↓ effects of levodopa

Drug classifications

Antacids: ↑ effects of levodopa

Anticholinergics, benzodiazepines, hydantoins: ↓ effects of levodopa

MAOIs: Hypertensive crisis

Food/drug

Protein: ↓ absorption of levodopa

Pyridoxine: ↓ levodopa effect

Herb/drug

Kava, octacosanol: ↑ Parkinson's symptoms

Indian snakeroot: ↓ action, ↑ extrapyramidal symptoms

Lab test interferences

False: ↑ Uric acid, urine protein, ↑ AST, ↑ ALT, ↑ bilirubin, ↑ LDH, ↑ alkaline phosphatase, ↓ VMA, ↑↓ BUN, ↓ creatinine

False positive: Urine ketones (dipstick)

False negative: Urine glucose

NURSING CONSIDERATIONS
Assessment

• Assess B/P, respiration, orthostatic B/P

• Monitor I&O ratio; retention commonly causes decreased urinary output, distention, frequency, incontinence; palpate bladder if retention occurs

• Assess for muscle twitching, blepharospasm that may indicate toxicity

• Monitor renal, liver, hematopoietic studies, also for diabetes, acromegaly during long-term therapy

• Assess for parkinsonism: shuffling gait, muscle rigidity, involuntary movements, pill rolling, muscle spasms, drooling before and during treatment

• Monitor for constipation, cramping, pain in abdomen, abdominal distention; increase fluids, bulk, exercise if this occurs

• Assess for tolerance over long-term therapy; dose may have to be increased or changed

• Assess for mental status: affect, mood, CNS depression, worsening of mental symptoms during early therapy

Nursing diagnoses

☑ Mobility, impaired physical (uses)

☑ Knowledge, deficient (teaching)

Implementation
PO route

• Give drug until NPO before surgery; check with prescriber for continuing drug

• Adjust dosage depending on patient response

• Give with meals or pc to prevent GI symptoms; limit protein taken with drug

• Give only after MAOIs have been discontinued for 2 wk; if previously on levodopa, discontinue for at least 8 hr before change to levodopa-carbidopa

🚫 • Controlled-release tabs should be swallowed whole, not crushed or chewed

Patient/family education

• Teach patient to change positions slowly to prevent orthostatic hypotension

• Teach patient to report side effects: twitching, eye spasms, grimacing, protrusion of tongue, personality changes that indicate overdose

• Instruct patient to use drug exactly as prescribed; if drug is discontinued abruptly, parkinsonian crisis may occur; do not double doses; take missed dose as soon as remembered up to 2 hr before next dose

• Teach patient that urine, sweat may darken and is harmless

• Advise patient to use physical activities to maintain mobility and lessen spasms

---

 Herb/drug   🚫 Do Not Crush   ◆ Alert   Key Drug   **G** Geriatric   **P** Pediatric

- Instruct patient that OTC medications should not be used unless approved by prescriber
- Advise patient that drowsiness, dizziness are common; to avoid hazardous activities until response is known
- Explain that sips of water, hard candy, or gum may lessen dry mouth
- Teach patient to take with meals to prevent GI symptoms; to limit protein intake, which impairs drug's absorption

Evaluation
Positive therapeutic outcome
- Decrease in akathisia
- Improved mood
- Decreased involuntary movements

⚠ HIGH ALERT

carboplatin (Rx)
(kar'boe'pla-tin)
Paraplatin, Paraplatin-AQ ✦
Func. class.: Antineoplastic alkylating agent
Chem. class.: Platinum coordination compound

Pregnancy category D

Action: Produces interstrand DNA cross-links and to a lesser extent DNA-protein cross-links; activity is not cell cycle phase specific

➡ **Therapeutic Outcome:** Prevention of rapidly growing malignant cells

Uses: Initial treatment of ovarian cancer in combination with other agents; palliative treatment of recurrent ovarian carcinoma after treatment with other antineoplastic agents, including cisplatin

Dosage and routes
(single agent)

Adult: **IV** inf initially 300 mg/m² given with cyclophosphamide, q4-6 wk; refractory tumors 360 mg/m² single dose, may repeat q4 wk, as needed

Renal dose
Adult: **IV** CCr 41-59 ml/min 250 mg/m², CCr 16-40 ml/min 200 mg/m²

Available forms: Inj 50, 150, 450 mg/vial

Adverse effects
(*italic* = common; **bold** = life-threatening)
CNS: **Seizures, central neurotoxicity,** peripheral neuropathy, dizziness, confusion
CV: Cardiac abnormalities

EENT: Tinnitus, hearing loss, *vestibular toxicity,* visual changes
GI: Severe nausea, vomiting, diarrhea, weight loss, mucositis, anorexia, constipation, taste change
GU: **Renal tubular damage,** renal insufficiency, impotence, sterility, amenorrhea, gynecomastia
HEMA: **Thrombocytopenia, leukopenia, pancytopenia, neutropenia, anemia,** bleeding
INTEG: Alopecia, dermatitis, rash, erythema, pruritus, urticaria
META: Hypomagnesemia, hypocalcemia, hypokalemia, hyponatremia, hyperuremia
SYST: **Anaphylaxis**

Contraindications: Hypersensitivity to this drug, platinum products, mannitol; severe bone marrow depression, significant bleeding, pregnancy **D**

Precautions: Radiation therapy within 1 mo, chemotherapy within 1 mo, lactation, liver disease

▧ Do Not Confuse:
carboplatin/cisplatin
Paraplatin/platinol

Pharmacokinetics	
Absorption	Complete
Distribution	Unknown
Metabolism	Liver
Excretion	Kidneys
Half-life	Initial 1-2 hr; postdistribution 2½-6 hr; increased in renal disease

Pharmacodynamics	
Onset	½ hr
Peak	Unknown
Duration	4-6 hr

Interactions
Individual drugs
Aspirin: ↑ risk of bleeding
Phenytoin: ↓ phenytoin level
Radiation: ↑ toxicity, bone marrow suppression
Drug classifications
Aminoglycosides: ↑ nephrotoxicity
Aminoglycosides, diuretics (loop): Ototoxicity
Antineoplastics: ↑ toxicity
Antineoplastics, bone marrow–suppressing drugs: ↑ bone marrow suppression
Live virus vaccines: ↓ or ↑ antibody reaction
Myelosuppressives: ↑ myelosuppression

Lab test interferences
↑ AST, ↑ BUN, ↑ alkaline phosphatase, ↑ bilirubin, ↑ creatinine

NURSING CONSIDERATIONS
Assessment
• Monitor CBC, differential, platelet count weekly; withhold drug if neutrophil count is <2000/mm³ or platelet count is <100,000/mm³; notify prescriber of results if WBC <20,000/mm³, platelets <150,000/mm³
• Assess for anaphylaxis: pruritus, wheezing, tachycardia; notify physician after discontinuing drugs; resuscitation equipment should be available
• Monitor renal function studies: BUN, creatinine, serum uric acid, urine CCr before and during therapy; I&O ratio; report fall in urine output to <30 ml/hr
• Monitor temp q4h (may indicate beginning of infection)
• Monitor liver function tests before and during therapy (bilirubin, AST, ALT, LDH) as needed or monthly; note jaundice of skin or sclera, dark urine, clay-colored stools, itchy skin, abdominal pain, fever, diarrhea
• Assess for bleeding: hematuria, stool guaiac, bruising or petechiae, mucosa or orifices q8h; inflammation of mucosa, breaks in skin
• Identify dyspnea, rales, unproductive cough, chest pain, tachypnea
• Identify effects of alopecia on body image; discuss feelings about body changes

Nursing diagnoses
☑ Injury, risk for (adverse reactions)
☑ Body image, disturbed (adverse reactions)
☑ Infection, risk for (adverse reactions)
☑ Knowledge, deficient (teaching)

Implementation
• Antiemetic 30-60 min before giving drug to prevent vomiting, and prn
IV **IV route**
• Give **IV** after diluting 10 mg/ml of sterile water for inj, D₅W, 0.9% NaCl (10 mg/ml); then further dilute with the same sol 1-4 mg/ml; give over 15 min or more (intermittent inf)
• Give **IV** inf over 5-6 hr; do not use needles or **IV** administration sets containing aluminum; may cause precipitate or loss of potency; diuretic (furosemide 40 mg **IV**) after inf
• Store protected from light at room temp; reconstituted sol is stable for 8 hr at room temp

Y-site compatibilities: Allopurinol, amifostine, aztreonam, cefepime, cladribine, DOXOrubicin liposome, filgrastim, fludarabine, granisetron, melphalan, ondansetron, paclitaxel, piperacillin/tazobactam, propofol, sargramostim, teniposide, thiotepa, vinorelbine

Additive compatibilities: Cisplatin, etoposide, floxuridine, ifosfamide, ifosfamide/etoposide, paclitaxel

Additive incompatibilities: Fluorouracil, mesna

Solution compatibilities: D₅/0.2% NaCl, D₅/0.45% NaCl, D₅/0.9% NaCl, 0.9% NaCl, D₅W, sterile water for inj

Solution incompatibilities: Sodium bicarbonate

Patient/family education
• Advise patient to report ringing/roaring in the ears, numbness, tingling in face, extremities, weight gain
• Teach patient to avoid use of products containing aspirin or ibuprofen, NSAIDs, alcohol, razors, commercial mouthwash, since bleeding may occur; to report symptoms of bleeding (hematuria, tarry stools)
• Instruct patient to report signs of anemia (fatigue, headache, irritability, faintness, shortness of breath); sore throat, bleeding, bruising, chills, back pain, blood in stools, dyspnea
• Instruct patient to report any changes in breathing or coughing even several months after treatment; to avoid crowds and persons with respiratory tract or other infections
• Advise patient that hair may be lost during treatment; a wig or hairpiece may make patient feel better; new hair may be different in color, texture
• Caution patient not to have any vaccinations without the advice of the prescriber; serious reactions can occur
• Teach patient that contraception is needed during treatment and for several months after the completion of therapy; not to breastfeed during treatment; to notify prescriber if pregnancy is planned or suspected

Evaluation
Positive therapeutic outcome
• Prevention of rapid division of malignant cells

---

carboprost (Rx)
(kar'boe-prost)
Hemabate, Prostin/15M ♣
Func. class.: Oxytocic, abortifacient
Chem. class.: Prostaglandin

Pregnancy category C

Action: Stimulates uterine contractions, causing complete abortion in approximately 16 hr

➡ **Therapeutic Outcome:** Loss of fetus; decreased postpartum bleeding

Uses: Abortion between 13-20 wk gestation; postpartum hemorrhage caused by uterine atony not controlled by other methods

Dosage and routes
To induce abortion
Adult: IM 250 mcg, then 250 mcg q1½-3½h, may increase to 500 mcg if no response, not to exceed 12 mg total dose

Postpartum hemorrhage
Adult: IM 250 mcg, repeat at 15-90 min intervals, max total dosage 2 mg

Available forms: Inj 250 mcg/ml

Adverse effects
(*italic* = common; **bold** = life-threatening)
CNS: Fever, chills, headache
GI: Nausea, vomiting, diarrhea

Contraindications: Hypersensitivity, severe hepatic disease, severe renal disease, PID, respiratory disease, cardiac disease

Precautions: Asthma, anemia, jaundice, diabetes mellitus, seizure disorders, past uterine surgery, pregnancy **C**

Pharmacokinetics	
Absorption	Well absorbed (nasal)
Distribution	Widely distributed (extracellular fluid)
Metabolism	Liver—rapidly
Excretion	Kidneys
Half-life	3-9 min

Pharmacodynamics	
Onset	Unknown
Peak	16 hr
Duration	Unknown

Interactions
Drug classifications
Oxytocics: ↑ effects

NURSING CONSIDERATIONS
Assessment
- Monitor B/P, pulse; watch for change that may indicate hemorrhage
- Monitor respiratory rate, rhythm, depth; notify physician of abnormalities
- For length, duration of contraction; notify physician of contractions lasting over 1 min or absence of contractions
- Assess for incomplete abortion, pregnancy must be terminated by another method; drug is teratogenic

Nursing diagnoses
✓ Knowledge, deficient (teaching)

Implementation
- Give IM inj in deep muscle mass; rotate inj sites if additional doses are given
- Have crash cart available on unit

Patient/family education
- Advise patient to report increased blood loss, abdominal cramps, increased temperature or foul-smelling lochia

Evaluation
Positive therapeutic outcome
- Loss of fetus
- Control of bleeding

carisoprodol (Rx)
(kar-i-soe-proe'dole)
carisoprodol, Soma, Vanadom
Func. class.: Skeletal muscle relaxant, central acting
Chem. class.: Meprobamate congener

Pregnancy category C

Action: Depresses CNS by blocking interneuronal activity in descending reticular formation of spinal cord, producing sedation

➡ **Therapeutic Outcome:** Relaxation of skeletal muscles

Uses: Relieving pain, stiffness in musculoskeletal disorders

Dosage and routes
🅟 *Adult and child >12 yr:* PO 350 mg tid and hs
🅟 *Child 6-12 yr:* PO 6.25 mg/kg qid

Available forms: Tabs 350 mg

Adverse effects
(*italic* = common; **bold** = life-threatening)
CNS: Dizziness, weakness, drowsiness, headache, tremor, depression, insomnia, ataxia, irritability
CV: Postural hypotension, tachycardia

EENT: Diplopia, temporary loss of vision
GI: Nausea, vomiting, hiccups, epigastric discomfort
HEMA: Eosinophilia
INTEG: Rash, pruritus, fever, facial flushing, **erythema multiforme**
RESP: Asthmatic attack
SYST: **Angioedema, anaphylaxis**

Contraindications: Hypersensitivity, P child <12 yr, intermittent porphyria

Precautions: Renal disease, hepatic disease, addictive personality, pregnancy **C**, G elderly

Do Not Confuse:
soma/soma compound

Pharmacokinetics

Absorption	Well absorbed
Distribution	Crosses placenta
Metabolism	Liver, partially
Excretion	Kidney, unchanged; breast milk
Half-life	8 hr

Pharmacodynamics

Onset	½ hr
Peak	4 hr
Duration	4-6 hr

Interactions
Individual drugs
Alcohol: ↑ CNS depression
Drug classifications
Antidepressants (tricyclic), barbiturates, opioids, sedative/hypnotics: ↑ CNS depression
Herb/drug
Chamomile, kava, skullcap, valerian: ↑ CNS depression
Lab test interferences
↑ AST, ↑ alkaline phosphatase, ↑ blood glucose

NURSING CONSIDERATIONS
Assessment
• Monitor ROM, atrophy, stiffness, and pain in muscles; assess throughout treatment
• Monitor ECG in seizure patients; poor seizure control has occurred with patients taking this drug
• Assess for idiosyncratic reaction within a few min or hr of administration (disorientation, restlessness, weakness, euphoria, blurred vision); patient should be reassured that reaction is temporary
• Check for allergic reactions: rash, fever

Nursing diagnoses
☑ Mobility, impaired (uses)
☑ Injury, risk for (adverse reactions)
☑ Knowledge, deficient (teaching)

Implementation
PO route
• Give with meals for GI symptoms
• Have patient use gum, frequent sips of water for dry mouth
• Store in tight container at room temp

Patient/family education
• Caution patient not to take with alcohol, other CNS depressants
• Advise patient to avoid altering activities while taking this drug
• Caution patient to avoid hazardous activities if drowsiness or dizziness occurs
• Caution patient to avoid using OTC medication such as cough preparations, antihistamines, unless directed by prescriber

Evaluation
Positive therapeutic outcome
• Decreased pain, spasticity

Treatment of overdose: Induce emesis of conscious patient, lavage, dialysis

---

! HIGH ALERT

carmustine (Rx)
(kar-mus'teen)
BiCNU, BCNU, Gliadel
Func. class.: Antineoplastic alkylating agent
Chem. class.: Nitrosourea

Pregnancy category D

Action: Alkylates DNA, RNA; inhibits enzymes that allow synthesis of amino acids in proteins; also responsible for cross-linking DNA strands; activity is not cell cycle phase specific

Therapeutic Outcome: Prevention of rapidly growing malignant cells

Uses: Brain tumors such as glioblastoma, medulloblastoma, astrocytoma, ependymoma, metastic brain tumors; multiple myeloma (with prednisone), Hodgkin's disease, other lymphomas; GI, breast, bronchogenic, and renal carcinomas, other lymphomas; wafer, as adjunct to surgery/radiation in newly diagnosed high-grade malignant glioma patients; in recurrent glioblastoma multiforme patients as adjunct to surgery

Investigational uses: Primary cutaneous T-cell lymphoma, malignant melanoma

---

Dosage and routes
Adult: **IV** 75-100 mg/m^2 over 1-2 hr × 2 days or 150-200 mg/m^2 × 1 dose q6-8 wk or 40 mg/m^2/day × 5 days q6 wk; if WBC 3000-3999/mm^3 give 50% of dose; if WBC is 2000-2999/mm^3 and platelet count is 25,000-75,000/mm^3 give 25% of dose; withhold dose if WBC <2000/mm^3 and platelets <25,000/mm^3

Adult: Intracavitary 8 wafers inserted into resection cavity

Available forms: Powder for inj 100 mg; wafer 7.7 mg intracavitary

Adverse effects
(*italic* = common; **bold** = life-threatening)
GI: *Nausea, vomiting, anorexia, stomatitis,* **hepatotoxicity**
GU: *Azotemia,* **renal failure**
HEMA: **Thrombocytopenia, leukopenia, myelosuppression, anemia**
INTEG: Burning, hyperpigmentation at inj site, alopecia
RESP: **Fibrosis, pulmonary infiltrate**

Contraindications: Hypersensitivity, leukopenia, thrombocytopenia, pregnancy **D**

Pharmacokinetics
Absorption	Completely absorbed
Distribution	Readily penetrates CSF
Metabolism	Liver, rapid
Excretion	Kidneys, breast milk
Half-life	Unknown

Pharmacodynamics
Unknown

Interactions
Individual drugs
Aspirin: ↑ risk of bleeding
Cimetidine, radiation: ↑ toxicity
Digoxin: ↓ effects of digoxin
Phenytoin: ↓ effects of phenytoin
Radiation: ↑ bone marrow suppression
Drug classifications
Anticoagulants: ↑ risk of bleeding
Antineoplastics: ↑ toxicity
Antineoplastics, bone marrow–suppressing drugs: ↑ bone marrow suppression
Live vaccines: ↑ adverse reactions, ↓ antibody reaction

NURSING CONSIDERATIONS
Assessment
• Assess buccal cavity q8h for dryness, sores or ulceration, white patches, pain, bleeding, dysphagia; obtain prescription for viscous lidocaine (Xylocaine)
• Assess symptoms indicating severe allergic reaction: rash, pruritus, urticaria, purpuric skin lesions, itching, flushing; drug should be discontinued
• Monitor CBC, differential, platelet count weekly; withhold drug if WBC <4000/mm^3 or platelet count is <100,000/mm^3; notify prescriber of results if WBC <20,000/mm^3, platelets <150,000/mm^3
• Monitor renal function studies: BUN, creatinine, urine CCr before and during therapy; I&O ratio; report fall in urine output to <30 ml/hr
• Monitor temp q4h (may indicate beginning of infection)
• Monitor liver function tests before and during therapy (bilirubin, AST, ALT, LDH) as needed or monthly; note yellowing of skin or sclera, dark urine, clay-colored stools, itchy skin, abdominal pain, fever, diarrhea; hepatotoxicity can be serious and fatal
• Assess for bleeding: hematuria, stool guaiac, bruising or petechiae, mucosa or orifices q8h; inflammation of mucosa, breaks in skin
• Monitor pulmonary function tests, chest x-ray films before, during therapy; chest film should be obtained q2wk during treatment; monitor for dyspnea, cough, pulmonary fibrosis; infiltrate occurs after high doses or several low dose courses
• Identify effects of alopecia on body image; discuss feelings about body changes

Nursing diagnoses
☑ Injury, risk for (adverse reactions)
☑ Body image, disturbed (adverse reactions)
☑ Infection, risk for (adverse reactions)
☑ Knowledge, deficient (teaching)

Implementation
• Blood transfusion or RBC colony-stimulating factors to counter anemia may be required
• Give fluids **IV** or PO before chemotherapy to hydrate patient
• Provide antiemetic 30-60 min before giving drug to prevent vomiting, and prn; antibiotics for prophylaxis of infection
• Provide liq diet (carbonated beverages); gelatin may be added if patient is not nauseated or vomiting
• Give all medications PO, if possible, avoid IM inj if platelets <100,000/mm^3
Wafer
• Foil pouches may be kept at room temp for 6 hr, if unopened
• If wafers are broken in several pieces, do not use

IV **IV route**
- Prepare in biologic cabinet wearing gown, gloves, mask; avoid contact with skin
- Administer after diluting 100 mg/3 ml ethyl alcohol (provided); then further dilute 27 ml sterile water for inj; then dilute with 100-500 ml 0.9% NaCl or D₅W; give over 1 hr or more; use only glass containers; reduce rate if discomfort is felt
- Flush **IV** line after carmustine with 10 ml 0.9% NaCl to prevent irritation at site
- Store reconstituted sol in refrigerator for 24 hr or room temp for 8 hr

Y-site compatibilities: Amifostine, aztreonam, cefepime, filgrastim, fludarabine, granisetron, melphalan, ondansetron, piperacillin/tazobactam, sargramostim, teniposide, thiotepa, vinorelbine

Additive incompatibilities: Sodium bicarbonate

Patient/family education
- Teach patient to avoid use of products containing aspirin or ibuprofen, razors, commercial mouthwash, since bleeding may occur; to report symptoms of bleeding (hematuria, tarry stools)
- Advise patient to avoid foods with citric acid, hot or rough texture if stomatitis is present
- Instruct patient to report signs of anemia (fatigue, headache, irritability, faintness, shortness of breath); avoid smoking
- Advise patient that hair may be lost during treatment; a wig or hairpiece may make patient feel better; new hair may be different in color, texture
- Caution patient not to have any vaccinations without the advice of the prescriber; serious reactions can occur
- Advise patient that contraception is needed during treatment and for several months after completion of therapy; drug has teratogenic properties

Evaluation
Positive therapeutic outcome
- Prevention of rapid division of malignant cells

---

carteolol (Rx)
(kar-tee′oe-lole)
Cartrol
Func. class.: Antihypertensive, antianginal
Chem. class.: Nonselective β-blocker

Pregnancy category C

Action: Produces fall in B/P without reflex tachycardia or significant reduction in heart rate through mixture of α-blocking, β-blocking effects and intrinsic sympathomimetic activity; elevated plasma renins are reduced; decreased intraocular pressure in glaucoma and intraocular hypertension

➡ **Therapeutic Outcome:** Decreased B/P, heart rate; decreased intraocular pressure

Uses: Mild to moderate hypertension; oph intraocular hypertension, open-angle glaucoma (see Appendix C)

Dosage and routes
Adult: PO 2.5 mg qd initially; may gradually increase to desired response, max 10 mg/day; ophth ĭ gtt bid

Renal dose
Adult: PO CCr >60 ml/min give dose q24h, CCr 20-60 ml/min give dose q48h, CCr <20 ml/min give dose q72h

Available forms: Tabs 2.5, 5 mg

Adverse effects
(*italic* = common; **bold** = life-threatening)
CNS: Dizziness, mental changes, drowsiness, fatigue, headache, catatonia, depression, anxiety, nightmares, paresthesia, lethargy, insomnia, decreased concentration
CV: Orthostatic hypotension, **bradycardia, CHF, chest pain, ventricular dysrhythmias, AV block, peripheral vascular insufficency,** palpitations
EENT: Tinnitus, visual changes, sore throat, double vision, dry, burning eyes
GI: Nausea, vomiting, diarrhea, dry mouth, flatulence, constipation, anorexia
GU: Impotence, dysuria, ejaculatory failure, urinary retention
HEMA: Agranulocytosis, thrombocytopenic purpura (rare)
INTEG: Rash, alopecia, urticaria, pruritus, fever
MISC: Facial swelling, decreased exercise tolerance, weight change, Raynaud's disease, lupuslike syndrome
MS: Joint pain, arthralgia, muscle cramps, pain
RESP: Bronchospasm, dyspnea, wheezing, nasal stuffiness, pharyngitis

---

Contraindications: Hypersensitivity to β-blockers, cardiogenic shock, heart block (2nd or 3rd degree), sinus bradycardia, bronchial asthma

Precautions: Major surgery, pregnancy **C**, lactation, CHF, diabetes mellitus, renal disease, thyroid disease, COPD, well-compensated heart failure, nonallergic bronchospasm

◼ Do Not Confuse:
Ocupress/Ocufen
Carteolol/Carvedilol

Pharmacokinetics

Absorption	80%-90%
Distribution	Unknown; protein binding 23%-30%
Metabolism	Liver to active metabolite
Excretion	Kidneys, unchanged (50%-75%)
Half-life	Carteolol (6-8 hr); metabolite (8-12 hr); ↑ renal disease

Pharmacodynamics

	PO	OPHTH
Onset	Unknown	Unknown
Peak	1-3 hr	Unknown
Duration	Unknown	Unknown

Interactions
Individual drugs
Alcohol, clonidine: ↑ hypotension (large amounts)
Dopamine, DOBUTamine: ↓ CV effect
Insulin: ↑ hypoglycemia
Phenytoin (**IV**), verapamil: ↑ myocardial depression
Thyroid agents: ↓ effectiveness of carteolol
Drug classifications
Amphetamines, anesthetics (general), MAOIs: ↑ hypertension
Antidiabetics, oral: ↑ hypoglycemia
Antihypertensives, nitrates: ↑ hypotension
β$_2$-Agonists, theophyllines: ↓ bronchodilatation
Cardiac glycosides: ↑ bradycardia
NSAIDs: ↓ antihypertensive action
▨ *Herb/drug*
Aconite: ↑ toxicity, death
Astragalus, cola tree: ↑ or ↓ antihypertensive effect
Barberry, betony, black catechu, black cohosh, bloodroot, broom, burdock, cat's claw, dandelion, goldenseal, Irish moss, Jamaican dogwood, kelp, khella, mistletoe, parsley: ↑ antihypertensive effect
Coltsfoot, guarana, khat, licorice: ↓ antihypertensive effect

Lab test interferences
↑ ANA titer, ↑ blood glucose, ↑ BUN, ↑ uric acid, ↑ lipoprotein, ↑ triglyceride

NURSING CONSIDERATIONS
Assessment
• Monitor B/P during beginning treatment, periodically thereafter; pulse q4h; note rate, rhythm, quality: apical/radial pulse before administration; notify prescriber of any significant changes (pulse <50 bpm)
• Monitor blood glucose in those taking insulin, oral antidiabetics, dosage adjustment may be needed
• Check for baselines in renal, liver function tests before therapy begins
• Assess for edema in feet, legs daily; monitor I&O, daily weight; check for jugular vein distention and rales bilaterally, dyspnea (CHF)
• Monitor skin turgor, dryness of mucous membranes for hydration status, especially ᴳelderly

Nursing diagnoses
✓Cardiac output, decreased (uses)
✓Injury, risk for (side effects)
✓Knowledge, deficient (teaching)
✓Noncompliance (teaching)

Implementation
PO route
• Give ac, hs; tab may be crushed or swallowed whole; give with food to prevent GI upset
• Store protected from light, moisture; placed in cool environment

Patient/family education
• Teach patient not to discontinue drug abruptly; taper over 2 wk; may cause precipitate dysrhythmias, hypertension, myocardial ischemia if stopped abruptly
• Teach patient not to use OTC products containing α-adrenergic stimulants (such as nasal decongestants, cold preparations); to avoid alcohol, smoking and to limit sodium intake as prescribed
• Teach patient how to take pulse and B/P at home; advise when to notify prescriber
• Instruct patient to comply with weight control, dietary adjustments, modified exercise program
• Advise patient to carry/wear emergency ID to identify drug being taken, allergies; tell patient drug controls symptoms but does not cure
• Caution patient to avoid hazardous activities if dizziness, drowsiness present
• Teach patient to report symptoms of CHF; difficult breathing, especially on exertion or

when lying down, night cough, swelling of extremities or bradycardia, dizziness, confusion, depression, fever
• Teach patient to take drug as prescribed, not to double doses, skip doses; take any missed doses as soon as remembered if at least 4 hr until next dose

Evaluation
Positive therapeutic outcome
• Decreased B/P in hypertension (after 1-2 wk)

Treatment of overdose: Lavage, **IV** atropine for bradycardia; **IV** theophylline for bronchospasm, digitalis, O_2, diuretic for cardiac failure; **IV** glucose for hypoglycemia; **IV** diazepam (or phenytoin) for seizures

---

carvedilol (Rx)
(kar-veh'dee-lol)
Coreg
Func. class.: Antihypertensive α/β-blocker

Pregnancy category C

Action: A mixture of nonselective β-blocking and α-blocking activity; decreases cardiac output, exercise-induced tachycardia, reflex orthostatic tachycardia; causes reduction in peripheral vascular resistance and vasodilatation

➡ Therapeutic Outcome: Decreased B/P in hypertension

Uses: Essential hypertension alone or in combination with other antihypertensives, CHF

Investigational uses: Angina pectoris, idiopathic cardiomyopathy

Dosage and routes
Essential hypertension
Adult: PO 6.25 mg bid × 7-14 days if tolerated well, then increase to 12.5 mg bid × 7-14 days if tolerated well, may be increased if needed to 25 mg bid, max 50 mg qd

Congestive heart failure
Adult: PO 3.125 mg bid × 2 wk; if well tolerated, give 6.25 mg bid × 2 wk, then double q2wk to max dose 25 mg bid <85 kg or 80 mg bid >85 kg

Angina pectoris
Adult: PO 25-50 mg bid

Idiopathic cardiomyopathy
Adult: PO 6.25-25 mg bid

Available forms: Tabs 3.125, 6.25, 12.5, 25 mg

Adverse effects
(*italic* = common; **bold** = life-threatening)
CNS: *Dizziness,* somnolence, insomnia, ataxia, hyperesthesia, paresthesia, vertigo, depression, fatigue, weakness
CV: *Bradycardia, postural hypotension,* dependent edema, peripheral edema, **AV block, extrasystoles,** hypertension, hypotension, palpitations, peripheral ischemia, **CHF,** pulmonary edema
GI: *Diarrhea,* abdominal pain, ↑ alkaline phosphatase, ↑ ALT/AST
GU: Decreased libido, *impotence*
MISC: Fatigue, injury, back pain, UTI, viral infection, hypertriglyceridemia, **thrombocytopenia,** *hyperglycemia*
RESP: Rhinitis, pharyngitis, dyspnea

Contraindications: Hypersensitivity, bronchial asthma, class IV decompensated cardiac failure, 2nd- or 3rd-degree heart block, cardiogenic shock, severe bradycardia, pulmonary edema

Precautions: Cardiac failure, hepatic injury, peripheral vascular disease, anesthesia, major surgery, diabetes mellitus, thyrotoxicosis, elderly, pregnancy **C**, lactation, children, emphysema, chronic bronchitis, renal disease

▧ Do Not Confuse:
Carvedilol/Captopril/Carteolol

Pharmacokinetics	
Absorption	Readily and extensively absorbed
Distribution	>98% protein binding
Metabolism	Extensively liver
Excretion	Via bile into feces
Half-life	Terminal half-life 7-10 hr, increased in the elderly, hepatic disease

Pharmacodynamics	
Unknown	

Interactions
Individual drugs
Alcohol (acute ingestion), cimetidine: ↑ toxicity
Clonidine: ↓ heart rate, B/P
Digoxin: ↑ concentrations of digoxin
Reserpine: ↑ hypotension, bradycardia
Rifampin: ↓ levels of carvedilol
Drug classifications
Antihypertensives, nitrates: ↑ toxicity
Antidiabetic agents: ↑ hypoglycemia
Calcium channel blockers: ↑ conduction disturbance
MAOIs: ↑ bradycardia, hypotension

NSAIDs, thyroid hormones: ↓ levels of carvedilol

🖉 *Herb/drug*
Aconite: ↑ toxicity, death

Astragalus, cola tree: ↑ or ↓ antihypertensive effect

Barberry, betony, black catechu, black cohosh, bloodroot, broom, burdock, cat's claw, dandelion, goldenseal, Irish moss, Jamaican dogwood, kelp, khella, mistletoe, parsley: ↑ antihypertensive effect

Coltsfoot, guarana, khat, licorice: ↓ antihypertensive effect

NURSING CONSIDERATIONS
Assessment
• Monitor renal studies including protein, BUN, creatinine; watch for increased levels that may indicate nephrotic syndrome; obtain baselines in renal and liver function studies before beginning treatment; if liver function studies are elevated, drug should be discontinued
• Monitor I&O, weight daily
• Monitor B/P during beginning treatment and periodically thereafter, pulse q4h, note rate, rhythm, quality
• Monitor apical/radial pulse before administration; notify prescriber of significant changes, pulse <50 bpm hold drug, notify prescriber
• Assess for edema in feet and legs daily, fluid overload: dyspnea, weight gain, jugular vein distention, fatigue, rales, crackles

Nursing diagnoses
✓ Cardiac output, decreased (uses)
✓ Injury, risk for (adverse reactions)
✓ Knowledge, deficient (teaching)
✓ Noncompliance (teaching)

Implementation
• Give PO ac, hs; tablets may be crushed or swallowed whole, give with food to decrease orthostatic hypotension
• Administer reduced dosage in renal dysfunction

Patient/family education
• Tell patient to comply with dosage schedule even if feeling better, that improvement may take several weeks
• Teach patient to rise slowly to sitting or standing position to minimize orthostatic hypotension
• Encourage patient to report bradycardia, dizziness, confusion, depression, fever, weight gain, shortness of breath, cold extremities, rash, sore throat, bleeding, bruising
• Teach patient to take pulse at home; advise when to notify prescriber
⬩• Encourage patient not to discontinue drug abruptly, taper over 1-2 wk
• Advise patient to avoid hazardous activities until stabilized on medication; dizziness may occur
• Advise patient to avoid all OTC medications unless approved by prescriber
• Advise patient to carry/wear emergency ID with drug name, prescriber at all times
• Advise patient to inform all health care providers of drugs, supplements taken

Evaluation
Positive therapeutic outcome
• Decreased B/P
• Decreased symptoms of CHF or angina

---

cascara sagrada/cascara sagrada aromatic fluid extract/cascara sagrada fluid extract (OTC)
(kas-kar′a)
Func. class.: Laxative
Chem. class.: Anthraquinone
Pregnancy category C

Action: Direct chemical irritation in colon; increases propulsion of stool; increases fluid in colon

➡ **Therapeutic Outcome:** Decreased constipation; removal of bowel contents before surgery or diagnostic tests

Uses: Constipation; bowel or rectal preparation for surgery or examination

Dosage and routes
Adult: PO 325 mg hs; fluid 1 ml qd; aromatic fluid 5 ml qd

P *Child 2-12 yr:* PO/fluid/aromatic fluid ½ adult dose

P *Child < 2 yr:* PO/fluid/aromatic fluid ¼ adult dose

Available forms: Tabs 325 mg; fluid extract 1 g/ml; aromatic fluid extract 1 g/ml

Adverse effects
(*italic* = common; **bold** = life-threatening)
GI: *Nausea, vomiting, anorexia, cramps, diarrhea*
META: Hypocalcemia, enteropathy, alkalosis, hypokalemia, **tetany**

Contraindications: Hypersensitivity, GI bleeding, obstruction, CHF, lactation, abdominal pain, nausea/vomiting, appendicitis, acute surgical abdomen, alcoholics (aromatic fluid extract)

Precautions: Pregnancy **C**

Pharmacokinetics

Absorption	Minimal
Distribution	Unknown
Metabolism	Liver, minimally
Excretion	Kidneys, feces, breast milk
Half-life	Not known

Pharmacodynamics

Onset	Unknown
Peak	6-12 hr
Duration	Unknown

Interactions
Individual drugs
Digitalis, nitrofurantoin: ↓ absorption
Drug classifications
Antibiotics, oral anticoagulants, salicylates, tetracyclines: ↓ absorption
☑ *Herb/drug*
Flax, lily of the valley, pheasant's eye, senna, squill: ↑ action, side effects

NURSING CONSIDERATIONS
Assessment
• Monitor blood, urine electrolytes if drug used often by patient; check I&O ratio to identify fluid loss
• Assess cramping, rectal bleeding, nausea, vomiting; if these symptoms occur, drug should be discontinued; identify cause of constipation; identify whether fluids, bulk, or exercise is missing from lifestyle

Nursing diagnoses
☑ Constipation (uses)
☑ Diarrhea
☑ Knowledge, deficient (teaching)
☑ Noncompliance (teaching)

Implementation
• Give alone with water only for better absorption; do not administer with food; do not take within 1 hr of antacids, milk, or cimetidine
☒ • Do not crush; swallow tabs whole
• Give in AM or PM (oral dose); evacuation will occur 6-12 hr later

Patient/family education
• Discuss with the patient that adequate fluid consumption is necessary
• Teach patient that normal bowel movements do not always occur daily
• Teach patient not to use in presence of abdominal pain, nausea, vomiting; tell patient to notify prescriber if constipation unrelieved or if symptoms of electrolyte imbalance occur: muscle cramps, pain, weakness, dizziness, excessive thirst

Evaluation
Positive therapeutic outcome
• Decreased constipation in 6-12 hr
• Removal of bowel contents

---

cefaclor
See cephalosporins—2nd generation
cefadroxil
See cephalosporins—1st generation
cefamandole
See cephalosporins—2nd generation
cefazolin
See cephalosporins—1st generation
cefdinir
See cephalosporins—3rd generation
cefditoren pivoxil
See cephalosporins—2nd generation
cefepime
cefixime
See cephalosporins—3rd generation
cefmetazole
cefonicid
See cephalosporins—2nd generation
cefoperazone
cefotaxime
See cephalosporins—3rd generation
cefotetan
cefoxitin
See cephalosporins—2nd generation
cefpodoxime
See cephalosporins—3rd generation
cefprozil
See cephalosporins—2nd generation
ceftazidime
ceftibuten
ceftizoxime
ceftriaxone
See cephalosporins—3rd generation
cefuroxime
See cephalosporins—2nd generation
cephalexin
See cephalosporins—1st generation

☑ Herb/drug   ☒ Do Not Crush   ◆ Alert   ☛ Key Drug   **G** Geriatric   **P** Pediatric

! HIGH ALERT

celecoxib (Rx)
(cel-eh-cox'ib)
Celebrex
Func. class.: Nonsteroidal antiinflammatory, antirheumatic
Chem. class.: COX-2 inhibitor

Pregnancy category C

Action: Inhibits prostaglandin synthesis by decreasing enzyme needed for biosynthesis; analgesic, antiinflammatory, antipyretic properties

⇒ **Therapeutic Outcome:** Decreased pain, inflammation

Uses: Acute, chronic rheumatoid arthritis, osteoarthritis, familial adenomatous polyposis (FAP), acute pain, primary dysmenorrhea

Investigational uses: Colorectal polyps

Dosage and routes
Do not exceed recommended dose, deaths have occurred

Acute pain/primary dysmenorrhea
Adult: PO 400 mg initially, then 200 mg on 1st day, then 200 mg bid prn on subsequent days, if needed

Osteoarthritis
Adult: PO 200 mg/day as a single dose or 100 mg bid

Rheumatoid arthritis
Adult: PO 100-200 mg bid

FAP
Adult: PO 400 mg bid

Colorectal polyps
Adult: PO 400 mg bid × 6 mo

Hepatic dose
(Child-Pugh class II)
Adult: PO reduce dose by 50%

Available forms: Caps 100, 200 mg

Adverse effects
(*italic* = common; **bold** = life-threatening)
CNS: Fatigue, anxiety, depression, nervousness, paresthesia, dizziness, insomnia
CV: **Stroke, MI, tachycardia,** angina, palpitations, dysrhythmias, hypertension, fluid retention
EENT: Tinnitus, hearing loss, blurred vision, glaucoma, cataract, conjunctivitis, eye pain
GI: Nausea, anorexia, vomiting, constipation, dry mouth, diverticulitis, gastritis, gastroenteritis, hemorrhoids, hiatal hernia, stomatitis, **GI bleeding**

GU: **Nephrotoxicity: dysuria, hematuria, oliguria, azotemia, cystitis, UTI**
HEMA: Blood dyscrasias, epistaxis, bruising, anemia
INTEG: Purpura, rash, pruritus, sweating, erythema, petechiae, photosensitivity, alopecia, **serious sometimes fatal Stevens-Johnson syndrome, toxic epidermal necrolysis**
RESP: Pharyngitis, shortness of breath, pneumonia, coughing

Contraindications: Hypersensitivity to aspirin, iodides, other NSAIDs, sulfonamides, 3rd trimester of pregnancy, asthma

Precautions: Pregnancy **C**, renal, hepatic, hypertension, severe dehydration, children <18 yr, lactation, bleeding, GI, cardiac disorders, hypersensitivity to other antiinflammatories, glucocorticoids, anticoagulants, elderly

Do Not Confuse:
Celebrex/Celexa/Cerebra/Cerebyx

Pharmacokinetics
Absorption	Well absorbed (PO)
Distribution	Crosses placenta, bound to plasma proteins
Metabolism	Liver
Excretion	Kidneys
Half-life	Unknown

Pharmacodynamics
Onset	Unknown
Peak	3 hr
Duration	Unknown

Interactions
Individual drugs
Aspirin: ↓ effectiveness, ↑ adverse reactions
Fluconazole: ↑ celecoxib level
Furosemide: ↓ effect of furosemide
Lithium: ↑ toxicity
Warfarin: ↑ anticoagulant effects
Drug classifications
ACE inhibitors: may ↓ effects of ACE inhibitors
Anticoagulants: ↑ risk of bleeding
Antineoplastics: ↑ risk of hematologic toxicity
Glucocorticoids, NSAIDs: ↑ adverse reactions
Thiazide diuretics: ↓ effectiveness of diuretics
Herb/drug
Arginine, gossypol: ↑ gastric irritation
Bearberry, bilberry: ↑ NSAID effect
Bogbean, chondroitin: ↑ bleeding risk

NURSING CONSIDERATIONS
Assessment
• Assess for pain of rheumatoid arthritis, osteoarthritis; check ROM, inflammation of joints, characteristics of pain

• Monitor blood counts during therapy; watch for decreasing platelets; if low, therapy may need to be discontinued, restarted after hematologic recovery; and for blood dyscrasias (thrombocytopenia): bruising, fatigue, bleeding, poor healing
• Assess FAP patient for decreasing number of polyps

Nursing diagnoses
☑ Pain (uses)
☑ Mobility, impaired physical (uses)
☑ Injury, risk for (side effects)
☑ Knowledge, deficient (teaching)

Implementation
PO route
• Administer with food or milk to decrease gastric symptoms
🚫 • Do not crush, dissolve, or chew caps; do not ↑ dose

Patient/family education
• Do not exceed recommended dose; notify prescriber immediately of chest pain, skin eruptions, stop drug
• Teach patient that drug must be continued for prescribed time to be effective; to avoid other NSAIDs, sulfonamides
• Caution patient to report bleeding, bruising, fatigue, malaise, since blood dyscrasias do occur; to report GI symptoms: black tarry stools, cramping
• Teach patient to take with a full glass of
🚫 water to enhance absorption; do not crush, break, or chew
• Teach patient to check with prescriber to determine when drug should be discontinued before surgery; advise patient to notify prescriber if pregnancy is planned or suspected

Evaluation
Positive therapeutic outcome
• Decreased pain in arthritic conditions
• Decreased inflammation in arthritic conditions
• Decreased number of polyps (FAP)

CEPHALOSPORINS—1ST GENERATION

cefadroxil (Rx)
(sef-a-drox′ill)
cefadroxil, Duricef
cefazolin (Rx)
(sef-a′zoe-lin)
Ancef, cefazolin, Kefzol
cephalexin (Rx)
(sef-a-lex′in)
Apo-Cephalex*, Biocef, cephalexin, Keflex, Keftab, Novo-Lexin*, Nu-Cephalex*
cephapirin (Rx)
(sef-a-pye′rin)
Cefadyl, cephapirin
cephradine (Rx)
(sef′ra-deen)
cephradine, Velosef
Func. class.: Antiinfective
Chem. class.: Cephalosporin (1st generation)

Action: Inhibits bacterial cell wall synthesis, rendering cell wall osmotically unstable, leading to cell death by binding to cell wall membrane

cefadroxil
➡ **Therapeutic Outcome:** Bactericidal effects for the following: gram-negative bacilli *Escherichia coli, Proteus mirabilis, Klebsiella* (UTI only); gram-positive organisms *Streptococcus pneumoniae, Streptococcus pyogenes, Staphylococcus aureus*

Uses: Upper, lower respiratory tract, urinary tract, skin infections; otitis media; tonsillitis, pharyngitis; particularly for UTI

cefazolin
➡ **Therapeutic Outcome:** Bactericidal effects for the following: gram-negative organisms *Enterobacter* sp., *Haemophilus influenzae, Escherichia coli, Proteus mirabilis, Klebsiella;* gram-positive organisms *Streptococcus pneumoniae, Streptococcus pyogenes, Staphylococcus aureus*

Uses: Upper, lower respiratory tract, urinary tract, skin infections; bone, joint, biliary, genital infections; endocarditis, surgical prophylaxis, septicemia

cephalexin
➡ **Therapeutic Outcome:** Bactericidal effects for the following: gram-negative organisms *Haemophilus influenzae, Escherichia coli, Proteus mirabilis, Klebsiella;* gram-

---

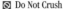 Herb/drug   🚫 Do Not Crush   ◆ Alert   ⊶ Key Drug   **G** Geriatric   **P** Pediatric

positive organisms *Streptococcus pneumoniae, Streptococcus pyogenes, Staphylococcus aureus*

Uses: Upper, lower respiratory tract, urinary tract, skin, bone infections; otitis media

cephapirin
⮞ **Therapeutic Outcome:** Bactericidal effects for the following: gram-negative bacilli *Haemophilus influenzae, Escherichia coli, Proteus mirabilis, Klebsiella;* gram-positive organisms *Streptococcus pneumoniae, Streptococcus viridans, Staphylococcus aureus*

Uses: Lower respiratory tract, urinary tract, skin infections; septicemia, endocarditis, bacterial peritonitis

cephradine
⮞ **Therapeutic Outcome:** Bactericidal effects for the following: gram-negative bacilli *Haemophilus influenzae, Escherichia coli, Proteus mirabilis, Klebsiella;* gram-positive organisms *Streptococcus pneumoniae, Streptococcus pyogenes, Staphylococcus aureus*

Uses: Serious respiratory tract, urinary tract, skin infections; otitis media

Dosage and routes
cefadroxil
Adult: PO 1-2 g qd or q12h in divided doses, give a loading dose of 1 g initially

🅟 *Child:* PO 30 mg/kg/day in divided doses bid

Renal dose:
Adult: PO CCr 25-50 ml/min, 500 mg q12h; CCr 10-24 ml/min 500 mg q24h, CCr <10 ml/min 500 mg q36h

Available forms: Caps 500 mg; tabs 1 g; oral susp 125, 250, 500 mg/5 ml

cefazolin
Life-threatening infections
Adult: IM/**IV** 1-2 g q6h

🅟 *Child >1 mo:* IM/**IV** 100 mg/kg in 3-4 divided doses

Mild/moderate infections
Adult: IM/**IV** 250 mg-1 g q8h

🅟 *Child >1 mo:* IM/**IV** 25-50 mg/kg in 3-4 equal doses

Renal dose
CCr 35-54 ml/min 250-1000 mg q12h; CCr 10-34 ml/min 125-500 mg q12h; CCr <10 ml/min 125-500 mg q18-24h

Available forms: Inj 250, 500 mg, 1, 5, 10, 20 g; infusion 500 mg, 1 g/50 ml vial

cephalexin
Renal dose
CCr <40 ml/min q8-12h; CCr 5-10 ml/min q12h; CCr <5 ml/min q24h

Moderate infections
Adult: PO 250-500 mg q6h

🅟 *Child:* PO 25-50 mg/kg/day in 4 equal doses

Moderate skin infections
Adult: PO 500 mg q12h

Endocarditis prophylaxis: 2 g 1 hr before procedure

Severe infections
Adult: PO 500 mg-1 g q6h

🅟 *Child:* PO 50-100 mg/kg/day in 4 equal doses

Available forms: Caps 250, 500 mg; tabs 250, 500 mg, 1 g; oral susp 125, 250 mg/5 ml

cephapirin
Adult: IM/**IV** 500 mg-1 g q4-6h

🅟 *Child:* IM/**IV** 40-80 mg/kg/day in divided doses q6h or 10-20 mg/kg q6h

Renal dose
CCr <10 ml/min give q12h

Available forms: Powder for inj 500 mg, 1, 2, 20 g; **IV** only 1, 2, 4 g

cephradine
Adult: PO 250 mg-1 g q6-12h

🅟 *Child >1 yr:* PO 6-12 mg/kg q6h

Renal dose
CCr >20 ml/min 500 mg q6h; CCr 5-20 ml/min 250 mg q6h

Available forms: Caps 250, 500 mg; oral susp 125, 250 mg/5 ml

Side effects/adverse reactions
(*italic* = common; **bold** = life-threatening)
CNS: Headache, dizziness, weakness, paresthesia, fever, chills, **seizures** (high doses)
GI: Nausea, vomiting, *diarrhea, anorexia,* pain, glossitis, bleeding; increased AST, ALT, bilirubin, LDH, alkaline phosphatase; abdominal pain, **pseudomembranous colitis**
GU: Proteinuria, vaginitis, pruritus, candidiasis, increased BUN, **nephrotoxicity, renal failure**
HEMA: Leukopenia, thrombocytopenia, agranulocytosis, anemia, neutropenia, lymphocytosis, eosinophilia, pancytopenia, hemolytic anemia
INTEG: Rash, urticaria, dermatitis
RESP: Dyspnea
SYST: Anaphylaxis, serum sickness, superinfection

Contraindications: Hypersensitivity to
P cephalosporins, infants <1 mo

Precautions: Hypersensitivity to penicillins,
pregnancy **B,** lactation, renal disease

N Do Not Confuse:
cephalexin/cefaclor, cephapirin/cephradine,
Kefzol/Cefzil

cefadroxil

Pharmacokinetics

Absorption	Well absorbed
Distribution	Widely distributed; crosses placenta
Metabolism	Not metabolized
Excretion	Unchanged by kidneys; enters breast milk
Half-life	1½-2 hr

Pharmacodynamics

	PO
Onset	Rapid
Peak	1½-2 hr
Duration	12-24 hr

cefazolin

Pharmacokinetics

Absorption	Well absorbed
Distribution	Widely distributed; crosses placenta
Metabolism	Not metabolized
Excretion	Unchanged by kidneys; enters breast milk
Half-life	1½-2½ hr

Pharmacodynamics

	IM	IV
Onset	Rapid	10 min
Peak	1-2 hr	Infusion's end
Duration	6-12 hr	

cephalexin

Pharmacokinetics

Absorption	Well absorbed
Distribution	Widely distributed; crosses placenta
Metabolism	Not metabolized
Excretion	Kidneys, unchanged; enters breast milk
Half-life	½-1 hr; increased in renal disease

Pharmacodynamics

Onset	15-30 min
Peak	1 hr
Duration	6-12 hr

cephapirin

Pharmacokinetics

Absorption	Well absorbed
Distribution	Widely distributed; crosses placenta
Metabolism	Not metabolized
Excretion	Kidneys, unchanged; enters breast milk
Half-life	½-1 hr

Pharmacodynamics

	IM	IV
Onset	Rapid	Immediate
Peak	½ hr	Infusion's end
Duration	4-6 hr	

cephradine

Pharmacokinetics

Absorption	Well absorbed
Distribution	Widely distributed; crosses placenta
Metabolism	Not metabolized
Excretion	Kidneys, unchanged; enters breast milk
Half-life	1-2 hr

Pharmacodynamics

	PO/IM	IV
Onset	Rapid	Immediate
Peak	1-2 hr	Infusion's end
Duration	6-12 hr	

Interactions
Individual drugs
Probenecid, vancomycin: ↑ toxicity
Drug classifications
Aminoglycosides, diuretics (loop), oral
contraceptives: ↑ toxicity
Herb/drug
Acidophilus: Do not use with antiinfectives
Lab test interferences
False positive: Urinary protein, direct
Coombs' test, urine glucose
Interference: Cross-matching
↑ AST, ↑ ALT, ↑ alkaline phosphatase, ↑ LDH,
↑ BUN, ↑ creatinine, ↑ bilirubin

NURSING CONSIDERATIONS
Assessment
• Assess patient for previous sensitivity reaction to penicillins or other cephalosporins;
cross-sensitivity between penicillins and
cephalosporins is common
• Assess patient for signs and symptoms of
infection including characteristics of wounds,

sputum, urine, stool, WBC >10,000/mm³, earache, fever; obtain baseline information and during treatment

• Obtain C&S before beginning drug therapy to identify if correct treatment has been initiated

• Assess for anaphylaxis: rash, urticaria, pruritus, chills, fever, joint pain; angioedema may occur a few days after therapy begins; epINEPHrine and resuscitation equipment should be available for anaphylactic reaction

• Identify urine output; if decreasing, notify prescriber (may indicate nephrotoxicity); also check for increased BUN, creatinine

• Monitor blood studies: AST, ALT, CBC, Hct, bilirubin, LDH, alkaline phosphatase, Coombs' test monthly if patient is on long-term therapy

• Monitor electrolytes: potassium, sodium, chloride monthly if patient is on long-term therapy

• Assess bowel pattern qd; if severe diarrhea occurs, drug should be discontinued; may indicate pseudomembranous colitis

• Monitor for bleeding: ecchymosis, bleeding gums, hematuria, stool guaiac daily if on long-term therapy

• Assess for superinfection: perineal itching, fever, malaise, redness, pain, swelling, drainage, rash, diarrhea, change in cough, sputum

Nursing diagnoses
✓ Infection, risk for (uses)
✓ Diarrhea (side effects)
✓ Fluid volume, risk for deficient (side effects)
✓ Injury, risk for (side effects)
✓ Knowledge, deficient (teaching)
✓ Noncompliance (teaching)

cefadroxil
Implementation
• Give in even doses around the clock; if GI upset occurs, give with food; drug must be given for 10-14 days to ensure organism death and prevent superinfection

• Shake susp, refrigerate, discard after 2 wk

cefazolin
Implementation
IM route
• Reconstitute 250-500 mg of drug with 2 ml sterile or bacteriostatic water for inj, or 0.9% NaCl; reconstitute 1 g of drug with 2.5 ml; give deep in large muscle mass, massage

IV route
• Check for irritation, extravasation, phlebitis daily, change site q72h

• For direct **IV** dilute in 10 ml of sterile water for inj; give over 5 min

• For intermittent inf dilute reconstituted sol

(500 mg or 1 mg) in 50-100 ml D₅W, D₁₀W, D₅/0.25% NaCl, D₅/0.45% NaCl, D₅/0.9% NaCl, D₅/LR, or LR, 0.9% NaCl; give over 30-60 min; may be refrigerated up to 96 hr or stored 24 hr at room temp

Syringe compatibilities: Heparin, vit B complex

Syringe incompatibilities: Ascorbic acid inj, cimetidine, lidocaine, vit B/C

Y-site compatibilities: Acyclovir, allopurinol, amifostine, atracurium, aztreonam, calcium gluconate, cyclophosphamide, diltiazem, enalaprilat, esmolol, famotidine, filgrastim, fluconazole, fludarabine, foscarnet, heparin, labetalol, lidocaine, magnesium sulfate, melphalan, meperidine, midazolam, morphine, multivitamins, ondansetron, perphenazine, pancuronium, regular insulin, sargramostim, tacrolimus, teniposide, theophylline, thiotepa, vecuronium, vit B/C

Y-site incompatibilities: Amiodarone, hetastarch, hydromorphone, idarubicin, vinorelbine tartrate

Additive compatibilities: Aztreonam, clindamycin, famotidine, fluconazole, metronidazole, verapamil

Additive incompatibilities: Amikacin, amobarbital, bleomycin, calcium gluceptate, calcium gluconate, colistimethate, erythromycin, kanamycin, oxytetracycline, pentobarbital, polymyxin B, tetracycline

cephalexin
Implementation
⊘ • Advise not to crush or chew caps
• Give in even doses around the clock; if GI upset occurs, give with food; drug must be taken for 10-14 days to ensure organism death and prevent superinfection

• Shake susp, refrigerate, discard after 2 wk

cephapirin
Implementation
IM route
• Reconstitute 1-2 g/1-2 ml of sterile water for inj; give deep in large muscle mass and massage

IV route
• Check for irritation, extravasation, phlebitis daily; change site q72h

• For intermittent inf, reconstitute 250 mg/2.4 ml, 500 mg/4.8 ml, 1 g/9.6 ml, 2 g/19.2 ml sterile water for inj, D₅W, 0.9% NaCl; do not use sol with benzyl alcohol for neonates; may be further diluted in 50-100 ml D₅W, D₁₀W, 0.9% NaCl, or LR; give over 30-60 min

• Store refrigerated 96 hr, room temp 24 hr

Y-site compatibilities: Acyclovir, cyclophosphamide, famotidine, heparin, hydrocortisone, hydromorphone, magnesium sulfate, meperidine, morphine, multivitamins, perphenazine, potassium chloride, vit B/C

Additive compatibilities: Bleomycin, calcium chloride, calcium gluconate, chloramphenicol, diphenhydrAMINE, ergonovine maleate, heparin, hydrocortisone, metaraminol, oxacillin, penicillin G potassium, pentobarbital, phenobarbital, phytonadione, potassium chloride, sodium bicarbonate, succinylcholine, verapamil, warfarin, vit B complex

Additive incompatibilities: Aminoglycosides, amikacin, ascorbic acid, epINEPHrine, gentamicin, kanamycin, mannitol, norepinephrine, oxytetracycline, phenytoin, tetracycline, thiopental

cephradine
Implementation
PO route
• May be given with food for GI symptoms
• When giving susp, shake well; refrigerate unused portion
IM route
• Reconstitute 250 mg/1.2 ml, 500 mg/ml, 1 g/4 ml sterile or bacteriostatic water for inj; give deep in large muscle mass, massage
IV **IV route**
• Check for irritation, extravasation, phlebitis daily; change site q72h
• For direct **IV** route, reconstitute 250-500 mg/5 ml sterile water, 0.9% NaCl, D_5W, or 1 g/10 ml, 2 g/20 ml; give over 3-5 min
• For intermittent inf, dilute 1 g/10 ml or more sterile water for inj, D_5W, $D_{10}W$, or D_5/0.9% NaCl; give over 30-60 min
• Store refrigerated 96 hr, room temp 24 hr

Additive incompatibilities: Other antibiotics, calcium salts, D_5W, epINEPHrine, lidocaine, Ringer's or LR sol, NormosolR, 0.9% NaCl, TPN #61, tetracycline

Patient/family education
• Teach patient to report sore throat, bruising, bleeding, joint pain; may indicate blood dyscrasias (rare)
• Advise patient to contact prescriber if vaginal itching, loose foul-smelling stools, furry tongue occur; may indicate superinfection
• Instruct patient to take all medication prescribed for the length of time ordered
• Advise patient to notify prescriber of diarrhea with blood, pus, mucus, which may indicate pseudomembranous colitis

Evaluation
Positive therapeutic outcome
• Absence of signs/symptoms of infection (WBC <10,000/mm³, temp WNL, absence of red draining wounds, earache)
• Reported improvement in symptoms of infection
• Negative C&S

Treatment of anaphylaxis: Epinephrine, antihistamines, resuscitate if needed

---

CEPHALOSPORINS—2ND GENERATION

cefaclor (Rx)
(sef'a-klor)
Ceclor
cefamandole (Rx)
(sef-a-man'dole)
Mandol
cefditoren pivoxil (Rx)
(sef-dit'oh-ren pih-vox'il)
Spectracef
cefmetazole (Rx)
(sef-met'a-zole)
Zefazone
cefonicid (Rx)
(se-fon'i-sid)
Monocid
cefotetan (Rx)
(sef'oh-tee-tan)
Cefotan
cefoxitin (Rx)
(se-fox'i-tin)
Mefoxin
cefprozil (Rx)
(sef-proe'zill)
Cefzil
cefuroxime (Rx)
(sef-yoor-ox'eem)
Ceftin, Cefuroxime, Kefurox, Zinacef
loracarbef (Rx)
(lor-a-kar'beff)
Lorabid
Func. class.: Antiinfective
Chem. class.: Cephalosporin (2nd generation)

Action: Inhibits bacterial cell wall synthesis, rendering cell wall osmotically unstable, leading to cell death by binding to cell wall membrane

---

cefaclor

➡ **Therapeutic Outcome:** Bactericidal effects for the following: gram-negative bacilli *Haemophilus influenzae, Escherichia coli, Proteus mirabilis, Klebsiella;* gram-positive organisms *Streptococcus pneumoniae, Staphylococcus* β-hemolytic; streptococci, anaerobes, *Bacteroides* sp.

Uses: Upper and lower respiratory tract, urinary tract, skin infections; otitis media; increased bone, joint, gynecologic infections; septicemia

cefamandole

➡ **Therapeutic Outcome:** Bactericidal effects for the following: anaerobes *Bacteroides* sp., *Clostridium* sp., *Fusobacterium* sp., *Peptococcus* sp., *Peptostreptococcus* sp.; gram negative organisms *Haemophilus influenzae, Escherichia coli, Proteus mirabilis, Klebsiella;* gram-positive organisms *Streptococcus pneumoniae, Streptococcus pyogenes, Staphylococcus aureus; Enterobacter* sp., *Morganella morganii, Proteus vulgaris, Providencia rettgeri*

Uses: Upper, lower respiratory tract, urinary tract, skin infections; peritonitis, septicemia, surgical prophylaxis

cefditoren pivoxil

➡ **Therapeutic Outcome:** Acute bacterial exacerbation of chronic bronchitis caused by *Haemophilus influenzae, Haemophilus parainfluenzae, Streptococcus pneumoniae, Moraxella catarrhalis;* pharyngitis/tonsillitis caused by *Streptococcus pyogenes;* uncomplicated skin, skin structure infections caused by *Staphylococcus aureus, S. pyogenes*

cefmetazole

➡ **Therapeutic Outcome:** Bactericidal effects for the following: anaerobes, *Clostridium, Bacteroides* sp., *Fusobacterium* sp.; gram-negative organisms *Morganella morganii, Haemophilus influenzae, Escherichia coli, Proteus, Klebsiella, Bacteroides fragilis;* gram-positive organisms *Streptococcus pneumoniae, Streptococcus pyogenes, Staphylococcus aureus*

Uses: Infections of lower respiratory tract, urinary tract, skin, bone; intraabdominal infections

cefonicid

➡ **Therapeutic Outcome:** Bactericidal effects for the following: gram-negative organ-isms *Morganella morganii, Proteus vulgaris, Providencia rettgeri, Haemophilus influenzae, Escherichia coli, Proteus mirabilis, Klebsiella;* gram-positive organisms *Streptococcus pneumoniae, Streptococcus pyogenes, Staphylococcus aureus*

Uses: Lower respiratory tract, urinary tract, skin, bone, joint infections; otitis media, peritonitis, septicemia, preoperative prophylaxis

cefotetan

➡ **Therapeutic Outcome:** Bactericidal effects for the following: gram-negative organ-isms *Haemophilus influenzae, Escherichia coli, Enterobacter aerogenes, Proteus mirabilis, Klebsiella, Morganella morganii, Proteus vulgaris, Providencia, Enterobacter, Salmonella, Shigella, Acinetobacter, Bacteroides fragilis, Neisseria, Serratia;* gram-positive organisms *Streptococcus pneumoniae, Streptococcus pyogenes, Staphylococcus aureus;* anaerobes *Bacteroides, Clostridium, Fusobacterium, Peptococcus, Peptostreptococcus*

Uses: Serious upper or lower respiratory tract, urinary tract, gynecologic, skin, bone, joint, gonococcal, intraabdominal infections

cefoxitin

➡ **Therapeutic Outcome:** Bactericidal effects for the following: gram-negative bacilli *Haemophilus influenzae, Escherichia coli, Proteus, Klebsiella, Providencia, Neisseria gonorrhoeae;* gram-positive organisms *Streptococcus pneumoniae, Streptococcus pyogenes, Staphylococcus aureus;* anaerobes including *Clostridium, Bacteroides, Peptococcus, Peptostreptococcus*

Uses: Lower respiratory tract, urinary tract, skin, bone, gynecologic, gonococcal infections; septicemia, peritonitis

cefprozil

➡ **Therapeutic Outcome:** Bactericidal effects for the following: gram-negative bacilli *Haemophilus influenzae, Escherichia coli;* gram-positive organisms *Streptococcus pneumoniae, Streptococcus pyogenes, Staphylococcus aureus*

Uses: Upper and lower respiratory tract, urinary tract, skin infections; otitis media

loracarbef

➡ **Therapeutic Outcome:** Bactericidal effects for the following: gram-negative organ-isms *Haemophilus influenzae, Escherichia*

C

coli, Proteus mirabilis, Klebsiella; gram-positive organisms *Streptococcus pneumoniae, Streptococcus pyogenes, Staphyloccus aureus*

Uses: Upper and lower respiratory tract, urinary tract, skin infections; otitis media, pharyngitis, tonsillitis

Dosage and routes
cefaclor
Adult: PO 250-500 mg q8h, not to exceed 4 g/day or 375-500 mg (ext rel) q12h × 7-10 days

 Child >1 mo: PO 20-40 mg/kg qd in divided doses q8h, or total daily dose may be divided and given q12h, not to exceed 1 g/day

Acute bacterial exacerbations of chronic bronchitis or acute bronchitis
Adult: 500 mg/12 hr × 1 wk (ext rel)

Pharyngitis/tonsillitis
Adult: 375 mg/12 hr × 10 days (ext rel)

Available forms: Caps 250, 500 mg; oral susp 125, 187, 250, 375 mg/5 ml; tabs, ext rel 375, 500 mg

cefamandole
Adult: IM/**IV** 500 mg-1 g q4-8h; may give up to 2 g q4h for severe infections

 Child >1 mo: IM/**IV** 8.3-16.7 mg/kg q4h, not to exceed adult dose

Renal dose
Dosage reduction indicated in renal impairment (CCr <50 ml/min)

Available forms: Inj 1, 2, 10 g

cefditoren pivoxil
Acute bacterial exacerbation of chronic bronchitis
Adult: PO 400 mg bid × 10 days

Pharyngitis/tonsillitis
Adult: PO 200 mg bid × 10 days

Uncomplicated skin, skin structure infections
Adult: PO 200 mg bid × 10 days

Renal dose
Adult: PO CCr 30-49 ml/min ≤200 mg bid × 10 days; CCr <30 ml/min give 200 mg qd × 10 days

Available forms:
Tabs 200 mg

cefmetazole
Adult: **IV** 2 g divided q6-12h × 5-14 days

Renal dose
CCr <50 ml/min 1-2 g q12h; CCr 10-29 ml/min 1-2 g q24-48h; CCr <10 ml/min 1-2 g q48hr

Available forms:
Powder for inj 1, 2 g/vial

cefonicid
Life-threatening infections

Adult: IM/**IV** bol or inf 0.5-2 g/24 hr; divide in two doses if giving 2 g

• Dosage reduction indicated in renal impairment

Available forms: Inj 500 mg, 1, 10 g

cefotetan
Adult: **IV**/IM 1-2 g q12h × 5-10 days

Renal dose
CCr 10-30 ml/min q24h; CCr <10 ml/min q48h

Perioperative proplylaxis
Adult: **IV** 1-2 g ½-1 hr before surgery

Available forms: Inj 1, 2, 10 g

cefoxitin
Adult: IM/**IV** 1-2 g q6-8h

Renal dose
CCr <50 ml/min q8-12h; CCr 10-29 ml/min q24h; CCr <10 ml/min q24-48h

• Uncomplicated gonorrhea 2 g IM as single dose with 1 g PO probenecid at same time

Severe infections
Adult: IM/**IV** 2 g q4h

 Child ≥3 mo: IM/**IV** 80-160 mg/kg/day divided q4-6h; max 12 g/day

Available forms: Powder for inj 1, 2, 10 g

cefprozil
Renal dose
CCr <30 ml/min 50% of dose

Upper respiratory infections
Adult: PO 500 mg q24h × 10 days

Otitis media
 Child 6 mo-12 yr: PO 15 mg/kg q12h × 10 days

Lower respiratory infections
Adult: PO 500 mg q12h × 10 days

Skin/skin structure infections
Adult: PO 250-500 mg q12h × 10 days

Available forms: Tabs 250, 500 mg; susp 125, 250 mg/5 ml *cefuroxime*

🅟 *Adult and child:* PO 250 mg q12h; may increase to 500 mg of q12h in serious infections

Adult: IM/**IV** 750 mg-1.5 g q8h for 5-10 days

Urinary tract infections
Adult: PO 125 mg q12h; may increase to 250 mg q12h if needed

Otitis media
🅟 *Child <2 yr:* PO 125 mg bid
🅟 *Child >2 yr:* PO 250 mg bid

Surgical prophylaxis
Adult: **IV** 1.5 g ½-1 hr preop

Severe infections
Adult: IM/**IV** 1.5 g q6h; may give up to 3 g q8h for bacterial meningitis

🅟 *Child >3 mo:* IM/**IV** 50-100 mg/kg/day; may give up to 200-240 mg/kg/day **IV** in divided doses for bacterial meningitis (not recommended)
• Dosage reduction indicated in severe renal impairment (CCr <20 ml/min)

Uncomplicated gonorrhea
Adult: 1.5 g IM as single dose with oral probenecid in 2 separate sites

Available forms: Tabs 125, 250, 500 mg: inj 150, 750 mg, 1.5, 7.5 g; inj 750 mg; 1.5 g powder, susp 125, 250 mg/5 ml

loracarbef
🅟 *Adult and child >13 yr:* PO 200-400 mg q12h

🅟 *Child to 12 yr:* PO 15-30 mg/kg/day in 2 divided doses q12h

Renal dose
CCr 10-49 ml/min 50% of dose; CCr <10 ml/min q3-5 days

Available forms: Caps 200, 400 mg; Oral susp 100, 200 mg/5 ml

Side effects/adverse reactions
(*italic* = common; **bold** = life-threatening)
CNS: Dizziness, headache, fatigue, paresthesia, fever, chills, confusion
GI: Diarrhea, nausea, vomiting, anorexia, dysgeusia, glossitis, bleeding; increased AST, ALT, bilirubin, LDH, alkaline phosphatase; abdominal pain, loose stools, flatulence, heartburn, stomach cramps, colitis, jaundice, **pseudomembranous colitis**
GU: Vaginitis, pruritus, candidiasis, increased BUN, **nephrotoxicity, renal failure,** pyuria, dysuria, reversible interstitial nephritis
HEMA: **Leukopenia, thrombocytopenia,** **agranulocytosis,** anemia, **neutropenia, lymphocytosis, eosinophilia, pancytopenia, hemolytic anemia, leukocytosis, granulocytopenia**
INTEG: Rash, urticaria, dermatitis, **Stevens-Johnson syndrome**
RESP: Dyspnea
SYST: **Anaphylaxis, serum sickness,** superinfection

Contraindications: Hypersensitivity to cephalosporins or related antibiotics, seizures

Precautions: Pregnancy **B,** lactation,
🅟 children, renal disease

◪ **Do Not Confuse:**
cefaclor/cephalexin, Cefotan/Ceftin, cefprozil/cefazolin, cefprozil/cefuroxime, Cefzil/Ceftin, Cefzil/Kefzol

cefaclor

Pharmacokinetics	
Absorption	Well absorbed
Distribution	Widely distributed; crosses placenta
Metabolism	Not metabolized
Excretion	Unchanged by kidneys (60%-80%); enters breast milk
Half-life	36-54 min; increased in renal disease

Pharmacodynamics	
Onset	15 min
Peak	½-1 hr

cefamandole

Pharmacokinetics	
Absorption	Well absorbed
Distribution	Widely distributed; crosses placenta
Metabolism	Not metabolized
Excretion	Unchanged by kidneys (60%-80%); enters breast milk
Half-life	½ to 1½ hr

Pharmacodynamics		
	IM	IV
Onset	Rapid	Immediate
Peak	½-2 hr	Infusion's end

C

cefditoren pivoxil

Pharmacokinetics

Absorption	Unknown
Distribution	Crosses placenta, enters breast-milk, poor penetration in CSF
Metabolism	Unknown
Excretion	Unknown
Half-life	½-1 hr

Pharmacodynamics

Onset	Unknown
Peak	1-1½ hr

cefmetazole

Pharmacokinetics

Absorption	Complete
Distribution	Widely distributed; crosses placenta
Metabolism	Not metabolized
Excretion	Kidneys, unchanged (85%); enters breast milk
Half-life	½-2 hr; increased in renal disease

Pharmacodynamics

Onset	Rapid
Peak	Infusion's end

cefonicid

Pharmacokinetics

Absorption	Well absorbed (IM)
Distribution	Widely distributed; crosses placenta
Metabolism	Not metabolized
Excretion	Kidneys, unchanged; enters breast milk
Half-life	4½ hr; increased in renal disease

Pharmacodynamics

	IM	IV
Onset	Rapid	5 min
Peak	1 hr	Infusion's end

cefotetan

Pharmacokinetics

Absorption	Well absorbed (IM)
Distribution	Widely distributed; crosses placenta
Metabolism	Not metabolized
Excretion	Kidneys, unchanged; enters breast milk
Half-life	5 hr; increased in renal disease

Pharmacodynamics

	IM	IV
Onset	Rapid	Immediate
Peak	1-3 hr	Infusion's end

cefoxitin

Pharmacokinetics

Absorption	Well absorbed (IM)
Distribution	Widely distributed; crosses placenta
Metabolism	Not metabolized
Excretion	Kidneys, unchanged; enters breast milk
Half-life	½-1 hr; increased in renal disease

Pharmacodynamics

	IM	IV
Onset	Rapid	Immediate
Peak	½ hr	Infusion's end

cefprozil

Pharmacokinetics

Absorption	Well absorbed (PO)
Distribution	Widely distributed; crosses placenta
Metabolism	Not metabolized
Excretion	Kidneys, unchanged; enters breast milk
Half-life	1-1½ hr; increased in renal disease

Pharmacodynamics

	PO
Onset	Unknown
Peak	Unknown

loracarbef

Pharmacokinetics

Absorption	Well absorbed
Distribution	Widely distributed; crosses placenta
Metabolism	Not metabolized
Excretion	Kidneys, unchanged; enters breast milk
Half-life	1 hr; increased in renal disease

Pharmacodynamics

Onset	Rapid
Peak	1 hr

 Herb/drug   Do Not Crush   Alert   Key Drug   Geriatric   Pediatric

Interactions

Individual drugs

Alcohol: Disulfiram reaction if ingested within 48-72 hr of cephalosporin
Plicamycin, valproic acid: ↑ bleeding
Probenecid: ↓ excretion of drug and ↑ blood levels
Sulfinpyrazone, furosemide, vancomycin: ↑ toxicity

Drug classifications

Aminoglycosides: ↑ toxicity
Anticoagulants, antiplatelets, NSAIDs, thrombolytics: ↑ bleeding

☑ Herb/drug

(cefotetan, cefamandole, cefmetazole)
Angelica, anise, arnica, bogbean, boldo, celery, chamomile, clove, fenugreek, feverfew, garlic, ginger, ginkgo, ginseng (Panax), horse chestnut, horseradish, licorice, meadowsweet, onion, papain, passion flower, prickly ash, red clover, turmeric, willow: ↑ bleeding risk
Acidophilus: Do not use with antiinfectives

Lab test interferences

False: ↑ Creatinine (serum urine), ↑ urinary 17-KS

False positive: Urinary protein, direct Coombs' test, urine glucose (clinitest)

Interference: Cross-matching

NURSING CONSIDERATIONS

Assessment

- Assess patient for previous sensitivity reaction to penicillins or other cephalosporins; cross-sensitivity between penicillins and cephalosporins is common
- Assess patient for signs and symptoms of infection including characteristics of wounds, sputum, urine, stool, WBC >10,000/mm³, earache, fever; obtain baseline information and during treatment
- Obtain C&S before beginning drug therapy to identify if correct treatment has been initiated
- Assess for anaphylaxis: rash, urticaria, pruritus, dyspnea, chills, fever, joint pain; angioedema may occur a few days after therapy begins; epINEPHrine and resuscitation equipment should be available for anaphylactic reaction
- Identify urine output; if decreasing, notify prescriber (may indicate nephrotoxicity); also check for increased BUN, creatinine
- Monitor blood studies: AST, ALT, CBC, Hct, bilirubin, LDH, alkaline phosphatase, Coombs' test monthly if patient is on long-term therapy
- Monitor electrolytes: potassium, sodium, chloride monthly if patient is on long-term therapy
- Assess bowel pattern qd; if severe diarrhea occurs, drug should be discontinued; may indicate pseudomembranous colitis
- Monitor for bleeding: ecchymosis, bleeding gums, hematuria, stool guaiac daily if on long-term therapy
- Assess for overgrowth of infection: perineal itching, fever, malaise, redness, pain, swelling, drainage, rash, diarrhea, change in cough, sputum

Nursing diagnoses

☑ Infection, risk for (uses)
☑ Diarrhea (side effects)
☑ Fluid volume, risk for deficient (side effects)
☑ Injury, risk for (side effects)
☑ Knowledge, deficient (teaching)
☑ Noncompliance (teaching)

Implementation

cefaclor

- Give in even doses around the clock; if GI upset occurs, give with food; drug must be given for 10-14 days to ensure organism death and prevent superinfection
- Shake susp, refrigerate, discard after 2 wk
- ⊘ Do not crush, cut, or chew ext rel tabs

cefamandole

IM route

- Reconstitute with 3 ml of sterile or bacteriostatic water for inj, 0.9% NaCl, or 0.5%-2.0% lidocaine HCl; give deep in large muscle mass, massage; check for redness, abscess at inj site

IV IV route

- Check for irritation, extravasation, phlebitis daily; change site q72h
- Direct **IV**: Dilute each g of drug with 10 ml of D₅W, 0.9% NaCl, or sterile water for inj; give over 5 min
- For intermittent inf further dilute with 100 ml of D₅W, D₁₀W, D₅/0.25% NaCl, D₅/0.45% NaCl, D₅/0.9% NaCl, D₅ LR, 0.9% NaCl; give over 15-30 min; may be refrigerated up to 96 hr or 24 hr at room temp
- For cont inf dilute with 500-1000 ml of above solutions; give over prescribed rate

Syringe compatibilities: Heparin

Syringe incompatibilities: Cimetidine, gentamicin, tobramycin

Y-site compatibilities: Acyclovir, cyclophosphamide, hydromorphone, magnesium sulfate, meperidine, morphine, perphenazine

Y-site incompatibilities: Amiodarone, hetastarch

Additive compatibilities: Clindamycin, floxacillin, furosemide, metronidazole, or verapamil

Additive incompatibilities: Aminoglycosides, calcium glucceptate, calcium gluconate, cimetidine, gentamicin

cefditoren pivoxil

- Give for 10 days to ensure organism death, prevent superinfection
- Give with food if needed for GI symptoms
- Give after C&S is completed

cefmetazole

- Check for irritation, extravasation, phlebitis daily; change site q72h
- For intermittent inf, reconstitute with sterile, bacteriostatic water for inj or 0.9% NaCl; may be further diluted with 0.9% NaCl, LR, D_5W (1-20 mg/ml); give over 30-60 min; may be refrigerated for 1 wk or stored 24 hr at room temp

Additive compatibilities: Famotidine, clindamycin, KCl

cefonicid

IM route
- Reconstitute 500 mg/2 ml of sterile water for inj (220 mg/ml) or 1000 mg/2.5 ml (325 mg/ml)
- Give deep in large muscle mass, massage

IV IV route
- Check for irritation, extravasation, phlebitis daily; change site q72h
- For direct **IV** give over 5 min
- For intermittent inf reconstituted sol should be further diluted in 50-100 ml of D_5W, $D_{10}W$, D_5/LR, D_5/0.25% NaCl, D_5/0.45% NaCl, D_5/0.9% NaCl, 0.9% NaCl; or Ringer's, LR; give over 30 min; may be refrigerated up to 96 hr or stored 24 hr at room temp

Y-site compatibilities: Acyclovir, amifostine, aztreonam, teniposide, thiotepa

Y-site incompatibilities: Hetastarch, sargramostim

Additive compatibilities: Clindamycin

Additive incompatibilities: Aminoglycosides

cefotetan

IM route
- Reconstitute 1 g/2 ml or 2 g/3 ml of sterile or bacteriostatic water for inj; may be diluted with 0.5% of 1% lidocaine to prevent pain; give deep in large muscle mass, massage

IV IV route
- May be stored 96 hr refrigerated or 24 hr room temp

- Check for irritation, extravasation, phlebitis daily; change site q72h
- For direct **IV** dilute in 1 g/10 ml or more and give over 5 min
- For intermittent inf further dilute in 50-100 ml of 0.9% NaCl or D_5W; give over 3-5 min; discontinue primary line while running intermittent inf

Syringe incompatibilities: Doxapram

Y-site compatibilities: Allopurinol, amifostine, aztreonam, diltiazem, famotidine, filgrastim, fluconazole, fludarabine, heparin, regular insulin, melphalan, meperidine, morphine, paclitaxel, sargramostim, tacrolimus, teniposide, theophylline, thiotepa

Additive incompatibilities: Aminoglycosides, tetracyclines, heparin

cefoxitin

IM route
- Reconstitute 1 g/2 ml of sterile water for inj; may be diluted with 0.5% or 1% lidocaine to prevent pain; give deep in large muscle mass, massage

IV IV route
- Check for irritation, extravasation, phlebitis daily; change site q72h
- For direct **IV**, dilute 1 g/10 ml or 2 g/20 ml of sterile water for inj; shake, let stand until clear; give over 3-5 min
- For intermittent inf further dilute with 50-100 ml of D_5W, $D_{10}W$, D_5/0.25% NaCl, D_5/0.45% NaCl, D_5/0.9% NaCl, 0.9% NaCl D_5/LR, D_5/0.02%, sodium bicarbonate, Ringer's, or LR; give over 15-30 min; may store 96 hr refrigerated or 24 hr room temp
- For cont inf dilute in 500-1000 ml; give over prescribed rate

Syringe incompatibilities: Heparin, insulin

Y-site compatibilities: Acyclovir, amifostine, aztreonam, cyclophosphamide, diltiazem, famotidine, fluconazole, foscarnet, hydromorphone, magnesium sulfate, meperidine, morphine, ondansetron, perphenazine, temiposide, thiotepa

Y-site incompatibilities: Hetastarch

Additive compatibilities: Amikacin, cimetidine, clindamycin, gentamicin, kanamycin, multivitamins, sodium bicarbonate, tobramycin, verapamil, vit B/C

Additive incompatibilities: Aztreonam

cefprozil

IM route
- Reconstitute with 1 g/2 ml or 2 g/3 ml of sterile or bacteriostatic water for inj; may be

diluted with 0.5% or 1% lidocaine to prevent pain; give deep in large muscle mass, massage

IV **IV route**
• Check for irritation, extravasation, phlebitis daily; change site q72h
• For direct **IV**, dilute 1 g/10 ml or more and give over 5 min
• For intermittent inf further dilute with 50-100 ml of 0.9% NaCl or D₅W; give over 3-5 min; discontinue primary line while running intermittent infusion

Syringe incompatibilities: Doxapram

Y-site compatibilities: Famotidine, fluconazole, fludarabine, regular insulin, meperidine, morphine, sargramostim

Additive incompatibilities: Aminoglycosides, tetracyclines, heparin

loracarbef
• Give on an empty stomach, 1 hr ac or 2 hr pc
⊘ • Do not crush, chew caps
• Oral susp should be shaken before administration; store for 2 wk at room temp, discard after 2 wk

Patient/family education
• Teach patient to report sore throat, bruising, bleeding, joint pain; may indicate blood dyscrasias (rare)
• Advise patient to contact prescriber if vaginal itching, loose foul-smelling stools, furry tongue occur; may indicate superinfection
• Instruct patient to take all medication prescribed for the length of time ordered; to use yogurt or buttermilk to maintain intestinal flora, decrease diarrhea
• Advise patient to notify prescriber of diarrhea with blood or pus, which may indicate pseudomembranous colitis
• Cefditoren can be taken with oral contraceptives

Evaluation
Positive therapeutic outcome
• Absence of signs/symptoms of infection (WBC <10,000/mm³, temp WNL, absence of red draining wounds, earache)
• Reported improvement in symptoms of infection
• Negative C&S

Treatment of anaphylaxis: EpINEPHrine, antihistamines, resuscitate if needed

CEPHALOSPORINS— 3RD GENERATION

C

cefdinir (Rx)
(sef′dih-ner)
Omnicef
cefepime (Rx)
(sef′e-peem)
Maxipime
cefixime (Rx)
(sef-icks′ime)
Suprax
cefoperazone (Rx)
(sef-oh-per′a-zone)
Cefobid
cefotaxime (Rx)
(sef-oh-taks′eem)
Claforan
cefpodoxime (Rx)
(sef-poe-docks′eem)
Vantin
ceftazidime (Rx)
(sef′tay-zi-deem)
Ceptaz, Fortaz, Tazicef, Tazidime
ceftibuten (Rx)
(sef-ti-byoo′tin)
Cedax
ceftizoxime (Rx)
(sef-ti-zox′eem)
Cefizox
ceftriaxone (Rx)
(sef-try-ax′one)
Rocephin
Func. class.: Broad-spectrum antibiotic
Chem. class.: Cephalosporin (3rd generation)

Action: Inhibits bacterial cell wall synthesis, rendering cell wall osmotically unstable, leading to cell death

cefdinir
→ **Therapeutic Outcome:** Bactericidal effects for the following: gram-negative organisms *Haemophilus influenzae*, gram-positive organisms *Streptococcus pneumoniae*, *Streptococcus pyogenes*, *Staphylococcus aureus*

Uses: Uncomplicated skin and skin structure infections, community-acquired pneumonia, acute exacerbations of chronic bronchitis, acute maxillary sinusitis, pharyngitis, tonsillitis

cefepime

➡ **Therapeutic Outcome:** Bactericidal effects for the following: gram-negative bacilli, *Escherichia coli, Proteus, Klebsiella*; gram-positive organisms *Streptococcus pneumoniae, Streptococcus pyogenes, Staphylococcus aureus*

Uses: Lower respiratory tract, urinary tract, skin, bone, gonococcal infections; septicemia, peritonitis

cefixime

➡ **Therapeutic Outcome:** Bactericidal effects for the following: *Escherichia coli, Proteus mirabilis, Streptococcus pyogenes, Streptococcus pneumoniae, Haemophilus influenzae, Moraxella catarrhalis*

Uses: Uncomplicated UTI, pharyngitis and tonsillitis, otitis media, acute bronchitis, and acute/exacerbations of chronic bronchitis

cefoperazone

➡ **Therapeutic Outcome:** Bactericidal effects for the following: gram-negative organisms *Acinetobacter, Morganella morganii, Neisseria gonorrhoeae, Proteus vulgaris*; gram-positive organisms *Staphylococci, Streptococci, Streptococci (β-hemolytic), Streptococcus pneumoniae, Haemophilus influenzae, Escherichia coli, Proteus mirabilis, Klebsiella, Enterobacter, Serratia, Citrobacter, Providencia, Pseudomonas aeruginosa*; anaerobes *Bacteroides, Clostridium, Eubacterium, Fusobacterium, Peptococcus, Peptostreptococcus*

Uses: Lower respiratory tract, urinary tract, skin, bone infections; bacterial septicemia, peritonitis, PID, endometritis

cefotaxime

➡ **Therapeutic Outcome:** Bactericidal effects for the following: gram-negative organisms *Haemophilus influenzae, Escherichia coli, Neisseria meningitidis, Proteus mirabilis, Klebsiella, Citrobacter, Serratia, Salmonella, Shigella*; gram-positive organisms *Streptococcus pneumoniae, Streptococcus pyogenes, Staphylococcus aureus*

Uses: Lower serious respiratory tract, urinary tract, skin, bone, gonococcal infections; bacteremia, septicemia, meningitis

cefpodoxime

➡ **Therapeutic Outcome:** Bactericidal effects for the following: gram-negative organisms *Neisseria gonorrhoeae, Haemophilus influenzae, Escherichia coli, Proteus mirabilis, Klebsiella*; gram-positive organisms *Streptococcus pneumoniae, Streptococcus pyogenes, Staphylococcus aureus*

Uses: Upper and lower respiratory tract, urinary tract, skin infections; otitis media, sexually transmitted diseases

ceftazidime

➡ **Therapeutic Outcome:** Bactericidal effects for the following: gram-negative organisms *Haemophilus influenzae, Escherichia coli, Enterobacter aerogenes, Proteus mirabilis, Klebsiella, Citrobacter, Enterobacter, Pseudomonas aeruginosa, Shigella, Acinetobacter, Bacteroides fragilis, Neisseria*; gram-positive organisms *Streptococcus pneumoniae, Streptococcus pyogenes, Staphylococcus aureus*

Uses: Serious upper or lower respiratory tract, urinary tract, skin, gynecologic, bone, joint, intraabdominal infections; septicemia, meningitis

ceftibuten

➡ **Therapeutic Outcome:** Bactericidal effects for the following: gram-negative bacilli *Haemophilus influenzae, Escherichia coli*; gram-positive organisms *Streptococcus pneumoniae, Streptococcus pyogenes, Staphylococcus aureus*

Uses: Upper and lower respiratory tract infections; otitis media

ceftizoxime

➡ **Therapeutic Outcome:** Bactericidal effects for the following: gram-negative organisms *Haemophilus influenzae, Escherichia coli, Enterobacter aerogenes, Proteus mirabilis, Klebsiella, Acinetobacter, Neisseria gonorrhoeae, Providencia rettgeri, Pseudomonas aeruginosa, Serratia, Enterobacter*; gram-positive organisms *Streptococcus pneumoniae, Streptococcus pyogenes, Staphylococcus aureus*; anaerobes *Bacteroides, Peptococcus, Peptostreptococcus*

Uses: Serious lower respiratory tract, urinary tract, skin, intraabdominal infections; septicemia, meningitis; bone, joint infections; PID caused by *Neisseria gonorrhoeae*

ceftriaxone

➡ **Therapeutic Outcome:** Bactericidal effects on the following: gram-negative organisms *Haemophilus influenzae, Escherichia coli, Enterobacter aerogenes, Proteus mirabilis, Klebsiella, Citrobacter, Enterobacter, Pseudomonas aeruginosa, Neisseria, Serratia*; gram-positive organisms *Streptococcus pneumoniae, Streptococcus pyo-*

---

genes, Staphylococcus aureus; anaerobes
Bacteroides

Uses: Serious lower respiratory tract, urinary tract, skin, gonococcal, intraabdominal infections; septicemia, meningitis; bone, joint infections

Dosage and routes
cefdinir
Uncomplicated skin and skin structure infections/community-acquired pneumonia
P *Adult and child ≥13 yr:* PO 300 mg q12h × 10 days

P *Child 6 mo-12 yr:* PO 7 mg/kg q12h or 14 mg/kg q24h × 10 days; max 60 mg qd

Acute exacerbations of chronic bronchitis/acute maxillary sinusitis
P *Adult and child ≥13 yr:* PO 300 mg q12h or 600 mg q24h × 10 days or 300 mg bid × 5 days in some infections

Pharyngitis/tonsillitis
P *Adult and child ≥13 yr:* PO 300 mg q12h or 600 mg q24h × 10 days

P *Child 6 mo-12 yr:* PO 7 mg/kg q12h × 5-10 days or 14 mg/kg q24h × 10 days

Renal dose
CCr <30 ml/min 300 mg qd (adult); 7 mg/kg
P qd (child)

Available forms: Caps 300 mg, oral susp 125 mg/5 ml

cefepime
Urinary tract infections (mild to moderate)
Adult: IV/IM 0.5-1 g q12h × 7-10 days

Urinary tract infections (severe)
Adult: IV 2 g q12h × 10 days

Pneumonia (moderate to severe)
Adult: IV 1-2 g q12h × 10 days
Dosage reduction indicated in renal impairment (CCr <50 ml/min)

Uncomplicated gonorrhea
• IM 2 g as a single dose with 1 g PO probenecid at the same time

Available forms: Powder for inj 500 mg, 1, 2 g

cefixime
Adult: PO 400 mg qd as a single dose or 200 mg q12h

P *Child >50 kg or >12 yr:* PO use adult dosage

P *Child <50 kg or <12 yr:* PO 8 mg/kg/day as a single dose or 4 mg/kg q12h

Renal dose
Adult: PO CCr 21-60 ml/min 75% of dose; CCr <20 ml/min 50% of dose

Available forms: Tabs 200, 400 mg; powder for oral susp 100 mg/5 ml

cefoperazone
Adult: IM/IV 1-2 g q12h

Severe infections
Adult: IM/IV 6-12 g/day divided in 2-4 equal doses

Hepatic dose: Give 50% of dose

Mild/moderate infections
Adult: IM/IV 1-2 g q12h
Available forms: Inj 1, 2 g

cefotaxime
Adult: IM/IV 1-2 g q12h as a single dose
P *Child 1 mo-12 yr:* IM/IV 50-180 mg/kg/day divided q6h

Severe infections
Adult: IM/IV 2 g q4h, not to exceed 12 g/day
P *Child 1 mo-12 yr:* IM/IV 50 mg/kg q6h

Uncomplicated gonorrhea
Adult: IM 1 g; dosage reduction indicated for severe renal impairment (CCr <30 ml/min)

Available forms: Powder for inj 1, 2, 10 g; frozen inj 20, 40 mg/ml

cefpodoxime
Adult >13 yr: Pneumonia: 200 mg q12h for 14 days; *uncomplicated gonorrhea:* 200 mg single dose; *skin and skin structure:* 400 mg q12h for 7-14 days; *pharyngitis and tonsillitis:* 100 mg q12h for 10 days; *uncomplicated UTI:* 100 mg q12h for 7 days; dosing interval increased in presence of severe renal impairment

Acute otitis media
P *Child 5 mo-12 yr:* 5 mg/kg q12h for 10 days; *pharyngitis/tonsillitis:* 5 mg/kg q12h (max 100 mg/dose or 200 mg/day) × 5-10 days

Renal dose: Reduce dose in renal disease

Available forms: Tabs 100, 200 mg/ granules for susp 50, 100 mg/5 ml

ceftazidime
Adult: IV/IM 1-2 g q8-12h × 5-10 days
P *Child:* IV 30-50 mg/kg q8h not to exceed 6 g/day
P *Neonate:* IV 30-50 mg/kg q12h

Renal dose
Adult: **IV** CCr <50 ml/min q12h; CCr 10-30 ml/min q24h; CCr <10 ml/min q48h

Available forms: Inj 500 mg, 1, 2, 6 g

ceftibuten
Adult: PO 400 mg qd × 10 days

P *Child 6 mo-12 yr:* PO 9 mg/kg qd × 10 days

Renal dose
Adult: PO CCr <50 ml/min 200 mg q24h; CCr 5-20 ml/min 100 mg q24h

Available forms: Caps 400 mg; susp 90, 180 mg/5 ml

ceftizoxime
Adult: IM/**IV** 1-2 g q8-12h, may give up to 4 g q8h in life-threatening infections

P *Child >6 mo:* IM/**IV** 50 mg/kg q6-8h

Renal dose
Adult: IM/**IV** CCr <80 ml/min 500-1500 mg q8h; CCr 10-49 ml/min 250-1000 mg q12h

PID
Adult: **IV** 2 g q8h, may increase to 4 g q8h in severe infections

Available forms: Powder for inj 500 mg, 1, 2, 10 g; premixed 1 g, 2 g/50 ml

ceftriaxone
Reduce dosage in severe renal impairment (CCr <10 ml/min)

Adult: IM/**IV** 1-2 g qd, max 2 g q12h

P *Child:* IM/**IV** 50-75 mg/kg/day in equal doses q12h

Uncomplicated gonorrhea
Adult: 250 mg IM as single dose

Meningitis
P *Adult and child:* IM/**IV** 100 mg/kg/day in equal doses q12h, max 4 g/day

Surgical prophylaxis
Adult: **IV** 1 g ½-2 hr preop

Available forms: Inj 500 mg, 1, 2, 10 g

Adverse effects
(*italic* = common; **bold** = life-threatening)
CNS: Headache, dizziness, weakness, paresthesia, fever, chills, **seizures**
GI: Nausea, vomiting, diarrhea, anorexia, pain, glossitis, **bleeding;** increased AST, ALT, bilirubin, LDH, alkaline phosphatase; abdominal pain, **pseudomembranous colitis**
GU: **Proteinuria,** vaginitis, pruritus, candidiasis, increased BUN, **nephrotoxicity, renal failure**

HEMA: **Leukopenia, thrombocytopenia, agranulocytosis,** anemia, **neutropenia,** lymphocytosis, eosinophilia, **pancytopenia, hemolytic anemia**
INTEG: Rash, urticaria, dermatitis
RESP: Dyspnea
SYST: **Anaphylaxis, serum sickness**

Contraindications: Hypersensitivity to
P cephalosporins, infants <1 mo

Precautions: Hypersensitivity to penicillins, pregnancy **B**, lactation, renal disease,
P children

◼ **Do Not Confuse:**
ceftazidime/ceftizoxime, Vantin/Ventolin

cefdinir

Pharmacokinetics	
Absorption	Well absorbed
Distribution	Widely distributed; crosses placenta
Metabolism	Not metabolized
Excretion	Kidneys, unchanged; enters breast milk
Half-life	Unknown

Pharmacodynamics	
	PO
Onset	Unknown
Peak	Unknown

cefepime

Pharmacokinetics	
Absorption	Well absorbed (IM)
Distribution	Widely distributed; crosses placenta
Metabolism	Not metabolized
Excretion	Kidneys, unchanged; enters breast milk
Half-life	2 hr; increased in renal disease

Pharmacodynamics		
	IM	IV
Onset	Rapid	Immediate
Peak	79 min	Infusion's end

cefixime

Pharmacokinetics

Absorption	40%-50% (PO: tab)
Distribution	Widely distributed
Metabolism	Not metabolized
Excretion	Kidneys, unchanged (50%); bile (10%); enters breast milk
Half-life	3-4 hr, increased in renal disease

Pharmacodynamics

Onset	15-30 min
Peak	1-2 hr

cefoperazone

Pharmacokinetics

Absorption	Well absorbed (IM)
Distribution	Widely distributed; crosses placenta
Metabolism	Not metabolized
Excretion	Bile; enters breast milk
Half-life	2 hr

Pharmacodynamics

	IM	IV
Onset	Rapid	5 min
Peak	1-2 hr	Infusion's end

cefotaxime

Pharmacokinetics

Absorption	Widely distributed
Distribution	Breast milk, small amounts
Metabolism	Liver, active metabolites
Excretion	40%-65% unchanged, kidney
Half-life	1 hr

Pharmacodynamics

	IV	IM
Onset	5 min	30 min
Peak	Unknown	Unknown
Duration	Unknown	Unknown

cefpodoxime

Pharmacokinetics

Absorption	Well absorbed (PO)
Distribution	Widely distributed; crosses placenta
Metabolism	Not metabolized
Excretion	Kidneys, unchanged; enters breast milk
Half-life	2-3 hr, increased in renal disease

Pharmacodynamics

	PO
Onset	Unknown
Peak	Unknown

ceftazidime

Pharmacokinetics

Absorption	Well absorbed (IM)
Distribution	Widely distributed; crosses placenta
Metabolism	Not metabolized
Excretion	Kidneys, unchanged; enters breast milk
Half-life	½-1 hr; increased in renal disease

Pharmacodynamics

	IM	IV
Onset	Rapid	Immediate
Peak	1 hr	Infusion's end

ceftibuten

Pharmacokinetics

Absorption	Well absorbed
Distribution	Widely distributed; crosses placenta
Metabolism	Not metabolized
Excretion	Kidneys, unchanged; enters breast milk
Half-life	1-1½ hr; increased in renal disease

Pharmacodynamics

Onset	Unknown
Peak	Unknown

ceftizoxime

Pharmacokinetics

Absorption	Well absorbed (IM)
Distribution	Widely distributed; crosses placenta
Metabolism	Not metabolized
Excretion	Kidneys, unchanged; enters breast milk
Half-life	1½-2 hr; increased in renal disease

Pharmacodynamics

	IM	IV
Onset	Rapid	Immediate
Peak	1 hr	Infusion's end

ceftriaxone

Pharmacokinetics

Absorption	Well absorbed
Distribution	Widely distributed; crosses placenta; enters CSF
Metabolism	Liver
Excretion	Kidneys, partly
Half-life	5-8 hr

Pharmacodynamics

	IM	IV
Onset	Rapid	Immediate
Peak	1 hr	Infusion's end

Interactions
Individual drugs
Furosemide, vancomycin: ↑ toxicity
Iron: ↓ absorption of cefdinir
Plicamycin, valproic acid: ↑ bleeding
Probenecid: ↓ excretion of drug and ↑ blood levels

Drug classifications
Aminoglycosides: ↑ toxicity
Anticoagulants, NSAIDs, thrombolytics: ↑ bleeding

▨ Herb/drug
Acidophilus: Do not use with antiinfectives
Angelica, anise, arnica, bogbean, boldo, celery, chamomile, clove, fenugreek, feverfew, garlic, ginger, ginkgo, ginseng (Panax), horse chestnut, horseradish, licorice, meadowsweet, onion, papain, passion flower, poplar, prickly ash, red clover, turmeric, willow: ↑ risk of bleeding when used with cefoperazone

Lab test interferences
False: ↑ Creatinine (serum urine), ↑ urinary 17-KS
False positive: Urinary protein, direct Coombs' test, urine glucose
Interference: Cross-matching ↑ AST, ↑ alkaline phosphatase, ↑ LDH, ↑ bilirubin, ↑ BUN, ↑ creatinine

NURSING CONSIDERATIONS
Assessment
• Assess patient for previous sensitivity reaction to penicillins or other cephalosporins; cross-sensitivity between penicillins and cephalosporins is common
• Assess patient for signs and symptoms of infection including characteristics of wounds, sputum, urine, stool, WBC >10,000/mm³, fever; obtain baseline information and during treatment
• Obtain C&S before beginning drug therapy to identify if correct treatment has been initiated

• Assess for anaphylaxis: rash, urticaria, pruritus, chills, fever, joint pain; angioedema may occur a few days after therapy begins; epINEPHrine and resuscitation equipment should be available for anaphylactic reaction
• Identify urine output; if decreasing, notify prescriber (may indicate nephrotoxicity); also check for increased BUN, creatinine
• Monitor blood studies: AST, ALT, CBC, Hct, bilirubin, LDH, alkaline phosphatase, Coombs' test monthly if patient is on long-term therapy
• Monitor electrolytes: potassium, sodium, chloride monthly if patient is on long-term therapy
• Assess bowel pattern qd; if severe diarrhea occurs, drug should be discontinued; may indicate pseudomembranous colitis
• Monitor for bleeding: ecchymosis, bleeding gums, hematuria, stool guaiac daily if on long-term therapy
• Assess for overgrowth of infection: perineal itching, fever, malaise, redness, pain, swelling, drainage, rash, diarrhea, change in cough, sputum

Nursing diagnoses
☑ Infection, risk for (uses)
☑ Injury, risk for (side effects)
☑ Diarrhea (side effects)
☑ Knowledge, deficient (teaching)

Implementation
cefdinir
PO route
• Give oral suspension after adding 39 ml water to the 60 ml bottle; 65 ml water to the 12.0 ml bottle; discard unused portion after 10 days

cefepime
IM route
• Reconstitute 1 g/2 ml of sterile water for inj; may be diluted with 0.5% or 1% lidocaine to prevent pain; give deep in large muscle mass, massage

Ⅳ IV route
• Check for irritation, extravasation, phlebitis daily; change site q72h
• For intermittent inf dilute with 50-100 ml of D₅W, give over 30 min

Solution compatibilities: 0.9% NaCl, D₅, 0.5, 1.0% lidocaine, bacteriostatic water for inj with parabens/benzyl alcohol

cefixime
• Give in even doses around the clock; if GI upset occurs, give with food; drug must be given for 10-14 days to ensure organism death and prevent superinfection
• Shake suspension

---

cefoperazone

IM route

- Reconstitute 1 g/2.8 ml of sterile or bacteriostatic water for inj, or 2 g/5.4 ml; may be diluted further with 1 ml or 1.8 ml of 2% lidocaine to prevent pain; give deep in large muscle mass, massage

IV IV route

- Check for irritation, extravasation, phlebitis daily; change site q72h
- For intermittent inf, reconstituted sol should be further diluted 1 g/20-40 ml of 0.9% NaCl, D_5W, D_5/0.9% NaCl, D_5/LR, or LR; give over 15-30 min; may be refrigerated up to 96 hr or stored 24 hr at room temp
- For cont inf, final concentration is 2-25 mg/ml, give at prescribed rate

Syringe compatibilities: Heparin

Syringe incompatibilities: Doxapram

Y-site compatibilities: Acyclovir, allopurinol, aztreonam, cyclophosphamide, enalaprilat, esmolol, famotidine, foscarnet, fludarabine, hydromorphone, magnesium sulfate, melphalan, morphine, teniposide, thiotepa

Y-site incompatibilities: Gentamicin, hetastarch, labetalol, meperidine, ondansetron, perphenazine, sargramostim, tobramycin, vinorelbine tartrate

Additive compatibilities: Cimetidine, clindamycin, furosemide

Additive incompatibilities: Aminoglycosides

cefotaxime

IV IV route

- Dilute 1 g/10 ml D_5W, NS, sterile H_2O for inj and give over 3-5 min by Y-tube or 3-way stopcock; may be diluted further with 50-100 ml of 0.9% NaCl or D_5W; run over ½-1 hr; discontinue primary inf during administration; or may be diluted in larger volume of sol and given as a cont inf over 6-24 hr
- Give for 10-14 days to ensure organism death, prevent superinfection

Syringe compatibilities: Heparin, oflaxacin

Y-site compatibilities: Acyclovir, amifostine, aztreonam, cyclophosphamide, diltiazem, famotidine, fludarabine, hydromorphone, lorazepam, magnesium sulfate, melphalan, meperidine, midazolam, morphine, ondansetron, perphenazine, sargramostim, teniposide, thiotepa, tolazoline, vinorelbine

Additive compatibilities: Clindamycin, metronidazole, verapamil

cefpodoxime

IM route

- Reconstitute 1 g/2 ml or 2 g/3 ml of sterile or bacteriostatic water for inj; may be diluted with 0.5% of 1% lidocaine to prevent pain; give deep in large muscle mass, massage

IV IV route

- Check for irritation, extravasation, phlebitis daily; change site q72h
- For direct **IV** dilute in 1 g/10 ml or more and give over 5 min
- For intermittent inf further dilute in 50-100 ml of 0.9% NaCl or D_5W; give over 3-5 min; discontinue primary line while running intermittent inf

Syringe incompatibilities: Doxapram

Y-site compatibilities: Famotidine, fluconazole, fludarabine, regular insulin, meperidine, morphine, sargramostim

Additive incompatibilities: Aminoglycosides, heparin, tetracyclines

ceftazidime

IM route

- Reconstitute 500 mg/1.5 ml or 1 g/3 ml of sterile or bacteriostatic water for inj; may be diluted with 0.5% or 1% lidocaine to prevent pain; give deep in large muscle mass, massage

IV IV route

- Check for irritation, extravasation, phlebitis daily; change site q72h
- For direct **IV** dilute 500 mg/5 ml or 1 g/10 ml sterile water for inj; give over 3-5 min; do **P** not use sol with benzyl alcohol for neonates
- For intermittent inf further dilute 1 g/10 ml or more 0.9% NaCl, D_5W, $D_{10}W$, D_5/0.25% NaCl, D_5/0.45% NaCl, D_5/0.9% NaCl, or LR; give over 30-60 min
- Store for 96 hr refrigerated, 24 hr room temp

Y-site compatibilities: Acyclovir, allopurinol, amifostine, aztreonam, ciprofloxacin, diltiazem, enalaprilat, esmolol, famotidine, filgrastim, fludarabine, foscarnet, granisetron, heparin, hydromorphone, labetalol, meperidine, melphalan, morphine, ondansetron, paclitaxel, rantidine, tacrolimus, teniposide, theophylline, thiotepa, vinorelbine tartrate, zidovudine

Y-site incompatibilities: Amsacrine, fluconazole, idarubicin, sargramostim

Additive compatibilities: Ciprofloxacin, clindamycin, fluconazole, metronidazole, ofloxacin

Additive incompatibilities: Aminoglycosides, sodium bicarbonate

ceftibuten
• Administer for 10 days to ensure organism death, prevent superimposed infection
• Administer after C&S

ceftizoxime
IM route
• Reconstitute 250 mg/0.9 ml, 500 mg/1.8 ml, 1 g/3.6 ml, 2 g/7.2 ml; may be diluted with 0.5% or 1% lidocaine to prevent pain; give deep in large muscle mass, massage

IV route
• Check for irritation, extravasation, phlebitis daily; change site q72h
• For intermittent inf reconstitute 250 mg/2.4 ml, 500 mg/4.8 ml, 1 g/9.6 ml/2 g/19.2 ml sterile water for inj, D_5W, or 0.9% NaCl; do not use sol with benzyl alcohol for neonates; may be further diluted in 50-100 ml of D_5W, $D_{10}W$, 0.9% NaCl, or LR; give over 30-60 min
• May store 96h refrigerated, 24h room temp

Y-site compatibilities: Acyclovir, allopurinol, amifostine, aztreonam, enalaprilat, esmolol, famotidine, fludarabine, foscarnet, hydromorphone, labetalol, melphalan, meperidine, morphine, ondansetron, sargramostim, teniposide, thiotepa, vinorelbine

Additive compatibilities: Clindamycin, metronidazole

Additive incompatibilities: Aminoglycosides

ceftriaxone
• Give for 10-14 days to ensure organism death, prevent superinfection
IV route
• Give **IV** after diluting 250 mg/2.4 ml of D_5W, H_2O for inj, 0.9% NaCl; may be further diluted with 50-100 ml of 0.9% NaCl, D_5W, $D_{10}W$, shake; run over ½-1 hr

Y-site compatibilities: Acyclovir, allopurinol, aztreonam, cisatracurium, diltiazem, DOXOrubicin liposome, fludarabine, foscarnet, heparin, melphalan, meperidine, methotrexate, morphine, paclitaxel, remifentanil, sargramostim, tacrolimus, teniposide, theophylline, vinorelbine, warfarin, zidovudine

Additive compatibilities: Amino acids or sodium bicarbonate, metronidazole

Patient/family education
• Teach patient to report sore throat, bruising, bleeding, joint pain; may indicate blood dyscrasias (rare)

• Advise patient to contact prescriber if vaginal itching, loose foul-smelling stools, furry tongue occur; may indicate superinfection
• Advise patient to notify prescriber of diarrhea with blood or pus, may indicate pseudomembranous colitis

Evaluation
Positive therapeutic outcome
• Absence of signs/symptoms of infection (WBC <10,000/mm^3, temp WNL, absence of red draining wounds, earache)
• Reported improvement in symptoms of infection
• Negative C&S

Treatment of anaphylaxis: EpINEPHrine, antihistamines, resuscitate if needed

---

cephapirin
cephradine
See cephalosporins—1st generation

---

cetirizine (Rx)
(se-tear'i-zeen)
Zyrtec
Func. class: Antihistamine, peripherally selective (2nd generation)
Chem. class.: Piperazine, H_1 histamine antagonist

Pregnancy category B

Action: Acts on blood vessels, GI, respiratory system by competing with histamine for H_1-receptor site; decreases allergic response by blocking pharmacologic effects of histamine; less sedation rate than with other antihistamines; causes increased heart rate, vasodilatation, increased secretions

Therapeutic Outcome: Absence of allergy symptoms and rhinitis

Uses: Rhinitis, allergy symptoms

Dosage and routes
Adult and child ≥6 yr: PO 5-10 mg qd

Child 2-6 yr: PO 2.5 mg qd, may increase to 5 mg qd or 2.5 mg bid

Elderly: PO 5 mg qd, may increase to 10 mg/day

Renal/hepatic dose
Adult: PO CCr 11-31 ml/min 5 mg qd

 Herb/drug   ⊗ Do Not Crush   ◆ Alert   ◆ₐ Key Drug   **G** Geriatric   **P** Pediatric

C

Available forms: Tabs 5, 10 mg; syr 5 mg/5 ml

Adverse effects
(*italic* = common; **bold** = life-threatening)

CNS: Headache, stimulation, *drowsiness,* sedation, *fatigue,* confusion, blurred vision, P tinnitus, restlessness, tremors, parodoxical G excitation in children or elderly

INTEG: Rash, eczema, photosensitivity, urticaria

RESP: Thickening of bronchial secretions; dry nose, throat

Contraindications: Hypersensitivity to P this drug or hydrOXYzine, newborn or premature infants, lactation, severe hepatic disease

P **Precautions:** Pregnancy **B**, children, respiratory disease, narrow-angle glaucoma, prostatic hypertrophy, bladder neck obstruction, asthma

🔊 **Do Not Confuse:**
Zyrtec/Xanax/Zantac

Pharmacokinetics	
Absorption	Well absorbed
Distribution	Protein binding 93%
Metabolism	Liver
Excretion	Kidneys
Half-life	8.3 hr, ↓ in children, ↑ in hepatic/renal disease

Pharmacodynamics	
Onset	½ hr
Peak	1-2 hr
Duration	24 hr

Interactions
Individual drugs
Alcohol: ↑ CNS depression
Drug classifications
CNS depressants, opioids, sedative/hypnotics: ↑ CNS depression
MAOIs: ↑ anticholinergic effect
🖉 *Herb/drug*
Corkwood: ↑ anticholinergic effect
Hops, Jamaican dogwood, kava, senna, valerian: ↑ CNS depression
Food/drug
↓ absorption by 1.7 hr
Lab test interferences
False negative: Skin allergy tests (discontinue antihistamine 3 days before testing)

NURSING CONSIDERATIONS
Assessment
• Assess respiratory status: rate, rhythm; increase in bronchial secretions, wheezing,

chest tightness; provide fluids to 2 L/day to decrease secretion thickness
• Assess for allergy symptoms: pruritus, urticaria, watering eyes, baseline and during treatment

Nursing diagnoses
✓ Airway clearance, ineffective (uses)
✓ Injury, risk for (side effects)
✓ Knowledge, deficient (teaching)
✓ Noncompliance (teaching overuse)

Implementation
• Give without regard to meals
• Store in tight, light-resistant container

Patient/family education
• Teach all aspects of drug uses; to notify prescriber if confusion, sedation, hypotension occur; to avoid driving or other hazardous activity if drowsiness occurs; to avoid alcohol or other CNS depressants that may potentiate effect
• Instruct patient to take 1 hr before or 2 hr pc to facilitate absorption
• Instruct patient not to exceed recommended dose; dysrhythmias may occur
• Advise patient to avoid using if breast feeding
• Advise patient to avoid exposure to sunlight; burns may occur
• Advise patient to use sugarless gum, candy, frequent sips of water to minimize dry mouth

Evaluation
Positive therapeutic outcome
• Absence of runny or congested nose, rashes

Treatment of overdose:
Lavage, diazepam, vasopressors, barbiturates (short acting)

---

cetrorelix (Rx)
(set-roe-ree′lix)
Cetrotide
Func. class.: Gonadotropin-releasing hormone antagonist
Chem. class.: Synthetic decapeptide

Pregnancy category X

Action: Inhibitor of pituitary gonadotropin secretion; initially increases LH and FSH, induces a rapid suppression of gonadotropin secretion

➔ **Therapeutic Outcome:** Pregnancy

Uses: For inhibition of premature LH surges in women undergoing controlled ovarian hyperstimulation

---

Dosage and routes
Single-dose regimen
Adult: SC 3 mg when serum estradiol level is at appropriate stimulation response, usually on stimulation day 7; if hCG has not been given within 4 days after inj of 3 mg cetrorelix, give 0.25 mg qd until day of hCG administration

Multiple-dose regimen
Adult: SC 0.25 mg is given on stimulation day 5 (either morning or evening) or 6 (morning) and continued qd until day hCG is given

Available forms: Inj 0.25, 3 mg

Adverse effects
(*italic* = common; **bold** = life-threatening)
CNS: Headache
ENDO: Ovarian hyperstimulation syndrome, abdominal pain (gyn)
GI: Nausea
INTEG: Pain on inj; local site reactions
SYST: Fetal death

Contraindications: Hypersensitivity, pregnancy **X**, latex allergy, lactation

Pharmacokinetics

Absorption	Unknown
Distribution	Protein binding 86%
Metabolism	Liver to metabolites
Excretion	Feces/urine
Half-life	Depends on dosage

Pharmacodynamics
Unknown

Interactions
None known

NURSING CONSIDERATIONS
Assessment
• Assess for suspected pregnancy; drug should not be used
• Assess for latex allergy; drug should not be used
• Monitor ALT, AST, GGT, alkaline phosphatase

Nursing diagnoses
☑ Knowledge, deficient (teaching)

Implementation
• Give SC using abdomen, around navel or upper thigh, swab inj area with disinfectant, clean a 2 in circle and allow to dry, pinch up area between thumb and finger, insert needle at 45-90° to surface; if blood is drawn into the syringe, reposition needle without removing it
• Do not administer if patient is pregnant
• Protect from light

Patient/family education
• Instruct to report abdominal pain, vaginal bleeding
• Teach self-administration technique if needed

Evaluation
Positive therapeutic outcome
• Pregnancy

---

chloral hydrate (Rx)
(klor′al hye′drate)
Aquachloral, chloral hydrate, Novo-Chlorhydrate ✦, PMS-Chloral Hydrate
Func. class.: Sedative/hypnotic
Chem. class.: Chloral derivative

Pregnancy category C

Controlled substance schedule IV (USA), schedule F (Canada)

Action: Reduced to product trichloroethanol, which produces mild cerebral depression, causing sleep; generalized CNS depression

Therapeutic Outcome: Ability to sleep, sedation

Uses: Sedation, short-term treatment of insomnia, preoperative reduction of anxiety

Dosage and routes
Sedation
Adult: PO/rec 250 mg tid pc
P **Child:** PO 25-50 mg/kg tid, not to exceed 500 mg tid

Procedure sedation
P **Child:** PO/REC 25-50 mg/kg, not to exceed 100 mg/kg or 2 g

Insomnia
Adult: PO/REC 500 mg-1 g 30 min before hs
P **Child:** PO/REC 50-75 mg/kg (one dose)

Renal dose
Adult: PO/REC CCr <50 ml/min avoid use

Available forms: Caps 250, 500, 650 mg; syr 250, 500 mg/5 ml; supp 325, 500 mg

Adverse effects
(*italic* = common; **bold** = life-threatening)
CNS: *Drowsiness,* dizziness, stimulation, nightmares, ataxia, hangover (rare), lightheadedness, headache, paranoia
CV: Hypotension, **dysrhythmias**
GI: *Nausea, vomiting, flatulence, diarrhea,* unpleasant taste, **gastric necrosis**
HEMA: Eosinophilia, leukopenia

 Herb/drug   🚫 Do Not Crush   ◆ Alert   ◆🚇 Key Drug   **G** Geriatric   **P** Pediatric

INTEG: Rash, urticaria, **angioedema,** fever, purpura, eczema
RESP: **Depression**

Contraindications: Hypersensitivity to this drug or triclofos, severe renal disease, severe hepatic disease, GI disorders (oral forms), gastritis

Precautions: Severe cardiac disease, depression, suicidal individuals, asthma, intermittent porphyria, pregnancy **C,** lactation, Ⓖ elderly

Pharmacokinetics

Absorption	Well absorbed (PO, rec)
Distribution	Widely distributed; crosses placenta
Metabolism	Liver to trichloroethanol
Excretion	Kidneys (inactive metabolite), feces, breast milk
Half-life	8-10 hr; active metabolite

Pharmacodynamics

	PO	REC
Onset	½-1 hr	Slow
Peak	Unknown	Unknown
Duration	4-8 hr	4-8 hr

Interactions
Individual drugs
Alcohol: ↑ CNS depression
Fluoxetine, propoxyphene: ↑ action
Furosemide: ↑ action of furosemide
Phenytoin: ↓ effect of phenytoin
Drug classifications
Analgesics (opioid), antidepressants, antihistamines, sedative/hypnotics: ↑ CNS depression
Anticoagulants (oral): ↑ action of anticoagulants
CNS depressants: ↑ action of both drugs
🌿*Herb/drug*
Catnip, chamomile, clary, cowslip, kava, lavender, mistletoe, nettle, pokeweed, poppy, Queen Anne's lace, senega, valerian: ↑ sedative effect
Black cohosh: ↑ hypotension
Lab test interferences
Interferences: Urine catecholamines, urinary 17-OHCS

NURSING CONSIDERATIONS
Assessment
• Assess patient's sleep pattern and note physical (sleep apnea, obstructed airway, pain/discomfort, urinary frequency) and psychologic (fear, anxiety) circumstances that interrupt sleep

• Assess patient's bedtime routine, presleep cues/props
• Assess potential for abuse; this drug may lead to physical and psychologic dependency; amount of drug should be limited
• Monitor blood studies: Hct, Hgb, RBCs, serum folate (if on long-term therapy), Pro-time in patients receiving anticoagulants since action of anticoagulant may be increased
• Monitor mental status: mood, sensorium, affect, memory (long, short)
• Monitor physical dependency: more frequent requests for medication, shakes, anxiety, pinpoint pupils
• Monitor respiratory dysfunction: respiratory depression, character, rate, rhythm; hold drug if respirations are <10/min or if pupils are dilated (rare)
• Assess for blood dyscrasias: fever, sore throat, bruising, rash, jaundice, epistaxis (rare)
• Assess previous history of substance abuse, cardiac disease, or gastritis

Nursing diagnoses
☑ Sleep pattern disturbance (uses)
☑ Anxiety (uses)
☑ Knowledge, deficient (teaching)
☑ Noncompliance (teaching)

Implementation
General
• Regulate environmental stimuli (light, noise, temperature), remove foods and fluids that interfere with sleep
• Place side rails up after giving medication for hypnotic; remove cigarettes/matches from patient's environment to prevent fires
PO route
• Give ½-1 hr before hs for sleeplessness; give on empty stomach with full glass of water or juice for best absorption and to decrease corrosion (do not chew); after meals to decrease GI symptoms if used for sedation; dilute syr in 4 oz water or juice
🚫• Do not crush, chew caps
⚠️• Check dose of syrup carefully, fatal overdoses have occurred
Rectal route
• Store supp in dark container, in refrigerator; remove outer wrapper before insertion

Patient/family education
• Caution patient to avoid driving and other activities requiring alertness; to avoid alcohol ingestion or CNS depressants; serious CNS depression may result plus tachycardia, flushing, headache, hypotension

- Instruct patient not to discontinue medication quickly after long-term use; drug should be tapered over 1-2 wk; that benefits may take 2 nights to be noticed; withdrawal symptoms include tremors, anxiety, hallucinations, delirium
- Teach patient alternative measures to improve sleep (reading, exercise several hours before hs, warm bath, warm milk, TV, self-hypnosis, deep breathing)
- Instruct the patient about factors that contribute to sleep pattern disturbances (lifestyle, shift work, long work hours, environmental factors, frequent napping)
- Teach patient to take drug as prescribed, not to double doses

Evaluation
Positive therapeutic outcome
- Ability to sleep at night
- Decreased amount of early morning awakening if taking drug for insomnia
- Sedation

Treatment of overdose: Lavage, activated charcoal; monitor electrolytes, VS

chlorambucil (Rx)
(klor-am′byoo-sil)
Leukeran
Func. class.: Antineoplastic alkylating agent
Chem. class.: Nitrogen mustard
Pregnancy category D

Action: Alkylates DNA, RNA; inhibits enzymes that allow synthesis of amino acids in proteins; activity is not cell cycle phase specific

➡ **Therapeutic Outcome:** Prevention of rapidly growing malignant cells

Uses: Chronic lymphocytic leukemia, Hodgkin's disease, other lymphomas, macroglobulinemia, nephrotic syndrome, breast carcinoma, choreocarcinoma, ovarian carcinoma

Dosage and routes
Adult: PO 0.1-0.2 mg/kg/day × 3-6 wk initially, then 2-6 mg/day; maintenance 0.2 mg/kg × 2-4 wk; course may be repeated at 2-4 wk intervals or 0.4 mg/kg (12 mg/m²) 2 ×/wk, may increase by 0.1 mg/kg (3 mg/m²) q2 wk, adjust as needed

G *Elderly:* PO initially ≤2-4 mg/day

P *Child:* PO 0.1-0.2 mg/kg/day (4.5 mg/m²/day) in divided doses or 4.5 mg/m²/day as 1 dose or in divided doses

Available forms: Tabs 2 mg

Adverse effects
(*italic* = common; **bold** = life-threatening)
CNS: Seizures
GI: *Nausea, vomiting, diarrhea, weight loss,* **hepatoxicity,** *jaundice*
GU: Hyperuremia
HEMA: **Thrombocytopenia, leukopenia, pancytopenia** (prolonged use), **permanent bone marrow suppression**
INTEG: Alopecia (rare), dermatitis, rash, **Stevens-Johnson syndrome**
RESP: **Fibrosis, pneumonitis**

Contraindications: Radiation therapy within 1 mo, chemotherapy within 1 mo, thrombocytopenia, recent smallpox vaccination, pregnancy **D,** lactation

Precautions: *Pneumococcus* vaccination

Do Not Confuse:
Leukeran/leucovorin, Leukeran/Leukine

Pharmacokinetics

Absorption	Rapidly, completely absorbed
Distribution	Crosses placenta
Metabolism	Liver, extensively
Excretion	Kidneys
Half-life	2 hr

Pharmacodynamics
Unknown

Interactions
Individual drugs
Radiation: ↑ toxicity, bone marrow suppression
Drug classifications
Anticoagulants, salicylates: ↑ risk of bleeding
Antineoplastics: ↑ toxicity
Antineoplastics, bone-marrow suppression: ↑ bone marrow suppression
Live vaccines: ↑ adverse reactions, ↓ antibody reaction
Lab test interferences
↑ Uric acid

NURSING CONSIDERATIONS
Assessment
- Monitor CBC, differential, platelet count weekly; withhold drug if WBC is <2000/mm³ or granulocyte count <1000/mm³ notify prescriber of results if WBC <20,000/mm³, platelets <50,000/mm³
- Monitor pulmonary function tests, chest x-ray films before, during therapy; chest film should be obtained q2 wk during treatment; check for dyspnea, rales, unproductive cough, chest pain, tachypnea

 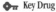

- Assess for increased uric acid levels, swelling, joint pain primarily in extremities; patient should be well hydrated to prevent urate deposits
- Monitor renal function studies: BUN, serum uric acid, urine CCr before, during therapy; I&O ratio; report fall in urine output of 30 ml/hr; monitor for decreased hyperuricemia
- Assess for jaundice of skin, sclera, dark urine, clay-colored stools, itchy skin, abdominal pain, fever, diarrhea
- Monitor for cold, fever, sore throat (may indicate beginning infection); identify edema in feet, joint, stomach pain, shaking; prescriber should be notified
- Assess for bleeding: hematuria, guaiac, bruising or petechiae, mucosa or orifices q8h, no rect temp

Nursing diagnoses
✓ Injury, risk for (adverse reactions)
✓ Body image, disturbed (adverse reactions)
✓ Infection, risk for (adverse reactions)
✓ Knowledge, deficient (teaching)

Implementation
- Give 1 hr ac or 2 hr pc to lessen nausea and vomiting or antacid before oral agent, give drug after evening meal, before hs or 1 hr before breakfast; antiemetic 30-60 min before giving drug to prevent vomiting
- Give allopurinol to maintain uric acid levels, alkalinization of urine; increase fluid intake to 2-3 L/day to prevent urate deposits, calculus formation
- Antibiotics for prophylaxis of infection may be prescribed, since infection potential is high
- Give all drugs PO if possible, avoid IM inj when platelets <100,000/mm³
- Store in tight container

Patient/family education
- Teach patient to avoid use of products containing aspirin or ibuprofen, razors, commercial mouthwash, since bleeding may occur; to report symptoms of bleeding (hematuria, tarry stools)
- Instruct patient to report signs of anemia (fatigue, headache, irritability, faintness, shortness of breath)
- Instruct patient to report any changes in breathing or coughing even several mo after treatment; to avoid crowds and persons with respiratory tract or other infections
- Advise patient hair loss is common; discuss the use of wigs or hairpieces
- Instruct patient to drink 2-3 L of fluid qd unless contraindicated
- Caution patient not to have any vaccinations

without the advice of the prescriber; serious reactions can occur
- Advise patient contraception is needed during treatment and for several months after the completion of therapy, may cause irreversible gonadal suppression

Evaluation
Positive therapeutic outcome
- Decreased size of tumor
- Decreased spread of malignancy
- Improved blood values
- Absence of sweating at night
- Increased appetite, increased weight

---

chloramphenicol (Rx)
(klor-am-fen′i-kole)
Ak-Chlor, Chloracol, Chlorofair, chloramphenicol, Chloromycetin, Chloroptic, EconoChlor, Fenicol ✤, I-Chlor, Novochlorocap ✤, Pentamycetin ✤
Func. class.: Antiinfective, misc.
Chem. class.: Dichloroacetic acid derivative

Pregnancy category C

Action: Binds to 50S ribosomal subunit, which interferes with or inhibits protein synthesis

Therapeutic Outcome: Bactericidal for *Haemophilus influenzae, Salmonella typhi, Rickettsia, Neisseria, Mycoplasma*

Uses: Meningitis, bacteremia, abdominal, skin, soft tissue infections; local infections of skin, ear, eye; not to be used if less-toxic drugs can be used

Dosage and routes
P *Adult/child:* PO/**IV** 50-75 mg/kg/day in divided doses q6h, 100 mg/kg/day (for meningitis only) max 4 g/day

P *Premature infants and neonates:* **IV**/PO 25 mg/kg/day in divided doses q12-24h

P *Adult and child:* OPHTH 1-2 gtt of sol or ointment q3-6 mo; otic 2-3 gtt bid or tid; top 1% cream tid or qid

Available forms: Inj **IV** 100 mg/ml in 1-g vial; caps 250 mg; OPHTH ointment 10 mg/g; OPHTH sol 25 mg/15 ml, 5 mg/ml; top cream 1%; otic sol 0.5%

Adverse effects
(*italic* = common; **bold** = life-threatening)
CNS: Headache, **depression,** confusion, peripheral neuritis

CV: **Gray syndrome in newborns: failure to feed, pallor, cyanosis, abdominal distention, irregular respiration, vasomotor collapse**
EENT: Optic neuritis, blindness
GI: Nausea, vomiting, diarrhea, abdominal pain, xerostomia, glossitis, colitis, pruritus ani
HEMA: **Anemia, bone marrow depression, thrombocytopenia, aplastic anemia, granulocytopenia, leukopenia** (rare)
INTEG: Itching, urticaria, contact dermatitis, rash

Contraindications: Hypersensitivity, severe renal disease, severe hepatic disease, minor infections

Precautions: Hepatic disease, renal disease, infants, children, bone marrow depression (drug-induced), pregnancy **C**, lactation

Pharmacokinetics

Absorption	Well absorbed (PO), Completely absorbed (**IV**)
Distribution	Wide
Metabolism	Liver
Excretion	Kidneys, unchanged
Half-life	1½-4 hr

Pharmacodynamics

	PO	IV	TOP	OPHTH	OTIC
Onset	15 min	Rapid	Unkn	Unkn	Unkn
Peak	1-2 hr	Inf end	Unkn	Unkn	Unkn

Interactions
Individual drugs
Folic acid: ↓ action of folic acid
Iron: ↑ action of iron
Phenytoin: ↑ action of phenytoin
Rifampin: ↓ action of rifampin
Vitamin B_{12}: ↓ action of vit B_{12}
Drug classifications
Anticoagulants: ↑ prothrombin time
Antidiabetics: ↑ action of antidiabetics
Barbiturates: ↑ levels of barbiturates
Penicillins: ↑ synergism
Herb/drug
Acidophilus: Do not use with antiinfectives

NURSING CONSIDERATIONS
Assessment
• Assess patient for previous sensitivity reaction to other antiinfectives; cross-sensitivity between penicillins and cephalosporins is common
• Assess patient for signs and symptoms of infection including characteristics of wounds, sputum, urine, stool, WBC >10,000/mm³, fever; obtain baseline information and during treatment
• Perform C&S testing before starting drug therapy to identify if correct treatment has been initiated
• Monitor drug level in impaired hepatic, renal systems; peak 15-20 mg/ml 3 hr after dose, trough 5-10 mg/ml before next dose
• Monitor blood studies: platelets q2 days, CBC
• Assess bowel pattern qd; if severe diarrhea occurs, drug should be discontinued
• Monitor for bleeding: ecchymosis, bleeding gums, hematuria, stool guaiac daily if on long-term therapy
• Assess for overgrowth of infection: perineal itching, fever, malaise, redness, pain, swelling, drainage, rash, diarrhea, change in cough, sputum

Nursing diagnoses
☑ Infection, risk for (uses)
☑ Diarrhea (adverse reaction)
☑ Injury, risk for (side effects)
☑ Knowledge, deficient (teaching)
☑ Noncompliance (teaching)

Implementation
Topical route
• Wash hands, clean area to be treated with soap and water before application
Ophthalmic route
• Apply a small amount of ointment in lower lid
• Have patient tilt head back before application
IV route
• Give after diluting 1 g/10 ml of sterile H_2O for inj or D_5W (10% sol); give >1 min
• May be further diluted in 50-100 ml of D_5W; give through Y-tube, 3-way stopcock, or additive infusion set; run over ½-1 hr; store reconstituted sol at room temp for up to 30 days

Syringe compatibilities: Ampicillin, cloxacillin, heparin, methicillin, penicillin G sodium

Y-site compatibilities: Acyclovir, cyclophosphamide, enalaprilat, esmolol, foscarnet, hydromorphone, labetalol, magnesium sulfate, meperidine, morphine, perphenazine, tacrolimus

Y-site incompatibilities: Fluconazole

Additive compatibilities: Amikacin, aminophylline, ascorbic acid, calcium chloride/gluconate, cephalothin, cephapirin,

---

☑ Herb/drug   ⓢ Do Not Crush   ◆ Alert   ◐ᴛᴛ Key Drug   Ⓖ Geriatric   Ⓟ Pediatric colistimethate, corticotropin, cyanocobalamin, dimenhyDRINATE, DOPamine, epHEDrine, heparin, hydrocortisone, kanamycin, lidocaine, magnesium sulfate, metaraminol, methicillin, methyldopa, methylPREDNISolone, metronidazole, nafcillin, oxacillin, oxytocin, penicillin G potassium, penicillin G sodium, pentobarbital, phenylephrine, phytonadione, plasma protein fraction, potassium chloride, promazine, ranitidine, sodium bicarbonate, thiopental, verapamil, vit B

PO route
• Give oral form on empty stomach with full glass of water
🚫 • Do not crush or chew caps
• Store cap in airtight container at room temp

Patient/family education
• Teach patient all aspects of drug therapy; need to complete entire course of medication to ensure organism death (10-14 days); culture may be taken after complete course of medication
• Advise patient to report sore throat, fever, fatigue, unusual bleeding, or bruising; could indicate bone marrow depression (may occur weeks or months after termination of drug)
• Tell patient that drug must be taken at regular intervals around the clock to maintain blood levels

Evaluation
Positive therapeutic outcome
• Decreased symptoms of infection

---

chlordiazepoxide (Rx)
(klor-dye-az-e-pox'ide)
Apo-Chlordiazepoxide ✣, chlordiazepoxide HCl, Libritabs, Librium, Novopoxide ✣
Func. class.: Antianxiety
Chem. class.: Benzodiazepine

Pregnancy category D
Controlled substance schedule IV

Action: Potentiates the actions of GABA, an inhibitory neurotransmitter, especially in the limbic system reticular formation, which depresses the CNS

➡️ **Therapeutic Outcome:** Decreased anxiety, successful alcohol withdrawal, relaxation

Uses: Short-term management of anxiety, acute alcohol withdrawal, preoperative relaxation

Dosage and routes
Mild anxiety
Adult: PO 5-10 mg tid-qid

🅟 *Child >6 yr:* PO 5 mg bid-qid, not to exceed 10 mg bid-tid

Severe anxiety
Adult: PO 20-25 mg tid-qid

Preoperatively
Adult: PO 5-10 mg tid-qid on day before surgery; IM 50-100 mg 1 hr before surgery

Alcohol withdrawal
Adult: PO/IM/**IV** 50-100 mg, not to exceed 300 mg/day

Available forms: Caps 5, 10, 25 mg; tabs 5, 10, 25 mg; IM inj 100 mg ampule

Adverse effects
(*italic* = common; **bold** = life-threatening)
CNS: Dizziness, drowsiness, confusion, headache, anxiety, tremors, stimulation, fatigue, depression, insomnia, hallucinations
CV: Orthostatic hypotension, **ECG changes, tachycardia,** hypotension
EENT: Blurred vision, tinnitus, mydriasis
GI: Constipation, dry mouth, nausea, vomiting, anorexia, diarrhea
INTEG: Rash, dermatitis, itching

Contraindications: Hypersensitivity to benzodiazepines, narrow-angle glaucoma, 🅟 psychosis, pregnancy **D**, child <6 yr

🅖 **Precautions:** Elderly, debilitated, hepatic disease, renal disease

🚫 **Do Not Confuse:**
Librium/Librax

Pharmacokinetics	
Absorption	Well absorbed (PO); slow, erratic (IM)
Distribution	Widely distributed; crosses placenta, blood-brain barrier
Metabolism	Liver extensively
Excretion	Kidneys, breast milk
🅖 **Half-life**	5-30 hr (increased in elderly)

Pharmacodynamics			
	PO	IM	IV
Onset	30 min	15-30 min	1-5 min
Peak	Within 2 hr	Unknown	Unknown
Duration	4-6 hr	Unknown	Up to 1 hr

Interactions
Individual drugs
Alcohol: ↑ CNS depression
Cimetidine, disulfiram, fluoxetine, ketoconazole, metoprolol, propranolol, rifampin, valproic acid: ↑ action of chlordiazepoxide
Isoniazid: ↑ action of isoniazid
Levodopa: ↓ action of levodopa
Drug classifications
Analgesics (opioid), antidepressants, antihistamines, CNS depressants: ↑ CNS depression
Barbiturates: ↓ effect of chlordiazepoxide
Contraceptives (oral): ↑ effect of contraceptive
 Herb/drug
Cowslip, kava, Queen Anne's lace, valerian: ↑ effect
Lab test interferences
17-OHCS
False positive: Pregnancy test (some methods)

NURSING CONSIDERATIONS
Assessment
• Assess anxiety reaction: inability to sleep, apprehension, dread, foreboding, or uneasiness related to unidentified source of danger
• Assess for previous drug dependence or tolerance; if drug dependent or tolerant, amount of medication should be restricted
• Monitor B/P (with patient lying, standing), pulse; if systolic B/P drops 20 mm Hg, hold drug, notify prescriber
• Monitor blood studies: CBC during long-term therapy; blood dyscrasias have occurred rarely
• Monitor hepatic studies: AST, ALT, bilirubin, creatinine, LDH, alkaline phosphatase during long-term therapy
• Monitor mental status: mood, sensorium, affect, sleeping patterns, drowsiness, dizziness, suicidal tendencies

Nursing diagnoses
☑ Anxiety (uses)
☑ Knowledge, deficient (teaching)
☑ Noncompliance (teaching)

Implementation
PO route
• Give with food or milk for GI symptoms, crushed if patient unable to swallow medication whole; do not open capsules; provide sugarless gum, hard candy, frequent sips of water for dry mouth
IM route
• Reconstitute with diluent provided (2 ml); agitate slowly, do not shake; give deep in large muscle mass to prevent severe pain; do not use IM diluent for **IV** route

IV route
• Reconstitute 100 mg/5 ml sterile water for inj or 0.9% NaCl; give over at least 1 min to prevent cardiac arrest, apnea, bradycardia
• Keep powder from light; refrigerate, mix when ready to use

Y-site compatibilities: Heparin, hydrocortisone, potassium chloride, vit B with C

Solution compatibilities: D₅W, 0.9% NaCl

Patient/family education
• Instruct patient that drug may be taken with food; if dose is missed take as soon as remembered; do not double doses
• Tell patient to avoid OTC preparations unless approved by prescriber; to avoid alcohol ingestion or other psychotropic medications unless directed by a prescriber
• Caution patient to avoid driving and activities requiring alertness, since drowsiness may occur; until medication response is known, tell patient that drowsiness may worsen at beginning of treatment
• Instruct patient not to discontinue medication abruptly after long-term use, drug should be tapered over 1 wk
• Caution patient to rise slowly or fainting may
 occur, especially in elderly
• Advise patient that drug should be avoided during pregnancy

Evaluation
Positive therapeutic outcome
• Increased well being
• Decreased anxiety, restlessness, sleeplessness, dread
• Successful alcohol withdrawal

Treatment of overdose: Lavage, VS, supportive care

---

chloroquine ⬥π (Rx)
(klor'oh-kwin)
Aralen HCl, Aralen Phosphate, chloroquine phosphate
Func. class.: Antimalarial
Chem. class.: Synthetic 4-aminoquinoline derivative

Pregnancy category C

Action: Inhibits parasite replications, transcription of DNA to RNA by forming complexes with DNA of parasite

---

 Herb/drug 🚫 Do Not Crush ⬥ Alert ⬥π Key Drug Ⓖ Geriatric Ⓟ Pediatric

→ **Therapeutic Outcome:** Decreased symptoms of malaria, amebiasis

Uses: Malaria caused by *Plasmodium vivax, Plasmodium malariae, Plasmodium ovale, Plasmodium falciparum* (some strains), amebiasis

Dosage and routes
Malaria suppression
P **Adult and child:** PO 5 mg base/kg/wk on same day of week, not to exceed 300 mg base; treatment should begin 1-2 wk before exposure and for 8 wk after; if treatment begins after exposure, 600 mg base for adult and 10 P mg base/kg for children in 2 divided doses 6 hr apart

Extraintestinal amebiasis
Adult: IM 160-200 mg base qd × 10-12 days or PO (HCl) 600 mg base qd × 2 days, then 300 mg base qd × 2-3 wk (phosphate)

P **Child:** IM/PO 10 mg/kg qd (HCl) × 2-3 wk, not to exceed 300 mg/day

Available forms: Tabs 250 mg (150 mg base), 500 mg (300 mg base) phosphate; inj 50 mg (40 mg base)/ml HCl

Adverse effects
(*italic* = common; **bold** = life-threatening)
CNS: Headache, stimulation, fatigue, **seizure,** psychosis
CV: Hypotension, **heart block, asystole with syncope,** ECG changes
EENT: *Blurred vision, corneal changes, retinal changes, difficulty focusing,* tinnitus, vertigo, deafness, photophobia, corneal edema
GI: *Nausea, vomiting, anorexia,* diarrhea, cramps
HEMA: **Thrombocytopenia, agranulocytosis, hemolytic anemia, leukopenia**
INTEG: Pruritus, pigmentary changes, skin eruptions, lichen planus–like eruptions, eczema, **exfoliative dermatitis**

Contraindications: Hypersensitivity, retinal field changes, porphyria

P **Precautions:** Pregnancy **C,** children, blood dyscrasias, severe GI disease, neurologic disease, alcoholism, hepatic disease, G6PD deficiency, psoriasis, eczema, lactation

Pharmacokinetics

Absorption	Well absorbed
Distribution	Widely
Metabolism	Liver
Excretion	Kidneys, feces
Half-life	3-5 days

Pharmacodynamics

	PO	IM
Onset	Rapid	Rapid
Peak	1-3 hr	30 min
Duration	6-8 hr	Unknown

Interactions
Individual drugs
Cimetidine: ↓ oral clearance, metabolism
Kaolin: ↓ absorption
Magnesium: ↓ action of chloroquine
Drug classifications
Antacids (aluminum): ↓ absorption

NURSING CONSIDERATIONS
Assessment
• Monitor liver studies weekly: ALT, AST, bilirubin; renal status: before exposure, monthly thereafter: BUN, creatinine, output, sp gr, urinalysis
• Assess mental status often: affect, mood, behavioral changes; psychosis may occur
• Assess hepatic status: decreased appetite, jaundice, dark urine, fatigue
• Assess for toxicity: blurring vision, difficulty focusing, headache, dizziness, decreased knee and ankle reflexes, drug should be discontinued immediately

Nursing diagnoses
✓ Infection, risk for (uses)
✓ Diarrhea (side effects)
✓ Knowledge, deficient (teaching)
✓ Noncompliance (teaching)
✓ Injury, risk for (side effects)

Implementation
PO route
• Give with meals to decrease GI symptoms; better to take on empty stomach 1 hr ac or 2 hr pc
• Give antiemetic if vomiting occurs
• Give after C&S is completed; monthly to detect resistance
IM route
• Give IM after aspirating to prevent inj into bloodstream

Additive compatibility: Promethazine

Patient/family education
• Advise patient that compliance with dosage schedule, duration is necessary

- Instruct patient that scheduled appointments must be kept or relapse may occur
- Caution patient to avoid alcohol while taking drug
- Instruct diabetic to use blood glucose monitor to obtain correct result
- Teach patient to report weakness, fatigue, loss of appetite, nausea, vomiting, yellowing of skin or eyes, tingling/numbness of hands/feet
- Advise patient that urine may turn rust brown color
- Instruct patient to use sunglasses in bright sunlight to prevent photophobia

Evaluation
Positive therapeutic outcome
- Decreased symptoms of malaria

Treatment of overdose: Induce vomiting, gastric lavage, administer barbiturate (ultrashort-acting), vasopressor; tracheostomy may be necessary

---

chlorothiazide (Rx)
(klor-oh-thye′a-zide)
Diuril
Func. class.: Diuretic, antihypertensive
Chem. class.: Thiazide; sulfonamide derivative

Pregnancy category B

Action: Acts on the distal tubule and thick ascending limb of the loop of Henle in the kidney, increasing excretion of sodium, water, chloride, magnesium, potassium, and bicarbonate

➡ **Therapeutic Outcome:** Decreased BP, decreased edema in tissues peripherally, diuresis

Uses: Edema in CHF, nephrotic syndrome; may be used alone or as adjunct with antihypertensives; also for edema in corticosteroids, estrogen therapy

Dosage and routes
Edema, hypertension
Adult: PO/**IV** 500 mg-2 g qd; may divide bid

Diuresis
Adult: **IV** 250 mg q6-12h

P *Child >6 mo:* PO 10-20 mg/kg/day may divide bid

P *Child <6 mo:* PO up to 40 mg/kg/day; may divide bid

Available forms: Tabs 250, 500 mg; oral susp 250 mg/5 ml; inj 500 mg

Adverse effects
(*italic* = common; **bold** = life-threatening)
CNS: Paresthesia, anxiety, depression, headache, *dizziness, fatigue, weakness, fever, insomnia*
CV: Irregular pulse, orthostatic hypotension, palpitations, volume depletion
EENT: Blurred vision
ELECT: *Hypokalemia,* hypercalcemia, hyponatremia, hypochloremia, hypophosphatemia, hypomagnesemia
GI: Nausea, vomiting, anorexia, constipation, diarrhea, cramps, pancreatitis, GI irritation, ***hepatitis***
GU: *Frequency,* polyuria, ***uremia,*** glucosuria, hematuria
HEMA: Aplastic anemia, hemolytic anemia, leukopenia, agranulocytosis, thrombocytopenia, neutropenia
INTEG: Rash, urticaria, purpura, photosensitivity, alopecia
META: Hyperglycemia, *hyperuricemia,* increased creatinine, BUN

Contraindications: Hypersensitivity to thiazides or sulfonamides, anuria, renal decompensation, lactation, hepatic coma

Precautions: Hypokalemia, renal disease, hepatic disease, gout, COPD, LE, **G** diabetes mellitus, pregnancy **B**, elderly, hyperlipidemia

▧ Do Not Confuse:
chlorothiazide/chlorproMAZINE,
chlorothiazide/chlorproPAMIDE,
chlorothiazide/chlorthalidone

Pharmacokinetics

	PO
Absorption	GI tract (10%-20%)
Distribution	Extracellular spaces; crosses placenta
Metabolism	Liver
Excretion	Urine, unchanged; breast milk
Half-life	1-2 hr

Pharmacodynamics

	PO	IV
Onset	2 hr	15 min
Peak	4 hr	½ hr
Duration	6-12 hr	2 hr

Interactions
Individual drugs
Alcohol: ↑ hypotension
Allopurinol, digitalis, lithium: ↑ toxicity

Amphotericin, mezlocillin, piperacillin, ticarcillin: ↑ hypokalemia

Cholestyramine, colestipol: ↓ absorption of chlorothiazide

Drug classifications
Antihypertensives: ↑ antihypertensive effect
Glucocorticoids: ↑ hypokalemia
Nitrates: ↑ hypotension
NSAIDs: ↓ diuretic action
Nondepolarizing skeletal muscle relaxants: ↑ toxicity

⊘ Herb/drug
Aloe, buckthorn, cascara sagrada, Chinese rhubarb, gossypol, licorice, nettle, senna: ↑ hypokalemia
St. John's wort: ↑ severe photosensitivity
Aloe, cucumber, dandelion, horsetail, pumpkin, Queen Anne's lace: ↑ diuretic effect

Lab test interferences
↑ BSP retention, ↑ calcium, ↑ amylase, ↑ parathyroid test
↓ PBI, ↓ PSP

False negative: Phentolamine and tyramine tests

Interference: Urine steroid tests

NURSING CONSIDERATIONS
Assessment
- Assess glucose in urine if patient is diabetic
- Monitor improvement in CVP q8h
- Check for rashes, temp elevation qd
- **G** • Assess for confusion, especially in elderly; take safety precautions if needed
- Monitor manifestations of hypokalemia; *RENAL:* acidic urine, reduced urine osmolality, nocturia; *CV:* hypotension, broad T wave, U wave, ectopy, tachycardia, weak pulse; *NEURO:* muscle weakness, altered LOC, drowsiness, apathy, lethargy, confusion, depression; *GI:* anorexia, nausea, cramps, constipation, distention, paralytic ileus; *RESP:* hypoventilation, respiratory muscle weakness
- Monitor for manifestations of hypomagnesemia; *CNS:* agitation, muscle twitching, paresthesias, hyperactive reflexes, positive Babinski's reflex, dysphagia, nystagmus, seizures, tetany; *GI:* nausea, vomiting, diarrhea, anorexia, abdominal distention; *CV:* ectopy, tachycardia, broad, flat, or inverted T waves, depressed ST segment, prolonged QT interval, decreased cardiac output, hypotension
- Monitor for manifestations of hyponatremia: *CV:* increased B/P, cold, clammy skin, hypovolemia or hypervolemia; *GI:* anorexia, nausea, vomiting, diarrhea, abdominal cramps; *NEURO:* lethargy, increased ICP, confusion, headache, seizures, coma, fatigue, tremors, hyperreflexia
- Monitor for manifestations of hyperchloremia: *NEURO:* weakness, lethargy, coma; *RESP:* coma, deep rapid breathing
- Assess fluid volume status: I&O ratios and record, count or weigh diapers as appropriate, weight, distended red veins, crackles in lung, color, quality and sp gr of urine, skin turgor, adequacy of pulses, moist mucous membranes, bilateral lung sounds, peripheral pitting edema; dehydration symptoms of decreasing output, thirst, hypotension, dry mouth and mucous membranes should be reported
- Monitor electrolytes: potassium, sodium, calcium, magnesium; also include BUN, blood pH, ABGs, uric acid, CBC, blood glucose
- Assess B/P before and during therapy with patient lying, standing, and sitting as appropriate; orthostatic hypotension can occur rapidly

Nursing diagnoses
- ☑ Urinary elimination, impaired (adverse reactions)
- ☑ Fluid volume deficient
- ☑ Fluid volume excess (uses)
- ☑ Knowledge, deficient (teaching)

Implementation
- Give in AM to avoid interference with sleep
- Potassium replacement if potassium level is 3.0 mg/dl
- Give whole, or use oral sol; drug may be crushed if patient is unable to swallow

PO route
- Give with food; if nausea occurs, absorption may be increased

IV IV route
- Do not use sol that is yellow, has a precipitate, or crystals
- Administer **IV** after diluting 0.5 g/18 ml or more of sterile water for inj; may be diluted further with dextrose or NaCl: give over 5 min; sol is stable at room temp for 24 hr

Additive compatibilities: Cimetidine, lidocaine, nafcillin, sodium bicarbonate

Additive incompatibilities: Amikacin, blood, blood products, chlorproMAZINE, codeine, hydrALAZINE, insulin, levorphanol, methadone, morphine, multivitamins, norepinephrine, polymyxin B, procaine, prochlorperazine, promazine, promethazine, streptomycin, tetracycline, triflupromazine, vancomycin

Patient/family education

- Teach patient to take medication early in the day to prevent nocturia
- Instruct patient to take with food or milk if GI symptoms of nausea and anorexia occur
- Teach patient to maintain a weekly record of weight and notify prescriber of weight loss >5 lb
- Caution patient that this drug causes a loss of potassium, so food rich in potassium should be added to the diet; refer to a dietician for assistance in planning
- Caution patient not to exercise in hot weather or stand for prolonged periods, since orthostatic hypotension will be enhanced; to use sunscreen to prevent burning
- Teach patient not to use alcohol or any OTC medications without prescriber's approval; serious drug reactions may occur
- Emphasize the need to contact prescriber immediately if muscle cramps, weakness, nausea, dizziness, or numbness occurs
- Teach patient to take own B/P and pulse and record
- Caution patient that orthostatic hypotension may occur; patient should rise slowly from sitting or reclining positions and lie down if dizziness occurs
- Teach patient to continue taking medication even if feeling better; this drug controls symptoms but does not cure the condition
- Advise the patient with hypertension to continue other medical treatment (exercise, weight loss, relaxation techniques, cessation of smoking)

Evaluation

Positive therapeutic outcome

- Decreased edema
- Decreased B/P
- Increased diuresis

Treatment of overdose: Lavage if taken orally, monitor electrolytes; administer dextrose in saline; monitor hydration, CV, renal status

---

chlorpheniramine (OTC, Rx)
(klor-fen-ir'a-meen)

Aller-Chlor, Allergy, Chlo-Amine, Chlorate, chlorpheniramine maleate, Chlor-Trimeton, Chlor-Tripolon ✦, Gen-Allerate, Novo-Pheniram ✦, PediaCare Allergy Formula, Phenetron, Teldrin

Func. class.: Antihistamine (1st generation, nonselective)

Chem. class.: Alkylamine, H_1-receptor antagonist

Pregnancy category B

Action: Acts on blood vessels, GI, respiratory system by competing with histamine for H_1-receptor site; decreases allergic response by blocking histamine

➔ **Therapeutic Outcome:** Absence of allergy symptoms and rhinitis

Uses: Allergy symptoms, rhinitis, allergic dermatoses, nasal allergies, hypersensitive reactions including blood transfusion reactions, anaphylaxis

Dosage and routes

P *Adult/child ≥12 yr:* PO 2-4 mg tid-qid, not to exceed 24 mg/day; time rel 8-12 mg bid-tid, not to exceed 24 mg/day; IM/**IV**/SC 5-40 mg/day, max 40 mg/day

P *Child 6-12 yr:* PO 2 mg q4-6h, not to exceed 12 mg/day; sus rel 8 mg hs or qd; sus rel not recommended for child <6 yr; SC 87.5 mcg/kg or 2.5 mg/m^2 q6h

P *Child 2-5 yr:* PO 1 mg q4-6h, not to exceed 4 mg/day

Available forms: Chewable tabs 2 mg; tabs 4, 8, 12 mg; time rel tabs 8, 12 mg; time rel caps 8, 12 mg; syr 1, 2, 2.5 mg/5 ml; inj 10, 100 mg/ml

Adverse effects

(*italic* = common; **bold** = life-threatening)

CNS: Dizziness, drowsiness, poor coordination, fatigue, anxiety, euphoria, confusion, paresthesia, neuritis

EENT: Blurred vision, dilated pupils, tinnitus, nasal stuffiness, dry nose, throat, mouth

GI: Nausea, anorexia, diarrhea

GU: Retention, dysuria, frequency

HEMA: **Thrombocytopenia, agranulocytosis, hemolytic anemia**

INTEG: Photosensitivity

RESP: Increased thick secretions, wheezing, chest tightness

Contraindications: Hypersensitivity to H_1-receptor antagonists, acute asthma attack, lower respiratory tract disease, stenosed peptic ulcers, bladder neck obstruction

Precautions: Increased intraocular pressure, renal disease, cardiac disease, hypertension, bronchial asthma, seizure disorder, hyperthyroidism, prostatic hypertrophy, 🛆 pregnancy **B**, elderly

🚫 Do Not Confuse:
Teldrin/Tedral

Pharmacokinetics

Absorption	Well absorbed (PO, SC, IM, **IV**)
Distribution	Widely distributed; crosses blood-brain barrier
Metabolism	Liver, mostly
Excretion	Kidneys, metabolite; breast milk (minimal)
Half-life	12-15 hr

Pharmacodynamics

	PO	PO-ER	SC	IM	IV
Onset	15-30 min	Unknown	Unknown	Unknown	Immediate
Peak	1-2 hr	Unknown	Unknown	Unknown	Unknown
Duration	4-12 hr	8-24 hr	4-12 hr	4-12 hr	4-12 hr

Interactions
Individual drugs
Alcohol: ↑ CNS depression
Atropine, disopyramide, haloperidol, quinidine: ↑ anticholinergic reactions
Drug classifications
Antidepressants (tricyclics), antihistamines, MAOIs, phenothiazines: ↑ anticholinergic reactions
CNS depressants, opiates, sedative/hypnotics: ↑ CNS depression
MAOIs: ↑ anticholinergic effect
🛆 *Herb/drug*
Corkwood, henbane leaf: ↑ anticholinergic effect
Hops, Jamaican dogwood, kava, khat, senega: ↑ sedative effect
Lab test interferences
False negative: Skin allergy tests (discontinue antihistamines 3 days before testing)

NURSING CONSIDERATIONS
Assessment
• Assess respiratory status: rate, rhythm, increase in bronchial secretions, wheezing, chest tightness; provide fluids to 2 L/day to decrease secretion thickness
• Monitor I&O ratio: be alert for urinary retention, frequency, dysuria, especially 🛆 elderly; drug should be discontinued if these occur
• **IV** administration may result in rapid drop in B/P, sweating, dizziness, especially in 🛆 elderly

Nursing diagnoses
✓ Airway clearance, ineffective (uses)
✓ Injury, risk for (side effects)
✓ Knowledge, deficient (teaching)
✓ Noncompliance (teaching, overuse)

Implementation
PO route
• May give with food to decrease GI upset; chewable tabs should be chewed and not swallowed whole; caps, time rel tabs should be swallowed whole
🚫 • Do not open or chew time rel tabs
• Store in tight, light-resistant container
SC/IM route
• Use only 20 and 100 mg/ml strengths; does not need to be reconstituted or diluted
IV IV route
Give undiluted by direct IV (10 mg/ml strength only); administer 10 mg over 1 min or more

Additive incompatibilities: Calcium chloride, kanamycin, norepinephrine, pentobarbital

Patient/family education
• Teach all aspects of drug use; to notify prescriber if confusion, sedation, hypotension, or difficulty voiding occurs; to avoid driving and other hazardous activity if drowsiness occurs; to avoid alcohol and other CNS depressants that may potentiate effect
• Teach patient not to exceed recommended dosage; dysrhythmias may occur
• Advise patient hard candy, gum, frequent rinsing of mouth may be used for dryness

Evaluation
Positive therapeutic outcome
• Absence of running or congested nose, rashes

Treatment of overdose: Administer ipecac syrup or lavage, diazepam, vasopressors, barbiturates (short acting)

*chlorproMAZINE (Rx)
(klor-proe'ma-zeen)

chlorproMAZINE HCl, Chlorpromanyl ✱, Largactil ✱, Novo-Chlorpromazine ✱, Thorazine, Thor-Prom

Func. class.: Antipsychotic/neuroleptic/antiemetic

Chem. class.: Phenothiazine, aliphatic

Pregnancy category C

Action: Depresses cerebral cortex, hypothalamus, limbic system, which control activity aggression; blocks neurotransmission produced by DOPamine at synapse; exhibits a strong α-adrenergic, anticholinergic blocking action; mechanism for antipsychotic effects is unclear

➡ **Therapeutic Outcome:** Decreased signs and symptoms of psychosis; control of nausea, vomiting, intractable hiccups, decreased anxiety preoperatively

Uses: Psychotic disorders, Tourette's syndrome, mania, schizophrenia, anxiety, intractable hiccups (adults), nausea, vomiting, preoperative relaxation, acute intermittent porphyria, behavioral problems in children, nonpsychotic patients with dementia

Investigational uses: Vascular headache

Dosage and routes
Psychosis
Adult: PO 10-50 mg q1-4h initially, then increase up to 2 g/day if necessary; IM 10-50 mg q1-4h, usual dose 300-800 mg/day

G *Elderly:* PO 10-25 mg qd-bid, ↑ by 10-25 mg/day q4-7 days, max 800 mg/day

P *Child >6 mo:* PO 0.5 mg/kg q4-6h; IM 0.5 mg/kg q6-8h; REC 1 mg/kg q6-8h

Nausea and vomiting
Adult: PO 10-25 mg q4-6h prn; IM 25-50 mg q3h prn; rec 50-100 mg q6-8h prn, not to exceed 400 mg/day; **IV** 25-50 mg qd-qid

P *Child ≥6 mo:* PO 0.55 mg/kg q4-6h; IM q6-8h; REC 1.1 mg/kg q6-8h, max IM ≤5 yr or ≤22.7 kg 40 mg; max IM 5-10 yr or 22.7-45.5 kg 75 mg; **IV** 0.55 mg/kg q6-8h

Intractable hiccups
Adult: PO 25-50 mg tid-qid; IM 25-50 mg (used only if PO dose does not work); **IV** 25-50 mg in 500-1000 ml saline (only for severe hiccups)

Available forms: Tabs 10, 25, 50, 100, 200 mg; sus rel caps 30, 75, 150, 200, 300 mg; syr 10, 25, 100 mg/5 ml; conc 30, 40, 100 mg/ml; supp 25, 100 mg; inj 25 mg/ml

Adverse effects
(*italic* = common; **bold** = life-threatening)

CNS: **Neuroleptic malignant syndrome,** dizziness, *extrapyramidal symptoms: pseudoparkinsonism, akathisia, dystonia, tardive dyskinesia,* seizures, *headache*

CV: *Orthostatic hypotension,* hypertension, **cardiac arrest,** ECG changes, **tachycardia**

EENT: Blurred vision, glaucoma, dry eyes

GI: *Dry mouth, nausea, vomiting, anorexia, constipation,* diarrhea, jaundice, weight gain

GU: Urinary retention, enuresis, impotence, amenorrhea, gynecomastia, breast engorgement

HEMA: Anemia, **leukopenia, leukocytosis, agranulocytosis**

INTEG: *Rash,* photosensitivity, dermatitis

RESP: **Laryngospasm,** dyspnea, **respiratory depression**

Contraindications: Hypersensitivity, circulatory collapse, liver damage, cerebral arteriosclerosis, coronary disease, severe hypertension/hypotension, blood dyscrasias, **P** coma, child <6 mo, brain damage, bone marrow depression, alcohol and barbiturate withdrawal, narrow-angle glaucoma

Precautions: Pregnancy **C**, lactation, seizure disorders, hypertension, hepatic **G** disease, cardiac disease, elderly, prostate enlargement

◪ **Do Not Confuse:**
chlorproMAZINE/chlorothiazide, chlorproMAZINE/chlorproPAMIDE, chlorproMAZINE/chlrothalidone, chlorproMAZINE/prochlorperazine

Pharmacokinetics

Absorption	Variable (PO); well absorbed (IM)
Distribution	Widely distributed; crosses placenta
Metabolism	Liver, GI mucosa extensively
Excretion	Kidneys
Half-life	30 hr

Pharmacodynamics

	PO	REC	IM	IV
Onset	½-1 hr	12 hr	Unkn	Rapid
Peak	Unkn	Unkn	Unkn	Unkn
Duration	4-6 hr*	3-4 hr	4-8 hr	Unkn

*Duration PO ext rel is 10-12 hr.

Interactions
Individual drugs
Alcohol: ↑ effects of both drugs, oversedation
Aluminum hydroxide, magnesium hydroxide: ↓ absorption
Bromocriptine, levodopa: ↓ antiparkinsonian activity
Disopyramide: ↑ anticholinergic effects
Epinephrine: ↑ toxicity
Guanethidine: ↓ antihypertensive response
Lithium: ↓ chlorproMAZINE levels, ↑ extrapyramidal symptoms (EPS), masking of lithium toxicity
Norepinephrine: ↓ vasoresponse, ↑ toxicity
Phenobarbital: ↓ effectiveness, ↑ metabolism
Valproic acid: ↑ valproic acid level
Warfarin: ↓ anticoagulant effect

Drug classifications
Antacids: ↓ absorption
Anticholinergics: ↑ anticholinergic effects
Anticonvulsants: ↓ seizure threshold
Antidepressants, antihistamines, barbiturate anesthetics, general anesthetics, MAOIs, opioids, sedative/hypnotics: ↑ CNS depression
Antidiarrheals, adsorbent: ↓ absorption
Antihypertensives: ↑ hypotension
Antiparkinsonian agents, β-adrenergic blockers: ↑ effect of both drugs
Antithyroid agents: ↑ agranulocytosis

Herb/drug
Cola tree, hops, kava, nettle, nutmeg: ↑ action
Henbane leaf: ↑ anticholinergic effect
Betel palm, kava: ↑ EPS

Lab test interferences
↑ Liver function tests, ↑ cardiac enzymes, ↑ cholesterol, ↑ blood glucose, ↑ prolactin, ↑ bilirubin, ↑ PBI, ↑ cholinesterase I, ↑ alkaline phosphatase, ↑ leukocytes, ↑ granulocytes, ↑ platelets, ↑^{131}I
↓ Hormones (blood and urine)
False positive: Pregnancy tests, PKU, urine bilirubin
False negative: Urinary steroids, 17-OHCS

NURSING CONSIDERATIONS
Assessment
• Assess mental status: orientation, mood, behavior, presence of hallucinations, and type before initial administration and monthly; this drug should significantly reduce psychotic behavior
• Assess any potentially reversible cause of behavior problems in the elderly before and during therapy
• Check for swallowing of PO medication; check for hoarding or giving of medication to other patients
• Monitor I&O ratio; palpate bladder if low urinary output occurs, especially in elderly; urinalysis recommended before, during prolonged therapy
• Monitor bilirubin, CBC, liver function studies monthly
• Assess affect, orientation, LOC, reflexes, gait, coordination, sleep pattern disturbances
• Monitor B/P with patient sitting, standing, and lying; take pulse and respirations q4h during initial treatment; establish baseline before starting treatment; report drops of 30 mm Hg; obtain baseline ECG, Q wave, and T wave changes
• Check for dizziness, faintness, palpitations, tachycardia on rising; severe orthostatic hypotension is common
• Identify for neuroleptic malignant syndrome: hyperpyrexia, muscle rigidity, increased CPK, altered mental status; drug should be discontinued
• Assess for EPS including akathisia (inability to sit still, no pattern to movements), tardive dyskinesia (bizarre movements of the jaw, mouth, tongue, extremities), pseudoparkinsonism (rigidity, tremors, pill rolling, shuffling gate); an antiparkinsonian drug should be prescribed
• Assess for constipation, urinary retention daily; if these occur, increase bulk, water in diet

Nursing diagnoses
☑ Thought processes, disturbed (uses)
☑ Coping, ineffective (uses)
☑ Knowledge, deficient (teaching)
☑ Noncompliance (teaching)

Implementation
PO route
• Give drug in liquid form mixed in glass of juice or cola if hoarding is suspected
• Periodically attempt dosage reduction in patients with behavioral problems
• Give with full glass of water, milk; or give with food to decrease GI upset
• Do not crush, break, or chew time rel caps
• Store in tight, light-resistant container, oral sol in amber bottle
Rectal route
• Give after placing in refrigerator for 30 min if too soft to insert; this route is used for nausea, vomiting, hiccups
IM route
• Inject in deep muscle mass; do not give SC; may be diluted with 0.9% NaCl, 2% procaine as prescribed; do not administer sol with a precipitate
IV route
• Give by direct **IV** by diluting with 0.9% NaCl

to a concentration of 1 mg/1 ml; administer at a rate of 1 mg/2 min

• Give by cont inf after diluting 50 mg/500-1000 ml of D₅W, D₁₀W, 0.9% NaCl, 0.45% NaCl, LR, Ringer's or combinations (used for intractable hiccups)

Syringe compatibilities:
Atropine, benztropine, butorphanol, diphenhydrAMINE, doxapram, droperidol, fentanyl, glycopyrrolate, hydromorphone, hydrOXYzine, meperidine, metoclopramide, midazolam, morphine, pentazocine, perphenazine, prochlorperazine, promazine, promethazine, scopolamine

Syringe incompatibilities:
Cimetidine, dimenhyDRINATE, heparin, pentobarbital, thiopental

Y-site compatibilities:
Amsacrine, cisatracurium, cisplatin, cladribine, cyclophosphamide, cytarabine, DOXOrubicin, DOXOrubicin liposome, famotidine, filgrastim, fluconazole, granisetron, heparin, hydrocortisone, ondansetron, potassium chloride, propofol, teniposide, thiotepa, vinorelbine

Additive compatibilities:
Ascorbic acid, ethacrynate, netilmicin, theophylline, vit B/C

Additive incompatibilities:
Aminophylline, amphotericin B, ampicillin, chloramphenicol, chlorothiazide, methicillin, methohexital, penicillin G, phenobarbital

Patient/family education

• Teach patient to use good oral hygiene; frequent rinsing of mouth, sugarless gum, candy or ice chips for dry mouth

• Caution patient to avoid hazardous activities until drug response is determined; dizziness, blurred vision may occur

• Inform patient that orthostatic hypotension occurs often and to rise from sitting or lying position gradually, to remain lying down after IM inj for at least 30 min; tell patient to avoid hot tubs, hot showers, tub baths, since hypotension may occur; tell patient that in hot weather heat stroke may occur; take extra precautions to stay cool

• Advise patient to avoid abrupt withdrawal of this drug, or extrapyramidal symptoms may result; drug should be withdrawn slowly

• Teach patient to avoid OTC preparations (cough, hay fever, cold) unless approved by prescriber, since serious drug interactions may occur; avoid use with alcohol, CNS depressants, since increased drowsiness may occur

• Caution patient to use sunscreen and sunglasses to prevent burns

• Teach patient about extrapyramidal symptoms and necessity of meticulous oral hygiene, since oral candidiasis may occur

• Instruct patient to take antacids 2 hr before or after taking this drug

• Instruct patient to report sore throat, malaise, fever, bleeding, mouth sores; if these occur, CBC should be drawn and drug discontinued

• Teach that urine may turn pink or red

• Teach patient to use contraceptive measures

Evaluation
Positive therapeutic outcome

• Decrease in emotional excitement, hallucinations, delusions, paranoia

• Reorganization of patterns of thought, speech

• Increase in target behaviors

Treatment of overdose: Lavage if orally ingested; provide airway, *do not induce vomiting or use epINEPHrine*

chlorthalidone (Rx)
(klor-tha'li-doan)
Apo-Chlorthalidone ✤, chlorthalidone, Hygroton, Thalitone, Uridon ✤
Func. class.: Diuretic, antihypertensive
Chem. class.: Thiazide-like phthalimindine derivative

Pregnancy category B

Action: Acts on the distal tubule and thick ascending limb of the loop of Henle in the kidney, increasing excretion of sodium, water, chloride, magnesium, potassium, and bicarbonate, possible arteriolar dilatation

➲**Therapeutic Outcome:** Decreased B/P, decreased edema in lung tissues and peripherally, diuresis

Uses: Edema in congestive heart failure, nephrotic syndrome; may be used alone or as adjunct with antihypertensives; also for edema in corticosteroid, estrogen therapy

Dosage and routes
Adult: PO 25-200 mg/day or 100 mg every other day

G *Elderly:* PO 12.5 mg qd, initially

P *Child:* PO 2 mg/kg or 60 mg/m² 3 ×/wk

Available forms: Tabs 25, 50, 100 mg

☑ Herb/drug   ⊗ Do Not Crush   ◆ Alert   ◆ₜₜ Key Drug   **G** Geriatric   **P** Pediatric

Adverse effects

(*italic* = common; **bold** = life-threatening)

CV: Irregular pulse, orthostatic hypotension, palpitations, volume depletion

CNS: Paresthesia, headache, *dizziness, fatigue, weakness,* fever

EENT: Blurred vision

ELECT: Hypokalemia, hypercalcemia, hyponatremia, hypochloremia, hypomagnesemia

GI: Nausea, vomiting, anorexia, constipation, diarrhea, cramps, pancreatitis, GI irritation, **hepatitis**

GU: Frequency, polyuria, **uremia,** glucosuria, impotence

HEMA: **Aplastic anemia, leukopenia, agranulocytosis, thrombocytopenia, neutropenia**

INTEG: Rash, urticaria, purpura, photosensitivity

META: Hyperglycemia, hyperuricemia, increased creatinine, BUN, gout

Contraindications: Hypersensitivity to thiazides or sulfonamides, anuria, renal decompensation, lactation

Precautions: Hypokalemia, hepatic disease, gout, COPD, LE, diabetes mellitus, elderly, pregnancy **B,** hyperlipidemia

◼ Do Not Confuse:

chlorthalidone/chlorothiazide, chlorthalidone/chlorproMAZINE, chlorthalidone/chlorproPAMIDE, Hygroton/Regroton, Uridon ✤/Vicodin

Pharmacokinetics

Absorption	Well absorbed
Distribution	Extracellular spaces; crosses placenta
Metabolism	Liver
Excretion	Urine, unchanged (30%-60%)
Half-life	40 hr

Pharmacodynamics

Onset	2 hr
Peak	6 hr
Duration	24-72 hr

Interactions

Individual drugs

Alcohol: ↑ hypotensive effect

Allopurinol, digitalis, lithium: ↑ toxicity

Amphotericin B: ↑ hypokalemia

Cholestyramine, colestipol: ↓ absorption of chlorthalidone

Diazoxide: ↑ hyperglycemia, hypotension

Drug classifications

Antihypertensives: ↑ antihypertensive effect

Nitrates: ↑ hypotension

Nondepolarizing skeletal muscle relaxants: ↑ toxicity

Glucocorticoids: ↑ hypokalemia

Sulfonylureas: ↓ effect of sulfonylurea

☑ Herb/drug

Aloe, buckthorn, cascara sagrada, Chinese rhubarb, gossypol, licorice, nettle, senna: ↑ hypokalemia

Cucumber, dandelion, horsetail, khella, pumpkin, Queen Anne's lace: ↑ hypotension

St. John's wort: Severe photosensitivity

Lab test interferences

↑ BSP retention, ↑ triglycerides, ↑ calcium, ↑ amylase, ↑ cholesterol

↓ PBI, ↓ PSP, ↓ parathyroid test

NURSING CONSIDERATIONS
Assessment

• Monitor manifestations of hypokalemia; *CV:* hypotension, broad T wave, U wave, ectopy, tachycardia, weak pulse; *GI:* anorexia, nausea, cramps, constipation, distention, paralytic ileus; *NEURO:* muscle weakness, altered LOC, drowsiness, apathy, lethargy, confusion, depression; *RENAL:* acidic urine, reduced urine, osmolality, nocturia; *RESP:* hypoventilation, respiratory muscle weakness

• Monitor for manifestations of hypomagnesemia; *CNS:* agitation, muscle twitching, paresthesias, hyperactive reflexes, positive Babinski's reflex, dysphagia, nystagmus seizures, tetany; *CV:* ectopy, tachycardia, broad, flat or inverted T waves, depressed ST segment, prolonged QT, decreased cardiac output, hypotension; *GI:* nausea, vomiting, diarrhea, anorexia, abdominal distention

• Monitor for manifestations of hyponatremia; *CV:* increased B/P, cold, clammy skin, hypovolemia or hypervolemia; *GI:* anorexia, nausea, vomiting, diarrhea, abdominal cramps; *NEURO:* lethargy, increased ICP, confusion, headache, seizures, coma, fatigue, tremors, hyperreflexia

• Monitor for manifestations of hyperchloremia; *NEURO:* weakness, lethargy, coma; *RESP:* coma, deep rapid breathing

• Assess fluid volume status: I&O ratios and record, count or weigh diapers as appropriate, weight, distended red veins, crackles in lung, color, quality and sp gr of urine, skin turgor, adequacy of pulses, moist mucous membranes, bilateral lung sounds, peripheral pitting edema; dehydration symptoms of decreasing output, thirst, hypotension, dry mouth, and mucous membranes should be reported

• Monitor electrolytes: potassium, sodium,

calcium, magnesium; also include BUN, blood pH, ABGs, uric acid, CBC, blood glucose
• Assess B/P before and during therapy with patient lying, standing, and sitting as appropriate; orthostatic hypotension can occur rapidly

Nursing diagnoses
☑ Fluid volume, deficient (adverse reactions)
☑ Fluid volume, excess (uses)
☑ Knowledge, deficient (teaching)
☑ Urinary elimination, impaired (side effect)

Implementation
• Brand names Thalitone/Hygroton should not be used interchangeably
• Give in AM to avoid interference with sleep
• Provide potassium replacement if potassium level is 3.0 mg/dl; give whole, or use oral solutions lightly; drug may be crushed if patient is unable to swallow
• Give with food; if nausea occurs, may crush tab and mix with fluids or applesauce for swallowing

Patient/family education
General
• Teach patient to take the medication early in the day to prevent nocturia
• Instruct patient to take with food or milk if GI symptoms of nausea and anorexia occur
• Teach patient to maintain weekly record of weight and notify prescriber of weight loss >5 lb
• Caution patient that this drug causes a loss of potassium, so foods rich in potassium should be added to the diet; refer to a dietician for assistance in planning
• Caution the patient not to exercise in hot weather or stand for prolonged periods, since orthostatic hypotension will be enhanced; to use sunscreen to prevent burns
• Teach patient not to use alcohol, or any OTC medications without prescriber's approval; serious drug reactions may occur
• Emphasize the need to contact prescriber immediately if muscle cramps, weakness, nausea, dizziness, or numbness occurs
• Teach patient to take own B/P and pulse and record
• Caution patient that orthostatic hypotension may occur; patient should rise slowly from sitting or reclining positions and lie down if dizziness occurs
• Teach patient to continue taking medication even if feeling better; this drug controls symptoms but does not cure the condition
• Advise patient with hypertension to continue other medical treatment (exercise, weight loss, relaxation techniques, cessation of smoking)

Evaluation
Positive therapeutic outcome
• Decreased edema
• Decreased B/P
• Increased diuresis

Treatment of overdose: Lavage if taken orally, monitor electrolytes; administer dextrose in saline; monitor hydration, CV, renal status

---

cholecalciferol
See vitamin D

---

cholestyramine (Rx)
(koe-less-tear'a-meen)
LoCHOLEST Light, Prevalite, Questran, Questran Light
Func. class.: Antilipemic
Chem. class.: Bile acid sequestrant

Pregnancy category C

Action: Absorbs, combines with bile acids to form an insoluble complex that is excreted through feces; loss of bile acids lowers cholesterol levels

▷ **Therapeutic Outcome:** Decreasing cholesterol levels and low-density lipoproteins, decreased pruritus

Uses: Primary hypercholesterolemia, pruritus associated with biliary obstruction, diarrhea caused by excess bile acid

Dosage and routes
Adult: PO 4 g qd-bid, max 24 g/day

🅿 *Child:* PO 240 mg/kg/day in 3 divided doses; administer with food or drink, max 8 g/day

Available forms: Powder for susp 4 g/ cholestyramine of 9 g/packet or scoop

Adverse effects
(*italic* = common; **bold** = life-threatening)
CNS: Headache, dizziness, drowsiness, vertigo, tinnitus, anxiety
GI: Constipation, abdominal pain, nausea, fecal impaction, hemorrhoids, flatulence, vomiting, steatorrhea, peptic ulcer
HEMA: **Bleeding,** increased Pro-time
INTEG: Rash, irritation of perianal area, tongue, skin
META: Decreased vit A, D, K, red cell folate content, **hyperchloremic acidosis**
MS: Muscle, joint pain

Contraindications: Hypersensitivity, biliary obstruction

Precautions: Pregnancy **C**, lactation, **P** children

Pharmacokinetics

Absorption	Not absorbed
Distribution	Not distributed
Metabolism	Not metabolized; LDL lowered in 4-7 days, serum cholesterol lowered in 1 mo
Excretion	Binds with bile acids, feces
Half-life	Unknown

Pharmacodynamics

Onset	24-48 hr
Peak	1-3 wk
Duration	2-4 wk

Interactions
Individual drugs
Clindamycin, clofibrate, gemfibrozil, glipizide, penicillin G, phenytoin, propranolol, iron, thyroid hormones: ↓ absorption of each specific drug
Drug classifications
Anticoagulants (oral), β-adrenergic blockers, cardiac glycosides, corticosteroids, NSAIDs, tetracyclines, thiazides, vit A, D, E, K: ↓ absorption
⊘ *Herb/drug*
Glucomannan: ↑ effect
Gotu kola: ↓ effect
Lab test interferences
Interference: Cholecystography
↑ AST, ALT, alkaline phosphatase
↓ Na, K

NURSING CONSIDERATIONS
Assessment
• Assess nutrition: fat, protein, carbohydrates; nutritional analysis should be completed by dietician
• Assess skin integrity after patient has been receiving drug; itching, pruritus often occur from bile deposits on skin
• Monitor cardiac glycoside level if both drugs are being administered; cardiac glycoside levels will be decreased
• Monitor for signs of vit A, D, E, K deficiency; fasting LDL, HDL, total cholesterol, triglyceride levels, electrolytes if on extended therapy
• Monitor bowel pattern daily; increase bulk, water in diet if constipation develops

Nursing diagnoses
☑ Constipation (adverse reactions)
☑ Knowledge, deficient (teaching)
☑ Noncompliance (teaching)

Implementation
• Give drug qd-bid, hs; give all other medications 1 hr before cholestyramine or 4-6 hr after cholestyramine to avoid poor absorption; do not take dry; mix drug with applesauce or stir into beverage (2-6 oz); let stand for 2 min; avoid inhaling powder
• Provide supplemental doses of vit A, D, E, K, if levels are low

Patient/family education
◆• Teach patient symptoms of hypoprothrombinemia: bleeding mucous membranes, dark tarry stools, hematuria, petechiae; report immediately
• Teach patient importance of compliance
• Teach patient that risk factors should be decreased: high-fat diet, smoking, alcohol consumption, absence of exercise
• Have patient mix drug with 6 oz of milk, water, fruit juice; do not mix with carbonated beverages; rinse glass to make sure all medication is taken or may mix drug in applesauce; allow to stand for 2 min before mixing

Evaluation
Positive therapeutic outcome
• Decreased cholesterol level (hyperlipidemia)
• Decreased diarrhea, pruritus (excess bile acids)

---

choline salicylate (Rx)
(koe'leen sa-lis'ih-late)
Arthropan
choline/magnesium salicylates (Rx)
CMT, Tricosal, Trilisate
Func. class.: Nonopioid analgesic
Chem. class.: Salicylate
Pregnancy category C

Action: Blocks pain impulses in CNS that occur in response to inhibition of prostaglandin synthesis; antipyretic action results from inhibition of hypothalamic heat-regulating center to produce vasodilatation to allow heat dissipation

➔ **Therapeutic Outcome:** Decreased pain, inflammation, fever

Uses: Mild to moderate pain or fever including arthritis, juvenile rheumatoid arthritis

Dosage and routes
Choline salicylate
P **Adult and child >12 yr:** PO 870-1740 mg qid; max 6×/day

Pain/fever
Adult: PO 435-870 mg q3-4h prn

Choline/magnesium salicylates
Adult: PO 2-3 g salicylate/day divided bid-tid
P **Child >37 kg:** PO 2.2 g of salicylate/day divided bid
P **Child <37 kg:** PO 50 mg of salicylate/kg/day divided bid

Available forms: Choline salicylate liq 870 mg/5 ml; choline/magnesium salicylate tabs 500, 750, 1000 mg; liq 500 mg/5 ml

Adverse effects
(*italic* = common; **bold** = life-threatening)
CNS: Stimulation, drowsiness, dizziness, confusion, **seizure,** headache, flushing, hallucinations, **coma**
CV: Rapid pulse, pulmonary edema
EENT: Tinnitus, hearing loss
ENDO: Hypoglycemia, hyponatremia, hypokalemia
GI: *Nausea, vomiting, GI bleeding, diarrhea, heartburn,* anorexia, **hepatitis, hepatotoxicity**
HEMA: **Thrombocytopenia, agranulocytosis, leukopenia, neutropenia, hemolytic anemia,** increased Pro-time
INTEG: *Rash,* urticaria, bruising, sweating
RESP: Wheezing, hyperpnea, hyperventilation

Contraindications: Hypersensitivity to salicylates, GI bleeding, bleeding disorders,
P children <3 yr, vit K deficiency, children with flulike symptoms

Precautions: Anemia, hepatic disease, renal disease, Hodgkin's disease, pregnancy **C,** lactation

Pharmacokinetics	
Absorption	Well absorbed
Distribution	Widely distributed; crosses placenta
Metabolism	Liver, extensively
Excretion	Kidney, active metabolites; breast milk
Half-life	2-3 hr (low doses); 15-30 hr (high doses)

Pharmacodynamics	
Onset	15-30 min
Peak	1-3 hr
Duration	3-6 hr

Interactions
Individual drugs
Alcohol, cefamandole, heparin, plicamycin: ↑ bleeding
Ammonium chloride, nizatidine: ↑ salicylate levels
Insulin, methotrexate, penicillins, phenytoin, valproic acid: ↑ effects
Probenecid, spironolactone, sulfinpyrazone: ↓ effects
Drug classifications
Antacids, steroids, urinary alkalizers: ↓ effects of choline salicylate
Anticoagulants, hypoglycemics (oral), thrombolytics: ↑ effects
β-blockers, sulfonamides: ↓ effects
Corticosteroids: ↓ salicylate effect
NSAIDs, steroids: ↑ gastric ulcers
Urinary acidifiers: ↑ salicylate levels
Food/drug
Foods that acidify the urine ↑ salicylate level
Herb/drug
Bilberry, bogbean, chondroitin, Irish moss, kelpware, pansy: ↑ bleeding risk
Lab test interferences
↑ Coagulation studies, ↑ liver function studies, ↑ serum uric acid, ↑ amylase, ↑ CO_2, ↑ urinary protein, ↓ serum potassium, ↓ PBI, ↓ cholesterol
Interference: Urine catecholamines, pregnancy test

NURSING CONSIDERATIONS
Assessment
• Monitor pain: location, duration, type, intensity, before dose and 1 hr after
• Monitor musculoskeletal status: ROM before dose
• Identify fever, length of time and related symptoms
• Monitor liver function studies: AST, ALT, bilirubin, creatinine if patient is on long-term therapy
• Monitor renal function studies: BUN, urine creatinine if patient is on long-term therapy
• Monitor blood studies: CBC, Hct, Hgb, Pro-time if patient is on long-term therapy
• Check I&O ratio; decreasing output may indicate renal failure (long-term therapy)
◆• Assess hepatotoxicity: dark urine, clay-colored stools, yellowing of the skin and sclera, itching, abdominal pain, fever, diarrhea if patient is on long-term therapy

• Assess for allergic reactions: rash, urticaria; if these occur, drug may have to be discontinued

• Assess for ototoxicity: tinnitus, ringing, roaring in ears; audiometric testing needed before, after long-term therapy

• Assess for visual changes: blurring, halos; corneal, retinal damage

• Check edema in feet, ankles, legs

• Identify prior drug history; there are many drug interactions

Nursing diagnoses
☑ Pain, acute (uses)
☑ Pain, chronic
☑ Mobility, impaired physical (uses)
☑ Knowledge, deficient (teaching)
☑ Injury, risk for (side effects)

Implementation
• Administer to patient crushed or whole

• Give with food or milk to decrease gastric symptoms; give 30 min ac or 2 hr pc; absorption may be slowed

• Give antacids 1-2 hr after enteric products

Patient/family education
• Teach patient to report any symptoms of hepatotoxicity, renal toxicity, visual changes, ototoxicity, allergic reactions, bleeding (long-term therapy)

• Advise patient to take with 8 oz of water and sit upright for 30 min after dose

• Caution patient not to exceed recommended dosage; acute poisoning may result

• Caution patient to read label on other OTC drugs; many contain aspirin products

• Inform patient that the therapeutic response takes 2 wk (arthritis)

• Teach patient to report tinnitus, confusion, diarrhea, sweating, hyperventilation

• Caution patient to avoid alcohol ingestion; GI bleeding may occur

• Teach patient that patients who have allergies may develop allergic reactions

• Caution patient to avoid buffered or effervescent products

P • Teach patient not to give to children; Reye's syndrome may develop

Evaluation
Positive therapeutic outcome
• Decreased pain
• Decreased inflammation
• Decreased fever
• Increased mobility

Treatment of overdose: Lavage, activated charcoal, monitor electrolytes, VS

cidofovir (Rx)
(si-doh-foh'veer)
Vistide
Func. class.: Antiviral
Chem. class.: Nucleotide analog

Pregnancy category C

Action: Suppresses cytomegalovirus (CMV) replication by selective inhibition of viral DNA synthesis

▷**Therapeutic Outcome:** Decreased symptoms of CMV

Uses: CMV retinitis in patients with HIV, used with probenecid

Dosage and routes
Dilute in 100 ml 0.9% NaCl sol before administration; probenecid must be given PO 2 g 3 hr before the cidofovir inf and 1 g at 2 and 8 hr after ending the cidofovir inf; give 1 L of 0.9% NaCl sol **IV** with each inf of cidofovir, give saline inf over 1-2 hr period immediately before cidofovir; patient should be given a second L if the patient can tolerate the fluid load; second L given at time of cidofovir or immediately afterward and should be given over a 1-3 hr period

Renal dose
Adult: **IV** CCr <50 ml/min reduce dose

Induction
Adult: **IV** inf initially 5 mg/kg given over 1 hr at a constant rate qwk × 2 consecutive wk;

Maintenance
Adult: **IV** inf 5 mg/kg given over 1 hr q2 wk

Available forms: Inj 75 mg/ml

Adverse effects
(*italic* = common; **bold** = life-threatening)
CNS: Fever, chills, **coma,** confusion, abnormal thought, *dizziness,* bizarre dreams, *headache,* psychosis, tremors, somnolence, paresthesia, *amnesia, anxiety, insomnia,* **seizures**
CV: **Dysrhythmias,** hypertension/hypotension
EENT: Retinal detachment in CMV retinitis
GI: Abnormal liver function tests, nausea, vomiting, anorexia, diarrhea, abdominal pain, **hemorrhage**
GU: **Hematuria,** increased creatinine, BUN, **nephrotoxicity**
HEMA: **Granulocytopenia, thrombocytopenia, irreversible neutropenia, anemia, eosinophilia**
INTEG: Rash, alopecia, pruritus, acne, urticaria, pain at inj site, phlebitis
RESP: Dyspnea

Contraindications: Hypersensitivity to this drug or probenecid, sulfa drugs

Precautions: Preexisting cytopenias, renal function impairment, pregnancy **C**, lactation, children <6 mo, elderly, platelet count <25,000/mm³

Pharmacokinetics
Unknown

Pharmacodynamics
Unknown

Interactions
Individual drugs
Amphotericin B, foscarnet, pentamidine **IV:** ↑ nephrotoxicity
Drug classifications
Aminoglycosides, NSAIDs: ↑ nephrotoxicity

NURSING CONSIDERATIONS
Assessment
- Obtain culture before treatment is initiated; cultures of blood, urine, and throat may all be taken; CMV is not confirmed by this method; the diagnosis is made by an ophthalmic exam
- Monitor renal, liver function, increased hematopoietic studies and BUN; serum creatinine, AST, ALT, creatinine, CCr, A-G ratio, baseline and drip treatment, blood counts should be done q2wk; watch for decreasing granulocytes, Hgb; if low, therapy may have to be discontinued and restarted after hematologic recovery; blood transfusions may be required
- Assess for GI symptoms: severe nausea, vomiting, diarrhea; severe symptoms may necessitate discontinuing drug
- Assess electrolytes and minerals: calcium, phosphorous, magnesium, sodium, potassium; watch closely for tetany during first administration
- Assess for symptoms of blood dyscrasias (anemia, granulocytopenia); bruising, fatigue, bleeding, poor healing
- Assess allergic reactions: flushing, rash, urticaria, pruritus
- Assess for leukopenia, neutropenia, thrombocytopenia: WBCs, platelets q2 days during 2×/day dosing and qwk thereafter; check for leukopenias, with qd WBC count in patients with prior leukopenia, with other nucleoside analogs, or for whom leukopenia counts are <1000 cells/mm³ at start of treatment
- Monitor serum creatinine or CCr at least q2

wk; give only to those with creatinine levels ≤1.5 mg/dl, CCr >55 ml/min, urine protein <100 mg/dl

Nursing diagnoses
☑ Infection, risk for (uses)

Implementation
- Mix under strict aseptic conditions using gloves, gown, and mask, and using precautions for antineoplastics
- Administer after diluting in 100 ml of 0.9% NaCl
- Give slowly; do not give by bolus **IV**, **IV**, SC inj
- Use diluted sol within 12 hr, do not refrigerate or freeze; do not use sol with particulate matter or discoloration

Patient/family education
- Advise to notify prescriber if sore throat, swollen lymph nodes, malaise, fever occur, may indicate other infections
- Advise to report perioral tingling, numbness in extremities, and paresthesias
- Teach that serious drug interactions may occur if OTC products are ingested; check first with prescriber
- Teach that drug is not a cure, but will control symptoms
- Advise that regular ophthalmic exams must be continued
- Advise that major toxicities may necessitate discontinuing drug
- Advise to use contraception during treatment and that infertility may occur; men should use barrier contraception for 90 days after treatment

Evaluation
Positive therapeutic outcome
- Decreased symptoms of CMV

Treatment of overdose: Discontinue drug; use hemodialysis, and increase hydration

---

cilastatin
See imipenem/cilastatin

---

cilostazol
(sil-oo-stay′zole)
Pletal
Func. class.: Platelet aggregation inhibitor
Chem. class.: Quinolinone derivative
Pregnancy category C

Action: Inhibits cellular phosphodiesterase; reversibly inhibits platelet aggregation induced

 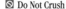

by thrombin, ADP, collagen, arachidonic acid, epINEPHrine, and shear stress

→ **Therapeutic Outcome:** Increased walking distance

Uses: Intermittent claudication

Dosage and routes
Adult: PO 100 mg bid taken ≥30 min ac or 2 hr pc breakfast and dinner or 50 mg bid, if using drugs that inhibit CYP3A4 and CYP2C19; 12 wk of treatment may be needed

Available forms: Tab 50, 100 mg

Adverse effects
(*italic* = common; **bold** = life-threatening)
CNS: *Dizziness,* headache
CV: *Palpitations, tachycardia,* **nodal dysrhythmia,** postural hypotension
EENT: Blindness, diplopia, ear pain, tinnitus, retinal hemorrhage
GI: *Nausea, vomiting, diarrhea, GI disorder,* colitis, cholelithiasis, ulcer, esophagitis, gastritis, anorexia, *flatulence, dyspepsia*
GU: Cystitis, frequency, vaginitis, **vaginal hemorrhage,** hematuria
HEMA: **Bleeding (epistaxis, hematuria, retinal hemorrhage, GI bleeding), thrombocytopenia,** anemia, polycythemia
INTEG: *Rash,* urticaria, dry skin
MISC: *Back pain, infection, myalgia, peripheral edema,* chills, fever, malaise, diabetes mellitus
RESP: *Cough, pharyngitis, rhinitis,* asthma, pneumonia

Contraindications: Hypersensitivity, CHF

Precautions: Past liver disease, renal
G disease, elderly, pregnancy **C,** lactation,
P children, increased bleeding risk, low platelet count, platelet dysfunction, active bleeding

⚊ **Do Not Confuse:**
Pletal/Plendil

Pharmacokinetics	
Absorption	Unknown
Distribution	95%-98% protein binding
Metabolism	Hepatic extensively by CYP450 enzymes
Excretion	Urine (74%), feces (20%)
Half-life	11-13 hrs

Pharmacodynamics
Unknown

Interactions
Individual drugs
Diltiazem, erythromycin: ↑ cilostazol levels
Fluconazole, fluoxetine, fluvoxamine, itraconazole, ketoconazole, nefazodone, omeprazole: May ↑ cilostazol levels; reduce dose to 50 mg bid
Drug classifications
Anticoagulants: May ↑ bleeding tendencies
Food/drug
• Do not use with grapefruit juice
⬚ *Herb/drug*
Agrimony, alfalfa, angelica, anise, basil, bay, bilberry, black haw, bogbean, bromelain, buchu, chondroitin, cinchona bark, dong quai, fenugreek, feverfew, garlic, ginger, ginkgo, ginseng, horse chestnut, Irish moss, kelp, kelpware, khella, lovage, lungwort, meadowsweet, motherwort, mugwort, nettle, papaya, parsley (large amounts), pau d'arco, pineapple, poplar, prickly ash, safflower, saw palmetto, tonka bean, turmeric, wintergreen, yarrow: ↑ risk of bleeding
Chamomile, coenzyme Q10, flax, glucomannan, goldenseal, guar gum: ↓ anticoagulant effect

NURSING CONSIDERATIONS
Assessment
• Assess for underlying CV disease since cardiovascular risk is great
• Assess for CV lesions with repeated oral administration
• Assess for CHF
• Monitor blood studies: CBC, Hct, Hgb, Pro-time if patient is on long-term therapy; thrombocytopenia, neutropenia may occur

Nursing diagnoses
✓ Injury, risk for (uses)
✓ Knowledge, deficient (teaching)

Implementation
• Give bid ≥1 hr ac or 2 hr pc; do not give with grapefruit juice

Patient/family education
• Advise patient to report any unusual bleeding to prescriber
• Caution patient to report side effects such as diarrhea, skin rashes, subcutaneous bleeding
• Teach patient that effects may take 2-4 wk, treatment of up to 12 wk may be required for necessary effect
• Teach patients with CHF about potential risks
• Advise patient to take ≥30 min ac or 2 hr pc
• Advise patient that reading patient package insert is necessary

Evaluation
Positive therapeutic outcome
• Increased walking distance and duration
• Decreased pain

cimetidine ◆═ (Rx, OTC)
(sye-met′i-deen)
Apo-Cimetidine ✤, cimetidine, Novocimetine ✤, Peptol ✤ Tagamet, Tagamet HB
Func. class.: H₂-receptor antagonist
Chem. class.: Imidazole derivative

Pregnancy category B

Action: Inhibits histamine at H₂-receptor site in the gastric parietal cells, which inhibits gastric acid secretion

⇒ **Therapeutic Outcome:** Healing of duodenal or gastric ulcers; prevention of duodenal ulcers; decreases symptoms of gastroesophageal reflux disease (GERD) and Zollinger-Ellison syndrome

Uses: Short-term treatment of duodenal and gastric ulcers and maintenance; management of GERD and Zollinger-Ellison syndrome

Investigational uses: Prevention of aspiration pneumonitis, stress ulcers, upper GI bleeding, herpes infection, hirsutism, urticaria, cutaneous/nongenital warts, weight loss

Dosage and routes
Treatment of active ulcers
P *Adult and child:* PO 300 mg qid with meals, hs × 8 wk or 400 mg bid, 800 mg hs; after 8 wk give hs dose only; **IV** bol 300 mg/20 ml 0.9% NaCl over 1-2 min q6h; **IV** inf 300 mg/50 ml D₅W over 15-20 min; IM 300 mg q6h, not to exceed 2400 mg

P *Child:* PO 20-40 mg/kg/day; IM/**IV** 5-10 mg/kg q6-8h

Prophylaxis of duodenal ulcer
P *Adult and child >16 yr:* 400 mg hs

GERD
Adult: PO 800-1600 mg/day in divided doses

Hypersecretory conditions (Zollinger-Ellison syndrome)
Adult: PO/IM/**IV** 300-600 mg q6h; may increase to 12 g/day if needed

Upper GI bleeding prophylaxis
Adult: **IV** 50 mg/hr; lowered in renal disease

Aspiration pneumonitis prophylaxis
Adult: IM/**IV** 300 mg IM 1 hr before anesthesia, then 300 mg **IV** q4h until patient is alert, max 2400 mg/day

Weight loss
Adult: PO 200-400 mg tid × 8-12 wk

Warts
Adult: PO 400-800 mg tid × 12 wk or 30-40 mg/kg/day given tid × 3 mo

Hirsutism
Adult: PO 300 mg qid × 5 day or 1600 mg qd up to 6 mo

Renal dose
Adult: PO CCr 20-40 ml/min 300 mg q8h; CCr <20 ml/min 300 mg q12h

Available forms: Tabs 100, 200, 300, 400, 800 mg; liq 200, 300 mg/5 ml; inj 300 mg/2 ml, 300 mg/50 ml 0.9% NaCl

Adverse effects
(*italic* = common; **bold** = life-threatening)
CNS: Confusion, headache, depression, dizziness, anxiety, weakness, psychosis, tremors, **seizures**
CV: Bradycardia, tachycardia, **dysrhythmias**
GI: Diarrhea, abdominal cramps, **paralytic ileus,** *jaundice*
GU: Gynecomastia, galactorrhea, impotence, increase in BUN, creatinine
***HEMA:* Agranulocytosis, thrombocytopenia, neutropenia, aplastic anemia, increase in Pro-time**
INTEG: Urticaria, rash, alopecia, sweating, flushing, **exfoliative dermatitis**

Contraindications: Hypersensitivity

P **Precautions:** Pregnancy **B**, lactation, child <16 yr, organic brain syndrome, hepatic
G disease, renal disease, elderly

Pharmacokinetics	
Absorption	Well absorbed (PO, IM); completely absorbed (**IV**)
Distribution	Widely distributed; crosses placenta
Metabolism	Liver (30%)
Excretion	Kidneys, unchanged (70%); breast milk
Half-life	1½-2 hr; increased in renal disease

Pharmacodynamics		
	PO	IV/IM
Onset	½ hr	10 min
Peak	45-90 min	½ hr
Duration	4-5 hr	4-5 hr

Interactions
Individual drugs
Carbamazepine, chloroquine, metronidazole, moricizine, quinine, valproic acid: ↑ toxicity (CYP450 pathway)
Ketoconazole: ↓ absorption of ketoconazole
Lidocaine, quinidine, warfarin: ↑ toxicity
Sucralfate: ↓ cimetidine absorption

☑ Herb/drug   Ⓢ Do Not Crush   ◆ Alert   ◆═ Key Drug   G Geriatric   P Pediatric

Drug classifications
Antacids: ↓ absorption of cimetidine
Antidepressants (tricyclic), benzodiazepines, β-adrenergic blockers, phenytoins, theophyllines: ↑ toxicity
Calcium channel blockers, sulfonylureas: ↑ toxicity (CYP450 pathway)

Lab test interferences
↑ Alkaline phosphatase, ↑ AST, ↑ creatinine, prolactin
False positive: Gastroccult, hemocult
False negative: Skin allergy tests

NURSING CONSIDERATIONS
Assessment
• Assess patient with ulcers or suspected ulcers: epigastric or abdominal pain, hematemesis, occult blood in stools, blood in gastric aspirate before and/or throughout treatment; monitor gastric pH (5 or > should be maintained)
• Monitor I&O ratio, BUN, creatinine, CBC with differential periodically

Nursing diagnoses
☑ Pain (uses)
☑ Knowledge, deficient (teaching)

Implementation
PO route
• Give with meals for lengthened drug effect; antacids 1 hr before or 1 hr after cimetidine

IV route
• Give by direct **IV** after diluting 300 mg/20 ml of 0.9% NaCl for inj; give over 5 min or more
• Give intermittent **IV** by diluting 300 mg/50 ml of D₅W; run over 15-20 min
• Give by cont inf after using total daily dose (900 mg) diluted in 100-1000 ml D₅W given over 24 hr
• Store diluted sol at room temp up to 48 hr

Syringe compatibilities: Atropine, butorphanol, cephalothin, diazepam, diphenhydrAMINE, doxapram, droperidol, fentanyl, glycopyrrolate, heparin, hydromorphone, hydrOXYzine, lorazepam, meperidine, midazolam, morphine, nafcillin, nalbuphine, penicillin G sodium, pentazocine, perphenazine, prochlorperazine, promazine, promethazine, scopolamine

Syringe incompatibilities: Cefamandole, cefazolin, chlorproMAZINE, pentobarbital, secobarbital

Y-site compatibilities: Acyclovir, amifostine, aminophylline, amrinone, atracurium, aztreonam, cisatracurium, cisplatin, cladribine, cyclosphosphamide, cytarabine, diltiazem, DOXOrubicin, DOXOrubicin liposome, enalaprilat, esmolol, filgrastim, fluconazole, fludarabine, foscarnet, gallium, granisetron, haloperidol, heparin, hetastarch, idarubicin, labetalol, melphalan, meropenem, methotrexate, midazolam, ondansetron, paclitaxel, pancuronium, piperacillin/tazobactam, propofol, sargramostim, tacrolimus, teniposide, theophylline, thiotepa, tolazoline, vecuronium, vinorelbine, zidovudine

Y-site incompatibilities: Amsacrine

Additive compatibilities: Acetazolamide, amikacin, aminophylline, atracurium, cefoperazone, cefoxitin, chlorothiazide, clindamycin, colistimethate, dexamethasone, digoxin, epINEPHrine, erythromycin, ethacrynate, floxacillin, flumazenil, furosemide, gentamicin, insulin, isoproterenol, lidocaine, lincomycin, meropenem, metaraminol, methylPREDNISolone, norepinephrine, penicillin G potassium, phytonadione, polymyxin B, potassium chloride, protamine, quinidine, tacrolimus, tetracycline, vancomycin, verapamil, vit B complex, vit B/C

Additive incompatibilities: Amphotericin B

Patient/family education
• Advise patient that any gynecomastia or impotence that develops is reversible after treatment is discontinued
• Caution patient to avoid driving, other hazardous activities until stabilized on this medication; drowsiness or dizziness may occur
• Advise patient to avoid black pepper, caffeine, alcohol, harsh spices, extremes in temp of food; tell patient to avoid OTC preparations: aspirin, cough, cold preparations; condition may worsen
• Advise patient that smoking decreases the effectiveness of the drug; smoking cessation should be considered
• Teach patient that drug must be continued for prescribed time to be effective and taken exactly as prescribed; doses are not to be doubled; to take missed dose when remembered up to 1 hr before next dose
• Instruct patient to report bruising, fatigue, malaise; blood dyscrasias may occur
• Have patient report to prescriber immediately any diarrhea, black tarry stools, sore throat, dizziness, confusion, or delirium

Evaluation
Positive therapeutic outcome
- Decreased pain in abdomen
- Healing of ulcers
- Absence of gastroesophageal reflux
- Gastric pH of ≥5

---

ciprofloxacin (Rx)
(sip-ro-floks'a-sin)
Cipro, Cipro IV
Func. class.: Urinary antiinfectives, broad-spectrum
Chem. class.: Fluoroquinolone

Pregnancy category C

Action: Interferes with conversion of intermediate DNA fragments into high-molecular-weight DNA in bacteria; DNA gyrase inhibitor

⇨ Therapeutic Outcome: Bactericidal action against the following: gram-positive organisms *Staphylococcus epidermidis,* methicillin-resistant strains of *Staphylococcus aureus, Streptococcus pyogenes, Streptococcus pneumoniae;* gram-negative organisms *Escherichia coli, Klebsiella* species, *Enterobacter, Salmonella, Shigella, Proteus vulgaris, Providencia stuartii, Providencia rettgeri, Morganella morganii, Pseudomonas aeruginosa, Serratia, Haemophilus, Acinetobacter, Neisseria gonorrhoeae, Neisseria meningitidis, Branhamella catarrhalis, Yersinia, Vibrio, Brucella, Campylobacter, Aeromonas*

Uses: Adult urinary tract infections (including complicated); chronic bacterial prostatitis; acute sinusitis; lower respiratory, skin, bone, joint infections; infectious diarrhea, exposure to inhalation anthrax; conjunctivitis, corneal ulcers (ophthalmic)

Dosage and routes
Uncomplicated urinary tract infections
Adult: PO 250 mg q12h; **IV** 200 mg q12h

Complicated/severe urinary tract infections
Adult: PO 500 mg q12h; **IV** 400 mg q12h

Respiratory, bone, skin, joint infections
Adult: PO 500 mg q12h

Corneal ulcers, conjunctivitis
Adult: Ophth 1-2 gtt q15-30 min until infection is controlled, then 1-2 gtt 4-6 times daily

Renal dose
Adult: PO CCr 30-50 ml/min PO 250-500 mg q12h; CCr 5-29 ml/min PO 250-500 mg q18h; **IV** 200-400 mg q18-24h

Available forms: Tabs 250, 500, 750 mg; inj 200 mg/20 ml, 400 mg/40 ml, 200 mg/100 ml D_5, 400 mg/200 ml D_5; oral susp 250, 500 mg/5 ml

Adverse effects
(*italic* = common; **bold** = life-threatening)
CNS: Headache, dizziness, fatigue, insomnia, depression, *restlessness,* **seizures,** confusion
GI: Nausea, constipation, increased ALT, AST, flatulence, insomnia, heartburn, *vomiting, diarrhea,* oral candidiasis, dysphagia, **pseudomembranous colitis,** dry mouth
INTEG: Rash, pruritus, urticaria, photosensitivity, flushing, fever, chills
MISC: **Anaphylaxis, Stevens-Johnson syndrome**
MS: Tremor, arthralgia, tendon rupture

Contraindications: Hypersensitivity to quinolones

Precautions: Pregnancy **C**, lactation, children, renal disease

⊠ Do Not Confuse:
ciprofloxacin/cephalexin

Pharmacokinetics
Absorption	Well absorbed (75%) (PO)
Distribution	Widely distributed
Metabolism	Liver (15%)
Excretion	Kidneys (40%-50%)
Half-life	3-4 hr; increased in renal disease

Pharmacodynamics
	PO	IV
Onset	Rapid	Immediate
Peak	1 hr	Infusion's end

Interactions
Individual drugs
Calcium, enteral feeding, sucralfate, zinc sulfate: ↓ ciprofloxacin absorption
Cyclosporine: ↑ nephrotoxicity
Probenecid: ↑ blood levels of ciprofloxacin, ↑ toxicity
Theophylline: ↑ theophylline levels
Warfarin: ↑ warfarin effect
Drug classifications
Aluminum, antacids, iron salts, magnesium: ↓ absorption of ciprofloxacin
⧄ Herb/drug
Acidophilus: Do not use with antiinfectives
Caffeine: ↑ caffeine levels

⧄ Herb/drug   Ⓢ Do Not Crush   ◆ Alert   ☎ Key Drug   G Geriatric   P Pediatric

Fennel: ↓ antiinfective effect
Yerba maté: ↑ toxicity
Food/drug
Dairy products, food: ↓ absorption
Lab test interferences
↑ AST, ↑ ALT, ↑ bilirubin, ↑ BUN, ↑ creatinine, ↑ alkaline phosphatase, ↑ LDH, ↑ or ↓ glucose, ↑ proteinuria, ↑ albuminuria ↓ WBC

NURSING CONSIDERATIONS
Assessment
• Assess patient for previous sensitivity reaction
• Assess patient for signs and symptoms of infection including characteristics of wounds, sputum, urine, stool, WBC >10,000/mm³, fever; obtain baseline information before and during treatment
• Obtain C&S before beginning drug therapy to identify if correct treatment has been initiated
• Assess for anaphylaxis: rash, urticaria, dyspnea, pruritus, chills, fever, joint pain; may occur a few days after therapy begins; epi-NEPHrine and resuscitation equipment should be available for anaphylactic reaction
• Identify urine output; if decreasing, notify prescriber (may indicate nephrotoxicity); also check for increased BUN, creatinine
• Monitor blood studies: AST, ALT, CBC, Hct, bilirubin, LDH, alkaline phosphatase, Coombs' test monthly if patient is on long-term therapy
• Monitor electrolytes: potassium, sodium, chloride monthly if patient is on long-term therapy
• Assess bowel pattern qd; if severe diarrhea occurs, drug should be discontinued
• Monitor for bleeding: ecchymosis, bleeding gums, hematuria, stool guaiac daily if on long-term therapy
• Assess for overgrowth of infection: perineal itching, fever, malaise, redness, pain, swelling, drainage, rash, diarrhea, change in cough, sputum

Nursing diagnoses
✓Infection, risk for (uses)
✓Diarrhea (side effects)
✓Injury, risk for (side effects)
✓Knowledge, deficient (teaching)
✓Noncompliance (teaching)

Implementation
PO route
• Give around the clock to maintain proper blood levels
• Administer 2 hr before or 2 hr after antacids, zinc, iron, calcium

IV route
• Check for irritation, extravasation, phlebitis daily
• For intermittent inf, dilute to 1-2 mg/ml of D₅W, 0.9% NaCl; give over 60 min; it will remain stable under refrigeration for 2 wk

Y-site compatibilities: Amifostine, amino acids, aztreonam, calcium gluconate, ceftazidime, cisatracurium, digoxin, diltiazem, diphenhydrAMINE, DOBUTamine, DOPamine, DOXOrubicin liposome, gallium, gentamicin, granisetron, hydrOXYzine, lidocaine, lorazepam, metoclopramide, midazolam, midodrine, piperacillin, potassium acetate, potassium chloride, potassium phosphates, predniso-LONE, promethazine, propofol, ranitidine, remifentanil, Ringer's, sodium chloride, tacrolimus, teniposide, thiotepa, tobramycin, verapamil

Y-site incompatibilities: Heparin, mezlocillin

Additive compatibilities: Amikacin, aztreonam, ceftazidime, cycloSPORINE, gentamicin, metronidazole, netilmicin, piperacillin, potassium acetate, potassium chloride, potassium phosphates, prednisoLONE, promethazine, propofol, ranitidine, Ringer's, sodium chloride, tobramycin, vit B/C

Additive incompatibilities: Aminophylline, amoxicillin, clindamycin, floxacillin, mezlocillin

Patient/family education
• Teach patient to report sore throat, bruising, bleeding, joint pain; may indicate blood dyscrasias (rare)
• Teach patient to contact prescriber if adverse reaction occurs or if inflammation or pain in tendon occurs
• Advise patient to contact prescriber if vaginal itching, loose foul-smelling stools, furry tongue occur; may indicate superinfection; report itching, rash, pruritus, urticaria
• Instruct patient to take all medication prescribed for the length of time ordered; drug must be taken around the clock to maintain blood levels; do not give medication to others
• Advise patient to notify prescriber of diarrhea with blood or pus
• Advise patient to rinse mouth frequently, use sugarless candy or gum for dry mouth

Evaluation
Positive therapeutic outcome
• Absence of signs/symptoms of infection (WBC <10,000/mm³, temp WNL, absence of red draining wounds)
• Reported improvement in symptoms of infection

cisatracurium (Rx)
(sis-a-tra-cyoor'ee-um)
Nimbex
Func. class.: Neuromuscular blocker (nondepolarizing)

Pregnancy category B

Action: Inhibits transmission of nerve impulses by binding with cholinergic receptor sites, antagonizing action of acetylcholine

⇒ **Therapeutic Outcome:** Paralysis of body for administration of anesthesia

Uses: Facilitation of endotracheal intubation, skeletal muscle relaxation during mechanical ventilation surgery, or general anesthesia

Dosage and routes
Adult: **IV** 0.15 and 0.2 mg/kg depending on desired time to intubate and length of surgery: use peripheral nerve stimulation to evaluate dosage

P *Child 2-12 yr:* **IV** 0.1 mg/kg over 5-10 sec with halothane or opioid anesthesia

Available forms: Inj 2, 10 mg/ml

Adverse effects
(*italic* = common; **bold** = life-threatening)
CV: Bradycardia, tachycardia; increased, decreased B/P
EENT: Increased secretions
RESP: Prolonged apnea, bronchospasm, cyanosis, respiratory depression
INTEG: Rash, flushing, pruritus, urticaria

Contraindications: Hypersensitivity

Precautions: Pregnancy **B**, cardiac disease,
P lactation, children <2 yr electrolyte imbalances, dehydration, neuromuscular disease, respiratory disease

Pharmacokinetics	
Unknown	

Pharmacodynamics	
Onset	1-3 min
Peak	2-5 min
Duration	30-40 min

Interactions
Individual drugs
Carbamazepine, phenytoin: ↓ duration of neuromuscular blockade
Lithium, isoflurane: ↑ neuromuscular blockade
Succinylcholine: ↓ neuromuscular blockade
Drug classifications
Aminoglycosides, antibiotics (polymix), β-adrenergic blockers, opioids: ↑ neuromuscular blockade

NURSING CONSIDERATIONS
Assessment
• Assess for electrolyte imbalances (K, Mg), may lead to increased action of this drug
• Assess vital signs (B/P, pulse, respirations, airway) until fully recovered; rate, depth, pattern of respirations; strength of handgrip
• Assess I&O ratio: check for urinary retention, frequency, hesitancy
• Assess recovery: decreased paralysis of face, diaphragm, legs, arms, rest of body
• Assess allergic reactions: rash, fever, respiratory distress, pruritus; drug should be discontinued

Nursing diagnoses
☑ Breathing pattern, ineffective (uses)
☑ Communication, impaired verbal (adverse reactions)
☑ Knowledge, deficient (teaching)

Implementation
Ⅳ **IV route**
• Use nerve stimulator by anesthesiologist to determine neuromuscular blockade
• Give anticholinesterase to reverse neuromuscular blockade
• Give by slow **IV** only by qualified person, do not administer IM
• Store in light-resistant area
• Reassure if communication is difficult during recovery from neuromuscular blockage

Evaluation
Positive therapeutic outcome
• Paralysis of jaw, eyelid, head, neck, rest of body

Treatment of overdose: Edrophonium or neostigmine, atropine, monitor VS; mechanical ventilation

---

! HIGH ALERT

cisplatin (Rx)
(sis'pla-tin)
Platinol, Platinol-AQ
Func. class.: Antineoplastic alkylating agent
Chem. class.: Inorganic heavy metal

Pregnancy category D

Action: Alkylates DNA, RNA; inhibits enzymes that allow synthesis of amino acids in proteins; activity is not cell cycle phase specific

➔ **Therapeutic Outcome:** Prevention of rapidly growing malignant cells

Uses: Advanced bladder cancer; adjunctive in metastatic testicular cancer and metastatic ovarian cancer; head, neck, esophageal, prostatic, lung, and cervical cancer; lymphoma

Dosage and routes
Dosage protocols may vary

Testicular cancer
Adult: **IV** 20 mg/m^2 qd × 5 days, repeat q3 wk for 3 cycles or more, depending on response

Bladder cancer
Adult: **IV** 50-70 mg/m^2 q3-4 wk

Metastatic ovarian cancer
Adult: **IV** 100 mg/m^2 q4 wk or 50 mg/m^2 q3 wk with cyclophosphamide therapy; mix with 2 L of NaCl and 37.5 g mannitol over 6 hr

Available forms: Inj 0.5 mg/ml ✤; 1 mg/ml powder for inj 10, 50 mg vials

Adverse effects
(*italic* = common; **bold** = life-threatening)
CNS: **Seizures,** peripheral neuropathy
CV: Cardiac abnormalities
EENT: Tinnitus, hearing loss, vestibular toxicity
GI: Severe nausea, vomiting, diarrhea, weight loss
GU: **Renal tubular damage,** renal insufficiency, impotence, sterility, amenorrhea, gynecomastia, hyperuremia
HEMA: **Thrombocytopenia, leukopenia, pancytopenia**
INTEG: Alopecia, dermatitis
META: Hypomagnesemia, hypocalcemia, hypokalemia, hypophosphatemia
RESP: **Fibrosis**
SYST: **Anaphylaxis**

Contraindications: Radiation therapy within 1 mo, chemotherapy within 1 mo, thrombocytopenia, recent smallpox vaccination, pregnancy **D**

Precautions: Pneumococcal vaccination, lactation

◼ Do Not Confuse:
cisplatin/carboplatin
Platinol/Paraplatin

C

Pharmacokinetics
Absorption	Complete
Distribution	Widely distributed, accumulates in body tissues for several months
Metabolism	Liver
Excretion	Kidneys
Half-life	30-100 hr

Pharmacodynamics
Unknown

Interactions
Individual drugs
Alcohol, aspirin, NSAIDs: ↑ risk of bleeding
Phenytoin: ↓ phenytoin effect
Radiation: ↑ toxicity, bone marrow suppression
Drug classifications
Aminoglycosides, diuretics (loop): ↑ nephrotoxicity
Antineoplastics: ↑ toxicity
Antineoplastics, bone marrow–suppressing drugs: ↑ bone marrow suppression
Diuretics (loop): ↑ ototoxicity
NSAIDs: ↑ risk of bleeding
Vaccines, live virus: ↓ antibody response
Lab test interferences
↑ Uric acid, ↑ BUN, ↑ creatinine, ↓ CCr, ↓ calcium, ↓ phosphate, ↓ potassium, ↓ magnesium
Positive: Coombs' test

NURSING CONSIDERATIONS
Assessment
• Monitor for bone marrow depression: CBC, differential, platelet count weekly; withhold drug if WBC count is <4000/mm^3 or platelet count is <100,000/mm^3; notify prescriber of results if WBC <20,000/mm^3, platelets <150,000/mm^3
• Monitor renal function studies: BUN, creatinine, serum uric acid, urine CCr before and during therapy; I&O ratio; report fall in urine output to <30 ml/hr; dose should not be given if BUN <25 mg/dl; creatinine <1.5 mg/dl
• Assess for anaphylaxis: wheezing, tachycardia, facial swelling, fainting; discontinue drug and report to prescriber, resuscitation equipment should be nearby
• Monitor temp q4h (may indicate beginning of infection)

- Monitor liver function tests before and during therapy (bilirubin, AST, ALT, LDH) as needed or monthly; note yellowing of skin or sclera, dark urine, clay-colored stools, itchy skin, abdominal pain, fever, diarrhea
- Assess for increased uric acid levels, swelling, joint pain primarily in extremities; patient should be well hydrated to prevent urate deposits
- Assess for bleeding: hematuria, stool guaiac, bruising or petechiae, mucosa or orifices q8h; note inflammation of mucosa, breaks in skin
- Identify dyspnea, rales, nonproductive cough, chest pain, tachypnea
- Identify effects of alopecia on body image; discuss feelings about body changes
- Identify edema in feet, joint pain, stomach pain, shaking; prescriber should be notified

Nursing diagnoses
☑ Injury, risk for (adverse reactions)
☑ Body image, disturbed (adverse reactions)
☑ Infection, risk for (adverse reactions)
☑ Knowledge, deficient (teaching)

Implementation
- Hydrate patient with 0.9% NaCl over 8-12 hr before treatment
- Give all medications PO, if possible; avoid IM inj when platelets <100,000/mm^3
- Give epINEPHrine, antihistamines, corticosteroids for hypersensitivity reaction; antiemetic 30-60 min before giving drug to prevent vomiting, and prn; allopurinol or sodium bicarbonate to maintain uric acid level, alkalinization of urine; antibiotics for prophylaxis of infection; diuretic (furosemide 40 mg **IV**) or mannitol after infusion
- After diluting 10 mg/10 ml or 50 mg/50 ml sterile water for inj; withdraw prescribed dose, dilute ½ dose with 1000 ml D$_5$ 0.2 NaCl or D$_5$ 0.45 NaCl with 37.5 g mannitol; **IV** inf is given over 3-4 hr; use a 0.45 μm filter; total dose 2000 ml over 6-8 hr; check site for irritation, phlebitis; do not use equipment containing aluminum
- Prepare in biologic cabinet using gown, gloves, mask; do not allow drug to come in contact with skin, use soap and water if contact occurs

Syringe compatibilities: Bleomycin, cyclophosphamide, doxapram, DOXOrubicin, droperidol, fluorouracil, furosemide, heparin, leucovorin, methotrexate, metoclopramide, mitomycin, vinBLAStine, vinCRIStine

Y-site compatibilities: Allopurinol, aztrenonam, bleomycin, chlorproMAZINE, cimetidine, cladribine, cyclophosphamide, dexamethasone, diphenhydrAMINE, doxapram, DOXOrubicin, DOXOrubicin liposome, droperidol, famotidine, filgrastim, fludarabine, fluorouracil, furosemide, ganciclovir, granisetron, heparin, hydromorphone, leucovorin, lorazepam, melphalan, methotrexate, methylPREDNISolone, metoclopramide, mitomycin, morphine, ondansetron, paclitaxel, prochlorperazine, promethazine, propofol, ranitidine, sargramostim, teniposide, vinBLAStine, vinCRIStine, vinorelbine

Additive compatibilities: Carboplatin, cyclophosphamide with etoposide, etoposide, etoposide with floxuridine, floxuridine, floxuridine with leucovorin, hydrOXYzine, ifosfamide, ifosfamide with etoposide, leucovorin, magnesium sulfate, mannitol, ondansetron

Additive incompatibilities: Fluorouracil, mesna, thiotepa

Solution compatibilities: D$_5$/0.225% NaCl, D$_5$/0.45% NaCl, D$_5$/0.9% NaCl, D$_5$/0.45% NaCl with mannitol 1.875%, D$_5$/0.33% NaCl with mannitol 1.875%, D$_5$/0.33% NaCl with KCl 20 mEq and mannitol 1.875%, 0.9% NaCl, 0.45% NaCl, 0.3% NaCl, 0.225% NaCl, water

Solution incompatibilities: Sodium bicarbonate 5%, 0.1% NaCl, water

Patient/family education
- Teach patient to avoid use of products containing aspirin or ibuprofen, NSAIDs, alcohol (may cause GI bleeding), razors, commercial mouthwash; to report symptoms of bleeding (hematuria, tarry stools, bruising, petechiae)
- Advise patient to report numbness, tingling in face or extremities, poor hearing or joint pain, swelling
- Instruct patient to report signs of anemia (fatigue, headache, irritability, faintness, shortness of breath)
- Instruct patient to report any changes in breathing or coughing even several months after treatment; to avoid crowds and persons with respiratory tract or other infections
- Advise patient that hair may be lost during treatment; a wig or hair piece may make patient feel better; new hair may be different in color, texture
- Tell patient not to have any vaccinations without the advice of the prescriber; serious reactions can occur
- Caution patient contraception is needed

---

during treatment and for several months after the completion of therapy

Evaluation
Positive therapeutic outcome
• Prevention of rapid division of malignant cells

---

citalopram (Rx)
(sigh-tal'oh-pram)
Celexa
Func. class.: Antidepressant
Chem class.: Selective serotonin reuptake inhibitor (SSRI)

Pregnancy category B

Action: Inhibits CNS neuron uptake of serotonin but not of norepinephrine; weak inhibitor of CYP450 enzyme system, making it more appealing than other drugs

Therapeutic Outcome: Decreased symptoms of depression after 2-3 wk

Uses: Major depressive disorder

Investigational uses: Fibromyalgia, premenstrual disorders, panic disorder, social phobia, impulsive aggression in children, obsessive-compulsive disorder in adolescents, treatment of psychotic symptoms in nondepressed, demented patients

Dosage and routes
Depression
Adult: PO 20 mg qd AM or PM, may increase if needed to 40 mg/day after 1 wk; maintenance: after 6-8 wk of initial treatment, continue for 24 wk (32 wk total), reevaluate long-term usefulness (max 60 mg/day)

Fibromyalgia
Adult: PO 20 mg qd × 4 wk, increase dose to 40 mg qd × 4 wk

G *Hepatic dose/elderly*
Adult: PO 20 mg/day, may increase to 40 mg/day if no response

Panic disorder
Adult: PO 20-30 mg/day
Child: Premenstrual dysphoria, social phobia, impulsive aggression in children

Adult: PO 20-40 mg/day used intermittently in premenstrual dysphoria

Available forms: Tabs 10, 20, 40 mg; oral sol 2 mg (as base)/ml

Adverse effects
(*italic* = common; **bold** = life-threatening)
CNS: *Headache, nervousness, insomnia, drowsiness, anxiety, tremor, dizziness, fatigue, sedation, poor concentration, abnormal dreams, agitation,* **seizures,** apathy, euphoria, hallucinations, delusions, psychosis, **suicidal attempts**
CV: *Hot flashes, palpitations,* angina pectoris, **hemorrhage,** hypertension, 1st-degree tachycardia, 1st-degree AV block, bradycardia, MI, thrombophlebitis
EENT: Visual changes, ear/eye pain, photophobia, tinnitus
GI: *Nausea, diarrhea, dry mouth, anorexia, dyspepsia, constipation, cramps, vomiting, taste changes, flatulence, decreased appetite*
GU: *Dysmenorrhea, decreased libido, urinary frequency, urinary tract infection,* amenorrhea, cystitis, impotence, urine retention
INTEG: *Sweating, rash, pruritus,* acne, alopecia, urticaria
MS: *Pain,* arthritis, twitching
RESP: *Infection, pharyngitis, nasal congestion, sinus headache, sinusitis, cough, dyspnea, bronchitis,* asthma, hyperventilation, pneumonia
SYST: *Asthenia, viral infection, fever, allergy, chills*

Contraindications: Hypersensitivity

P Precautions: Pregnancy **C,** lactation, **G** children, elderly

Do Not Confuse:
celexa/celebrex/cerebyx/cerebra

Pharmacokinetics
Absorption	Well absorbed
Distribution	Unknown
Metabolism	Liver
Excretion	Kidneys, steady state 28-35 days
Half-life	Unknown

Pharmacodynamics
Onset	Unknown
Peak	Unknown
Duration	Unknown

Interactions
Individual drugs
Alcohol: ↑ CNS depression
Carbamazepine: ↑ toxicity, ↓ citalopram levels
Lithium: ↑ serotonergic effects
Drug classifications
Antidepressants, tricyclics: ↑ effect, use cautiously

Antifungals (azole), macrolides: ↑ citalopram levels

Barbiturates, benzodiazepines, CNS depressants, sedative/hypnotics: ↑ CNS depression

β-Adrenergic blockers: ↑ plasma levels of β-blockers

MAOIs: Hypertensive crisis, seizures, fatal reactions, do not use together

☑ *Herb/drug*
SAM-e, St. John's wort: do not use with citalopram, fatal reaction may occur
Yohimbe: ↑ CNS stimulation

Lab test interferences: ↑ Serum bilirubin, ↑ blood glucose, ↑ alkaline phosphatase, ↓ VMA, ↓ 5-HIAA
False: ↑ Urinary catecholamines

NURSING CONSIDERATIONS
Assessment
• Monitor B/P (lying, standing), pulse q4h; if systolic B/P drops 20 mm Hg, hold drug and notify prescriber; take vital signs q4h in patients with cardiovascular disease
• Monitor blood studies: CBC, leukocytes, differential, cardiac enzymes if patient is receiving long-term therapy; check platelets, bleeding can occur
• Monitor hepatic studies: AST, ALT, bilirubin
• Check weight qwk; appetite may increase with drug
• Assess ECG for flattening of T wave, bundle branch block, AV block, dysrhythmias in cardiac patients
G • Assess extrapyramidial symptoms (EPS) primarily in elderly: rigidity, dystonia, akathisia
• Assess mental status: mood, sensorium, affect, suicidal tendencies; increase in psychiatric symptoms: depression, panic
• Monitor urinary retention, constipation;
P constipation is more likely to occur in children **G** or elderly
◆ • Assess for withdrawal symptoms: headache, nausea, vomiting, muscle pain, weakness; usually do not occur unless drug is discontinued abruptly
• Identify patient's alcohol consumption; if alcohol is consumed, hold dose until AM

Nursing diagnoses
☑ Coping, ineffective (uses)
☑ Injury, risk for (side effects)
☑ Knowledge, deficient (teaching)
☑ Noncompliance (teaching)

Implementation
• Give with food or milk for GI symptoms

• Give dosage hs if oversedation occurs during day
• Store at room temp; do not freeze

Patient/family education
• Teach patient that therapeutic effects may take 2-3 wk
• Instruct patient to use caution in driving or other activities requiring alertness because of drowsiness, dizziness, blurred vision; to avoid rising quickly from sitting to standing, **G** especially elderly
• Caution patient to avoid alcohol ingestion, other CNS depressants
• Advise patient not to discontinue medication quickly after long-term use: may cause nausea, headache, malaise
• Instruct patient to increase fluids, bulk in diet if constipation, urinary retention occur, **G** especially elderly
• Advise patient to take gum, hard sugarless candy, or frequent sips of water for dry mouth

Evaluation
Positive therapeutic outcome
• Decrease in depression
• Absence of suicidal thoughts

---

clarithromycin (Rx)
(clare-i-thro-mye'sin)
Biaxin, Biaxin XL
Func. class.: Antiinfective
Chem. class.: Macrolide

Pregnancy category C

Action: Binds to 50S ribosomal subunits of susceptible bacteria and suppresses protein synthesis

➔ **Therapeutic Outcome:** Bactericidal action against the following: *Streptococcus pneumoniae, Streptococcus pyogenes, Mycoplasma pneumoniae, Corynebacterium diphtheriae, Bordetella pertussis, Listeria monocytogenes, Haemophilus influenzae, Staphylococcus aureus, Mycobacterium avium (MAC), Mycobacterium intracellulare,* complex infections in AIDS patients, *Helicobacter pylori* in combination with omeprazole

Uses: Mild to moderate infections of the upper respiratory tract, lower respiratory tract; uncomplicated skin and skin structure infections

Dosage and routes
Adult: PO 250-500 mg q12h × 7-14 days; 500 mg q12h continues for MAC

P *Child:* PO 15 mg/kg/day (max 1000 mg) divided q12h × 10 days

H. pylori *infection*
Adult: PO 500 mg qd plus omeprazole 2 × 20 mg q AM (day 1-14) then omeprazole 20 mg q AM (days 15-28)

Acute maxillary sinusitis/acute bacterial bronchitis
Adult: PO 500 mg q12h × 10 days

Available forms: Tabs 250, 500 mg; granules for oral susp 125, 250 mg/5 ml; ext rel tab 500 mg

Adverse effects
(*italic* = common; **bold** = life-threatening)
CV: Ventricular dysrhythmias
GI: Nausea, vomiting, diarrhea, **hepatotoxicity**, abdominal pain, stomatitis, heartburn, anorexia, abnormal taste, **pseudomembranous colitis**
GU: Vaginitis, moniliasis
HEMA: Leukopenia, thrombocytopenia, increased INR
INTEG: Rash, urticaria, pruritus, **Stevens-Johnson syndrome**
MISC: Headache

Contraindications: Hypersensitivity to this drug or other macrolides

Precautions: Pregnancy **C**, lactation, hepatic/renal disease

Pharmacokinetics	
Absorption	50%
Distribution	Widely distributed
Metabolism	Liver
Excretion	Kidneys, unchanged (20%-30%)
Half-life	4-6 hr

Pharmacodynamics	
Onset	Unknown
Peak	2 hr

Interactions
Individual drugs
Carbamazepine: ↑ toxicity, from ↑ levels of carbamazepine
Digoxin: ↑ blood levels of digoxin, ↑ digoxin effects
Fluconazole: ↑ clarithromycin levels
Pimozide: ↑ effect, ↑ dysrhythmias
Theophylline: ↑ toxicity from ↑ levels of theophylline
Zidovudine: ↓ action
Drug classifications
Oral anticoagulants: ↑ effects of oral anticoagulants

Herb/drug
Acidophilus: Do not use with antiinfectives
Lab test interferences
↑ 17-OHCS/17-KS, ↑ AST, false ↑ ALT, BUN, creatinine, LDH, total bilirubin
↓ Folate assay, ↓ WBC

C

NURSING CONSIDERATIONS
Assessment
• Assess patient for signs and symptoms of infection including characteristics of wounds, sputum, urine, stool, WBC >10,000/mm^3, earache, fever; obtain baseline information before and during treatment
• Obtain C&S before beginning drug therapy to identify if correct treatment has been initiated
• Monitor blood studies: AST, ALT, CBC, Hct, bilirubin, LDH, alkaline phosphatase, Coombs' test monthly if patient is on long-term therapy
• Assess bowel pattern qd; if severe diarrhea occurs, drug should be discontinued
• Assess for overgrowth of infection: perineal itching, fever, malaise, redness, pain, swelling, drainage, rash, diarrhea, change in cough, sputum

Nursing diagnoses
✓ Infection, risk for (uses)
✓ Diarrhea (side effects)
✓ Knowledge, deficient (teaching)
✓ Noncompliance (teaching)

Implementation
• Ensure adequate fluid intake (2 L) during diarrhea episodes
• Give q12h to maintain serum level

Patient/family education
• Advise patient to contact physician if vaginal itching, loose foul-smelling stools, furry tongue occur; may indicate superinfection
• Instruct patient to take all medication prescribed for the length of time ordered, do
🚫 not crush
• Advise prescriber if pregnancy is planned or suspected

Evaluation
Positive therapeutic outcome
• Absence of signs/symptoms of infection (WBC <10,000/mm^3, temp WNL, absence of red draining wounds)
• Reported improvement in symptoms of infection

clavulanate
See amoxicillin/clavulanate, ticarcillin/clavulanate

clemastine (Rx)
(klem'as-teen)
Antihist-1, Contac Allergy 12 Hour, Tavist
Func. class.: Antihistamine
Chem. class.: Ethanolamine derivative, H_1-receptor antagonist

Pregnancy category B

Action: Acts on blood vessels, GI, respiratory system by competing with histamine for H_1-receptor site; decreases allergic response by blocking histamine

→ **Therapeutic Outcome:** Absence of allergy symptoms and rhinitis

Uses: Allergy symptoms, rhinitis, allergic dermatoses, nasal allergies, hypersensitive reactions including blood transfusion reactions, anaphylaxis

Dosage and routes
P *Adult and child >12 yr:* PO 1.34-2.68 mg bid-tid, not to exceed 8.04 mg/day

Available forms: Tabs 1.34, 2.68 mg; syr 0.67 mg/ml

Adverse effects
(*italic* = common; **bold** = life-threatening)
CNS: Dizziness, drowsiness, poor coordination, fatigue, anxiety, euphoria, confusion, paresthesia, neuritis, paradoxic excitement
P (child)
CV: Hypotension, palpitations, tachycardia
EENT: Blurred vision, dilated pupils, tinnitus, nasal stuffiness, dry nose, throat, *mouth*
GI: Constipation, dry mouth, nausea, vomiting, anorexia, diarrhea
GU: Retention, dysuria, frequency
HEMA: **Thrombocytopenia, agranulocytosis, hemolytic anemia**
INTEG: Rash, urticaria, photosensitivity, sweating
RESP: Increased thick secretions, wheezing, chest tightness

Contraindications: Hypersensitivity to H_1-receptor antagonists, acute asthma attack, lower respiratory tract disease

Precautions: Increased intraocular pressure, renal disease, cardiac disease, hypertension, bronchial asthma, seizure disorder, stenosed peptic ulcers, hyperthyroidism, prostatic hypertrophy, bladder neck
G obstruction, pregnancy **B**, elderly

Pharmacokinetics
Absorption	Well absorbed
Distribution	Widely distributed
Metabolism	Liver, extensively
Excretion	Kidneys, breast milk (high)
Half-life	Unknown

Pharmacodynamics
Onset	15-60 min
Peak	1-2 hr
Duration	12 hr

Interactions
Individual drugs
Alcohol: ↑ CNS depression
Drug classifications
CNS depressants, opioids, sedative/hypnotics: ↑ CNS depression
MAOIs: ↑ anticholinergic effect
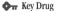 *Herb/drug*
Corkwood, henbane leaf: ↑ anticholinergic effect
Hops, Jamaican dogwood, kava, khat, senega: ↑ sedative effect
Lab test interferences
False negative: Skin allergy tests (discontinue antihistamines 3 days before testing)

NURSING CONSIDERATIONS
Assessment
• Assess respiratory status: rate, rhythm, increase in bronchial secretions, wheezing, chest tightness; provide fluids to 2 L/day to decrease secretion thickness
• Monitor I&O ratio: be alert for urinary retention, frequency, dysuria, especially
G elderly; drug should be discontinued if these occur

Nursing diagnoses
☑ Airway clearance, ineffective (uses)
☑ Injury, risk for (side effects)
☑ Knowledge, deficient (teaching)
☑ Noncompliance (teaching, overuse)

Implementation
• May give with food to decrease GI upset
🚫 • Do not crush or chew caps
• Store in tight, light-resistant container

Patient/family education
• Teach all aspects of drug uses; to notify prescriber if confusion, sedation, hypotension occur; to avoid driving and other hazardous activity if drowsiness occurs; to avoid alcohol and other CNS depressants that may potentiate effect
• Instruct patient to take 1 hr ac or 2 hr pc to facilitate absorption

---

 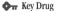 Herb/drug   🚫 Do Not Crush   ◆ Alert   ☏ Key Drug   **G** Geriatric   **P** Pediatric

- Caution patient not to exceed recommended dosage; dysrhythmias may occur
- Teach patient hard candy, gum, frequent rinsing of mouth may be used for dryness
- Tell patient if EENT or CNS symptoms occur (blurred vision, severe dry mouth, dry throat, confusion, dizziness, poor coordination, euphoria), prescriber should be notified

Evaluation
Positive therapeutic outcome
- Absence of running or congested nose, rashes

Treatment of overdose: Administer ipecac syrup or lavage, diazepam, vasopressors, barbiturates (short acting)

---

clindamycin HCl (Rx)
(klin-dah-my'sin)
Cleocin HCl
clindamycin palmitate (Rx)
Cleocin Pediatric, Dalacin C Palmitate
clindamycin phosphate (Rx)
Cleocin Phosphate, Dalacin C, Dalacin C Phosphate
Func. class.: Antiinfective—misc.
Chem. class.: Lincomycin derivative

Pregnancy category B

Action: Binds to 50S subunit of bacterial ribosomes; suppresses protein synthesis

Therapeutic Outcome: Absence of infection

Uses: Infections caused by staphylococci, streptococci, *Rickettsia, Fusobacterium, Actinomyces, Peptococcus, Clostridium*

Dosage and routes
Adults: PO 150-450 mg q6h, max 1.8 g/day; IM/**IV** 1.2-1.8 g/day in 2-4 divided doses q6-12h, not to exceed 4800 mg/day

P *Child <1 mo:* 15-20 mg/kg/day divided q6-8h

P *Child >1 mo:* PO 8-25 mg/kg/day in divided doses q6-8h; IM/**IV** 20-40 mg/kg/day in divided doses q6-8h in 3-4 equal doses

Vaginal route
Adult: 5 g applicatorful at bedtime × 1 wk

Topical route
Adult: Sol 1% apply bid

PID
Adult: **IV** 600 mg q6h plus gentamicin or 900 mg q8h

Bacterial endocarditis prophylaxis
Adult: 600 mg 1 hr before procedure

Available forms: Phosphate: inj 150, 300, 600 mg base/4 ml; 900 mg base/ml; 900 mg base/60 ml; inj inf in D_5 300, 600, 900 mg; HCl: caps 75, 150, 300 mg; palmitate: oral sol 75 mg/ml

Adverse effects
(*italic* = common; **bold** = life-threatening)
INTEG: Rash, urticaria, pruritus, erythema, pain, abscess at inj site
GI: Nausea, vomiting, abdominal pain, diarrhea, **pseudomembranous colitis,** *anorexia, weight loss,* increased AST, ALT, bilirubin, alkaline phosphatase, jaundice
GU: Vaginitis, urinary frequency
HEMA: **Leukopenia, eosinophilia, agranulocytosis, thrombocytopenia, polyarthritis**

Contraindications: Hypersensitivity to this drug or lincomycin, tartrazine dye, ulcerative colitis/enteritis

Precautions: Renal disease, liver disease, GI disease, elderly, pregnancy **B,** lactation, tartrazine sensitivity, pseudomembranous colitis

Pharmacokinetics
Absorption	Well absorbed (PO, IM), minimal (top)
Distribution	Widely distributed; crosses placenta
Metabolism	Liver, extensively
Excretion	Kidneys, breast milk
Half-life	2½ hr

Pharmacodynamics
	PO	IM	IV	TOP	VAG
Onset	Rapid	Rapid	Rapid	Rapid	Rapid
Peak	½-1 hr	1½ hr	Infusion's end	Unknown	Unknown

Interactions
Individual drugs
Erythromycin: ↓ action of clindamycin
Kaolin: ↓ absorption
Drug classifications
Neuromuscular blockers: ↑ neuromuscular blockade
Herb/drug
Acidophilus: Do not use with antiinfectives
Lab test interferences
↑ Alkaline phosphatase, ↑ bilirubin, ↑ CPK, ↑ AST, ↑ ALT

NURSING CONSIDERATIONS
Assessment
• Assess any patient with compromised renal system; drug is excreted slowly in poor renal system function; toxicity may occur rapidly
• Assess patient for signs and symptoms of infection including characteristics of wounds, sputum, urine, stool, WBC >10,000/mm^3, fever; obtain baseline information before and during treatment
• Complete C&S testing before beginning drug therapy; this will identify if correct treatment has been initiated
• Assess for allergic reactions: rash, urticaria, pruritus, chills, fever, joint pain; may occur a few days after therapy begins; epINEPHrine and resuscitation equipment should be available in case of an anaphylactic reaction
• Identify urine output; if decreasing, notify prescriber (may indicate nephrotoxicity); also look for increased BUN and creatinine levels
• Monitor blood studies: AST, ALT, CBC, Hct, bilirubin, LDH, alkaline phosphatase, Coombs' test monthly if patient is on long-term therapy
• Monitor electrolytes: potassium, sodium, chloride monthly if patient is on long-term therapy
• Assess bowel pattern qd; if severe diarrhea occurs, drug should be discontinued; may indicate pseudomembranous colitis
• Monitor for bleeding: ecchymosis, bleeding gums, hematuria, stool guaiac daily if on long-term therapy
• Assess for overgrowth of infection: perineal itching, fever, malaise, redness, pain, swelling, drainage, rash, diarrhea, change in cough, sputum

Nursing diagnoses
✓ Infection, risk for (uses)
✓ Diarrhea (adverse reactions)
✓ Injury, risk for (adverse reaction)
✓ Knowledge, deficient (teaching)
✓ Noncompliance (teaching)

Implementation
PO route
• Give with 8 oz of water; give with meals for GI symptoms
• Shake liquids well
• Do not refrigerate oral preparations; stable at room temperature for 2 wk
🚫 • Do not crush, chew caps
IM route
• If more than 600 mg must be given, divide into 2 inj
• Give deeply in large muscle mass; rotate sites

ⅣⅤ **IV route**
• Give by inf only; do not administer bolus dose; dilute 300 mg or more/50 ml or more of D$_5$W, 0.9% NaCl
• May be further diluted in greater amounts of D$_5$W, 0.9% NaCl and given as a cont inf in acute PID; give first dose 10 mg/min over ½ hr, then 0.75 mg/min; increased rates may be used to keep serum blood levels higher; run over >10 min; no more than 1200 mg in a 1 hr inf

Syringe compatibilities: Amikacin, aztreonam, gentamicin, heparin

Syringe incompatibilities: Tobramycin

Y-site compatibilities: Amifostine, amiodarone, amphotericin B cholesteryl, amsacrine, aztreonam, cisatracurium, cyclophosphamide, diltiazem, DOXOrubicin liposome, enalaprilat, esmolol, fludarabine, foscarnet, granisetron, heparin, hydromorphone, labetolol, magnesium sulfate, melphalan, meperidine, midazolam, morphine, multivitamins, odansetron, perphenazine, piperacillin/tazobactam, propofol, remifentanil, sargramostim, tacrolimus, teniposide, theophylline, thiotepa, vinorelbine, vit B/C, zidovudine

Y-site incompatibilities: Idarubicin

Additive compatibilities: Amikacin, ampicillin, aztreonam, cefamandole, cefazolin, cefepine, cefonicid, cefoperazone, cefotaxime, cefoxitin, ceftazidime, ceftizoxime, cefuroxime, cephalothin, cimetidine, fluconazole, heparin, hydrocortisone, kanamycin, methylPREDNISolone, metoclopramide, metronidazole, netilmicin, ofloxacin, penicillin G, pipercillin, potassium chloride, sodium bicarbonate, tobramycin, verapamil, vit B/C

Additive incompatibilities: Ciprofloxacin
Topical route
• Avoid contact with eyes, mucous membranes, and open cuts during topical application; if accidental contact occurs, rinse with cool water
• Wash affected areas with warm water and soap, rinse, pat dry before application

Patient/family education
• Tell patient to take oral drug with full glass of water; may take with food if GI symptoms occur; antiperistaltic drugs may worsen diarrhea

---

- Teach patient aspects of drug therapy: need to complete entire course of medication to ensure organism death (10-14 days); culture may be taken after medication course has been completed
- Advise patient to report sore throat, fever, fatigue; may indicate superimposed infection
- Advise patient that drug must be taken at equal intervals around clock to maintain blood levels

Evaluation
Positive therapeutic outcome
- Decreased temperature, negative C&S

Treatment of hypersensitivity:
Withdraw drug; maintain airway; administer epINEPHrine, aminophylline, O₂, **IV** corticosteroids

---

*clomiPHENE (Rx)
(kloe′mi-feen)
Clomid, clomiPHENE citrate, Milophene, Serophene
Func. class.: Ovulation stimulant
Chem. class.: Nonsteroidal antiestrogenic

Pregnancy category   X

Action: Increases LH, FSH release from the pituitary, which increases maturation of ovarian follicle, ovulation, development of corpus luteum

➡ **Therapeutic Outcome:** Pregnancy

Uses: Female infertility (ovulatory failure)

Dosage and routes
Adult: PO 50-100 mg qd × 5 days or 50-100 mg qd beginning on day 5 of cycle; may be repeated until conception occurs or 3 cycles of therapy have been completed

Available forms: Tabs 50 mg

Adverse effects
(*italic* = common; **bold** = life-threatening)
CNS: *Headache, depression,* restlessness, anxiety, nervousness, fatigue, insomnia, dizziness, flushing
CV: Vasomotor flushing, phlebitis, **deep vein thrombosis**
EENT: Blurred vision, diplopia, photophobia
GI: *Nausea, vomiting, constipation,* abdominal pain, bloating
GU: Polyuria, frequency of urination, **birth defects, spontaneous abortions,** multiple ovulation, breast pain, oliguria, abnormal uterine bleeding
INTEG: *Rash, dermatitis,* urticaria, alopecia

Contraindications: Hypersensitivity, pregnancy **X,** hepatic disease, undiagnosed uterine bleeding, uncontrolled thyroid or adrenal dysfunction, intracranial lesion, ovarian cysts

Precautions: Hypertension, depression, seizures, diabetes mellitus

◤ Do Not Confuse:
clomiPHENE/clomiPRAMINE

Pharmacokinetics	
Absorption	Well distributed
Distribution	Unknown
Metabolism	Liver, extensively
Excretion	Feces
Half-life	5 days

Pharmacodynamics
Unknown

Interactions: None
Lab test interferences
↑ FSH/LH, ↑ BSP, ↑ thyroxine, ↑ TBG

NURSING CONSIDERATIONS
Assessment
- Determine liver function tests before therapy: AST, ALT, alkaline phosphatase
- Monitor serum progesterone, urinary excretion of pregnanediol to identify occurrence of ovulation
- Pelvic examination should be done to determine ovarian size, cervical condition
- Endometrial biopsy may be done in women over 35 to rule out endometrial carcinoma

Nursing diagnoses
☑ Sexual dysfunction (uses)
☑ Knowledge, deficient (teaching)

Implementation
- Give after discontinuing estrogen therapy
- Give at same time qd to maintain drug level; begin on 5th day of menstrual cycle

Patient/family education
- Advise patient that multiple births are common after drug is taken
- Instruct patient to notify prescriber immediately if low abdominal pain occurs; may indicate ovarian cyst, cyst rupture
- Advise patient to notify prescriber of photophobia, blurred vision, diplopia
- Teach patient if dose is missed, double at next time; if more than one dose is missed, call prescriber
- Instruct patient that response usually occurs 4-10 days after last day of treatment
- Teach patient method for taking, recording

---

basal body temp to determine whether ovulation has occurred; if ovulation can be determined (there is a slight decrease in temp, then a sharp increase for ovulation), to attempt coitus 3 days before and qod until after ovulation
• Teach patient if pregnancy is suspected, to notify prescriber immediately

Evaluation
Positive therapeutic outcome
• Fertility

---

*clomiPRAMINE (Rx)
(klom-ip'ra-meen)
Anafranil
Func. class.: Tricyclic antidepressant
Chem. class.: Tertiary amine
Pregnancy category C

Action: Potent inhibitor of serotonin and norepinephrine uptake; also increases dopamine metabolism

⮑ **Therapeutic Outcome:** Decreased signs and symptoms of obsessive-compulsive disorder, decreased depression

Uses: Obsessive-compulsive disorder, depression, dysphoria, anxiety, agoraphobia and other phobias

Dosage and routes
Obsessive-compulsive disorder
Adult: PO 25 mg hs; increase gradually over 4 wk to a dosage of 75-250 mg/day in divided doses
P *Child 10-18 yr:* PO 25-50 mg/day gradually increased or 3 mg/kg/day whichever is smaller; not to exceed 200 mg/day

Depression
Adult: PO 50-150 mg/day in a single or divided dose

Anxiety/agoraphobia
Adult: PO 25-75 mg/day

Available forms: Caps 25, 50, 75 mg

Adverse effects
(*italic* = common; **bold** = life-threatening)
CNS: Dizziness, tremors, mania, **seizures,** aggressiveness, drowsiness, headache, extrapyramidial symptoms (EPS)
CV: Hypotension, tachycardia, **cardiac arrest**
ENDO: Galactorrhea, hyperprolactinemia
GI: Constipation, dry mouth, nausea, dyspepsia, weight gain
GU: Delayed ejaculation, anorgasmia, retention, decreased libido

HEMA: **Agranulocytosis, neutropenia, pancytopenia**
INTEG: Diaphoresis, photosensitivity
META: Hyponatremia
EENT: Blurred vision

Contraindications: Hypersensitivity, immediately after MI

Precautions: Seizures, suicidal patients,
G elderly, cardiac disease, pregnancy **C**

◨ **Do Not Confuse:**
clomiPRAMINE/clomiPHENE, clomiPRAMINE/desipramine/norpramin

Pharmacokinetics
Absorption	Well absorbed
Distribution	Widely distributed
Metabolism	Liver, extensively
Excretion	Kidneys, breast milk
Half-life	19-37 hr; steady state 1-2 wk

Pharmacodynamics
Onset	≥2 wk
Peak	2-6 hr

Interactions
Individual drugs
Alcohol: ↑ CNS depression
Carbamazepine: ↓ clomiPRAMINE action
Cimetidine, fluoxetine, fluvoxamine, sertraline: ↑ clomiPRAMINE level; do not use together
Clonidine, epINEPHrine, norepinephrine: Severe hypertension; avoid use
Phenytoin: ↓ clomiPRAMINE action
Drug classifications
Barbiturates: ↓ clomiPRAMINE levels
CNS depressants: ↑ effects; do not use together
MAOIs: Hypertensive crisis, seizures; do not use together
▨ *Herb/drug*
SAM-e, St. John's wort: serotonin syndrome, do not use together
Belladonna, henbane leaf: ↑ anticholinergic effect
Hops, kava, lavender: ↑ sedative effect
Corkwood, jimsonweed, scopolia: ↑ clomiPRAMINE effect
Lab test interferences
↑ Prolactin, ↑ TBG
↑ Serum thyroid hormones

NURSING CONSIDERATIONS
Assessment
• Monitor B/P (with patient lying, standing), pulse q4h; if systolic B/P drops 20 mm Hg hold drug, notify prescriber; take VS q4h in patients with cardiovascular disease

---

- Monitor blood studies: CBC, leukocytes, differential, cardiac enzymes if patient is receiving long-term therapy
- Monitor hepatic studies: AST, ALT, bilirubin
- Check weight weekly; appetite may increase with drug
- Assess ECG for flattening of T wave, QTc prolongation bundle branch block, AV block, dysrhythmias in cardiac patients
G • Assess for EPS primarily in elderly: rigidity, dystonia, akathisia
- Assess mental status: mood, sensorium, affect, suicidal tendencies; increase in psychiatric symptoms: depression, panic, frequency of obsessive-compulsive behaviors
- Monitor urinary retention, constipation;
P constipation is more likely to occur in children
G or elderly
- Assess for withdrawal symptoms: headache, nausea, vomiting, muscle pain, weakness; do not usually occur unless drug was discontinued abruptly
- Identify alcohol consumption; if alcohol is consumed, hold dose until morning

Nursing diagnoses
☑ Coping, ineffective (uses)
☑ Injury, risk for physical (side effects)
☑ Knowledge, deficient (teaching)
☑ Noncompliance (teaching)

Implementation
- Give with food or milk for GI symptoms
Ⓢ • Do not crush, chew caps
- Store at room temp; do not freeze

Patient/family education
- Teach patient that therapeutic effects may take 2-3 wk
- Teach patient to use caution in driving or other activities requiring alertness because of drowsiness, dizziness, blurred vision; to avoid rising quickly from sitting to standing, especially elderly
- Teach patient to avoid alcohol ingestion, other CNS depressants
- Teach patient not to discontinue medication quickly after long-term use: may cause nausea, headache, malaise
- Teach patient to wear sunscreen or large hat, since photosensitivity occurs
- Teach patient to increase fluids, bulk in diet if constipation, urinary retention occur, especially elderly
- Teach patient to take gum, hard sugarless candy, or frequent sips of water for dry mouth
- Advise patient to notify prescriber if pregnancy is planned or suspected

Evaluation
Positive therapeutic outcome
- Decrease in depression
- Absence of suicidal thoughts

Treatment of overdose: ECG monitoring, induce emesis, lavage, activated charcoal, administer anticonvulsant

clonazepam (Rx)
(kloe-na′zi-pam)
Klonopin, Rivotril, Syn-Clonazepam ♣
Func. class.: Anticonvulsant
Chem. class.: Benzodiazepine derivative

Pregnancy category C

Controlled substance schedule IV

Action: Inhibits spike, wave formation in absence seizures (petit mal), decreases amplitude, frequency, duration, spread of discharge in minor motor seizures

Therapeutic Outcome: Decreased frequency, severity of seizures

Uses: Absence, atypical absence, akinetic, myoclonic seizures, Lennox-Gastaut syndrome

Investigational uses: Parkinsonian dysarthrias, acute mania, adjunct in schizophrenia, neuralgias, multifocal tic disorders, restless leg syndrome, rectal administration

Dosage and routes
Adult: PO not to exceed 1.5 mg/day in 3 divided doses; may be increased 0.5-1 mg q3 days until desired response; not to exceed 20 mg/day; rec 0.02 mg/kg
P *Child <10 yr or 30 kg:* PO 0.01-0.03 mg/kg/day in divided doses q8h, not to exceed 0.05 mg/kg/day; may be increased 0.25-0.5 mg q3 days until desired response; not to exceed 0.1-0.2 mg/kg/day; rec 0.05-0.1 mg/kg

Available forms: Tabs 0.5, 1, 2 mg; oral susp; **IV** sol

Adverse effects
(*italic* = common; **bold** = life-threatening)
CNS: Drowsiness, dizziness, confusion, behavioral changes, tremors, insomnia, headache, suicidal tendencies, slurred speech
CV: Palpitations, bradycardia, tachycardia
EENT: Increased salivation, nystagmus, diplopia, abnormal eye movements
GI: Nausea, constipation, polyphagia, anorexia, xerostomia, diarrhea, gastritis, sore gums
GU: Dysuria, enuresis, nocturia, retention, libido changes

HEMA: **Thrombocytopenia, leukocytosis, eosinophilia**
INTEG: Rash, alopecia, hirsutism
RESP: **Respiratory depression,** dyspnea, congestion

Contraindications: Hypersensitivity to benzodiazepines, acute narrow-angle glaucoma, psychosis, severe liver disease

Precautions: Open-angle glaucoma, chronic respiratory disease, renal/hepatic
🄶 disease, elderly, pregnancy **C**

🚫 **Do Not Confuse:**
Klonopin/clonidine
clonazepam/lorazepam/clorazepate

Pharmacokinetics	
Absorption	Well absorbed
Distribution	Crosses blood-brain barrier, placenta
Metabolism	Liver
Excretion	Kidneys
Half-life	18-50 hr

Pharmacodynamics	
Onset	½-1 hr
Peak	1-2 hr
Duration	6-12 hr

Interactions
Individual drugs
Alcohol: ↑ CNS depression
Carbamazepine: ↓ effectiveness
Metoprolol: ↓ metabolism, ↑ action
Phenytoin: ↓ clonazepam levels
Valproic acid: ↑ seizures
Drug classifications
Antidepressants, anticonvulsants, antihistamines, barbiturates, general anesthetics, opiates, sedative/hypnotics: ↑ CNS depression
Barbiturates: ↓ effect of clonazepam
🗷 *Herb/drug*
Ginseng, ginkgo, santonica: ↓ clonazepam effect
Kava: ↑ sedative effect
Lab test interferences
↑ AST, ↑ alkaline phosphatase

NURSING CONSIDERATIONS
Assessment
• Assess mental status: mood, sensorium, affect, memory (long, short), especially
🄶 elderly
• Assess for blood dyscrasias: fever, sore throat, bruising, rash, jaundice, epistaxis (long-term treatment only)
• Monitor blood level: therapeutic level 20-80 ng/ml

• Assess seizure activity including type, location, duration, and character; provide seizure precaution
• Assess renal studies: urinalysis, BUN, urine creatinine
• Monitor blood studies: RBCs, Hct, Hgb, reticulocyte counts weekly for 4 wk then monthly
• Monitor hepatic studies: ALT, AST, bilirubin, creatinine
• Monitor drug levels during initial treatment
• Assess for signs of physical withdrawal if medication suddenly discontinued
• Assess eye problems: need for ophthalmic examinations before, during, after treatment (slit lamp, fundoscopy, tonometry)
• Assess allergic reaction: red raised rash; if this occurs, drug should be discontinued
• Monitor for toxicity: bone marrow depression, nausea, vomiting, ataxia, diplopia, cardiovascular collapse

Nursing diagnoses
☑ Injury, risk for (side effects)
☑ Knowledge, deficient (teaching)

Implementation
PO route
• Give on empty stomach for best absorption
Rectal route
• **IV** sol may be used rectally, 1 ml syringe inserted 3 cm into rectum
• Oral susp may be used rectally (1 mg/ml of drug with 1 ml of water), use plastic tube (volume 2.2-3.3 ml)

Patient/family education
• Teach patient to carry/wear emergency ID card stating patient's name, drugs taken, condition, physician's name, phone number
• Caution patient to avoid driving, other activities that require alertness
• Caution patient to avoid alcohol ingestion or CNS depressants; increased sedation may occur
• Teach patient not to discontinue medication quickly after long-term use; taper off over several weeks

Evaluation
Positive therapeutic outcome
• Decreased seizure activity

Treatment of overdose: Lavage, activated charcoal, VS, monitor electrolytes

---

🗷 Herb/drug   🚫 Do Not Crush   ◆ Alert   ◆₋ Key Drug   🄶 Geriatric   🄿 Pediatric

clonidine ⚛ (Rx)

(klon'i-deen)

Catapres, Catapres-TTS, clonidine HCl, Dixarit ♣, Duraclon

Func. class.: Antihypertensive, centrally acting analgesic

Chem. class.: Centrally acting α-adrenergic agonist

Pregnancy category C

Action: Inhibits sympathetic vasomotor center in CNS, which reduces impulses in sympathetic nervous system; B/P, pulse rate, cardiac output decreased; prevents pain signal transmission in CNS by α-adrenergic receptor stimulation of the spinal cord

➡ **Therapeutic Outcome:** Decreased B/P in hypertension

Uses: Mild to moderate hypertension; used alone or in combination

Investigational uses: Opioid withdrawal, prevention of vascular headaches, treatment of menopausal symptoms, dysmenorrhea, attention deficit hyperactivity disorder (ADHD)

Dosage and routes
Hypertension

Adult: PO/trans 0.1 mg bid, then increase by 0.1-0.2 mg/day at weekly intervals, until desired response; range 0.2-0.6 mg/day in divided doses

G *Elderly:* PO 0.1 mg hs, may increase gradually

P *Child:* PO 5-10 mcg/kg/day in divided doses q8-12h, max 0.9 mg/day

Opioid withdrawal (unlabeled use)

Adult: PO 0.3-1.2 mg/day; may decrease by 50% × 3 days then decrease by 0.1-0.2 mg/day or discontinue

Severe pain

Adult: Cont epidural inf 30 mcg/hr

Menopausal symptoms (unlabeled use)

Adult: TD 0.1 mg patch q1 wk; PO 0.05-0.4 mg qd

ADHD (unlabeled use)

P *Child:* PO 5 mcg/kg/day × 8 wk

Available forms: Tabs 0.025 ♣, 0.1, 0.2, 0.3 mg; trans sys 2.5, 5, 7.5 mg delivering 0.1, 0.2, 0.3 mg/24 hr, respectively; inj 100, 500 mcg/ml

Adverse effects

(*italic* = common; **bold** = life-threatening)

CNS: *Drowsiness, sedation, headache,* *fatigue,* nightmares, insomnia, mental changes, anxiety, depression, hallucinations, delirium

CV: *Orthostatic hypotension, palpitations,* **CHF,** ECG abnormalities

EENT: Taste change, parotid pain

ENDO: Hyperglycemia

GI: *Nausea, vomiting, malaise,* constipation, *dry mouth*

GU: Impotence, dysuria, *nocturia,* gynecomastia

INTEG: *Rash,* alopecia, facial pallor, pruritus, hives, edema, burning papules, excoriation (trans patches)

MISC: *Withdrawal symptoms*

MS: Muscle, joint pain, leg cramps

Contraindications: Hypersensitivity; (epidural) bleeding disorders, anticoagulants

Precautions: MI (recent), diabetes mellitus, chronic renal failure, Raynaud's disease, **P** thyroid disease, depression, COPD, child <12 yr (transdermal), asthma, pregnancy **C,** **G** lactation, elderly, noncompliant patients

🔃 **Do Not Confuse:**

Catapres/Cataflam/catarase, clonidine/ Klonopin/clonazepam

Pharmacokinetics	
Absorption	Well absorbed (PO, trans)
Distribution	Widely distributed; crosses blood-brain barrier
Metabolism	Liver, extensively
Excretion	Kidneys, unchanged (30%)
Half-life	12-21 hr

Pharmacodynamics		
	PO	TD
Onset	½-1 hr	3 days
Peak	2-4 hr	Unknown
Duration	8-12 hr	8 hr (after removal)

Interactions
Individual drugs

Alcohol: ↑ CNS depression

Levodopa: ↓ levodopa effect

Prazosin: ↓ hypotensive effects

Verapamil: AV block

Drug classifications

Amphetamines, appetite suppressants, MAOIs: ↓ hypotensive effects

Anesthetics, opiates, sedatives/hypnotics: ↑ CNS depression

Antidepressants (tricyclic), β-adrenergic blockers: life-threatening ↑ B/P

Cardiac glycosides: ↑ bradycardia

Diuretics, nitrates: ↑ hypotensive effects

Herb/drug

Aconite: ↑ toxicity, death

Astragalus, cola tree: ↑ or ↓ antihypertensive effect

Barberry, betony, black catechu, black cohosh, bloodroot, broom, burdock, cat's claw, dandelion, goldenseal, Irish moss, Jamaican dogwood, kelp, khella, mistletoe, parsley: ↑ antihypertensive effect

Coltsfoot, guarana, khat, licorice: ↓ antihypertensive effect

Lab test interferences

↑ Blood glucose

↓ VMA, ↓ urinary catecholamines, ↓ aldosterone

NURSING CONSIDERATIONS
Assessment

• Assess pain: location, intensity, character, alleviating, aggravation factors, baseline and frequency

• Perform blood studies: neutrophils, decreased platelets

• Perform renal studies: protein, BUN, creatinine; watch for increased levels that may indicate nephrotic syndrome: polyuria, oliguria, frequency

• Monitor baselines for renal, liver function tests before therapy begins; check potassium levels, although hyperkalemia rarely occurs

• Monitor B/P, pulse if the drug is being used for hypertension; notify prescriber of changes

• Assess for opiate withdrawal in patients receiving the drug for opioid withdrawal, including fever, diarrhea, nausea, vomiting, cramps, insomnia, shivering, dilated pupils, weakness

• Check for edema in feet, legs daily; monitor I&O; check for decreasing output

• Note allergic reaction: rash, fever, pruritus, urticaria; drug should be discontinued if antihistamines fail to help

• Note allergic reaction from patches: rash, urticaria, angioedema; should not continue to use

• Assess for symptoms of CHF: edema, dyspnea, wet rales, B/P, weight gain, report significant changes

Nursing diagnoses

☑ Injury, risk for physical (side effects)

☑ Knowledge, deficient (teaching)

☑ Noncompliance (teaching)

Implementation
PO route

• PO: give last dose at hs

Transdermal route

• Apply patch weekly; remove old patch and wash off residue; apply to site without hair; best absorption over chest or upper arm; rotate sites with each application; clean site before application; apply firmly, especially around edges

• Store patches in cool environment, tabs in tight container

Patient/family education

• Instruct patient not to discontinue drug abruptly, or withdrawal symptoms may occur: anxiety, increased B/P, headache, insomnia, increased pulse, tremors, nausea, sweating

• Caution patient not to use OTC (cough, cold, or allergy) products unless directed by prescriber

• Teach patient to comply with dosage schedule even if feeling better; drug controls symptoms, does not cure

• Caution patient to change position slowly, to rise slowly to sitting or standing position to minimize orthostatic hypotension, especially **G** elderly

• Instruct patient to notify physician of mouth sores, sore throat, fever, swelling of hands or feet, irregular heartbeat, chest pain, signs of angioedema, increased weight

• Teach patient about excessive perspiration, dehydration, vomiting; diarrhea may lead to fall in B/P; consult prescriber if these occur

• Tell patient that drug may cause dizziness, fainting; light-headedness may occur during 1st few days of therapy; use hard candy, saliva product, or frequent rinsing of mouth for dry mouth

• Advise patient that compliance is necessary; not to skip or stop drug unless directed by prescriber

• Teach patient that drug may cause skin rash or impaired perspiration

• Teach patient that response may take 2-3 days if drug is given TD; instruct on administration of patch; return demonstration

• Teach patient to avoid hazardous activities, since drug may cause drowsiness, dizziness

• Teach patient to administer 1 hr ac

Evaluation
Positive therapeutic outcome

• Decrease in B/P in hypertension

• Decrease in withdrawal symptoms

• Decrease in pain

• Decrease in vascular headaches

• Decrease in dysmenorrhea

• Decrease in menopausal symptoms

Treatment of overdose: Supportive treatment; administer tolazoline, atropine, DOPamine prn

clopidogrel (Rx)
(klo-pid'oh-grel)
Plavix
Func. class.: Platelet aggregation inhibitor
Chem. class.: Thienopyridine derivative

Pregnancy category B

Action: Inhibits first and second phases of ADP-induced effects in platelet aggregation

➡ Therapeutic Outcome: Decreased possibility of stroke, MI by decreasing platelet aggregation

Uses: Reducing the risk of stroke, MI, peripheral arterial disease in high-risk patients, acute coronary syndrome

Dosage and routes
Adult: PO 75 mg qd with or without food

Acute coronary syndrome
Adult: PO 300 mg then 75 mg qd

Available forms: Tabs 75 mg

Adverse effects
(*italic* = common; **bold** = life-threatening)
CNS: Headache, dizziness, depression, syncope, hyperesthesia, neuralgia
CV: Edema, hypertension
GI: Nausea, vomiting, diarrhea, GI discomfort, **GI bleeding**
HEMA: Epistaxis, purpura, **bleeding, neutropenia**
INTEG: Rash, pruritus
MISC: UTI, hypercholesterolemia, chest pain, fatigue, **intracranial hemorrhage**
MS: Arthralgia, back pain
RESP: Upper respiratory tract infection, dyspnea, rhinitis, bronchitis, cough

Contraindications: Hypersensitivity, active bleeding

Precautions: Past liver disease, pregnancy B, lactation, children, increased bleeding risk, neutropenia, agranulocytosis

Pharmacokinetics
Absorption	Rapidly absorbed
Distribution	Unknown
Metabolism	Liver, extensively, protein binding 95%
Excretion	Kidneys, unchanged drug
Half-life	8 hr

Pharmacodynamics
Onset	Unknown
Peak	1-3 hr
Duration	Unknown

Interactions
Individual drugs
Abciximab, aspirin, eptifibatide, ticlopidine, tirofiban: ↑ bleeding tendencies
Fluvastatin, phenytoin, tamoxifen, TOLBUTamide, torsemide, warfarin: ↑ action of each specific drug

Drug classifications
Anticoagulants, NSAIDs, thrombolytics: ↑ bleeding tendencies
NSAIDs: ↑ action of some NSAIDs

Herb/drug
Agrimony, alfalfa, angelica, anise, basil, bay, bilberry, black haw, bogbean, bromelain, buchu, chondroitin, cinchona bark, dong quai, fenugreek, feverfew, garlic, ginger, ginkgo, ginseng, horse chestnut, Irish moss, kelp, kelpware, khella, lovage, lungwort, meadowsweet, motherwort, mugwort, nettle, papaya, parsley (large amounts), pau d'arco, pineapple, poplar, prickly ash, safflower, saw palmetto, tonka bean, turmeric, wintergreen, yarrow: ↑ risk of bleeding
Chamomile, coenzyme Q10, flax, glucomannan, goldenseal, guar gum: ↓ anticoagulant effect

NURSING CONSIDERATIONS
Assessment
• Assess for symptoms of stroke, MI during treatment
• Monitor liver function studies: AST, ALT, bilirubin, creatinine if patient is on long-term therapy (4 mo or more)
• Monitor blood studies: CBC, Hct, Hgb, Pro-time, cholesterol if patient is on long-term therapy; thrombocytopenia, neutropenia may occur

Nursing diagnoses
✓ Injury, risk for (uses)
✓ Knowledge, deficient (teaching)

Implementation
• Give with food to decrease gastric symptoms

Patient/family education
• Advise patient that blood work will be necessary during treatment
• Advise patient to report any unusual bleed-

ing to prescriber, that it may take longer to stop bleeding
• Instruct patient to take with food or just after eating to minimize GI discomfort
• Caution patient to report diarrhea, skin rashes, subcutaneous bleeding, chills, fever, sore throat
• Teach patient to tell all health care providers that clopidogrel is used

Evaluation
Positive therapeutic outcome
• Absence of stroke

---

clorazepate (Rx)
(klor-az'e-pate)
APO-Clorazepate ✤, clorazepate, Gen-XENE, Novo-Clopate ✤, Tranxene, Tranxene-SD
Func. class.: Antianxiety, anticonvulsant, sedative/hypnotic
Chem. class.: Benzodiazepine

Pregnancy category D

Controlled substance schedule IV

Action: Potentiates the actions of GABA; especially in limbic system, reticular formation has anticonvulsant effects

➡ **Therapeutic Outcome:** Decreased anxiety, restlessness, insomnia

Uses: Anxiety, acute alcohol withdrawal, adjunct in seizure disorders

Dosage and routes
Anxiety
Adult: PO 15-60 mg/day or 7.5-15 mg 2-4×/day or 11.25-22.5 mg at hs

G Elderly: PO 7.5 mg qd bid

Alcohol withdrawal
Adult: PO 30 mg then day 1, 30-60 mg in divided doses; day 2, 45-90 mg in divided doses; day 3, 22.5-45 mg in divided doses; day 4, 15-30 mg in divided doses; then reduce daily dose to 7.5-15 mg

Seizure disorders
P Adult and child >12 yr: PO 7.5 mg tid; may increase by 7.5 mg/wk or less, not to exceed 90 mg/day

P Child 9-12 yr: PO 3.75-7.5 mg bid; may increase by 3.75 mg/wk or less, not to exceed 60 mg/day

Available forms: Caps 3.75, 7.5, 15 mg; tabs 3.75, 7.5, 15 mg

Adverse effects
*(italic = common; **bold** = life-threatening)*
CNS: *Dizziness, drowsiness,* confusion, headache, anxiety, tremors, stimulation, fatigue, depression, insomnia, hallucinations, lethargy
CV: *Orthostatic hypotension,* **ECG changes, tachycardia,** hypotension, chest pain
EENT: *Blurred vision,* tinnitus, mydriasis
GI: Constipation, dry mouth, nausea, vomiting, anorexia, diarrhea
INTEG: Rash, dermatitis, itching

Contraindications: Hypersensitivity to benzodiazepines, narrow-angle glaucoma, **P** psychosis, pregnancy **D**, lactation, child <9 yr

G Precautions: Elderly, debilitated, hepatic disease, renal disease

◥ Do Not Confuse:
clorazapate/clonazepam

Pharmacokinetics	
Absorption	Well absorbed
Distribution	Widely distributed; crosses placenta
Metabolism	Liver
Excretion	Kidneys, breast milk
Half-life	30-100 hr

Pharmacodynamics	
Onset	1 hr
Peak	1-2 hr
Duration	Up to 24 hr

Interactions
Individual drugs
Alcohol: ↑ CNS depression
Cimetidine, disulfiram, fluoxetine, isoniazid, ketoconazole, propoxyphene, valproic acid: ↑ effects of clorazepate
Rifampin: ↓ action of clorazepate
Drug classifications
Antidepressants, β-blockers (some), MAOIs, oral contraceptives: ↑ clorazepate action
Barbiturates: ↓ clorazepate effect
CNS depressants: ↑ CNS depression
☑ Herb/drug
Catnip, chamomile, clary, cowslip, kava, mistletoe, nettle, pokeweed, poppy, senega, Queen Anne's lace, valerian: ↑ CNS depression
Black cohosh: ↑ hypotension
Lab test interferences
↑ AST/ALT, ↓ HCT

NURSING CONSIDERATIONS
Assessment
• Assess seizures: duration, location, intensity, aura

- Monitor B/P (with patient lying, standing), pulse; if systolic B/P drops 20 mm Hg, hold drug, notify prescriber
- Monitor blood studies: CBC during long-term therapy; blood dyscrasias have occurred rarely
- Monitor hepatic studies: AST, ALT, bilirubin, creatinine, LDH, alkaline phosphatase
- Monitor I&O; may indicate renal dysfunction
- Monitor mental status: mood, sensorium, affect, sleeping pattern, drowsiness, dizziness, physical dependency; withdrawal symptoms: headache, nausea, vomiting, muscle pain, weakness after long-term use; suicidal tendencies

Nursing diagnoses
☑ Coping, ineffective (uses)
☑ Knowledge, deficient (teaching)
☑ Noncompliance (teaching)

Implementation
- Give with food or milk for GI symptoms
- Do not chew, crush caps
- Use sugarless gum, hard candy, frequent sips of water for dry mouth
- Check to see PO medication has been swallowed

Patient/family education
- Teach patient that drug may be taken with food
- Teach patient not to use for everyday stress or longer than 4 mo, unless directed by a prescriber; not to take more than prescribed amount; may be habit forming
- Caution patient to avoid OTC preparations unless approved by a prescriber
- Caution patient to avoid driving, activities that require alertness; drowsiness may occur, especially in elderly
- Advise patient to avoid alcohol ingestion or other psychotropic medications, unless prescribed
- Advise patient not to discontinue medication abruptly after long-term use
- Advise patient to rise slowly or fainting may occur
- Teach patient that drowsiness may worsen at beginning of treatment

Evaluation
Positive therapeutic outcome
- Decreased anxiety, restlessness
- Decreased seizure activity

Treatment of overdose: Lavage, VS, supportive care, flumazenil

cloxacillin (Rx)
(klox-a-sill'in)
Apo-Cloxi ✤, cloxacillin, Cloxapen, Novo-cloxin ✤, Nu-Clox ✤, Orbenin ✤
Func. class.: Broad-spectrum antiinfective
Chem. class.: Penicillinase-resistant penicillin

Pregnancy category B

Action: Interferes with cell wall replication of susceptible organisms; the cell wall, rendered osmotically unstable, swells, bursts from osmotic pressure; resists the penicillinase action that inactivates penicillins

Therapeutic Outcome: Bactericidal effects for the following: gram-positive cocci *Staphylococcus aureus, Staphylococcus epidermidis,* penicillinase-producing staphylococci

Uses: Penicillinase-producing staphylococci, streptococci; respiratory tract, skin, skin structure infections; sinusitis

Dosage and routes
Adult: PO 1-4 g/day in divided doses q6h
Child: PO 50-100 mg/kg in divided doses q6h, max 4 g/day

Available forms: Caps 250, 500 mg; oral sol 125 mg/5 ml

Adverse effects
(*italic* = common; **bold** = life-threatening)
CNS: Lethargy, hallucinations, anxiety, depression, muscle twitching, **coma, seizures**
GI: Nausea, vomiting, diarrhea, increased AST, ALT, abdominal pain, glossitis, **pseudomembranous colitis,** colitis
GU: **Oliguria, proteinuria,** hematuria, *vaginitis, moniliasis,* **glomerulonephritis**
HEMA: Anemia, **increased bleeding time, bone marrow depression, granulocytopenia**
SYST: **Anaphylaxis, serum sickness**

Contraindications: Hypersensitivity to penicillins; neonates, severe renal, hepatic disease

Precautions: Pregnancy **B,** hypersensitivity to cephalosporins

Pharmacokinetics	
Absorption	Moderate (35%-60%)
Distribution	Widely distributed; crosses placenta
Metabolism	Liver (up to 22%)
Excretion	Breast milk; kidneys, unchanged (30%-45%)
Half-life	0.5-1.1 hr, increased in hepatic/renal disease

Pharmacodynamics	
Onset	½ hr
Peak	½-2 hr

Interactions
Individual drugs
Probenecid: ↑ cloxacillin concentrations, ↓ renal excretion
Drug classifications
Anticoagulants (oral): ↑ anticoagulant effects
Food/drug
Food, carbonated drinks, citrus fruit juices: ↓ absorption
☑ Herb/drug
Acidophilus: Do not use with antiinfectives
Khat: ↓ absorption, separate by ≥2 hr
Lab test interferences
False positive: Urine glucose, urine protein

NURSING CONSIDERATIONS
Assessment
• Assess patient for previous sensitivity reaction to penicillins or other cephalosporins; cross-sensitivity between penicillins and cephalosporins is common
• Assess patient for signs and symptoms of infection including characteristics of wounds, sputum, urine, stool, WBC >10,000/mm³, fever; obtain baseline information and during treatment
• Obtain C&S before beginning drug therapy to identify if correct treatment has been initiated
• Assess for anaphylaxis: rash, urticaria, pruritus, chills, fever, joint pain may occur a few days after therapy begins; epINEPHrine and resuscitation equipment should be available for anaphylactic reaction
◆● Identify urine output; if decreasing, notify prescriber (may indicate nephrotoxicity); also check for increased BUN, creatinine
• Monitor blood studies: AST, ALT, CBC, Hct, Hgb, bilirubin, LDH, alkaline phosphatase, Coombs' test monthly if patient is on long-term therapy
• Monitor electrolytes: potassium, sodium, chloride monthly if patient is on long-term therapy

• Assess bowel pattern qd; if severe diarrhea occurs, drug should be discontinued; may indicate pseudomembranous colitis
• Monitor for bleeding: ecchymosis, bleeding gums, hematuria, stool guaiac daily if on long-term therapy
• Assess for overgrowth of infection: perineal itching, fever, malaise, redness, pain, swelling, drainage, rash, diarrhea, change in cough, sputum

Nursing diagnoses
☑ Infection, risk for (uses)
☑ Diarrhea (side effects)
☑ Injury, risk for (side effects)
☑ Knowledge, deficient (teaching)
☑ Noncompliance (teaching)

Implementation
• Give in even doses around the clock; if GI upset occurs, give with food; drug must be given for 10-14 days to ensure organism death and prevent superinfection; store in airtight container
🚫● Do not crush, chew caps
• Shake susp well before each dose; store in refrigerator for 2 wk, 3 days at room temp

Patient/family education
• Teach patient to report sore throat, bruising, bleeding, joint pain; may indicate blood dyscrasias (rare)
• Advise patient to contact prescriber if vaginal itching, loose foul-smelling stools, furry tongue occur; may indicate superinfection
• Instruct patient to take all medications prescribed for the length of time ordered
• Advise patient to notify prescriber of diarrhea with blood or pus, which may indicate pseudomembranous colitis
• Advise patient to wear or carry emergency ID if allergic to penicillins

Evaluation
Positive therapeutic outcome
• Absence of signs/symptoms of infection (WBC <10,000/mm³, temp WNL, absence of red, draining wounds)
• Reported improvement in symptoms of infection

Treatment of anaphylaxis: Withdraw drug, maintain airway, administer epINEPHrine, aminophylline, O₂, **IV** corticosteroids

---

☑ Herb/drug   🚫 Do Not Crush   ◆ Alert   ◆ₜₜ Key Drug   G Geriatric   P Pediatric

clozapine (Rx)

(kloz'a-peen)

clozapine, Clozaril

Func. class.: Antipsychotic

Chem. class.: Tricyclic dibenzodiazepine derivative

Pregnancy category B

Action: Interferes with dopamine receptor binding with lack of extrapyramidal symptoms and tardive dyskinesia; also acts as an adrenergic, cholinergic, histaminergic, serotonergic antagonist

➡ **Therapeutic Outcome:** Decreased psychotic behavior

Uses: Management of psychotic symptoms in schizophrenic patients for whom other antipsychotics have failed

Dosage and routes

Adult: PO 25 mg qd or bid; may increase by 25-50 mg/day; normal range 300-450 mg/day after 2 wk; do not increase dosage more than 2 times/wk; do not exceed 900 mg/day; use lowest dosage to control symptoms

Available forms: Tabs 25, 100 mg

Adverse effects

(*italic* = common; **bold** = life-threatening)

CNS: Sedation, salivation, dizziness, headache, tremors, sleep problems, akinesia, fever, **seizures,** *sweating, akathisia, confusion, fatigue, insomnia, depression, slurred speech, anxiety,* **neuroleptic malignant syndrome,** agitation

CV: Tachycardia, hypotension, hypertension, chest pain, ECG changes, orthostatic hypotension

GI: Drooling or excessive salivation, constipation, nausea, abdominal discomfort, vomiting, diarrhea, anorexia, weight gain, dry mouth, heartburn

GU: Urinary abnormalities, incontinence, ejaculation dysfunction, frequency, urgency, retention, dysuria

HEMA: **Leukopenia, neutropenia, agranulocytosis, eosinophilia, thrombocytopenia**

MS: Weakness; pain in back, neck, legs; spasm

RESP: Dyspnea, nasal congestion, throat discomfort

EENT: Blurred vision

Contraindications: Hypersensitivity, myeloproliferative disorders, severe granulocytopenia (WBC <3500/mm³ before therapy), CNS depression, coma

Precautions: Pregnancy **B,** lactation, ▣ children <16 yr, hepatic, renal, cardiac disease, ⬚ seizures, prostatic enlargement, elderly, narrow-angle glaucoma

◪ **Do Not Confuse:**
Clozaril/Clinoril/Colazal

Pharmacokinetics	
Absorption	Well absorbed
Distribution	Widely distributed; crosses blood-brain barrier, placenta; 95% bound to plasma proteins
Metabolism	Liver
Excretion	Kidneys, feces (metabolites)
Half-life	8-12 hr

Pharmacodynamics	
Onset	Unknown
Peak	Steady state 2½ hr
Duration	4-12 hr

Interactions

Individual drugs

Alcohol: ↑ effects of both drugs, oversedation

Cimetidine: ↑ clozapine levels

Digoxin: ↑ plasma concentration of digoxin

Erythromycin: ↑ erythromycin levels

Phenytoin: ↓ phenytoin action

Warfarin: ↑ plasma concentrations

Drug classifications

Antacids: ↓ absorption

Anticholinergics: ↑ anticholinergic effects

Antidepressants, antihistamines, CNS depressants, psychoactives: ↑ CNS depression

Antihypertensives, nitrates: ↑ hypotension

Antineoplastics: ↑ bone marrow suppression

Food/drug

Caffeine: ↓ clozapine levels

▨ *Herb/drug*

Kava, St. John's wort: ↑ CNS depression

Cola tree, hops, nettle, nutmeg: ↑ clozapine action

Betel palm, kava: ↑ extrapyramidal symptoms (EPS)

Lab test interferences

↑ Liver function tests, ↑ cardiac enzymes, ↑ cholesterol, ↑ blood glucose, ↑ bilirubin, ↑ PBI, ↑ cholinesterase, ↑ ¹³¹I

False positive: Pregnancy tests, PKU

False negative: Urinary steroids, 17-OHCS

NURSING CONSIDERATIONS

Assessment

• Assess mental status: orientation, mood, behavior, presence of hallucinations, and type before initial administration and monthly; this drug should significantly reduce psychotic behavior

- Check for swallowing of PO medication; check for hoarding or giving of medication to other patients
- **G** Monitor I&O ratio, palpate bladder if low urinary output occurs, especially in elderly; urinalysis recommended before, during prolonged therapy
- Monitor bilirubin, CBC, liver function studies monthly; discontinue treatment if WBC <3000/mm^3 or if ANC <1500/mm^3; test qwk; may resume when normal; if WBC <2000/mm^3 or ANC <1000/mm^3, discontinue
- Assess affect, orientation, LOC, reflexes, gait, coordination, sleep pattern disturbances
- Monitor B/P with patient sitting, standing, and lying; take pulse and respirations q4h during initial treatment; establish baseline before starting treatment; report drops of 30 mm Hg
- Check for dizziness, faintness, palpitations, tachycardia on rising
- Assess for neuroleptic malignant syndrome: hyperpyrexia, muscle rigidity, increased CPK, altered mental status; drug should be discontinued
- Assess for EPS including akathisia (inability to sit still, no pattern to movements), tardive dyskinesia (bizarre movements of the jaw, mouth, tongue, extremities), pseudoparkinsonism (rigidity, tremors, pill rolling, shuffling gate)
- Assess for constipation, urinary retention daily; if these occur, increase bulk, water in diet

Nursing diagnoses
☑ Thought processes, disturbed (uses)
☑ Coping, ineffective (uses)
☑ Knowledge, deficient (teaching)
☑ Noncompliance (teaching)

Implementation
- **G** Decrease dosage in elderly since metabolism is slowed
- Give with full glass of water, milk; or give with food to decrease GI upset
- Store in tight, light-resistant container; oral sol in amber bottle

Patient/family education
- Teach patient to use good oral hygiene; frequent rinsing of mouth, sugarless gum for dry mouth
- Caution patient to avoid hazardous activities until drug response is determined
- Inform patient that orthostatic hypotension occurs often and to rise from sitting or lying position gradually
- Caution patient to avoid hot tubs, hot showers, tub baths, since hypotension may occur
- Teach patient to avoid OTC preparations (cough, hay fever, cold) unless approved by prescriber, since serious drug interactions may occur; avoid use with alcohol, CNS depressants; increased drowsiness may occur
- Teach patient about EPS and necessity of meticulous oral hygiene, since oral candidiasis may occur
- Teach patient to report sore throat, malaise, fever, bleeding, mouth sores; if these occur, CBC should be performed and drug discontinued
- Advise patient that in hot weather, heat stroke may occur; take extra precautions to stay cool
- Teach patient symptoms of agranulocytosis and need for blood test qwk for 6 mo, then q2wk; report flulike symptoms

Evaluation
Positive therapeutic outcome
- Decrease in emotional excitement, hallucinations, delusions, paranoia
- Reorganization of patterns of thought, speech

Treatment of anaphylaxis: Withdraw drug, maintain airway

! HIGH ALERT

coagulation factor VIIa, recombinant (Rx)
NovoSeven
Func. class.: Antihemophilic

Pregnancy category C

Action: Promotes hemostasis by activating the intrinsic pathway of coagulation

Uses: Bleeding in hemophilia A or B, with inhibitors to factor VIII or IX

Dosage and routes
Adult: **IV** bol 90 mcg/kg q2h until hemostasis occurs, or until therapy is deemed to be inadequate; posthemostatic doses q3-6h may be required

Available forms: Lyophilized powder 1.2 mg/vial (1200 mcg/vial) recombinant human coagulation factor VIIa (rFVIIa); 4.8 mg/vial (4800 mcg/vial) recombinant human coagulation factor VIIa (rFVIIa)

Adverse effects
(*italic* = common; **bold** = life-threatening)
CNS: Fever, headache

INTEG: Pain, redness at inj site, pruritus, purpura, rash

SYST: **Hemorrhage not otherwise specified, hemarthrosis, fibrinogen plasma decreased,** hypertension, bradycardia, **DIC, coagulation disorder, thrombosis**

Contraindications: Hypersensitivity to this product or mouse, hamster, or bovine products

Precautions: Pregnancy **C**, lactation, P children

Pharmacokinetics
Half-life   2-3 hr

Pharmacodynamics
Unknown

Interactions
Individual drugs
Activated prothrombin complex concentrate, prothrombin complex concentrate: Do not use together

NURSING CONSIDERATIONS
Assessment
• Assess VS, B/P, pulse, respirations, neurologic signs, temp at least q4h, temperature 104° F (40° C) or indicators of internal bleeding, cardiac rhythm
• Monitor Pro-time, APTT, plasma FVII clotting
• Monitor for thrombosis, dose should be reduced or stopped

Implementation
IV **IV route**
• Bring to room temp; for 1.2 mg vial/2.2 ml sterile water for inj; 4.8 mg vial/8.5 ml sterile water for inj; remove caps from stopper, cleanse stopper with alcohol, allow to dry, draw back plunger of sterile syringe and allow air into syringe, insert needle of syringe into sterile water for inj, inject the air and withdraw amount required, insert syringe needle with diluent into drug vial, aim to side so liquid runs down vial wall, gently swirl until dissolved, use within 3 hr, give by bol over 3-5 min
• Do not admix, keep refrigerated until ready to use, avoid sunlight

Evaluation
Positive therapeutic outcome
• Therapeutic response: hemostasis

codeine ⊙ₙ **(Rx)**
(koe′deen)
Paveral ♣, Codeine, opiate analgesics
Func. class.: Opiate, phenanthrene derivative

Pregnancy category C

Controlled substance schedule II, III, IV, V
(depends on route)

Action: Depresses pain impulse transmission at the spinal cord level by interacting with opioid receptors; decreases cough reflex, GI motility

➡ **Therapeutic Outcome:** Pain relief, decreased cough, decreased diarrhea depending on route

Uses: Moderate to severe pain, nonproductive cough

Investigational uses: Diarrhea

Dosage and routes
Pain
Adult: PO 15-60 mg q4h prn; IM/SC 15-60 mg q4h prn

P *Child:* PO 3 mg/kg/day in divided doses q4h prn

Cough
Adult: PO 10-20 mg q4-6h, not to exceed 120 mg/day

P *Child:* PO 1-1.5 mg/kg/day in 4 divided doses, not to exceed 60 mg/day

Diarrhea
Adult: PO 30 mg; may repeat qid prn

Renal dose
Adult: PO CCr 10-50 ml/min 75% of dose; CCr <10 ml/min 50% of dose

Available forms: Inj 30, 60 mg/ml; tabs 15, 30, 60 mg; oral sol 10 mg/5 ml, 15 mg/5 ml

Adverse effects
(*italic* = common; **bold** = life-threatening)
CNS: Drowsiness, sedation, dizziness, agitation, dependency, lethargy, restlessness, euphoria, **seizures**
CV: Bradycardia, palpitations, orthostatic hypotension, tachycardia, **circulatory collapse**
GI: Nausea, vomiting, anorexia, constipation
GU: Urinary retention
INTEG: Flushing, rash, urticaria, pruritus

C

RESP: **Respiratory depression, respiratory paralysis**
SYST: **Anaphylaxis**

Contraindications: Hypersensitivity to opiates, respiratory depression, increased intracranial pressure, seizure disorders, severe respiratory disorders

G Precautions: Elderly, cardiac dysrhythmias, pregnancy **C**, prostatic hypertrophy, lactation

N Do Not Confuse:
codeine/Lodine/Iodine/Cardene

Pharmacokinetics

Absorption	Complete (IM)
Distribution	Widely distributed; crosses placenta
Metabolism	Liver, extensively
Excretion	Kidneys (up to 15%), breast milk
Half-life	3-4 hr

Pharmacodynamics

	PO	IM	SC
Onset	30-45 min	15-30 min	15-30 min
Peak	1-2 hr	30-60 min	Unknown
Duration	4 hr	4 hr	4 hr

Interactions
Individual drugs
Alcohol: ↑ respiratory depression, hypotension, ↑ sedation
Drug classifications
Antihistamines, CNS depressants, phenothiazines, sedative/hypnotics: ↑ respiratory depression, hypotension
Antipsychotics, opiates, sedative/hypnotics, skeletal muscle relaxants: ↑ CNS depression
MAOIs: ↑ toxicity
☑ *Herb/drug*
Jamaican dogwood, kava, lavender, mistletoe, nettle, pokeweed, poppy, senega, valerian: ↑ CNS depression
Corkwood: ↑ anticholinergic effects
Lab test interferences
↑ Amylase, ↑ lipase

NURSING CONSIDERATIONS
Assessment
• Assess pain: intensity, type, alleviating factors
• Assess GI function: nausea, vomiting, constipation
• Monitor VS after parenteral route; note muscle rigidity, drug history, liver, kidney function tests, respiratory dysfunction: respiratory depression, character, rate, rhythm; notify prescriber if respirations are <10/min

• Monitor CNS changes: dizziness, drowsiness, hallucinations, euphoria, LOC, pupil reaction
• Monitor allergic reactions: rash, urticaria

Nursing diagnoses
✓ Pain (uses)
✓ Sensory perceptual, disturbed: visual, auditory (adverse reactions)
✓ Breathing pattern, ineffective (adverse reactions)
✓ Knowledge, deficient (teaching)

Implementation
• Give with antiemetic if nausea, vomiting occur
• Administer when pain is beginning to return, determine dosage interval by patient response; continuous dosing of medication is more effective given prn; explain analgesic effect
• Medication should be slowly withdrawn after long-term use to prevent withdrawal symptoms
• Store in light-resistant container at room temp
PO route
• May be given with food or milk to lessen GI upset
IM/SC route
• Do not give if cloudy, or a precipitate has formed
IV IV route
• Give slowly by direct inj

Syringe compatibilities: Glycopyrrolate, hydrOXYzine

Y-site compatibilities: Cefmetazole

Additive incompatibilities: Aminophylline, amobarbital, chlorothiazide, heparin, methicillin, pentobarbital, phenobarbital, phenytoin, secobarbital, thiopental

Patient/family education
• Teach patient to report any symptoms of CNS changes, allergic reactions; to avoid CNS depressants: alcohol, sedative/hypnotics for at least 24 hr after taking this drug
• Discuss with patient that dizziness, drowsiness, and confusion are common
• Advise patient to avoid getting up without assistance
• Discuss in detail all aspects of the drug

Evaluation
Positive therapeutic outcome
• Decreased pain
• Decreased cough
• Decreased diarrhea

☑ Herb/drug   **◎** Do Not Crush   **◆** Alert   **◆ₙ** Key Drug   **G** Geriatric   **P** Pediatric

Treatment of overdose: Naloxone 0.2-0.8 **IV**, O_2, **IV** fluids, vasopressors

colchicine ☦ (Rx)
(kol'chi-seen)
Func. class.: Antigout agent
Chem. class.: Colchicum autumnale alkaloid

Pregnancy category
C (PO), D (IV)

Action: Inhibits microtubule formation of lactic acid in leukocytes, which decreases phagocytosis and inflammation in joints

→ **Therapeutic Outcome:** Decreased pain, inflammation of joints

Uses: Gout, gouty arthritis (prevention, treatment); to arrest progression of neurologic disability in multiple sclerosis

Investigational uses: Hepatic cirrhosis, familial Mediterranean fever, pericarditis

Dosage and routes
Prevention
Adult: PO 0.6-1.8 mg qd depending on severity; **IV** 0.5-1 mg qd-bid

Treatment
Adult: PO 0.6-1.2 mg, then 0.5-1.2 mg q1h, until pain decreases or side effects occur; **IV** 2 mg, then 0.5 mg q6h, not to exceed 4 mg/24 hr

Available forms: Tabs 0.6 mg; inj **IV** 0.5 mg/ml

Adverse effects
(*italic* = common; **bold** = life-threatening)
GI: Nausea, vomiting, anorexia, malaise, metallic taste, cramps, peptic ulcer, diarrhea
GU: Hematuria, **oliguria, renal damage**
HEMA: **Agranulocytosis, thrombocytopenia, aplastic anemia, pancytopenia**
INTEG: Chills, dermatitis, pruritus, purpura, erythema
MISC: Myopathy, alopecia, reversible azoospermia, peripheral neuritis

Contraindications: Hypersensitivity; serious GI, renal, hepatic, cardiac disorders; blood dyscrasias, pregnancy **D (IV)**

Precautions: Severe renal disease, blood dyscrasias, pregnancy **C** (PO), hepatic disease, elderly, lactation, children

Pharmacokinetics
Absorption	Well absorbed
Distribution	WBCs
Metabolism	Deacetylates in liver
Excretion	Feces (metabolites/active drug)
Half-life	20 min

Pharmacodynamics
	PO
Onset	Unknown
Peak	½-2 hr
Duration	Unknown

Interactions
Individual drugs
CycloSPORINE, radiation: ↑ bone marrow depression
CycloSPORINE: toxicity
Vitamin B_{12}: ↓ action of vit B_{12}; may cause reversible malabsorption
Drug classifications
Acidifiers: ↓ action of colchicine
Alkalinizers: ↑ action of colchicine
Bone marrow depressants: ↑ bone marrow depression
CNS depressants: ↑ action of CNS depressants
NSAIDs: ↑ GI effects
Sympathomimetics: ↑ action of sympathomimetics
Lab test interferences
↑ Alkaline phosphatase, ↑ AST
False positive: Urine, RBC, Hgb
Interference:
Urinary 17-hydroxycorticosteroids

NURSING CONSIDERATIONS
Assessment
• Assess pain and mobility of joints
• Monitor I&O ratio; observe for decrease in urinary output; CBC, platelets, reticulocytes before, during therapy (q3 mo), may cause aplastic anemia, agranulocytosis, decreased platelets
• Assess for toxicity: weakness, abdominal pain, nausea, vomiting, diarrhea

Nursing diagnoses
✓ Pain, chronic (uses)
✓ Mobility, impaired (uses)
✓ Knowledge, deficient (teaching)

Implementation
PO route
• Give with food for GI symptoms
IV route
• Give **IV** undiluted or diluted 1 mg/10-20 ml normal saline or sterile water for inj; give over 2-5 min
• Do not give IM or SC

- Do not dilute in D_5W or change in **IV** line that is running or contains D_5W
- Wait ≥1 wk after giving a full course of **IV** colchicine, before giving more doses

Patient/family education
- Caution patient to avoid alcohol, OTC preparations that contain alcohol
- Instruct patient to report any pain, redness, or hard area, usually in legs; rash, sore throat, fever, bleeding, bruising, weakness, numbness, tingling
- Teach patient importance of complying with medical regimen (diet, weight loss, drug therapy); bone marrow depression may occur

Evaluation
Positive therapeutic outcome
- Decreased stone formation on x-ray
- Decreased pain in kidney region
- Absence of hematuria
- Decreased pain in joints

Treatment of overdose: D/C medication, may need opioids to treat diarrhea

---

colesevelam (Rx)
(coal-see-vel'am)
Welchol
Func. class.: Antilipemic
Chem. class.: Bile acid sequestrant
Pregnancy category C

Action: Absorbs, combines with bile acids to form insoluble complex that is excreted through feces; loss of bile acids lowers cholesterol levels

➡ **Therapeutic Outcome:** Decreasing LDL cholesterol

Uses: Elevated LDL cholesterol, alone or in combination with HMG-CoA reductase inhibitor

Dosage and routes
Adult: PO monotherapy: 3 625 mg tabs bid with meals or 6 tabs qd with a meal; may increase to 7 tabs if needed

Combination therapy
3 tabs bid with meals or 6 tabs qd with a meal given with an HMG-CoA reductase inhibitor

Available forms: Tabs 625 mg

Adverse effects
(*italic* = common; **bold** = life-threatening)
CNS: Headache, dizziness, drowsiness, vertigo, tinnitus

GI: Constipation, abdominal pain, nausea, fecal impaction, hemorrhoids, flatulence, vomiting, steatorrhea, peptic ulcer
INTEG: Rash, irritation of perianal area, tongue, skin
META: Decreased vit A, D, K, **hyperchloremic acidosis**
HEMA: Red cell folate content; ***bleeding***, ↓ Pro-time
MS: Muscle, joint pain

Contraindications: Hypersensitivity, biliary obstruction

Precautions: Pregnancy **C**, lactation, P children

Pharmacokinetics

Absorption	Unknown
Distribution	Unknown
Metabolism	Unknown
Excretion	Feces
Half-life	Unknown

Pharmacodynamics
LDL ↓ in 4-7 days

Interactions
Individual drugs
Cephalexin, chenodiol, clindamycin, digitalis, folic acid, iron, penicillin G, phenobarbital, phenylbutazone, trimethoprim, warfarin: ↓ absorption of each specific drug
Corticosteroid: ↓ corticosteroid action
Thyroid hormones: ↓ absorption of thyroid
Drug classifications
Tetracyclines: ↓ absorption of tetracyclines
Thiazides: ↓ absorption of thiazides
Vitamins (fat-soluble): ↓ absorption of fat-soluble vitamins
▨ *Herb/drug*
Glucomannan: ↑ effect
Gotu kola: ↓ effect
Lab test interferences
↑ Liver function studies, ↑ Cl, ↑ PO_4

NURSING CONSIDERATIONS
Assessment
- Assess cardiac glycoside level if both drugs are being administered
- Assess for signs of vit A, D, K deficiency
- Monitor fasting LDL, HDL, total cholesterol,

 Herb/drug   Do Not Crush   Alert   Key Drug   Geriatric   Pediatric

triglyceride levels, electrolytes if on extended therapy
• Monitor bowel pattern daily; increase bulk, H_2O in diet for constipation

Nursing diagnoses
✓ Constipation (adverse reactions)
✓ Knowledge, deficient (teaching)
✓ Noncompliance (teaching)

Implementation
• Give drug qd, bid with meals; give all other medications 1 hr before colesevelam or 4 hr after colesevelam to avoid poor absorption, take with liquid
• Give supplemental doses of vit A, D, K, if levels are low

Patient/family education
◆ Teach the symptoms of hypoprothrombinemia: bleeding mucous membranes, dark tarry stools, hematuria, petechiae; report immediately
• Teach the importance of compliance; toxicity may result if doses missed
• Teach that risk factors should be decreased: high-fat diet, smoking, alcohol consumption, absence of exercise
• Advise not to discontinue suddenly

Evaluation
Positive therapeutic outcome
• Decreased cholesterol level (hyperlipidemia); diarrhea, pruritus (excess bile acids)

---

colestipol (Rx)
(koe-les'ti-pole)
Colestid
Func. class.: Antilipemic
Chem. class.: Bile acid sequestrant

Pregnancy category B

Action: Absorbs, combines with bile acids to form an insoluble complex that is excreted through feces; loss of bile acids lowers cholesterol levels

➡ **Therapeutic Outcome:** Decreasing cholesterol levels and low-density lipoproteins, decreased pruritus

Uses: Primary hypercholesterolemia, xanthomas

Investigational uses: Digitalis toxicity

Dosage and routes
Adult: PO tabs 2 g qd-bid, may increase by 1 g/mo, max 16 g/day; granules 5 g qd-bid, may increase qmo, max 30 g/day

Available forms: Granules 300, 450 g, 500 g bottles, 5, 7.5 g packets, tabs 1 g

Adverse effects
(*italic* = common; **bold** = life-threatening)
GI: *Constipation, abdominal pain, nausea,* fecal impaction, hemorrhoids, flatulence, vomiting, steatorrhea, peptic ulcer
HEMA: **Bleeding, increased Pro-time**
INTEG: *Rash,* irritation of perianal area, tongue, skin
META: *Decreased vit A, D, E, K,* red folate content; **hyperchloremic acidosis**

Contraindications: Hypersensitivity, biliary obstruction

Precautions: Pregnancy **B,** lactation, children, bleeding disorders

Pharmacokinetics
Absorption	Not absorbed
Distribution	Not distributed
Metabolism	Not metabolized
Excretion	Binds with bile acids, feces
Half-life	Unknown

Pharmacodynamics
Onset	24-48 hr
Peak	30 days
Duration	30 days

Interactions
Individual drugs
Acetaminophen, amiodarone, methotrexate, naproxen, piroxicam, propranolol, ursodiol: ↓ absorption of each specific drug
Clindamycin, digoxin, folic acid, gemfibrozil, glipizide, iron, penicillin G, propranolol, tetracycline, warfarin: ↓ action of each specific drug
Phenytoin, tolbutamide: ↓ effect of each specific drug
Drug classifications
Anticoagulants (oral), cardiac glycosides, diuretics (thiazide): ↓ absorption
Corticosteroids: ↓ corticosteroid action
Vitamins A, D, E, K: ↓ absorption
⊘ *Herb/drug*
Glucomannan: ↑ effect
Gotu kola: ↓ effect
Lab test interferences
↑ Liver function studies, ↑ Cl, ↑ PO_4, ↑ AST, ↑ ALT, ↑ Alkaline phosphatase, ↓ Na, ↓ K, ↓ Ca

---

NURSING CONSIDERATIONS
Assessment

• Assess nutrition: fat, protein, carbohydrates; nutritional analysis should be completed by dietician

• Assess skin integrity after patient has been receiving drug; itching, pruritus often occur from bile deposits on skin

• Monitor cardiac glycoside level, if both drugs are being administered; cardiac glycoside levels will be decreased

• Monitor for signs of vit A, D, E, K deficiency; check serum cholesterol, triglyceride levels, electrolytes if on extended therapy

• Monitor bowel pattern daily; increase bulk, water in diet if constipation develops

Nursing diagnoses

☑ Constipation (adverse reactions)
☑ Knowledge, deficient (teaching)
☑ Noncompliance (teaching)

Implementation

• Give drug qd or bid; give all other medications 1 hr before or 4 hr after colestipol to avoid poor absorption; give drug mixed with applesauce or stirred into beverage (2-6 oz), let stand for 2 min; do not take dry

• Provide supplemental doses of vit A, D, E, K, if levels are low

🚫 • Tabs should be swallowed whole; do not crush, chew

Patient/family education

• Teach patient symptoms of hypoprothrombinemia: bleeding mucous membranes, dark, tarry stools, hematuria, petechiae; report immediately

• Teach patient importance of compliance, not to miss or double doses

• Teach patient that risk factors should be decreased: high-fat diet, smoking, alcohol consumption, absence of exercise

• Tell patient to mix drug with 6 oz of milk, water, fruit juice; may be mixed with carbonated beverages; rinse glass to make sure all medication is taken or may mix drug in applesauce; allow to stand for 2 min before mixing

Evaluation

Positive therapeutic outcome

• Decreased cholesterol level (hyperlipidemia)

---

cortisone ⊶π (Rx)
(kor'ti-sone)
Cortone ✦, cortone acetate
Func. class.: Corticosteroid, synthetic
Chem. class.: Short-acting glucocorticoid

Pregnancy category D

Action: Decreases inflammation by suppression of migration of polymorphonuclear leukocytes, fibroblasts, reversal of increased capillary permeability, and lysosomal stabilization; suppresses adrenal function with long-term use

➡ **Therapeutic Outcome:** Replacement of cortisol in adrenal insufficiency

Uses: Inflammation, severe allergy, adrenal insufficiency, collagen disorders, respiratory and dermatologic, rheumatic disorders

Dosage and routes
Adult: PO/IM 25-300 mg qd or q2 days, titrated to patient response

🅟 *Child:* PO 2.5-10 mg/kg/day; IM 1-5 mg/kg/day

Available forms: Tabs 5, 10, 25 mg; inj 50 mg/ml

Adverse effects
(*italic* = common; **bold** = life-threatening)
CNS: Depression, flushing, sweating, headache, mood changes
CV: Hypertension, **circulatory collapse, thrombophlebitis, embolism,** tachycardia, **necrotizing angiitis, CHF,** edema
EENT: Fungal infections, increased intraocular pressure, blurred vision
GI: Diarrhea, nausea, abdominal distention, **GI hemorrhage,** increased appetite, **pancreatitis**
META: Sodium fluid retention; potassium loss
HEMA: **Thrombocytopenia**
INTEG: Acne, poor wound healing, ecchymosis, bruising, petechiae
MS: Fractures, osteoporosis, weakness, loss of muscle mass

Contraindications: Psychosis, hypersensitivity, idiopathic thrombocytopenia, acute glomerulonephritis, amebiasis, fungal infections, nonasthmatic bronchial disease, child <2 yr, AIDS, TB, pregnancy **D**

  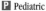

Precautions: Diabetes mellitus, glaucoma, osteoporosis, seizure disorders, ulcerative colitis, CHF, myasthenia gravis, renal disease, esophagitis, peptic ulcer

Pharmacokinetics	
Absorption	Slowly IM
Distribution	Widely, crosses placenta
Metabolism	Liver
Excretion	Unknown
Half-life	½ hr

Pharmacodynamics		
	PO	IM
Onset	Unknown	Unknown
Peak	2 hr	20-48 hr
Duration	1½ days	1½ days

Interactions
Individual drugs
Alcohol: ↑ side effects
Amphotericin, mezlocillin: ↑ hypokalemia
Indomethacin: ↑ GI symptoms, ↑ side effects
Insulin: ↑ need for insulin
Ketoconazole: ↑ cortisone action
Phenobarbital, phenytoin: ↓ effectiveness of cortisone
Rifampin, theophylline: ↓ cortisone action
Drug classifications
Anticoagulants: ↓ anticoagulant effect
Antidiabetics: ↓ antidiabetic effect
Antiinfectives (macrolide), estrogens: ↑ cortisone action
Barbiturates: ↓ cortisone action
Contraceptives (oral): blocked metabolism of cortisone
Diuretics (potassium-wasting), salicylates: ↑ side effects
NSAIDs: ↑ GI symptoms
Salicylates: ↑ GI symptoms, ↓ salicylate effect, ↑ cortisone effects
Toxoids: ↓ toxoid effect
Vaccines: ↓ vaccine effect
⬛ Herb/drug
Aloe, buckthorn bark/berry, cascara sagrada bark, Chinese rhubarb, rhubarb root, senna leaf/fruits: ↑ potassium deficiency
Aloe, licorice, perilla: ↑ steroid effect
Lab test interferences
↑ Cholesterol, ↑ sodium, ↑ blood glucose, ↑ uric acid, ↑ calcium, ↑ urine glucose
↓ Calcium, ↓ potassium, ↓ T_4, ↓ T_3, ↓ thyroid ^{131}I uptake test, ↓ urine 17-OHCS, ↓ 17-KS, ↓ PBI
False negative: Skin allergy tests

NURSING CONSIDERATIONS
Assessment
• Assess for adrenal insufficiency symptoms: weakness, nausea, vomiting, confusion, anxiety, restlessness, decreased B/P, weight loss; check before and during treatment
• Monitor potassium, blood/urine glucose for patient on long-term therapy; hypokalemia and hyperglycemia can occur
• Check B/P, pulse q4h; notify prescriber if chest pain occurs
• Monitor I&O ratio and weight daily; be alert for decreasing urinary output and increasing edema with bilateral rales, dyspnea, weight gain
• Monitor plasma cortisol levels during long-term therapy (normal level: 138-635 nmol/L if checked at 8 AM)
• Assess for symptoms of infection: increased temp, WBC even after withdrawal of medication; drug masks symptoms of infection
• Monitor for potassium depletion: paresthesias, fatigue, nausea, vomiting, depression, polyuria, dysrhythmias, weakness, edema, hypertension, cardiac symptoms, weight daily; notify prescriber of weekly gain >5 lb
• Assess for mental changes: affect, mood, behavioral changes, aggression; depression, psychoses may occur

Nursing diagnoses
☑ Infection, risk for (adverse reactions)
☑ Injury, risk for (adverse reactions)
☑ Knowledge, deficient (teaching)

Implementation
PO route
• Administer with food or milk to decrease GI symptoms
IM route
• Give after shaking susp (parenteral); titrate dose; use lowest effective dosage
• Give IM inj deep in large muscle mass; rotate sites; avoid deltoid; use a 21-G needle
• Administer in 1 dose in AM to prevent adrenal suppression; avoid SC administration; damage may be done to tissue; do not give **IV**

Patient/family education
• Advise patient to carry/wear emergency ID as steroid user at all times
• Instruct patient to notify prescriber if therapeutic response decreases; dosage adjustment may be needed; teach not to discontinue this medication abruptly or adrenal crisis can result; teach all aspects of drug usage, including cushingoid symptoms
• Caution patient to avoid OTC products: salicylates, potassium, alcohol in cough

products, cold preparations unless directed by prescriber

• Teach patient symptoms of adrenal insufficiency: nausea, anorexia, fatigue, dizziness, dyspnea, weakness, joint pain, tarry stools, bruising, blurred vision

• Advise patient to avoid persons with known infections; report probable infection rapidly; drug masks infection

• Caution patient that diet modification is necessary if on long-term treatment: increased calcium, potassium, and protein; also low sodium and carbohydrates

• Advise the patient to avoid exposure to chickenpox, measles

• Advise the patient to take PO dose in AM with food or fluid (milk)

Evaluation
Positive therapeutic outcome
• Ease of respirations, decreased inflammation

---

cotrimoxazole
See trimethoprim/sulfamethoxazole

---

cyclobenzaprine (Rx)
(sye-kloe-ben′za-preen)
cyclobenzaprine HCl, Cycloflex, Flexeril
Func. class.: Skeletal muscle relaxant, central acting
Chem. class.: Tricyclic amine salt
Pregnancy category B

Action: Unknown; may be related to antidepressant effects

➡ **Therapeutic Outcome:** Relaxation of skeletal muscle

Uses: Adjunct for relief of muscle spasm and pain in musculoskeletal conditions

Dosage and routes
Musculoskeletal disorders
Adult: PO 10 mg tid × 1 wk, not to exceed 60 mg/day × 3 wk

Fibromyalgia
Adult: PO 10-40 mg hs

Available forms: Tabs 10 mg

Adverse effects
(*italic* = common; **bold** = life-threatening)
CNS: *Dizziness, weakness, drowsiness,* headache, tremor, depression, insomnia, confusion, paresthesia

CV: Postural hypotension, tachycardia, **dysrhythmias**

EENT: Diplopia, temporary loss of vision

GI: *Nausea,* vomiting, hiccups, dry mouth, constipation

GU: Urinary retention, frequency, change in libido

INTEG: Rash, pruritus, fever, facial flushing, sweating

Contraindications: Acute recovery phase of MI, dysrhythmias, heart block, CHF, hypersensitivity, child <12 yr, intermittent porphyria, thyroid disease

Precautions: Renal disease, hepatic disease, addictive personality, pregnancy **B**, elderly, lactation

Do Not Confuse:
cyclobenzaprine/cyproheptadine

Pharmacokinetics	
Distribution	Well
Metabolism	Liver, partially
Excretion	Kidney (unchanged)
Half-life	1-3 days

Pharmacodynamics	
Onset	1 hr
Peak	3-8 hr
Duration	12-24 hr

Interactions
Individual drugs
Alcohol: ↑ CNS depression
Drug classifications
Antidepressants (tricyclic), antihistamines, barbiturates, opiates, sedative/hypnotics: ↑ CNS depression
MAOIs: Do not use within 14 days
Herb/drug
Kava: ↑ CNS depression

NURSING CONSIDERATIONS
Assessment
• Assess pain periodically: location, duration, mobility, stiffness, baseline
• Monitor ECG in epileptic patients; poor seizure control has occurred in patients taking this drug
• Check for allergic reactions: rash, fever, respiratory distress
• Check for severe weakness, numbness, in extremities
• Assess for CNS depression: dizziness, drowsiness, psychiatric symptoms

Nursing diagnoses
☑ Mobility, impaired physical
☑ Injury, risk for (adverse reactions)
☑ Knowledge, deficient (teaching)

Implementation
• Give with meals for GI symptoms
• Store in airtight container at room temp

Patient/family education
• Teach patient not to discontinue medication quickly; insomnia, nausea, headache, spasticity, tachycardia will occur; drug should be tapered off over 1-2 wk
• Caution patient not to take with alcohol, other CNS depressants
• Advise to avoid altering activities while taking this drug
• Caution patient to avoid hazardous activities if drowsiness/dizziness occurs
• Caution patient to avoid using OTC medication: cough preparations, antihistamines, unless directed by prescriber
• Teach patient to use gum, frequent sips of water for dry mouth

Evaluation
Positive therapeutic outcome
• Decreased pain, spasticity; muscle spasms of acute, painful musculoskeletal conditions are generally short term; long-term therapy is seldom warranted

Treatment of overdose: Empty stomach with emesis, gastric lavage, then administer activated charcoal; use anticonvulsants if indicated; monitor cardiac function

---

! HIGH ALERT

cyclophosphamide ⊙π (Rx)
(sye-kloe-foss'fa-mide)
Cytoxan, Neosar, Procytox ✢
Func. class.: Antineoplastic alkylating agent
Chem. class.: Nitrogen mustard

Pregnancy category D

Action: Alkylates DNA, RNA; inhibits enzymes that allow synthesis of amino acids in proteins; is also responsible for cross-linking DNA strands; activity is not cell cycle phase specific

⇒ **Therapeutic Outcome:** Prevention of rapidly growing malignant cells

Uses: Hodgkin's disease, lymphomas, leukemia, multiple myeloma, neuroblastoma, retinoblastoma, Ewing's sarcoma, cancer of female reproductive tract, breast, lung, prostate

Dosage and routes
Adult: PO initially 1-5 mg/ kg over 2-5 days; maintenance 1-5 mg/kg; **IV** initially 40-50 mg/kg in divided doses over 2-5 days; maintenance 10-15 mg/kg q7-10 days, or 3-5 mg/kg q3 days

P *Child:* PO/**IV** 2-8 mg/kg or 60-250 mg/m² in divided doses × 6 or more days; maintenance **IV** 10-15 mg/kg q7-10 days or 30 mg/kg q3-4 wk; dose should be reduced by half when bone marrow suppression occurs

Renal dose
Adult: PO/**IV** CCr 25-50 ml/min 50% of dose; CCr <25 ml/min avoid use

Available forms: Powder for inj **IV** 100, 200, 500, 750 mg, 1, 2 g; tabs 25, 50 mg

Adverse effects
(*italic* = common; **bold** = life-threatening)
CNS: Headache, dizziness
CV: **Cardiotoxicity** (high doses)
ENDO: Syndrome of inappropriate antidiuretic hormone (SIADH), gonadal suppression
GI: Nausea, vomiting, diarrhea, weight loss, colitis, **hepatotoxicity**
GU: **Hemorrhagic cystitis, hematuria, neoplasms, amenorrhea, azoospermia, sterility, ovarian fibrosis**
HEMA: **Thrombocytopenia, leukopenia, pancytopenia, myelosuppression**
INTEG: Alopecia, dermatitis
META: Hyperuricemia
MISC: Secondary neoplasms
RESP: **Fibrosis**

Contraindications: Lactation, pregnancy **D**

Precautions: Radiation therapy

⊠ **Do Not Confuse:**
cyclophosphamide/cycloSPORINE, Cytoxan/Cytosar, Cytoxan/Cytotec/centoxin/Cytarabine

Pharmacokinetics	
Absorption	Well absorbed (PO)
Distribution	Widely distributed; crosses placenta, blood-brain barrier (50%)
Metabolism	Liver to active drug
Excretion	Kidneys, unchanged (30%)
Half-life	4-6½ hr

Pharmacodynamics	
Unknown	

Interactions
Individual drugs
Allopurinol, radiation, rifampin: ↑ bone marrow suppression

Chloramphenicol: ↓ cyclophosphamide
Digoxin: ↓ digoxin levels
Insulin: ↑ hypoglycemia
Phenobarbital, radiation, rifampin: ↑ toxicity
Succinylcholine: ↑ neuromuscular blockade
Warfarin: ↑ warfarin action

Drug classifications
Aminoglycosides: ↑ nephrotoxicity
Anticoagulants (oral): ↑ bleeding
Antineoplastics: ↑ toxicity
Antineoplastics, bone marrow–suppressing drugs, diuretics (thiazides): ↑ bone marrow suppression
Barbiturates: ↑ toxicity of cyclophosphamide
Corticosteroids: ↓ cyclophosphamide effect
Diuretics (loop): ↑ ototoxicity
Live virus vaccines: ↓ antibody reaction

Lab test interferences
↑ Uric acid
↓ Pseudocholinesterase
False positive: Pap smear
False negative: PPD, mumps trichophytin, *Candida*

NURSING CONSIDERATIONS
Assessment
◆• Assess symptoms indicating severe allergic reaction: rash, pruritus, urticaria, purpuric skin lesions, itching, flushing
• Assess for tachypnea, ECG changes, dyspnea, edema, fatigue
• Monitor CBC, differential, platelet count weekly; withhold drug if WBC count is <2500/mm³ or platelet count is <75,000/mm³; notify prescriber of results
• Assess for hemorrhagic cystitis: renal function studies including BUN, creatinine, serum uric acid, urine CCr before and during therapy; I&O ratio; report fall in urine output to <30 ml/hr
• Monitor temp q4h (elevated temp may indicate beginning of infection)
• Monitor liver function tests before and during therapy (bilirubin, AST, ALT, LDH) as needed or monthly; note jaundice of skin or sclera, dark urine, clay-colored stools, itchy skin, abdominal pain, fever, diarrhea
• Assess for bleeding: hematuria, stool guaiac, bruising or petechiae, mucosa or orifices q8h
• Identify dyspnea, rales, unproductive cough, chest pain, tachypnea
• Identify effects of alopecia on body image; discuss feelings about body changes

Nursing diagnoses
☑ Injury, risk for (adverse reactions)
☑ Body image, disturbed (adverse reactions)
☑ Infection, risk for (adverse reactions)
☑ Knowledge, deficient (teaching)

Implementation
• Give fluids **IV** or PO before chemotherapy to hydrate patient
• Give antacid before oral agent, pc PM, before hs; antiemetic 30-60 min before giving drug to prevent vomiting, and prn; antibiotics for prophylaxis of infection
• Give top or syst analgesics for pain; give in AM so drug can be eliminated before hs

IV **IV route**
• Give **IV** after diluting 100 mg/5 ml of sterile or bacteriostatic water; shake; let stand until clear; may be further diluted in up to 250 ml D₅ 0.9% NaCl, 0.45% NaCl, LR, Ringer's; give 100 mg or less/min through 3-way stopcock of glucose or saline inf
• Use 21-, 23-, or 25-G needle; check site for irritation, phlebitis

Syringe compatibilities: Bleomycin, cisplatin, doxapram, DOXOrubicin, droperidol, fluorouracil, furosemide, heparin, leucovorin, methotrexate, metoclopramide, mitomycin, mitoxantrone, vinBLAStine, vinCRIStine

Y-site compatibilities: Amifostine, amikacin, ampicillin, azlocillin, aztreonam, bleomycin, cefamandole, cefazolin, cefepime, cefoperazone, cefotaxime, cefoxitin, cefuroxime, cephalothin, cephapirin, chloramphenicol, chlorproMAZINE, cimetidine, cisplatin, cladribine, clindamycin, dexamethasone, diphenhydrAMINE, DOXOrubicin, doxycycline, droperidol, erythromycin, famotidine, filgrastim, fludarabine, fluorouracil, furosemide, gallium, ganciclovir, gentamicin, granisetron, heparin, hydromorphone, idarubicin, kanamycin, leucovorin, lorazepam, melphalan, methotrexate, methylPREDNISolone, metoclopramide, metronidazole, mezlocillin, minocycline, mitomycin, moxalactam, nafcillin, ondansetron, oxacillin, paclitaxel, penicillin G potassium, piperacillin, piperacillin/tazobactam, prochlorperazine, promethazine, propofol, ranitidine, sargramostim, sodium bicarbonate, teniposide, tetracycline, thiotepa, ticarcillin, ticarcillin-clavulanate, tobramycin, trimethoprim-sulfamethoxazole, vancomycin, vinBLAStine, vinCRIStine, vinorelbine

Additive compatibilities: Cisplatin with etoposide, hydrOXYzine, methotrexate, methotrexate with fluorouracil, mitoxantrone, ondansetron

Solution compatibilities: Amino acids 4.25%/D₂₅, D₅/0.9% NaCl, D₅W, 0.9% NaCl

Patient/family education
- Teach patient to avoid use of products containing aspirin or ibuprofen, razors, commercial mouthwash, since bleeding may occur; to report symptoms of bleeding (hematuria, tarry stools, bruising)
- Instruct patient to report signs of anemia (fatigue, headache, faintness, shortness of breath)
- Teach patient to report any changes in breathing or coughing even several months after treatment
- Advise patient that hair may be lost during treatment; a wig or hairpiece may make patient feel better; new hair may be different in color, texture
- Teach patient not to have any vaccinations without the advice of the prescriber; serious reactions can occur
- Advise patient contraception is needed during treatment and for several months after the completion of therapy

Evaluation
Positive therapeutic outcome
- Prevention of rapid division of malignant cells
- Increased appetite, increased weight

---

*cycloSPORINE (Rx)
(sye-kloe-spor′een)
Neoral, Sandimmune, SangCya
Func. class.: Immunosuppressant
Chem. class.: Fungus-derived peptide

Pregnancy category C

Action: Produces immunosuppression by inhibiting T lymphocytes

Therapeutic Outcome: Absence of transplant rejection

Uses: Organ transplants (liver, kidney, heart) to prevent rejection, rheumatoid arthritis, psoriasis

Investigational uses: Recalcitrant ulcerative colitis

Dosage and routes
Prevention of transplant rejection
Adult and child: PO 15 mg/kg several hr before surgery, daily for 2 wk, reduce dosage by 2.5 mg/kg/wk to 5-10 mg/kg/day; **IV** 5-6 mg/kg several hr before surgery, daily, switch to PO form as soon as possible

Rheumatoid arthritis
Adult: PO 2.5 mg/kg/day divided bid, may increase 0.5-0.75 mg/kg/day after 8-12 wk, max 4 mg/kg/day

Psoriasis
Adult: PO 2.5 mg/kg/day divided bid × 4 wk, then increase by 0.5 mg/kg/day q2 wk, max 4 mg/kg/day

Available forms: Microemulsion oral sol (Neoral) 100 mg/ml; microemulsion soft gel cap (Neoral) 25, 100 mg; soft gel caps 25, 100 mg; oral sol 100 mg/ml; inj 50 mg/ml

Adverse effects
(*italic* = common; **bold** = life-threatening)
CNS: Tremors, *headache,* **seizures**
GI: Nausea, vomiting, diarrhea, *oral Candida, gum hyperplasia,* **hepatotoxicity,** pancreatitis
GU: **Albuminuria, hematuria, proteinuria, renal failure**
INTEG: Rash, acne, *hirsutism*
META: Hyperkalemia, hypomagnesemia, hyperlipidemia, hyperuricemia
MISC: *Infection*

Contraindications: Hypersensitivity

Precautions: Severe renal disease, severe hepatic disease, pregnancy **C**

⚠ Do Not Confuse:
cycloSPORINE/CycloSERINE,
cycloSPORINE/cyclophosphamide

Pharmacokinetics
Absorption	Poorly absorbed (PO)
Distribution	Crosses placenta
Metabolism	Liver to mercaptopurine
Excretion	Kidney, minimal
Half-life	Biphasic 1.2 hr, 25 hr

Pharmacodynamics
	PO
Onset	Unknown
Peak	4 hr
Duration	Unknown

Interactions
Individual drugs
Amiodarone, amphotericin B, carvedilol, cimetidine, colchicine, fluconazole, foscarnet, imipenem-cilastatin, ketoconazole, melphalan, metoclopramide: ↑ cycloSPORINE toxicity
Carbamazepine, phenobarbital, phenytoin, trimethoprim/sulfamethoxazole: ↓ cycloSPORINE action
Digoxin: ↑ digoxin level
Etoposide: ↑ etoposide level
Tacrolimus: Do not use with cycloSPORINE

Drug classifications:
Androgens, antifungals (azole), calcium channel blockers, corticosteroids: ↑ cyclo-SPORINE levels
Live virus vaccines: ↓ antibody reaction
Macrolides, NSAIDs, contraceptives (oral): ↑ cycloSPORINE toxicity
Neoral products: ↓ absorption
Rifamycins: ↓ cycloSPORINE levels
Food/drug
Grapefruit juice: ↑ slowed metabolism of drug
☑ *Herb/drug*
Ginseng, maitake, mistletoe, schisandra, St. John's wort, turmeric: ↓ effect
Safflower: ↑ effect

NURSING CONSIDERATIONS
Assessment
• Monitor renal studies: BUN, creatinine at least monthly during treatment, 3 mo after treatment
• Monitor liver function studies: alkaline phosphatase, AST, ALT, bilirubin
• Monitor drug blood levels during treatment
• Assess for hepatotoxicity: dark urine, jaundice, itching, light-colored stools; drug should be discontinued
• Assess for nephrotoxicity: 6 wk postop, CyA trough level >200 ng/ml, intracapsular pressure <40 mm Hg, rise in creatinine 0.15 mg/dl/day

Nursing diagnoses
☑ Mobility, impaired (uses)
☑ Infection, risk for (uses)
☑ Knowledge, deficient (teaching)

Implementation
PO route
• Use pipette provided to draw up oral sol; may mix with milk or juice, wipe pipette, do not wash
• Give for several days before transplant surgery with corticosteroids
• Microemulsion products (Neoral) and other products are not interchangeable
• Give with meals for GI upset or drug placed in chocolate milk
🚫 • Do not crush, chew caps
• Give with oral antifungal for *Candida* infections
IV IV route
• Give **IV** after diluting each 50 mg/20-100 ml of 0.9% NaCl or D₅W; run over 2-6 hr; use an infusion pump, glass inf bottles only; may give as cont inf over 24 hr

Additive compatibilities: Ciprofloxacin

Y-site compatibility: Cefmetazole, propofol, sargramostim

Solution compatibilities: D_5W, NaCl 0.9%
• Give for several days before transplant surgery
• Give with corticosteroids

Patient/family education
• Advise patient to report fever, rash, severe diarrhea, chills, sore throat, fatigue, since serious infections may occur; also to report clay-colored stools, cramping (may indicate hepatotoxicity); tremors, bleeding gums, increased B/P
• Caution patient to use contraceptive measures during treatment and for 12 wk after ending therapy; drug is teratogenic
• Caution patient to avoid crowds and persons with known infections to reduce risk of infection

Evaluation
Positive therapeutic outcome
• Absence of graft rejection

---

cyproheptadine (Rx)
(si-proe-hep'ta-deen)
cyproheptadine HCl, Periactin, PMS-Cyproheptadine
Func. class.: Antihistamine, H₁-receptor antagonist
Chem. class.: Piperidine
Pregnancy category B

Action: Acts on blood vessels, GI, respiratory system by competing with histamine for H₁-receptor site; decreases allergic response by blocking histamine; blocks serotonin to increase appetite and relieve vascular headaches

➔ **Therapeutic Outcome:** Absence of allergy symptoms and rhinitis

Uses: Allergy symptoms, rhinitis, pruritus, cold urticaria

Investigational uses: Appetite stimulant, management of vascular headache, nightmares, posttraumatic stress disorder

Dosage and routes
Adult: PO 4 mg tid-qid, not to exceed 0.5 mg/kg/day
P *Child 7-14 yr:* PO 4 mg bid-tid, not to exceed 16 mg/day
P *Child 2-6 yr:* PO 2 mg bid-tid, not to exceed 12 mg/day

Nightmares, posttraumatic stress disorder
Adult: PO 4-12 mg qhs, max 32 mg

Available forms: Tabs 4 mg; syr 2 mg/5 ml

Adverse effects
(*italic* = common; **bold** = life-threatening)
CNS: Dizziness, drowsiness, poor coordination, fatigue, anxiety, euphoria, confusion, paresthesia, neuritis
CV: Hypotension, palpitations, tachycardia
EENT: Blurred vision, dilated pupils; tinnitus; nasal stuffiness; dry nose, throat, mouth
GI: Constipation, dry mouth, nausea, vomiting, anorexia, diarrhea, weight gain, increased appetite
GU: Retention, dysuria, frequency
HEMA: Hemolytic anemia, leukopenia, thrombocytosis, agranulocytosis
INTEG: Rash, urticaria, photosensitivity
MISC: Anaphylaxis
RESP: Increased thick secretions, wheezing, chest tightness

Contraindications: Hypersensitivity to H_1-receptor antagonist, acute asthma attack, lower respiratory tract disease

Precautions: Increased intraocular pressure, renal disease, cardiac disease, hypertension, bronchial asthma, seizure disorder, stenosed peptic ulcers, hyperthyroidism, prostatic hypertrophy, bladder neck obstruction, pregnancy **B**, elderly

Do Not Confuse:
cyproheptadine/cyclobenzaprine

Pharmacokinetics	
Absorption	Well absorbed
Distribution	Unknown
Metabolism	Liver, complete
Excretion	Kidneys
Half-life	Unknown

Pharmacodynamics	
Onset	15-60 min
Peak	1-2 hr
Duration	8 hr

Interactions
Individual drugs
Alcohol: ↑ CNS depression
Drug classifications
Antidepressants (tricyclics), barbiturates, CNS depressants, opiates, sedative/hypnotics: ↑ CNS depression
MAOIs: ↑ anticholinergic effect

Herb/drug
Corkwood, henbane leaf: ↑ anticholinergic effect
Hops, Jamaican dogwood, kava, khat, senega: ↑ CNS depression
Lab test interferences
False negative: Skin allergy tests (discontinue antihistamine 3 days before testing)

NURSING CONSIDERATIONS
Assessment
• Assess respiratory status: rate, rhythm, increase in bronchial secretions, wheezing, chest tightness; provide fluids to 2 L/day to decrease secretion thickness
• Monitor I&O ratio: be alert for urinary retention, frequency, dysuria, especially elderly; drug should be discontinued if these occur; monitor food intake, weight if using as an appetite stimulant

Nursing diagnoses
☑ Airway clearance, ineffective (uses)
☑ Injury, risk for (side effects)
☑ Knowledge, deficient (teaching)
☑ Noncompliance (teaching, overuse)

Implementation
• May give with food to decrease GI upset
• Syrup may be used for patients with difficulty swallowing or children
• Store in tight, light-resistant container

Patient/family education
• Teach all aspects of drug uses; tell patient to notify prescriber if confusion, sedation, hypotension occur; to avoid driving and other hazardous activity if drowsiness occurs; to avoid alcohol and other CNS depressants that may potentiate effect
• Caution patient not to exceed recommended dosage; dysrhythmias may occur
• Teach patient hard candy, gum, frequent rinsing of mouth may be used for dryness

Evaluation
Positive therapeutic outcome
• Absence of runny or congested nose, rashes

Treatment of overdose: Administer ipecac syrup or lavage, diazepam, vasopressors, barbiturates (short acting)

⚠ HIGH ALERT

cytarabine (Rx)
(sye-tare´a-been)
Ara-C, Cytosar ✤, Cytosar-U, cytosine arabinoside, Depo Cyt, Tarabine PFS
Func. class.: Antineoplastic, antimetabolite
Chem. class.: Pyrimidine nucleoside

Pregnancy category D

Action: Competes with physiologic substrate of DNA synthesis, thus interfering with cell replication in the S phase of the cell cycle (before mitosis)

➡ **Therapeutic Outcome:** Prevention of rapidly growing malignant cells

Uses: Acute myelocytic leukemia, acute lymphocytic leukemia, chronic myelocytic leukemia, lymphomatous meningitis (IT), and in combination for non-Hodgkin's lymphomas Ⓟ in children

Dosage and routes
Acute myelocytic leukemia
Adult: **IV** inf 200 mg/m²/day × 5 days q2 wk as single agent or 2-6 mg/kg/day (100-200 mg/m²/day) as single dose or 2-3 divided doses for 5-10 days until remission, used in combination; maintenance 70-200 mg/m²/day for 2-5 days qmo; SC maintenance 1 mg/kg 1-2×/wk

Lymphomatous meningitis Liposomal (DepoCyt)
Adult: IT 50 mg q14 days × 2 doses (wk 1, 3) then 50 mg q14 days × 3 doses (wk 5, 7, 9) followed by 1 dose wk 13; then 50 mg q28 days × 4 doses (wk 17, 21, 25, 29); if neurotoxicity occurs, reduce dose to 25 mg, if it persists, discontinue use

In combination
Ⓟ *Child:* **IV** inf 100 mg/m²/day × 5-10 days

Available forms: Powder for inj 100, 500 mg, 1, 2 g; liposomal for IT use 10 mg/ml

Adverse effects
(*italic* = common; **bold** = life-threatening)
CNS: Neuritis, dizziness, headache, personality changes, ataxia, mechanical dysphasia, **coma; chemical arachnoiditis** (IT)
CV: Chest pain, **cardiopathy**
CYTARABINE SYNDROME: Fever, myalgia, bone pain, chest pain, rash, conjunctivitis, malaise (6-12 hr after administration)
EENT: Sore throat, conjunctivitis
GI: Nausea, vomiting, anorexia, diarrhea, stomatitis, **hepatotoxicity**, abdominal pain, hematemesis, **GI hemorrhage**

GU: Urinary retention, **renal failure, hyperuricemia**
HEMA: **Thrombophlebitis, bleeding, thrombocytopenia, leukopenia, myelosuppression, anemia**
INTEG: Rash, fever, freckling, cellulitis
META: Hyperuricemia
RESP: **Pneumonia**, dyspnea, **pulmonary edema** (high doses)
SYST: **Anaphylaxis**

Contraindications: Hypersensitivity, Ⓟ infants, pregnancy **D**

Precautions: Renal disease, hepatic disease, lactation

◨ Do Not Confuse:
Cytosar/Cytovene, Cytosar/Cytoxan

Pharmacokinetics
Absorption	Complete
Distribution	Widely distributed; crosses blood-brain barrier, placenta
Metabolism	Liver, extensively
Excretion	Kidneys
Half-life	1-3 hr; IT 100-236 hr

Pharmacodynamics
Unknown

Interactions
Individual drugs
Digoxin oral: ↓ digoxin effects
Radiation: ↑ toxicity, bone marrow suppression
Drug classifications
Antineoplastics: ↑ toxicity, bone marrow suppression

NURSING CONSIDERATIONS
Assessment
- Assess buccal cavity q8h for dryness, sores or ulceration, white patches, pain, bleeding, dysphagia; obtain prescription for viscous lidocaine (Xylocaine)
- Assess symptoms indicating anaphylaxis: rash, pruritus, urticaria, purpuric skin lesions, itching, flushing, resuscitation equipment should be nearby
◆- Assess for chemical arachnoiditis (IT): headache, nausea, vomiting, fever; neck rigidity/pain, meningism, CSF pleocytosis; may be decreased by dexamethasone
- Assess tachypnea, dyspnea, edema, fatigue; identify dyspnea, rales, unproductive cough, chest pain, tachypnea; pulmonary edema may be fatal (rare)
◆- Assess for cytarabine syndrome 6-12 hr after inf: fever, myalgia, bone pain, chest pain,

rash, conjunctivitis, malaise; corticosteroid may be ordered

• Monitor CBC, differential, platelet count weekly; withhold drug if WBC count is <1000/mm³ or platelet count is <50,000/mm³

• Assess for increased uric acid levels, swelling, joint pain primarily in extremities; patient should be well hydrated to prevent urate deposits

• Monitor renal function studies: BUN, creatinine, serum uric acid, urine CCr before and during therapy; I&O ratio; report fall in urine output to <30 ml/hr

• Monitor temp q4h (may indicate beginning of infection)

• Monitor liver function tests before and during therapy (bilirubin, AST, ALT, LDH) as needed or monthly; note yellowing of skin or sclera, dark urine, clay-colored stools, pruritus, abdominal pain, fever, diarrhea; an antispasmodic may be used for GI symptoms

• Assess for bleeding: hematuria, stool guaiac, bruising or petechiae, mucosa or orifices q8h; identify inflammation of mucosa, breaks in skin

Nursing diagnoses

✓ Injury, risk for (adverse reactions)
✓ Body image, disturbed (adverse reactions)
✓ Infection, risk for (adverse reactions)
✓ Knowledge, deficient (teaching)

Implementation

• Avoid contact with skin; very irritating; wash completely to remove

• Give fluids **IV** or PO before chemotherapy to hydrate patient

• Give antiemetic 30-60 min before giving drug to prevent vomiting, and prn; antibiotics for prophylaxis of infection

• Give top or syst analgesics for pain

• Give in AM so drug can be eliminated before hs

• Provide liquid diet: carbonated beverages; gelatin may be added if patient is not nauseated or vomiting

• Provide rinsing of mouth tid-qid with water, club soda; brushing of teeth bid-qid with soft brush or cotton-tipped applicators for stomatitis; use unwaxed dental floss

• Give **IV** direct after diluting 100 mg/5 ml of sterile water for inj; give by direct **IV** over 1-3 min through free-flowing tubing

IV **IV infusion**

• May be further diluted in 50-100 ml 0.9% NaCl or D₅W and given over 30 min to 24 hr depending on dosage; may be given by cont inf also

Syringe compatibilities: Metoclopramide

Y-site compatibilities: Amifostine, amsacrine, aztreonam, cefepime, chlorproMAZINE, cimetidine, cladribine, dexamethasone, diphenhydrAMINE, droperidol, famotidine, filgrastim, fludarabine, gentamicin, granisetron, heparin, hydrocortisone, hydromorphone, idarubicin, lorazepam, melphalan, methotrexate, methylPREDNISolone, metoclopramide, morphine, ondansetron, paclitaxel, piperacillin/tazobactam, prochlorperazine, promethazine, propofol, ranitidine, sargramostim, sodium bicarbonate, teniposide, thiotepa, vinorelbine

Additive compatibilities: Corticotropin, DAUNOrubicin with etoposide, etoposide, hydrOXYzine, lincomycin, mitoxantrone, potassium chloride, prednisoLONE, ondansetron, sodium bicarbonate, vinCRIStine

Additive incompatibilities: Carbenicillin, fluorouracil, heparin, regular insulin, nafcillin, oxacillin, penicillin G sodium

Solution compatibilities: Amino acids, 4.25%/D₂₅, D₅/LR, D₅/0.2% NaCl, D₅/0.9% NaCl, D₁₀/0.9% NaCl, D₅W, invert glucose 10% in electrolyte #1, Ringer's LR, 0.9% NaCl, sodium lactate 1/6 mol/L, TPN #57

Intrathecal route

• Liposomal: withdraw drug immediately before use; use within 4 hr, do not save unused portions, or use in-line filter; give directly into CSF by intraventricular reservoir or by direct inj into lumbar site

• Give slowly over 1-5 min, follow with lumbar puncture, instruct patient to lie flat, give dexamethasone 4 mg bid PO or **IV** × 5 days beginning on day of liposomal inj

SC/IM route

• Reconstitute 100 mg/5 ml or 500 mg/10 ml with bacteriostatic water for inj with benzyl alcohol 0.9%; do not use sol with precipitate; stable for 48 hr

Patient/family education

• Advise patient that contraceptive measures are recommended during and 4 mo after therapy

• Teach patient to avoid use of products containing aspirin or ibuprofen, NSAIDs, razors, commercial mouthwash, since bleeding may occur; to report symptoms of bleeding (hematuria, tarry stools)

• Advise patient to continue using dexamethasone with IT administration, that fever, headache, nausea, vomiting are likely to occur

• Advise patient to report signs of anemia

(fatigue, headache, irritability, faintness, shortness of breath)

• Advise patient to avoid foods with citric acid, hot or rough texture if stomatitis is present, use sponge brush and rinse with water after each meal; to report stomatitis: any bleeding, white spots, ulcerations in mouth; tell patient to examine mouth qd, report any symptoms

• Instruct patient to report any changes in breathing or coughing even several months after treatment; to avoid crowds and persons with respiratory tract or other infections; neurotoxicity

• Caution patient not to have any vaccinations without the advice of the prescriber; serious reactions can occur

• Advise patient to take fluids 3 L/day to prevent renal damage

Evaluation
Positive therapeutic outcome

• Prevention of rapid division of malignant cells

❗ HIGH ALERT

dacarbazine (Rx)
(da-kar′ba-zeen)
dacarbazine, DTIC ✤, DTIC-Dome
Func. class.: Antineoplastic—misc agent
Chem. class.: Imidazole

Pregnancy category C

Action: Alkylates DNA, RNA; inhibits enzymes that allow synthesis of amino acids in proteins; also responsible for cross-linking DNA strands; activity is not cell cycle phase specific

➡ **Therapeutic Outcome:** Prevention of rapidly growing malignant cells

Uses: Hodgkin's disease, sarcomas, neuroblastoma, malignant melanoma

Investigational uses: Metastatic sarcoma

Dosage and routes
Malignant melanoma
Adult: IV 2-4.5 mg/kg or 250 mg/m² qd × 5 days; repeat q3 wk depending on response

Hodgkin's disease
Adult: IV 150 mg/m² qd × 5 days with other agents, repeat q4 wk or 375 mg/m² on day 1 when given in combination, repeat q15 days

Available forms: Inj 100, 200 mg

Adverse effects
(*italic* = common; **bold** = life-threatening)
CNS: Facial paresthesia, flushing, fever, malaise
GI: *Nausea, anorexia, vomiting,* **hepatotoxicity** (rare)
HEMA: **Thrombocytopenia, leukopenia,** anemia
INTEG: *Alopecia,* dermatitis, pain at inj site
SYST: **Anaphylaxis**

Contraindications: Lactation

Precautions: Radiation therapy, pregnancy (1st trimester) **C**

Pharmacokinetics

Absorption	Complete bioavailability (**IV**)
Distribution	Widely distributed; concentrates in liver
Metabolism	Liver (50%, 5% protein bound)
Excretion	Kidneys, unchanged (50%)
Half-life	Initial 35 min, terminal 5 hr

Pharmacodynamics
Unknown

Interactions
Individual drugs
Phenobarbital, radiation: ↑ toxicity
Phenytoin: ↑ metabolism, ↓ effect
Radiation: Bone marrow suppression
Drug classifications
Aminoglycosides: ↑ nephrotoxicity
Anticoagulants, salicylates: ↑ risk of bleeding
Antineoplastics, bone marrow–suppressing drugs: ↑ toxicity, bone marrow suppression
Diuretics, loop: ↑ ototoxicity
Live virus vaccines: ↑ adverse reactions, ↓ antibody reaction

NURSING CONSIDERATIONS
Assessment

• Assess symptoms indicating severe allergic reaction: rash, pruritus, urticaria, purpuric skin lesions, itching, flushing; drug should be discontinued

• Monitor CBC, differential, platelet count weekly; withhold drug if WBC is <4000/mm³ or platelet count is <100,000/mm³

• Monitor renal function studies: BUN, creatinine, urine CCr before and during therapy; I&O ratio; report fall in urine output to <30 ml/hr

• Monitor temp q4h (may indicate beginning of infection)

• Monitor liver function tests before and during therapy (bilirubin, AST, ALT, LDH) as needed or monthly; note jaundice of skin or

---

sclera, dark urine, clay-colored stools, itchy skin, abdominal pain, fever, diarrhea; hepatotoxicity can be serious and fatal
• Assess for bleeding: hematuria, stool guaiac, bruising or petechiae, mucosa or orifices q8h; check for inflammation of mucosa, breaks in skin
• Identify effects of alopecia on body image; discuss feelings about body changes

Nursing diagnoses
☑ Injury, risk for (adverse reactions)
☑ Body image, disturbed (adverse reactions)
☑ Infection, risk for (adverse reactions)
☑ Knowledge, deficient (teaching)

Implementation
• Give fluids **IV** or PO before chemotherapy to hydrate patient
• Give antiemetic 30-60 min before giving drug to prevent vomiting, and prn; antibiotics for prophylaxis of infection
• Provide liquid diet: carbonated beverages; gelatin may be added if patient is not nauseated or vomiting
• After diluting 100 mg/9.9 ml of sterile water for inj (10 mg/ml), give by direct **IV** over 1 min through Y-tube or 3-way stopcock
• May be further diluted in 50-250 ml of D_5W or normal saline for inj and given over 30 min
• Watch for extravasation; give 3-5 ml of mixture of 4 ml sodium thiosulfate 10% plus 5 ml of sterile water SC as prescribed

Y-site compatibilities:
Amifostine, aztreonam, filgrastim, fludarabine, granisetron, melphalan, ondansetron, paclitaxel, sargramostim, teniposide, thiotepa, vinorelbine

Additive compatibilities:
Bleomycin, carmustine, cyclophosphamide, cytarabine, dactinomycin, DOXOrubicin, fluorouracil, mercaptopurine, methotrexate, ondansetron, vinBLAStine

Additive incompatibilities:
Hydrocortisone sodium succinate, cysteine

Patient/family education
• Teach patient to avoid use of products containing aspirin or ibuprofen, razors, commercial mouthwash, since bleeding may occur; to report symptoms of bleeding (hematuria, tarry stools)
• Instruct patient to report signs of anemia (fatigue, headache, irritability, faintness, shortness of breath)
• Advise patient that hair may be lost during treatment; a wig or hairpiece may make patient feel better; new hair may be different in color, texture

• Caution patient not to have any vaccinations without the advice of prescriber; serious reactions can occur
• Advise patient contraception is needed during treatment and for several months after the completion of therapy; drug has teratogenic properties

Evaluation
Positive therapeutic outcome
• Prevention of rapid division of malignant cells

！HIGH ALERT

daclizumab (Rx)
(dah-kliz′uh-mab)
Zenapax
Func. class.: Immunosuppressant
Chem class.: Humanized IgGl monoclonal antibody

Pregnancy category C

Action: Binds to the IL-2 receptor antagonist

Therapeutic Outcome: Prevention of graft rejection

Uses: Acute allograft rejection in renal transplant patients

Dosage and routes
Adult: **IV** 1 mg/kg as part of a regimen that includes cycloSPORINE and corticosteroids, mix calculated vol with 50 ml of 0.9% NaCl and give via peripheral/central vein over 15 min

Available forms: Inj 25 mg/ml

Adverse effects
(*italic* = common; **bold** = life-threatening)
CNS: Chills, tremors, headache, prickly sensation
CV: Hypertension, **tachycardia, thrombosis, bleeding**
GI: Vomiting, nausea, diarrhea, constipation, abdominal pain, pyrosis
GU: Oliguria, dysuria, **renal tubular necrosis, renal damage, hydronephrosis**
INTEG: Impaired wound healing
RESP: *Dyspnea, wheezing,* **pulmonary edema,** coughing, atelectasis, congestion, hypoxia

Contraindications: Hypersensitivity

Precautions: Pregnancy C, child <2 yr, lactation, elderly

Pharmacokinetics

Unknown

Pharmacodynamics

Unknown

Interactions
Herb/drug
Ginseng, maitake, mistletoe, schisandra, St. John's wort, turmeric: ↓ effect
Safflower: ↑ effect

NURSING CONSIDERATIONS
Assessment
- Monitor blood studies: Hgb, WBC, platelets during treatment qmo; if leukocytes are <3000/mm³, drug should be discontinued
- Monitor liver function studies: alkaline phosphatase, AST, ALT, bilirubin
- Assess for hepatotoxicity: dark urine, jaundice, itching, light-colored stools; drug should be discontinued
- Assess for anaphylaxis: have corticosteroids, epINEPHrine available

Nursing diagnoses
☑ Injury, risk for (uses)
☑ Knowledge, deficient (teaching)

Implementation
- Give all other medications PO if possible; avoid IM inj, since infection may occur

IV IV route
- Solution compatibilities 0.9% NaCl
- Protect undiluted sol from direct light; should be used with drugs for immunosuppression

Patient/family education
- Teach patient to report fever, chills, sore throat, fatigue, since serious infection may occur
- Instruct patient to use contraception (women), before, during, and for 4 mo after treatment
- Advise patient to avoid vaccinations during treatment
- Advise patient to drink fluids during treatment

Evaluation
Positive therapeutic outcome
- Absence of graft rejection

! HIGH ALERT

dactinomycin (Rx)
(dak-ti-noe-mye′sin)
Cosmegen
Func. class.: Antineoplastic, antibiotic
Pregnancy category C

Action: Inhibits DNA, RNA, protein synthesis; derived from *Streptomyces parvulus;* replication is decreased by binding to DNA, which causes strand splitting; cell cycle nonspecific; a vesicant

➡ Therapeutic Outcome: Prevention of rapidly growing malignant cells, immunosuppression

Uses: Sarcomas, melanomas, trophoblastic tumors in women, testicular cancer, Wilms' tumor, rhabdomyosarcoma

Dosage and routes
Adult: **IV** 500 mcg/m²/day × 5 days; stop drug for 2-4 wk; then repeat cycle

P *Child:* **IV** 15 mcg/kg/day × 5 days, not to exceed 500 mcg/day; stop drug until bone marrow recovery, then repeat cycle

Available forms: Inj 0.5 mg/vial

Adverse effects
(*italic* = common; **bold** = life-threatening)
CNS: Malaise, fatigue, lethargy, fever
EENT: Cheilitis, dysphagia, esophagitis
GI: Nausea, vomiting, anorexia, stomatitis, **hepatotoxicity,** abdominal pain, diarrhea
HEMA: **Thrombocytopenia, leukopenia, aplastic anemia**
INTEG: Rash, alopecia, pain at inj site, folliculitis, acne, desquamation, *extravasation*
MS: Myalgia

Contraindications: Hypersensitivity,
P herpes infections, child <6 mo

Precautions: Renal, hepatic disease, pregnancy **C**, lactation, bone marrow suppression

Pharmacokinetics

Absorption	Complete bioavailability
Distribution	Widely distributed; crosses placenta
Metabolism	Unknown
Excretion	Bile; feces, unchanged (50%); kidneys (10%)
Half-life	36 hr

Pharmacodynamics

Unknown

 Herb/drug   Do Not Crush   Alert   Key Drug   **G** Geriatric   **P** Pediatric

Interactions

Individual drugs
Radiation: ↑ toxicity, bone marrow suppression

Drug classifications
Antineoplastics: ↑ toxicity
Antineoplastics, bone marrow–suppressing drugs: ↑ bone marrow suppression
Live virus vaccines: ↓ antibody reaction

Lab test interferences
↑ Uric acid

NURSING CONSIDERATIONS
Assessment
• Assess buccal cavity q8h for dryness, sores or ulceration, white patches, pain, bleeding, dysphagia; obtain prescription for viscous lidocaine (Xylocaine)

• Assess symptoms indicating severe allergic reaction: rash, pruritus, urticaria, purpuric skin lesions, itching, flushing; drug should be discontinued

• Monitor CBC, differential, platelet count weekly; withhold drug if WBC is <4000/mm^3 or platelet count is <100,000/mm^3; notify prescriber of results if WBC <20,000/mm^3, platelets <150,000/mm^3

• Monitor renal function studies: BUN, creatinine, serum uric acid, urine CCr before and during therapy; I&O ratio; report fall in urine output to <30 ml/hr

• Monitor temp q4h (may indicate beginning of infection)

• Monitor liver function tests before and during therapy (bilirubin, AST, ALT, LDH) as needed or monthly; note jaundice of skin or sclera, dark urine, clay-colored stools, itchy skin, abdominal pain, fever, diarrhea

• Assess for bleeding: hematuria, stool guaiac, bruising or petechiae, mucosa or orifices q8h; check for inflammation of mucosa, breaks in skin

• Identify effects of alopecia on body image; discuss feelings about body changes

Nursing diagnoses
✓ Injury, risk for (adverse reactions)
✓ Body image, disturbed (adverse reactions)
✓ Oral mucous membranes, impaired (adverse reactions)
✓ Infection, risk for (adverse reactions)
✓ Knowledge, deficient (teaching)

Implementation
• Provide antacid before oral agent; give drug pc PM, before hs; antiemetic 30-60 min before giving drug to prevent vomiting, and prn; antibiotics for prophylaxis of infection

• Provide liquid diet: carbonated beverages; gelatin may be added if patient is not nauseated or vomiting

• Help patient rinse mouth tid-qid with water, club soda, brush teeth bid-qid with soft brush or cotton-tipped applicators for stomatitis, use unwaxed dental floss

• Drug should be prepared by experienced personnel using proper precautions

• Give after diluting 0.5 mg/1.1 ml of sterile water for inj without preservative; use 2.2 ml (0.25 mg/ml), give by direct **IV** at 0.5 mg or less/min through Y-tube or 3-way stopcock of inf in progress

Intermittent infusion
• May be further diluted in 50 ml of D$_5$W or 0.9% NaCl for inf; run over 10-15 min

• Give hydrocortisone, sodium thiosulfate to infiltration area, and ice compress after stopping inf

• Store in darkness in cool environment

Y-site compatibilities: Allopurinol, amifostine, aztreonam, cefepime, fludarabine, granisetron, melphalan, ondansetron, sargramostim, teniposide, thiotepa, vinorelbine

Patient/family education
• Teach patient to avoid use of products containing aspirin or ibuprofen, razors, commercial mouthwash, since bleeding may occur; to report symptoms of bleeding (hematuria, tarry stools)

• Instruct patient to report signs of anemia (fatigue, headache, irritability, faintness, shortness of breath)

• Advise patient that hair may be lost during treatment; a wig or hairpiece may make patient feel better; new hair may be different in color, texture

• Caution patient not to have any vaccinations without the advice of the prescriber, serious reactions can occur

• Advise patient that contraception is needed during treatment and for several months after the completion of therapy

• Advise patient to increase fluids to 3 L/day

Evaluation
Positive therapeutic outcome
• Prevention of rapid division of malignant cells

⚠ HIGH ALERT

dalteparin (Rx)
(dahl'ta-pear-in)
Fragmin
Func. class.: Anticoagulant
Chem. class.: Low molecular weight heparin

Pregnancy category B

Action: Prevents conversion of fibrinogen to fibrin and prothrombin to thrombin by enhancing inhibitory effects of antithrombin III

➔ **Therapeutic Outcome:** Absence of deep vein thrombosis

Uses: Unstable angina/non-Q-wave MI; prevention of deep vein thrombosis in abdominal surgery, hip replacement patients

Investigational uses: Systemic anticoagulation in venous/arterial thromboembolic complications

Dosage and routes
*Hip replacement surgery/
DVT prophylaxis*
Adult: SC 2500 international units 2 hr before surgery and 2nd dose in the evening the day of surgery, then 5000 international units SC 1st postop day and qd 5-10 days

*Unstable angina/
non-Q-wave MI*
Adult: SC 120 international units/kg, do not exceed 10,000 international units q12h with concurrent aspirin, continue until stable

Systemic anticoagulation
Adult: SC 200 international units/kg qd or 100 international units/kg bid

Deep vein thrombosis, prophylaxis for abdominal surgery
Adult: SC 2500 international units qd, 1-2 hr before abdominal surgery and repeat qd × 5-10 days; in high-risk patients 5000 international units may be used

Available forms: Prefilled syringes, 2500, 5000 international units/0.2 ml; 10,000 international units multidose vials; 7500 international units/0.3 ml, 10,000 international units/ml

Adverse effects
(*italic* = common; **bold** = life-threatening)
CNS: **Intracranial bleeding**
HEMA: **Thrombocytopenia**
INTEG: Pruritus, superficial wound infection
SYST: Hypersensitivity, **hemorrhage, anaphylaxis** possible

Contraindications: Hypersensitivity to this drug, heparin, pork products, benzyl alcohol; hemophilia, leukemia with bleeding, thrombocytopenic purpura, cerebrovascular hemorrhage, cerebral aneurysm, severe hypertension, other severe cardiac disease, those undergoing regional anesthesia for unstable angina, non-Q-wave MI

G Precautions: Elderly, pregnancy **B**, hepatic disease, severe renal disease, blood dyscrasias, subacute bacterial endocarditis, acute nephri-**P** tis, lactation, child, recent childbirth, peptic ulcer disease, pericarditis, pericardial effusion, recent lumbar puncture, vasculitis, other diseases where bleeding is possible

Pharmacokinetics
Absorption	87%
Distribution	Unknown
Metabolism	Liver
Excretion	Kidney
Half-life	3-5 hr elimination

Pharmacodynamics
Onset	Unknown
Peak	4 hr
Duration	Unknown

Interactions
Drug classifications
Anticoagulants, NSAIDs, platelet inhibitors, salicylates, thrombolytics: ↑ risk of bleeding
Herb/drug
Agrimony, alfalfa, angelica, anise, basil, bay, bilberry, black haw, bogbean, bromelain, buchu, chondroitin, cinchona bark, dong quai, fenugreek, feverfew, garlic, ginger, ginkgo, ginseng, horse chestnut, Irish moss, kelp, kelpware, khella, lovage, lungwort, meadowsweet, motherwort, mugwort, nettle, papaya, parsley (large amounts), pau d'arco, pineapple, poplar, prickly ash, safflower, saw palmetto, tonka bean, turmeric, wintergreen, yarrow: ↑ risk of bleeding
Chamomile, coenzyme Q10, flax, glucomannan, goldenseal, guar gum: ↓ anticoagulant effect

NURSING CONSIDERATIONS
Assessment
• Assess for bleeding (Hct, occult blood in stools) during treatment since bleeding can occur
• Assess for bleeding gums, petechiae, ecchymosis, black tarry stools, hematuria, epistaxis, decrease in Hct, B/P; may indicate bleeding,

possible hemorrhage; notify prescriber immediately, drug should be discontinued
• Assess for hypersensitivity: fever, skin rash, urticaria; notify prescriber immediately
• Assess for needed dosage change q1-2 wk; dose may need to be decreased if bleeding occurs

Nursing diagnoses
✓ Injury, risk for (uses, adverse reactions)
✓ Tissue perfusion, ineffective (uses) altered
✓ Knowledge, deficient (teaching)

Implementation
SC route
• Cannot be used interchangeably (unit for unit with unfractionated heparin or LMWHs)
• Do not give IM or **IV** drug route; approved in SC only; do not mix with other inj or sol
• Give by SC only; have patient sit or lie down; SC inj may be 2 in from umbilicus in a U-shape, upper outer side of thigh, around navel, or upper outer quadrangle of the buttocks; rotate inj sites
• Changing needles is not recommended; change inj site qd, use at same time of day

Patient/family education
• Advise patient to avoid OTC preparations that contain aspirin, other anticoagulants; serious drug interaction may occur
• Advise patient to use soft-bristle toothbrush to avoid bleeding gums, avoid contact sports, use electric razor, avoid IM inj
• Instruct patient to report any signs of bleeding: gums, under skin, urine, stools; unusual bruising

Evaluation
Positive therapeutic outcome
• Absence of deep vein thrombosis

Treatment of overdose: Protamine sulfate 1% given **IV**; 1 mg protamine/100 anti-Xa international units of dalteparin given

---

⚠ HIGH ALERT

danaparoid (Rx)
(dan-a-pair′oid)
orgaran
Func. class.: Anticoagulant, antithrombotic
Chem. class.: Glycosaminoglycan

Pregnancy category B

Action: Prevents conversion of fibrinogen to fibrin and prothrombin to thrombin by enhancing inhibitory effects of antithrombin III

⤏ Therapeutic Outcome: Absence of deep vein thrombosis

Uses: Prevention of vein thrombosis in hemodialysis, stroke, elective surgery for malignancy or total hip replacement, hip fracture surgery

Dosage and routes
Prevention of venous thrombosis
Adult: SC 750 anti-Xa units bid × 7-10 days, begin 1-4 hr presurgery and restart 2 hr after surgery; use lower dose in renal failure

Hemodialysis
Adult: IV 2400-4800 anti-Xa units given predialysis

Available forms: Inj 750 anti-Xa units in 0.6 ml H$_2$O

Adverse effects
(*italic* = common; **bold** = life-threatening)
CNS: Insomnia, headache
GI: Nausea, vomiting, constipation
HEMA: **Thrombocytopenia**
INTEG: Rash, pruritis, inj site pain
MS: Asthenia
SYST: Hypersensitivity, **hemorrhage**

Contraindications: Hypersensitivity to this drug, sulfites, pork; hemophilia, leukemia with bleeding; thrombocytopenia purpura; cerebrovascular hemorrhage, cerebral aneurysm, other severe cardiac disease

Precautions: Hypersensitivity to heparin, severe hypertension, elderly, pregnancy **B,** severe renal disease, blood dyscrasias, subacute bacterial endocarditis, acute nephritis, lactation, child, recent childbirth, peptic ulcer disease, pericarditis, pericardial effusion, recent lumbar puncture, vasculitis, other diseases where bleeding is possible

Pharmacokinetics	
Absorption	100%
Distribution	Unknown
Metabolism	Unknown
Excretion	Kidneys
Half-life	24 hr

Pharmacodynamics	
Onset	Unknown
Peak	4 hr
Duration	Unknown

Interactions
Individual drugs
Aspirin, dextran, penicillin: ↑ risk of bleeding

Drug classifications
Anticoagulants (oral), NSAIDs, platelet inhibitors, salicylates: ↑ risk of bleeding

 Herb/drug
Agrimony, alfalfa, angelica, anise, basil, bay, bilberry, black haw, bogbean, bromelain, buchu, chondroitin, cinchona bark, dong quai, fenugreek, feverfew, garlic, ginger, ginkgo, ginseng, horse chestnut, Irish moss, kelp, kelpware, khella, lovage, lungwort, meadowsweet, motherwort, mugwort, nettle, papaya, parsley (large amounts), pau d'arco, pineapple, poplar, prickly ash, safflower, saw palmetto, tonka bean, turmeric, wintergreen, yarrow: ↑ risk of bleeding
Chamomile, coenzyme Q10, flax, glucomannan, goldenseal, guar gum: ↓ anticoagulant effect

NURSING CONSIDERATIONS
Assessment
• Monitor blood studies (Hct, CBC, occult blood in stools) during treatment since bleeding can occur; APTT, ACT, antifactor Xa test, platelets
• Assess for bleeding gums, petechiae, ecchymosis, black tarry stools, hematuria, epistaxis, decrease in Hct, B/P; may indicate bleeding, possible hemorrhage; notify prescriber immediately, drug should be discontinued
• Assess for hypersensitivity: fever, skin rash, urticaria; notify prescriber immediately
• Assess for needed dosage change q1-2 wk; dose may need to be decreased if bleeding occurs

Nursing diagnoses
☑ Tissue perfusion, ineffective (uses)
☑ Injury, risk for (adverse reactions)
☑ Knowledge, deficient (teaching)

Implementation
• Cannot be used interchangeably (unit for unit) with heparin, LMWHs or heparinoids
SC route
• Use SC only
• Have patient sit or lie down; SC inj may be around the navel in a U shape, upper outer side of thigh or upper outer quadrangle of the buttocks; rotate inj sites
• Changing needles is not recommended

Patient/family education
• Advise patient to avoid OTC preparations that may cause serious drug interactions unless directed by prescriber; may contain aspirin, other anticoagulants
• Advise patient to use soft-bristle toothbrush to avoid bleeding gums, avoid contact sports, use electric razor, avoid IM inj

• Advise patient to report any signs of bleeding: gums, under skin, urine, stools; unusual bruising

Evaluation
Positive therapeutic outcome
• Absence of deep vein thrombosis

Treatment of overdose: Discontinue drug; protamine sulfate 1% given **IV**; 1 mg protamine/100 anti-Xa international units of dalteparin sodium given

---

danazol (Rx)
(da'na-zole)
Cyclomen ✤, danazol, Danocrine
Func. class.: Androgen, anabolic steroid
Chem. class.: α-Ethinyl testosterone derivative

Pregnancy category X

Action: Atrophy of endometrial tissue; decreases FSH, LH, which are controlled by pituitary; this leads to amenorrhea/anovulation; has weak androgen, anabolic activity

➡ **Therapeutic Outcome:** Decreased pain and nodules/fibrocystic breast disease; correction in hereditary angioedema; atrophy of endometrial tissue (ectopic)

Uses: Endometriosis, prevention of hereditary angioedema, fibrocystic breast disease

Dosage and routes
Endometriosis
Adult: PO 100-500 mg bid, uninterrupted for 3-9 mo

Fibrocystic breast disease
Adult: PO 100-400 mg qd in 2 divided doses × 2-6 mo

Hereditary angioedema prevention
Adult: PO 200 mg bid-tid until desired response, then decrease dose to 100 mg at 1-3 mo intervals

Available forms: Caps 50, 100, 200 mg

Adverse effects
(*italic* = common; **bold** = life-threatening)
CNS: Dizziness, headache, fatigue, tremors, paresthesias, flushing, sweating, anxiety, *lability,* insomnia
CV: Increased B/P
EENT: Conjunctival edema, nasal congestion, voice weakness
ENDO: Abnormal GTT
GI: Nausea, vomiting, constipation, *weight gain,* **cholestatic jaundice**

GU: Hematuria, *amenorrhea,* atrophic vaginitis, decreased libido, *decreased breast size,* clitoral hypertrophy, testicular atrophy
INTEG: Rash, *acneiform lesions,* oily hair and skin, flushing, sweating, acne vulgaris, alopecia, *hirsutism,* pruritus
MS: Cramps, spasms, joint swelling

Contraindications: Severe renal disease, severe cardiac disease, severe hepatic disease, hypersensitivity, genital bleeding (abnormal), P pregnancy **X**, children

Precautions: Migraine headaches, seizure disorders

N **Do Not Confuse:**
danazol/Dantrium

Pharmacokinetics	
Absorption	GI absorption
Distribution	Unknown
Metabolism	Liver
Excretion	Kidneys
Half-life	4½ hr

Pharmacodynamics
Unknown

Interactions
Individual drugs
Cyclosporine: ↑ risk of nephrotoxicity
Insulin: ↑ action
Drug classifications
Anticoagulants: ↑ anticoagulant action
Antidiabetics, corticosteroids: ↑ action
Lab test interferences
↑ Cholesterol, ↓ cholesterol, ↓ T$_4$, ↓ T$_3$, ↓ thyroid ^{131}I uptake test, ↓ 17-KS, ↓ PBI
Interferences: GTT

NURSING CONSIDERATIONS
Assessment
• Assess for pain before and after treatment in endometriosis, fibrocystic breast disease; tenderness, nodules in fibrocystic breast disease
• Monitor potassium, blood, urine glucose while patient is on long-term therapy; liver function tests, periodically; semen volume, sperm count, motility in hereditary angioedema
• Assess breast for fibrocystic nodules; check for pain, tenderness before therapy and throughout to identify if treatment is effective
• Monitor weight daily; notify prescriber if weekly weight gain is >5 lb; I&O ratio; be alert for decreasing urinary output, increasing

edema, hypertension, cardiac symptoms, jaundice
• Assess for mental status: affect, mood, behavioral changes, aggression, sleep disorders, depression; change may be extreme
• Assess for signs of virilization: deepening of voice, decreased libido, facial hair (may not be reversible)

Nursing diagnoses
✓ Infection, risk for (adverse reactions)
✓ Injury, risk for (adverse reactions)
✓ Knowledge, deficient (teaching)

Implementation
• Start treatment during menstruation in endometriosis, fibrocystic breast disease
• Store in airtight container at room temp
• Provide ROM exercise for patients who are immobile
• Give with food or milk to decrease GI symptoms
⊘ • Do not crush, chew caps

Patient/family education
• Teach patient to notify prescriber if therapeutic response decreases; advise that endometriosis tends to recur after drug is discontinued; not to discontinue medication abruptly but to taper over several weeks
• Advise patient that nonhormonal contraceptive measures are needed during treatment; amenorrhea may occur with higher dosages
• Teach patient to report menstrual irregularities; that amenorrhea usually occurs but menstruation resumes 2-3 mo after termination of therapy; that drug should induce anovulation; reversible within 60-90 days after drug is discontinued
• Teach patient about routine breast self-exam technique, to report any increase in nodule size
• Instruct patient to report masculinization: deepening voice, facial hair growth, body hair growth
• Advise patient to use sunscreen or stay out of the sun to prevent burns

Evaluation
Positive therapeutic outcome
• Decreased pain in endometriosis
• Decreased size, pain in fibrocystic breast disease
• Decreased signs of angioedema (hereditary)

dantrolene (Rx)
(dan'troe-leen)
Dantrium
Func. class.: Skeletal muscle relaxant, direct acting
Chem. class.: Hydantoin

Pregnancy category C

Action: Interferes with intracellular release from the sarcoplasmic reticulum of calcium necessary to initiate contraction; slows catabolism in malignant hyperthermia

➡ **Therapeutic Outcome:** Decreased muscle spasticity; absence of malignant hyperthermia

Uses: Spasticity in multiple sclerosis, stroke, spinal cord injury, cerebral palsy, prevention and treatment of malignant hyperthermia

Dosage and routes
Spasticity
Adult: PO 25 mg/day; may increase by 25-100 mg bid-qid, not to exceed 400 mg/day × 1 wk

🅿 *Child:* PO 1 mg/kg/day given in divided doses bid-tid; may increase gradually, not to exceed 100 mg qid

Malignant hyperthermia
🅿 *Adult and child:* **IV** 1 mg/kg; may repeat to total dose of 10 mg/kg; PO 4-8 mg/kg/day in 4 divided doses × 3 days to prevent further hyperthermia; postcrisis follow-up 4-8 mg/kg/day for 1-3 days

Prevention of malignant hyperthermia
🅿 *Adult and child:* PO 4-8 mg/kg/day in 3-4 divided doses × 1-2 days before procedures; give last dose 4 hr preoperatively; **IV** 2.5 mg/kg prior to anesthesia

Available forms: Caps 25, 50, 100 mg; powder for inj 20 mg/vial

Adverse effects
(*italic* = common; **bold** = life-threatening)
CNS: Dizziness, weakness, fatigue, drowsiness, headache, disorientation, insomnia, paresthesias, tremors, **seizures**
CV: Hypotension, chest pain, palpitations
EENT: Nasal congestion, blurred vision, mydriasis
GI: **Hepatic injury,** *nausea,* constipation, vomiting, increased AST and alkaline phosphatase, abdominal pain, dry mouth, anorexia, hepatitis, dyspepsia
GU: Urinary frequency, nocturia, impotence, crystalluria

HEMA: Eosinophilia
INTEG: Rash, pruritus, photosensitivity

Contraindications: Hypersensitivity, compromised pulmonary function, active hepatic disease, impaired myocardial function

Precautions: Peptic ulcer disease, renal disease, hepatic disease, stroke, seizure disorder, diabetes mellitus, pregnancy **C,**
🅖 elderly

🔲 **Do Not Confuse:**
Dantrium/danazol

Pharmacokinetics	
Absorption	PO (30%-35%)
Distribution	Unknown
Metabolism	Liver, extensively
Excretion	Kidney
Half-life	9 hr

Pharmacodynamics		
	PO	IV
Onset	Unknown	Immediate
Peak	5 hr	5 hr
Duration	Dose related	Dose related

Interactions
Individual drugs
Alcohol: ↑ CNS depression
Verapamil: ↑ dysrhythmias
Drug classifications
Antidepressants (tricyclic), antihistamines, barbiturates, opiates, sedative/hypnotics: ↑ CNS depression
Estrogens, hepatotoxic agents: ↑ hepatotoxicity

NURSING CONSIDERATIONS
Assessment
• Monitor I&O ratio; check for urinary retention, frequency, hesitancy, especially
🅖 elderly
• Monitor ECG in epileptic patients; poor seizure control has occurred with patients taking this drug; assess for increased seizure activity in epilepsy patient
• Monitor hepatic function by frequent determination of AST, ALT, bilirubin, alkaline phosphatase, GGTP, renal function studies, CBC
• Assess for allergic reactions: rash, fever, respiratory distress
• Monitor for severe weakness, numbness in extremities
• Assess for CNS depression: dizziness, drowsiness, psychiatric symptoms
🔶• Assess for signs of hepatotoxicity: jaundice, yellow sclera, pain in abdomen, nausea, fever;

drug should be discontinued if these signs and symptoms occur

Nursing diagnoses
✓ Pain, chronic (uses)
✓ Mobility, impaired physical (uses)
✓ Injury, risk for (adverse reactions)
✓ Knowledge, deficient (teaching)

Implementation
PO route
• Give with meals for GI symptoms; capsules may be opened and mixed with liquid; patient should drink after mixing
• Store in airtight container at room temp
ⅣIV route
• Administer **IV** after reconstituting 20 mg/60 ml sterile water for inj without bacteriostatic agent (333 mcg/ml); shake until clear; give by rapid **IV** push through Y-tube or 3-way stopcock; follow by prescribed doses immediately; may also give by intermittent inf over 1 hr before anesthesia; assess site for extravasation, phlebitis
• Protect diluted sol from light; use reconstituted sol within 6 hr
• Considered incompatible in sol or syringe, compatibility unknown

Patient/family education
• Notify prescriber of abdominal pain, jaundiced sclera, clay-colored stools, change in color of urine, rash, itching
• Caution patient not to take with alcohol, other CNS depressants; severe CNS depression can occur; avoid using OTC medication: cough preparations, antihistamines, unless directed by prescriber
• Tell patient that if improvement does not occur within 6 wk, prescriber may discontinue
• Caution patient to avoid hazardous activities if drowsiness, dizziness, blurred vision occurs; wait several days to identify patient response to medication
• Teach patient to use sunscreen, protective clothing for photosensitivity
• Instruct patient to take medication as prescribed; do not double doses; take missed dose within 1 hr of scheduled time

Evaluation
Positive therapeutic outcome
• Decreased pain, spasticity
• Absence or decreased symptoms of malignant hyperthermia

Treatment of overdose: Induce emesis of conscious patient; lavage, dialysis

---

darbepoetin alfa (Rx)
(dar'bee-poh'-eh-tin al'fah)
Aranesp
Func. class.: Hematopoietic agent
Chem. class.: Recombinant human erythropoietin

Pregnancy category C   **D**

Action: Stimulates erythropoiesis by the same mechanism as endogenous erythropoietin; in response to hypoxia, erythropoietin is produced in the kidney and released into the bloodstream, where it interacts with progenitor stem cells to increase red cell production

⇥**Therapeutic Outcome:** Decreased anemia with increased RBCs

Uses: Anemia associated with chronic renal failure in patients on and not on dialysis and anemic in nonmyeloid malignancies receiving coadministered chemotherapy

Dosage and routes
Correction of anemia
Adult: SC/**IV** 0.45 mcg/kg as a single inj, titrate not to exceed a target Hgb of 12 g/dl

Conversion from epoetin alfa to darbepoetin
Adult: SC/**IV** estimate starting dose based on weekly epoetin alfa dose; because of longer serum half-life, darbepoetin must be administered less frequently than epoetin alfa; if epoetin was given 2-3×/wk, give darbepoetin 1×/wk; if epoetin was given 1×/wk, give darbepoetin 1× q2 wk; do not increase doses more often than 1×/mo

Available forms: Sol for inj 25, 40, 60, 100, 150, 200, 300, 500 mcg/ml

Adverse effects
(*italic* = common; **bold** = life-threatening)
CNS: **Seizures**, sweating, headache, dizziness
CV: Hypertension, hypotension, **cardiac arrest,** *angina pectoris,* **thrombosis, CHF, stroke, acute MI, dysrhythmias,** chest pain, transient ischemic attacks
GI: Diarrhea, vomiting, nausea, abdominal pain, constipation
MISC: Infection, fatigue, fever, **death,** *fluid overload,* **vascular access hemorrhage**
MS: Bone pain, myalgia, limb pain, back pain
RESP: Upper respiratory infection, dyspnea, cough, bronchitis
SYST: Allergic reactions, **anaphylaxis**

Contraindications: Hypersensitivity to mammalian cell–derived products or human albumin, uncontrolled hypertension

---

Precautions: Seizuredisorder, porphyria, **P** pregnancy **C,** hypertension, lactation, children

Pharmacokinetics

Absorption	Slow, rate-limiting (SC)
Distribution	Vascular space
Metabolism	Metabolized in body (**IV**), extent unknown
Excretion	Unknown
Half-life	49 hr

Pharmacodynamics

Onset	Onset of increased reticulocyte count 1-6 wk
Peak	34 hr
Duration	Unknown

Interactions
Drug classifications
Anticoagulants: ↑ anticoagulants needed during hemodialysis

NURSING CONSIDERATIONS
Assessment
• Assess for serious allergic reactions: rash, urticaria; if anaphylaxis occurs, stop drug, administer emergency treatment (rare)
• Assess blood studies: ferritin, transferrin monthly; transferrin sat ≥20%, ferritin ≥100 ng/ml; Hgb 2×/wk until stabilized in target range (30%-33%) then at regular intervals; those with endogenous erythropoietin levels of <500 units/L respond to this agent
• Assess renal studies: urinalysis, protein, blood, BUN, creatinine
• Assess B/P, Hct; check for rising B/P as Hct rises, antihypertensives may be needed
• Assess CV status: hypertension may occur rapidly leading to hypertensive encephalopathy
• Assess I&O ratio; report drop in output to <50 ml/hr
• Assess for seizures if Hgb is increased within 2 wk by 4 pts
• Assess CNS symptoms: cold sensation, sweating, pain in long bones
• Assess dialysis patients for thrill, bruit of shunts; monitor for circulation impairment

Nursing diagnoses
✓ Fatigue (uses)
✓ Activity intolerance (uses)
✓ Knowledge, deficient (teaching)

Implementation
IV **IV/SC**
• Do not shake, do not dilute, do not mix with other drugs or solutions
• Check for discoloration, particulate matter; do not use if present, discard unused portion, do not pool unused portion

Patient/family education
• Caution patient to avoid driving or hazardous activity during beginning of treatment
• Advise patient to monitor B/P
• Advise patient to take iron supplements, vit B₁₂, folic acid as directed
• Advise patient to report side effects to prescriber, to comply with treatment regimen
• Teach home administration and review information for patients and caregivers if home administration is deemed appropriate

Evaluation
Positive therapeutic outcome
• Increased reticulocyte count, Hgb/Hct
• Increased appetite
• Enhanced sense of well-being

Treatment of overdose: If polycythemia occurs, discontinue drug temporarily; perform phlebotomy if clinically indicated

---

❗HIGH ALERT

*DAUNOrubicin (Rx)
(daw-noe-roo'bi-sin)
Cerubidine
*DAUNOrubicin citrate liposome (Rx)
DaunoXome
Func. class.: Antineoplastic, antibiotic
Chem. class.: Anthracycline glycoside

Pregnancy category D

Action: Inhibits DNA synthesis, primarily; derived from *Streptomyces coeruleorubidus;* replication is decreased by binding to DNA, which causes strand splitting; cell cycle specific (S phase); a vesicant

Therapeutic Outcome: Prevention of rapidly growing malignant cells; immunosuppression

Uses: Myelogenous, monocytic leukemia, acute nonlymphocytic leukemia, Ewing's sarcoma, Wilms' tumor, neuroblastoma, rhabdomyosarcoma; DAUNOrubicin citrate liposome: advanced Kaposi's sarcoma in HIV

Dosage and routes
G Use decreased dose for those >60 yr

Single agent
Adult: **IV** 60 mg/m²/day × 3-5 day q4 wk

In combination
Adult: **IV** 45 mg/m²/day × 3 days, then 2 days of subsequent courses in combination

---

P *Child:* **IV** 25-60 mg/m² depending on cycle

DAUNOrubicin citrate liposome
Adult: **IV** 40 mg/m² q2 wk

Renal dose
Adult: **IV** serum Cr >3 mg/dl reduce dose by 50%

Hepatic dose
Adult: **IV** serum bilirubin 1.2-3 mg/dl reduce dose by 25%; bilirubin >3 mg/dl reduce dose by 50%

Available forms: Inj 20 mg powder/vial, sol for inj 5 mg/ml; liposome: dispersion for inj 2 mg/ml

Adverse effects
(*italic* = common; **bold** = life-threatening)
DAUNOrubicin
CNS: Fever, chills
CV: **Dysrhythmias, CHF, pericarditis, myocarditis,** peripheral edema
GI: *Nausea, vomiting, anorexia, mucositis,* **hepatotoxicity**
GU: Impotence, sterility, amenorrhea, gynecomastia, hyperuricemia
HEMA: **Thrombocytopenia, leukopenia, anemia**
INTEG: *Rash, extravasation,* dermatitis, reversible alopecia, cellulitis, thrombophlebitis at inj site
MISC: **Anaphylaxis**

DAUNOrubicin citrate liposome
CNS: Fatigue, headache, depression, insomnia, dizziness, malaise, neuropathy
CV: Chest pain, edema
GI: Cramps, diarrhea, constipation, stomatitis
INTEG: Sweating, pruritus
MS: Arthralgia, back pain

Contraindications: Hypersensitivity, pregnancy **D**, lactation, systemic infections, cardiac disease

Precautions: Renal, hepatic disease, gout, bone marrow suppression

⚠ Do Not Confuse:
DAUNOrubicin/DOXOrubicin

Pharmacokinetics	
Absorption	Complete
Distribution	Widely distributed; crosses placenta
Metabolism	Liver, extensively
Excretion	Biliary (40%-50%)
Half-life	18½ hr, liposome 55½ hr

Pharmacodynamics
Unknown

Interactions
Individual drugs
Cyclophosphamide: ↑ cardiotoxicity, CHF
Radiation: ↑ toxicity, bone marrow suppression
Drug classifications
Antineoplastics: ↑ toxicity, bone marrow suppression
Live virus vaccines: ↓ antibody reaction
NSAIDs, salicylates: ↑ risk of bleeding
Lab test interferences
↑ Uric acid

D

NURSING CONSIDERATIONS
Assessment
• Assess buccal cavity q8h for dryness, sores or ulceration, white patches, pain, bleeding, dysphagia; obtain prescription for viscous lidocaine (Xylocaine)
• Assess symptoms indicating severe allergic reaction: rash, pruritus, urticaria, purpuric skin lesions, itching, flushing; drug should be discontinued
• Assess chest x-ray, echocardiography, radionuclide angiography, ECG; watch for ST-T wave changes, low QRS and T, possible dysrhythmias (sinus tachycardia, heart block, PVCs); watch for CHF (jugular vein distention, weight gain, edema, rales or crackles), may occur after 2-6 mo of treatment
• Monitor CBC, differential, platelet count weekly, leukocyte nadir within 2 wk after administration, recovery within 3 wk; do not administer if absolute granulocyte count is <750/mm³ (liposome)
• Assess for increased uric acid levels, swelling, joint pain primarily in extremities; patient should be well hydrated to prevent urate deposits
• Monitor renal function studies: BUN, creatinine, serum uric acid, urine CCr baseline and before each dose; I&O ratio; report fall in urine output to <30 ml/hr
• Monitor temp q4h (may indicate beginning of infection)
• Monitor liver function tests baseline and before each dose (bilirubin, AST, ALT, LDH) as needed or monthly; note jaundice of skin or sclera, dark urine, clay-colored stools, itchy skin, abdominal pain, fever, diarrhea; hepatotoxicity can be severe
• Assess for bleeding: hematuria, stool guaiac, bruising or petechiae, mucosa or orifices q8h; check for inflammation of mucosa, breaks in skin
• Identify effects of alopecia on body image; discuss feelings about body changes

Nursing diagnoses

✓ Injury, risk for (adverse reactions)
✓ Cardiac output, decreased (adverse reactions)
✓ Body image, disturbed (adverse reactions)
✓ Infection, risk for (adverse reactions)
✓ Knowledge, deficient (teaching)

Implementation

- Avoid contact with skin; very irritating; wash completely to remove
- Give fluids **IV** or PO before chemotherapy to hydrate patient; give antiemetic 30-60 min before giving drug to prevent vomiting, and prn; antibiotics for prophylaxis of infection
- Provide liquid diet: carbonated beverages; gelatin may be added if patient is not nauseated or vomiting
- Help patient rinse mouth tid-qid with water, club soda, brush teeth bid-qid with soft brush or cotton-tipped applicators for stomatitis, use unwaxed dental floss
- Drug should be prepared by experienced personnel using proper precautions

IV **IV route: Cerubidine**

- Give after diluting 20 mg/4 ml sterile water for inj (5 mg/ml); rotate; further dilute in 10-15 ml 0.9% NaCl; give over 3-5 min by direct **IV** through Y-tube or 3-way stopcock of inf of D_5W or 0.9% NaCl

Intermittent infusion

- Dilute further in 50-100 ml 0.9% NaCl, LR, D_5W; give over 15 min (50 ml), 30 min (100 ml)

Y-site compatibilities: Amifostine, filgrastim, granisetron, melphalan, methotrexate, ondansetron, sodium bicarbonate, teniposide, thiotepa, vinorelbine

Y-site incompatibilities: Fludarabine

Additive compatibilities: Cytarabine with etoposide, hydrocortisone; not recommended for admixing

Additive incompatibilities: Dexamethasone, heparin

Solution compatibilities: $D_{3.3}/0.3\%$ NaCl, D_5W, Normosol-R, Ringer's, 0.9% NaCl

IV **IV route: DaunoXome**

- Dilute with D_5W (1 mg/ml), give over 60 min, do not use in-line filter, reconstituted sol may be stored ≤6 hr refrigerated; do not admix

Patient/family education

- Teach patient to avoid use of products containing aspirin or ibuprofen, razors, commercial mouthwash, since bleeding may occur; to report symptoms of bleeding (hematuria, tarry stools)

- Instruct patient to report signs of anemia (fatigue, headache, irritability, faintness, shortness of breath); signs of infection; bleeding, bruising, shortness of breath, swelling, change in heart rate; to avoid crowds, those with known infections
- Advise patient that hair may be lost during treatment; a wig or hairpiece may make patient feel better; new hair may be different in color, texture
- Caution patient not to have any vaccinations without the advice of the prescriber; serious reactions can occur
- Advise patient that contraception is needed during treatment and for 4 mo after the completion of therapy
- Advise patient to avoid alcohol, aspirin, NSAIDs

Evaluation

Positive therapeutic outcome

- Prevention of rapid division of malignant cells

---

delavirdine (Rx)

(de-la-veer′deen)
Rescriptor
Func. class.: Antiretroviral
Chem. class.: Nonnucleoside reverse transcriptase inhibitor (NNRII)

Pregnancy category C

Action: Binds directly to reverse transcriptase and blocks RNA, DNA causing a disruption of the enzyme's site

➡ **Therapeutic Outcome:** Improvement of HIV-1 infection

Uses: HIV-1 in combination with other antiretrovirals

Dosage and routes

P *Adult and child ≥16 yr:* 400 mg tid

Available forms: Tabs 100, 200 mg

Adverse effects

(*italic* = common; **bold** = life-threatening)

CNS: Headache, fatigue
GI: Diarrhea, anorexia, abdominal pain, nausea, vomiting, dyspepsia, **hepatotoxicity**
GU: **Nephrotoxicity**
HEMA: **Neutropenia, leukopenia, thrombocytopenia, anemia, granulocytopenia**
INTEG: Rash
MS: Pain, myalgia

Contraindications: Hypersensitivity to this drug or atevirdine

Precautions: Liver disease, pregnancy **C**, P lactation, children, renal disease, myelosuppression

Pharmacokinetics

Absorption	Well
Distribution	Highly protein bound
Metabolism	Liver, extensively
Excretion	Kidneys, feces
Half-life	2-11 hr

Pharmacodynamics

Onset	Unknown
Peak	1 hr
Duration	8 hr

Interactions
Individual drugs

Alprazolam, amprenavir, clarithromycin, dapsone, felodipine, indinavir, midazolam, nifidepine, saquinavir: ↑ level of each specific drug

Clarithromycin, fluoxetine, ketoconazole: ↑ level of delavirdine

Pimozide: life-threatening reactions; do not combine

Quinidine: ↑ level of both drugs

Drug classifications

Amphetamines, benzodiazepines, calcium channel blockers, ergots, sildenafil: ↑ serious life-threatening adverse reaction

Antacids, anticonvulsants, protease inhibitors: ↓ delavirdine levels

Antidysrhythmics, sedative/hypnotics: life-threatening reactions; do not combine

Contraceptives (oral): ↓ action of oral contraceptives

NURSING CONSIDERATIONS
Assessment

• Assess signs of infection, anemia
• Assess liver studies: ALT, AST; renal studies
• Assess C&S before drug therapy; drug may be taken as soon as culture is taken; repeat C&S after treatment; determine the presence of other sexually transmitted disease
• Assess bowel pattern before, during treatment; if severe abdominal pain with bleeding occurs, drug should be discontinued; monitor hydration
• Assess skin eruptions; rash, urticaria, itching

• Assess allergies before treatment, reaction to each medication; place allergies on chart
• Assess plasma delavirdine concentrations (trough 10 µm)
• Assess CBC, blood chemistry, plasma HIV RNA, absolute CD4$^+$/CD8$^+$/cell counts/%, serum β_2 microglobulin, serum ICD+24 antigen levels
• Assess for signs of delavirdine toxicity: severe nausea, vomiting, maculopapular rash

Nursing diagnoses
☑ Infection, risk for (uses)
☑ Diarrhea (side effects)
☑ Knowledge, deficient (teaching)

Implementation
• Add 4 tabs/3-4 oz of water, let stand, stir, swallow, rinse glass, swallow; use only 100 mg tabs for dispersion

Patient/family education
• Advise patient to take as prescribed; if dose is missed, take as soon as remembered up to 1 hr before next dose; do not double dose
• Advise patient that drug must be taken in equal intervals around the clock to maintain blood levels for duration of therapy
• Advise patient that tabs may be dissolved, drink right away, rinse cup with water, and drink that to get all medication
• Instruct patient to make sure health care provider knows of all the medications being taken
• Advise patient that if severe rash, mouth sores, swelling, aching muscles/joints, or eye redness occur, stop taking and notify health care provider
• Advise patient not to breastfeed if taking this drug

Evaluation
Positive therapeutic outcome
• Increased CD4$^+$ cell count
• Decreased viral load
• Improvement in symptoms of HIV

---

denileukin diftitox (Rx)
(den-ih-loo'kin dif'tih-tox)
Ontak
Func. class.: Antineoplastic misc agent

Pregnancy category C

Action: A recombinant DNA-derived cytotoxic protein; inhibits cellular protein synthesis

→ **Therapeutic Outcome:** Prevention of rapidly growing malignant cells

Uses: Cutaneous T-cell lymphoma that express CD25 component of the IL-2 receptor

Dosage and routes
Adult: **IV** 9-18 mcg/kg/day given for 5 days q21 days, give over ≥15 min

Available forms: Sol for inj, frozen 150 mcg/ml

Adverse effects
(*italic* = common; **bold** = life-threatening)
CNS: Dizziness, paresthesia, nervousness, confusion, insomnia
CV: Hypotension, vasodilatation, tachycardia, thrombosis, hypertension, dysrhythmia
GI: Nausea, anorexia, vomiting, diarrhea, constipation, dyspepsia, dysphagia
GU: Hematuria, albuminuria, pyuria, creatinine increase
HEMA: **Thrombocytopenia, leukopenia,** anemia
INTEG: Rash, pruritus, sweating
META: Hypoalbuminemia, edema, hypocalcemia, weight decrease, dehydration, hypokalemia
MISC: Fever, chills, asthenia, infection, pain, headache, chest pain, flulike symptoms
MS: Myalgia, arthralgia
RESP: Dyspnea, cough, pharyngitis, rhinitis

Contraindications: Hypersensitivity to denileukin, diphtheria toxin, interleukin-2

G **Precautions:** Radiation therapy, pregnancy
P C, elderly, lactation, children

Pharmacokinetics	
Absorption	Complete bioavailability (**IV**)
Distribution	Widely distributed; concentrates in liver/kidneys
Metabolism	Proteolytic degradation
Excretion	Unknown
Half-life	Unknown

Pharmacodynamics
Unknown

Interactions
Antineoplastics, bone marrow-suppressing drugs, radiation: ↑ bone marrow suppression
Live virus vaccines: ↑ adverse reactions, ↓ antibody reaction

NURSING CONSIDERATIONS
Assessment
• Assess symptoms indicating severe allergic reaction: rash, pruritus, urticaria, purpuric skin lesions, itching, flushing; drug should be discontinued
• Assess for vascular leak syndrome after 2 wk of treatment: hypotension, edema, hypoalbuminemia; monitor weight, B/P, serum albumin, edema
• Obtain CD25 expression on skin biopsy samples
• Monitor CBC, differential, platelet count weekly; withhold drug if WBC count is <4000/mm^3 or platelet count is <100,000/mm^3
• Monitor renal function studies: BUN, creatinine, urine CCr before and during therapy; I&O ratio; report fall in urine output to <30 ml/hr
• Monitor temp q4h (may indicate beginning of infection)
• Monitor liver function tests before and during therapy (bilirubin, AST, ALT, LDH) as needed or monthly; note jaundiced skin or sclera, dark urine, clay-colored stools, itchy skin, abdominal pain, fever, diarrhea; hepatotoxicity can be serious and fatal
• Assess for bleeding: hematuria, stool guaiac, bruising or petechiae, mucosa or orifices q8h; check for inflammation of mucosa, breaks in skin

Nursing diagnoses
✓ Injury, risk for (adverse reactions)
✓ Body image, disturbed (adverse reactions)
✓ Infection, risk for (adverse reactions)
✓ Knowledge, deficient (teaching)

Implementation
• Give fluids **IV** or PO before chemotherapy to hydrate patient
• Give antiemetic 30-60 min before giving drug to prevent vomiting, and prn; antibiotics for prophylaxis of infection
• Provide liquid diet: carbonated beverages; gelatin may be added if patient is not nauseated or vomiting
• Prepare and hold sol in plastic syringes or soft plastic **IV** bags only
• Draw calculated dose from vial, inject into empty **IV** infusion bag, for each 1 ml of drug removed from vial, no more than 9 ml of sterile saline without preservative should be added to **IV** bag; infuse over ≥15 min; do not give by bolus; do not admix with other drugs; do not use a filter
• Use within 6 hr, discard unused portions
• Watch for extravasation; give 3-5 ml of

---

mixture of 4 ml sodium thiosulfate 10% plus 5 ml sterile water SC as prescribed

Patient/family education

• Teach patient to avoid use of products containing aspirin or NSAIDs, razors, commercial mouthwash, since bleeding may occur; to report symptoms of bleeding (hematuria, tarry stools)

• Instruct patient to report signs of anemia (fatigue, headache, irritability, faintness, shortness of breath)

• Caution patient not to have any vaccinations without the advice of prescriber; serious reactions can occur

• Advise patient contraception is needed during treatment and for several months after the completion of therapy; drug has teratogenic properties

Evaluation

Positive therapeutic outcome

• Prevention of rapid division of malignant cells

desirvdin
Iprivask
See Appendix A, Selected New Drugs

desloratadine (Rx)
(des-lor-at'ah-deen)
Clarinex
Func. class.: Antihistamine, 2nd generation
Chem. class.: Selective histamine (H_1-) receptor antagonist

Pregnancy category C

Action: Binds to peripheral histamine receptors, providing antihistamine action without sedation

Therapeutic Outcome: Decreased nasal stuffiness, itching, swollen eyes

Uses: Seasonal allergic rhinitis

Dosage and routes
Adult and child ≥12 yr: PO 5 mg qd

Hepatic/renal dose
Adult: PO 5 mg qod

Available forms: Tabs 5 mg

Adverse effects
(*italic* = common; **bold** = life-threatening)
CNS: Sedation (more common with increased doses), headache

Contraindications: Hypersensitivity, acute asthma attacks, lower respiratory tract disease

Precautions: Pregnancy **C,** bronchial asthma, liver or renal impairment

Pharmacokinetics
Absorption	Unknown
Distribution	Bound to plasma proteins (82%-87%)
Metabolism	Liver (active metabolites)
Excretion	Urine, feces (metabolites)
Half-life	8½-28 hr

Pharmacodynamics
Onset	1 hr
Peak	1½ hr
Duration	24 hr

Interactions
None significant

NURSING CONSIDERATIONS
Assessment
• Assess for allergy: hives, rash, rhinitis; monitor respiratory status

Nursing diagnoses
✓ Airway clearance, ineffective (uses)
✓ Knowledge, deficient (teaching)
✓ Noncompliance (teaching, overuse)

Implementation
• May administer without regard to meals
• Store in airtight container at room temp

Patient/family education
• Advise patient to avoid driving, other hazardous activities if drowsiness occurs; to observe caution until drug's effects are known
• Advise patient that drug may cause photosensitivity; use sunscreen or stay out of the sun to prevent burns
• Caution patient to avoid use of other CNS depressants

Evaluation
Positive therapeutic outcome
• Absence of running or congested nose, other allergy symptoms

desmopressin (Rx)
(des-moe-press'in)
DDAVP, Stimate
Func. class.: Pituitary hormone
Chem. class.: Synthetic antidiuretic hormone

Pregnancy category B

Action: Promotes reabsorption of water by action on renal tubular epithelium in the kidney; causes smooth muscle constriction and increase in plasma factor VIII levels, which increases platelet aggregation resulting in vasopressor effect; similar to vasopressor

⮞ Therapeutic Outcome: Prevention of nocturnal enuresis, decreased bleeding in hemophilia A, von Willebrand's disease type 1, control and stabilization of water in diabetes insipidus

Uses: Hemophilia A, von Willebrand's disease type 1, nonnephrogenic diabetes insipidus, symptoms of polyuria/polydipsia caused by pituitary dysfunction, nocturnal enuresis

Dosage and routes
Primary nocturnal enuresis
P *Adult and Child ≥6 yr:* Intranasal 20 mcg (10 mcg in each nostril) hs, may increase to 40 mcg; PO 0.2 mg hs, may be increased to max 0.6 mg hs

Diabetes insipidus
Adult: Intranasal 0.1-0.4 ml qd in divided doses (1-4 sprays with pump); **IV**/SC 0.5-1 ml qd in divided doses
P *Child 3 mo-12 yr:* Intranasal 0.05-0.3 ml qd in divided doses

Hemophilia/von Willebrand's disease
P *Adult and child >3 mo:* **IV** 0.3 mcg/kg in NaCl over 15-30 min; may repeat if needed

Antihemorrhagic
P *Adult and child >3 mo:* **IV** 0.3 mcg/kg
P *Adult and child <50 kg:* Intranasal 1 spray in one nostril
P *Adult and child >50 kg:* 1 spray each nostril

Available forms: Inj 4, 15 mcg/ml, Rhinal Tube del 2.5 mcg/vial (0.1 mg/ml); tabs 0.1, 0.2 mg; nasal spray pump 10 mcg/spray (0.1 mg/ml); nasal sol 1.5 mg/ml (150 mcg/dose)

Adverse effects
(*italic* = common; **bold** = life-threatening)
CNS: Drowsiness, headache, lethargy, flushing

CV: Increased B/P
EENT: Nasal irritation, congestion, rhinitis
GI: Nausea, heartburn, cramps
GU: *Vulval pain*
SYST: Anaphylaxis **(IV)**

Contraindications: Hypersensitivity, nephrogenic diabetes insipidus

Precautions: Pregnancy **B,** CAD, lactation, hypertension

Pharmacokinetics
Absorption	Nasal (up to 20%)
Distribution	Unknown
Metabolism	Unknown
Excretion	Unknown; breast milk
Half-life	8 min (initial), 76 min (terminal)

Pharmacodynamics
	PO	INTRANASAL	IV/SC
Onset	1 hr	1 hr	Rapid
Peak	4-7 hr	1-4 hr	15-30 min
Duration	Unknown	8-20 hr	3 hr

Interactions
Individual drugs
Carbamazepine, chlorpropamide, clofibrate: ↑ antidiuretic action
Demeclocycline, epinephrine (large doses), heparin, lithium: ↓ antidiuretic action

NURSING CONSIDERATIONS
Assessment
• Monitor I&O ratio, urine osmolality, sp gr, weight daily; check for edema in extremities; if water retention is severe, diuretic may be prescribed; check pulse, B/P when giving drug **IV** or SC
• Assess for water intoxication: lethargy, behavioral changes, disorientation, neuromuscular excitability, dehydration, poor skin turgor, severe thirst, dry skin, tachycardia
• Assess intranasal use: nausea, congestion, cramps, headache; usually decreased with decreased dosage
• Monitor for enuresis during treatment (nocturnal enuresis)
• Assess for allergic reaction including anaphylaxsis (**IV** route)
• Assess for nasal mucosa changes: congestion, edema, discharge, scarring (nasal route)
• Monitor urine volume osmolality and plasma osmolality (diabetes insipidus)
• Monitor factor VIII coagulant activity before using for hemostasis

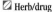

Nursing diagnoses
☑ Fluid volume, deficient (uses)
☑ Fluid volume, excess (side effects)
☑ Knowledge, deficient (teaching)

Implementation
• Store in refrigerator or cool environment

IV IV route
Direct IV
• Give undiluted over 1 min in diabetes insipidus or **IV** for hemophilia

Intermittent infusion
• Give single dose diluted in 50 ml of 0.9% **P** NaCl (adult and child >10 kg); a single dose/10 ml as an **IV** inf over 15-30 min in von Willebrand's disease or hemophilia A

Patient/family education
• Use demonstration, return demonstration to teach technique for nasal instillation: draw medication into tube, insert tube into nostril to instill drug and blow on other end to deliver sol into nasal cavity; rinse after use
• Teach patient to notify prescriber of dyspnea, vomiting, cramping, drowsiness, headache, nasal congestion
• Caution patient to avoid OTC products (cough, hay fever), since these preparations may contain epINEPHrine and decrease drug response; do not use with alcohol
• Advise patient to carry/wear emergency ID or other identification specifying disease and medication used
• Advise patient if dose is missed, take when remembered up to 1 hr before next dose; do not double doses

Evaluation
Positive therapeutic outcome
• Absence of severe thirst
• Decreased urine output, osmolality
• Absence of bleeding (hemophilia)

---

desoxyribonuclease
See fibrinolysin/desoxyribonuclease

---

dexamethasone (Rx)
(dex-ah-meth'ah-sone)
Decadron, Deronil ♣, Dexasone ♣, Dexon, Hexadrol, Mymethasone
dexamethasone acetate (Rx)
Dalalone DP, Dalalone LA, Decadron-LA, Decaject-LA, Dexacen LA-8, Dexasone-LA, Dexone LA, Solurex-LA
dexamethasone sodium phosphate (Rx)
Dalalone, Decadron Phosphate, Decaject, Dexacen-4, Dexone, Hexadrol Phosphate, Solurex
Func. class.: Corticosteroid
Chem. class.: Glucocorticoid, long-acting
Pregnancy category C

Action: Decreases inflammation by suppression of migration of polymorphonuclear leukocytes, fibroblasts, reversal of increased capillary permeability and lysosomal stabilization

Uses: Inflammation, allergies, neoplasms, cerebral edema, septic shock, collagen disorders

Dosage and routes
Inflammation
Adult: PO 0.75-9 mg/day, in divided doses q6-12h or phosphate IM 0.5-9 mg/day; or acetate IM 4-16 mg q1-3 wk
P *Child:* PO 0.08-0.3 mg/kg/day in divided doses q6-12h

Shock
Adult: IV (phosphate) single dose 1-6 mg/kg or IV 40 mg q2-6h as needed up to 72 hr

Cerebral edema
Adult: IV (phosphate) 10 mg, then 4-6 mg IM q6h × 2-4 days, then taper over 1 wk
P *Child:* PO 0.2 mg/kg/day in divided doses

Adrenocortical insufficiency
P *Child:* 23.3 mcg/kg/day in 3 divided doses

Suppression test
Adult: PO 1 mg at 11 PM or 0.5 mg q6h × 48 hr

Available forms: Dexamethasone: tabs 0.25, 0.5, 0.75, 1, 1.5, 2, 4, 6 mg; elix 0.5 mg/5 ml; oral sol 0.5 mg/5 ml, 1 mg/1 ml; inj acetate 8, 16 mg/ml; inj phosphate 4, 10, 20, 24 mg/ml

Adverse effects

(*italic* = common; **bold** = life-threatening)

CNS: *Depression, flushing, sweating,* headache, mood changes, euphoria, psychosis, **seizures,** insomnia

CV: *Hypertension,* **circulatory collapse, thrombophlebitis, embolism,** tachycardia, edema

EENT: Fungal infections, increased intraocular pressure, blurred vision

ENDO: Hypothalmic-pituitary-adrenal axis suppression, hyperglycemia, sodium, fluid retention

GI: *Diarrhea, nausea, abdominal distention,* **GI hemorrhage,** *increased appetite,* **pancreatitis**

HEMA: **Thrombocytopenia**

INTEG: Acne, poor wound healing, ecchymosis, petechiae, hirsutism

META: Hypokalemia

MS: Fractures, osteoporosis, weakness

Contraindications: Psychosis, hypersensitivity, idiopathic thrombocytopenia, acute glomerulonephritis, amebiasis, fungal infections, nonasthmatic bronchial disease, child <2 yr, AIDS, TB

Precautions: Pregnancy **C**, lactation, diabetes mellitus, glaucoma, osteoporosis, seizure disorders, ulcerative colitis, CHF, myasthenia gravis, renal disease, peptic ulcer, esophagitis

◼ **Do Not Confuse:**
Decadron/Percodan

Pharmacokinetics

Absorption	Unknown
Distribution	Unknown
Metabolism	Liver
Excretion	Kidneys
Half-life	3-4½ hr

Pharmacodynamics

	PO	IM
Onset	1 hr	Unknown
Peak	1-2 hr	8 hr
Duration	2½ days	6 days

Interactions
Individual drugs

Alcohol, amphotericin B, cycloSPORINE, digoxin, indomethacin: ↑ side effects
Ambemonium, isoniazid, neostigmine, sometrem: ↓ effects of each specific drug
Cholestyramine, colestipol, epHEDrine, phenytoin, rifampin, theophylline: ↓ action of dexamethasone

Indomethacin, ketoconazole: ↑ action of dexamethasone

Drug classifications

Antacids, barbiturates: ↓ action of dexamethasone
Antibiotics (macrolide), contraceptives (oral), estrogens, salicylates: ↑ action of dexamethasone
Anticholinesterases, anticoagulants, anticonvulsants, antidiabetics, toxoids/vaccines: ↓ effects of each specific drug
Diuretics, salicylates: ↑ side effects
Salicylates: ↑ action of dexamethasone

◩ **Herb/drug**

Aloe, buckthorn bark/berry, cascara sagrada, senna pod/leaf: ↑ hypokalemia
Aloe, licorice, perilla: ↑ corticosteroid effect

Lab test interferences

↑ Cholesterol, ↑ Na, ↑ blood glucose, ↑ uric acid, ↑ Ca, ↑ urine glucose
↓ Ca, ↓ K, ↓ T_4, ↓ T_3, ↓ thyroid ^{131}I uptake test, ↓ urine 17-OHCS, ↓ 17-KS, ↓ PBI
False negative: Skin allergy tests

NURSING CONSIDERATIONS
Assessment

- Monitor K, blood, urine glucose while on long-term therapy; hypokalemia and hyperglycemia
- Monitor weight daily; notify prescriber of weekly gain >5 lb
- Monitor B/P q4h, pulse; notify prescriber of chest pain
- Monitor I&O ratio; be alert for decreasing urinary output, increasing edema
- Monitor plasma cortisol levels during long-term therapy (normal: 138-635 nmol/L SI units when assessed at 8 AM)
- Assess infection: fever, WBC even after withdrawal of medication; drug masks infection
- Assess potassium depletion: paresthesias, fatigue, nausea, vomiting, depression, polyuria, dysrhythmias, weakness
- Assess edema, hypertension, cardiac symptoms
- Assess mental status: affect, mood, behavioral changes, aggression

Nursing diagnoses

☑ Infection, risk for (adverse reaction)
☑ Knowledge, deficient (teaching)
☑ Mobility, impaired (uses)

Implementation
▣ IV route
- **IV** undiluted direct over 1 min or less or diluted with 0.9% NaCl or D₅W and give as an **IV** inf at prescribed rate
- After shaking susp (parenteral); do not give susp **IV**
- Titrated dose; use lowest effective dose

Dexamethasone sodium phosphate
Syringe compatibilities: Granisetron, metoclopramide, ranitidine, sufentanil

Y-site compatibilities: Acyclovir, allopurinol, amifostine, amikacin, amphotericin B cholesteryl, amsacrine, aztreonam, cefepime, cisatracurium, cisplatin, cladribine, cyclophosphamide, cytarabine, DOXOrubicin, DOXOrubicin liposome, famotidine, filgrastim, fluconazole, fludarabine, foscarnet, heparin, melphalan, meperidine, meropenem, morphine, ondansetron, paclitaxel, piperacillin/tazobactam, potassium chloride, propofol, remifentanil, sargramostim, sodium bicarbonate, sufentanil, tacrolimus, teniposide, theophylline, vinorelbine, vit B/C, zidovudine

Additive compatibilities: Aminophylline, bleomycin, cimetidine, floxacillin, furosemide, lidocaine, meropenem, nafcillin, netilmicin, ondansetron, prochlorperazine, ranitidine, verapamil

PO route
- Give with food or milk to decrease GI symptoms
- Provide assistance with ambulation in patient with bone tissue disease to prevent fractures

IM route
- IM inj deep in large muscle mass; rotate sites; avoid deltoid; use 21-G needle
- In one dose in AM to prevent adrenal suppression; avoid SC administration, may damage tissue

Patient/family education
- Advise that emergency ID as steroid user should be carried or worn
- Teach to notify prescriber if therapeutic response decreases; dosage adjustment may be needed
- Teach not to discontinue abruptly or adrenal crisis can result
- Teach to avoid OTC products: salicylates, alcohol in cough products, cold preparations unless directed by prescriber
- Instruct patient to contact prescriber if surgery, trauma, stress occurs, dose may need to be adjusted
- Teach patient all aspects of drug usage, including cushingoid symptoms
- Instruct patient to notify prescriber of infection
- Teach symptoms of adrenal insufficiency: nausea, anorexia, fatigue, dizziness, dyspnea, weakness, joint pain
- Advise patient to avoid exposure to chickenpox or measles, persons with infections

Evaluation
Positive therapeutic outcome
Ease of respirations, decreased inflammation

D

---

dexmedetomidine (Rx)
(deks-med-ee-tome′a-dine)
Precedex
Func. class.: Sedative, α₂-adrenoceptor agonist

Pregnancy category C

Action: Produces α₂ activity as seen at low and moderate doses; also, α₁ at high doses

Uses: Sedation in mechanically ventilated, intubated patients in ICU

Dosage and routes
Adult: **IV** Loading dose of 1 mcg/kg over 10 min, then 0.2-0.7 mcg/kg/hr, do not use for more than 24 hr

Available forms: Inj 100 mcg/ml

Adverse effects
(*italic* = common; **bold** = life-threatening)
CV: *Bradycardia, hypotension, hypertension,* **atrial fibrillation, infarction**
GI: *Nausea,* thirst
GU: Oliguria
HEMA: Leukocytosis, anemia
RESP: **Pulmonary edema, pleural effusion, hypoxia**

Contraindications: Hypersensitivity

⬛ Precautions: Elderly, renal disease, respiratory depression, severe respiratory disorders, cardiac dysrhythmias, pregnancy **C**, **⬛** lactation, children

Pharmacokinetics	
Half-life	8 min

Interactions
Drug classifications
Anesthetics, antipsychotics, opiates, sedative/

---

hypnotics, skeletal muscle relaxants: ↑ CNS depression

NURSING CONSIDERATIONS
Assessment
- Assess inj site: phlebitis, burning, stinging
- Monitor ECG for changes: atrial fibrillation
- Assess CNS changes: movement, jerking, tremors, dizziness, LOC, pupil reaction
- Assess respiratory dysfunction: respiratory depression, character, rate, rhythm; notify prescriber if respirations are <10/min

Implementation
IV IV route
- Give after diluting with D₅W, 0.9% NaCl, withdraw 2 ml of drug and add to 48 ml of 0.9% NaCl to a total of 50 ml, shake to mix well
- Give only with resuscitative equipment available
- Give only by qualified persons trained in management of ICU sedation

Solution compatibilities: LR, D₅W, 0.9% NaCl, 20% mannitol

Additive compatibilities: Atracurium, atropine, etomidate, fentanyl, glycopyrrolate, midazolam, mivacurium, morphine, pancuronium, phenylephrine, succinylcholine, thiopental, vecuronium
- Provide safety measures: side rails, nightlight, call bell within easy reach

Evaluation
- Therapeutic response: induction of sedation

---

dexmethylphenidate (Rx)
(dex′meth-ul-fen′ih-dayt)
Focalin
Func. class.: Central nervous system (CNS) stimulant

Pregnancy category C

Controlled substance schedule II

Action: Increases release of norepinephrine and dopamine into the extraneuronal space, also blocks reuptake of norepinephrine and dopamine into the presynaptic neuron; mode of action in treating attention deficit hyperactivity disorder (ADHD) is unknown

➡ **Therapeutic Outcome:** Increased alertness, decreased fatigue, ability to stay awake (narcolepsy), increased attention span, decreased hyperactivity (ADHD)

Uses: ADHD

Dosage and routes
P *Child >6 yr:* PO 2.5 mg bid with doses at least 4 hr apart, gradually increase to a maximum of 20 mg/day (10 mg bid); for those taking methylphenidate, use ½ of methylphenidate dose initially, then increase as needed to a maximum of 20 mg/day

Available forms: Tabs 2.5, 5, 10 mg

Adverse effects
(*italic* = common; **bold** = life-threatening)
CNS: Dizziness, headache, drowsiness, **toxic psychosis, neuroleptic malignant syndrome (rare),** Gilles de la Tourette's syndrome
CV: Palpitations, B/P changes, angina, **dysrhythmias**
GI: Nausea, anorexia, abnormal liver function, **hepatic coma,** abdominal pain
HEMA: **Leukopenia, anemia, thrombocytopenic purpura**
INTEG: **Exfoliative dermatitis,** urticaria, rash, erythema multiforme
MISC: Fever, arthralgia, scalp hair loss

Contraindications: Hypersensitivity to methylphenidate, anxiety, history of Gilles de la
P Tourette's syndrome; children <6 yr, glaucoma, concurrent treatment with MAOIs or within 14 days of discontinuing treatment with MAOIs

Precautions: Hypertension, depression, pregnancy **C,** seizures, lactation, drug abuse, psychosis, cardiovascular disorders

Pharmacokinetics	
Absorption	Readily absorbed
Distribution	Unknown
Metabolism	Liver
Excretion	Kidneys
Half-life	2.2 hr

Pharmacodynamics	
Onset	½-1 hr
Peak	1-1 ½ hr
Duration	4 hr

Interactions
Drug classifications
Anticoagulants (coumarin) (e.g., warfarin), anticonvulsants, SSRIs, tricyclics: ↑ effects
Antihypertensives: ↓ effects
Decongestants: ↑ sympathomimetic effect
MAOIs: Hypertensive crisis if coadministered or given within 14 days
Vasoconstrictors: ↑ sympathomimetic effect
Vasopressors: Hypertensive crisis

⬛ Herb/drug   ⓢ Do Not Crush   ◆ Alert   ◆π Key Drug   Ⓖ Geriatric   Ⓟ Pediatric

☢ Herb/drug

Horsetail, yohimbe: ↑ stimulant effect
Melatonin: ↑ synergistic effect

NURSING CONSIDERATIONS
Assessment

• Assess VS, B/P; may reverse antihypertensives; check patients with cardiac disease more often for increased B/P
• Assess CBC, urinalysis in diabetes; blood/urine glucose; insulin changes may have to be made, since eating will decrease
• Assess height, growth rate q3 mo in 🅿 children; growth rate may be decreased
• Assess mental status: mood, sensorium, affect, stimulation, insomnia, aggressiveness
◆• Assess withdrawal symptoms: headache, nausea, vomiting, muscle pain, weakness
• Assess appetite, sleep, speech patterns
• Assess for attention span, decreased hyperactivity in persons with ADHD

Nursing diagnoses

☑ Thought processes, disturbed (uses, adverse reactions)
☑ Coping, ineffective (uses)
☑ Knowledge, deficient (teaching)
☑ Coping, disabled family (uses)

Implementation
Administer

• Twice daily at least 4 hr apart
• Without regard to meals

Patient/family education

• Advise patient to decrease caffeine consumption (coffee, tea, cola, chocolate); may increase irritability, stimulation
🚫• Caution patient not to break, crush, or chew time rel medication
• Advise patient to avoid OTC preparations unless approved by prescriber
• Caution patient to taper off drug over several wk to avoid depression, increased sleeping, lethargy
• Caution patient to avoid alcohol ingestion
• Caution patient to avoid hazardous activities until stabilized on medication
• Advise patient to get needed rest; patients will feel more tired at end of day

Evaluation
Positive therapeutic outcome

• Decreased hyperactivity or ability to stay awake

Treatment of overdose: Administer fluids; hemodialysis or peritoneal dialysis; antihypertensive for increased B/P; administer short-acting barbiturate before lavage

---

dextroamphetamine (Rx)
(dex-troe-am-fet'a-meen)
Dexedrine, dextroamphetamine, Dextrostat
dextroamphetamine sulfate
Dextrostat
Func. class.: Cerebral stimulant
Chem. class.: Amphetamine

Pregnancy category C

Controlled substance schedule II

Action: Increases release of norepINEPHrine, dopamine in cerebral cortex to reticular activating system

➡ **Therapeutic Outcome:** Increased alertness, decreased fatigue, ability to stay awake (narcolepsy); increased attention span, decreased hyperactivity (ADHD)

Uses: Narcolepsy, attention deficit disorder with hyperactivity

Dosage and routes
Narcolepsy
Adult: PO 5-60 mg qd in divided doses

🅿 *Child >12 yr:* PO 10 mg qd increasing by 10 mg/day at weekly intervals

🅿 *Child 6-12 yr:* PO 5 mg qd increasing by 5 mg/wk (max 60 mg/day)

ADHD
Adult: PO 5-60 mg/day in divided doses

🅿 *Child >6 yr:* PO 5 mg qd-bid increasing by 5 mg/day at weekly intervals

🅿 *Child 3-6 yr:* PO 2.5 mg qd increasing by 2.5 mg/day at weekly intervals

Available forms: Tabs 5, 10 mg; sus rel caps 5, 10, 15 mg

Adverse effects
(*italic* = common; **bold** = life-threatening)
CNS: Hyperactivity, insomnia, restlessness, talkativeness, dizziness, headache, chills, stimulation, dysphoria, irritability, aggressiveness, tremor, dependence, addiction
CV: Palpitations, **tachycardia,** hypertension, decrease in heart rate, **dysrhythmias**
GI: Anorexia, dry mouth, diarrhea, constipation, weight loss, metallic taste
GU: Impotence, change in libido
INTEG: Urticaria

Contraindications: Hypersensitivity to sympathomimetic amines, hyperthyroidism, hypertension, glaucoma, severe arteriosclerosis, drug abuse, cardiovascular disease, anxiety

Precautions: Gilles de la Tourette's 🅿 disorder, pregnancy **C,** lactation, child <3 yr

---

Pharmacokinetics

Absorption	Well absorbed
Distribution	Widely distributed; crosses placenta
Metabolism	Liver
Excretion	Kidneys, pH dependent: increased pH, increased reabsorption
Half-life	10-30 hr; increased when urine is alkaline

Pharmacodynamics

Onset	½ hr
Peak	1-3 hr
Duration	4-10 hr

Interactions

Individual drugs
Acetazolamide, sodium bicarbonate: ↑ effect of dextroamphetamine
Ammonium chloride, ascorbic acid: ↓ effect of dextroamphetamine
Haloperidol: ↑ CNS effect
Phenytoin: ↓ absorption of phenytoin

Drug classifications
Adrenergic blockers: ↓ adrenergic blocking effect
Antacids: ↑ effect of dextroamphetamine
Antidepressants (tricyclic), phenothiazines: ↑ CNS effect
Antidiabetics: ↓ antidiabetic effect
Barbiturates: ↓ absorption of barbiturate
MAOIs: Hypertensive crisis if used within 14 days

Food/drug
Caffeine: ↑ amine effect

▨ Herb/drug
Eucalyptus: ↓ stimulant effect
Khat: ↑ stimulant effect
St. John's wort: ↑ serotonin syndrome

NURSING CONSIDERATIONS
Assessment
• Monitor VS, B/P, since this drug may reverse antihypertensives; check patients with cardiac disease more often for increased B/P
• Monitor CBC, urinalysis; for diabetic patients monitor blood, urine glucose; insulin changes may be required, since eating will decrease
• Monitor height and weight q3 mo since
P growth rate in children may be decreased; appetite is suppressed so weight loss is common during the first few months of treatment
• Monitor mental status: mood, sensorium, affect, stimulation, insomnia; aggressiveness may occur; depression with crying spells may occur after drug has worn off

• Assess for physical dependency; should not be used for extended time except in ADHD; dosage should be decreased gradually to prevent withdrawal symptoms
• Assess for narcoleptic symptoms before medication and after; ability to stay awake should increase significantly
P • In children or adults with ADHD, monitor for improved organizational skills, attention span, attending to tasks, impulse control, socialization, and ability to get along better with others
• Assess for withdrawal symptoms: headache, nausea, vomiting, muscle pain, weakness; drug tolerance develops after long-term use; dosage should not be increased if tolerance develops; this medication has a high abuse potential

Nursing diagnoses
☑ Thought processes, disturbed (uses, adverse reactions)
☑ Coping, impaired (uses)
☑ Coping, compromised family (uses)
☑ Knowledge, deficient (teaching)

Implementation
• Give at least 6 hr before hs to avoid sleeplessness; titrate to patient's response; lowest dosage should be used to control symptoms
• Give gum, hard candy, frequent sips of water for dry mouth at beginning of treatment; these symptoms tend to lessen with time
Ⓢ • Do not crush, chew sus rel forms

Patient/family education
• Advise patient to decrease caffeine consumption (coffee, tea, cola, chocolate), which may increase irritability and stimulation; to avoid OTC preparations unless approved by prescriber; to avoid alcohol ingestion; these may cause serious drug interactions
• Caution patient to taper off drug over several weeks, or depression, increased sleeping, lethargy may occur
• Caution patient to avoid hazardous activities until patient is stabilized on medication
• Instruct patient not to double doses if medication is missed; prescriber may suggest drug holidays (ADHD) during the school year to assess progress and determine continued drug necessity
• Instruct patient/family to notify prescriber if significant side effects occur: tremors, insomnia, palpitations, restlessness, drug changes may be needed
• Inform patient that if dry mouth occurs to use frequent sips of water, sugarless gum, hard candy during beginning therapy; dry mouth lessens with continued treatment

- Advise patient to get needed rest; patients will feel more tired at end of day; to give last dose at least 6 hr before hs to avoid insomnia

Evaluation
Positive therapeutic outcome
- Decreased activity in ADHD
- Absence of sleeping during day in narcolepsy

Treatment of overdose: Administer fluids, hemodialysis, peritoneal dialysis, antihypertensives for increased B/P; ammonium chloride for increased excretion

dextromethorphan (OTC)
(dex-troe-meth-or'fan)
Balminil DM ✤, Benylin DM, Broncho-Grippol-DM ✤, Children's Hold, Creo-Terpin, Delsym, Hold DM, Koffex ✤, Neo-DM ✤, Ornex-DM ✤, Pertussin, Pertussin ES, Robidex ✤, Robitussin Cough Calmers, Robitussin Pediatric, Sedatuss ✤, St. Joseph Cough Suppressant, Scot-Tussin DM, Sucrets Cough Control, Suppress, Vicks Formula 44
Func. class.: Antitussive, nonopioid
Chem. class.: Levorphanol derivative

Pregnancy category C

Action: Depresses cough center in medulla by direct effect related to levorphanol

➥**Therapeutic Outcome:** Absence of cough

Uses: Nonproductive cough carried by minor respiratory tract infections or irritants that might be inhaled

Investigational uses: Neuropathy

Dosage and routes
P *Adult and Child ≥12 yr:* PO 10-20 mg q4h, or 30 mg q6-8h, not to exceed 120 mg/day; sus rel liq 60 mg q12h, not to exceed 120 mg/day

P *Child 6-12 yr:* PO 5-10 mg q4h; sus rel liq 30 mg bid, not to exceed 60 mg/day

P *Child 2-6 yr:* PO 2.5-5 mg q4h, or 7.5 mg q6-8h, not to exceed 30 mg/day

Neuropathy
Adult: PO doses vary widely

Available forms: Loz 2.5, 5, 7.5, 15 mg; sol; liq 3.5 mg, 7.5, 15 mg/5 ml, 3.5, 5, 7.5, 10, 15 mg/5 ml; syr 15 mg/15 ml, 10 mg/5 ml; sus action liq equivalent to 30 mg/5 ml; caps 30 mg; ext rel susp 30 mg/5 ml

Adverse effects
(*italic* = common; **bold** = life-threatening)
CNS: *Dizziness,* sedation
GI: *Nausea*

Contraindications: Hypersensitivity, asthma/emphysema, productive cough

Precautions: Nausea/vomiting, increased temp, persistent headache, pregnancy **C**

Pharmacokinetics
Absorption	Rapid (PO); slow (sus rel)
Distribution	Unknown
Metabolism	Liver
Excretion	Kidneys
Half-life	Unknown

Pharmacodynamics
	PO	PO-SUS
Onset	15-30 min	Unknown
Peak	Unknown	Unknown
Duration	3-6 hr	12 hr

Interactions
Individual drugs
Alcohol: ↑ CNS depression
Amiodarone, fluoxetine, quinidine: ↑ adverse reactions
Drug classifications
Antihistamines, antidepressants, opiates, sedative/hypnotics: ↑ CNS depression
MAOIs: ↑ hypotension, hyperpyrexia, do not give within 2 wk of MAOI

NURSING CONSIDERATIONS
Assessment
- Assess cough: type, frequency, character including sputum; provide adequate hydration to 2 L/day to decrease viscosity of secretions

Nursing diagnoses
☑ Airway clearance, ineffective (uses)
☑ Knowledge, deficient (teaching)

Implementation
- Administer decreased dosage to elderly patients; their metabolism may be slowed; do not provide water within 30 min of administration because it dilutes drug
- Shake susp before administration

Patient/family education
- Caution patient to avoid driving or other hazardous activities until stabilized on this medication; may cause drowsiness, dizziness in some individuals
- Advise patient to avoid smoking, smoke-filled rooms, perfumes, dust, environmental pollutants, cleaners, which increase cough; may use gum, hard candy to prevent dry mouth

- Advise patient to avoid alcohol or other CNS depressants while taking this medication; drowsiness will be increased
- Caution patient that any cough lasting over a few days should be assessed by prescriber

Evaluation
Positive therapeutic outcome
- Absence of dry, irritating cough

---

dextrose (D-glucose) (Rx)
Glucose, Glutose, Insta-Glucose
Func. class.: Caloric agent

Pregnancy category D

Action: Needed for adequate utilization of amino acids; decreases protein, nitrogen loss; prevents ketosis

Therapeutic Outcome: Provides calories, prevents severe hypoglycemia

Uses: Increases intake of calories; increases fluids in patients unable to take adequate fluids, calories orally; 2.5%-11.5% forms provide calories, increased hydration; 20%-70% forms used to treat severe hypoglycemia

Dosage and routes
Adult and child: IV, depends on individual requirements

Available forms: Inj IV 2.5%, 5%, 10%, 20%, 30%, 40%, 50%, 60%, 70%; oral gel 40%; chewable tabs 5 g

Adverse effects
(*italic* = common; **bold** = life-threatening)
CNS: Confusion, **loss of consciousness,** dizziness
CV: Hypertension, **CHF, pulmonary edema**
ENDO: Hyperglycemia, rebound hypoglycemia, hyperosmolar syndrome, hyperglycemic nonketolytic syndrome
GU: Glycosuria, osmotic diuresis
INTEG: Chills, flushing, warm feeling, rash, urticaria, extravasation necrosis

Contraindications: Hyperglycemia, delirium tremens, hemorrhage (cranial/spinal), CHF, pregnancy **D**

Precautions: Renal, liver, cardiac disease, diabetes mellitus

Pharmacokinetics
Absorption	Well absorbed (PO); completely absorbed (**IV**)
Distribution	Widely distributed
Metabolism	Unknown
Excretion	Unknown
Half-life	Unknown

Pharmacodynamics
	IV	PO
Onset	Immediate	Rapid
Peak	Immediate	Rapid
Duration	Immediate	Rapid

Interactions
Individual drugs
Insulin: ↑ need for insulin
Drug classifications
Corticosteroids: ↑ fluid retention/electrolyte excretion
Hypoglycemics, oral: ↑ need for hypoglycemic

NURSING CONSIDERATIONS
Assessment
- Assess I&O, skin turgor, edema, electrolytes (potassium, sodium, calcium, chloride, magnesium), blood glucose, ammonia, phosphate
- Monitor inj site for extravasation: redness along vein, edema at site, necrosis, pain, hard tender area; site should be changed immediately
- Monitor temp q4h for increased fever, indicating infection; if infection suspected, inf is discontinued and tubing, bottle, catheter tip cultured
- Monitor serum glucose in patients receiving hypertonic glucose 5% and over
- Assess nutritional status: calorie count by dietician; GI system function

Nursing diagnoses
☑ Nutrition: less than body requirements, imbalanced (uses)
☑ Fluid volume, excess (adverse reactions)
☑ Knowledge, deficient (teaching)

Implementation
PO route
- Oral glucose preparations (gel, chewable tabs) are to be used for conscious patients only; serum blood glucose should be monitored after first oral dose; if glucose has not increased by 20 mg/100 ml in 20-30 min, dose should be repeated and serum glucose checked again
IV IV route
- Give only protein (4%) and dextrose (up to

12.5%) via peripheral vein; stronger sol requires central **IV** administration
• May be given undiluted via prepared sol; give 10% sol (5 ml/15 sec), 20% sol (1000 ml/3 hr or more), 50% sol (500 ml/30-60 min); too rapid **IV** administration may cause fluid overload and hyperglycemia
• After changing **IV** catheter, change dressing q24h with aseptic technique

Patient/family education
• Teach patient reason for dextrose infusion
• Provide literature and information on when and how to use oral products for hypoglycemia
• Review hypoglycemia/hyperglycemia symptoms
• Review blood glucose monitoring procedure

Evaluation
Positive therapeutic outcome
• Increased weight
• Blood glucose level at normal limits for patient
• Adequate hydration

---

diazepam ⊶π (Rx)
(dye-az′e-pam)
Apo-Diazepam ✦, Diastat, diazepam, Diazemuls ✦, Novo-Diapam ✦, PMS-Diazepam ✦, Valium, Valrelease, Vivol ✦
Func. class.: Antianxiety, anticonvulsant, skeletal muscle relaxant, central acting
Chem. class.: Benzodiazepine

Pregnancy category D

Controlled substance schedule IV

Action: Potentiates the actions of GABA, especially in limbic system, reticular formation; enhances presympathetic inhibition, inhibits spinal polysynaptic afferent paths

➔ **Therapeutic Outcome:** Decreased anxiety, restlessness, insomnia

Uses: Anxiety, acute alcohol withdrawal, adjunct in seizure disorders; preoperative skeletal muscle relaxation; rectally for acute repetitive seizures

Investigational uses: Panic attacks

Dosage and routes
Anxiety/convulsive disorders
Adult: PO 2-10 mg bid-qid; ext rel 15-30 mg qd
G *Elderly:* PO 1-2 mg qd-bid, increase slowly as needed
P *Child >6 mo:* PO 1-2.5 mg tid-qid

Muscle relaxation
Adult: PO 2-10 mg tid-qid or ext rel 15-30 mg qd; **IV**/IM 5-10 mg repeat in 2-4 hr
G *Elderly:* PO 2-5 mg bid-qid; **IV**/IM 2-5 mg, may repeat in 2-4 hr

Tetanic muscle spasms
P *Child >5 yr:* IM/**IV** 5-10 mg q3-4h prn
P *Infants >30 days:* IM/**IV** 1-2 mg q3-4h prn

Status epilepticus
Adult: **IV**/IM 5-10 mg, 2 mg/min, may repeat q10-15 min, not to exceed 30 mg; may repeat in 2-4 hr if seizures reappear
P *Child >5 yr:* **IV**/IM 1 mg q2-5 min, max 10 mg, may repeat in 2-4 hr
P *Child 1 mo-5 yr:* **IV**/IM 0.05-0.3 mg/kg/dose given over 2-3 min q15-30, max 5 mg
Adult: REC 0.2 mg/kg, may repeat 4-12 hr later
P *Child 6-11 yr:* REC 0.3 mg/kg, may repeat 4-12 hr later
P *Child 2-5 yr:* REC 0.5 mg/kg, may repeat 4-12 hr later

Alcohol withdrawal
Adult: PO 10 mg tid-qid in 1st 24 hr, then 5 mg tid-qid; IM/**IV** 10 mg, then 5-10 mg after 3 hr

Available forms: Tabs 2, 5, 10 mg; caps ext rel 15 mg; inj emulsified 5 mg/ml; oral sol 5 mg/5 ml; gel, rectal delivery system 2.5, 5, 10, 15, 20 mg, twin packs

Adverse effects
(*italic* = common; **bold** = life-threatening)
CNS: *Dizziness, drowsiness,* confusion, headache, anxiety, tremors, stimulation, fatigue, depression, insomnia, hallucinations
CV: *Orthostatic hypotension,* **ECG changes, tachycardia,** hypotension
EENT: *Blurred vision,* tinnitus, mydriasis, nystagmus
GI: Constipation, dry mouth, nausea, vomiting, anorexia, diarrhea
HEMA: **Neutropenia**
INTEG: Rash, dermatitis, itching
RESP: **Respiratory depression**

Contraindications: Hypersensitivity to benzodiazepines, narrow-angle glaucoma, psychosis, pregnancy **D,** coma, respiratory
P depression, child <6 mo
G **Precautions:** Elderly, debilitated, hepatic disease, renal disease, addiction
N **Do Not Confuse:**
diazepam/Ditropan/lorazepam

Pharmacokinetics

Absorption	Rapid (PO); erratic (IM)
Distribution	Widely distributed; crosses blood-brain barrier, placenta
Metabolism	Liver, extensively
Excretion	Kidneys, breast milk
Half-life	20-80 hr

Pharmacodynamics

	PO	IM	IV
Onset	½ hr	15 min	Immediate
Peak	1-2 hr	½-1½ hr	15 min
Duration	2-3 hr	1-1½ hr	15 min-1 hr

Interactions
Individual drugs
Alcohol: ↑ CNS depression
Cimetidine, valproic acid: ↑ toxicity
Disulfiram, isoniazid, propranolol, valproic acid: ↓ metabolism of diazepam
Drug classifications
Barbiturates, CNS depressants, SSRIs: ↑ toxicity
CNS depressants: ↑ CNS depression
Opiates: ↓ diazepam effects
Oral contraceptives: ↓ metabolism of diazepam
⬛ *Herb/drug*
Cowslip, goldenseal, kava, melatonin, mistletoe, pokeweed, poppy, Queen Anne's lace, valerian: ↑ diazepam effect
Cola tree: ↓ diazepam effect
Lab test interferences
↑ AST/ALT, ↑ serum bilirubin
↓ Radioactive iodine uptake
False: ↑ 17-OHCS

NURSING CONSIDERATIONS
Assessment
• Assess degree of anxiety; what precipitates anxiety and whether drug controls symptoms; other signs of anxiety: dilated pupils, inability to sleep, restlessness, inability to focus
• Assess for alcohol withdrawal symptoms, including hallucinations (visual, auditory), delirium, irritability, agitation, fine to coarse tremors
• Monitor B/P (with patient lying, standing), pulse, respiratory rate; if systolic B/P drops 20 mm Hg, hold drug, notify prescriber; monitor respirations q5-15 min if given **IV**
• Monitor blood studies: CBC during long-term therapy; blood dyscrasias have occurred (rarely)
• Monitor for seizure control; type, duration, and intensity of seizures; what precipitates seizures
• Monitor hepatic studies: AST, ALT, bilirubin, creatinine, LDH, alkaline phosphatase
• Assess mental status: mood, sensorium, affect, sleeping pattern, drowsiness, dizziness, suicidal tendencies, and ability of drug to control these symptoms; check for tolerance, withdrawal symptoms: headache, nausea, vomiting, muscle pain, weakness after long-term use

Nursing diagnoses
✓ Anxiety (uses)
✓ Injury, risk for (uses, adverse reactions)
✓ Coping, ineffective (uses)
✓ Knowledge, deficient (teaching)
✓ Noncompliance (teaching)

Implementation
PO route
• Give with food or milk for GI symptoms; crush tab if patient is unable to swallow
🚫 medication whole; do not crush ext rel caps; use sugarless gum, hard candy, frequent sips of water for dry mouth
• Reduce opioid dosage by ⅓ if given concomitantly with diazepam
• Check to see PO medication has been swallowed
IV route
• Administer **IV** into large vein; do not dilute or mix with any other drug; give **IV** 5 mg or less/1 min or total dose over 3 min or more
🅿 (children, infants); cont inf is not recommended
• Check **IV** site for thrombosis or phlebitis, which may occur rapidly

Syringe compatibilities: Cimetidine

Syringe incompatibilities: Benzquinamide, doxapram, glycopyrrolate, heparin, nalbuphine

Y-site compatibilities: Cefmetazole, DOBUTamine, nafcillin, quinidine, sufentanil

Y-site incompatibilities: Hydromorphone, fluconazole, foscarnet, heparin, pancuronium, potassium chloride, vecuronium, vit B with C

Additive compatibilities: Netilmicin, verapamil
Sterile emulsion for injection
• Use **IV** only, within 6 hr, flush line after use and after 6 hr
Rectal route
• Do not use more than 5×/mo or for an episode q5 days

⬛ Herb/drug   🚫 Do Not Crush   ◆ Alert   ◆⚏ Key Drug   🅖 Geriatric   🅿 Pediatric

Patient/family education
- Advise patient that drug may be taken with food; that drug is not to be used for everyday stress or used longer than 4 mo unless directed by prescriber; take no more than prescribed amount; may be habit forming
- Caution patient to avoid OTC preparations unless approved by a prescriber; to avoid alcohol, other psychotropic medications unless prescribed; that smoking may decrease diazepam effect; not to discontinue medication abruptly after long-term use
- Inform patient to avoid driving, activities that require alertness; drowsiness may occur; to rise slowly or fainting may occur, especially 🅖 in elderly
- Advise patient not to become pregnant while using this drug
- Inform patient that drowsiness may worsen at beginning of treatment

Evaluation
Positive therapeutic outcome
- Decreased anxiety, restlessness, insomnia

Treatment of overdose: Lavage, VS, supportive care, flumazenil

---

diazoxide (Rx)
(dye-az-ox'ide)
Hyperstat IV, diazoxide parenteral
Func. class.: Antihypertensive
Chem. class.: Vasodilator

Pregnancy category C

Action: Decreases release of insulin from β-cells in pancreas, resulting in an increase in blood glucose; relaxes vascular smooth muscle (peripheral arterioles)

➡ **Therapeutic Outcome:** Decreased B/P, increased blood glucose

Uses: Hypoglycemia caused by hyperinsulinism; emergency treatment of hypertension

Dosage and routes
Hypoglycemia
🅟 **Adult and child:** PO 3-8 mg/kg/day in 2-3 divided doses q8-12h

🅟 **Infants and neonates:** PO 8-15 mg/kg/day in 2-3 divided doses 8-12h

Hypertension
Adult: IV bol 1-3 mg/kg rapidly up to a max of 150 mg in a single inj; dose may be repeated until desired response is achieved; give **IV** in 30 sec or less

🅟 **Child:** **IV** bol 1-2 mg/kg rapidly: administration same as adult, not to exceed 150 mg

Available forms: Caps 50 mg; oral susp 50 mg/ml; inj 15 mg/ml, 300 mg/20 ml

Adverse effects
(*italic* = common; **bold** = life-threatening)
CNS: Headache, weakness, malaise, anxiety, dizziness, insomnia, paresthesia, **seizures, cerebral ischemia, paralysis,** sleepiness, euphoria, anxiety, extrapyramidal symptoms (EPS), confusion, tinnitus, blurred vision, malaise
CV: Palpitations, hypotension, **shock, MI,** T-wave changes, angina pectoris, **supraventricular tachycardia, edema,** rebound hypertension
EENT: Diplopia, cataracts, ring scotoma, subconjunctival hemorrhage, lacrimation
ENDO: Hyperglycemia in diabetics, transient hyperglycemia in nondiabetics, increased uric acid
GI: Nausea, vomiting, dry mouth
GU: Reversible nephrotic syndrome, decreased urinary output, hematuria, breast tenderness, increased BUN, fluid, electrolyte imbalances, Na, water retention
HEMA: **Thrombocytopenia,** decreased Hgb, Hct
INTEG: Rash

Contraindications: Hypersensitivity to this drug or thiazides, sulfonamides, hypertension of aortic coarctation or AV shunt, pheochromocytoma, dissecting aortic aneurysm

Precautions: Pregnancy **C,** lactation, renal disease, diabetes mellitus, CV disease, gout

Pharmacokinetics
Absorption	Well absorbed (PO); completely absorbed (**IV**)
Distribution	Crosses blood-brain barrier, placenta, protein binding >90%
Metabolism	Liver (50%)
Excretion	Kidneys, unchanged (50%)
Half-life	20-36 hr

Pharmacodynamics
	PO	IV
Onset	1 hr	1-2 min
Peak	8-12 hr	5 min
Duration	8 hr	3-12 hr

Interactions
Individual drugs
Warfarin: ↑ effects
Drug classifications
Antihypertensives: severe hypotension

Diuretics (thiazides): ↑ hyperuricemic, antihypertensive effects of diazoxide
Hydantoins: ↓ anticonvulsant effect
Sulfonylureas: ↑ hyperglycemia

Herb/drug
Aconite: ↑ toxicity, death

NURSING CONSIDERATIONS
Assessment
• Assess for allergies to sulfonamide; cross-sensitivity may occur
• Assess B/P q5 min until stabilized
• Monitor electrolytes, blood studies: potassium, sodium, chloride, carbon dioxide, CBC, serum glucose
• Monitor weight daily, I&O; edema in feet, legs daily; check skin turgor, dryness of mucous membranes for hydration status
• Assess for rales, dyspnea, orthopnea; peripheral edema, fatigue, weight gain, jugular vein distention (CHF)
• Assess for signs of hyperglycemia: acetone breath, increased urinary output, severe thirst, lethargy, dizziness

Nursing diagnoses
✓ Cardiac output, decreased (adverse reactions)
✓ Injury, risk for (side effects)
✓ Knowledge, deficient (teaching)

Implementation
PO route
• Shake susp before using
• Store protected from light and heat
IV IV route
• Give by direct **IV** over 30 sec or less; may repeat q5-15 min until desired response; do not administer dark solution
• Give to patient in recumbent position; keep in that position for 1 hr after

Syringe compatibility: Heparin

Y-site incompatibilities: Hydralazine, propranolol

Evaluation
Positive therapeutic outcome
• Decreased B/P in hypertension

Treatment of overdose: Administer levarterenol, DOPamine, or norepinephrine for hypotension, dialysis

---

diclofenac potassium (Rx)
(dye-kloe'fen-ak)
Cataflam, Voltaren Rapide ✦
diclofenac sodium
Apo-Dilo ✦, Novo-Difenac ✦, Nu-Diclo, Voltaren, Voltaren XR
Func. class.: Nonsteroidal antiinflammatory (NSAIDs), nonopioid analgesic
Chem. class.: Phenylacetic acid

Pregnancy category B

Action: Inhibits prostaglandin synthesis by decreasing enzyme needed for biosynthesis; analgesic, antiinflammatory, antipyretic properties

➔**Therapeutic Outcome:** Decreased pain, inflammation

Uses: Acute, chronic rheumatoid arthritis, osteoarthritis, ankylosing spondylitis, analgesia, primary dysmenorrhea

Dosage and routes
Osteoarthritis
Adult: PO 100-150 mg/day in 2-3 divided doses

Rheumatoid arthritis
Adult: PO 100-200 mg/day in 2-4 divided doses (potassium); 50 mg tid-qid, then reduce to lowest dose needed (25 mg tid) (sodium)

Ankylosing spondylitis
Adult: PO 100-125 mg/day in 4-5 divided doses; give 25 mg qid and 25 mg hs if needed (potassium)

Postcataract surgery
Adult: Ophth 1 gtt of 0.1% sol qid × 2 wk 24 hr postsurgery

Analgesia/primary dysmenorrhea
Adult: PO 50 mg tid, max 150 mg/day (potassium)

Available forms: Potassium: tabs 50, 75 mg; sodium: tabs delayed rel (enteric-coated) 25, 50, 75 mg; ext rel tabs 75, 100 mg; supp 50, 100 mg

Adverse effects
(*italic* = common; **bold** = life-threatening)
CNS: Dizziness, headache, drowsiness, fatigue, tremors, confusion, insomnia, anxiety, depression, nervousness, paresthesia, muscle weakness
CV: **CHF,** tachycardia, peripheral edema, palpitations, dysrhythmias, hypotension, hypertension, fluid retention
EENT: Tinnitus, hearing loss, blurred vision, **laryngeal edema**
GI: Nausea, anorexia, vomiting, diarrhea,

---

jaundice, **cholestatic hepatitis**, constipation, flatulence, cramps, dry mouth, peptic ulcer, GI bleeding, **hepatotoxicity**
GU: **Nephrotoxicity: dysuria, hematuria, oliguria, azotemia, cystitis, UTI**
HEMA: **Blood dyscrasias**, epistaxis, bruising
INTEG: Purpura, rash, pruritus, sweating, erythema, petechiae, photosensitivity, alopecia
RESP: Dyspnea, hemoptysis, pharyngitis, **bronchospasm, laryngeal edema,** rhinitis, shortness of breath
SYST: Anaphylaxis

Contraindications: Hypersensitivity to aspirin, iodides, other NSAIDs, asthma, pregnancy (3rd trimester)

Precautions: Pregnancy **B** (1st trimester), not recommended in 2nd half of pregnancy, lactation, children, bleeding disorders, GI disorders, cardiac disorders, hypersensitivity to other antiinflammatory agents, CCr <30 ml/min

◼ Do Not Confuse:
Cataflam/Catapres

Pharmacokinetics

Absorption	Well absorbed (PO, ophth)
Distribution	Crosses placenta; 90% bound to plasma proteins
Metabolism	Liver (50%)
Excretion	Breast milk
Half-life	1-2 hr

Pharmacodynamics

	PO	OPHTH
Onset	Unknown	Unknown
Peak	2-3 hr	Unknown
Duration	Unknown	Unknown

Interactions
Individual drugs
Aspirin: ↑ GI side effects
Cyclosporine, lithium, methotrexate, phenytoin: ↑ toxicity
Drug classifications
Anticoagulants: ↑ risk of bleeding
Antidiabetics: ↑ need for dosage adjustment
β-blockers, diuretics: ↓ antihypertensive effect
Diuretics (potassium-sparing): Hyperkalemia
NSAIDs: ↑ GI side effects, adverse reactions
Herb/drug
Arginine, gossypol: ↑ gastric irritation
Bearberry, bilberry: ↑ NSAIDs effect
Bogbean, chondroitin, saw palmetto, turmeric: ↑ bleeding risk
St. John's wort: ↑ severe photosensitivity

NURSING CONSIDERATIONS
Assessment
• Assess for pain of rheumatoid arthritis, osteoarthritis, ankylosing spondylitis; check ROM, inflammation of joints, characteristics of pain
• Assess ophth patients for pain, inflammation, redness, swelling
◆• Monitor blood counts during therapy; watch for decreasing platelets; if low, therapy may need to be discontinued, restarted after hematologic recovery
• Assess for asthma, aspirin hypersensitivity, nasal polyps; may develop hypersensitivity
• Monitor liver function tests (may be elevated) and uric acid (may be decreased—serum; increased—urine) periodically; also BUN, creatinine, electrolytes (may be elevated)
◆• Monitor for blood dyscrasias (thrombocytopenia): bruising, fatigue, bleeding, poor healing

Nursing diagnoses
☑ Pain, chronic (uses)
☑ Mobility, impaired physical (uses)
☑ Injury, risk for (side effects)
☑ Knowledge, deficient (teaching)

Implementation
PO route
• Administer with food or milk to decrease gastric symptoms;
🚫• Do not crush, dissolve, or chew enteric coated or sus rel caps
Ophthalmic route
• Administer with patient recumbent or tilting head back; pull down on lower lid; when conjunctival sac is exposed, instill 1 drop; wait a few minutes before instilling other drops

Patient/family education
• Teach patient that drug must be continued for prescribed time to be effective; to avoid aspirin, NSAIDs, acetaminophen, or other OTC medications unless approved by prescriber, alcoholic beverages; to contact prescriber before surgery regarding when to discontinue this drug
• Caution patient to report bleeding, bruising, fatigue, malaise, since blood dyscrasias do occur
• Advise patient to report hepatotoxicity: flulike symptoms, nausea, vomiting, jaundice, pruritus, lethargy
• Instruct patient to use sunscreen to prevent photosensitivity
• Teach patient to avoid use in 3rd trimester of pregnancy
• Instruct patient to use caution when driving; drowsiness, dizziness may occur

• Teach patient to take with a full glass of water to enhance absorption; remain upright for ½ hr; if dose is missed, take as soon as remembered within 2 hr if taking 1-2 ×/day, do not double doses; do not crush, break, or chew

Evaluation
Positive therapeutic outcome
• Decreased pain in arthritic conditions
• Decreased inflammation in arthritic conditions
• Decreased ocular irritation

---

dicloxacillin (Rx)
(dye-klox-a-sill'in)
dicloxacillin sodium, Dycill, Dynapen, Pathocil
Func. class.: Antiinfective
Chem. class.: Penicillinase-resistant penicillin

Pregnancy category B

Action: Interferes with cell wall replication of susceptible organisms; osmotically unstable cell wall swells, bursts from osmotic pressure

➡ **Therapeutic Outcome:** Bactericidal effects for the following: gram-positive cocci *Staphylococcus aureus, Streptococcus pyogenes, Streptococcus viridans, Streptococcus faecalis, Streptococcus bovis, Streptococcus pneumoniae;* infections caused by penicillinase-producing *Staphylococcus* organisms

Uses: Penicillinase-producing staphylococci, streptococci; respiratory tract, skin, skin structure infections; sinusitis

Dosage and routes
P *Adult and Child ≥40 kg:* PO 0.5-4 g/day in divided doses q6h, max 4 g/day

P *Child ≤40 kg:* PO 12.5-50 mg/kg in divided doses q6h, max 4 g/d

Available forms: Caps 125, 250, 500 mg; powder for oral susp 62.5 mg/5 ml

Adverse effects
(*italic* = common; **bold** = life-threatening)
CNS: Lethargy, hallucinations, anxiety, depression, twitching, **coma, seizures**
GI: Nausea, vomiting, diarrhea, increased AST, ALT, abdominal pain, glossitis, pseudomembranous colitis
GU: **Oliguria, proteinuria, hematuria, vaginitis, moniliasis, glomerulonephritis**
HEMA: Anemia, increased bleeding time, **bone marrow depression, granulocytopenia**
SYST: **Anaphylaxis**

Contraindications: Hypersensitivity to **P** penicillins; neonates

Precautions: Hypersensitivity to cephalosporins, pregnancy **B**, severe renal or hepatic disease

Do Not Confuse:
Pathocil/Bactocil

Pharmacokinetics	
Absorption	Rapid, incomplete (35%-75%)
Distribution	Widely distributed; crosses placenta
Metabolism	Liver (6%-10%)
Excretion	Kidneys, unchanged (60%); breast milk
Half-life	½-1 hr, increased in hepatic renal disease

Pharmacodynamics	
Onset	½ hr
Peak	½-2 hr

Interactions
Individual drugs
Aspirin: ↑ dicloxacillin concentrations
Probenecid: ↑ dicloxacillin levels
Drug classifications
Oral anticoagulants: ↓ anticoagulant effects
Oral contraceptives: ↑ dicloxacillin concentration
Food/drug
Food, carbonated drinks, citrus fruit juices: ↓ absorption
Herb/drug
Acidophilus: Do not use with antiinfectives
Khat: ↓ absorption; separate by 2 hr
Lab test interferences
False positive: Urine glucose, urine protein

NURSING CONSIDERATIONS
Assessment
• Assess patient for previous sensitivity reaction to penicillins or other cephalosporins; cross-sensitivity between penicillins and cephalosporins is common
• Assess patient for signs and symptoms of infection including characteristics of wounds, sputum, urine, stool, WBC >10,000/mm³, fever; obtain baseline information and during treatment
• Obtain C&S before beginning drug therapy to identify if correct treatment has been initiated
• Assess for anaphylaxis: rash, urticaria,

---

pruritus, chills, fever, joint pain may occur a few days after therapy begins; epINEPHrine and resuscitation equipment should be available for anaphylactic reaction

◆• Identify urine output; if decreasing, notify prescriber (may indicate nephrotoxicity); check for increased BUN, creatinine
• Monitor blood studies: AST, ALT, CBC, Hct, bilirubin, LDH, alkaline phosphatase, Coombs' test monthly if patient is on long-term therapy
• Monitor electrolytes: potassium, sodium, chloride monthly if patient is on long-term therapy
• Assess bowel pattern qd; if severe diarrhea occurs, drug should be discontinued; may indicate pseudomembranous colitis
• Monitor for bleeding: ecchymosis, bleeding gums, hematuria, stool guaiac daily if on long-term therapy
• Assess for overgrowth of infection: perineal itching, fever, malaise, redness, pain, swelling, drainage, rash, diarrhea, change in cough, sputum

Nursing diagnoses
☑ Infection, risk for (uses)
☑ Diarrhea (side effects)
☑ Knowledge, deficient (teaching)
☑ Noncompliance (teaching)
☑ Injury, risk for (side effects)

Implementation
• Give in even doses around the clock; if GI upset occurs, give with food; drug must be given for 10-14 days to ensure organism death and prevent superinfection; store in airtight container
🚫• Do not crush, chew caps
• Shake susp well before each dose; store in refrigerator for 2 wk or 1 wk at room temp

Patient/family education
• Teach patient to report sore throat, bruising, bleeding, joint pain; may indicate blood dyscrasias (rare)
• Advise patient to contact prescriber if vaginal itching, loose, foul-smelling stools, furry tongue occur; may indicate superinfection
• Instruct patient to take all medication prescribed for the length of time ordered, carry/wear emergency ID if allergic to penicillins
• Advise patient to notify prescriber of diarrhea with blood or pus, which may indicate pseudomembranous colitis

Evaluation
Positive therapeutic outcome
• Absence of signs/symptoms of infection

(WBC <10,000/mm^3, temp WNL, absence of red draining wounds)
• Reported improvement in symptoms of infection

Treatment of anaphylaxis: Withdraw drug, maintain airway, administer epINEPHrine, aminophylline, O$_2$, **IV** corticosteroids

D

---

didanosine (Rx)
(dye-dan'oh-seen)
DDL, dideoxyinosine, Videx, Videx EC
Func. class.: Antiretroviral
Chem. class.: Synthetic purine nucleoside reverse transcriptase inhibitor

Pregnancy category B

Action: Nucleoside analog incorporating into cellular DNA by viral reverse transcriptase, thereby terminating the cellular DNA chain that prevents viral replication

➡ **Therapeutic Outcome:** Antiviral against the retroviruses, primarily HIV

Uses: HIV infection in combination with other antiretrovirals

Dosage and routes
Renal dose
Adult: PO reduce dosage CCr <60 ml/min

Adult: PO >60 kg, 200 mg bid tabs, or 250 mg bid buffered powder; caps, del rel 400 mg qd; <60 kg, 125 mg bid tabs, or 167 mg bid buffered powder; caps del rel 250 mg qd

🅟 *Child:* PO tabs 90-120 mg/m^2 q12h; buffered powder packets 112.5-150 mg/m^2 q12h; PO (child BSA 1.1-1.4 m^2) tab 100 mg q8-12h; reconstituted pediatric powder 125 mg q8-12h; PO (child BSA 0.8-1 m^2) tabs 75 mg q8-12h; reconstituted pediatric powder 94 mg q8-12h; PO (child BSA 0.5-0.7 m^2) tabs 50 mg q8-12h; reconstituted pediatric powder 62 mg q8-12h; PO (child BSA <0.4 m^2) tabs 25 mg q8-12h; reconstituted pediatric powder 31 mg q8-12h

Available forms: Tabs, buffered, chewable/dispersible 25, 50, 100, 150 mg; powder for oral sol, buffered 100, 167, 250, 375 mg/packet; powder for oral sol, pediatric 10 mg, 20 mg/ml; caps del rel 125, 200, 250, 400

Adverse effects
(*italic* = common; **bold** = life-threatening)
CNS: **Peripheral neuropathy, seizures,** confusion, *anxiety,* hypertonia, abnormal

---

thinking, asthenia, *insomnia, CNS depression,* pain, dizziness, chills, fever
CV: Hypertension, vasodilatation, **dysrhythmia,** syncope, **CHF,** palpitations
EENT: Ear pain, otitis, photophobia, visual impairment, retinal depigmentation
GI: **Pancreatitis,** *diarrhea, nausea,* vomiting, *abdominal pain,* constipation, stomatitis, dyspepsia, liver abnormalities, flatulence, taste perversion, dry mouth, oral thrush, melena, increased ALT, AST, alkaline phosphatase, amylase, **hepatic failure**
GU: Increased bilirubin, uric acid
HEMA: **Leukopenia, granulocytopenia, thrombocytopenia, anemia**
INTEG: Rash, *pruritus,* alopecia, ecchymosis, hemorrhage, petechiae, sweating
MS: Myalgia, arthritis, myopathy, muscular atrophy
RESP: Cough, pneumonia, dyspnea, asthma, epistaxis, hypoventilation, sinusitis
SYST: **Lactic acidosis, anaphylaxis**

Contraindications: Hypersensitivity

Precautions: Renal, hepatic disease, pregnancy **B,** lactation, children, sodium-restricted diets, elevated amylase, preexistent peripheral neuropathy, phenylketonuria, hyperuricemia

Pharmacokinetics

Absorption	Rapidly absorbed (up to 40%)
Distribution	Unknown
Metabolism	Not metabolized
Excretion	Kidneys (55%)
Half-life	0.8-1.6 hr, shorter in children

Pharmacodynamics

Onset	Unknown
Peak	Up to 1 hr, del rel 2 hr
Duration	Unknown

Interactions
Individual drugs
Allopurinol, tenofovir: ↑ didanosine level
Dapsone, itraconazole, ketoconazole: ↓ absorption of each specific drug
Disopyramide: ↑ anticholinergic effects
Drug classifications
Antacids, magnesium, aluminum: ↑ side effects
Antiretrovirals, other: ↓ concentration
Fluoroquinolones, tetracyclines: ↓ absorption of each specific drug

Food/drug
↓ Absorption
• Do not use with acidic juices

NURSING CONSIDERATIONS
Assessment
• Assess for peripheral neuropathy: tingling or pain in hands and feet, distal numbness; onset usually occurs 2-6 mo after beginning treatment, if these occur during therapy, drug may be decreased or discontinued
• Assess for pancreatitis: abdominal pain, nausea, vomiting, elevated liver enzymes; drug should be discontinued, since condition can be fatal
• Assess children by dilated retinal examination q6 mo to rule out retinal depigmentation
• Monitor CBC, differential, platelet count monthly; withhold drug if WBC is <4000/mm³ or platelet count is <75,000 mm³, viral load, CD4⁺ count; notify prescriber of results
• Monitor renal function studies: BUN, serum uric acid, urine CCr before, during therapy; these may be elevated throughout treatment
• Assess for anaphylaxis, lactic acidosis
• Monitor temp q4h; may indicate beginning of infection
• Monitor liver function tests before, during therapy (bilirubin, AST, ALT, amylase, alkaline phosphatase) as needed or monthly

Nursing diagnoses
✓ Infection, risk for (uses)
✓ Injury, risk for (adverse reactions)
✓ Knowledge, deficient (teaching)

Implementation
• Give on empty stomach, 1 hr ac or 2 hr pc, q12h; food decreases effectiveness of drug; adjust dose in renal impairment
• Patient should chew tabs; may be crushed and mixed with water
• Pediatric powder for oral sol should be prepared in the pharmacy; shake before using
• Packets for oral sol must be mixed with ½ glass of water; stir until dissolved
• Store tabs, caps in tightly closed bottle at room temp; store oral sol after dissolving at room temp ≤4 hr

Patient/family education
• Advise patient to take on empty stomach; not to take dapsone at same time as DDL; not to mix powder with fruit juice; to chew tab or crush and dissolve in water; to drink powder immediately after mixing; to use exactly as prescribed
• Instruct patient to report signs of infection: increased temp, sore throat, flulike symptoms; to avoid crowds and those with known infections

---

 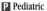

- Instruct patient to report signs of anemia: fatigue, headache, faintness, shortness of breath, irritability
- Advise patient to report numbness/tingling in extremities
- Instruct patient to report bleeding; avoid use of razors and commercial mouthwash
- Advise patient that hair may be lost during therapy; a wig or hairpiece may make patient feel better
- Caution patient to avoid OTC products and other medications without approval of prescriber; to avoid alcohol
- Teach patient not to have any sexual contact without use of a condom; needles should not be shared; blood from infected individual should not come in contact with another's mucous membranes

Evaluation
Positive therapeutic outcome
- Absence of opportunistic infection, symptoms of HIV

---

difenoxin with atropine
See diphenoxylate with atropine

! HIGH ALERT

digoxin ⊖π (Rx)
(di-jox'in)
digoxin, Lanoxicaps, Lanoxin
Func. class.: Inotropic antidysrhythmic, cardiac glycoside
Chem. class.: Digitalis preparation

Pregnancy category C

Action: Inhibits sodium-potassium ATPase, which makes more calcium available for contractile proteins, resulting in increased cardiac output; increases force of contraction (positive inotropic effect); decreases heart rate (chronotropic effect); decreases AV conduction speed

▸Therapeutic Outcome: Decreased edema, pulse, respiration, rales

Uses: Rapid digitalization in acute and chronic CHF, atrial fibrillation, atrial flutter, atrial tachycardia; cardiogenic shock, paroxysmal atrial tachycardia

Dosage and routes
Adult: **IV** *digitalizing dose* 0.6-1.0 mg given as 50% of the dose initially, additional fractions given at 4-8 hr intervals; PO *digitalizing dose* 0.75-1.25 mg given as 50% of the dose ini-

tially, additional fractions given at 4-8 hr intervals; *maintenance* 0.063-0.5 mg/day (tabs), or 0.350-0.5 mg/day (gelatin cap)

P *Child >10 yr:* **IV** *digitalizing dose* 8-12 mcg/kg given as 50% of the dose initially, additional fractions given at 4-8 hr intervals; PO *digitalizing dose* 0.01-0.015 mg/kg given as 50% of the dose initially, additional fractions given at 6-8 hr intervals; maintenance 25%-35% of the loading dose qd as a single dose

P *Child 5-10 yr:* **IV** *digitalizing dose* 0.015-0.03 mg/kg given as 50% of the dose initially, additional fractions given at 4-8 hr intervals; PO *digitalizing dose* 0.02-0.035 mg/kg given as 50% of the dose initially, additional fractions given at 6-8 hr intervals; *maintenance* 25%-35% of the loading dose qd in 2 divided doses

P *Child 2-5 yr:* **IV** *digitalizing dose* 0.025-0.035 mg/kg given as 50% of the dose initially, additional fractions given at 4-8 hr intervals; PO *digitalizing dose* 0.03-0.04 mg/kg given as 50% of the dose initially, additional fractions given at 6-8 hr intervals; *maintenance* 25%-35% of the loading dose qd in 2 divided doses

P *Child 1-2 yr:* **IV** *digitalizing dose* 0.03-0.05 mg/kg given as 50% of the dose initially, additional fractions given at 4-8 hr intervals; PO *digitalizing dose* 0.035-0.06 mg/kg given as 50% of the dose initially, additional fractions given at 4-8 hr intervals; *maintenance* 25%-35% of the loading dose qd in 2 divided doses

P *Infants:* **IV** *digitalizing dose* 0.02-0.03 mg/kg given as 50% of the dose initially, additional fractions given at 4-8 hr intervals; PO *digitalizing dose* 0.025-0.035 mg/kg given as 50% of the dose initially, additional fractions given at 6-8 hr intervals; *maintenance* 25%-35% of the loading dose qd in 2 divided doses

P *Infants, premature:* **IV** *digitalizing dose* 0.015-0.025 mg/kg given as 50% of the dose initially, additional fractions given at 4-8 hr intervals; PO *digitalizing dose* 0.02-0.03 mg/kg given as 50% of the dose initially, additional fractions given at 6-8 hr intervals; *maintenance* 20%-30% of the loading dose qd in 2 divided doses

Available forms: Caps 0.05, 0.1, 0.2 mg; elix 0.05 mg/ml; tabs 0.125, 0.25, 0.5 mg; inj 0.5 ✤, 0.25 mg/ml; pediatric inj 0.1 mg/ml

Adverse effects
(*italic* = common; **bold** = life-threatening)
CNS: **Headache**, drowsiness, apathy, confusion, disorientation, fatigue, depression, hallucinations

---

CV: **Dysrhythmias, hypotension,** bradycardia, **AV block**
EENT: Blurred vision, yellow-green halos, photophobia, diplopia
GI: Nausea, vomiting, anorexia, abdominal pain, diarrhea

Contraindications: Hypersensitivity to digitalis, ventricular fibrillation, ventricular tachycardia, carotid sinus syndrome, 2nd- or 3rd-degree heart block

Precautions: Renal disease, acute MI, AV block, severe respiratory disease, hypothyroidism, elderly, pregnancy **C**, sinus nodal disease, lactation, hypokalemia

Do Not Confuse:
Lanoxin/Lasix/Lonox,
Lanoxin/Lomotil,
Lanoxin/Xanax/Levoxine

Pharmacokinetics

Absorption	Unknown
Distribution	Widely distributed; 20%-25% protein bound
Metabolism	Liver, small amount; also intestinal bacteria
Excretion	Urine
Half-life	1½ days

Pharmacodynamics

	PO	IV
Onset	½-1½ hr	5-30 min
Peak	2-6 hr	1-5 hr
Duration	After steady state	6-8 days

Interactions
Individual drugs
Amiodarone: ↑ digoxin levels, bradycardia
Amphotericin B, carbenicillin, ticarcillin: ↑ hypokalemia
Amphotericin B, propafenone: ↑ toxicity
Calcium IV: ↑ hypercalcemia, hypomagnesemia, digoxin toxicity
Carbenicillin, ticarcillin: Digitalis toxicity
Cholestyramine, colestipol, metoclopramide, thyroid hormones: ↓ digoxin levels
Diltiazem: ↑ blood levels
Kaolin/pectin: ↓ absorption
Nifedipine, propafenone, quinidine, verapamil: ↑ digoxin levels
Verapamil: ↓ positive inotropic effect
Drug classifications
Antacids: ↓ digoxin absorption
Anticholinergics: ↑ digoxin blood levels
Antidysrhythmics, β-adrenergic blockers: ↑ bradycardia

Diuretics (thiazide): ↑ hypokalemia, hypercalcemia, hypomagnesemia, digitalis toxicity
Sympathomimetics: ↑ cardiac dysrhythmia risk
Herb/drug
Aconite, hawthorn, horsetail: ↑ toxicity
Aloe, betel palm, broom, buckthorn, cascara sagrada castor, Chinese rhubarb, figwort, fumitory, hawthorn, khat, licorice, lily of the valley, Mayapple, mistletoe, motherwort, night blooming cereus, oleander, pheasant's eye, purple foxglove, Queen Anne's lace, rhubarb, rue, senna, Siberian ginseng, squill, yellow dock : ↑ digoxin action
Bethroot, goldenseal: ↓ digoxin effect
Blackroot: Forms insoluble complex
Cocoa, cola, guarana, horsetail, licorice, yerba maté: ↑ hypokalemia
Indian snakeroot: ↑ bradycardia
Psyllium: ↓ digoxin absorption
Lab test interferences
↑ CPK

NURSING CONSIDERATIONS
Assessment
• Assess and document apical pulse for 1 min before giving drug; if pulse <60 in adult or <90 in an infant or is significantly different, take again in 1 hr; if <60 in adult, call prescriber; note rate, rhythm, character
• Monitor electrolytes: potassium, sodium, chloride, magnesium, calcium; renal function studies: BUN, creatinine; other blood studies: ALT, AST, bilirubin, Hct, Hgb, drug levels (therapeutic level 0.5-2 ng/ml) before initiating treatment and periodically thereafter
• Monitor I&O ratio, daily weights; monitor turgor, lung sounds, edema
• Monitor cardiac status: apical pulse, character, rate, rhythm; resolution of atrial dysrhythmias by ECG; if tachydysrhythmia develops, hold drug; delay cardioversion while drug levels are determined
• Monitor ECG continuously during parenteral loading doses and for patients with suspected toxicity; provide hemodynamic monitoring for patients with heart failure or administer multiple cardiac drugs
Nursing diagnoses
☑ Cardiac output, decreased (uses)
☑ Gas exchange, impaired (adverse reactions)
☑ Knowledge, deficient (teaching)
Implementation
• Do not give at same time as antacids or other drugs that decrease absorption
PO route
• Give PO with or without food; may crush tabs

• Give potassium supplements if ordered for potassium levels <3, or give foods high in potassium: bananas, orange juice

IV **IV route**
• Give **IV** undiluted or 1 ml of drug/4 ml sterile water, D_5, or 0.9% NaCl; give over >5 min through Y-tube or 3-way stopcock; during digitalization close monitoring is necessary
• Store protected from light

Syringe compatibilities: Heparin, milrinone

Syringe incompatibility: Doxapram

Y-site compatibilities: Amrinone, cefmetazole, ciprofloxacin, cisatracurium, diltiazem, famotidine, meperidine, meropenem, midazolam, milrinone, morphine, potassium chloride, propofol, remifentanil, tacrolimus, vit B/C

Y-site incompatibilities: Fluconazole, foscarnet

Additive compatibilities: Bretylium, cimetidine, floxacillin, furosemide, lidocaine, ranitidine, verapamil

Additive incompatibility: Dobutamine

Patient/family education
• Caution patient to avoid OTC medications including cough, cold, allergy preparations, antacids, since many adverse drug interactions may occur; do not take antacid at same time
• Instruct patient to notify prescriber of any loss of appetite, lower stomach pain, diarrhea, weakness, drowsiness, headache, blurred or yellow-green vision, rash, depression; teach toxic symptoms of this drug and when to notify prescriber
• Advise patient to maintain a sodium-restricted diet as ordered; to take potassium supplements as ordered to prevent toxicity
• Instruct patient to report shortness of breath, difficulty breathing, weight gain, edema, persistent cough
• Teach patient purpose of drug is to regulate the heart's functioning
• Teach patient as outpatient to check and record pulse for 1 min before taking dose; if there is a change of >15 bpm from usual pulse, prescriber should be notified
• Teach patient to take medication at the same time each day, take missed doses within 12 hr; do not double doses; notify prescriber if doses are missed for 2 days or more; how to monitor heart rate

• Advise patient to carry/wear emergency ID describing dosage and reason for digoxin

Evaluation
Positive therapeutic outcome
• Decreased weight, edema, pulse, respiration, rales
• Increased urine output
• Serum digoxin level 0.5-2 ng/ml

D

Treatment of overdose: Discontinue drug, administer potassium, monitor ECG, administer an adrenergic blocking agent, digoxin immune Fab

---

digoxin immune Fab (ovine) ⚷π (Rx)
(di-jox'in)
Digibind
Func. class.: Antidote, digoxin specific
Pregnancy category C

Action: Antibody fragments bind to free digoxin or to reverse toxicity by not allowing digoxin or digitoxin to bind to sites of action

➔**Therapeutic Outcome:** Correction of digoxin toxicity

Uses: Reversal of life-threatening digoxin or digitoxin toxicity, including severe bradycardia, ventricular tachycardia/fibrillation, severe hypertension

Dosage and routes
Digoxin toxicity (known amount) (tabs, oral sol, IM)
P *Adult/child:* **IV** dose (mg) = dose ingested (mg) $\times$ 0.8/1000 $\times$ 38; if ingested amount is unknown, give 760 mg **IV**

Toxicity (known amount) (cap, IV)
P *Adult/child:* **IV** dose = dose ingested (mg)/0.5 $\times$ 38

Toxicity (known amount) by serum digoxin concentrations (SDCs)
P *Adult/child:* **IV** SDC (nanograms/ml) $\times$ kg of weight/100 $\times$ 38

Skin test
Adult: **ID** 9.5 mcg

Available forms: Inj 38 mg/vial (binds 0.5 mg of digoxin), 40 mg/vial (binds 0.5 mg digoxin)

Adverse effects
(*italic* = common; **bold** = life-threatening)
CV: **Worsening of CHF,** *ventricular rate increase,* **atrial fibrillation,** *low cardiac output*

INTEG: *Hypersensitivity,* allergic reactions, facial swelling, redness
META: *Hypokalemia*
MISC: **Anaphylaxis** (rare)
RESP: **Impaired respiratory function, rapid respiratory rate**

Contraindications: Mild digoxin toxicity, hypersensitivity to this product or papain

P **Precautions:** Children, lactation, cardiac disease, renal disease, pregnancy **C**, allergy to **G** ovine proteins, elderly

Pharmacokinetics

Absorption	Complete
Distribution	Widely distributed into plasma, interstitial fluids
Metabolism	Unknown
Excretion	Kidneys
Half-life	Biphasic (14-20 hr); increased in renal disease

Pharmacodynamics

Onset	30 min (variable)
Peak	Unknown
Duration	Unknown

Interactions
Individual drugs
Digitoxin, digoxin, lanatoside C: ↓ effect of each specific drug
Lab test interferences
Interference: Immunoassay (digoxin)

NURSING CONSIDERATIONS
Assessment
• Assess for hypokalemia: ST depression, flat T waves, presence of U wave, ventricular dysrhythmias
• Obtain information on previous allergies: previous exposure to sheep (ovine) proteins; scratch test may be performed before use of this product; hypersensitive reactions are more common in persons with previous exposure
• Monitor VS before, during, and after infusion
• Monitor heart rate, B/P q10 min during inf and after completion until stabilized; hemodynamic monitoring is used for unstable or hypotensive patients; check potassium levels until toxicity is resolved
• Assess for oxygen or perfusion deficit: hypotension, chest pain, dizziness, loss of consciousness
• Assess respiratory status: auscultate lung fields for bibasilar crackles in patients with advanced CHF

Nursing diagnoses
☑ Injury, risk for (uses)
☑ Knowledge, deficient (teaching)

Implementation
• Test doses have proven to be ineffective in the general population; only use test dose in those with known allergies or those previously treated with digoxin immune FAB
• For test dose dilute 0.1 ml or reconstituted drug (9.5 mg/ml) in 9.9 ml sterile isotonic saline, inj 0.1 ml (1:100 dilution) ID and observe for wheal with erythema; read in 20 min
• For scratch test place 1 gtt of sol on skin and make a scratch through the drop with a sterile needle; read in 20 min
• Give after diluting 40 mg/4 ml of sterile water (10 mg/ml), mix gently; may be further diluted with 0.9% NaCl; sol should be clear, colorless
• Give by bol if cardiac arrest is imminent or **IV** over 30 min using a 0.22-μm filter
• Store reconstituted sol for up to 4 hr in refrigerator; do not freeze DigiFab

Patient/family education
• Teach that purpose of medication is to bind excess digoxin and reduce high blood levels
• Instruct patients to report fever, chills, itching, sweating, dyspnea, delayed hypersensitivity
• Advise other prescribers that this medication has been used previously

Evaluation
Positive therapeutic outcome
• Correction of digoxin toxicity
• Digoxin blood level 0.5-2 ng/ml
• Digitoxin blood level 9-25 ng/ml

---

dihydroergotamine
See ergotamine

---

dihydrotachysterol (Rx)
(dye-hye-droh-tak-iss'ter-ole)
DHT Intensol ✦, Hytakerol
Func. class.: Parathyroid agent (calcium regulator)
Chem. class.: Vitamin D analog

Pregnancy category C

Action: Increases intestinal absorption of calcium, increases renal tubular absorption of phosphorus; is able to regulate calcium levels by regulation of calcitonin, parathyroid hormone

→ **Therapeutic Outcome:** Prevention of continued calcium loss in bones

Uses: Renal osteodystrophy, hypoparathyroidism, pseudohypoparathyroidism, familial hypophosphatemia, postoperative tetany

Investigational uses: Renal osteodystrophy

Dosage and routes
Hypophosphatemia
🅟 **Adult and child:** PO 0.5-2 mg qd; maintenance 0.2-1.5 mg qd

*Hypoparathyroidism/
pseudohypoparathyroidism*
Adult: PO 0.8-2.4 mg qd × 4 days, maintenance 0.2-2 mg qd regulated by serum calcium levels

🅟 **Neonates:** PO 0.05-0.1 mg/day

🅟 **Infants-young child:** PO 0.1-0.5 mg/day

🅟 **Older child:** PO 0.5-1 mg/day

Renal osteodystrophy
Adult: PO 0.25-0.375 mg/day

🅟 **Child:** PO 0.125-0.5 mg/day

Rickets (vit D resistant)
🅟 **Child:** PO 0.25-1 mg/day

Available forms: Tab 0.125, 0.2, 0.4 mg; cap 0.125 mg; oral sol 0.2, 0.25 mg/5 ml, 0.2 mg/ml ♣ (Intensol)

Adverse effects
(*italic* = common; **bold** = life-threatening)
CNS: Drowsiness, headache, vertigo, fever, lethargy, depression
CV: **Dysrhythmias,** hypertension
EENT: Tinnitus
GI: Nausea, diarrhea, vomiting, jaundice, anorexia, dry mouth, constipation, cramps, metallic taste, thirst
GU: **Polyuria,** hypercalciuria, hyperphosphatemia, **hematuria,** nocturia, renal calculi
MS: Myalgia, arthralgia, decreased bone development, weakness, ataxia

Contraindications: Hypersensitivity, renal disease, hyperphosphatemia, hypercalcemia

Precautions: Pregnancy **C**, renal calculi, lactation, CV disease

Pharmacokinetics

Absorption	Well absorbed from small intestine
Distribution	Liver, fat
Metabolism	Liver
Excretion	Feces (inactive, active metabolites)
Half-life	Unknown

Pharmacodynamics

Onset	2 wk
Peak	2 wk
Duration	2 wk

Interactions
Individual drugs
Cholestyramine, colestipol, mineral oil: ↓ absorption of dihydrotachysterol
Phenytoin: ↓ effect of dihydrotachysterol
Verapamil: ↑ dysrhythmias
Drug classifications
Barbiturates, corticosteroids: ↓ effect of dihydrotachysterol
Calcium supplements, diuretics (thiazide): ↑ hypercalcemia
Cardiac glycosides: ↑ dysrhythmias
Lab test interferences
False: ↑ cholesterol

NURSING CONSIDERATIONS
Assessment
● Monitor BUN, urinary calcium, AST, ALT, cholesterol, alkaline phosphatase, creatinine, uric acid, chloride, magnesium, electrolytes, urine pH, phosphate; may increase calcium; should be kept at 9-10 mg/dl; keep vit D at 50-135 international units/dl, phosphate at 70 mg/dl; these tests should be checked before and throughout treatment
● Monitor for increased blood level, since toxic reaction may occur rapidly
● Monitor for dry mouth, metallic taste, polyuria, bone pain, muscle weakness, headache, fatigue, tinnitus, change in LOC, irregular pulse, dysrhythmias, increased respirations, anorexia, nausea, vomiting, cramps, diarrhea, constipation; may indicate hypercalcemia; if these occur, discontinue drug, give laxatives, low-calcium diet
● Monitor renal status: decreased urinary output (oliguria, anuria), edema in extremities, weight gain >5 lb, periorbital edema
● Assess nutritional status; check diet for sources of vit D (milk, some seafood), calcium (dairy products, dark green vegetables); phosphates (dairy products) must be avoided

Nursing diagnoses
✓ Nutrition: Less than body requirements, imbalanced (uses)
✓ Knowledge, deficient (teaching)

Implementation
⊘ ● Do not crush, chew caps
● May be increased q4 wk depending on blood level; give with meals for GI symptoms
● Store in tight, light-resistant containers at room temp

- Restrict sodium, potassium if required
- Restriction of fluids may be required for chronic renal failure

Patient/family education
- Teach symptoms of hypercalcemia and when to report symptoms to prescriber
- Teach patient about foods rich in calcium, vit D; provide list of calcium-rich foods; renal failure patients are given a renal diet
- Caution patient not to double doses, take exactly as prescribed

Evaluation
Positive therapeutic outcome
- Prevention of bone deficiencies
- Calcium, phosphorus at normal levels

⚠ HIGH ALERT

diltiazem (Rx)
(dil-tye′a-zem)
Apo-Diltiaz ✤, Cardizem, Cardizem SR, Cardizem CD, diltiazem, Dilacor-XR, Tiazac
Func. class.: Calcium channel blocker, antianginal
Chem. class.: Benzothiazepine

Pregnancy category C

Action: Inhibits calcium ion influx across cell membrane during cardiac depolarization, produces relaxation of coronary vascular smooth muscle, dilates coronary arteries, slows SA/AV node conduction times, dilates peripheral arteries

➔ **Therapeutic Outcome:** Decreased angina pectoris, dysrhythmias, B/P

Uses
Oral: Angina pectoris due to coronary insufficiency, hypertension, coronary artery spasm
Parenteral: Atrial fibrillation, flutter
Investigational use: Raynaud's syndrome

Dosage and routes
Hypertension
Adult: PO 60-120 mg bid (sus rel), max 360 mg/day, or 180-240 mg (ext rel) qd

Prinzmetal's or variant angina, chronic stable angina
Adult: PO 30 mg qid, increasing dose gradually to 180-360 mg/day in divided doses or 60-120 mg bid; may increase to 240-360 mg/day or 120 or 180 mg ext rel PO qd

Atrial fibrillation, flutter, paroxysmal supraventricular tachycardia
Adult: **IV** 0.25 mg/kg as bol over 2 min initially, then 0.35 mg/kg may be given after 15 min; if no response, may give cont inf 5-15 mg/hr for up to 24 hr

Available forms: Tab 30, 60, 90, 120 mg; tab ext rel 120, 180, 240 mg; caps sus rel 60, 90, 120, 180, 240, 300, 360, 420 mg; caps ext rel 60, 90, 120, 180, 240, 300, 360, 420 mg; inj **IV** 5 mg/ml (5, 10 ml); inj 25 mg; inj for **IV** only 100 mg

Adverse effects
(*italic* = common; **bold** = life-threatening)
CNS: Headache, fatigue, drowsiness, dizziness, depression, weakness, insomnia, tremor, paresthesia
CV: **Dysrhythmia,** *edema,* **CHF,** bradycardia, hypotension, palpitations, **heart block**
GI: Nausea, vomiting, diarrhea, gastric upset, *constipation,* increased liver function studies
GU: Nocturia, polyuria, **acute renal failure**
INTEG: Rash, pruritus, flushing, photosensitivity
RESP: Rhinitis, dyspnea, pharyngitis

Contraindications: Sick sinus syndrome, 2nd- or 3rd-degree heart block, hypotension less than 90 mm Hg systolic, acute MI, pulmonary congestion

Precautions: CHF, hypotension, hepatic [P] injury, pregnancy C, lactation, children, renal disease

◼ Do Not Confuse:
Cardizem/Cardene, Cardizem CD/Cardizem SR, Cardizem SR/Cardene SR

Pharmacokinetics	
Absorption	Well absorbed
Distribution	Not known
Metabolism	Liver, extensively
Excretion	Metabolites (96%)
Half-life	3½-9 hr

Pharmacodynamics			
	PO	PO–SUS REL	IV
Onset	½ hr	Unknown	Unknown
Peak	2-3 hr	Unknown	Unknown
Duration	6-8 hr	12 hr	Unknown

Interactions
Individual drugs
Carbamazepine, lithium: ↑ effects of each specific drug
Cimetidine: ↑ effects of diltiazem

Cyclosporine: ↑ cycloSPORINE effect
Digoxin: ↑ digoxin levels

Drug classifications
Anesthetics: ↑ effects of anesthetics
Antihypertensives: ↑ hypotension
β-Adrenergic blockers: ↑ bradycardia, CHF, ↑
β-blocker effect

Food/drug
Grapefruit juice: ↑ hypotension

Herb/drug
Barberry, betel palm, burdock, goldenseal,
khat, khella, lily of the valley, plantain:
↑ diltiazem effect
Yohimbe: ↓ diltiazem effect

NURSING CONSIDERATIONS
Assessment
• Assess fluid volume status: I&O ratio and
record, weight, distended red veins, crackles
in lung, color, quality, and sp gr of urine, skin
turgor, adequacy of pulses, moist mucous
membranes, bilateral lung sounds, peripheral
pitting edema; dehydration symptoms of
decreasing output, thirst, hypotension, dry
mouth and mucous membranes should be
reported
• Monitor B/P and pulse, respiration, ECG and
intervals (PR, QRS, QT); PCWP, CVP often
during infusion; if B/P drops 30 mm Hg, stop
inf and call prescriber
• Monitor ALT, AST, bilirubin daily; if these are
elevated, hepatotoxicity is suspected
• If platelets are <150,000/mm³, drug is
usually discontinued and another drug started
• Assess for extravasation: change site q48h

Nursing diagnoses
✓ Cardiac output, decreased (uses)
✓ Knowledge, deficient (teaching)

Implementation
PO route
• Give with meals for GI symptoms; may be
crushed and mixed with food/fluids for swal-
lowing difficulty
⊘ • Do not chew or crush sus rel caps
• Store in airtight container at room temp

IV route
• Give direct **IV** undiluted over 2 min
• For continuous inf dilute 125 mg/100 ml
(1.25 mg/ml) or 250 mg/250 ml (1 mg/ml) or
250 mg/500 ml (0.5 mg/ml) of D₅W, 0.9%
NaCl, D₅/0.45% NaCl; give 10 mg/hr; may
increase by 5 mg/hr to 15 mg/hr; may continue inf up to 24 hr

Y-site compatibilities: Albumin, amikacin, amphotericin B, aztreonam, bretylium,
bumetanide, cefazolin, cefotaxime, cefotetan,
cefoxitin, ceftazidime, ceftriaxone, cefuroxime,
cimetidine, ciprofloxacin, clindamycin, digoxin, DOBUTamine, DOPamine, doxycycline,
epINEPHrine, erythromycin, esmolol, fentanyl,
fluconazole, gentamicin, hetastarch, hydromorphone, imipenem-cilastatin, labetalol,
lidocaine, lorazepam, meperidine, metoclopramide, metronidazole, midazolam, milrinone, morphine, multivitamins, niCARDipine,
nitroglycerin, norepinephrine, oxacillin,
penicillin G potassium, pentamidine, piperacillin, potassium chloride, potassium phosphates,
ranitidine, sodium nitroprusside, theophylline,
ticarcillin, ticarcillin/clavulanate, tobramycin,
trimethoprim-sulfamethoxazole, vancomycin,
vecuronium

Patient/family education
• Caution patient to avoid hazardous activities
until stabilized on drug and dizziness is no
longer a problem
• Instruct patient to limit caffeine consumption; to avoid alcohol and OTC drugs unless
directed by prescriber
◆• Tell patient to comply in all areas of medical
regimen; diet, exercise, stress reduction, drug
therapy; to notify prescriber of irregular heart
beat, shortness of breath, swelling of feet and
hands, pronounced dizziness, constipation,
nausea, hypotension
• Teach patient to use as directed even if
feeling better; may be taken with other cardiovascular drugs (nitrates, β-blockers)

Evaluation
Positive therapeutic outcome
• Decreased anginal pain
• Decreased B/P
• Absence of dysrhythmias

Treatment of overdose: Atropine for
AV block, vasopressor for hypotension

*dimenhyDRINATE (OTC, Rx)
(dye-men-hye'dri-nate)

Apo-Dimenhydrinate ✦, Calm-X, Children's Dramamine, dimenhyDRINATE, Dimentabs, Dinate, Dramamine, Dramanate, Dymenate, Gravol ✦, Gravol L/A ✦, Hydrate, Nauseatol ✦, Novo-Dimenate ✦, PMS-Dimenhydrinate ✦, Travamine ✦, Triptone Caplets

Func. class.: Antiemetic, antihistamine, anticholinergic

Chem. class.: H₁-receptor antagonist, ethanolamine derivative

Pregnancy category B

Action: Vestibular stimulator is decreased; anticholinergic, antiemetic, antihistamine response

➡ **Therapeutic Outcome:** Absence of motion sickness

Uses: Motion sickness, nausea, vomiting

Dosage and routes
Adult: PO 50-100 mg q4h; IM/**IV** 50 mg as needed

P *Child:* IM/PO 5 mg/kg divided in 4 equal doses

Available forms: Tab 50 mg; inj 50 mg/ml; elix 15 mg/5 ml ✦, chew tab 50 mg

Adverse effects
(*italic* = common; **bold** = life-threatening)

CNS: *Drowsiness,* restlessness, headache, dizziness, insomnia, confusion, nervousness, tingling, vertigo

CV: Hypertension, *hypotension,* palpitations

EENT: Dry mouth, blurred vision, diplopia, nasal congestion, photosensitivity

GI: Nausea, anorexia, vomiting, *constipation*

INTEG: Rash, urticaria, fever, chills, flushing

MISC: **Anaphylaxis**

Contraindications: Hypersensitivity to opioids, shock

P **Precautions:** Children, cardiac dysrhyth-**G** mias, elderly, asthma, pregnancy **B**, prostatic hypertrophy, bladder neck obstruction, narrow-angle glaucoma, stenosing peptic ulcer, pyloroduodenal obstruction

N **Do Not Confuse:**
dimenhyDRINATE/diphenhydrAMINE

Pharmacokinetics
Absorption	Well absorbed (PO, IM)
Distribution	Unknown; crosses placenta
Metabolism	Liver
Excretion	Kidneys, breast milk
Half-life	Unknown

Pharmacodynamics
	PO	IM	IV
Onset	15-60 min	30 min	Immediate
Peak	1-2 hr	1-2 hr	Unknown
Duration	4-6 hr	4-6 hr	4-6 hr

Interactions
Individual drugs
Alcohol: ↑ CNS depression
Drug classifications
CNS depressants, opiates, sedative/hypnotics: ↑ CNS depression
⊘ *Herb/drug*
Corkwood, henbane leaf: ↑ anticholinergic effect
Jamaican dogwood, khat, senega: ↑ effect
Lab test interferences
False negative: Skin allergy tests (discontinue antihistamines 3 days before testing)

NURSING CONSIDERATIONS
Assessment
- Assess for signs of toxicity to other drugs or masking of symptoms of disease (brain tumor, intestinal obstruction); monitor GI symptoms including nausea, vomiting, abdominal pain, increased bowel sounds
- Monitor VS, B/P; check patients with cardiac disease more often
- Monitor I&O; check for dehydration (poor skin turgor, increased sp gr, tachycardia, **G** severe thirst) especially in the elderly

Nursing diagnoses
✓ Injury, risk for (side effects)
✓ Knowledge, deficient (teaching)

Implementation
PO route
- Tabs may be swallowed whole, chewed, or allowed to dissolve; give 1-2 hr before activity that may cause motion sickness; use measuring device for liq for correct dosing
IM route
- Give IM inj in large muscle mass; aspirate to avoid **IV** administration; massage
IV **IV route**
- Give **IV** directly after diluting 50 mg/10 ml or NaCl inj; give 50 mg or less over 2 min

---

 Herb/drug   Do Not Crush   Alert   Key Drug   Geriatric   Pediatric

Syringe compatibilities: Atropine, diphenhydrAMINE, droperidol, fentanyl, heparin, hydromorphone, meperidine, metoclopramide, morphine, pentazocine, perphenazine, ranitidine, scopolamine

Syringe incompatibilities: Butorphanol, chlorproMAZINE, glycopyrrolate, hydrOXYzine, midazolam, pentobarbital, prochlorperazine, promazine, promethazine, thiopental

Y-site compatibilities: Acyclovir

Y-site incompatibilities: Aminophylline, heparin, hydrocortisone sodium succinate, hydrOXYzine, phenobarbital, phenytoin, prednisoLONE, prochlorperazine, promazine, promethazine

Additive compatibilities: Amikacin, calcium gluconate, chloramphenicol, corticotropin, erythromycin, heparin, hydrOXYzine, methicillin, norepinephrine, penicillin G potassium, pentobarbital, phenobarbital, potassium chloride, prochlorperazine, vancomycin, vit B/C

Additive incompatibilities: Tetracycline, thiopental

Patient/family education

• Teach all aspects of drug uses; to notify prescriber if confusion, sedation, hypotension occur; to avoid driving and other hazardous activity if drowsiness occurs; to avoid alcohol and other CNS depressants that may potentiate effect

• Tell patient not to exceed recommended dosage

• Inform patient hard candy, gum, frequent rinsing of mouth may be used for dryness

• Advise patient that a false negative result may occur with skin testing; these procedures should not be scheduled until 4 days after discontinuing use

• Caution patient to avoid hazardous activities, activities requiring alertness; dizziness may occur; instruct patient to request assistance with ambulation

• Caution patient to avoid alcohol, other CNS depressants when taking this medication; response will be increased

Evaluation

Positive therapeutic outcome

• Absence of motion sickness

• Absence of nausea, vomiting

---

dinoprostone (Rx)

(dye-noe-prost'one)

Cervidil Vaginal Insert, Prepidil, Endocervical Gel, Prostin E Vaginal Suppository

Func. class.: Oxytocic, abortifacient
Chem. class.: Prostaglandin E_2

Pregnancy category C

D

Action: Stimulates uterine contractions similar to labor by myometrium stimulation, causing abortion; acts within 30 hr for complete abortion; GI smooth muscle stimulation, effacement, dilatation of the cervix

⇒**Therapeutic Outcome:** Beginning of labor, fetal expulsion

Uses: Abortion during 2nd trimester, benign hydatidiform mole, expulsion of uterine contents in fetal deaths to 28 wk, missed abortion, cervical effacement and dilatation in term pregnancy when they have not occurred spontaneously

Dosage and routes

Abortifacient

Adult: VAG SUPP 20 mg; repeat q3-5h until abortion occurs; max dose is 240 mg

Cervical ripening

Adult: GEL; warm to room temperature; choose correct length shielded catheter (10 or 20 mm), fill catheter by pushing plunger; have patient recumbent for 15-30 min; insert one 10 mg insert

Available forms: Vag supp 20 mg; gel 0.5 mg/3 g (prefilled syringe); gel 0.5 mg; 10 mg insert

Adverse effects

(*italic* = common; **bold** = life-threatening)

CNS: Headache, dizziness, chills, fever
CV: Hypotension, **dysrhythmias**
EENT: Blurred vision
GI: Nausea, vomiting, diarrhea
GU: Vaginitis, vaginal pain, vulvitis, vaginismus
INTEG: Rash, skin color changes
MS: Leg cramps, joint swelling, weakness
Insert: Uterine hyperstimulation, fever, nausea, vomiting, diarrhea, abdominal pain
Gel: Uterine contractile abnormality, GI side effects, back pain, fever
Fetal: Bradycardia (i.e., deceleration)
Suppository: Uterine rupture, anaphylaxis

Contraindications: Hypersensitivity, uterine fibrosis, cervical stenosis, pelvic surgery, PID, respiratory disease

---

Precautions: Hepatic, renal, cardiac disease, asthma, anemia, jaundice, diabetes mellitus, seizure disorders, hypertension, hypotension, pregnancy **C**

Do Not Confuse:
Prepidil/bepridil

Pharmacokinetics

Absorption	Rapidly absorbed
Distribution	Unknown
Metabolism	Enzymes
Excretion	Kidneys
Half-life	Unknown

Pharmacodynamics

	GEL	SUPP
Onset	Rapid	10 min
Peak	30-45 min	Unknown
Duration	Unknown	2-3 hr

Interactions
Individual drugs
Alcohol: ↓ oxytoxic effect
Oxytocin: ↑ effect

NURSING CONSIDERATIONS
Assessment
• Assess dilatation and effacement of the cervix, uterine contractions, fetal heart tones; watch for contractions lasting over 1 min, hypertonus, fetal distress; drug should be slowed or discontinued
• Assess for fever that occurs approximately 30 min after supp insertion (abortion)
• Monitor for nausea, vomiting, diarrhea; these may require medication
• Assess for hypersensitivity reaction: dyspnea, rash, chest discomfort
• Assess respiratory rate, rhythm, depth; notify prescriber of abnormalities, in pulse, B/P
• Check vaginal discharge; itching, irritation indicates vaginal infection

Nursing diagnoses
✓ Injury, high risk for (side effects)
✓ Knowledge, deficient (teaching)

Implementation
Suppository route
• Warm supp by running warm water over package; insert high in vagina, wear gloves to prevent absorption; have patient recumbent for at least 10 min
Gel route
• Do not allow to come in contact with skin; use soap and water to wash after use
• Gel should be at room temp

• Place patient in dorsal or lithotomy position to insert gel into cervical canal; remove catheter; discard all items after use; keep supine 15-30 min

Patient/family education
• Teach patient all aspects of treatment including purpose of medication and expected results
• Tell patient that gel may produce warmth in her vagina
• Caution patient that if contractions are longer than 1 min to notify nurse or prescriber
• Advise patient to notify prescriber of cramping, pain, increased bleeding, chills, increased temp, or foul-smelling discharge; these symptoms may indicate uterine infection
• Advise patient to remain supine 10-15 min after insertion of suppository; 2 hr after insert, 15-30 min after gel

Evaluation
Positive therapeutic outcome
• Progression of labor
• Abortion

---

*diphenhydrAMINE ◆π
(OTC, Rx)
(dye-fen-hye′dra-meen)
Allerdryl ✦, AllerMax, Allermed, Banophen, Benadryl, Benadryl 25, Benadryl Kapseals, Benahist 10, Benahist 50, Ben-Allergin-50, Benoject-10, Benoject-50, Benylin Cough, Bydramine, Compoz, Diphenadryl, Diphen Cough, Diphenhist, diphenhydrAMINE HCl, Dormin, Genahist, Hydramine, Hydramyn, Hydril, Hyrexin-50, Insomnal ✦, Nidryl, Nighttime Sleep Aid, Nordryl, Nordryl Cough, Nytol, Phendry, Siladril, Sleep-Eze 3, Sominex 2, Tusstat, Twilite, Uni-Bent Cough, Wehdryl
Func. class.: Antihistamine (1st generation, nonselective), antitussive
Chem. class.: Ethanolamine derivative, H₁-receptor antagonist

Pregnancy category B

Action: Acts on blood vessels, GI, respiratory system by competing with histamine for H₁-receptor site; decreases allergic response by blocking histamine; causes increased heart rate, vasodilatation, secretions

⇒ **Therapeutic Outcome:** Absence of allergy symptoms and rhinitis, decreased dystonic symptoms, absence of motion sickness, absence of cough, ability to sleep

Uses: Allergy symptoms, rhinitis, motion sickness, antiparkinsonism, nighttime sedation, infant colic, nonproductive cough, anaphylaxis, nasal allergies, allergic dermatoses, dystonic reactions

Dosage and routes
Adult: PO 25-50 mg q4-6h, not to exceed 400 mg/day; IM/**IV** 10-50 mg, not to exceed 400 mg/day

P *Child >12 kg:* PO/IM/**IV** 5 mg/kg/day in 4 divided doses, not to exceed 300 mg/day

Nighttime sleep aid
P *Adult and child ≥12 yr:* PO 25-50 mg hs

Antitussive (syrup only)
P *Adult and child ≥12 yr:* 25 mg q4h, max 100 mg/24 hr

P *Child 6-12 yr:* 12.5 mg q4h, max 50 mg/24 hr

P *Child 2-6 yr:* 6.25 mg q4h, max 25-50 mg/24 hr

Renal dose
Adult: PO CCr 10-50 ml/min dose q6-12h; CCr <10 ml/min dose q12-18h

Available forms: Caps 25, 50 mg; tabs 25, 50 mg; chew tabs 25 mg; elix 12.5 mg/5 ml; syr 12.5 mg/5 ml; inj 10, 50 mg/ml

Adverse effects
(*italic* = common; **bold** = life-threatening)
CNS: *Dizziness, drowsiness,* poor coordination, fatigue, anxiety, euphoria, confusion, paresthesia, neuritis, **seizures**
EENT: Blurred vision, dilated pupils, tinnitus, nasal stuffiness, dry nose, throat, mouth
GI: Nausea, anorexia, diarrhea
GU: *Retention,* dysuria, frequency
HEMA: **Thrombocytopenia, agranulocytosis, hemolytic anemia**
INTEG: Photosensitivity
MISC: Anaphylaxis
RESP: Increased thick secretions, wheezing, chest tightness

Contraindications: Hypersensitivity to H_1-receptor antagonist, acute asthma attack, lower respiratory tract disease

Precautions: Increased intraocular pressure, renal disease, cardiac disease, hypertension, bronchial asthma, seizure disorder, stenosed peptic ulcers, hyperthyroidism, prostatic hypertrophy, bladder neck obstruction, pregnancy **B**

🔲 **Do Not Confuse:**
diphenhydrAMINE/dicyclomine
diphenhydrAMINE/dimenhyDRINATE

Pharmacokinetics
Absorption	Well absorbed (PO, IM); completely absorbed (**IV**)
Distribution	Widely distributed; crosses placenta
Metabolism	Liver (95%)
Excretion	Kidneys, breast milk
Half-life	2½-7 hr

Pharmacodynamics
	PO	IM	IV
Onset	15-60 min	30 min	Immediate
Peak	1-4 hr	1-4 hr	Unknown
Duration	4-8 hr	4-8 hr	4-8 hr

Interactions
Individual drugs
Alcohol: ↑ CNS depression
Drug classifications
Antidepressants (tricyclic), barbiturates, CNS depressants, opiates, sedative/hypnotics: ↑ CNS depression
MAOIs: ↑ effect of diphenhydrAMINE
🔲 *Herb/drug*
Corkwood, henbane leaf: ↑ anticholinergic effect
Hops, Jamaican dogwood, khat, senega: ↑ effect
Lab test interferences
False negative: Skin allergy tests (discontinue antihistamines 3 days before testing)

NURSING CONSIDERATIONS
Assessment
• Assess respiratory status: rate, rhythm, increase in bronchial secretions, wheezing, chest tightness; provide fluids to 2 L/day to decrease secretion thickness
• Monitor I&O ratio: be alert for urinary retention, frequency, dysuria, especially
G elderly; drug should be discontinued if these occur
• Monitor CBC during long-term therapy; blood dyscrasias may occur but are rare
• If giving for dystonic reactions, assess type of involuntary movements and evaluate response to this medication
• Assess cough characteristics including type, frequency, thickness of secretions, and evaluate response to this medication if using for cough

Nursing diagnoses
☑ Injury, risk for (side effects)
☑ Sleep pattern, disturbed (uses)
☑ Knowledge, deficient (teaching)

Implementation
• Give 20 min before hs if using for sleep aid

PO route
- Give with meals if GI symptoms occur; absorption may be slightly decreased; cap may be opened and drug mixed with food/fluids for patients with swallowing difficulties

IM route
- Give IM inj in large muscle mass; aspirate to avoid **IV** administration; rotate sites

IV **IV route**
- Give **IV** undiluted 25 mg/min; may be diluted with 0.9% NaCl, D_5W, $D_{10}W$, 0.45% NaCl, D_5/0.9% NaCl, D_5/0.45% NaCl, D_5/0.25% NaCl, LR, Ringer's, give 25 mg/min or less

Syringe compatibilities: Atropine, butorphanol, chlorproMAZINE, cimetidine, cisatracurium, dimenhyDRINATE, DOXOrubicin liposome, droperidol, fentanyl, fluphenazine, glycopyrrolate, hydromorphone, hydrOXYzine, meperidine, metoclopramide, midazolam, morphine, nalbuphine, pentazocine, perphenazine, prochlorperazine, promazine, promethazine, ranitidine, remifentanil, scopolamine, sufentanil, thiothixene

Syringe incompatibilities: Pentobarbital, phenytoin, thiopental

Y-site compatibilities: Acyclovir, aldesleukin, amifostine, amsacrine, aztreonam, ciprofloxacin, cisplatin, cladribine, cyclophosphamide, cytarabine, DOXOrubicin, famotidine, filgrastim, fluconazole, fludarabine, gallium, granisetron, heparin, hydrocortisone, idarubicin, melphalan, meperidine, meropenem, methotrexate, ondansetron, paclitaxel, piperacillin/tazobactam, potassium chloride, propofol, sargramostim, sufentanil, tacrolimus, teniposide, thiotepa, vinorelbine, vit B/C

Y-site incompatibilities: Foscarnet

Additive compatibilities: Amikacin, aminophylline, ascorbic acid, bleomycin, cephapirin, erythromycin, hydrocortisone, lidocaine, methicillin, methyldopate, nafcillin, netilmicin, penicillin G potassium, penicillin G sodium, polymyxin B, vit B/C

Additive incompatibilities: Amobarbital, cephalothin, thiopental

Patient/family education
- Tell patient that a false-negative result may occur with skin testing; these procedures should not be scheduled until 3 days after discontinuing use
- Caution patient to avoid hazardous activities and activities requiring alertness, since dizziness may occur; instruct patient to request assistance with ambulation
- Teach patient to use sunscreen to prevent photosensitivity
- Advise patient to avoid alcohol, other depressants; CNS depression may occur
- Teach all aspects of drug uses; to notify prescriber if confusion, sedation, hypotension occur; to avoid driving and other hazardous activity if drowsiness occurs; to avoid alcohol or other CNS depressants that may potentiate effect

Evaluation
Positive therapeutic outcome
- Absence of motion sickness
- Absence of nausea, vomiting
- Ability to sleep
- Absence of cough
- Decrease in involuntary movements

Treatment of overdose:
- Administer ipecac syrup or lavage, diazepam, vasopressors, barbiturates (short acting)

diphenoxylate with atropine (Rx)
(dye-fen-ox'i-late)
Logen, Lomanate, Lomotil, Lonox
Func. class.: Antidiarrheal
Chem. class.: Phenylpiperidine derivative, opiate agonist

Pregnancy category C
Controlled substance schedule V

Action: Inhibits gastric motility by acting on mucosal receptors responsible for peristalsis; related to opioid analgesics as adjunct

→ **Therapeutic Outcome:** Decreased loose stools

Uses: Diarrhea (cause undetermined)

Dosage and routes
Adult: 2.5-5 mg qid, titrated to patient response, not to exceed 8 tabs/24 hr

P *Child 2-12 yr:* PO 0.3-0.4 mg/kg/day in divided doses

Available forms: Tab 2.5 mg diphenoxylate/0.025 mg atropine; liq 2.5 mg diphenoxylate/0.025 mg atropine/5 ml

Adverse effects
(*italic* = common; **bold** = life-threatening)
CNS: *Dizziness, drowsiness, lightheadedness, headache,* fatigue, nervousness, insomnia, confusion, flushing
EENT: Blurred vision, burning eyes

GI: *Nausea, vomiting, dry mouth, epigastric distress,* constipation, **paralytic ileus**
RESP: **Respiratory depression**
MISC: **Anaphylaxis, angioedema**

Contraindications: Hypersensitivity, pseudomembranous enterocolitis, jaundice, glaucoma, child <2 yr, severe electrolyte imbalances, diarrhea associated with organisms that penetrate intestinal mucosa

Precautions: Hepatic, renal disease, ulcerative colitis, pregnancy **C**, lactation, severe liver disease

Do Not Confuse:
Diphenatol/diphenidol, Lomotil/Lamictal, Lomotil/Lanoxin, Lomotil/Lasix

Pharmacokinetics

Absorption	Well absorbed
Distribution	Unknown
Metabolism	Liver, active metabolite
Excretion	Kidneys
Half-life	2½ hr

Pharmacodynamics

Onset	45-60 min
Peak	2 hr
Duration	3-4 hr

Interactions
Individual drugs
Alcohol: ↑ action of alcohol
Drug classifications
Anticholinergics: ↑ anticholinergic effect
Barbiturates: ↑ action of barbiturates
CNS depressants: ↑ action of CNS depressants
MAOIs: Hypertensive crisis; do not use together
Opiates: ↑ action of opioids
Sedative/hypnotics: ↑ CNS depression
Herb/drug
Nutmeg: ↑ antidiarrheal effect

NURSING CONSIDERATIONS
Assessment
• Monitor electrolytes (potassium, sodium, chloride) if on long-term therapy; fluid status, skin turgor
• Assess bowel pattern before, during treatment; check for rebound constipation after termination of medication; check bowel sounds
• Check response after 48 hr; if no response, drug should be discontinued and other treatment initiated
• Assess for abdominal distention and toxic

megacolon, which may occur in ulcerative colitis
• Assess hepatic function if on long-term therapy

Nursing diagnoses
✓ Diarrhea (uses)
✓ Constipation (adverse reactions)
✓ Knowledge, deficient (teaching)
✓ Noncompliance (teaching)

Implementation
• Give for 48 hr only; tabs may be given with food, crushed and mixed with fluids; liq should be measured accurately

Patient/family education
• Advise patient to avoid alcohol and OTC products unless directed by prescriber; may cause increased CNS depression
• Caution patient not to exceed recommended dosage; that drug may be habit forming
• Advise patient that drug may cause drowsiness; to avoid hazardous activities until response to drug is determined
• Teach patient that dry mouth can be decreased by frequent sips of water, hard candy, sugarless gum

Evaluation
Positive therapeutic outcome
• Decreased diarrhea

dipyridamole (Rx)
(dye-peer-id′a-mole)
Apo-Dipyridamole ✤, dipyridamole, Novo-Dipiradol ✤, Persantine, Persantine IV
Func. class.: Coronary vasodilator, antiplatelet agent
Chem. class.: Nonnitrate

Pregnancy category B

Action: Inhibits adenosine uptake, which produces coronary vasodilatation; increases oxygen saturation in coronary tissues, coronary blood flow; acts on small vessels with little effect on vascular resistance; may increase development of collateral circulation; decreased platelet aggregation by the inhibition of phosphodiesterases (enzymes)

Therapeutic Outcome: Inhibition of platelet aggregation; absence of ischemic attacks, reinfarction

Uses: Prevention of transient ischemic attacks, inhibition of platelet adhesion to prevent myocardial reinfarction, thromboembolism, with warfarin in prosthetic heart valves, prevention of coronary bypass graft occlusion with aspirin; **IV** form used to evaluate coronary artery disease; used as alternative to exercise in thallium myocardial perfusion imaging to evaluate coronary artery disease

Dosage and routes
Transient ischemic attacks
Adult: PO 50 mg tid, 1 hr ac, not to exceed 400 mg qd

Inhibition of platelet adhesion
Adult: PO 50-75 mg qid in combination with aspirin or warfarin

Thallium myocardial perfusion imaging
Adult: **IV** 570 mcg/kg

Available forms: Tabs 25, 50, 75 mg; inj 10 mg/2 ml

Adverse effects
(*italic* = common; **bold** = life-threatening)
CNS: *Headache, dizziness, weakness, fainting, syncope;* **IV**: transient cerebral ischemia, weakness

CV: *Postural hypotension;* **IV**: **MI**

GI: *Nausea, vomiting,* anorexia, diarrhea

INTEG: *Rash,* flushing

RESP: **IV**: **Bronchospasm**

Contraindications: Hypersensitivity

Precautions: Pregnancy **B**, hypotension

Pharmacokinetics
Absorption	30%-50% (PO)
Distribution	Widely distributed; crosses placenta
Metabolism	Liver
Excretion	Bile, undergoes enterohepatic recirculation; enters breast milk
Half-life	10 hr

Pharmacodynamics
	PO	IV
Onset	Unknown	Unknown
Peak	1.25 hr	6 min
Duration	6 hr	½ hr
Therapeutic effect	Several mo	

Interactions
Individual drugs
Aspirin, cefamandole, cefotetan, cefoperazone, plicamycin, sulfinpyrazone, valproic acid: ↑ risk of bleeding
Theophylline: ↓ effects of disopyramide (thallium)
Drug classifications
Anticoagulants, NSAIDs, thrombolytics: ↑ risk of bleeding

☑ Herb/drug
Arginine: ↑ gastric irritation
Bilberry, saw palmetto: ↓ antiplatelet effect
Bogbean, dong quai, feverfew, ginger, ginkgo: ↑ antiplatelet effect

NURSING CONSIDERATIONS
Assessment
• Monitor B/P, pulse baseline and during treatment until stable; take B/P with patient lying, standing; orthostatic hypotension is common
• Assess cardiac status: chest pain, what aggravates or ameliorates condition
• If using by **IV** route, monitor VS before, during, and after infusion; monitor for chest pain, bronchospasm; use ECG for identifying dysrhythmias; use aminophylline up to 250 mg **IV** for bronchospasm and chest pain if chest pain is unrelieved with the 250 mg dose of aminophylline; give SL dose of nitroglycerin

Nursing diagnoses
☑ Cardiac output, decreased (uses)
☑ Pain, acute (uses)
☑ Knowledge, deficient (teaching)

Implementation
PO route
• Give with 8 oz of water; to improve absorption give on an empty stomach; if GI symptoms occur may give with meals
• Tabs may be crushed, mixed with food or fluids for swallowing difficulty or swallowed whole
• Store at room temp
☑ Intermittent **IV** infusion
• Give by **IV** after diluting to at least 1:2 ratio using D₅W, 0.45% NaCl, or 0.9% NaCl; 20-50 ml should be given; give over 4 min; do not give undiluted

Patient/family education
• Teach patient that this medication is not a cure; that drug may have to be taken continuously in evenly spaced doses only as directed; if a dose is missed, take one when remembered up to 4 hr; do not double doses
• Advise patient to rise slowly from sitting or lying down to prevent orthostatic hypotension
• Caution patient not to use alcohol or OTC medication unless approved by prescriber
• Caution patient to avoid hazardous activities until stabilized on medication; dizziness may occur

Evaluation
Positive therapeutic outcome
• Absence of reinfarction, ischemic attacks

Treatment of overdose: Administer **IV** phenylephrine

---

dirithromycin (Rx)
(die-rith-roe-mie'sin)
Dynabac
Func. class.: Antibacterial
Chem. class.: Macrolide

Pregnancy category C

Action: Binds to 50S ribosomal subunits of susceptible bacteria; suppresses protein synthesis

Therapeutic Outcome: Bactericidal action against *Moraxella catarrhalis, Streptococcus pneumoniae, Streptococcus pyogenes, Streptococcus viridans, Legionella pneumophila, Mycoplasma pneumoniae, Staphylococcus aureus, Staphylococcus agalactiae, Bordetella pertussis*

Uses: Infections of upper and lower respiratory tract

Dosage and routes
Adult: PO 500 mg qd, given for 7-14 days depending on infections

Available forms: Tab, enteric coated 250 mg

Adverse effects
(*italic* = common; **bold** = life-threatening)
CNS: Headache, dizziness, insomnia
GI: Abdominal pain, nausea, diarrhea, vomiting, dyspepsia, GI disorders, flatulence, abnormal stools, anorexia, constipation, **pseudomembranous colitis**
HEMA: Increased platelet count, increased eosinophils
INTEG: Pruritus, urticaria
RESP: Cough, dyspnea

Contraindications: Hypersensitivity to this drug or any other macrolide or to erythromycin, bacteremias

Precautions: Pregnancy C, lactation, children, hepatic, renal disease

Do Not Confuse:
Dynabac/DynaCirc

Pharmacokinetics

Absorption	Rapidly absorbed
Distribution	Widely distributed
Metabolism	No hepatic metabolism
Excretion	Bile, feces (up to 97%)
Half-life	Plasma half-life 8 hr, terminal 44 hr

Pharmacodynamics
Unknown

Interactions
Drug classifications
Antacids, H₂ antagonists: Slightly enhanced absorption of dirithromycin
Theophylline: May alter effect
Food/drug
↑ Absorption
Herb/drug
Acidophilus: Do not use with antiinfectives

NURSING CONSIDERATIONS
Assessment
• Assess I&O ratio; report hematuria, oliguria in renal disease
• Monitor liver function studies: AST, ALT if on long-term therapy
• Monitor renal studies: urinalysis, protein, blood
• Monitor C&S before drug therapy; drug may be given as soon as culture is taken; C&S may be repeated after treatment
• Assess bowel pattern before, during treatment; pseudomembranous colitis may occur
• Assess for skin eruptions, itching
• Assess respiratory status: rate, character, wheezing, tightness in chest; discontinue drug

Nursing diagnoses
✓ Infection, risk for (uses)
✓ Diarrhea (side effects)
✓ Knowledge, deficient (teaching)
✓ Noncompliance (teaching)

Implementation
• Give adequate intake of fluids (2 L) during diarrhea episodes
• Administer whole; do not cut, crush, chew tablets
• Give with food or within 1 hr of food at same time each day
• Store at room temp in tight container

Patient/family education
• Teach patient to take with full glass of water; give with food
• Instruct patient to report sore throat, fever, fatigue; may indicate superinfection
• Teach patient to notify nurse of diarrhea, dark urine, pale stools, yellow discoloration of eyes or skin, severe abdominal pain
• Instruct patient to take at evenly spaced intervals; complete dosage regimen

---

♣ Canada Only   ◼ Do Not Confuse   * "Tall Man" lettering (See Preface)

Evaluation

Positive therapeutic outcome
- C&S negative for infection

Treatment of hypersensitivity:

Withdraw drug, maintain airway, administer epINEPHrine, aminophylline, O_2, **IV** corticosteroids

---

disopyramide (Rx)

(dye-soe-peer'a-mide)

disopyramide, Norpace, Norpace CR, Rhythmodan

Func. class.: Antidysrhythmic (class IA)
Chem. class.: Nonnitrate

Pregnancy category C

Action: Prolongs action potential duration and effective refractory period; reduces disparity in refractory period between normal and infarcted myocardium; prevents increased myocardial excitability and conduction contractility

⇒ **Therapeutic Outcome:** Suppression of supraventricular dysrhythmias

Uses: PVCs, ventricular tachycardia, supraventricular tachycardia, atrial flutter, fibrillation

Investigational uses: Supraventricular tachycardia (prevention, treatment)

Dosage and routes
Adult: PO 100-200 mg q6h; in renal dysfunction 100 mg q6h; sus rel cap 200-400 mg q12h

P *Child 12-18 yr:* PO 6-15 mg/kg/day, in divided doses q6h

P *Child 4-12 yr:* PO 10-15 mg/kg/day in divided doses q6h

P *Child 1-4 yr:* PO 10-20 mg/kg/day in divided doses q6h

P *Child <1 yr:* PO 10-30 mg/kg/day, in divided doses q6h

Renal dose
Adult: PO CCr 30-40 ml/min dose q8h; CCr 15-30 ml/min dose q12h; CCr <15 ml/min dose q24h

Available forms: Caps 100, 150 mg; cont rel caps 100, 150 mg; tabs, sus rel 250 mg ✤

Adverse effects
(*italic* = common; **bold** = life-threatening)
CNS: *Headache, dizziness,* psychosis, fatigue, depression, paresthesias, insomnia
CV: *Hypotension, bradycardia,* angina, PVCs, tachycardia, increases in QRS and QT segments, **cardiac arrest,** edema, weight gain, AV block, ***CHF,*** syncope, chest pain
EENT: *Blurred vision, dry nose, throat, eyes,* narrow-angle glaucoma
GI: *Dry mouth, constipation,* nausea, anorexia, flatulence, diarrhea, vomiting
GU: *Retention, hesitancy,* impotence
HEMA: **Thrombocytopenia, agranulocytosis,** anemia (rare), decreased Hgb, Hct
INTEG: Rash, pruritus, urticaria
META: Hypoglycemia, hypokalemia
MS: Weakness, pain in extremities

Contraindications: Hypersensitivity, 2nd- or 3rd-degree heart block, cardiogenic shock, CHF (uncompensated), sick sinus syndrome, QT prolongation

Precautions: Pregnancy **C**, lactation, diabetes mellitus, renal, hepatic disease,
P children, myasthenia gravis, narrow-angle glaucoma, cardiomyopathy, conduction abnormalities, potassium imbalance

Pharmacokinetics

Absorption	Well absorbed
Distribution	Widely distributed
Metabolism	Liver
Excretion	Kidneys
Half-life	4-10 hr

Pharmacodynamics

	PO	PO–SUS REL
Onset	½-3½ hr	Unknown
Peak	2 hr	Unknown
Duration	1½-8 hr	12 hr

Interactions

Individual drugs
Atenolol, erythromycin, lidocaine, procainamide, propranolol: ↑ effects of disopyramide
Phenobarbital, phenytoin: ↓ effects of disopyramide
Quinidine: ↑ levels, toxicity
Rifampin: ↓ disopyramide levels

Drug classifications
Anticholinergics: ↑ side effects, urinary retention of disopyramide

⧄ *Herb/drug*
Aconite: ↑ toxicity, death
Aloe, broom, buckthorn (chronic use), cascara sagrada (chronic use), Chinese rhubarb, figwort, fumitory, goldenseal, kudzu, licorice: ↑ effect
Coltsfoot: ↓ effect
Horehound: ↑ serotonin effect

Lab test interferences
↑ Liver enzymes
↑ Lipids, ↑ BUN, ↑creatinine
↓ Hgb/Hct, ↓ blood glucose

NURSING CONSIDERATIONS
Assessment
• Assess respiratory status: auscultate lung fields for bibasilar crackles in patients with advanced CHF
• Monitor I&O ratio and electrolytes: potassium, sodium, chloride; watch for decreasing urinary output, possible retention
• Monitor liver function studies: AST, ALT, bilirubin, alkaline phosphatase
• Monitor ECG to determine drug effectiveness, measure PR, QRS, QT intervals; check for PVCs, other dysrhythmias; monitor B/P for hypotension; check for prolonged widening QT intervals, QRS complex; if QT or QRS increase by 50% or more, withhold next dose, notify prescriber
• Monitor for dehydration or hypovolemia
• Monitor for CNS symptoms: psychosis, numbness, depression; if these occur, drug should be discontinued

Nursing diagnoses
✓ Cardiac output, decreased (uses)
✓ Knowledge, deficient (teaching)

Implementation
⊘ • Do not crush or break sus rel caps
• Give 1 hr ac or 2 hr pc
• If changing from regular release to sus rel cap, give sus rel 6 hr after last dose of regular release

Patient/family education
• Teach patient to report side effects immediately to prescriber; to take exactly as prescribed; if dose is missed take when remembered if within 3-4 hr of next dose; do not double doses
• Teach patient to complete follow-up appointment with prescriber including pulmonary function studies, chest x-ray
• Instruct patient that dry mouth may be relieved by frequent sips of water, hard candy, sugarless gum
• Caution patient to make position changes from lying to standing slowly to prevent orthostatic hypotension

Evaluation
Positive therapeutic outcome
• Decreased PVCs, ventricular tachycardia

Treatment of overdose: Administer O_2, artificial ventilation, ECG; administer DOPamine for circulatory depression; administer diazepam or thiopental for seizures, isoproterenol

---

divalproex sodium
See valproate

---

*DOBUTamine (Rx)
(doe-byoo'ta-meen)
DOBUTamine, Dobutrex
Func. class.: Adrenergic direct-acting β_1-agonist, inotropic agent, cardiac stimulant
Chem. class.: Catecholamine

Pregnancy category B

Action: Causes increased contractility, increased cardiac output without marked increase in heart rate by acting on β_1-receptors in heart; minor α/β_2 effects

→**Therapeutic Outcome:** Cardiac output increased with decreased fatigue and dyspnea

Uses: Cardiac decompensation due to organic heart disease or cardiac surgery

Investigational uses: Cardiogenic shock in children, congenital heart disease in children undergoing cardiac catherization

Dosage and routes
Adult: **IV** inf 2.5-10 mcg/kg/min; may increase to 40 mcg/kg/min if needed

P *Child:* **IV** inf 5-20 mcg/kg/min over 10 min for cardiac cath

Available forms: Inj 12.5 mg/ml

Adverse effects
(*italic* = common; **bold** = life-threatening)
CNS: Anxiety, headache, dizziness
CV: Palpitations, tachycardia, hypertension, PVCs, angina, hypotension
GI: Heartburn, nausea, vomiting
MS: Muscle cramps (leg)

Contraindications: Hypersensitivity, idiopathic hypertrophic subaortic stenosis

Precautions: Pregnancy **B**, lactation, children, hypertension

⊠ **Do Not Confuse:**
DOBUTamine/DOPamine, Dobutrex/Diamox

Pharmacokinetics

Absorption	Complete
Distribution	Unknown
Metabolism	Liver
Excretion	Kidneys
Half-life	2 min

Pharmacodynamics

Onset	1-5 min
Peak	10 min
Duration	<10 min

Interactions
Individual drugs
Bretylium, oxytocin: ↑ dysrhythmias
Guanethidine: ↑ severe hypertension
Oxytocin: ↑ pressor effects
Drug classifications
Anesthetics, MAOIs: ↑ dysrhythmias
Antidepressants (tricyclic): ↑ pressor response
β-blockers: ↓ action of DOBUTamine
MAOIs: ↑ pressor effect

NURSING CONSIDERATIONS
Assessment
• Assess for hypovolemia; if present, correct before beginning treatment with DOBUTamine; avoid use in patients with atrial fibrillation before digitalization
• Monitor ECG for dysrhythmias, ischemia during treatment; some patients may not need continuous ECG monitoring; also monitor PCWP, CVP, CO_2, urinary output; notify prescriber if <30 ml/hr
• Assess for heart failure: bibasilar crackles, S_3 gallop, dyspnea, neck vein distention in patients with cardiomyopathy or CHF
• Assess for oxygenation or perfusion deficit: decreased B/P, chest pain, dizziness, loss of consciousness
• Monitor B/P and pulse q5 min during inf; if B/P drops 30 mm Hg, stop inf and call prescriber
• Monitor ALT, AST, bilirubin daily
• Monitor for sulfite sensitivity, which may be life threatening

Nursing diagnoses
☑ Cardiac output, decreased (uses)
☑ Knowledge, deficient (teaching)

Implementation
IV IV route
• Reconstitute 250 mg/10 ml of D_5W or sterile water for inj; may add another 10 ml to dissolve completely if needed, then dilute in 50 ml or more of D_5W, 0.9% NaCl, 0.45% NaCl, D_5/0.45% NaCl, D_5/0.9% NaCl, D_5/LR, LR; titrate to patient response; use infusion pump for correct dose
• Use a CVP catheter or large peripheral vein, use infusion pump, titrate to patient response
• Change **IV** site q48h

Syringe compatibilities: Heparin, ranitidine

Syringe incompatibility: Doxapram

Y-site compatibilities: Amifostine, amrinone, atracurium, aztreonam, bretylium, calcium chloride, calcium gluconate, ciprofloxacin, cladribine, diazepam, diltiazem, DOPamine, enalaprilat, epINEPHrine, famotidine, fentanyl, fluconazole, granisetron, haloperidol, hydromorphone, regular insulin, labetalol, lidocaine, lorazepam, magnesium sulfate, meperidine, milrinone, morphine, nicARDipine, nitroglycerin, norepinephrine, pancuronium, potassium chloride, propofol, ranitidine, sodium nitroprusside, streptokinase, tacrolimus, theophylline, thiotepa, tolazoline, vecuronium, verapamil, zidovudine

Y-site incompatibilities: Acyclovir, alteplase, aminophylline, foscarnet, phytonadione

Additive compatibilities: Amiodarone, atracurium, atropine, DOPamine, enalaprilat, epINEPHrine, flumazenil, hydrALAZINE, isoproterenol, lidocaine, meperidine, meropenem, metaraminol, morphine, nitroglycerin, norepinephrine, phentolamine, phenylephrine, procainamide, propranolol, ranitidine, verapamil

Additive incompatibilities: Acyclovir, aminophylline, bumetanide, calcium gluconate, diazepam, digoxin, furosemide, insulin, magnesium sulfate, phenytoin, potassium phosphate, sodium bicarbonate

Patient/family education
• Teach patient reason for medication and expected results, reason for all monitoring and procedures
• Advise patient to report dyspnea, headache, **IV** site discomfort, chest pain, numbness of extremities

Evaluation
Positive therapeutic outcome
• Increased cardiac output
• Decreased PCWP, adequate CVP
• Decreased dyspnea, fatigue, edema, ECG
• Increased urine output

Treatment of overdose: Discontinue drug, support circulation

 Herb/drug   Do Not Crush   Alert   Key Drug   Geriatric   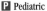 Pediatric

docusate calcium (OTC)
(dok'yoo-sate)
DC Softgels, Pro-Cal-Sof, Sulfalax Calcium, Surfak

docusate sodium (OTC)
Colace, Correctol Extra Gentle, Dialose Dok, Diocto, Dioeze, Disonate, Di-Sosal, D-S-S, Ex-Lax, Modane, Regulex SS, Regulex ♣, Silace
Func. class.: Laxative, emollient
Chem. class.: Anionic surfactant

Pregnancy category C

Action: Increases water, fat penetration in intestine; allows for easier passage of stool; increases electrolyte, water secretion in colon

➡ **Therapeutic Outcome:** Passage of softened stool, absence of constipation

Uses: To soften stools, prevent constipation, soften fecal impaction (rec route)

Dosage and routes
Adult: PO 50-300 mg qd (docusate sodium) or 240 mg (docusate calcium or docusate potassium) prn; enema 5 ml (docusate sodium)

P *Child >12 yr:* Enema 2 ml (docusate sodium)

P *Child 6-12 yr:* PO 40-120 mg qd (docusate sodium)

P *Child 3-6 yr:* PO 20-60 mg qd (docusate sodium)

P *Child <3 yr:* PO 10-40 mg qd (docusate sodium)

Available forms
Docusate calcium: Caps 50, 240 mg
Docusate sodium: Caps 50, 100, 240, 250 mg; tabs 50, 100 mg; syr 20 mg/5 ml, 50, 60 mg/15 ml; liq 150 mg/15 ml; oral sol 10, 50 mg/ml; enema 283 mg/3.9 g cap

Adverse effects
(*italic* = common; **bold** = life-threatening)
EENT: Bitter taste, throat irritation
GI: Nausea, anorexia, cramps, diarrhea
INTEG: Rash

Contraindications: Hypersensitivity, obstruction, fecal impaction, nausea/vomiting

Precautions: Pregnancy C

Pharmacokinetics
Absorption	Minimal (PO)
Distribution	Unknown
Metabolism	Not metabolized
Excretion	Bile
Half-life	Unknown

Pharmacodynamics
	PO	REC
Onset	24-72 hr	4-6 hr
Peak	Unknown	Unknown
Duration	Unknown	Unknown

Interactions
Mineral oil: toxicity
▨ *Herb/drug*
Flax, senna: ↑ laxative action

NURSING CONSIDERATIONS
Assessment
• Assess cramping, rectal bleeding, nausea, vomiting; if these symptoms occur, drug should be discontinued; identify cause of constipation; identify whether fluids, bulk, or exercise is missing from lifestyle

Nursing diagnoses
✓ Constipation (uses)
✓ Diarrhea (side effects)
✓ Knowledge, deficient (teaching)
✓ Noncompliance (teaching)

Implementation
PO route
• Dilute oral sol in juice or other fluid to disguise taste
• Give tabs or caps with 8 oz of liq; give on empty stomach for increased absorption, results

Patient/family education
• Discuss with patient that adequate fluid consumption is as necessary as bulk, exercise for adequate bowel function
• Teach patient that normal bowel movements do not always occur daily
• Advise patient not to use in presence of abdominal pain, nausea, vomiting; tell patient to notify prescriber if unrelieved constipation or if symptoms of electrolyte imbalance occur: muscle cramps, pain, weakness, dizziness, excessive thirst
• Advise patient that drug may take up to 3 days to soften stools
• Instruct patient to take oral preparation with a full glass of water and increase fluid intake unless on fluid restrictions
• Caution patients with heart disease to avoid

using the Valsalva maneuver to expedite evacuation

Evaluation
Positive therapeutic outcome
- Decreased constipation within 3 days

---

dofetilide
(doff-ee-till'-lide)
Tikosyn
Func. class.: Antidysrhythmic (Class III)

Pregnancy category C

Action: Blocks cardiac ion channel carrying the rapid component of delayed potassium current, no effect on sodium channels

➡ **Therapeutic Outcome:** Absence of atrial fibrillation

Uses: Atrial fibrillation, flutter, maintenance of normal sinus rhythm

Dosage and routes
Adult: PO 125-500 mcg bid depending on CCr, may be adjusted q2-3h to get appropriate increase in QTc

Renal dose: PO initial dose for CCr > 60 mg/ml 500 mcg bid; CCr 40-60 mg/min 250 mcg bid; CCr 20-39 mg/min 125 mcg bid; CCr <20 mg/min do not use

Available forms: Caps 125, 250, 500 mcg

Adverse effects
(*italic* = common; **bold** = life-threatening)
CNS: *Syncope, dizziness,* headache
CV: *Hypotension, postural hypotension, bradycardia,* chest pain, angina, PVCs, substernal pressure, precipitation of angina transient hypertension
GI: *Nausea, vomiting,* severe diarrhea, anorexia

Contraindications: Hypersensitivity, digitalis toxicity, aortic stenosis, pulmonary [P] hypertension, children, QT syndromes, severe renal disease

Precautions: Renal disease, pregnancy **C**, lactation

Pharmacokinetics

Absorption	>90%
Distribution	Steady state 2-3 days
Metabolism	Not metabolized
Excretion	Kidneys 80%
Half-life	10 hr

Pharmacodynamics
Unknown

Interactions
Individual drugs
Amiloride, cimetidine, ketoconazole, megestrol, metformin, prochlorperazine, triamterene, trimethoprim/sulfamethoxazole, verapamil: Do not use together
Diuretics, potassium depletion: ↑ hypokalemia
☑ *Herb/drug*
Aconite: ↑ toxicity, death
Aloe, broom, buckthorn (chronic use), cascara sagrada (chronic use), Chinese rhubarb, figwort, fumitory, goldenseal, kudzu, licorice: ↑ effect
Coltsfoot: ↓ effect
Horehound: ↑ serotonin effect

NURSING CONSIDERATIONS
Assessment
- Monitor ECG continuously to determine drug effectiveness; measure PR, QRS, QT intervals; check for PVCs, other dysrhythmias; monitor B/P continuously; this drug is available only to facilities that have been educated in its administration; patient must be hospitalized
- Before administration, QTc must be determined using an average of 5-10 beats, if the QTc >440 msec or 500 msec in ventricular conduction abnormalities, do not use; do not use if heart rate <60 bpm
- Before dosing, identify CCr, using CCr to determine dosing

Nursing diagnoses
☑ Cardiac output, decreased (uses)
☑ Gas exchange, impaired (adverse reactions)
☑ Knowledge, deficient (teaching)

Implementation
PO route
- Give for 3 days with patient hospitalized
- Give dofetilide after withholding class I or III antidysrhythmic for 3 half-lives of dofetilide before starting dofetilide

Patient/family education
- Notify prescriber if fast heartbeats with fainting or dizziness occur
- Notify all prescribers of all medications and supplements taken
- Teach patient that if a dose is missed, do not double, take next dose at usual time

Evaluation
Positive therapeutic outcome
- Increased control in atrial fibrillation

---

dolasetron (Rx)
(do-la'se-tron)
Anzemet
Func. class.: Antiemetic
Chem. class.: 5-HT receptor antagonist

Pregnancy category C

Action: Prevents nausea, vomiting by blocking serotonin peripherally, centrally, and in the small intestine

→Therapeutic Outcome: Control of nausea, vomiting

Uses: Prevention of nausea, vomiting associated with cancer chemotherapy and prevention of postoperative nausea, vomiting

Investigational uses: Radiotherapy-induced nausea/vomiting

Dosage and routes
Prevention of nausea/vomiting associated with cancer chemotherapy
P *Adult and child 2-16 yr :* **IV** 1.8 mg/kg as a single dose ½ hr before chemotherapy

Adult: PO 100 mg 1 hr before chemotherapy

P *Child 2-16 yr:* PO 1.8 mg/kg 1 hr before chemotherapy, max 100 mg

Prevention of postoperative nausea/vomiting
Adult: **IV** 12.5 mg as a single dose 15 min before cessation of anesthesia; PO 100 mg 2 hr before surgery (prevention only)
P *Child 2-16 yr:* **IV** 0.35 mg/kg as a single dose 15 min before cessation of anesthesia; PO 1.2 mg/kg within 2 hr before surgery (prevention only)

Available forms: Tabs 50, 100 mg; inj 20 mg/ml (12.5 mg/0.625 ml)

Adverse effects
(*italic* = common; **bold** = life-threatening)
CNS: Headache, dizziness, fatigue, drowsiness
CV: **Dysrhythmias,** ECG changes, hypotension, tachycardia, hypertension, bradycardia
GI: Diarrhea, constipation, increased AST, ALT, abdominal pain, anorexia
GU: Urinary retention, oliguria
MISC: Rash, **bronchospasm**

Contraindications: Hypersensitivity

P **Precautions:** Pregnancy **C,** lactation, **G** children, elderly

Pharmacokinetics
Absorption	Completely absorbed
Distribution	Unknown
Metabolism	Liver, extensively
Excretion	Kidneys
Half-life	Unknown

Pharmacodynamics
Unknown

Interactions
Individual drugs
Cimetidine: ↑ dolasetron levels
Rifampin: ↓ dolasetron levels
Drug classifications
Antidysrhythmics: ↑ dysrhythmias

NURSING CONSIDERATIONS
Assessment
• Assess for absence of nausea, vomiting during chemotherapy
• Assess for hypersensitivity reaction: rash, bronchospasm
• Assess for cardiac conditions, electrolyte imbalances or dysrhythmias

Nursing diagnoses
☑ Knowledge, deficient (teaching)
☑ Noncompliance (teaching)

Implementation
IV **IV route**
• Administer by inj 100 mg/30 sec or less or diluted in 50 ml of compatible sol; give over 15 sec
• Store at room temp for 24 hr after dilution

Patient/family education
• Instruct patient to report diarrhea, constipation, rash, or changes in respirations; may cause headache, use analgesic
• Teach patient reason for medication and expected results

Evaluation
Positive therapeutic outcome
• Absence of nausea, vomiting during cancer chemotherapy

donepezil (Rx)
(don-ep-ee'zill)
Aricept
Func. class.: Reversible cholinesterase inhibitor

Pregnancy category C

Action: Elevates acetylcholine concentrations (cerebral cortex) by slowing degradation of acetylcholine released in cholinergic neurons; does not alter underlying dementia

→ **Therapeutic Outcome:** Decreased symptoms of Alzheimer's disease

Uses: Treatment of mild to moderate dementia in Alzheimer's disease

Dosage and routes
Adult: PO 5 mg qd hs; may increase to 10 mg qd after 4-6 wk

Available forms: Tabs 5, 10 mg

Adverse effects
(*italic* = common; **bold** = life-threatening)
CNS: Dizziness, insomnia, somnolence, headache, fatigue, abnormal dreams, syncope, **seizures**
CV: **Atrial fibrillation,** hypotension or hypertension
GI: *Nausea, vomiting,* anorexia, *diarrhea*
GU: Frequency, UTI, incontinence
INTEG: Rash, flushing
MS: Cramps, arthritis
RESP: Rhinitis, URI, cough, pharyngitis

Contraindications: Hypersensitivity to this drug or piperidine derivatives

Precautions: Sick sinus syndrome, history of ulcers, GI bleeding, hepatic disease, bladder obstruction, asthma, pregnancy **C**, lactation, **P** children, seizures, asthma, COPD

Pharmacokinetics	
Absorption	Well
Distribution	Unknown
Metabolism	Liver to metabolites
Excretion	Unknown
Half-life	10 hr (single dose)

Pharmacodynamics
Unknown

Interactions
Individual drugs
Carbamazepine, dexamethasone, phenobarbital, phenytoin, rifampin: ↓ donepezil effect
Succinylcholine: Synergistic effects
Drug classification
Anticholinergics: ↓ activity
Cholinergic agonists, cholinesterase inhibitors: Synergistic effects
NSAIDs: ↑ gastric acid secretions

NURSING CONSIDERATIONS
Assessment
• Monitor B/P: hypotension, hypertension
• Assess mental status: affect, mood, behavioral changes, depression, complete suicide assessment
• Assess GI status: nausea, vomiting, anorexia, diarrhea
• Assess GU status: urinary frequency, incontinence

Nursing diagnoses
✓ Confusion, chronic (uses)
✓ Memory, impaired (uses)

Implementation
• Give between meals; may be given with meals for GI symptoms
• Administer dosage adjusted to response no more than q6 wk
• Provide assistance with ambulation during beginning therapy; dizziness, ataxia may occur

Patient/family education
• Advise patient to report side effects: twitching, nausea, vomiting, sweating; indicates overdose
• Advise patient to use drug exactly as prescribed; at regular intervals, preferably between meals; may be taken with meals for GI upset
• Advise patient to notify prescriber of nausea, vomiting, diarrhea (dose increase or beginning treatment), or rash
• Advise patient not to increase or abruptly decrease dose, serious consequences may result
• Instruct patient that drug is not a cure

Evaluation
Positive therapeutic outcome
• Decrease in confusion; improved mood

Treatment of overdose:
Withdraw drug, administer tertiary anticholinergics, provide supportive care

!HIGH ALERT

*DOPamine (Rx)
(doe'pa-meen)
DOPamine HCl, Intropin, Revimine ♣
Func. class.: Agonist, vasopressor, inotropic agent
Chem. class.: Catecholamine

Pregnancy category C

Action: Causes increased cardiac output; acts on β_1- and α-receptors, causing vasoconstriction in blood vessels; when low doses are administered, causes renal and mesenteric vasodilatation; β_1 stimulation produces inotropic effects with increased cardiac output

➡ **Therapeutic Outcome:** Increased B/P, cardiac output

Uses: Shock; to increase perfusion; hypotension

Investigational uses: COPD, RDS in ☐ infants

Dosage and routes
Shock
Adult: **IV** inf 2-5 mcg/kg/min, not to exceed 50 mcg/kg/min; titrate to patient's response

☐ *Child:* **IV** 5-20 mcg/kg/min adjust depending on response

COPD
Adult: **IV** 4 mcg/kg/min

CHF
Adult: **IV** 2-5 mcg/kg/min

RDS
☐ *Infants:* **IV** 5 mcg/kg/min

Available forms: Inj 40, 80, 160 mg/ml; conc for **IV** inf 0.8, 1.6, 3.2 mg/ml in D_5W

Adverse effects
(*italic* = common; **bold** = life-threatening)
CNS: Headache
CV: Palpitations, **tachycardia,** *hypertension,* **ectopic beats,** *angina,* **wide QRS complex,** peripheral vasoconstriction
GI: Nausea, vomiting, diarrhea
INTEG: Necrosis, tissue sloughing with extravasation, **gangrene**
RESP: Dyspnea

Contraindications: Hypersensitivity, ventricular fibrillation, tachydysrhythmias, pheochromocytoma

Precautions: Pregnancy **C**, lactation, arterial embolism, peripheral vascular disease

▨ **Do Not Confuse:**
DOPamine/DOBUTamine

Pharmacokinetics	
Absorption	Complete
Distribution	Widely
Metabolism	Liver
Excretion	Kidney, plasma
Half-life	2 min

Pharmacodynamics	
Onset	2-5 min
Peak	Unknown
Duration	<10 min

Interactions
Individual drugs
Phenytoin: Do not use within 2 wk, hypertensive crisis may result
Drug classifications
α-Adrenergic blockers: ↓ action of dopamine
Anesthetics: ↑ dysrhythmias
Antidepressants (tricyclic): ↑ pressor response
β-Adrenergic blockers: ↓ cardiac response
Cardiac glycosides: ↑ inotropic effect
Ergots: Severe hypertension
MAOIs: ↑ hypertension (severe), do not use within 2 wk, ↑ pressor effect
Oxytocics: ↑ B/P
Lab test interferences
↑ Urinary catecholamine, ↑ serum glucose

D

NURSING CONSIDERATIONS
Assessment
• Monitor ECG for dysrhythmias, ischemia during treatment; some patients may not need continuous ECG monitoring; also monitor PCWP, CVP, CO_2, urinary output; notify prescriber if <30 ml/hr
• Assess for heart failure: bibasilar crackles, S_3 gallop, dyspnea, neck vein distention in patients with cardiomyopathy or CHF
• Assess for oxygenation or perfusion deficit: decreased B/P, chest pain, dizziness, loss of consciousness
• Monitor B/P and pulse q5 min during inf; if B/P drops 30 mm Hg, stop inf and call prescriber
• Check for extravasation: change site q48h

Nursing diagnoses
☑ Cardiac output, decreased (uses)
☑ Tissue perfusion, ineffective (uses)
☑ Fluid volume, excess (uses)
☑ Knowledge, deficient (teaching)

Implementation
• Give by continuous inf; dilute 200-400 mg/250-500 ml of D_5W, 0.9% NaCl, D_5/LR, D_5/0.45% NaCl, D_5/0.9% NaCl, LR; do not use discolored sol; sol is stable for 24 hr; give 0.5-5 mcg/kg/min; may increase by 1-4 mcg/kg/min q15-30 min until desired patient response; use infusion pump

Syringe compatibilities: Doxapram, heparin, ranitidine

Y-site compatibilities: Aldesleukin, amifostine, amiodarone, amrinone, atracurium, aztreonam, cefmetazole, cefpirome, ciprofloxacin, cladribine, diltiazem, DOBUTamine, enalaprilat, epINEPHrine, esmolol, famotidine, fentanyl, fluconazole, foscarnet, granisetron, haloperidol, heparin, hydrocortisone, hydromorphone, labetalol, lidocaine, lorazepam, meperidine, methylPREDNISolone, metronidazole, midazolam, milrinone, morphine, niCARDipine, nitroglycerin, norepinephrine, ondansetron, pancuronium, piperacillin/tazobactam, potassium chloride, propofol, ranitidine, sargramostim, sodium nitroprusside, streptokinase, tacrolimus, theophylline, thiotepa, tolazoline, vecuronium, verapamil, vit B/C, warfarin, zidovudine

Additive compatibilities: Aminophylline, atracurium, bretylium, calcium chloride, cephalothin, chloramphenicol, DOBUTamine, enalaprilat, flumazenil, heparin, hydrocortisone, kanamycin, lidocaine, meropenem, methylPREDNISolone, nitroglycerin, oxacillin, potassium chloride, ranitidine, verapamil

Patient/family education
• Teach patient reason for medication, expected results, reason for all monitoring, and procedures
• Advise patient to report all side effects

Evaluation
Positive therapeutic outcome
• Increased cardiac output

Treatment of overdose: Discontinue drug, support circulation; give a short-acting α-blocker

---

doxapram (Rx)
(dox'a-pram)
Dopram
Func. class.: Analeptic (respiratory/cerebral stimulant)

Pregnancy category B

Action: Respiratory stimulation through activation of peripheral carotid chemoreceptor in low dosages; with higher dosages medullary respiratory centers are stimulated, with progressive general CNS stimulation

➡ **Therapeutic Outcome:** Ease of breathing, ABGs at normal limits

Uses: COPD, postanesthesia CNS and respiratory depression, prevention of acute hypercapnia, drug-induced CNS depression

Investigational uses: Treatment of apnea in premature infants when methylxanthines have failed

Dosage and routes
Postanesthesia stimulation
Adult: **IV** inj 0.5-1 mg/kg, not to exceed 1.5 mg/kg total as a single inj; **IV** inf 250 mg in 250 ml sol, not to exceed 4 mg/kg; run at 1-3 mg/min

Drug-induced CNS depression
Adult: **IV** priming dose of 2 mg/kg, repeated in 5 min; repeat q1-2h until patient awakens; **IV** inf priming dose 2 mg/kg at 1-3 mg/min, not to exceed 3 g/day

COPD (hypercapnia)
Adult: **IV** inf 1-2 mg/min, not to exceed 3 mg/min for no longer than 2 hr

Apnea of premature infant
P *Infant:* **IV** 1-1.5 mg/kg/hr loading dose followed by inf of 0.5-2.5 mg/kg/hr

Available forms: Inj **IV** 20 mg/ml

Adverse effects
(*italic* = common; **bold** = life-threatening)
CNS: **Seizures** (clonus/generalized), *headache*, restlessness, dizziness, confusion, paresthesias, flushing, sweating, bilateral Babinski's sign, rigidity, depression
CV: Chest pain, hypertension, change in heart rate, lowered T waves, tachycardia, dysrhythmias
EENT: Pupil dilation, sneezing
GI: Nausea, vomiting, diarrhea, desire to defecate
GU: Retention, incontinence, elevation of BUN, albuminuria
INTEG: Pruritus, irritation at inj site
RESP: **Laryngospasm, bronchospasm,** rebound hypoventilation, dyspnea, cough, tachypnea, hiccups

Contraindications: Hypersensitivity, seizure disorders, severe hypertension, severe bronchial asthma, severe dyspnea, severe cardiac disorders, pneumothorax, pulmonary embolism, severe respiratory disease

Precautions: Bronchial asthma, pheochromocytoma, severe tachycardia, dysrhythmias, **P** pregnancy **B**, hypertension, lactation, children

Pharmacokinetics
Absorption	Complete
Distribution	Unknown
Metabolism	Liver
Excretion	Kidneys, metabolites
Half-life	2.5-4 hr

Pharmacodynamics
Onset	20-40 sec
Peak	1-2 min
Duration	5-10 min

Interactions
Individual drugs
Cyclopropane, enflurane, halothane:
↑ dysrhythmias; delay use of doxapram
for 10 min
Drug classifications
MAOIs, sympathomimetics: Synergistic pressor
effect

NURSING CONSIDERATIONS
Assessment
• Monitor B/P, heart rate, deep tendon reflexes, level of consciousness, ABGs before
administration q30 min; check for Po_2, Pco_2,
O_2 saturation during treatment
• Monitor ECG; watch for hypertension,
increased pulse, increased pulmonary artery
pressures
• Monitor for hypertension: dysrhythmias,
tachycardia, dyspnea, skeletal muscle hyperactivity; may indicate overdosage; discontinue
if these occur
• Assess for respiratory stimulation: increased
respiratory rate, depth, abnormal rhythm;
check for patent airway; elevate head of bed to
45 degrees or higher, position patient on side
• Check for extravasation: redness, inflammation, pain; may cause phlebitis; change **IV** site
q48h

Nursing diagnoses
☑ Breathing pattern, ineffective (uses)
☑ Gas exchange, impaired (uses)
☑ Knowledge, deficient (teaching)

Implementation
• May give **IV** diluted with equal parts of
sterile water for inj; may be diluted 250
mg/250 ml (1 mg/ml) of D_5W, $D_{10}W$ (dilute
400 mg/180 ml of compatible **IV** sol [2
mg/ml] and run as inf over 2 hr)
• Give **IV** undiluted over 5 min; **IV** inf at
1-3 mg/min; adjust for desired respiratory
response, using infusion pump **IV**; if an inf
is used after initial dose, start at 1-3 mg/min;
adjust for desired respiratory response, using
infusion pump **IV**; if an inf is used after initial
dose, start at 1-3 mg/min depending on patient
response; discontinue after 2 hr; wait 1-2 hr
and repeat
• Give only after adequate airway is established; ensure O_2, **IV** barbiturates, resuscitative equipment available
• Discontinue inf if side effects occur; narrow
margin of safety

Syringe compatibilities: Amikacin,
bumetadine, chlorproMAZINE, cimetidine,
cisplatin, cyclophosphamide, DOPamine,
doxycycline, epINEPHrine, hydrOXYzine,
imipramine, isoniazid, lincomycin, methotrexate, netilmicin, phytonadione, pyridoxine,
terbutaline, thiamine, tobramycin, vinCRIStine

Syringe incompatibilities: Aminophylline, ascorbic acid, cefoperazone, cefotaxime,
cefotetan, cefuroxime, dexamethasone, diazepam, digoxin, DOBUTamine, folic acid, furosemide, hydrocortisone, ketamine, methylPRED-
NISolone, minocycline, thiopental, ticarcillin

Patient/family education
• Teach all aspects of drug, purpose, expected
reactions
• Caution patient if difficulty breathing or
shortness of breath occurs to notify nurse or
prescriber

Evaluation
Positive therapeutic outcome
• Increased breathing capacity
• ABGs WNL for patient

---

doxazosin (Rx)
(dox-ay′zoe-sin)
Cardura
Func. class.: Peripheral α-adrenergic
blocker, antihypertensive
Chem. class.: Quinazoline
Pregnancy category B

Action: Peripheral blood vessels are dilated,
peripheral resistance lowered; reduction in
B/P results from α-adrenergic receptors being
blocked

▸**Therapeutic Outcome:** Decreased B/P,
decreased symptoms of benign prostatic
hypertrophy (BPH)

Uses: Hypertension alone or as an adjunct,
urinary outflow obstruction, symptoms of
benign prostatic hyperplasia

Investigational uses: CHF with digoxin
and diuretics

Dosage and routes
BPH
Adult: PO 1 mg qd, increase in stepwise
manner to 2, 4, 8 mg qd as needed at 1-2 wk
intervals, max 8 mg

Hypertension
Adult: PO 1 mg qd, increasing up to 16 mg
qd if required; usual range 4-16 mg/day

🄶 *Elderly:* PO 0.5 mg qhs, gradually increase
Available forms: Tabs 1, 2, 4, 8 mg

Adverse effects
(*italic* = common; **bold** = life-threatening)
CNS: *Dizziness,* headache, drowsiness, anxiety, depression, vertigo, weakness, fatigue, asthenia
CV: Palpitations, *orthostatic hypotension,* **tachycardia,** edema, **dysrhythmias,** chest pain
EENT: Epistaxis, tinnitus, dry mouth, red sclera, pharyngitis, rhinitis
GI: Nausea, vomiting, diarrhea, constipation, abdominal pain
GU: Incontinence, polyuria

Contraindications: Hypersensitivity to quinazolines

P **Precautions:** Pregnancy **C**, children, lactation, hepatic disease

N **Do Not Confuse:**
Cardura/Coumadin/Cardene, Cardura/Ridaura

Pharmacokinetics	
Absorption	Well absorbed
Distribution	Not known; 98% plasma protein bound
Metabolism	Liver, extensively (<63%)
Excretion	Kidneys
Half-life	22 hr

Pharmacodynamics	
Onset	2 hr
Peak	2-6 hr
Duration	6-12 hr

Interactions
Individual drugs
Clonidine: ↓ antihypertensive effect
Indomethacin: ↓ hypotensive effects
Verapamil: ↑ hypotensive effects
Drug classifications
β-Adrenergic blockers: ↑ postural hypotension
NSAIDs: ↓ hypotensive effects
☑ *Herb/drug*
Angelica: ↑ doxazosin effect
Butcher's broom, capsicum peppers: ↓ doxazosin effect
Yohimbe: ↑ toxicity

NURSING CONSIDERATIONS
Assessment
• Monitor B/P (lying, standing) and pulse, syncope; check for edema in feet, legs daily; I&O; monitor for weight daily; notify prescriber of changes
• Assess skin turgor, dryness of mucous membranes for hydration status
• Assess for orthostatic hypotension; tell patient to rise slowly from sitting or lying position; assess pulse, jugular venous distention q4h, rales, dyspnea, orthopnea with B/P

Nursing diagnoses
☑ Cardiac output, decreased (uses)
☑ Injury, risk for physical (side effects)
☑ Knowledge, deficient (teaching)
☑ Noncompliance (teaching)

Implementation
• Store in tight container at 86° F (30° C) or less
• May be used in combination with other antihypertensives
• May be given with food to prevent GI symptoms

Patient/family education
• Teach patient not to discontinue drug abruptly; emphasize the importance of complying with dosage schedule, even if feeling better; if dose is missed take as soon as remembered; take at same time each day
• Instruct patient to take 1st dose at hs to decrease orthostatic B/P changes
• Teach patient not to use OTC products (cough, cold, allergy) unless directed by prescriber; also to avoid large amounts of caffeine
• Emphasize the need to rise slowly to sitting or standing position to minimize orthostatic hypotension
• Teach patient to notify prescriber of mouth sores, sore throat, fever, swelling of hands or feet, irregular heartbeat, chest pain
• Caution patient to report excessive perspiration, dehydration, vomiting, diarrhea; may lead to fall in B/P
• Caution patient that drug may cause dizziness, fainting, lightheadedness; may occur during 1st few days of therapy; to avoid hazardous activities
• Teach patient how to take B/P, and normal readings for age-group; to take B/P q7 days

Evaluation
Positive therapeutic outcome
• Decreased B/P in hypertension
• Decreased symptoms of BPH

Treatment of overdose: Administer volume expanders or vasopressors; discontinue drug; place in supine position

---

☑ Herb/drug   Ⓢ Do Not Crush   ◆ Alert   ◆π Key Drug   G Geriatric   P Pediatric

doxepin (Rx)

(dox'e-pin)

Adepin, doxepin HCl, Novo-Doxepin ✦, Sinequan, Sinequan Concentrate, Triadapin ✦, Zonolon Topical Cream

Func. class.: Antidepressant, tricyclic; antianxiety

Chem. class.: Dibenzoxepin, tertiary amine

Pregnancy category C

Action: Blocks reuptake of norepinephrine, serotonin into nerve endings, increasing action of norepinephrine, serotonin in nerve cells; has anticholinergic effects

➡ **Therapeutic Outcome:** Decreased symptoms of depression after 2-3 wk

Uses: Major depression, anxiety

Investigational uses: Chronic pain management; topical—pruritus

Dosage and routes

Oral conc should be diluted with 120 ml of water, milk, or orange, grapefruit, tomato, prune, pineapple juice; do not mix with grape juice.

Depression/anxiety

Adult: PO 25-75 mg/day, may increase to 300 mg/day for severely ill

G *Elderly:* PO 10-25 mg hs, increase qwk by 10-25 mg to desired dose

Pruritus

Adult: PO 10 mg hs, may increase to 25 mg hs; top apply a thin film qid ≥3 hr apart

Available forms: Caps 10, 25, 50, 75, 100, 150 mg; oral conc 10 mg/ml; cream 5%

Adverse effects

(*italic* = common; **bold** = life-threatening)

CNS: *Dizziness, drowsiness,* confusion, headache, anxiety, tremors, stimulation,
G weakness, insomnia, nightmares, extrapyramidal symptoms (EPS) (elderly), increased psychiatric symptoms, paresthesia

CV: *Orthostatic hypotension, ECG changes,* **tachycardia,** *hypertension,* palpitations, **dysrhythmias**

EENT: *Blurred vision,* tinnitus, mydriasis, ophthalmoplegia, glossitis

GI: *Diarrhea, dry mouth,* nausea, vomiting, **paralytic ileus,** increased appetite, cramps, epigastric distress, jaundice, **hepatitis,** stomatitis, constipation

GU: *Retention,* **acute renal failure**

HEMA: **Agranulocytosis, thrombocytopenia, eosinophilia, leukopenia**

INTEG: Rash, urticaria, sweating, pruritus, photosensitivity

Contraindications: Hypersensitivity to tricyclic antidepressants, urinary retention, narrow-angle glaucoma, prostatic hypertrophy

G **Precautions:** Suicidal patients, elderly, pregnancy C (PO), seizures

Do Not Confuse:
Sinequan/Serentil/Sarafem

Pharmacokinetics	
Absorption	Well absorbed
Distribution	Widely distributed; crosses placenta
Metabolism	Liver, extensively
Excretion	Kidneys, breast milk
Half-life	8-24 hr

Pharmacodynamics
Unknown

Interactions

Individual drugs

Alcohol: ↑ CNS depression

Cimetidine, fluoxetine, sertraline: ↑ doxepin effect

Clonidine: Severe hypotension; avoid use

EpINEPHrine, norepinephrine: ↑ hypertensive action

Drug classifications

Barbiturates, benzodiazepines, CNS depressants, sedative/hypnotics: ↑ CNS depression

MAOIs: Hypertensive crisis, seizures, hyperpyretic crisis

✏ *Herb/drug*

Belladonna, corkwood, henbane, jimsonweed: ↑ anticholinergic effect

Hops, kava, lavender, scopolia: ↑ action of doxepin

SAM-e, St. John's wort: ↑ serotonin syndrome

Yohimbe: ↑ hypertension

Lab test interferences

↑ Serum bilirubin, ↑ blood glucose, ↑ alkaline phosphatase

NURSING CONSIDERATIONS

Assessment

• Monitor B/P (with patient lying, standing), pulse q4h; if systolic B/P drops 20 mm Hg, hold drug, notify prescriber; take VS q4h in patients with CV disease

• Monitor blood studies: CBC, leukocytes, differential, cardiac enzymes if patient is receiving long-term therapy

• Monitor hepatic studies: AST, ALT, bilirubin

• Check weight weekly; appetite may increase with drug

- Assess ECG for flattening of T wave, bundle branch block, AV block, dysrhythmias in cardiac patients; drug should be discontinued gradually several days before surgery

G • Assess for (EPS) primarily in elderly: rigidity, dystonia, akathisia

- Assess mental status: mood, sensorium, affect, suicidal tendencies; increase in psychiatric symptoms: depression, panic
- Monitor urinary retention, constipation; **P** constipation is more likely to occur in children **G** or elderly
- Assess for withdrawal symptoms: headache, nausea, vomiting, muscle pain, weakness; do not usually occur unless drug was discontinued abruptly
- Identify alcohol consumption; if alcohol is consumed, hold dose until AM

Nursing diagnoses
✓ Coping, ineffective (uses)
✓ Injury, risk for (side effects)
✓ Knowledge, deficient (teaching)

Implementation
- Give with food or milk for GI symptoms; do not give with carbonated beverages
- Give dosage hs if oversedation occurs **G** during day; may take entire dose hs; elderly may not tolerate once/day dosing
- Store at room temp; do not freeze
- Provide safety measures, primarily for **G** elderly

Patient/family education
- Tell patient that therapeutic effects of decreased depression may take 2-3 wk, antianxiety effects sooner; to use caution in driving and other activities requiring alertness because of drowsiness, dizziness, blurred vision
- Advise patient to avoid rising quickly from **G** sitting to standing, especially elderly
- Teach patient to avoid alcohol ingestion, other CNS depressants; not to discontinue medication quickly after long-term use: may cause nausea, headache, malaise
- Teach patient to wear sunscreen or large hat, since photosensitivity occurs
- Teach patient to increase fluids, bulk in diet **G** if constipation occurs, especially elderly; to take gum, hard sugarless candy, or frequent sips of water for dry mouth
- Teach patient to report urinary retention immediately

Evaluation
Positive therapeutic outcome
- Decrease in depression
- Absence of suicidal thoughts

Treatment of overdose: ECG monitoring, induce emesis, lavage, activated charcoal, administer anticonvulsant

doxercalciferol (Rx)
(dox-er-kal'-cif-er-ol)
Hectorol
Func. class.: Parathyroid agent (calcium regulator)
Chem. class.: Vitamin D hormone
Pregnancy category C

➡ **Therapeutic Outcome:** Calcium at normal level

Uses: To lower high parathyroid hormone levels in patients undergoing chronic kidney dialysis, postmenopausal osteoporosis, prostate cancer

Dosage and routes
Adult: PO 10 mcg 3×/wk at dialysis

Adults: **IV** 4 mcg 3×/wk at end of dialysis, max 18 mcg/dose

Available forms: Caps 2.5 mcg; inj 2 mcg/ml

Adverse effects
(*italic* = common; **bold** = life-threatening)
CNS: Drowsiness, headache, lethargy
GI: Nausea, diarrhea, vomiting, anorexia, dry mouth, constipation, cramps, metallic taste
GU: Polyuria, hypercalciuria, hyperphosphatemia, hematuria
MS: Myalgia, arthralgia, decreased bone development
RESP: Shortness of breath

Contraindications: Hypersensitivity, hyperphosphatemia, hypercalcemia, vit D toxicity

Precautions: Pregnancy **C**, renal calculi, lactation, CV disease

Pharmacokinetics	
Absorption	Unknown
Distribution	Unknown
Metabolism	Liver
Excretion	Unknown
Half-life	96 hr, Terminal

Pharmacodynamics
Unknown

⧄ Herb/drug　Ⓢ Do Not Crush　⬥ Alert　☌π Key Drug　**G** Geriatric　**P** Pediatric

Interactions
Individual drugs
Cholestyramine, magnesium antacids, mineral oil: ↓ doxercalciferol levels, do not use together

NURSING CONSIDERATIONS
Assessment
- Assess GI symptoms, polyuria, flushing, head swelling, tingling, headache; may indicate hypercalcemia
- Identify nutritional status; check diet for sources of vit D (milk, some seafood), calcium (dairy products, dark green vegetables), phosphates
- Monitor BUN, creatinine, uric acid, chloride electrolytes, urine pH, urinary calcium, magnesium, phosphate, urinalysis (calcium should be kept at 9-10 mg/dl; vit D 50-135 international units/dl), alkaline phosphatase baseline and q3-6 mo
- Assess for increased drug level, since toxic reactions occur rapidly; have calcium chloride on hand if calcium level drops too low; check for tetany

Nursing diagnoses
✓ Injury, risk for (adverse reactions)
✓ Pain, chronic (uses)
✓ Knowledge, deficient (teaching)

Implementation
- Give with meals for GI symptoms
- Do not crush or chew caps

Patient/family education
- Teach patient the symptoms of hypercalcemia and about foods rich in calcium
- Advise patient to avoid products with sodium: cured meats, dairy products, cold cuts, olives, beets, pickles, soups, meat tenderizers in chronic renal failure
- Advise patient to avoid products with potassium: oranges, bananas, dried fruit, peas, dark green leafy vegetables, milk, melons, beans in chronic renal failure
- Advise patient to avoid OTC products containing calcium, potassium, or sodium in chronic renal failure
- Instruct patient to avoid all preparations containing vit D
- Instruct patient to monitor weight weekly

Evaluation
Positive therapeutic outcome
- Calcium levels 9-10 mg/dl

⚠ HIGH ALERT

***DOXOrubicin** (Rx)
(dox-oh-roo'bi-sin)
Adriamycin PFS, Adriamycin RDF, Rubex
***DOXOrubicin liposome** (Rx)
Doxil
Func. class.: Antineoplastic, antibiotic
Chem. class.: Anthracycline glycoside

Pregnancy category D

Action: Inhibits DNA synthesis primarily; derived from *Streptomyces peucetius;* replication is decreased by binding to DNA, which causes strand splitting; active throughout entire cell cycle; a vesicant

➔ Therapeutic Outcome: Prevention of rapidly growing malignant cells

Uses: Wilms' tumor; bladder, breast, cervical, head, neck, liver, lung, ovarian, prostatic, stomach, testicular, thyroid cancer; Hodgkin's disease; acute lymphoblastic leukemia; myeloblastic leukemia; neuroblastomas; lymphomas; sarcomas

Dosage and routes
DOXOrubicin
Adult: **IV** 60-75 mg/m² q3 wk, or 30 mg/m² on days 1-3 of 4-wk cycle, not to exceed 550 mg/m² cumulative dose

P *Child:* **IV** 30 mg/m²/day × 3 days, may repeat q4 wk

DOXOrubicin liposome
Adult: **IV** 20 mg/m² q3 wk

Available forms: Inj 10, 20, 50, 100, 150 mg; Doxil: liposomal dispersion for inj: 20 mg/ml

Adverse effects
(*italic* = common; **bold** = life-threatening)
CV: Increased B/P, **sinus tachycardia, PVCs,** chest pain, **bradycardia, extrasystole**
GI: Nausea, vomiting, anorexia, mucositis, **hepatotoxicity**
GU: Impotence, sterility, amenorrhea, gynecomastia, hyperuricemia
HEMA: **Thrombocytopenia, leukopenia, anemia**
INTEG: Rash, necrosis at inj site, dermatitis, reversible alopecia, cellulitis, thrombophlebitis at inj site

Contraindications: Hypersensitivity, pregnancy **D** (1st trimester), lactation, systemic infections, cardiac disorders

---

Precautions: Renal, hepatic, cardiac disease, gout, bone marrow suppression (severe)

🔊 **Do Not Confuse:**
Adriamycin/Aredia, Adriamycin/Idamycin, DOXOrubicin/DAUNOrubicin, DOXOrubicin/idarubicin

Pharmacokinetics

Absorption	Complete bioavailability
Distribution	Widely distributed; crosses placenta
Metabolism	Liver, extensively
Excretion	Bile (40%-50%)
Half-life	12 min; 3½ hr; 29⅔ hr

Pharmacodynamics
Unknown

Interactions
Individual drugs
Cyclophosphamide: ↑ cardiotoxicity
Mercaptopurine, radiation: ↑ toxicity
Radiation: ↑ bone marrow suppression
Drug classifications
Antineoplastics: ↑ toxicity, bone marrow suppression
Live virus vaccines: ↓ antibody response
Lab test interferences
↑ Uric acid

NURSING CONSIDERATIONS
Assessment
• Monitor ECG; watch for ST-T wave changes, low QRS and T; possible dysrhythmias (sinus tachycardia, heart block, PVCs); signs of irreversible cardiomyopathy
• Assess buccal cavity q8h for dryness, sores or ulceration, white patches, pain, bleeding, dysphagia; obtain prescription for viscous lidocaine (Xylocaine)
• Assess symptoms indicating severe allergic reaction: rash, pruritus, urticaria, purpuric skin lesions, itching, flushing; drug should be discontinued
• Assess tachypnea, ECG changes, dyspnea, edema, fatigue
• Monitor CBC, differential, platelet count weekly; withhold drug if WBC is <4000/mm³ or platelet count is <100,000/mm³; notify prescriber of results if WBC <20,000/mm³, platelets <150,000/mm³
• Assess for increased uric acid levels, swelling, joint pain, primarily extremities; patient should be well hydrated to prevent urate deposits

• Monitor renal function studies: BUN, creatinine, serum uric acid, urine CCr before and during therapy; I&O ratio; report fall in urine output to <30 ml/hr
• Monitor temp q4h (may indicate beginning of infection)
• Monitor liver function tests before and during therapy (bilirubin, AST, ALT, LDH) as needed or monthly; note jaundice of skin or sclera, dark urine, clay-colored stools, itchy skin, abdominal pain, fever, diarrhea
• Assess for bleeding: hematuria, stool guaiac, bruising or petechiae, mucosa or orifices q8h; inflammation of mucosa, breaks in skin
• Identify effects of alopecia on body image; discuss feelings about body changes

Nursing diagnoses
☑ Injury, risk for (adverse reactions)
☑ Body image, disturbed (adverse reactions)
☑ Infection, risk for (adverse reactions)
☑ Knowledge, deficient (teaching)

Implementation
• Avoid contact with skin; very irritating; wash completely to remove; give fluids **IV** or PO before chemotherapy to hydrate patient
• Give antiemetic 30-60 min before giving drug to prevent vomiting and prn; give antibiotics for prophylaxis of infection
• Provide liq diet: carbonated beverages; gelatin may be added if patient is not nauseated or vomiting
• Help patient to rinse mouth tid-qid with water or club soda, brush teeth bid-qid with soft brush or cotton-tipped applicators for stomatitis, use unwaxed dental floss
• Drug should be prepared by experienced personnel using proper precautions
• Do not interchange DOXOrubicin with DOXOrubicin liposome
• Give **IV** after diluting 10 mg/5 ml of NaCl for inj; another 5 ml of diluent/10 mg is recommended; shake; give over 3-5 min; give through Y-tube or 3-way stopcock through free-flowing D₅ inf or 0.9% NaCl
• **IV** liposome inj (Doxil): dilute dose up to 90 mg/250 ml of D₅W, give over ½ hr; do not admix with other solution medications
• Use hydrocortisone, dexamethasone, or sodium bicarbonate (1 mEq/1 ml) for extravasation: apply ice compress

Syringe compatibilities: Bleomycin, cisplatin, cyclophosphamide, droperidol, fluorouracil, leucovorin, methotrexate, metoclopramide, mitomycin, vinCRIStine

Syringe incompatibilities: Furosemide, heparin

Y-site compatibilities: Amifostine, aztreonam, bleomycin, chlorproMAZINE, cimetidine, cisplatin, cladribine, cyclophosphamide, dexamethasone, diphenhydrAMINE, droperidol, famotidine, filgrastim, fludarabine, fluorouracil, granisetron, hydromorphone, leucovorin calcium, lorazepam, melphalan, methotrexate, methylPREDNISolone, metoclopramide, mitomycin, morphine, ondansetron, paclitaxel, prochlorperazine, promethazine, propofol, ranitidine, sargramostim, sodium bicarbonate, teniposide, thiotepa, vinBLAStine, vinCRIStine, vinorelbine

Y-site incompatibilities: Furosemide, heparin

Additive compatibilities: Ondansetron

Additive incompatibilities: Aminophylline, cephalothin, dexamethasone, diazepam, fluorouracil, hydrocortisone

Patient/family education
• Advise patient to add 2-3 L of fluids unless contraindicated prior to and for 24-48 hr after, to decrease possible hemorrhagic cystitis
• Tell patient that urine and other body fluids may be red-orange for 48 hr; contraceptive measures are recommended during and 4 mo after therapy; drug is teratogenic to fetus
• Advise patient to avoid use of products containing aspirin or ibuprofen, razors, commercial mouthwash, since bleeding may occur; to report symptoms of bleeding (hematuria, tarry stools)
• Instruct patient to report signs of anemia (fatigue, headache, irritability, faintness, shortness of breath)
• Inform patient that hair may be lost during treatment; a wig or hairpiece may make patient feel better; new hair may be different in color, texture
• Caution patient not to have any vaccinations without the advice of the prescriber; serious reactions can occur

Evaluation
Positive therapeutic outcome
• Prevention of rapid division of malignant cells

doxycycline (Rx)
(dox-i-sye′kleen)
Apo-Doxy ✤, Atridox, Doryx, Doxy, Doxycin ✤, doxycycline, Monodox, Novodoxyclin ✤, Periostat, Vibramycin, Vibra-Tabs
Func. class.: Antiinfective
Chem. class.: Tetracycline

Pregnancy category D

Action: Inhibits protein synthesis, phosphorylation in microorganisms by binding to 30S ribosomal subunits, reversibly binding to 50S ribosomal subunits; bacteriostatic

➡ **Therapeutic Outcome:** Bactericidal action against the following: gram-positive pathogens *Bacillus anthracis, Clostridium perfringens, Clostridium tetani, Listeria monocytogenes, Nocardia, Propionibacterium acnes, Actinomyces israelii;* gram-negative pathogens *Haemophilus influenzae, Legionella pneumophila, Yersinia enterocolitica, Yersinia pestis, Neisseria gonorrhoeae, Neisseria meningitidis, Mycoplasma, Chlamydia, Rickettsia*

Uses: Syphilis, gonorrhea, *Chlamydia,* lymphogranuloma venereum, uncommon gram-negative or -positive organisms, malaria prophylaxis, acne, anthrax

Investigational uses: Traveler's diarrhea, Lyme disease, prevention of chronic bronchitis

Dosage and routes
Adult: PO/**IV** 100 mg q12h on day 1, then 100 mg/day; **IV** 200 mg in 1-2 inf on day 1, then 100-200 mg/day

▣ *Child >8 yr (>45 kg):* PO/**IV** 2.2-4.4 mg/kg/day in divided doses q12h

Gonorrhea (uncomplicated) (patients allergic to penicillin)
Adult: Uncomplicated, PO 200 mg, then 100 mg hs and 100 mg bid × 3 days or 300 mg, then 300 mg in 1 hr; disseminated, 100 mg PO bid × at least 7 days

Malaria prophylaxis
Adult: 100 mg qd 1-2 days prior to travel and daily during travel

Chlamydia trachomatis
Adult: PO 100 mg bid × 7days

Syphilis
Adult: PO 300 mg/day in divided doses × 10 days

Periodontitis

Adult: 20 mg bid after sealing and root planing for ≤9 mo; give ≥1 hr before meal AM or PM

Available forms: Tabs 50, 75, 100 mg; caps 50, 100 mg; cap, coated pellets 75, 100 mg; syr 50 mg/5 ml; powder for inj 100, 200 mg; powder for oral susp 25 mg/5 ml; inj 42.5 mg

Adverse effects
(*italic* = common; **bold** = life-threatening)
CNS: Fever
CV: Pericarditis
EENT: Dysphagia, glossitis, decreased calcification of deciduous teeth, oral candidiasis
GI: Nausea, abdominal pain, vomiting, diarrhea, anorexia, enterocolitis, **hepatotoxicity,** flatulence, abdominal cramps, gastric burning, stomatitis
GU: Increased BUN
HEMA: **Eosinophilia, neutropenia, thrombocytopenia, hemolytic anemia**
INTEG: Rash, urticaria, photosensitivity, increased pigmentation, **exfoliative dermatitis,** pruritus, **angioedema**

Contraindications: Hypersensitivity to **P** tetracyclines, children <8 yr, pregnancy **D**

Precautions: Hepatic disease, lactation

Do Not Confuse:
doxycycline/doxepin

Pharmacokinetics

Absorption	Well absorbed
Distribution	Widely distributed, crosses placenta
Metabolism	Some hepatic recycling
Excretion	Bile, feces; kidneys unchanged (20%-40%), enters breast milk
Half-life	14-17 hr; increased in severe renal disease

Pharmacodynamics

	PO	IV
Onset	1½-4 hr	Immediate
Peak	1½-4 hr	Infusion's end

Interactions
Individual drugs
Carbamazepine, cimetidine, cholestyramine, colestipol, kaolin/pectin, NaHCO₃, phenytoin, sucralfate: ↓ effect of doxycycline
Iron: Forms chelates, ↓ absorption
Penicillins: ↓ effects of penicillins
Warfarin: ↑ effect of warfarin

Drug classifications
Alkali products, antacids, barbiturates: ↓ effect of doxycycline
Anticoagulants (oral): ↑ effect of anticoagulants
Contraceptives (oral): ↓ effect of oral contraceptive
Food/drug
↓ Absorption with dairy products
Herb/drug
Bromelain: ↑ action
Acidophilus: Do not use with antiinfectives
Lab test interferences
False ↑ Urinary catecholamines, ↑ ALT, ↑ AST

NURSING CONSIDERATIONS
Assessment
• Assess patient for previous sensitivity reaction
• Assess patient for signs and symptoms of infection including characteristics of wounds, sputum, urine, stool, WBC >10,000/mm³, fever; obtain baseline information before and during treatment
• Obtain C&S before beginning drug therapy to identify if correct treatment has been initiated
• Assess for allergic reactions: rash, urticaria, pruritus, chills, fever, joint pain; angioedema may occur a few days after therapy begins
• Assess bowel pattern daily; if severe diarrhea occurs, drug should be discontinued
• Monitor for bleeding: ecchymosis, bleeding gums, hematuria, stool guaiac daily if on long-term therapy; blood dyscrasias may occur
• Assess for overgrowth of infection: perineal itching, fever, malaise, redness, pain, swelling, drainage, rash, diarrhea, change in cough, sputum

Nursing diagnoses
✓ Infection, risk for (uses)
✓ Diarrhea (side effects)
✓ Injury, risk for (side effects)
✓ Knowledge, deficient (teaching)
✓ Noncompliance (teaching)

Implementation
PO route
⊘ • Do not crush, chew caps
• Give around the clock to maintain proper blood levels; give with food to increase absorption of drug; do not give within 3 hr of other agents; drug reactions may occur
• Give with 8 oz of water, 1 hr before hs to prevent ulceration
• Shake liq preparation well before giving; use calibrated device for proper dosing
• Do not give with iron, calcium, magnesium

products or antacids, which decrease absorption and form insoluble chelate

IV IV route
- Check for irritation, extravasation, phlebitis daily; change site q72h
- For intermittent inf, dilute each 100 mg/10 ml of 0.9% NaCl, sterile water for inj; further dilute in at least 100 ml of 0.9% NaCl, D₅W, Ringer's, LR, D₅/LR; protect from direct light; keep at room temp; give over 1-4 hr; **IV** sol stable for 12 hr at room temp, 72 hr refrigerated, discard if precipitate forms

Syringe compatibilities: Doxapram

Y-site compatibilities: Acyclovir, amifostine, amiodarone, aztreonam, cyclophosphamide, diltiazem, filgrastim, fludarabine, granisetron, hydromorphone, magnesium sulfate, melphalan, meperidine, morphine, ondansetron, perphenazine, propofol, sargramostim, tacrolimus, teniposide, theophylline, thiotepa, vinorelbine

Y-site incompatibilities: Hetastarch

Additive compatibilities: Ranitidine

Patient/family education
- Teach patient to report sore throat, bruising, bleeding, joint pain; may indicate blood dyscrasias (rare)
- Advise patient to contact prescriber if vaginal itching, loose foul-smelling stools, furry tongue occur; may indicate superinfection; report itching, rash, pruritus, urticaria
- Instruct patient to take all medication prescribed for the length of time ordered; drug must be taken around the clock to maintain blood levels; do not give medication to others
- Advise patient to notify prescriber of diarrhea with blood or pus

Evaluation
Positive therapeutic outcome
- Absence of signs/symptoms of infection (WBC <10,000/mm³, temp WNL, absence of red draining wounds)
- Reported improvement in symptoms of infection

! HIGH ALERT

droperidol (Rx)
(droe-per'i-dole)
droperidol, Inapsine
Func. class.: Neuroleptic, tranquilizer, antiemetic
Chem. class.: Butyrophenone derivative

Pregnancy category C

Action: Acts on CNS at subcortical levels, producing tranquilization, sleep; antiemetic; mild α-blockade

Therapeutic Outcome: Maintenance of anesthesia

Uses: Premedication for surgery; induction, maintenance in general anesthesia; postoperatively for nausea and vomiting

Dosage and routes
Induction
Adult: **IV**/IM 0.22-0.275 mg/kg given with analgesic or general anesthetic; may give 1.25-2.5 mg additionally

Child 2-12 yr: **IV** 88-165 mcg/kg, titrated to response needed

Premedication
Adult: IM 2.5-10 mg ½-1 hr before surgery, may give 1.25-2.5 mg additionally

Child 2-12 yr: IM 88-165 mcg/kg

Maintaining general anesthesia
Adult: **IV** 1.25-2.5 mg

Regional anesthesia adjunct
Adult: IM/**IV** 2.5-5 mg

Diagnostic procedures without general anesthesia
Adult: IM 2.5-10 mg ½-1 hr before procedure; 1.25-2.5 mg may be needed additionally

Antiemetic
Adult: **IV** 0.5-1.25 mg q4h prn (unlabeled)

Available forms: Inj 2.5 mg/ml

Adverse effects
(*italic* = common; **bold** = life-threatening)
CNS: Dystonia, akathisia, flexion of arms, fine tremors, dizziness, anxiety, drowsiness, restlessness, hallucinations, depression, **seizures,** extrapyramidal symptoms, **neuroleptic malignant syndrome**
CV: **Tachycardia,** *hypotension*
EENT: Upward rotation of eyes, oculogyric crisis
INTEG: Chills, *facial sweating, shivering*
RESP: **Laryngospasm, bronchospasm**

Contraindications: Hypersensitivity, child <2 yr

Precautions: Elderly, CV disease (hypotension, bradydysrhythmias), renal, liver disease, Parkinson's disease, pregnancy **C**, pheochromocytoma

Pharmacokinetics

Absorption	Well absorbed (IM)
Distribution	Crosses blood-brain barrier, placenta
Metabolism	Liver
Excretion	Kidneys, unchanged (10%)
Half-life	2-3 hr

Pharmacodynamics

	IM/IV
Onset	3-10 min
Peak	30 min
Duration	3-6 hr

Interactions
Individual drugs
Alcohol: ↑ CNS depression
Lithium: ↑ side effects of lithium
Drug classifications
Antihistamines, antipsychotics, barbiturates, CNS depressants, opiates: ↑ CNS depression
Antihypertensives, hypotension: ↑ hypotension
Herb/drug
Kava: ↑ action

NURSING CONSIDERATIONS
Assessment
• Check VS q10 min during **IV** administration, q30 min after IM dose; for increasing heart rate or decreasing B/P, notify prescriber at once; do not place patient in Trendelenburg's position, sympathetic blockade may occur, causing respiratory arrest
• Assess extrapyramidal reactions: dystonia, akathisia, extended neck, restlessness, tremors; if these occur, an anticholinergic should be given
• If given for nausea or vomiting, monitor for significant loss of fluids, bowel sounds before and during administration

Nursing diagnoses
☑ Injury, risk for (adverse reactions)
☑ Knowledge, deficient (teaching)

Implementation
IM route
• Give deeply in large muscle mass

IV route
• Give direct **IV** undiluted; give through Y-tube or 3-way stopcock at 10 mg or less/min; titrate to patient response
• Intermittent inf may be given by adding dose to 250 ml of LR, D₅W, 0.9% NaCl; give slowly, titrate to patient response
• Give anticholinergics (benztropine, diphenhydrAMINE) for extrapyramidal reaction
• Give only with resuscitative equipment nearby

Syringe compatibilities: Atropine, bleomycin, butorphanol, chlorproMAZINE, cimetidine, cisplatin, cyclophosphamide, dimenhyDRINATE, diphenhydrAMINE, DOXOrubicin, fentanyl, glycopyrrolate, hydrOXYzine, meperidine, metoclopramide, midazolam, mitomycin, morphine, nalbuphine, pentazocine, perphenazine, prochlorperazine, promazine, promethazine, scopolamine, vinBLAStine, vinCRIStine

Syringe incompatibilities: Fluorouracil, furosemide, heparin, leucovorin, methotrexate, pentobarbital

Y-site compatibilities: Amifostine, aztreonam, bleomycin, cisatracurium, cisplatin, cladribine, cyclophosphamide, cytarabine, DOXOrubicin, DOXOrubicin liposome, famotidine, filgrastim, fluconazole, fludarabine, granisetron, hydrocortisone sodium succinate, idarubicin, melphalan, meperidine, metoclopramide, mitomycin, ondansetron, paclitaxel, potassium chloride, propofol, remifentanil, sargramostim, teniposide, thiotepa, vinBLAStine, vinCRIStine, vinorelbine, vit B/C

Y-site incompatibilities: Fluorouracil, foscarnet, furosemide, leucovorin, methotrexate, nafcillin

Additive incompatibilities: Barbiturates

Patient/family education
• Advise patient that orthostatic hypotension is common; to rise from lying or sitting position slowly; to avoid ambulation without assistance
• Caution patient that drowsiness may occur; to call for assistance for ambulation

Evaluation
Positive therapeutic outcome
• Decreased anxiety
• Absence of vomiting during and after surgery

drotrecogin alfa (Rx)

(droh'treh-koh-jin al'fah)

Xigris

Func. class.: Thrombolytic agent

Chem. class.: Recombinant human activated protein C

Pregnancy category C

Action: Activated protein C exerts an anti-thrombotic effect by inhibiting factor Va/VIIIa

➡ **Therapeutic Outcome:** Reduction of mortality in adult patients with severe sepsis who have a high risk of death

Uses: Severe sepsis (sepsis associated with acute organ dysfunction)

Dosage and routes

Adult: **IV** inf 24 mcg/kg/hr × 96 hr

Available forms: Powder for inj, lyophilized, 5 mg, 20 mg

Adverse effects

(*italic* = common; **bold** = life-threatening)

HEMA: Decreased Hct, **bleeding**

SYST: **GI, GU, intracranial, intraabdominal, intrathoracic, retroperitoneal bleeding; surface bleeding**

Contraindications: Hypersensitivity, internal active bleeding, intraspinal surgery, CNS neoplasms, ulcerative colitis, enteritis, hepatic disease, hypocoagulation, hemorrhagic stroke, epidural catheter in place, cerebral embolism/thrombosis/hemorrhage, recent major surgery, trauma

Precautions: Recent GI bleeding, prothrombin time −INR >3, pregnancy **C**, lactation, children, use >96 hr

Pharmacokinetics

Absorption	Rapid
Distribution	Plasma
Metabolism	Unknown
Excretion	Unknown
Half-life	Unknown

Pharmacodynamics

Onset	Within 2 hr of beginning infusion
Peak	96 hr
Duration	2 hr postinfusion

Interactions

Drug classifications

Anticoagulants, glycoprotein IIb/IIIa inhibitors, salicylates, thrombolytics: ↑ bleeding risk

Herb/drug

Agrimony, alfalfa, angelica, anise, basil, bay, bilberry, black haw, bogbean, bromelain, buchu, chondroitin, cinchona bark, dong quai, fenugreek, feverfew, garlic, ginger, ginkgo, ginseng, horse chestnut, Irish moss, kelp, kelpware, khella, lovage, lungwort, meadowsweet, motherwort, mugwort, nettle, papaya, parsley (large amounts), pau d'arco, pineapple, poplar, prickly ash, safflower, saw palmetto, tonka bean, turmeric, wintergreen, yarrow: ↑ risk of bleeding

Chamomile, coenzyme Q10, flax, glucomannan, goldenseal, guar gum: ↓ anticoagulant effect

Lab test interferences

Possible variably prolonged APTT, possible altered one-stage coagulation assays based on APTT (factor VIII, IX, XI assays)

NURSING CONSIDERATIONS

Assessment

◆• Assess for bleeding during treatment; hematuria, hematemesis, bleeding from mucous membranes, epistaxis, ecchymosis; may require transfusion (rare), continue to assess for bleeding

• Assess blood studies (Hct, platelets, PTT, PT, TT, APTT) before starting therapy; PT or APTT must be less than 2× control before starting therapy; PTT or PT q3-4h during treatment

• Assess VS, B/P, pulse, respirations, neurologic signs, temp at least q4h; temp >104° F (40° C) indicates internal bleeding; systolic pressure increase >25 mm Hg should be reported to prescriber

◆• Assess for neurologic changes that may indicate intracranial bleeding

◆• Assess for retroperitoneal bleeding: back pain, leg weakness, diminished pulses

Nursing diagnoses

☑ Knowledge, deficient (teaching)

Implementation

• Store in refrigerator at 2°-8° C (36°-46° F); do not freeze

• Protect unreconstituted vials from light; keep in carton until time of use

IV IV route

• Reconstitute 5 mg vial/2.5 ml; 20 mg vial/10 ml sterile water for inj to a concentration of 2 mg/ml; slowly add sterile water for inj; do not shake or invert, gently swirl until dissolved

• Further dilute with 0.9% NaCl, slowly withdraw prescribed amount and add to bag of 0.9% NaCl, direct stream to side of bag, gently invert bag; do not transport infusion bag

between locations using mechanical delivery systems
• Use immediately after reconstituting, may be held for only 3 hr at controlled room temp 59°-86° F and must complete inf within 12 hr after preparation
• Do not use if discolored or if particulate is present
• If using an infusion pump, usual concentration is 100-200 mcg/ml; if using a syringe pump, usual concentration is 100-1000 mcg/ml
• Use a dedicated **IV** line, or dedicated lumen of central venous catheter, may use only 0.9% NaCl, LR, dextrose, or dextrose/saline mixtures through same line
• Do not expose to heat or direct sunlight
• Discontinue 2 hr prior to invasive surgery or procedures introducing risk of bleeding

Evaluation
Positive therapeutic outcome
• Decreasing symptoms of sepsis, lack of mortality

---

dutasteride (Rx)
(doo-tass'ter-ide)
Duagen
Func. class.: Sex hormone, 5α-reductase inhibitor
Chem. class.: Synthetic 4-azasteroid compound

Pregnancy category X

Action: Inhibits both types 1 and 2 forms of a steroid enzyme that converts testosterone to 5 μ-dihydrotestosterone (DHT), which is responsible for the initial growth of prostatic tissue

➧**Therapeutic Outcome:** Decreased symptoms of benign prostatic hyperplasia (BPH)

Uses: Treatment of symptomatic BPH in men with an enlarged prostate gland

Dosage and routes
Adult: PO 0.5 mg qd

Available forms: Cap 0.5 mg

Adverse effects
(*italic* = common; **bold** = life-threatening)
GU: Decreased libido, impotence, gynecomastia, ejaculation disorders (rare)

Contraindications: Hypersensitivity, pregnancy **X**, lactation, women, children

Precautions: Hepatic disease

Pharmacokinetics

Absorption	Absolute bioavailability ~60%
Distribution	Protein binding 99%
Metabolism	Liver (CYP3A4)
Excretion	Feces
Half-life	5 wk at steady state

Pharmacodynamics

Onset	Rapid
Peak	2-3 hr
Duration	Levels detectable 4-6 mo posttreatment

Interactions
Individual drugs
Cimetidine, ciprofloxacin, diltiazem, ketoconazole, ritonavir, verapamil: ↑ dutasteride concentrations
Drug classifications
CYP3A4-metabolized drugs: ↑ dutasteride concentrations
Lab test interferences
↑ TSH
↓ Prostate-specific antigen (PSA)

NURSING CONSIDERATIONS
Assessment
• Assess for decreasing symptoms in BPH: decreasing urinary retention, frequency, urgency, nocturia
• Assess PSA levels, digital rectal exam, urinary obstruction; determine the absence of urinary cancer before starting treatment
• Assess liver function studies: ALT, AST, bilirubin

Nursing diagnoses
☑ Knowledge, deficient (teaching)
☑ Body image, disturbed (adverse reactions)

Implementation
• May be given without regard to meals
Ⓢ• Administer caps whole; do not break, open, or chew

Patient/family education
• Advise patient to notify prescriber if therapeutic response decreases, if edema occurs
• Caution patient not to discontinue drug abruptly
• Inform patient about changes in sex characteristics
• Caution patient not to donate blood for at least 6 mo after last dose to prevent possible blood administration to pregnant female
• Advise patient and family that caps should not be handled by pregnant women since this drug can be absorbed through the skin

---

- Inform patient that ejaculate volume may decrease during treatment, that drug rarely interferes with sexual function
- Advise patient to read patient information leaflet before starting therapy and reread it upon prescription renewal

Evaluation
Positive therapeutic outcome
- Decreased levels of DHT (5 α-dihydrotestosterone)
- Decreased urinary frequency
- Decreased urinary retention
- Decreased urinary urgency
- Decreased nocturia

---

dyphylline (Rx)
(dye'fi-lin)
Dilor, Dyflex-200, Dylline, dyphylline, Lufyllin, Neothylline
Func. class.: Bronchodilator, phosphodiesterase inhibitor
Chem. class.: Xanthine, theophylline derivative

Pregnancy category B

Action: Relaxes smooth muscle of respiratory system by blocking phosphodiesterase, which increases cyclic AMP; cyclic AMP results in positive inotropic, chronotropic effects, bronchodilatation, stimulation of CNS

➔ **Therapeutic Outcome:** Bronchodilatation with ease of breathing

Uses: Bronchial asthma, bronchospasm in chronic bronchitis and emphysema, COPD

Dosage and routes
Adult: PO 200-800 mg q6h; IM 250-500 mg q6h injected slowly, max 15 mg/kg/q6h

P *Child > 6 yr:* PO 4-7 mg/kg/day in 4 divided doses

Available forms: Tabs 200, 400 mg; elix 33.3, 53.3 mg/5 ml; inj 250 mg/ml

Adverse effects
(*italic* = common; **bold** = life-threatening)
CNS: Anxiety, restlessness, insomnia, dizziness, **seizures,** headache, lightheadedness, muscle twitching
CV: Palpitations, sinus tachycardia, hypotension, flushing, **dysrhythmias, circulatory failure**
GI: Nausea, diarrhea, *vomiting, anorexia,* dyspepsia, epigastric pain, rectal irritation, bleeding
INTEG: Flushing, urticaria

OTHER: Fever, dehydration, **albuminuria,** hyperglycemia, increased diuresis
RESP: Tachypnea, **respiratory arrest**

Contraindications: Hypersensitivity to xanthines, active peptic ulcer disease, seizure disorder

G **Precautions:** Elderly, CHF, cor pulmonale, hepatic disease, diabetes mellitus, P hypertension, children, renal disease, pregnancy **B,** glaucoma, hyperthyroidism

Pharmacokinetics
Absorption	Well absorbed (PO)
Distribution	Unknown
Metabolism	Liver
Excretion	Kidneys (85%), breast milk
Half-life	2 hr; increased in renal disease

Pharmacodynamics
	PO	IM
Onset	Unknown	Unknown
Peak	1 hr	Unknown
Duration	6 hr	Unknown

Interactions
Individual drugs
Cimetidine, erythromycin, propranolol, troleandomycin: ↑ action of dyphylline
Phenytoin: ↓ levels of phenytoin, metabolism of dyphylline
Drug classifications
Barbiturates: ↑ metabolism of dyphilline
β-Adrenergic blockers: ↑ cardiotoxicity
Uricosurics: ↓ elimination of dyphylline

NURSING CONSIDERATIONS
Assessment
- Monitor dyphylline blood levels (therapeutic level is <20 mcg/ml); toxicity (dysrhythmias, seizures, diuresis, flushing, headache) may occur with small increase above 20 mcg/ml,
G especially elderly; determine whether theophylline was given recently (24 hr)
- Monitor I&O; an increase in diuresis
G occurs; dehydration may result in elderly or
P children
- Assess respiratory rate, rhythm, depth; before and during treatment auscultate lung fields bilaterally; notify prescriber of abnormalities
- Assess for allergic reactions: rash, urticaria; if these occur, drug should be discontinued
- Assess for drug toxicity: nausea, vomiting, anorexia, cramping, diarrhea, confusion

---

Nursing diagnoses
☑ Injury, risk for (uses, adverse reactions)
☑ Airway clearance, ineffective (uses)
☑ Activity intolerance (uses)
☑ Knowledge, deficient (teaching)

Implementation
PO route
• Give around the clock to maintain blood levels, qd dose each AM
• Give 1 hr ac and 2 hr pc to increase absorption; elix should be measured accurately
IM route
• Inject slowly; do not give by **IV** route; do not administer if cloudy or a precipitate occurs, avoid this route, do not give **IV**

Patient/family education
• Teach patient to take doses as prescribed, not to skip doses or double dose; patient should check OTC medications and current prescription medications for epHEDrine, which increases CNS stimulation; tell patient not to drink alcohol or caffeine products (tea, coffee, chocolate, colas) or CV effects may occur, not to change brands
• Advise patient to avoid hazardous activities; dizziness may occur
• Caution patient if GI upset occurs, to take drug with 8 oz of water and food
• Teach patient to notify prescriber of change in smoking habit; a change in dosage may be required
• Instruct patient to report nausea, vomiting, insomnia, tachycardia, dysrhythmias, seizures, or restlessness; can indicate toxicity
• Teach patient to increase fluids to 2 L/day to decrease viscosity of secretions
• Advise patient to obtain drug level q6-12 mo

Evaluation
Positive therapeutic outcome
• Decreased dyspnea
• Clear lung fields bilaterally

---

edrophonium (Rx)
(ed-roe-fone'ee-yum)
Enlon, Reversol, Tensilon
Func. class.: Cholinergics, anticholinesterase
Chem. class.: Quaternary ammonium compound

Pregnancy category C

Action: Inhibits destruction of acetylcholine, which increases concentration at sites where acetylcholine is released; this facilitates transmission of impulses across myoneural junction

⇒ **Therapeutic Outcome:** Reversal of nondepolarizing neuromuscular blockers; absence of difficulty with muscular function in myasthenia gravis

Uses: Diagnosis of myasthenia gravis; curare antagonist; differentiation of myasthenic crisis from cholinergic crisis; reversal of nondepolarizing neuromuscular blockers

Dosage and routes
Tensilon test (myasthenia gravis diagnosis)
Adult: **IV** 1-2 mg over 15-30 sec, then 8 mg if no response; IM 10 mg; if cholinergic reaction occurs, retest after ½ hr with 2 mg IM

P *Child >34 kg:* **IV** 2 mg; if no response in 45 sec, then 1 mg q45 sec, not to exceed 10 mg; IM 5 mg

P *Child <34 kg:* **IV** 1 mg; if no response in 45 sec, then 1 mg q45 sec, not to exceed 5 mg; IM 2 mg

P *Infant:* **IV** 0.5 mg

Reversal of nondepolarizing neuromuscular blockers
Adult: **IV** 10 mg over 30-45 sec, may repeat, not to exceed 40 mg

Differentiation of myasthenic crisis from cholinergic crisis
Adult: **IV** 1 mg, if no response in 1 min, may repeat

Available forms: Inj 10 mg/ml

Adverse effects
(*italic* = common; **bold** = life-threatening)
CNS: Dizziness, headache, sweating, weakness, **seizures,** uncoordination, **paralysis,** drowsiness, **loss of consciousness**
CV: Dysrhythmias, bradycardia, hypotension, **AV block,** ECG changes, **cardiac arrest,** syncope
EENT: Miosis, blurred vision, lacrimation, visual changes
GI: Nausea, diarrhea, vomiting, cramps, increased salivary and gastric secretions, dysphagia, increased peristalsis
GU: Frequency, incontinence, urgency
INTEG: Rash, urticaria
RESP: **Respiratory depression, bronchospasm, constriction, laryngospasm, respiratory arrest,** dyspnea, increased bronchial secretions

Contraindications: Obstruction of intestine, renal system, hypersensitivity

Precautions: Seizure disorders, bronchial asthma, coronary occlusion, hyperthyroidism, dysrhythmias, peptic ulcer, megacolon, poor GI motility, pregnancy **C**, bradycardia, hypotension

Pharmacokinetics

Absorption	Unknown
Distribution	Unknown
Metabolism	Unknown
Excretion	Unknown
Half-life	Unknown

Pharmacodynamics

	IM	IV
Onset	2-10 min	30-60 sec
Peak	Unknown	Unknown
Duration	12-45 min	6-25 min

Interactions
Individual drugs
Atropine, haloperidol, magnesium, procainamide, quinidine: ↓ action of edrophonium
Digitalis: ↑ bradycardia
Drug classifications
Anesthetics, antidysrhythmics, antihistamines, corticosteroids, phenothiazines: ↓ action of edrophonium
Muscle relaxants, depolarizing: ↑ action of muscle relaxant

NURSING CONSIDERATIONS
Assessment
• Assess vital signs, respiration during test
• Monitor diabetic patient carefully, this drug lowers blood glucose
Nursing diagnoses
✓ Breathing pattern, ineffective (uses)
✓ Knowledge, deficient (teaching)
Implementation
IV route
• Administer undiluted 2 mg or less over 15-30 sec, or give as continuous inf in myasthenia crisis
• Give only after ensuring that atropine sulfate is available for cholinergic crisis
• Give only after all other cholinergics have been discontinued
• Store at room temp

Y-site compatibilities: Heparin, hydrocortisone, potassium chloride, vit B/C

Patient/family education
• Instruct patient to carry/wear emergency ID specifying myasthenia gravis and drugs taken

Evaluation
Positive therapeutic outcome
• Increased muscle strength, hand grasp; improved gait; absence of labored breathing (if severe)

Treatment of overdose: Respiratory support, atropine 1-4 mg (**IV**)

efalizumab
Raptiva
See Appendix A, Selected New Drugs

efavirenz (Rx)
(ef-ah-veer'enz)
Sustiva
Func. class.: Antiretroviral
Chem. class.: Nonnucleoside reverse transcriptase inhibitor (NNRTI)
Pregnancy category C

Action: Binds directly to reverse transcriptase and blocks RNA, DNA causing a disruption of the enzyme's site

Therapeutic Outcome: Improvement of HIV-1 infection

Uses: HIV-1 in combination with other antiretrovirals

Dosage and routes
Given in combination with protease inhibitor or nucleoside analog reverse transcriptase inhibitors (NRTIs)
Adult and child >40 kg: PO 600 mg qd hs
Child:
10-15 kg: PO 200 mg qd hs
15-20 kg: PO 250 mg qd hs
20-25 kg: PO 300 mg qd hs
25-32.5 kg: PO 350 mg qd hs
32.5-40 kg: PO 400 mg qd hs

Available forms: Caps 50, 100, 200, 600 mg

Adverse effects
(*italic* = common; **bold** = life-threatening)
CNS: Headache, dizziness, fatigue, impaired concentration, insomnia, abnormal dreams, depression
GI: *Diarrhea,* abdominal pain, *nausea,* hyperlipidemia
GU: Hematuria, kidney stones
INTEG: *Rash,* **erythema multiforme,**

Stevens-Johnson syndrome, toxic epidermal necrolysis

Contraindiations Hypersensitivity

Precautions: Liver disease, pregnancy **C**, **P** lactation, children <3 yr, renal disease, myelo-suppression

Pharmacokinetics	
Absorption	Well
Distribution	Highly protein bound (99%)
Metabolism	Liver
Excretion	Kidneys, feces
Half-life	Terminal 52-76 hr

Pharmacodynamics
Unknown

Interactions
Individual drugs
Alcohol: ↑ CNS depression
Clarithromycin, saquinavir: ↓ level of each specific drug
Indinavir, warfarin: ↑ level of each specific drug
Midazolam, triazolam: Do not give together
Ritonavir: ↑ levels of both drugs
Drug classifications
Antidepressants, antihistamines, opioids: ↑ CNS depression
Benzodiazepines, ergots: Do not give together
Estrogens: ↑ levels of both drugs
Rifamycins: ↓ efavirenz action
Herb/drug
St. John's wort: Do not use together
Food/drug
↑ Absorption of high fat foods
Lab test interferences
↑ ALT
False positive: Cannabinoids

NURSING CONSIDERATIONS
Assessment
• Assess signs of infection, anemia
• Assess liver studies: ALT, AST; renal studies
• Assess bowel pattern before, during treatment; if severe abdominal pain with bleeding occurs, drug should be discontinued; monitor hydration
• Assess skin eruptions; rash, urticaria, itching
• Assess allergies before treatment, reaction to each medication
• Assess CBC, blood chemistry, plasma HIV RNA, absolute $CD4^+/CD8^+$/cell counts/%, serum β_2 microglobulin, serum ICD+24 antigen levels, cholesterol, hepatic enzymes

• Assess for signs of toxicity: severe nausea/vomiting, maculopapular rash

Nursing diagnoses
☑ Infection, risk for (uses)
☑ Diarrhea (side effects)
☑ Knowledge, deficient (teaching)

Implementation
• Give hs to decrease CNS side effects, give on empty stomach

Patient/family education
• Inform patient that drug does not cure disease but controls symptoms, HIV still can be transmitted to others
• Advise patient to take as prescribed; if dose is missed, take as soon as remembered; do not double dose, take with water/juice; may be taken with or without food
• Instruct patient to make sure health care provider knows of all the medications being taken, supplements, herbs, OTC drugs
• Advise patient that if severe rash occurs, stop taking and notify health care provider
• Advise patient not to breastfeed or become pregnant if taking this drug
• Advise patient that adverse reactions: rash, dizziness, abnormal dreams, insomnia, lessen after a month
• Teach patient to avoid hazardous activities if dizziness, drowsiness occurs

Evaluation
Positive therapeutic outcome
• Increased CD4, cell counts
• Decreased viral load
• Improvement in symptoms and progression of HIV-1 infection

---

eletriptan (Rx)
(el-ee-trip′tan)
Relpax
Func. class.: Antimigraine agent
Pregnancy category C

Action: Binds selectively to the vascular $5\text{-}HT_1$-receptor subtype, exerts antimigraine effect; causes vasoconstriction in cranial arteries

⮕ **Therapeutic Outcome:** Decreased severity of migraine

Uses: Acute treatment of migraine with or without aura

Dosage and routes
Adult: **PO** 20 mg, may increase if needed, max 40 mg (single dose); may repeat in 2 hr if

 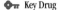

headache improves but returns, max 80 mg/day

Available forms: Tabs 20, 40 mg

Adverse effects

(*italic* = common; **bold** = life-threatening)

CNS: *Dizziness,* headache, anxiety, paresthesia, asthenia, somnolence, flushing, fatigue, hot/cold sensation

CV: Chest pain, palpitations, hypertension

GI: Nausea, dry mouth

MS: *Weakness*

RESP: Chest tightness, pressure

Contraindications: Concurrent use of ergotamine-containing preparations, uncontrolled hypertension, hypersensitivity, basilar or hemiplegic migraine; ischemic bowel disease; severe hepatic disease

Precautions: Postmenopausal women, men >40 yr, risk factors of CAD, MI, or other cardiac disease, hypercholesterolemia, obesity, �**P** diabetes, impaired hepatic or renal function, �**G** pregnancy C, lactation, children, elderly

Pharmacokinetics

Absorption	Unknown
Distribution	Unknown
Metabolism	Liver
Excretion	Urine, feces
Half-life	Unknown

Pharmacodynamics

Onset	Of pain relief 2 hr
Peak	Unknown
Duration	Unknown

Interactions

Drug classifications

CYP3A4 inhibitors: ↑ concentration of eletriptan

Herb/drug

Butterbur: ↑ effect

NURSING CONSIDERATIONS

Assessment

• Monitor B/P; signs/symptoms of coronary vasospasms

• Assess for tingling, hot sensation, burning, feeling of pressure, numbness, flushing

• Assess stress level, activity, recreation, coping mechanisms

• Assess neurologic status: LOC, blurring vision, nausea, vomiting, tingling in extremities preceding headache

• Identify ingestion of tyramine foods (pickled products, beer, wine, aged cheese), food additives, preservatives, colorings, artificial sweeteners, chocolate, caffeine, which may precipitate these types of headaches

Nursing diagnoses

☑ Pain, acute (uses)

☑ Knowledge, deficient (teaching)

Implementation

⊘ • Swallow whole

• Provide quiet, calm environment with decreased stimulation from noise, bright light, excessive talking

Patient/family education

• Have patient report any side effects to prescriber

• Teach patient to use contraception while taking drug

• Teach patient to have dark, quiet environment

• Teach patient that drug does not prevent or reduce number of migraine attacks

Evaluation

Positive therapeutic outcome

• Decrease in severity of migraine

emtricitabine

Emtriva

See Appendix A, Selected New Drugs

enalapril/enalaprilat (Rx)

(e-nal'april/e-nal'a-pril-at)

Vasotec, Vasotec IV

Func. class.: Antihypertensive

Chem. class.: Angiotensin-converting enzyme (ACE) inhibitor

Pregnancy category

D (2nd/3rd trimesters),

C (1st trimester)

Action: Selectively suppresses renin-angiotensin-aldosterone system; inhibits ACE; prevents conversion of angiotensin I to angiotensin II, resulting in dilatation of arterial and venous vessels

⮕ **Therapeutic Outcome:** Decreased B/P in hypertension; decreased preload, afterload in CHF

Uses: Hypertension, CHF, left ventricular dysfunction

Dosage and routes

Hypertension

Adult: PO 5 mg/day, may increase or decrease to desired response; range 10-40 mg/day

Adult: **IV** 1.25 mg q6h over 5 min

🅿 *Child:* PO 0.08 mg/kg/day in 1-2 divided doses, max 0.58 mg/kg/day

🅿 *Child:* **IV** 5-10 mcg/kg/dose q8-24h

Patients on diuretics
Adult: **IV** 0.625 mg over 5 min, may give additional doses of 1.25 mg q6h

Renal dose
Adult: PO 2.5 mg qd (CCr <30 ml/min) increase gradually; **IV** CCr >30 ml/min 1.25 mg q6h; CCr <30 ml/min 0.625 mg as one-time dose, increase as per B/P

CHF
Adult: PO 2.5-20 mg/day in 2 divided doses, max 40 mg qd in divided doses

Available forms: Enalapril: tabs 2.5, 5, 10, 20 mg; enalaprilat: inj 1.25 mg/ml

Adverse effects
(*italic* = common; **bold** = life-threatening)
CNS: *Insomnia, dizziness,* paresthesias, headache, fatigue, anxiety
CV: *Hypotension,* chest pain, tachycardia, **dysrhythmias,** syncope, angina, **MI,** orthostatic hypotension
EENT: *Tinnitus,* visual changes, sore throat, double vision, dry burning eyes
GI: Nausea, vomiting, colitis, cramps, diarrhea, constipation, flatulence, dry mouth, loss of taste
GU: **Proteinuria, renal failure,** increased frequency of polyuria or oliguria
HEMA: **Agranulocytosis, neutropenia**
INTEG: Rash, purpura, alopecia, hyperhidrosis, photosensitivity
META: Hyperkalemia
RESP: Dyspnea, dry cough, rales, angioedema

Contraindications: Hypersensitivity, history of angioedema, pregnancy **D** (2nd/3rd trimesters)

Precautions: Renal disease, hyperkalemia, hepatic failure, dehydration, bilateral renal artery stenosis, pregnancy **C** (1st trimester), lactation

🔌 **Do Not Confuse:**
enalapril/Eldepryl, enalapril/ramipril/Anafranil

Pharmacodynamics		
	PO	IV
Onset	1 hr	15 min
Peak	4-6 hr	1-4 hr
Duration	24 hr	6 hr

Interactions
Individual drugs
Alcohol: ↑ hypotension (large amounts)
Allopurinol: ↑ hypersensitivity
CycloSPORINE: ↑ potassium levels
Digoxin, lithium: ↑ serum levels
Indomethacin: ↓ antihypertensive effect
Rifampin: ↓ effects of enalapril
Drug classifications
α-Adrenergic blockers, diuretics, general anesthesia, nitrates, phenothiazines: ↑ hypotension
Antacids: ↓ absorption
Diuretics (potassium-sparing), potassium supplements, sympathomimetics: ↑ toxicity
Salt substitutes: ↑ potassium levels
⬜ *Herb/drug*
Arginine: Fatal hypokalemia
Pill-bearing spurge: ↑ effect
Pineapple, yohimbe: ↓ effect
St. John's wort: Severe photosensitivity
Lab test interferences
↑ ALT, ↑ AST, ↑ bilirubin, ↑ alkaline phosphatase, ↑ glucose, ↑ uric acid
False positive: ANA titer

NURSING CONSIDERATIONS
Assessment
• Monitor blood studies: neutrophils, decreased platelets with differential baseline and q3 mo if neutrophils <1000/mm³, discontinue treatment
• Monitor B/P, orthostatic hypotension, syncope; if changes occur dosage change may be required; obtain peak/trough levels
• Monitor electrolytes: K, Na, Cl during 1st 2 wk of therapy
• Monitor renal studies: protein, BUN, creatinine; increased levels may indicate nephrotic syndrome and renal failure
• Monitor renal symptoms: polyuria, oliguria, frequency, dysuria
• Establish baselines in renal, liver function tests before therapy begins and 1 wk into therapy
• Check potassium levels throughout treatment, although hyperkalemia rarely occurs
• Check for edema in feet, legs daily
• Assess for allergic reactions: rash, fever, pruritus, urticaria; drug should be discontinued if antihistamines fail to help

⬜ Herb/drug   🚫 Do Not Crush   ◆ Alert   ◆ᴛ Key Drug   🅖 Geriatric   🅿 Pediatric

Nursing diagnoses
☑ Cardiac output, decreased (uses)
☑ Injury, risk for (adverse reactions)
☑ Knowledge, deficient (teaching)
☑ Noncompliance (teaching)

Implementation
PO route
• Store in air-tight container at 86° F (30° C) or less
• Severe hypotension may occur after 1st dose of this medication; decreased hypotension may be prevented by reducing or discontinuing diuretic therapy 3 days before beginning benazepril therapy
• Give by **IV** inf of 0.9% NaCl (as ordered) to expand fluid volume if severe hypotension occurs

IV IV route
• Give **IV** direct over 5 min
• Dilute in 50 ml of 0.9% NaCl, D$_5$W, D$_5$/0.9% NaCl, D$_5$/LR; diluted solution may be used for 24 hr

Y-site compatibilities: Allopurinol, amifostine, amikacin, aminophylline, ampicillin, ampicillin/sulbactam, aztreonam, butorphanol, calcium gluconate, cefazolin, cefoperazone, ceftazidime, ceftizoxime, chloramphenicol, cimetidine, cladribine, clindamycin, dextran 40, DOBUTamine, DOPamine, erythromycin lactobionate, esmolol, famotidine, fentanyl, filgrastim, ganciclovir, gentamicin, granisetron, heparin, hetastarch, hydrocortisone, labetalol, lidocaine, magnesium sulfate, melphalan, meropenem, methylPREDNISolone, metronidazole, morphine, nafcillin, niCARdipine, penicillin G potassium, phenobarbital, piperacillin, piperacillin/tazobactam, potassium chloride, potassium phosphate, propofol, ranitidine, teniposide, thiotepa, tobramycin, trimethoprim/sulfamethoxazole, vancomycin, vinorelbine

Y-site incompatibilities: Amphotericin B, phenytoin

Additive compatibilities: DOBUTamine, DOPamine, heparin, meropenem, nitroglycerin, nitroprusside, potassium chloride

Patient/family education
• Advise patient not to discontinue drug abruptly; advise patient to tell all persons associated with health care that drug is being taken
• Teach patient not to use OTC products (cough, cold, allergy medications) unless directed by physician, to avoid potassium, salt substitutes; serious side effects can occur; xanthines, such as coffee, tea, chocolate, cola can prevent action of drug
• Instruct patient on the importance of complying with dosage schedule, even if feeling better; to continue with medical regimen to decrease B/P: exercise, cessation of smoking, decreasing stress, diet modifications
• Emphasize the need to rise slowly to sitting or standing position to minimize orthostatic hypotension; not to exercise in hot weather, which can cause increased hypotension
• Advise patient to notify prescriber of mouth sores, sore throat, fever, swelling of hands or feet, irregular heartbeat, chest pain, coughing, shortness of breath
• Caution patient to report excessive perspiration, dehydration, vomiting, diarrhea; may lead to fall in B/P
• Caution patient that drug may cause skin rash or impaired perspiration; that angioedema may occur and to discontinue if it occurs
• Caution patient that drug may cause dizziness, fainting, light-headedness; may occur during 1st few days of therapy; to avoid activities that may be hazardous
• Teach patient how to take B/P, and normal readings for age-group

Evaluation
Positive therapeutic outcome
• Decreased B/P in hypertension

Treatment of overdose: Lavage, **IV** atropine for bradycardia; **IV** theophylline for bronchospasm, digitalis, O$_2$; diuretic for cardiac failure, hemodialysis

---

enfuvirtide
Fuzeon
See Appendix A, Selected New Drugs

---

enoxacin (Rx)
(en-ox′a-sin)
Penetrex
Func. class.: Antiinfective
Chem. class.: Fluoroquinolone

Pregnancy category C

Action: Interferes with conversion of intermediate DNA fragments into high molecular weight DNA in bacteria; DNA gyrase inhibitor

→ Therapeutic Outcome: Bactericidal against the following organisms: staphylococci, *Enterobacter* sp, *Escherichia coli, Klebsiella* sp, *Neisseria gonorrhoeae, Pseudomonas aeruginosa*

Uses: Uncomplicated urethral or cervical gonorrhea, uncomplicated and complicated UTI

Dosage and routes
Gonorrhea
Adult: PO 400 mg as a single dose

Uncomplicated UTI
Adult: PO 200 mg q12h × 7 days

Complicated UTI
Adult: PO 400 mg q12h × 14 days

Renal dose
Adult: PO CCr <30 ml/min give initial dose, then give 50% of dose q12h

Available forms: Tabs 200, 400 mg

Adverse effects
(*italic* = common; **bold** = life-threatening)
CNS: Dizziness, headache, fatigue, somnolence, depression, insomnia, anxiety, **seizures**
EENT: Visual disturbances, dizziness
GI: Diarrhea, nausea, vomiting, anorexia, flatulence, heartburn, abdominal pain, dry mouth, increased AST, ALT, **pseudomembranous colitis**
INTEG: Rash, pruritus, photosensitivity
SYST: **Anaphylaxis, Stevens-Johnson syndrome**

Contraindications: Hypersensitivity to quinolones

P Precautions: Pregnancy **C**, lactation, **G** children, elderly, renal disease, seizure disorders

⊠ Do Not Confuse:
enoxacin/enoxaparin

Pharmacokinetics	
Absorption	Well absorbed
Distribution	Widely
Metabolism	Liver 20%
Excretion	Kidneys 50%-80%
Half-life	3-6 hr, increased in renal disease

Pharmacodynamics	
Onset	Unknown
Peak	Unknown

Interactions
Individual drugs
Aluminum, iron salts, sucralfate: ↓ enoxacin absorption

Aminophylline: ↑ level of aminophylline
Bismuth subsalicylate: ↓ enoxacin level, ↓ effects of enoxacin
Cyclosporine: ↑ nephrotoxicity
Digoxin: ↑ digoxin levels
Theophylline: ↑ toxicity
Drug classifications
Antacids, magnesium: ↓ enoxacin absorption
Oral anticoagulants: ↑ anticoagulation
Food/drug
↓ Absorption, dairy products
⊠ Herb/drug
Acidophilus: Do not use with antiinfectives

NURSING CONSIDERATIONS
Assessment
• Assess patient for previous sensitivity reaction to quinolones
• Assess patient for signs and symptoms of infection including WBC >10,000/mm^3, hematuria, foul-smelling urine; obtain baseline information before and during treatment
• Complete C&S testing before beginning drug therapy; this will identify if correct treatment has been initiated
• Assess for anaphylaxis: rash, urticaria, pruritus; may occur a few days after therapy begins, emergency equipment should be available
• Identify urine output; also monitor increases in BUN, creatinine
• Monitor blood studies: AST, ALT, alkaline phosphatase

Nursing diagnoses
✓ Infection, risk for (uses)
✓ Diarrhea (adverse reactions)
✓ Knowledge, deficient (teaching)
✓ Noncompliance (teaching)

Implementation
• Give 1 hr ac or 2 hr pc to maintain proper blood levels
• Give with 8 oz of water, 1 hr before hs to prevent ulceration
• Do not give 4 hr before or 2 hr after medication
• Give 2 hr before or 2 hr after antacids, zinc, iron, or calcium

Patient/family education
• Instruct patient to increase fluids to 2 L/day to prevent crystallization in the kidney
• Instruct patient to report itching, rash, pruritus, urticaria
• Instruct patient to contact prescriber if adverse reactions occur or if inflammation or pain of tendon occurs
• Instruct patient to take all medication

 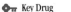

prescribed for the length of time ordered; drug must be taken as ordered

- Advise patient to limit intake of alkaline foods and drugs: milk, dairy products, peanuts, vegetables, alkaline antacids, sodium bicarbonate, not to double or miss doses
- Advise patient to ambulate, perform activities with assistance, do not perform hazardous activities
- Advise to avoid OTC medications unless approved by prescriber

Evaluation

Positive therapeutic outcome

- Reported improvement in symptoms of infection
- Negative C&S test results

! HIGH ALERT

enoxaparin (Rx)
(ee-nox'a-par-in)
Lovenox
Func. class.: Anticoagulant, antithrombotic
Chem. class.: Unfractionated porcine heparin (low molecular weight heparin)
Pregnancy category B

Action: Prevents conversion of fibrinogen to fibrin and prothrombin to thrombin by enhancing inhibitory effects of antithrombin III; produces higher ratio of anti-factor Xa to anti-factor IIa

➡ **Therapeutic Outcome:** Prevention of deep vein thrombosis

Uses: Prevention of deep vein thrombosis, pulmonary emboli in hip and knee replacement, abdominal surgery at risk for thrombosis; unstable angina/non–Q-wave MI

Dosage and routes
Hip/knee replacement
Adult: SC 30 mg bid given 12-24 hr postoperatively for 7-10 days, provided that hemostasis has been established

Abdominal surgery
Adult: SC 40 mg qd × 7-10 days to prevent thromboembolic complications, start 2 hr before surgery

DVT/PE
Adult: SC (outpatient without PE) 1 mg/kg q12h or 1.5 mg/kg qd (outpatient/inpatient) initiate warfarin therapy usually within 72 hr of enoxaparin, continue enoxaparin for ≥5 days until INR is 2-3

Prevention of ischemic complications in unstable angina/ non–Q-wave MI with aspirin
Adult: SC 1 mg/kg q12h until stable with aspirin 100-325 mg qd

Available forms: Inj 30 mg/0.3 ml, 40 mg/0.4 ml, 60 mg/0.6 ml, 80 mg/0.8 ml, 100 mg/1 ml, 120 mg/0.8 ml, 150 mg/ml, 300 mg/3 ml

Adverse effects
(*italic* = common; **bold** = life-threatening)
CNS: Fever, confusion
GI: Nausea
SYST: Edema, peripheral edema
HEMA: **Hemorrhage, hypochromic anemia, thrombocytopenia,** bleeding
INTEG: Ecchymosis, inj site hematoma

Contraindications: Hypersensitivity to this drug, heparin, or pork; hemophilia; leukemia with bleeding; peptic ulcer disease; thrombocytopenic purpura, heparin-induced thrombocytoparia

🅖 **Precautions:** Alcoholism, elderly, pregnancy **B,** hepatic disease (severe), renal disease (severe), blood dyscrasias, severe hypertension, subacute bacterial endocarditis,
🅟 acute nephritis, lactation, children, recent burn, spinal surgery

◼ **Do Not Confuse:**
enoxaparin/enoxacin
Lovenox/Lotronex

Pharmacokinetics

Absorption	Well absorbed (90%)
Distribution	Unknown
Metabolism	Unknown
Excretion	Kidneys
Half-life	4½ hr

Pharmacodynamics

Onset	Unknown
Peak	3-5 hr
Duration	Unknown

Interactions
Drug classifications
Anticoagulants, antiplatelets, NSAIDs, salicylates, thrombolytics: ↑ bleeding
Plicamycin, valproic acid: ↑ hypoprothrombinemia

🗹 *Herb/drug*
Agrimony, alfalfa, angelica, anise, basil, bay, bilberry, black haw, bogbean, bromelain, buchu, chondroitin, cinchona bark, dong quai, fenugreek, feverfew, garlic, ginger, ginkgo,

ginseng, horse chestnut, Irish moss, kelp, kelpware, khella, lovage, lungwort, meadowsweet, motherwort, mugwort, nettle, papaya, parsley (large amounts), pau d'arco, pineapple, poplar, prickly ash, safflower, saw palmetto, tonka bean, turmeric, wintergreen, yarrow: ↑ risk of bleeding

Chamomile, coenzyme Q10, flax, glucomannan, goldenseal, guar gum: ↓ anticoagulant effect

Lab test interferences
↑ AST/ALT
↓ platelets

NURSING CONSIDERATIONS
Assessment
• Monitor blood studies (Hct, CBC, coagulation studies, occult blood in stools), anti-Xa levels q3 mo; platelet count q2-3 days; thrombocytopenia may occur
• Assess patient for bleeding gums, petechiae, ecchymosis, black tarry stools, hematuria, epistaxis, decrease in B/P; indicate bleeding and possible hemorrhage; notify prescriber immediately
• Assess for neurosymptoms in patients that have received spinal anesthesia

Nursing diagnoses
☑ Injury, risk for (uses, adverse reactions)
☑ Tissue perfusion, ineffective (uses)
☑ Knowledge, deficient (teaching)

Implementation
• Give at same time each day to maintain steady blood levels
• Administer SC deeply; do not give IM, begin 2 hr before surgery, do not aspirate, do not expel bubble from syringe before administration; sol is clear to yellow; do not use sol with precipitate; apply gentle pressure for 1 min
• Leave vascular access sheath in place for 6 hr after dose, then give next dose, 6 hr after sheath removed
• Give to recumbent patient, rotate sites (left/right anterolateral, left/right posterolateral abdominal wall)
◆• Only this drug when ordered; not interchangeable with heparin or LMWHs

Patient/family education
• Warn patient to avoid OTC preparations unless directed by prescriber because they could cause serious drug interactions
• Instruct patient to use soft-bristled toothbrush to avoid bleeding gums; to avoid contact sports; to use electric razor; to avoid IM inj
• Advise patient to report any signs of bleeding, bruising: gums, under skin, urine, stools

Evaluation
Positive therapeutic outcome
• Absence of deep vein thrombosis

---

entacapone (Rx)
(en-ta'-ka-pone)
Comtan
Func. class.: Antiparkinsonian agent
Chem. class.: COMT

Pregnancy category C

Action: Inhibits COMT (catechol-*O*-methyltransferase) and alters the plasma pharmacokinetics of levodopa; given with levodopa/carbidopa

➡**Therapeutic Outcome:** Decreased symptoms of Parkinson's disease (involuntary movements)

Uses: Parkinsonism in those experiencing end of dose, decreased effect as an adjunct to levodopa/carbidopa

Dosage and routes
Adult: PO 200 mg given with carbidopa/levodopa, max 1600 mg/day

Available forms: Tabs 200 mg film coated

Adverse effects
(*italic* = common; **bold** = life-threatening)
CNS: *Involuntary choreiform movements, dyskinesia, hypokinesia, hyperkinesia, hand tremors, fatigue, headache, anxiety, twitching, numbness, weakness, confusion, agitation, nightmares,* psychosis, hallucinations, hypomania, severe depression, dizziness, **neuroleptic malignant syndrome**
CV: *Orthostatic hypotension*
GI: *Nausea, vomiting, anorexia, abdominal distress, dry mouth, flatulence, dyspepsia,* gastritis, GI disorder, *diarrhea, constipation,* bitter taste
INTEG: Rash, sweating, alopecia
MISC: Dark urine, back pain, dyspnea, purpura, fatigue, asthenia, infection-bacterial, **rhabdomyolysis**

Contraindications: Hypersensitivity

Precautions: Renal, hepatic disease, pregnancy **C,** affective disorders, psychosis, P lactation, children

---

Pharmacokinetics

Absorption	Well absorbed
Distribution	Protein binding 98%
Metabolism	Liver extensively
Excretion	Kidneys, feces; breast milk
Half-life	0.5 hr initial, 2.5 hr second

Pharmacodynamics

Onset	Unknown
Peak	Unknown
Duration	≤8 hr

Interactions
Individual drugs
Ampicillin, chloramphenicol, erythromycin, rifampin: ↓ excretion of entacapone
Apomorphine, bitolterol, DOBUTamine, DOPamine, epINEPHrine, isoetharine, methyldopa, norepinephrine: ↑ CV reactions, avoid use
Cholestyramine: ↓ excretion
Probenecid: May decrease excretion of entacapone
Drug classifications
MAOIs: Prevents catecholamine metabolism, do not use together
⊘ Herb/drug
Kava: ↓ effect

NURSING CONSIDERATIONS
Assessment
• Assess for neuroleptic malignant syndrome: high temp, increased CPK, rigidity, change in consciousness
• Monitor B/P, respiration during initial treatment; hypotension should be reported
• Assess mental status: affect, mood, behavioral changes, depression; complete suicide assessment
• Monitor liver function enzymes: AST, ALT, alkaline phosphatase; also check LDH, bilirubin, CBC
• Assess for involuntary movements in parkinsonism: akinesia, tremors, staggering gait, muscle rigidity, drooling; these symptoms should improve with therapy when given with levodopa/carbidopa

Nursing diagnoses
☑ Mobility, impaired (uses)
☑ Injury, risk for (uses)
☑ Knowledge, deficient (teaching)
☑ Noncompliance (teaching)

Implementation
• Adjust dosage to patient response
• Give with meals to decrease GI upset; limit protein taken with drug

• Give only after MAOIs have been discontinued for 2 wk
Patient/family education
• Advise patient that hallucinations, mental changes, nausea, dyskinesia can occur
• Caution patient to change positions slowly to prevent orthostatic hypotension; not to drive or operate machinery until stabilized on medication and mental performance is not affected
• Instruct patient to use drug exactly as prescribed
• Inform patient that urine, sweat may darken
• Inform patient to notify prescriber if pregnancy is suspected; if lactating, drug is excreted in breast milk

Evaluation
Positive therapeutic outcome
• Decreased akathisia, other involuntary movements when used with levodopa/carbidopa
• Increased mood when used with levodopa/carbidopa

❗ HIGH ALERT

*epHEDrine (Rx, OTC)
(e-fed'rin)
epHEDrine sulfate, Neorespin, Kondon's Nasal Jelly, Pretz-D, Vicks Vatronel
Func. class.: Bronchodilator, nonselective, adrenergic, mixed direct and indirect effects; bronchodilator, nasal decongestant, vasopressor
Chem. class.: Phenylisopropylamine
Pregnancy category C

Action: Increases contractility and heart rate by acting on β-receptors in the heart; also acts on α-receptors, causing vasoconstriction in blood vessels

⇥ Therapeutic Outcome: Decreased nasal congestion, bronchodilatation, stimulation, increased B/P

Uses: Shock; increased perfusion; hypotension, bronchodilatation; nasal congestion; orthostatic hypotension, depression, narcolepsy; vasopressor

Dosage and routes
Vasopressor
Adult: IM/SC 25-50 mg, not to exceed 150 mg/24 hr; **IV** 10-25 mg, not to exceed 150 mg/24 hr
P *Child:* SC/**IV** 3 mg/kg/day or 25-100 mg/m^2/day in divided doses q4-6h or 16.7 mg/m^2 q4-6h

Bronchodilator

P *Adult and child ≥12 yr:* PO 25-50 mg bid-qid, not to exceed 400 mg/day; IM/SC 12½-25 mg

P *Child 6-12 yr:* 6.25-12.5 mg q4h, max 75 mg/24 hr

P *Child >2 yr:* PO 2-3 mg/kg/day or 100 mg/m²/day in 4-6 divided doses

Nasal decongestant

P *Adult and child >6 yr:* Nasal 1-2 sprays in each nostril prn q4h for <3-4 days

Stimulation
Adult: PO 25-50 mg q3-4h prn

P *Child:* PO 3 mg/kg/day or 100 mg/m²/day in 4-6 divided doses

Orthostatic hypotension
Adult: PO 25 mg qd-qid

P *Child:* PO 3 mg/kg/day in 4-6 divided doses

Labor
Adult: Administer dose to maintain B/P at or <130/80 mm Hg

Available forms: Inj 25, 30, 50 mg/ml; caps 25, 50 mg; nasal spray 0.25%; nasal drops 0.5%; nasal jelly 1%

Adverse effects
(*italic* = common; **bold** = life-threatening)
CNS: *Tremors, anxiety,* insomnia, sweating, headache, dizziness, confusion, hallucinations, **seizures, CNS depression, cerebral hemorrhage**
CV: Palpitations, tachycardia, hypertension, chest pain, **dysrhythmias**
EENT: Rebound congestion (nasal)
GI: *Anorexia, nausea, vomiting*
GU: Dysuria, urinary retention
RESP: *Dyspnea*

Contraindications: Hypersensitivity to sympathomimetics, narrow-angle glaucoma, nonanaphylactic shock during general anesthesia

Precautions: Pregnancy **C**, cardiac disorders, hyperthyroidism, diabetes mellitus, prostatic hypertrophy, hypertension

** Do Not Confuse:**
epHEDrine/epINEPHrine

Pharmacokinetics	
Absorption	Well absorbed (PO/IM/SC) complete (**IV**)
Distribution	Unknown
Metabolism	Liver
Excretion	Kidneys—unchanged
Half-life	3-5 hr

Pharmacodynamics					
	PO	SC	IM	IV	NASAL
Onset	¼-1 hr	Unkn	15-30 min	5 min	Unkn
Peak	Unkn	Unkn	Unkn	Unkn	Unkn
Duration	2-4 hr	1 hr	1 hr	2 hr	6 hr

Interactions
Drug classifications
α-Adrenergic blockers, antidepressants (tricyclic), diuretics, methyldopa, rauwolfia alkaloids, urinary acidifiers: ↓ effect of epHEDrine
Anesthetics (halothane), cardiac glycosides, levodopa: ↑ dysrhythmias
Guanethidine: ↓ effect of guanethedine
MAOIs: ↑ chance of hypertensive crisis, do not use together
Oxytoxics: ↑ severe hypertension
Sympathomimetics: ↑ adrenergic side effects
Urinary alkalizers: ↑ effect of epHEDrine

NURSING CONSIDERATIONS
Assessment
• Monitor respiratory function: vital capacity, forced expiratory volume, ABGs, lung sounds, heart rate, baseline rhythm (bronchodilator)
• Monitor for evidence of allergic reactions; paradoxical bronchospasm; withhold dose; notify prescriber
• Monitor ECG, B/P, pulse, q5 min when using **IV** route (shock)
• Assess for paresthesias and coldness of extremities; peripheral blood flow may decrease; long-term use may produce pseudo anxiety state requiring sedatives, increased lactic acid with severe metabolic acidosis
• Assess nasal congestion to identify factors contributing to ongoing congestion (nasal use)
• Assess mental status and sleeping patterns; mood, sensorium, ability to stay awake

Nursing diagnoses
✓ Airway clearance, ineffective (uses)
✓ Gas exchange, impaired (uses)
✓ Sleep pattern, disturbed (uses)
✓ Knowledge, deficient (teaching)

Implementation
PO route
• Administer several hr (up to 6 hr) before hs to prevent sleeplessness
** IV route**
• Give **IV** directly undiluted using 3-way

stopcock or Y-site; give 10-25 mg slowly, may repeat in 5-10 min

• Use clear sol without precipitate; unused sol should be discarded, protect from light

Syringe compatibilities: Pentobarbital

Y-site compatibilities: Etomidate, propofol

Additive compatibilities: Chloramphenicol, lidocaine, metaraminol, nafcillin, penicillin G potassium

Solution compatibilities: 0.9% NaCl, 0.45% NaCl, D_5W, $D_{10}W$, Ringer's, LR

Patient/family education

• Advise patient to avoid use of OTC medications; extra stimulation may occur, and not to use alcohol

Evaluation

Positive therapeutic outcome

• Increased B/P (vasopressor)
• Ability to stay awake (absence of narcolepsy) or improved mood (absence of depression)
• Absence of bronchospasm
• Decreased nasal congestion

---

epinastine
Elastat
See Appendix A, Selected New Drugs

⚠ HIGH ALERT

*epINEPHrine (Rx, OTC)
(ep-i-nef'rin)
Adrenalin, Ana-Guard, AsthmaHaler Mist, AsthmaNefrin (racepinephrine), Bronitin Mist, Bronkaid Mist, epINEPHrine, Epinal, Epitrate, Eppy/N, Epinephrine Pediatric, EpiPen, EpiPen Jr., microNefrin, Nephron, Primatene Mist, S-2, Sus-Phrine, Vaponefrin (racepinephrine)
Func. class.: Bronchodilator, nonselective adrenergic agonist, cardiac stimulant, vasopressor
Chem. class.: Catecholamine

Pregnancy category C

Action: β_1- and β_2-agonist causing increased levels of cyclic AMP producing bronchodilatation, cardiac and CNS stimulation; large doses cause vasoconstriction via α-receptors; small doses can cause vasodilatation via β_2-vascular receptors

→ **Therapeutic Outcome:** Vasoconstrictor, cardiac stimulator, bronchodilator, decreased aqueous humor

Uses: Acute asthmatic attacks, hemostasis, bronchospasm, anaphylaxis, allergic reactions, cardiac arrest, adjunct in anesthesia, shock

Dosage and routes
Asthma
P **Adult and child:** INH 1-2 puffs of 1:100 or 2.25% racemic q15 min

Bronchodilator
Adult: SC 0.2-0.5 mg, q20 min-4 hr max 1 mg/dose

Anaphylactic shock/vasopressor
Adult: SC/IM 0.1-0.5 mg, repeat q5 min if needed, then **IV** 0.1-0.25 mg, repeat q5-15 min or inf 1 mcg/min, increase to 4 mcg/min

P **Child <30 kg:** SC/IM/**IV** 10 mcg/kg, repeat q5-15 min, up to 0.3 mg

Anaphylactic reaction/asthma
Adult: SC/IM 0.1-0.5 mg, repeat q10-15 min, not to exceed 1 mg/dose; epINEPHrine susp 0.5 mg SC, may repeat 0.5-1.5 mg q6h

P **Child:** SC 0.01 mg/kg, repeat q15 min × 2 doses, then q4h as needed, up to 0.5 mg/dose; epINEPHrine susp 0.025 mg/kg SC, may repeat q6h, max 0.75 mg in child ≤30 kg

Cardiac arrest
Adult: IC, **IV**, endotracheal 0.1-1 mg repeat q5 min prn

P **Child:** IC, **IV**, endotracheal 5-10 mcg q5 min, may use 0.1 mcg/kg/min **IV** inf after initial dose

Available forms: Aerosol 0.16, 0.2, 0.25 mg/spray, inj 1:1000 (1 mg/ml), 1:200 (5 mg/ml), 0.01 mg/ml (1:100,000), 0.1 mg/ml (1:10,000), 0.5 mg/ml (1:2,000); sol for nebulization 1:100, 1.25% 2.25% (base)

Adverse effects
(*italic* = common; **bold** = life-threatening)
CNS: *Tremors, anxiety,* insomnia, headache, dizziness, weakness, drowsiness, confusion, hallucinations, **cerebral hemorrhage**
CV: *Palpitations, tachycardia,* hypertension, *dysrhythmias,* increased T-wave
GI: *Anorexia, nausea, vomiting*
RESP: *Dyspnea*

Contraindications: Hypersensitivity to sympathomimetics, narrow-angle glaucoma, nonanaphylactic shock during general anesthesia, organic brain syndrome, local anesthesia of certain areas, labor, cardiac dilatation, coronary insufficiency, cerebral arteriosclerosis, organic heart disease

E

Precautions: Pregnancy **C**, cardiac disorders, hyperthyroidism, diabetes mellitus, prostatic hypertrophy, elderly, lactation, hypertension

Do Not Confuse:
epINEPHrine/ephEDrine

Pharmacokinetics

Absorption	Well absorbed (PO), complete **(IV)**
Distribution	Unknown, crosses placenta
Metabolism	Liver
Excretion	Breast milk
Half-life	Unknown

Pharmacodynamics

	SC	IM	IV	INH
Onset	3-5 min	5-10 min	Immediate	1 min
Peak	Unknown	Unknown	Unknown	Unknown
Duration	1-4 hr	1-4 hr	Unknown	1-4 hr

Interactions
Individual drugs
Bretylium: ↑ dysrhythmias
Guanethidine, levothyroxine: ↑ pressor response
Drug classifications
α-Adrenergic blockers: ↓ hypertensive effects
Anesthetics (halothane), cardiac glycosides: ↑ dysrhythmias
Antidepressants, tricyclic: ↑ chance of hypertensive crisis; do not use together
Antihistamines: ↑ pressor response
Diuretics, ergots, phenothiazines: ↓ vascular response
MAOIs: ↑ chance of hypertensive crisis, do not use together
Other sympathomimetics: Toxicity
Oxytocics: Severe hypertension

NURSING CONSIDERATIONS
Assessment
• Monitor respiratory function: vital capacity, forced expiratory volume, ABGs, lung sounds, heart rate, rhythm (baseline); amount, color of sputum
• Monitor ECG during administration continuously; if B/P increases, drug should be decreased; check B/P, pulse q5 min after parenteral route; CVP, PCWP, SVR; inadvertent high arterial B/P can result in angina, aortic rupture, cerebral hemorrhage

• Check inj site for tissue sloughing; if this occurs, administer phentolamine mixed with 0.9% NaCl
• Monitor for evidence of allergic reactions, paradoxical bronchospasm, withhold dose, notify prescriber; sulfite sensitivity, which may be life threatening

Nursing diagnoses
☑ Airway clearance, ineffective (uses)
☑ Gas exchange, impaired (uses)
☑ Cardiac output, decreased (uses)
☑ Sensory perception, disturbed, visual (uses) (ophth)
☑ Knowledge, deficient (teaching)

Implementation
• Check for correct concentration, route, dosage before administration
IV route
• Give after diluting 1 mg of 1:1000 sol/10 ml or more; 0.9% NaCl yields 1:10,000 sol, give 1 mg/min
• Give by continuous inf after further diluting in 0.9% NaCl, D$_5$W, D$_{10}$W, D$_5$/LR, LR via 3-way stopcock; for Y-site, use infusion pump, protect from light; increase dose of insulin in diabetic patients

Syringe compatibilities: Doxapram, heparin, milrinone

Y-site compatibilities: Amrinone, atracurium, calcium chloride, calcium gluconate, diltiazem, DOBUTamine, DOPamine, famotidine, fentanyl, furosemide, heparin, hydrocortisone sodium succinate, hydromorphone, labetalol, lorazepam, midazolam, milrinone, morphine, niCARdipine, nitroglycerin, norepinephrine, pancuronium, phytonadione, potassium chloride, propofol, ranitidine, vecuronium, vit B/C

Y-site incompatibilities: Ampicillin

Additive compatibilities: Amikacin, cimetidine, DOBUTamine, floxacillin, furosemide, metaraminol, ranitidine, verapamil

Additive incompatibilities: Aminophylline, mephentermine, sodium bicarbonate, warfarin
SC/IM route
• Rotate inj sites, massage well, do not use gluteal (IM) site
• Shake susp before using
Inhalation route
• Use 2.25% sol diluted in nebulizer/respirator

- 10 gtt of a 1% sol should be placed in nebulizer
- Dilute racepinephrine 2.25% sol
Endotracheal route
- Only used in intubated patient; use **IV** dose that should be injected by endotracheal tube into bronchi

Patient/family education
- Tell patient not to use OTC medications; extra stimulation may occur; to use this medication before other medications and allow at least 5 min between each, to prevent overstimulation
- Teach patient that paradoxical broncho-spasm may occur and to stop drug immediately and notify prescriber; to limit caffeine products such as chocolate, coffee, tea, and colas
- Patient should rinse mouth after inh
- Patient should report blurred vision, irritation with ophth preparations

Evaluation
Positive therapeutic outcome
- Absence of dyspnea, wheezing
- Improved airway exchange, improved ABGs
- Decreased aqueous humor
- Stabilization of heart rate and cardiac output

Treatment of overdose: Administer a β_2-adrenergic blocker, vasodilators, α-blocker

---

⚠ HIGH ALERT

epirubicin (Rx)
(ep-i-roo′-bi-sin)
Ellence
Func. class.: Antineoplastic, antibiotic
Chem. class.: Anthracycline
Pregnancy category D

Action: Inhibits DNA synthesis primarily; replication is decreased by binding to DNA, which causes strand splitting; maximum cytotoxic effects at S and G_2 phases; a vesicant

➔ **Therapeutic Outcome:** Prevention of rapidly growing malignant cells

Uses: Breast cancer as an adjuvant therapy, with axillary node involvement, after resection

Dosage and routes
Adult: **IV** inf 100-120 mg/m^2 initially given with other antineoplastics; given in repeated cycles; 3-4 wk cycles

Hepatic Dose
Adult: **IV**, bilirubin 1.2-3 mg/dl or AST 2-4 × normal upper limit, 50% of starting dose; bilirubin >3 mg/dl or AST >4 × normal upper limit, 25% of starting dose

Available forms: Inj 2 mg/ml

Adverse effects
(*italic* = common; **bold** = life-threatening)
CV: Increased B/P, **sinus tachycardia, PVCs,** chest pain, **bradycardia, extrasystole, CHF**
GI: Nausea, vomiting, diarrhea, anorexia, mucositis
GU: Hot flashes, amenorrhea, hyperuricemia
HEMA: Thrombocytopenia, leukopenia, anemia, neutropenia, secondary AML
INTEG: Rash, necrosis at inj site, reversible alopecia
MISC: Infection, febrile neutropenia, lethargy, fever, conjunctivitis

Contraindications: Hypersensitivity to this drug, anthracyclines, anthracenediones, pregnancy **D,** lactation, systemic infections, severe hepatic disease, baseline neutrophil count <1500 cell/mm^3, severe myocardial insufficiency, recent MI

Precautions: Renal, hepatic, cardiac disease, gout, bone marrow suppression (severe), elderly, children

---

Pharmacokinetics

Absorption	Complete bioavailability
Distribution	Widely distributed, crosses placenta
Metabolism	Liver, extensively
Excretion	Bile (60%)
Half-life	3 min; 2.5 hr; 33 hr

Pharmacodynamics
Unknown

Interactions
Individual drugs
Cimetidine, radiation: ↑ toxicity
Drug classifications
Antineoplastics: ↑ toxicity
Live virus vaccines: ↓ antibody response

NURSING CONSIDERATIONS
Assessment
- Monitor left ventricular ejection fraction, multigated acquisition scan or echocardio-gram, ECG; watch for ST-T wave changes, low QRS and T; possible dysrhythmias (sinus tachycardia, heart block, PVCs) may occur; assess tachypnea, ECG changes, dyspnea,

edema, fatigue; cardiac status: B/P, pulse, character, rhythm, rate, ABGs

• Assess for bone marrow depression, infection

• Assess symptoms indicating severe allergic reaction: rash, pruritus, urticaria, purpuric skin lesions, itching, flushing; drug should be discontinued

• Monitor CBC, differential, platelet count weekly; withhold drug if baseline neutrophil count is <1500/mm^3; notify prescriber of results if WBC <20,000/mm^3, platelets <150,000/mm^3; leukocyte nadir occurs 10-14 days after administration, recovery by 21st day

• Assess for increased uric acid levels, swelling, joint pain, primarily extremities; patient should be well hydrated to prevent urate deposits

• Monitor renal function studies: BUN, creatinine, serum uric acid, urine CCr before and during therapy; I&O ratio; report fall in urine output to <30 ml/hr; dosage adjustment is needed if serum creatinine >5 mg/dl

• Monitor liver function tests before and during therapy (bilirubin, AST, ALT, LDH) as needed or monthly; note jaundice of skin or sclera, dark urine, clay-colored stools, itchy skin, abdominal pain, fever, diarrhea

• Assess for bleeding: hematuria, stool guaiac, bruising or petechiae, mucosa or orifices q8h; inflammation of mucosa, breaks in skin

• Identify effects of alopecia on body image; discuss feeling about body changes

Nursing diagnoses

☑ Injury, risk for (adverse reactions)
☑ Body image, disturbed (adverse reactions)
☑ Infection, risk for (adverse reactions)
☑ Knowledge, deficient (teaching)

Implementation

• Avoid contact with skin; very irritating; wash completely to remove; give fluids **IV** or PO before chemotherapy to hydrate patient

• Give antiemetic 30-60 min before giving drug to prevent vomiting and prn

• Administer prophylactic antibiotic with a fluoroquinolone or trimethoprim/ sulfamethoxazole if dose of epirubicin is 120 mg/m^2

• Provide liq diet: carbonated beverages; gelatin may be added if patient is not nauseated or vomiting

• Drug should be prepared by experienced personnel using proper precautions

• Give into tubing of free-flowing **IV** inf 0.9% NaCl or D$_5$ over 3-5 min; do not admix with other drugs in syringe

• Use hydrocortisone, dexamethasone, or sodium bicarbonate (1 mEq/1 ml) for extravasation: apply ice compress

🚫 • Do not break, crush, or chew; only chewable tabs should be chewed

Patient/family education

• Advise patient to avoid use of products containing aspirin or NSAIDs, razors, commercial mouthwash, since bleeding may occur; to report symptoms of bleeding (hematuria, tarry stools)

• Instruct patient to report signs of anemia (fatigue, headache, irritability, faintness, shortness of breath)

• Inform patient that hair may be lost during treatment; a wig or hairpiece may make patient feel better; new hair may be different in color, texture

• Caution patient not to have any vaccinations without the advice of the prescriber; serious reactions can occur

• Advise patient to use contraception during treatment and 4 mo afterward

• Advise patient that urine may appear red for 2 days

• Instruct patient to avoid crowds, persons with known infection

• Caution patient to avoid OTC medications, supplements unless approved by prescriber

Evaluation

Positive therapeutic outcome

• Prevention of rapid division of malignant cells

---

eplerenone (Rx)

(ep-ler-ee´known)
Inspra
Func. class.: Antihypertensive

Pregnancy category C

Action: Binds to mineralocorticoid receptor and blocks the binding of aldosterone, a component of the renin-angiotensin-aldosterone system (RAAS)

➔ **Therapeutic Outcome:** Absence of hypertension

Uses: Hypertension, alone or in combination with thiazide diuretics

Dosage and routes

Adult: **PO** 50 mg qd initially, may increase to 50 mg bid after 4 wk; start dose at 25 mg qd if patient is taking CYP3A4 inhibitors

Available forms: Tabs 25, 50, 100 mg

☑ Herb/drug   🚫 Do Not Crush   ◆ Alert   ◆╥ Key Drug   Ⓖ Geriatric   Ⓟ Pediatric

Adverse effects
(*italic* = common; **bold** = life-threatening)
CNS: Headache, dizziness, fatigue
CV: Angina, **MI**
GI: Increased GGT diarrhea, abdominal pain, increased ALT
GU: Increased BUN, creatinine, gynecomastia, mastodynia (males), abnormal vaginal bleeding
META: Hyperkalemia, hyponatremia, hypercholesteremia, hypertriglyceridemia, increased uric acid
RESP: Cough

Contraindications: Hypersensitivity, lactation, children, increased serum creatinine >2 mg/dl (male) or >8 mg/dl (female), potassium >5.5 mEq/L, type 2 diabetes with microalbuminuria, hepatic disease, CCr >50 ml/min

Precautions: Impaired renal, liver function; elderly; pregnancy **B**; hyperkalemia; lactation

Pharmacokinetics
Absorption	Unknown
Distribution	Protein binding 50%
Metabolism	Liver (CYP3A4 inhibitor)
Excretion	Urine
Half-life	4-6 hr

Pharmacodynamics
Onset	Unknown
Peak	1½ hr
Duration	Unknown

Interactions
Individual drugs
Erythromycin, fluconazole, itraconazole, ketoconazole, saquinavir, verapamil: ↑ levels of eplerenone
Lithium: ↑ serum lithium levels
Drug classifications
ACE inhibitors, angiotensin II inhibitors, NSAIDs, potassium supplements: ↑ hyperkalemia
CYP3A4 inhibitors: ↑ levels of eplerenone
NSAIDs: ↓ antihypertensive effect
Food/drug
Grapefruit juice: ↑ drug level by 25%
Herb/drug
Aconite: ↑ toxicity, death
Astragalus, cola tree: ↑ or ↓ antihypertensive effect
Barberry, betony, black catechu, black cohosh, bloodroot, broom, burdock, cat's claw, dandelion, goldenseal, Irish moss, Jamaica dog-

wood, kelp, khella, mistletoe, parsley: ↑ antihypertensive effect
Coltsfoot, guarana, khat, licorice: ↓ antihypertensive effect
St. John's wort: ↓ levels of eplerenone

NURSING CONSIDERATIONS
Assessment
• Monitor B/P at peak/trough level of drug, orthostatic hypotension, syncope when used with diuretic
• Monitor renal studies: protein, BUN, creatinine; increased liver function tests; uric acid may be increased
• Monitor potassium levels, hyperkalemia may occur

Nursing diagnoses
☑ Tissue perfusion, ineffective (uses)
☑ Cardiac output, decreased (uses)
☑ Diarrhea (side effects)
☑ Knowledge, deficient (teaching)
☑ Noncompliance (teaching)

Implementation
• Store in tight container at 86° F (30° C) or less

Patient/family education
• Advise not to discontinue drug abruptly
• Advise not to use OTC products (cough, cold, allergy) unless directed by prescriber; do not use salt substitutes containing potassium without consulting prescriber
• Teach the importance of complying with dosage schedule, even if feeling better
• Teach that drug may cause dizziness, fainting, light-headedness; may occur during first few days of therapy
• Teach how to take B/P, and normal readings for age-group

Evaluation
Positive therapeutic outcome
• Decrease in B/P

epoetin (Rx)
(ee-poe'e-tin)
Epogen, rHU-EPO, Eprex ✤, Procrit
Func. class.: Antianemic, biologic modifier, hormone
Chem. class.: Amino acid polypeptide

Pregnancy category C

Action: Erythropoietin is one factor controlling rate of red cell production; drug is developed by recombinant DNA technology

⇒ **Therapeutic Outcome:** Decreased anemia with increased RBCs

Uses: Anemia caused by reduced endogenous erythropoietin production, primarily end-stage renal disease; to correct hemostatic defect in uremia; anemia caused by AZT (zidovudine) treatment in HIV-positive patients; anemia caused by chemotherapy; reduction of allogeneic blood transfusion in surgery patients

Investigational uses: Pruritus, anemia **P** in premature preterm infants, anemia in myelodysplastic syndrome, anemia in chronic inflammatory disorders

Dosage and routes
Anemia secondary to chemotherapy
Adult: SC 150 units/kg 3×/wk, may increase after 2 mo up to 300 units/kg 3×/wk

Anemia in chronic renal failure
Adult: SC/**IV** 50-100 units/kg 3×/wk, then adjust to maintain the target Hct of 30%-36%

P *Child:* **IV**/SC 50 units/kg 3×/wk

Anemia secondary to zidovudine treatment
Adult: SC/**IV** 100 units/kg 3×/wk × 2 mo; may increase by 50-100 units/kg q1-2 mo, up to 300 units/kg 3×/wk

Surgery
Adult: SC 300 units/kg/day × 10 days before surgery, the day of surgery and for 4 days postsurgery or 600 units/kg 3, 2, 1 wk before and on day of surgery

Available forms: Inj 2000, 3000, 4000, 10,000, 20,000, 40,000 units/ml

Adverse effects
(*italic* = common; **bold** = life-threatening)
CNS: **Seizures,** coldness, sweating, headache
CV: *Hypertension,* **hypertensive encephalopathy**
MS: Bone pain

Contraindications: Hypersensitivity to mammalian cell-derived products, or human albumin, uncontrolled hypertension

Precautions: Seizure disorder, porphyria, **P** pregnancy **C** , children <1 mo, lactation, multidose preserved formulation contains benzyl alcohol and should not be used in premature infants

Pharmacokinetics
Absorption	Well absorbed (SC), completely absorbed (**IV**)
Distribution	Unknown
Metabolism	Unknown
Excretion	Unknown
Half-life	5-14 hr

Pharmacodynamics
	SC/IV
Onset	Unknown
Peak	Unknown
Duration	Unknown
Increased RBC count	2-6 wk

Interactions
Drug classifications
Anticoagulants: Need for ↑ anticoagulants during hemodialysis

NURSING CONSIDERATIONS
Assessment
• Monitor renal studies: urinalysis, protein, blood, BUN, creatinine; I&O; report drop in output to <50 ml/hr
• Monitor blood studies: ferritin, transferrin monthly, transferrin sat ≥20%; ferritin ≥100 ng/ml; Hct 2×/wk until stabilized in target range (30%-36%) then at regular intervals; those with endogenous erythropoietin levels of <500 units/L respond to this agent; check for symptoms of anemia: fatigue, pallor, dyspnea; monitor Hct 2×/wk in chronic renal failure; those being treated with zidovudine or cancer patients should be monitored wk, then periodically after stabilization
• Assess for CNS symptoms: coldness, sweating, pain in long bones
• Assess CV status: B/P before and during treatment; hypertension may occur rapidly leading to hypertensive encephalopathy, antihypertensives may be needed
• Assess patient during hemodialysis for bruits, thrills, or shunts; drug prevents severe anemia in chronic renal failure; clotting may need to be treated with increased anticoagulant
• Assess for seizures if Hct is increased within 2 wk by 4 points
• Monitor serum iron levels, ferritin, transferrin levels; iron therapy may be needed to prevent recurring anemia
• Monitor B/P, check for rising B/P as Hct rises
• Monitor blood studies: BUN, creatinine, uric acid, platelets, WBC, phosphorus, potassium,

 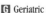

bleeding time; Hct, Hgb, RBCs, reticulocytes should be checked in chronic renal failure
- For hypersensitivity reactions: Skin rashes, urticaria (rare), antibody development does not occur
◆• For pure cell aplasia (PRCA) in absence of other causes, evaluate by testing sera for recombinant erythropoietin antibodies; any loss of response to epoetin should be evaluated

Nursing diagnoses
✓ Fatigue (uses)
✓ Activity intolerance (uses)
✓ Knowledge, deficient (teaching)

Implementation
IV IV route
- Administer by direct route at end of dialysis by venous line, do not shake vial
- If Hct increases by 4% in 2 wk, decrease dose by 25 units/kg; increase dose if Hct does not increase by 5-6 pts after 8 wk of therapy, suggested target Hct range 30%-36%
- Give additional heparin to lower chance of clots

Solution compatibilities: Do not dilute or administer with other solutions
SC route
- Before injecting, preservative-free, single dose formulation may be admixed by using 0.9% NaCl, USP, with benzyl alcohol 0.9% at a 1:1 ratio to reduce injection site discomfort

Patient/family education
- Teach patient how to take B/P
- Advise patients to take iron supplements, vit B_{12}, folic acid as directed
- Teach patient to avoid driving or hazardous activity during treatment
- Teach patients with renal disease to include high-iron and low-potassium foods in their diets (meat, dark green leafy vegetables, eggs, enriched breads)
- Teach patient the reason for treatment, expected results
- Advise patient to use contraception

Evaluation
Positive therapeutic outcome
- Increased appetite
- Enhanced sense of well-being
- Increase in reticulocyte count in 2-6 wk, Hgb, Hct

---

eprosartan (Rx)
(ep-roh-sar′tan)
Teveten HCT
Func. class.: Antihypertensive
Chem. class.: Angiotensin II receptor antagonist (Subtype AT_1)

Pregnancy category
C (1st trimester),
D (2nd/3rd trimesters)

E

Action: Blocks the vasoconstrictor and aldosterone-secreting effects of angiotensin II; selectively blocks the binding of angiotensin II to the AT_1 receptor found in tissues

➔ **Therapeutic Outcome:** Decreased B/P

Uses: Hypertension, alone or in combination with other antihypertensives

Dosage and routes
Adult: PO 600 mg qd; dose may be divided and given bid with total daily doses ranging from 400-800 mg

Available forms: Tabs 600 mg eprosartan/12.5 mg hydrochlorothiazide, 600 mg eprosartan/25 mg hydrochlorothiazide

Adverse effects
(*italic* = common; **bold** = life-threatening)
CNS: Dizziness, depression, fatigue, headache
CV: Chest pain
EENT: Sinusitis
GI: Diarrhea, dyspepsia, abdominal pain
GU: UTI
META: Hypertriglyceridemia
MS: Myalgia, arthralgia
RESP: Cough, upper respiratory infection, rhinitis, pharyngitis, viral infection

Contraindications: Hypersensitivity, pregnancy **D** 2nd/3rd trimesters

Precautions: Hypersensitivity to ACE inhibitors; pregnancy **C** 1st trimester, lactation, children, elderly; renal, hepatic disease

Pharmacokinetics	
Absorption	Absolute bioavailability ~13%; food delays absorption
Distribution	Protein binding 98%
Metabolism	Moderate renal impairment increases drug levels by 30%, hepatic impairment increases levels by 40%
Excretion	Urine, feces
Half-life	5-9 hr

Pharmacodynamics	
Onset	Unknown
Peak	1-2 hr
Duration	Unknown

Interactions
⊘ Herb/drug
Aconite: ↑ toxicity, death
Astragalus, cola tree: ↑ or ↓ antihypertensive effect
Barberry, betony, black catechu, black cohosh, bloodroot, broom, burdock, cat's claw, dandelion, goldenseal, Irish moss, Jamaican dogwood, kelp, khella, mistletoe, parsley: ↑ antihypertensive effect
Coltsfoot, guarana, khat, licorice: ↓ antihypertensive effect
Lab test interferences
↓ Hgb
↑ ALT, ↑ AST, ↑ alkaline phosphatase

NURSING CONSIDERATIONS
Assessment
• Assess B/P with position changes, pulse q4h; note rate, rhythm, quality
• Assess electrolytes: K, Na, Cl
• Assess baselines in renal, liver function tests before therapy begins
• Assess for edema in feet, legs qd
• Assess skin turgor, dryness of mucous membranes for hydration status

Nursing diagnoses
✓ Fluid volume, deficient (adverse reactions)
✓ Noncompliance (teaching)
✓ Knowledge, deficient (teaching)
✓ Injury, risk for (adverse reactions)

Implementation
• May be given without regard to meals

Patient/family education
• Advise patient to comply with dosage schedule, even if feeling better
• Advise patient to notify prescriber of fever, swelling of hands or feet, chest pain
• Inform patient that excessive perspiration, dehydration, diarrhea may lead to fall in blood pressure; consult prescriber if these occur
• Inform patient that drug may cause dizziness; advise to avoid hazardous activities until effect is known
• Advise patient not to take this medication if pregnant or breastfeeding, or if allergic reaction to this drug has occurred
• Advise patient to take missed dose as soon as possible, unless within 1 hr of next dose

Evaluation
Positive therapeutic outcome
• Decreased B/P

! HIGH ALERT

eptifibatide (Rx)
(ep-tih-fib′ah-tide)
Integrilin
Func. class.: Antiplatelet agent
Chem. class.: Glycoprotein IIb/IIIa inhibitor

Pregnancy category B

Action: Platelet glycoprotein antagonist; reversibly prevents fibrinogen, von Willebrand's factor from binding to the glycoprotein IIb/IIIa receptor, inhibiting platelet aggregation

➡ **Therapeutic Outcome:** Decreased platelets

Uses: Acute coronary syndrome including those undergoing percutaneous coronary intervention (PCI)

Dosage and routes
Acute coronary syndrome
Adult: IV BOL 180 mcg/kg as soon as diagnosed, then **IV** cont inf 2 mcg/kg/min until discharge or coronary artery bypass graft (CABG) up to 72 hr; allowing up to 96 hr of treatment

PCI in patients without acute coronary syndrome
Adult: IV BOL 180 mcg/kg given immediately before PCI; then 2 mcg/kg/min × 18 hr and a second 180 mcg/kg bolus, 10 min after 1st bolus; continue inf for up to 18-24 hr

Renal dose
CCr <50 ml/min 2-4 mg/dl same loading dose, then ½ usual inf dose

Available forms: Sol for inj 2 mg/ml (10 ml), 0.75 mg/ml (100 ml)

Adverse effects
(*italic* = common; **bold** = life-threatening)
CV: **Stroke,** hypotension
HEMA: **Thrombocytopenia**
SYST: **Bleeding, anaphylaxis**

Contraindications: Hypersensitivity, active internal bleeding; history of bleeding, stroke within 1 mo; major surgery with severe trauma, severe hypertension, history of intracranial bleeding, current or planned use of another parenteral GPIIb/IIIa inhibitor, dependence on renal dialysis

---

 Herb/drug   Do Not Crush   Alert   Key Drug   Geriatric   **P** Pediatric

P Precautions: Bleeding, pregnancy **B**,
G lactation, children, elderly, renal function
impairment

Pharmacokinetics	
Absorption	Unknown
Distribution	Unknown
Metabolism	Limited
Excretion	Kidneys
Half-life	2.5 hr

Pharmacodynamics	
Onset	Unknown
Peak	Unknown
Duration	Unknown

Interactions
Individual drugs
Abciximab, aspirin, clopidogrel, dipyridamole,
heparin, plicamycin, ticlopidine, valproate:
↑ bleeding
Drug classifications
Anticoagulants, NSAIDs, thrombolytics:
↑ bleeding
Platelet receptor inhibitors IIb, IIIa: Do not
give together

NURSING CONSIDERATIONS
Assessment
• Monitor platelets, Hgb, Hct, creatinine,
PT/APTT baseline, INR, within 6 hr of loading
dose and qd thereafter; patients undergoing
PCI should have ACT monitored; maintain
APTT 50-70 sec unless PCI is to be performed;
during PCI, ACT should be 200-300 sec; if
platelets drop <100,000/mm^3, obtain addi-
tional platelet counts; if thrombocytopenia is
confirmed, discontinue drug; also draw Hct,
Hgb, serum creatinine
• Assess for bleeding: gums, bruising, ecchymosis, petechiae; from GI, GU tract, cardiac
catheter sites, IM inj sites
Nursing diagnoses
☑ Tissue perfusion, ineffective (uses)
☑ Knowledge, deficient (teaching)
Implementation
• Aspirin and heparin may be given with this
drug
• Discontinue heparin before removing
femoral artery sheath after PCI
IV **IV route**
• After withdrawing the bolus dose from
10-ml vial, give **IV** push over 1-2 min; follow
bolus dose with cont inf using infusion pump,
give drug undiluted directly from the 100-ml
vial, spike the 100-ml vial with a vented

infusion set, use caution when centering the
spike on the circle of the stopper top
• Do not use discolored sol or those with
particulate

Y-site compatibilities: Alteplase, atropine, DOBUTamine, heparin, lidocaine,
meperidine, metoprolol, midazolam, morphine, nitroglycerin, verapamil

Solution compatibilities: 0.9% NaCl,
D$_5$/0.9% NaCl
• Discontinuing drug before CABG
• Give all medications PO if possible, avoid IM
inj and catheters

Patient/family education
• Teach patient to report bruising, bleeding,
chest pain immediately
• Inform patient of reason for medication and
expected results

Evaluation
Positive therapeutic outcome
• Decreased platelets

---

ergocalciferol
See vitamin D

---

ergonovine (Rx)
(er-goe-noe'veen)
Ergometrine, ergotrate
Func. class.: Oxytocic
Chem. class.: Ergot alkaloid
Pregnancy category N/A

Action: Stimulates uterine and vascular
smooth muscle contractions, decreases
bleeding

➙ **Therapeutic Outcome:** Uterine contraction, decreases bleeding

Uses: Treatment of postpartum or postabor-
tion hemorrhage

Investigational uses: To induce a
coronary artery spasm for diagnostic purposes

Dosage and routes
Oxytoxic
Adult: PO/SL 0.2-0.4 mg q6-12h; IM 0.2 mg
q2-4h, not to exceed 5 doses; **IV** 0.2 mg given
over 1 min

Induced coronary artery spasm
Adult: **IV** 50 mg q5 min up to 400 mcg or
until chest pain occurs

Available forms: Inj 0.2, 0.25 mg/ml

Adverse effects

(*italic* = common; **bold** = life-threatening)
CNS: *Headache, dizziness,* fainting
CV: Hypertension, chest pain
EENT: Tinnitus
GI: *Nausea, vomiting,* diarrhea
GU: Cramping
INTEG: Sweating
RESP: Dyspnea

Contraindications: Hypersensitivity to ergot medication, augmentation of labor, before delivery of placenta, spontaneous abortion (threatened), PID

Precautions: Hepatic, renal, cardiac disease, asthma, anemia, seizure disorders, hypertension, glaucoma, obliterative vascular disease

Pharmacokinetics

Absorption	Well absorbed (IM), completely absorbed (**IV**)
Distribution	Unknown
Metabolism	Liver
Excretion	Kidneys
Half-life	Unknown

Pharmacodynamics

	IM	IV
Onset	2-5 min	Immediate
Peak	Unknown	Unknown
Duration	3 hr	45 min

Interactions

Drug classifications
Ergots, sympathomimetics: ↑ hypertension
Herb/drug
Horehound: ↑ serotonin effect

NURSING CONSIDERATIONS
Assessment

- Monitor B/P, pulse; watch for change that may indicate hemorrhage; check respiratory rate, rhythm, depth; notify prescriber of abnormalities
- Assess fundal tone, nonphasic contractions; check for relaxation or severe cramping
- Assess for ergotism or overdose: nausea, vomiting, weakness, muscular pain, insensitivity to cold, paresthesia of extremities; drug should be decreased or inf discontinued
- Before administering ergonovine, calcium levels should be checked; if hypocalcemia is present, correction should be made to increase effectiveness of this drug
- Monitor prolactin levels and decreased breast milk production

Nursing diagnoses

✓ Tissue perfusion, ineffective (uses)
✓ Injury, risk for (adverse reactions)
✓ Knowledge, deficient (teaching)

Implementation
IM route
- Contractions begin in 2-5 min, drug is given q2-4h for contractions to continue; give deeply in large muscle mass; rotate inj sites if additional doses are given

IV IV route
- Give **IV** directly after dilution with 5 ml of 0.9% NaCl, give over >1 min through Y-site of free-running **IV** of 0.9% NaCl or D$_5$W

Additive compatibilities: Amikacin, cephapirin, sodium bicarbonate

Patient/family education
- Advise patient to report increased blood loss, increased temp or foul-smelling lochia; need for pad count
- Inform patient that cramping is normal; pad count should be done to determine amount of bleeding
- Tell patient not to smoke during treatment to prevent excessive vasoconstriction

Evaluation
Positive therapeutic outcome
- Absence of severe bleeding

Treatment of overdose: Stop drug; give vasodilators, heparin, dextran

---

ergotamine (Rx)
(er-got′a-meen)
Ergostat, Ergomar ✤, Gynergen
dihydroergotamine
(dy-hy′droh-er-got′ah-meen)
DHE 45, Dihydroergotamine Sandoz ✤, Migranal
Func. class.: α-Adrenergic blocker, vascular headache suppressant
Chem. class.: Ergot alkaloid–amino acid

Pregnancy category X

Action: Constricts smooth muscle in peripheral, cranial blood vessels; relaxes uterine muscle; blocks serotonin release

Therapeutic Outcome: Absence of headache

Uses: Vascular headache (migraine, histamine, cluster)

Dosage and routes
Ergotamine
Adult: SL 1 tab, may use q30 min, max 3 tabs/24 hr

Dihydroergotamine
Adult: SC/IM 1 mg, may repeat in 1 hr to 3 mg, max 3 mg/day or 6 mg/ wk; **IV** 0.5 mg, may repeat in 1 hr, max 2 mg/day or 6 mg/wk

P *Child ≥6 yr:* SC/IM 0.5 mg, may repeat in 1 hr; **IV** 0.25 mg, may repeat in 1 hr

Severe acute migraine
P *Child 12-16 yr:* **IV** 0.25-0.5 mg, may repeat q20 min for 1-2 doses

Available forms: Ergotamine: SL tab 2 mg; dihydroergotamine: inj 1 mg/ml; nasal spray 4 mg/ml

Adverse effects
(*italic* = common; **bold** = life-threatening)
CNS: Numbness in fingers, toes, headache, weakness
CV: Transient tachycardia, chest pain, bradycardia, edema, claudication, increase or decrease in B/P, **MI**
GI: Nausea, vomiting, diarrhea, abdominal cramps
MS: Muscle pain

Contraindications: Hypersensitivity to ergot preparations, occlusion (peripheral, vascular), CAD, hepatic, renal disease, peptic ulcer, hypertension, Raynaud's disease, peripheral vascular disease, intermittent claudication, pregnancy **X**

G **Precautions:** Lactation, elderly, children, **P** anemia

Pharmacokinetics
Absorption	Erratic (PO), poor (SL), rapidly (SC, IM)
Distribution	Crosses blood-brain barrier
Metabolism	Liver—extensively
Excretion	Kidneys (metabolites)
Half-life	Biphasic 2.7 hr, 21 hr

Pharmacodynamics
	PO	SL	IM/SC	IV
Onset	1-2 hr	Unknown	Unknown	Unknown
Peak	½-3 hr	Unknown	Unknown	¼-2 hr
Duration	Unknown	Unknown	8 hr	8 hr

Interactions
Drug classifications
Antiinfectives (macrolide): ↑ ergot toxicity
β-blockers: ↑ vasoconstriction
Herb/drug
Horehound: ↑ serotonin effect

NURSING CONSIDERATIONS
Assessment
• Assess characteristics of pain: duration, intensity, location, frequency, alleviating factors; also identify if halos, nausea, vomiting, blurred vision occur with headache; assess before and during treatment
• Assess for ergotism or overdose: nausea, vomiting, weakness, muscular pain, insensitivity to cold, paresthesia of extremities; drug should be decreased or infusion discontinued
• Check for hypertension: B/P, pulse, monitor all peripheral pulses; if hypertension occurs, notify prescriber; also check for tachycardia or bradycardia

Nursing diagnoses
☑ Pain, acute (uses)
☑ Injury, risk for (adverse reactions)
☑ Knowledge, deficient (teaching)

Implementation
SL route
• Have patient place tab under tongue; patient should not chew, crush, or swallow SL tab
• Patient should not drink, eat, or smoke until tab has dissolved
Inhalation route
• Teach patient how to use inhaler, protect ampules from heat/light
IV **IV route**
• Give dihydroergotamine undiluted over 1 min

Patient/family education
• Caution patient not to smoke during treatment to prevent excessive vasoconstriction
• Advise patient to avoid alcohol or OTC medications unless approved by prescriber
• Tell patient to inform prescriber if pregnancy occurs

Treatment of overdose: Stop drug, give vasodilators, heparin, dextran

ertapenem (Rx)
(er-tah-pen'em)
Invanz
Func. class.: Antiinfective—misc.
Chem. class.: Carbapenem

Pregnancy category B

Action: Interferes with cell wall replication of susceptible organisms; osmotically unstable cell wall swells, bursts from osmotic pressure

→ **Therapeutic Outcome:** Bactericidal action against the following organisms: *Bacteroides fragilis, Bacteroides distasonis, Bacteroides ovatus, Bacteroides thetaiotaomicron, Bacteroides uniformis; Clostridium clostridioforme, Escherichia coli, Eubacterium lentum, Haemophilus influenzae* (beta-lactamase-negative), *Klebsiella pneumoniae, Moraxella catarrhalis, Peptostreptococcus* sp., *Porphyromonas asaccharolytica, Prevotella bivia, Staphylococcus aureus* (methicillin-susceptible); *Streptococcus agalactiae, Streptococcus pneumoniae* (penicillin-susceptible), *Streptococcus pyogenes*

Uses: Adult patients with moderate to severe intraabdominal infections, complicated skin/skin structure infections, community-acquired pneumonia, complicated UTI, acute pelvic infections

Dosage and routes
Complicated intraabdominal infections
Adult: **IV**/IM 1 g qd × 5-14 days

Complicated skin/skin structure infections
Adult: **IV**/IM 1 g qd × 7-14 days

Community-acquired pneumonia
Adult: **IV**/IM 1 g qd × 10-14 days

Complicated UTI
Adult: **IV**/IM 1 g qd × 10-14 days

Acute pelvic infections
Adult: **IV**/IM 1 g qd × 3-10 days

Available forms: Powder, lyophilized, 1 g

Adverse effects
(*italic* = common; **bold** = life-threatening)
CNS: Insomnia, **seizures**, dizziness, *headache*
GI: Diarrhea, nausea, vomiting,
pseudomembranous colitis
GU: Vaginitis
INTEG: Rash, urticaria, *pruritus,* pain at inj site, *infused vein complication, phlebitis/thrombophlebitis,* erythema at inj site

RESP: Dyspnea, cough, pharyngitis, rales, respiratory distress
SYST: **Anaphylaxis**

Contraindications: Hypersensitivity to this drug or its components, to amide-type local anesthetics (IM only); anaphylactic reactions to beta-lactams

P G Precautions: Pregnancy **B**, lactation, elderly, children, renal disease

Do Not Confuse:
Invanz/Aninza

Pharmacokinetics

Absorption	Almost completely absorbed (IM); completely (**IV**)
Distribution	85%-95% plasma protein bound
Metabolism	Liver (IM, **IV**)
Excretion	Urine (80%), feces (10%), breast milk (IM, **IV**)
Half-life	4 hr (**IV**)

Pharmacodynamics

	IM	IV
Onset	Unknown	Immediate
Peak	2.3 hr	Dose-dependent
Duration	Unknown	Unknown

Interactions
Individual drugs
Probenecid: ↑ ertapenem plasma levels; do not coadminister
☑ *Herb/drug*
Acidophilus: Do not use with antiinfectives

NURSING CONSIDERATIONS
Assessment
• Assess for sensitivity to carbapenem antibiotics, other beta-lactam antibiotics, penicillins
• Assess for renal disease: lower dose may be required
• Assess bowel pattern qd: if severe diarrhea occurs, drug should be discontinued; may indicate pseudomembranous colitis
• Assess for infection: temp, sputum, characteristics of wound before, during, after treatment
◆• Assess for allergic reactions, anaphylaxis: rash, urticaria, pruritus; may occur a few days after therapy begins
• Assess for overgrowth of infection: perineal itching, fever, malaise, redness, pain, swelling, drainage, rash, diarrhea, change in cough or sputum

Nursing diagnoses
☑ Infection, risk for (uses)
☑ Diarrhea (adverse reaction)

 Herb/drug   Do Not Crush   ◆ Alert   Key Drug   Geriatric   Pediatric

☑ Injury, risk for (adverse reactions)
☑ Knowledge, deficient (teaching)
☑ Noncompliance (teaching)

Implementation
- Administer by **IV** or IM
- Give after C&S is taken

IM route
- Reconstitute 1 g vial of ertapenem with 3.2 ml of 1% lidocaine HCl without epinephrine, shake well
- Withdraw contents, administer deep IM in large muscle mass, use within 1 hr

IV IV route
- Do not co-infuse or mix with other medications; do not use diluents containing dextrose
- Reconstitute 1 gm vial of ertapenem with either 10 ml of water for inj, 0.9% NaCl, or bacteriostatic water for inj
- Shake well to dissolve, transfer contents of reconstituted vial to 50 ml 0.9% NaCl inj
- Complete inf within 6 hr

Patient/family education
- Advise patient to report severe diarrhea; may indicate pseudomembranous colitis
- Advise patient to report overgrowth of infection: black, furry tongue, vaginal itching, foul-smelling stools
- Caution patient to avoid breastfeeding; drug is excreted in breast milk

Evaluation
Positive therapeutic outcome
- Negative C&S, absence of signs and symptoms of infection

Treatment of overdose: Administer epinephrine, antihistamines; resuscitate if needed (anaphylaxis)

---

erythromycin base (Rx)
(eh-rith-roh-my'sin)
Apo Erythro ✤, E-base, E-Mycin, Eramycin, Erybid ✤, Ery C, Ery-Tab, Erythromid ✤, Erythromycin Base Filmtab, Erythromycin Delayed-Release, Novo-Rythro Encap ✤, PCE

erythromycin estolate (Rx)
Ilosone, Novo-Rythro ✤

erythromycin ethylsuccinate (Rx)
Apo-Erythro-ES ✤, EES, Ery Ped, Novo-Rythro ✤

erythromycin glucceptate (Rx)

erythromycin lactobionate (Rx)
Erythrocin

erythromycin stearate (Rx)
Apo-Erythro-s ✤, Novo-Rythro ✤

Func. class.: Antiinfective
Chem. class.: Macrolide

Pregnancy category C

Action: Binds to 50S ribosomal subunits of susceptible bacteria and suppresses protein synthesis

➡ **Therapeutic Outcome:** Bactericidal action against the following organisms: *Neisseria gonorrhoeae, Streptococcus pneumoniae, Mycoplasma pneumoniae, Corynebacterium diphtheriae, Bordetella pertussis, Borrelia burgdorferi, Listeria monocytogenes;* syphilis, Legionnaire's disease; streptococci, staphylococci; gram-positive bacilli: *Clostridium, Corynebacterium;* gram-negative pathogens: *Neisseria, Haemophilus influenzae, Legionella pneumophila, Mycoplasma, Chlamydia trachomatis, Entamoeba histolytica*

Uses: Mild to moderate respiratory tract, skin, soft tissue infections

Dosage and routes
Soft tissue infections
Adult: PO 250-500 mg q6-12h (base, estolate, stearate); PO 400-800 mg q6-12h (ethylsuccinate); **IV** inf 15-20 mg/kg/day (lactobionate) divided q6h

P *Child:* PO 30-50 mg/kg/day in divided doses q6h (salts); **IV** 20-40 mg/kg/day in divided doses q6h (lactobionate)

N. gonorrhoeae/*PID*
Adult: **IV** 500 mg q6h × 3 days (glucceptate, lactobionate), then PO 250 mg (base, estolate,

---

stearate) or 400 mg (ethylsuccinate) q6h ×
1 wk

Syphilis
Adult: PO 30 g in divided doses over 15 days
(base, estolate, stearate)

Chlamydia
Adult: PO 500 mg q6h × 1 wk or 250 mg
qid × 2 wk

P *Infant:* PO 50 mg/kg/day in 4 divided
doses × 3 wk or more

P *Newborn:* PO 50 mg/kg/day in 4 divided
doses × 2 wk or more

Intestinal amebiasis
Adult: PO 250 mg q6h × 10-14 days (base,
estolate, stearate)

P *Child:* PO 30-50 mg/kg/day in divided doses
q6h × 10-14 days (base, estolate, stearate)

Available forms: Base: tab, enteric-
coated 250, 333 mg; tabs, film-coated 250,
500 mg; caps, enteric-coated 125, 250 mg;
estolate: tabs, chewable 125, 250 mg; tab 500
mg; caps 125, 250 mg; drops 100 mg/ml; susp
125, 250 mg/5 ml; stearate: tabs, film-coated
250, 500 mg; ethylsuccinate: tabs, chewable
200, 400 mg; 100 mg/2.5 ml, 200, 400 mg/5
ml; susp 200, 400 mg; powder for susp 100
mg/2.5 ml, 200, 400 mg/ 5 ml; powder for inj
500 mg, 1 g (lactobionate); 250 mg, 500 mg,
1 g (as gluceptate)

Adverse effects
(*italic* = common; **bold** = life-threatening)
CV: **Dysrhythmias**
EENT: Hearing loss, tinnitus
GI: *Nausea, vomiting, diarrhea,* **hepatotox-
icity,** abdominal pain, stomatitis, heartburn,
anorexia, pruritus ani
GU: *Vaginitis, moniliasis*
INTEG: Rash, urticaria, pruritus, thrombo-
phlebitis (**IV** site)
SYST: **Anaphylaxis**

Contraindications: Hypersensitivity,
preexisting liver disease (estolate), hepatic
disease

Precautions: Pregnancy **B**, hepatic disease,
lactation

Pharmacokinetics

Absorption	Well absorbed (PO)
Distribution	Widely distributed; minimally distributed (CSF); crosses placenta
Metabolism	Liver, partially
Excretion	Bile, unchanged; kidneys (minimal), unchanged
Half-life	1-3 hr

Pharmacodynamics

	PO	IV
Onset	1 hr	Rapid
Peak	4 hr	Infusion's end

Interactions
Individual drugs
Bromocriptine, clindamycin, cycloSPORINE,
dihydropyridine, disopyramide, lovastatin,
methylPREDNISolone, midazolam, simvastatin,
triazolam: ↑ toxicity
Bromocriptine, cycloSPORINE, disopyramide,
methylPREDNISolone: ↑ action
Carbamazepine, theophylline: ↑ toxicity, from
↑ levels
Clindamycin, digoxin, dihydropyridine, disopy-
ramide, lovastatin, midazolam, simvastatin:
↑ action of each specific drug
Digoxin: ↑ blood levels of digoxin
Pimozide, sparfloxacin: ↑ serious dysrhyth-
mias, do not use together
Triazolam: ↑ effects of triazolam
Drug classifications
Calcium antagonists: ↑ action of calcium
antagonists
Calcium antagonists, ergots: ↑ toxicity
Ergots: ↑ action
Oral anticoagulants: ↑ effects of oral antico-
agulants
⊘ *Herb/drug*
Acidophilus: Do not use with antiinfectives
Lab test interferences
↑ AST/ALT
↓ Folate assay
False ↑ 17-OHCS/17-KS

NURSING CONSIDERATIONS
Assessment
- Assess patient for previous sensitivity reaction
- Assess patient for signs and symptoms of
infection including characteristics of wounds,
sputum, urine, stool, WBC >10,000/mm³,
earache, fever; obtain baseline information
before and during treatment
- Obtain C&S test results before beginning
drug therapy to identify if correct treatment
has been initiated
- Assess for allergic reactions: rash, urticaria
may occur a few days after therapy begins
- Identify urine output; if decreasing, notify
prescriber (may indicate nephrotoxicity); also
monitor increases in BUN, creatinine

- Monitor blood studies: AST, ALT, CBC, Hct, bilirubin, LDH, alkaline phosphatase, Coombs' test monthly if patient is on long-term therapy
- Monitor electrolytes: potassium, sodium, chloride monthly if patient is on long-term therapy
- Assess bowel pattern qd; if severe diarrhea occurs, drug should be discontinued
- Assess for overgrowth of infection: perineal itching, fever, malaise, redness, pain, swelling, drainage, rash, diarrhea, change in cough, sputum

Nursing diagnoses
✓ Infection, risk for (uses)
✓ Diarrhea (adverse reactions)
✓ Knowledge, deficient (teaching)
✓ Noncompliance (teaching)
✓ Injury, risk for (adverse reactions)

Implementation
PO route
- Give around the clock on an empty stomach, at least 1 hr ac or 2 hr pc; may be taken with food if GI upset occurs; do not take with juices; take dose with a full glass of water: use calibrated measuring device for drops or susp; shake well
- Store susp in refrigerator
- Chewable tab may be crushed or chewed, not swallowed whole
⊘ - Do not open, crush, or chew time-release cap or tab, enteric-coated tab may be given

Ⓘ IV route
- Add 10 ml of sterile water for inj without preservatives to 250- or 500-mg vials and 20 ml to 1-g vial; sol is stable for 1 wk after reconstitution if refrigerated
- Intermittent inf: dilute further in 100-250 ml of 0.9% NaCl or D_5W
- Give over 20-60 min to avoid phlebitis; assess for pain along vein; slow inf if pain occurs; apply ice to site and notify prescriber if unable to relieve pain
- Cont inf: may also be administered as an infusion in a dilution of 1 g/L of 0.9% NaCl, D_5W, over 4 hr

Syringe incompatibilities: Heparin

Additive compatibilities: Calcium gluconate, hydrocortisone, lidocaine, methicillin, penicillin G potassium, potassium chloride, sodium bicarbonate

Additive incompatibilities: Aminophylline, cephapirin, pentobarbital, secobarbital, streptomycin, tetracycline

Erythromycin lactobionate
Syringe compatibilities: Methicillin

Syringe incompatibilities: Ampicillin, heparin

Y-site compatibilities: Acyclovir, amiodarone, cyclophosphamide, enalaprilat, esmolol, famotidine, foscarnet, hydromorphone, idarubicin, labetalol, lorazepam, magnesium sulfate, merperidine, midazolam, morphine, multivitamins, perphenazine, vit B/C, zidovudine

Y-site incompatibilities: Fluconazole

Additive compatibilities: Aminophylline, ampicillin, cimetidine, diphenhydrAMINE, hydrocortisone, lidocaine, methicillin, penicillin G potassium, penicillin G sodium, pentobarbital, polymyxin B, potassium chloride, prednisoLONE, prochlorperazine, promazine, ranitidine, sodium bicarbonate, verapamil

Additive incompatibilities: Cephalothin, colistimethate, floxacillin, furosemide, heparin, metaraminol, metoclopramide, tetracycline, vit B/C

Patient/family education
- Teach patient to report sore throat, bruising, bleeding, joint pain; may indicate blood dyscrasias (rare)
- Advise patient to contact prescriber if vaginal itching, loose foul-smelling stools, furry tongue occur; may indicate superimposed infection
- Instruct patient to take all medication prescribed for the length of time ordered

Evaluation
Positive therapeutic outcome
- Absence of signs/symptoms of infection (WBC <10,000/mm^3, temp WNL, absence of red, draining wounds, earache)
- Reported improvement in symptoms of infection

Treatment of overdose: Withdraw drug, maintain airway, administer epINEPHrine, aminophylline, O_2, **IV** corticosteroids

escitalopram (Rx)

(es-sit-tal'oh-pram)

Lexapro

Func. class.: Antidepressant, SSRI (selective serotonin reuptake inhibitor)

Pregnancy category C

Action: Inhibits CNS neuron uptake of serotonin but not of norepinephrine

⇨ Therapeutic Outcome: Decreased symptoms of depression

Uses: Major depressive disorder

Dosage and routes

Adult: **PO** 10 mg qd in AM or PM; after 1 wk if no clinical improvement is noted, dose may be increased to 20 mg qd PM; maintenance 10-20 mg/day, reassess to determine need for treatment

G *Geriatric/hepatic dose:* **PO** 10 mg/day

Available forms: Tabs 10, 20 mg; oral sol 5 mg (as base)/5 ml

Adverse effects

(*italic* = common; **bold** = life-threatening)

CNS: Headache, nervousness, insomnia, drowsiness, anxiety, tremor, dizziness, fatigue, sedation, poor concentration, abnormal dreams, agitation, **seizures,** apathy, euphoria, hallucinations, delusions, psychosis

CV: Hot flashes, palpitations, angina pectoris, **hemorrhage,** hypertension, **tachycardia,** 1st-degree AV block, **bradycardia, MI, thrombophlebitis,** postural hypotension

EENT: Visual changes, ear/eye pain, photophobia, tinnitus

GI: Nausea, diarrhea, dry mouth, anorexia, dyspepsia, constipation, cramps, vomiting, taste changes, flatulence, decreased appetite

GU: Dysmenorrhea, decreased libido, urinary frequency, UTI, amenorrhea, cystitis, impotence, urine retention

INTEG: Sweating, rash, pruritus, acne, alopecia, urticaria, photosensitivity

MS: Pain, arthritis, twitching

RESP: Infection, pharyngitis, nasal congestion, sinus headache, sinusitis, cough, dyspnea, bronchitis, asthma, hyperventilation, pneumonia

SYST: Asthenia, viral infection, fever, allergy, chills

Contraindications: Hypersensitivity

P Precautions: Pregnancy **C,** lactation,
G children, elderly, renal disease, history of seizures

Pharmacokinetics

Absorption	Unknown
Distribution	Unknown
Metabolism	Liver
Excretion	Urine
Half-life	Unknown

Pharmacodynamics

Unknown

Interactions

Individual drugs

Alcohol: ↑ CNS depression

Amantadine, bromocriptine, buspirone, lithium: ↑ serotonin syndrome

Buspirone: ↑ symptoms of OCD

Carbamazepine, lithium, phenytoin, warfarin: ↑ levels or toxicity of each specific drug

Cyproheptadine: ↓ escitalopram effect

Diazepam: ↑ half-life of diazepam

Haloperidol: ↑ effect of haloperidol

Drug classifications

Antidepressants: ↑ serotonin syndrome

MAOIs: Do not use with or 14 days before escitalopram

Opioids, sedatives: ↑ CNS depression

Phenothiazines: ↑ levels of phenothiazines

Tricyclics: ↑ levels of tricyclics

☑ Herb/drug

Corkwood, jimsonweed: ↑ anticholinergic effect

Hops, kava, lavender: ↑ CNS effect

SAM-e, St. John's wort: Do not use together

Yohimbe: ↑ hypertension

NURSING CONSIDERATIONS

Assessment

• Assess mental status: mood, sensorium, affect, suicidal tendencies, increase in psychiatric symptoms, depression, panic

• Assess appetite in bulimia nervosa, weight qd, increase nutritious foods in diet, watch for bingeing and vomiting

• Assess allergic reactions: itching, rash, urticaria; drug should be discontinued, may need to give antihistamine

• Monitor B/P (lying/standing), pulse q4h; if systolic B/P drops 20 mm Hg, hold drug, notify prescriber; take VS q4h in patients with cardiovascular disease

• Monitor blood studies: CBC, leukocytes, differential, cardiac enzymes if patient is

 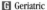

receiving long-term therapy; check platelets; bleeding can occur
• Montior liver function tests: AST, ALT, bilirubin, creatinine
• Monitor weight qwk; appetite may decrease with drug
• Monitor ECG for flattening of T wave, bundle branch, AV block, dysrhythmias in cardiac patients
• Monitor alcohol consumption; if alcohol is consumed, hold dose until AM

Nursing diagnoses
✓ Coping, ineffective (uses)
✓ Risk for injury (uses/adverse reactions)
✓ Knowledge, deficient (teaching)

Implementation
• Give with food or milk for GI symptoms
• Give crushed if patient is unable to swallow medication whole
• Give dosage hs if oversedation occurs during the day
• Give gum, hard candy, frequent sips of water for dry mouth
• Store at room temperature; do not freeze
• Provide assistance with ambulation during therapy, because drowsiness, dizziness occur
• Provide safety measures primarily in elderly
• Check to see if PO medication swallowed

Patient/family education
• Teach that therapeutic effect may take 1-4 wk
• Advise to use caution in driving, other activities requiring alertness because of drowsiness, dizziness, blurred vision
• Advise to use sunscreen to prevent photosensitivity
• Advise to avoid alcohol ingestion, other CNS depressants
• Advise patient to notify prescriber if pregnant or plan to become pregnant or breastfeed
• Advise patient to change positions slowly, orthostatic hypotension may occur
• Teach to avoid all OTC drugs unless approved by prescriber
• To report immediately signs of urinary retention

Evaluation
Positive therapeutic outcome
• Decreased depression

esmolol (Rx)
(ez'moe-lole)
Brevibloc
Func. class.: β-Adrenergic blocker (antidysrhythmic II)

Pregnancy category C

Action: Competitively blocks stimulation of β_1-adrenergic receptors in the myocardium; produces negative chronotropic, inotropic activity (decreases rate of SA node discharge, increases recovery time), slows conduction of AV node, decreases heart rate, decreases O_2 consumption in myocardium; also decreases renin-aldosterone-angiotensin system at high doses; inhibits β_2-receptors in bronchial system at higher doses

→**Therapeutic Outcome:** Decreased supraventricular tachycardia

Uses: Supraventricular tachycardias, noncompensatory sinus tachycardia, hypertensive crisis, intraoperative and postoperative tachycardia, hypertension

Dosage and routes
Adult: **IV** loading dose 500 mcg/kg/min over 1 min; maintenance 50 mcg/kg/min for 4 min; if no response in 5 min, give 2nd loading dose; then increase inf to 100 mcg/kg/min for 4 min; if no response, repeat loading dose, then increase maintenance inf by 50 mcg/kg/min (max of 200 mcg/kg/min); titrate to patient response

P *Child:* **IV** 50 mcg/kg/min, may increase q10 min, max 300 mcg/kg/min

Available forms: Inj 10 mg, 250 mg/ml

Adverse effects
(*italic* = common; **bold** = life-threatening)
CNS: Confusion, light-headedness, paresthesia, somnolence, fever, dizziness, fatigue, headache, depression, anxiety, **seizures**
CV: Hypotension, bradycardia, chest pain, peripheral ischemia, shortness of breath, CHF, conduction disturbances 1st-, 2nd-, 3rd-degree heart block
GI: Nausea, vomiting, anorexia, gastric pain, flatulence, constipation, heartburn, bloating
GU: Urinary retention, impotence, dysuria
***INTEG:** Induration, inflammation at inj site,* discoloration, edema, erythema, burning pallor, flushing, rash, pruritus, dry skin, alopecia
RESP: **Bronchospasm,** dyspnea, cough, wheezing, nasal stuffiness

Contraindications: Heart block (2nd- or 3rd-degree), cardiogenic shock, CHF, cardiac failure, hypersensitivity

Precautions: Hypotension, pregnancy **C**, peripheral vascular disease, diabetes, hypoglycemia, thyrotoxicosis, renal disease, lactation

🛇 **Do Not Confuse:**
Brevibloc/Brevital
esmolol/Osmitrol

Pharmacokinetics	
Absorption	Complete
Distribution	Unknown
Metabolism	Liver
Excretion	Kidneys
Half-life	9 min

Pharmacodynamics	
Onset	Rapid
Peak	Unknown
Duration	1-2 min

Interactions
Individual drugs
Amphetamine, epHEDrine, epINEPHrine, norepinephrine, phenylephrine, pseudoephedrine: ↑ α-adrenergic stimulation
Digoxin: ↑ digoxin levels
Thyroid hormones: ↓ effect of esmolol
Drug classifications
MAOIs: Avoid use
⌷ *Herb/drug*
Aloe, buckthorn, cascara sagrada, senna: ↑ hypokalemia
Betel palm, butterbur, cola tree, figwort, fumitory, guarana, hawthorn, lily of the valley, motherwort, plantain: ↑ β-blocking effect
Jamborandi tree: ↑ CV reactions
Lab test interferences
Interference: Glucose/insulin tolerance test

NURSING CONSIDERATIONS
Assessment
• Monitor B/P during beginning treatment, periodically thereafter; pulse q4h; note rate, rhythm, quality; apical/radial pulse before administration; notify prescriber of any significant changes (pulse <50 bpm)
• Check for baselines in renal, liver function tests before therapy begins
• Assess for edema in feet, legs daily, monitor I&O, daily weight; check for jugular vein distention, rales bilaterally, dyspnea (CHF)
• Monitor skin turgor, dryness of mucous membranes for hydration status, especially
🝆 elderly

Nursing diagnoses
✓ Cardiac output, decreased (uses)
✓ Injury, risk for (adverse reactions)
✓ Knowledge, deficient (teaching)
✓ Noncompliance (teaching)

Implementation
• Give by intermittent inf after diluting 5 g/500 ml of D$_5$W, 0.9% NaCl, D$_5$/0.45% NaCl, D$_5$/LR, D$_5$/0.9% NaCl, 0.45% NaCl, LR (10 mg/ml)
• Give loading dose over 1 min, then maintenance dose over 4 min, may repeat loading dose q5 min with increased maintenance dose; maintenance dose should not be >200 mcg/kg/min and be administered up to 48 hr; dosage should be tapered at a rate of 25 mcg/kg/min
• Store at room temp for 24 hr; sol should be clear

Y-site compatibilities: Amikacin, aminophylline, ampicillin, amiodarone, atracurium, butorphanol, calcium chloride, cefazolin, cefmetazole, cefoperazone, ceftazidime, ceftizoxime, chloramphenicol, cimetidine, cisatracurium, clindamycin, diltiazem, DOPamine, enalaprilat, erythromycin, famotidine, fentanyl, gentamicin, heparin, hydrocortisone, regular insulin, labetalol, magnesium sulfate, methyldopate, metronidazole, midazolam, morphine, nafcillin, nitroglycerin, norepinephrine, nitroprusside, pancuronium, penicillin G potassium, phenytoin, piperacillin, polymyxin B, potassium chloride, potassium phosphate, propofol, ranitidine, remifentanil, streptomycin, tacrolimus, tobramycin, trimethoprim/sulfamethoxazole, vancomycin, vecuronium

Y-site incompatibilities: Furosemide

Additive compatibilities: Aminophylline, atracurium, bretylium, heparin

Additive incompatibilities: Diazepam, procainamide, sodium bicarbonate, thiopental

Patient/family education
• Teach patient need for medication and expected results
• Caution patient to rise slowly to prevent orthostatic hypotension
• Advise patient to notify if pain, swelling occurs at **IV** site

Evaluation
Positive therapeutic outcome
• Absence of dysrhythmias

Treatment of overdose: Defibrillation, vasopressor for hypotension

---

esomeprazole (Rx)
(es'oh-mep'rah-zohl)
Nexium
Func. class.: Anti-ulcer, proton pump inhibitor
Chem. class.: Benzimidazole

Pregnancy category B

Action: Suppresses gastric secretion by inhibiting hydrogen/potassium ATPase enzyme system in the gastric parietal cell; characterized as gastric acid pump inhibitor, since it blocks final step of acid production

➔ **Therapeutic Outcome:** Absence of duodenal ulcers; decreased gastroesophageal reflux

Uses: Gastroesophageal reflux disease (GERD), severe erosive esophagitis; treatment of active duodenal ulcers in combination with antiinfectives for *Helicobacter pylori* infection

Dosage and routes
Active duodenal ulcers associated with H. pylori
Adult: PO 40 mg qd × 10 days in combination with clarithromycin 500 mg bid × 10 days and amoxicillin 1000 mg bid × 10 days

GERD
Adult: PO 20 or 40 mg qd × 4-8 wk

Available forms: Caps 20, 40 mg

Adverse effects
(*italic* = common; **bold** = life-threatening)
CNS: Headache, dizziness
GI: Diarrhea, flatulence, anorexia, dry mouth
GU: UTI, urinary frequency
INTEG: Rash, dry skin
MISC: Fatigue
RESP: Cough

Contraindications: Hypersensitivity

🅿 **Precautions:** Pregnancy **B,** lactation, 🅖 children, elderly

Pharmacokinetics
Absorption	Unknown
Distribution	97% plasma protein bound
Metabolism	Liver (metabolites)
Excretion	Urine (metabolites), feces 🅖 (metabolites); in elderly, elimination rate ↓, bioavailability ↑
Half-life	1-1½ hr

Pharmacodynamics
Onset	Unknown
Peak	1½ hr
Duration	Unknown

E

Interactions
Individual drugs
Diazepam: Possible ↓ diazepam clearance resulting in ↑ diazepam serum concentrations
Flurazepam, triazolam: ↑ serum levels of esomeprazole
Warfarin: Possible ↑ bleeding

NURSING CONSIDERATIONS
Assessment
• Assess GI system: bowel sounds q8h, abdomen for pain, swelling, anorexia
• Assess hepatic enzymes: AST, ALT, alkaline phosphatase during treatment

Nursing diagnoses
☑ Pain, acute (uses)
☑ Pain, chronic (uses)
☑ Knowledge, deficient (teaching)

Implementation
• Administer at least 1 hr before eating
🚫 • Make sure capsule is swallowed whole; do not break, crush, or chew

Patient/family education
• Instruct patient to report severe diarrhea; drug may have to be discontinued
• Advise diabetic patients that hypoglycemia may occur
• Advise patient to avoid hazardous activities; dizziness may occur
• Advise patient to avoid alcohol, salicylates, ibuprofen; may cause GI irritation

Evaluation
Positive therapeutic outcome
• Absence of epigastric pain, swelling, fullness

---

estradiol (Rx)

(ess-tra-dye′ole)

Estrace

estradiol cypionate

depGynogen, Depo-Estradiol, Depogen, Dura-Estrin, E-Cypionate, Estragyn LAS, Estro-Cyp, Estrofem, Estroject-LA, Estro-L.A.

estradiol valerate

Clinagen LA, Delestrogen, Dioval, Duragan, Estra-L, Estro-span, Femogex ✤, Gynogen LA, Menaval, Valergen

estradiol transdermal system

Alora, Climara, Esclim, Estraderm, FemPatch, Vivelle

estradiol vaginal tablet

Vagifem

estradiol vaginal ring

Estring

Func. class.: Estrogen, progestin

Chem. class.: Nonsteroidal synthetic estrogen

Pregnancy category X

Action: Needed for adequate functioning of female reproductive system; affects release of pituitary gonadatropins, inhibits ovulation, promotes adequate calcium use in bone structure

➲ **Therapeutic Outcome:** Decreased tumor size in prostatic cancer; increased estrogen levels in menopause, female hypogonadism

Uses: Symptoms associated with menopause, breast cancer, prostatic cancer, atrophic vaginitis, kraurosis vulvae, hypogonadism, castration, primary ovarian failure, prevention of osteoporosis

Dosage and routes

Hormone replacement

Adult: TD 0.05-0.1 mg/24 hr apply 2×/wk

Menopause/hypogonadism/ castration/ovarian failure

Adult: PO 1-2 mg qd 3 wk on, 1 wk off or 5 days on, 2 days off; IM 1-5 mg q3-4 wk (cypionate), 10-20 mg q4 wk (valerate); top Estraderm 0.05 mg/24 hr applied 2×/wk, Climara 0.05 mg/hr applied 1×/wk in a cyclic regimen, women with hysterectomy may use continuously

Prostatic cancer

Adult: IM 30 mg q1-2wk (valerate); PO 1-2 mg tid (oral estradiol)

Breast cancer

Adult: PO 10 mg tid × 3 mo or longer

Atropic vaginitis/kraurosis vulvae

Adult: Vag cream 2-4 g qd × 1-2 wk, then 1 g 1-3 ×/wk cycled; vag tab 1 qd × 2 wk, maintenance 1 tab 2×/wk; vag ring inserted and left in place continuously for 3 mo

Available forms: Estradiol tabs 0.5, 1, 2 mg; valerate inj 10, 20, 40 mg/ml; TD 0.025, 0.0375, 0.05, 0.075, 0.1 mg/24-hr release rate; vag cream 100 mcg/g; vag ring 2 mg/90 days; vag tab 25 mcg

Adverse effects

(*italic* = common; **bold** = life-threatening)

CNS: Dizziness, headache, migraine, depression, **seizures**

CV: Hypotension, thrombophlebitis, edema, **thromboembolism, stroke, pulmonary embolism, MI**

EENT: Contact lens intolerance, increased myopia, astigmatism

GI: Nausea, vomiting, diarrhea, anorexia, pancreatitis, cramps, constipation, increased appetite, increased weight, **cholestatic jaundice, hepatic adenoma**

GU: Amenorrhea, cervical erosion, breakthrough bleeding, dysmenorrhea, vaginal candidiasis, breast changes, *gynecomastia, testicular atrophy, impotence,* **increased risk of breast, endometrial cancer,** changes in libido

INTEG: Rash, urticaria, acne, hirsutism, alopecia, oily skin, seborrhea, purpura, melasma

META: Folic acid deficiency, hypercalcemia, hyperglycemia

Contraindications: Breast cancer, thromboembolic disorders, reproductive cancer, genital bleeding (abnormal, undiagnosed), pregnancy **X**, lactation

Precautions: Hypertension, asthma, blood dyscrasias, gallbladder disease, CHF, diabetes mellitus, bone disease, depression, migraine headache, seizure disorders, hepatic, renal disease, family history of cancer of breast or reproductive tract, smoking

Pharmacokinetics	
Absorption	Well absorbed
Distribution	Widely distributed, crosses placenta
Metabolism	Unknown
Excretion	Unknown
Half-life	Unknown

Pharmacodynamics

	PO	IM	IV
Onset	Rapid	Slow	Rapid
Peak	Unknown	Unknown	Unknown
Duration	Unknown	Unknown	Unknown

Interactions
Individual drugs
Calcium, phenylbutazone, rifampin: ↓ estradiol action
Cyclosporine, dantrolene: ↑ toxicity
Tamoxifen: ↓ tamoxifen action
Drug classifications
Anticoagulants: ↓ action of anticoagulants
Anticonvulsants, barbiturates: ↓ estradiol action
Corticosteroids: ↑ action of corticosteroids
Food/drug
Grapefruit juice: ↑ estrogen level
⬚ Herb/drug
Alfalfa, hops: ↑ estrogen effect
Saw palmetto: ↓ estrogen effect
Black cohosh, DHEA: Altered estrogen effect
Lab test interferences
↑ BSP retention test; ↑ PBI; ↑ T_4; ↑ serum sodium; ↑ platelet aggregation; ↑ thyroxine-binding globulin (TBS); ↑ prothrombin; ↑ factors VII, VIII, IX, X; ↑ triglycerides
↓ serum folate, ↓ serum triglyceride, ↓ T_3 resin uptake test, ↓ glucose tolerance test, ↓ antithrombin III, ↓ pregnanediol, ↓ metyrapone test
False positive: LE prep, ANA titer

NURSING CONSIDERATIONS
Assessment
• Monitor blood glucose in patient with diabetes; hyperglycemia may occur
• Monitor B/P q4h; watch for increase caused by water and sodium retention
• Monitor I&O ratio; be alert for decreasing urinary output and increasing edema; monitor weight daily; notify prescriber if weekly weight gain is >5 lb; if increased, diuretic may be ordered
• Obtain liver function studies baseline, periodically, including AST, ALT, bilirubin, alkaline phosphatase
• Assess edema, hypertension, cardiac symptoms, jaundice
• Assess mental status: affect, mood, behavioral changes, aggression; depression may occur, drug may need to be discontinued
• Assess female patient for intact uterus, if so, progesterone should be added to estrogen therapy to decrease risk of endometrial cancer

Nursing diagnoses
✓ Sexual dysfunction (uses)
✓ Injury, risk for (adverse reactions)
Implementation
PO route
• Give titrated dose, use lowest effective dose
• Give with food or milk to decrease GI symptoms
IM route
• Administer deeply in large muscle mass; drug is painful
• Rotate syringe to mix oil and medication
TD route
• Apply to area free of hair to ensure adhesion on trunk of body 2×/wk; press firmly and hold in place for 10 sec to ensure good contact
• Start TD dose 7 days before last PO dose if routes are to be changed
Vaginal route
• Place cream in applicator by attaching tube to applicator; squeeze cream into tube to mark; insert with patient reclining
• Applicator should be washed after each use

Patient/family education
• Tell patient to take exactly as prescribed; do not double doses
◆• Advise patient that increased weight gain and symptoms of fluid retention should be reported to prescriber: edema of feet, ankles, sacral area; abnormal vaginal bleeding; breast lumps; hepatic disease (dark urine, clay-colored stools, jaundice of skin, sclera, pruritus)
◆• Caution patient that thromboembolic symptoms should be reported: tenderness in legs, chest pain, dyspnea, headaches, blurred vision
• Inform patient to use sunscreen and protective clothing because sunburns may occur
• Advise patient to stop smoking; smokers have a greater chance of thromboembolic disorder
• Tell patient to use nonhormonal birth control, and to notify prescriber if pregnancy is suspected

Evaluation
Positive therapeutic outcome
• Reversal of menopausal symptoms
• Decrease in tumor size in prostatic or breast cancer
• Decrease in itching, inflammation of vagina
• Absence of symptoms of osteoporosis

E

estrogens, conjugated
◆ㅠ (Rx)

Cenestin, C.E.S ✦, Congest ✦, conjugated estrogens, Premarin, Premarin Intravenous

estrogens, conjugated synthetic A

Cenestin

Func. class.: Estrogen hormone
Chem. class.: Nonsteroidal synthetic estrogen

Pregnancy category X

Action: Needed for adequate functioning of female reproductive system; affects release of pituitary gonadotropins; inhibits ovulation; promotes adequate calcium use in bone structures

⬗ Therapeutic Outcome: Decreased tumor size in prostatic cancer; increased estrogen levels in menopause, female hypogonadism

Uses: Symptoms associated with menopause, breast cancer, prostatic cancer, abnormal uterine bleeding, hypogonadism, castration, primary ovarian failure, prevention of osteoporosis

Dosage and routes
Menopause
Adult: PO 0.3-1.25 mg qd 3 wk on, 1 wk off

Prevention of osteoporosis
Adult: PO 0.625 mg qd or in a cycle

Atrophic vaginitis
Adult: Vag 2-4 g cream qd × 21 days, off 7 days, repeat

Prostatic cancer
Adult: PO 1.25-2.5 mg tid

Breast cancer
Adult: PO 10 mg tid × 3 mo or longer

Abnormal uterine bleeding
Adult: IV/IM 25 mg, repeat in 6-12 hr

Ovariectomy/primary ovarian failure/castration
Adult: PO 1.25 mg qd 3 wk on, 1 wk off

Hypogonadism
Adult: PO 2.5 mg bid-tid × 20 days/mo

Available forms: Tabs 0.3, 0.625, 0.9, 1.25, 2.5 mg; inj 25 mg/vial; vag cream 0.625 mg/g; synthetic A tabs 0.625, 0.9 mg

Adverse effects
(*italic* = common; **bold** = life-threatening)
CNS: Dizziness, headache, migraine, depression, **seizures**

CV: Hypotension, thrombophlebitis, edema, **thromboembolism, stroke, pulmonary embolism, MI**
EENT: Contact lens intolerance, increased myopia, astigmatism
GI: Nausea, vomiting, diarrhea, anorexia, pancreatitis, cramps, constipation, increased appetite, increased weight, **cholestatic jaundice, hepatic adenoma**
GU: Amenorrhea, cervical erosion, breakthrough bleeding, dysmenorrhea, vaginal candidiasis, breast changes, *gynecomastia, testicular atrophy, impotence,* **increased risk of breast, endometrial cancer,** libido changes
INTEG: Rash, urticaria, acne, hirsutism, alopecia, oily skin, seborrhea, purpura, melasma
META: Folic acid deficiency, hypercalcemia, hyperglycemia

Contraindications: Breast cancer, thromboembolic disorders, reproductive cancer, genital bleeding (abnormal, undiagnosed), pregnancy **X,** lactation

Precautions: Hypertension, asthma, blood dyscrasias, gallbladder disease, CHF, diabetes mellitus, bone disease, depression, migraine headache, seizure disorders, hepatic, renal disease, family history of cancer of breast or reproductive tract, smoking

⬔ Do Not Confuse:
Premarin/Provera

Pharmacokinetics	
Absorption	Well absorbed (PO), completely absorbed (**IV**)
Distribution	Widely distributed, crosses placenta
Metabolism	Liver—exclusively; hepatic recirculation
Excretion	Kidney
Half-life	Unknown

Pharmacodynamics			
	PO	IM	IV
Onset	Rapid	Slow	Immediate
Peak	Unknown	Unknown	Unknown
Duration	Unknown	Unknown	Unknown

Interactions
Individual drugs
Cyclosporine, dantrolene: ↑ toxicity
Phenylbutazone, rifampin: ↓ action of estrogens
Tamoxifen: ↓ tamoxifen action

E

Drug classifications
Anticoagulants: ↓ action of anticoagulants
Anticonvulsants, barbiturates: ↓ action of estrogens
Corticosteroids: ↑ action of corticosteroids
Oral hypoglycemics: ↓ action of hypoglycemics
Food/drug
Grapefruit juice: ↑ estrogen level
Herb/drug
Alfalfa, hops: ↑ estrogen level
Black cohosh, DHEA: Altered estrogen effect
Saw palmetto: ↓ estrogen level
Lab test interferences
↑ BSP retention test; ↑ PBI, ↑ T₄; ↑ serum sodium; ↑ platelet aggressability; ↑ thyroxine-binding globulin (TBG); ↑ prothrombin; ↑ factors VII, VIII, IX, X; ↑ triglycerides ↓ Serum folate, ↓ serum triglyceride, ↓ T₃ resin uptake test, ↓ glucose tolerance test, ↓ antithrombin III, ↓ pregnanediol, ↓ metyrapone test
False positive: LE prep, ANA titer

NURSING CONSIDERATIONS
Assessment
• Monitor blood glucose in patient with diabetes; hyperglycemia may occur
• Monitor B/P q4h; watch for increase caused by water and sodium retention
• Monitor I&O ratio; be alert for decreasing urinary output and increasing edema; monitor weight daily; notify prescriber if weekly weight gain is >5 lb; if increased, diuretic may be ordered
• Obtain liver function studies, including AST, ALT, bilirubin, alkaline phosphatase
• Assess edema, hypertension, cardiac symptoms, jaundice
• Assess mental status: affect, mood, behavioral changes, aggression; depression may occur, drug may need to be discontinued
• Assess female patient for intact uterus; if so, progesterone should be added to estrogen therapy to decrease risk of endometrial cancer

Nursing diagnoses
☑ Sexual dysfunction (uses)
☑ Injury, risk for (adverse reactions)

Implementation
PO route
• Give titrated dose, use lowest effective dose
• Give in 1 dose in AM for prostatic cancer, vaginitis, hypogonadism
• Give with food or milk to decrease GI symptoms
IM route
• Reconstitute after withdrawing at least 5 ml

of air from container and inject sterile diluent on vial side, rotate to dissolve
• Give IM inj deeply in large muscle
IV route
• Direct **IV**: reconstitute as for IM, inject into distal port of running **IV** line of D₅W, 0.9% NaCl, LR, at a rate of 5 mg/min or less

Y-site compatibilities: Heparin/hydrocortisone, potassium chloride, vit B/C
Vaginal route
• Place cream in applicator by attaching tube to applicator, squeeze cream into tube to mark, insert with patient recumbent
• Applicator should be washed after each use

Patient/family education
• Caution patient to take exactly as prescribed and not to double doses
• Advise patient that increased weight gain and symptoms of fluid retention should be reported to prescriber: edema of feet, ankles, sacral area; abnormal vaginal bleeding; breast lumps; hepatic disease (dark urine, clay-colored stools, jaundice of skin, sclera, pruritus)
• Caution patient that thromboembolic symptoms should be reported: pain, redness, tenderness in legs; chest pain, dyspnea, headaches, blurred vision
• Inform patient that sunburns may occur and to use sunscreen and protective clothing
• Advise patient to stop smoking; smokers have a greater chance of thromboembolic disorder
• Tell patient to use nonhormonal birth control, and to notify prescriber if pregnancy is suspected

Evaluation
Positive therapeutic outcome
• Reversal of menopause symptoms
• Decrease in tumor size in prostatic, breast cancer
• Decrease in itching, inflammation of vagina
• Absence of symptoms of osteoporosis

etanercept (Rx)
(eh-tan′er-sept)
Enbrel
Func. class.: Antirheumatic agent (disease-modifying)
Pregnancy category B

Action: Binds to tumor necrosis factor (TNF), which decreases inflammation and immune response

➔ **Therapeutic Outcome:** Decreased pain, inflammation

Uses: Acute, chronic rheumatoid arthritis that has not responded to other disease-modifying agents; polyarticular course juvenile rheumatoid arthritis (JRA)

Investigational uses: CHF, psoriasis/psoriatic arthritis

Dosage and routes
Osteoarthritis
Adult: SC 25 mg 2×/wk, may be given with other drugs for rheumatoid arthritis

P *Child 4-17 yr:* SC 0.4 mg/kg 2×/wk, max 25 mg/dose

CHF
Adult: SC 5-12 mg/m² 2×/wk × 3 mo

Psoriasis/psoriatic arthritis
Adult: SC 25 mg 2×/wk × 12 wk

Available forms: Powder for inj: 25 mg

Adverse effects
(*italic* = common; **bold** = life-threatening)
CNS: Headache, asthenia, dizziness
GI: Abdominal pain, dyspepsia
INTEG: Rash, *inj site reaction*
RESP: Pharyngitis, rhinitis, *cough, URI,* non-URI sinusitis

Contraindications: Hypersensitivity, sepsis

P **Precautions:** Pregnancy **B**, lactation,
G children <4 yr, elderly

Pharmacokinetics	
Absorption	Rapidly (60%)
Distribution	Unknown
Metabolism	Unknown
Excretion	Unknown
Half-life	115 hr

Pharmacodynamics	
Onset	Unknown
Peak	Unknown
Duration	Unknown

Interactions
Drug classifications
Immunizations: Should be brought up to date before treatment
Immunizations, vaccines: Do not give concurrently

NURSING CONSIDERATIONS
Assessment
• Assess for pain of rheumatoid arthritis;

check ROM, inflammation of joints, characteristics of pain
• Assess inj site for pain, swelling, usually occurs after 2 inj (4-5 days)

Nursing diagnoses
✓ Pain, chronic (uses)
✓ Mobility, impaired physical (uses)
✓ Injury, risk for (side effects)
✓ Knowledge, deficient (teaching)

Implementation
SC route
• Administer after reconstituting 1 ml of supplied diluent, slowly inject diluent into vial, swirl contents, do not shake, sol should be clear/colorless, do not use if cloudy or discolored
• Do not admix with other sol or medications; do not use filter
• May be injected SC into upper arm, abdomen, thigh; rotate inj sites

Patient/family education
• Teach patient that drug must be continued for prescribed time to be effective; to avoid aspirin, alcoholic beverages
• Instruct patient to use caution when driving; dizziness may occur
• Teach patient about self-administration, if appropriate: inj should be made in thigh, abdomen, upper arm; rotate sites at least 1 in from old site

Evaluation
Positive therapeutic outcome
• Decreased pain in arthritic conditions
• Decreased inflammation in arthritic conditions

---

ethambutol (Rx)
(e-tham'byoo-tole)
Etibi ✤, Myambutol
Func. class.: Antitubercular
Chem. class.: Diisopropylethylene diamide derivative

Pregnancy category B

Action: Inhibits RNA synthesis, decreases tubercle bacilli replication

➔ **Therapeutic Outcome:** Resolution of TB infection

Uses: Pulmonary TB, as an adjunct, other mycobacterial infections

Dosage and routes
P *Adult and child >13 yr:* PO 15-25 mg/kg/day as a single dose or 50 mg/kg 2×/wk or 25-30 mg/kg 3×/wk

---

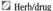 Herb/drug   Ⓢ Do Not Crush   ◆ Alert   ◆ᴛ Key Drug   G Geriatric   P Pediatric

Renal dose
Adult: PO CCr 10-50 ml/min dose q24-36h; CCr <10 ml/min dose q48h

Retreatment
Adult: PO 25 mg/kg/day as single dose × 2 mo with at least 1 other drug, then decrease to 15 mg/kg/day as single dose, max 2.5 g/day

P *Child:* PO 15 mg/kg/day

Available forms: Tabs 100, 400 mg

Adverse effects
(*italic* = common; **bold** = life-threatening)
CNS: *Headache, confusion,* fever, malaise, dizziness, *disorientation,* hallucinations
EENT: Blurred vision, optic neuritis, photophobia, decreased visual acuity
GI: *Abdominal distress, anorexia, nausea, vomiting*
INTEG: Dermatitis, pruritus, **toxic epidermal necrolysis**
META: *Elevated uric acid, acute gout,* liver function impairment
MISC: **Thrombocytopenia,** joint pain, bloody sputum, **anaphylaxis**

Contraindications: Hypersensitivity,
P optic neuritis, child <13 yr

Precautions: Renal disease, diabetic retinopathy, cataracts, ocular defects, hepatic and hematopoietic disorders, pregnancy **B**, lactation

N Do Not Confuse:
ethambutol/Ethmozine

Pharmacokinetics	
Absorption	Rapidly absorbed
Distribution	Widely distributed, crosses blood-brain barrier, placenta
Metabolism	Liver
Excretion	Kidneys—unchanged
Half-life	3 hr, increased in liver, kidney disease

Pharmacodynamics	
Onset	Rapid
Peak	2-4 hr

Interactions
Drug classifications
Antacids, aluminum: ↓ absorption
Neurotoxic agents, other: ↑ neurotoxicity

NURSING CONSIDERATIONS
Assessment
• Obtain C&S tests including sputum tests before initiating treatment; monitor qmo to detect resistance

• Monitor liver function studies qwk × 2 wk, then q2 mo: ALT, AST, bilirubin; renal studies: before, qmo: BUN, creatinine, output, sp gr, urinalysis, uric acid
• Assess patient's mental status often: affect, mood, behavioral changes; psychosis may occur with hallucinations, confusion
• Assess patient's hepatic status: decreased appetite, jaundice, dark urine, fatigue
• Assess patient for visual disturbance that may indicate optic neuritis: blurred vision, change in color perception; may lead to blindness

Nursing diagnoses
✓ Infection, risk for (uses)
✓ Diarrhea (adverse reactions)
✓ Sensory perception, disturbed (adverse reactions)
✓ Knowledge, deficient (teaching)
✓ Noncompliance (teaching)

Implementation
• Give with meals to decrease GI symptoms, at same time each day to maintain blood level
• Give 2 hr before antacids
• Give antiemetic if vomiting occurs

Patient/family education
• Advise patient that compliance with dosage schedule and duration is necessary to eradicate disease; to keep scheduled appointments including ophthalmic appointments or relapse may occur
• Caution patient to report weakness, fatigue, loss of appetite, nausea, vomiting, yellowing of skin or eyes, tingling/numbness of hands/feet, weight gain, or decreased urine output
• Instruct patient to report any visual changes; rash; hot, swollen, painful joints; numbness or tingling of extremities to physician
• Caution patient to inform prescriber if pregnancy is suspected

Evaluation
Positive therapeutic outcome
• Decreased symptoms of TB
• Decrease in acid-fast bacteria

etidronate (Rx)
(eh-tih-droe'nate)
Didronel, Didronel IV
Func. class.: Bone resorption inhibitor
Chem. class.: Bisphosphonate

Pregnancy category C

Action: Decreases bone resorption and new bone development (accretion)

⇒ Therapeutic Outcome: Decreased bone reabsorption, calcium levels WNL

Uses: Paget's disease, heterotopic ossification, hypercalcemia of malignancy

Dosage and routes
Paget's disease
Adult: PO 5-10 mg/kg/day, 2 hr ac with water, not to exceed 20 mg/kg/day, max 6 mo or 11-20 mg/kg/day for max of 3 mo

Heterotopic ossification
Adult: PO 20 mg/kg qd × 2 wk, then 10 mg/kg/day for 10 wk, total 12 wk

Hypercalcemia
Adult: **IV** 7.5 mg/kg/day × 3 days, then 20 mg/kg/day (PO)

Heterotopic ossification/hip replacement
Adult: PO 20 mg/kg/day × 4 wk before and 3 mo after surgery

Available forms: Tabs 200, 400 mg; inj 50 mg/ml

Adverse effects
(*italic* = common; **bold** = life-threatening)
GI: *Nausea,* constipation, metallic taste (**IV**)
GU: Nephrotoxicity
MISC: Dyspnea; low magnesium, phosphorous
MS: *Bone pain,* hypocalcemia, decreased mineralization of nonaffected bones

Contraindications: Pathologic fractures, clinically overt osteomalacia, severe renal disease with creatinine >5 mg/dl

Precautions: Pregnancy **C**, renal disease, **P** lactation, restricted vit D/Ca, children

🠖 Do Not Confuse:
etidronate/etomidate, etidronate/etretinate

Pharmacokinetics

Absorption	Poorly absorbed (PO), completely absorbed (**IV**)
Distribution	50% bond to crystals in osteogenesis
Metabolism	None
Excretion	Feces (unabsorbed), kidney (unchanged)
Half-life	5-7 hr; in bone >3 mo

Pharmacodynamics

	PO	IV
Onset	4 wk	24 hr
Peak	Unknown	3-4 days
Duration	Up to 1 yr	10-12 days

Interactions
Individual drugs
Warfarin: ↑ Pro-time
Drug classifications
Antacids, mineral supplements with magnesium, calcium, iron products, or aluminum: ↓ absorption of etidronate
Food/drug
Dairy products: ↓ absorption of etidronate

NURSING CONSIDERATIONS
Assessment
- Assess for GI symptoms, polyuria, flushing, head swelling, tingling, headache, may indicate hypercalcemia; nervousness, irritability, twitching, seizures, spasm, paresthesia indicates hypocalcemia at start of treatment
- Identify nutritional status; evaluate diet for sources of vit D (milk, some seafood), calcium (dairy products, dark green vegetables), phosphates
- Monitor BUN, creatinine, uric acid, chloride, electrolytes, urine pH, urinary calcium, magnesium, phosphate, urinalysis (calcium should be kept at 9-10 mg/dl), albumin, alkaline phosphatase baseline and q3-6 mo; check urine sediment for casts throughout treatment
- Assess for increased drug level; toxic reactions occur rapidly; have calcium chloride or gluconate on hand if calcium level drops too low; check for tetany

Nursing diagnoses
☑ Injury, risk for (adverse reactions)
☑ Pain, chronic (uses)
☑ Knowledge, deficient (teaching)

Implementation
PO route
- Administer on empty stomach to improve absorption (2 hr ac)
IV IV route
- Used in hypercalcemias; give by intermittent inf after diluting 300 mg/250 ml or more 0.9% NaCl; run over 2-3 hr, therapy should not last >6 mo

Patient/family education
- Teach method of inj if patient will be responsible for self-medication
- Caution patient to notify prescriber if hypercalcemia recurs: renal calculi, nausea, vomiting, thirst, lethargy, deep bone or flank pain, heat over bone, restricted mobility
- Teach patient that warmth and flushing occur and last 1 hr
- Teach patient to follow a low-calcium diet as prescribed (Paget's disease, hypercalcemia)

 Herb/drug   Do Not Crush   Alert   Key Drug   Geriatric   **P** Pediatric

• Advise patient to notify prescriber of diarrhea, nausea; dose may be divided to lessen these symptoms

• Inform patient that metallic taste may occur with **IV** dosing

Evaluation
Positive therapeutic outcome
• Calcium levels 9-10 mg/dl
• Decreasing symptoms of Paget's disease including pain
• Decreased bone loss in osteoporosis

---

etodolac (Rx)
(ee-toe-doe'lak)
Lodine, Lodine XL
Func. class.: Nonsteroidal antiinflammatory, nonopioid analgesic

Pregnancy category C

Action: Inhibits prostaglandin synthesis by decreasing enzyme needed for biosynthesis; analgesic, antiinflammatory properties

⟶ **Therapeutic Outcome:** Decreased pain, inflammation

Uses: Mild to moderate pain, osteoarthritis

Dosage and routes
Osteoarthritis
Adult: PO 800-1200 mg/day in divided doses q6-8h initially, then adjust to 600-1200 mg/day in divided doses; do not exceed 1200 mg/day; patients <60 kg not to exceed 20 mg/kg

Analgesia
Adult: PO 200-400 mg q6-8h prn for acute pain; do not exceed 1200 mg/day; patients <60 kg not to exceed 20 mg/kg

Available forms: Caps 200, 300 mg; tabs 400, 500 mg; ext rel tabs 400, 600 mg

Adverse effects
(*italic* = common; **bold** = life-threatening)
CNS: Dizziness, headache, drowsiness, fatigue, tremors, confusion, insomnia, anxiety, depression, light-headedness, vertigo
CV: Tachycardia, peripheral edema, fluid retention, palpitations, dysrhythmias, CHF
EENT: Tinnitus, hearing loss, blurred vision, photophobia
GI: Nausea, anorexia, vomiting, diarrhea, jaundice, **cholestatic hepatitis,** constipation, flatulence, cramps, dry mouth, peptic ulcer, dyspepsia, **GI bleeding**
GU: **Nephrotoxicity, dysuria, hematuria, oliguria, azotemia, cystitis, UTI**
HEMA: **Blood dyscrasias**
INTEG: Erythema, urticaria, purpura, rash, pruritus, sweating, **Stevens-Johnson syndrome**
SYST: **Angioedema, anaphylaxis**

Contraindications: Hypersensitivity; patients in whom aspirin, iodides, or other NSAIDs have produced asthma, rhinitis, urticaria, nasal polyps, angioedema, bronchospasm

Precautions: Pregnancy **C,** avoid in 2nd half of pregnancy, lactation, children, bleeding, GI, cardiac disorders, elderly; renal, hepatic disorders

Do Not Confuse:
Lodine/codeine/iodine

Pharmacokinetics
Absorption	Well absorbed
Distribution	Highly bound to plasma protein
Metabolism	Unknown
Excretion	Unknown
Half-life	7 hr

Pharmacodynamics
Onset	½ hr
Peak	1-2 hr
Duration	4-12 hr

Interactions
Individual drugs
Aspirin: May ↑ GI toxicity
Cyclosporine, digoxin, lithium, methotrexate, phenytoin: ↑ toxicity
Digoxin: ↑ levels
Drug classifications
Antacids: Delayed etodolac effect
β-Adrenergic blockers: ↓ effect
Diuretics: ↓ effectiveness of diuretics
Herb/drug
Arginine, gossypol: ↑ gastric irritation
Bearberry, bilberry: ↑ NSAIDs action
Bogbean, chondroitin, saw palmetto, turmeric: ↑ bleeding risk
St. John's wort: Severe photosensitivity

NURSING CONSIDERATIONS
Assessment
• Assess pain: location, frequency, characteristics; relief after medication
• Assess for GI bleeding: black stools, hematemesis
• Assess for asthma, aspirin hypersensitivity, nasal polyps that may be hypersensitive to etodolac
• Monitor blood counts during therapy; watch for decreasing platelets; if low, therapy may need to be discontinued, then restarted after

---

hematologic recovery; watch for blood dyscrasia (thrombocytopenia): bruising, fatigue, bleeding, poor healing

Nursing diagnoses
✓ Pain, acute (uses)
✓ Pain, chronic (uses)
✓ Mobility, impaired physical (uses)
✓ Knowledge, deficient (teaching)
✓ Injury, risk for (adverse reactions)

Implementation
• Administer with food or milk to decrease gastric symptoms; food will slow absorption slightly, will not decrease absorption.
🚫 • Do not crush, chew ext rel tabs

Patient/family education
• Inform patient that drug must be continued for prescribed time to be effective; to avoid aspirin, alcoholic beverages, NSAIDs
• Caution patient to report bleeding, bruising, fatigue, malaise because blood dyscrasias can occur
• Instruct patient to use caution when driving; drowsiness, dizziness may occur
• Teach patient to take with a full glass of
🚫 water to enhance absorption; do not crush, break, or chew medication

Evaluation
Positive therapeutic outcome
• Decreased pain
• Decreased inflammation
• Increased mobility

! HIGH ALERT

etoposide (VP-16) (Rx)
(e-toe′poe-side)
Etopophos, VePesid
Func. class.: Antineoplastic—misc.
Chem. class.: Semisynthetic podophyllotoxin

Pregnancy category D

Action: Inhibits mitotic activity through metaphase to mitosis; also inhibits cells from entering mitosis, depresses DNA, RNA synthesis, cell cycle specific S and G_2

➔ **Therapeutic Outcome:** Prevention of rapid growth of malignant cells

Uses: Leukemias, lung, testicular cancer, lymphomas, neuroblastoma, melanoma, ovarian cancer; being investigated for use in leukemia, lymphoma

Dosage and routes
Testicular cancer
Adult: **IV** 50-100 mg/m^2/day × 3-5 days

given q3-5 wk or 200-250 mg/m^2/wk, or 125-140 mg/m^2/day 3 × wk, q5 wk

Lung cancer
Adult: PO 35 mg/m^2/day × 4 days, repeated q3-4 wk; **IV** 35 mg/m^2/day × 4 days

Available forms: Inj 20 mg/ml; 113.6 etoposide phosphate = 100 etoposide; caps 50, 100 mg

Adverse effects
(*italic* = common; **bold** = life-threatening)
CNS: Headache, *fever,* peripheral neuropathy, paresthesia, confusion
CV: Hypotension, **MI,** dysrhythmia
GI: Nausea, vomiting, anorexia, **hepatotoxicity,** dyspepsia, diarrhea, constipation
GU: **Nephrotoxicity**
HEMA: **Thrombocytopenia, leukopenia, myelosuppression, anemia**
INTEG: Rash, alopecia, phlebitis at **IV** site, radiation recall
RESP: **Bronchospasm,** pleural effusion
SYST: **Anaphylaxis**

Contraindications: Hypersensitivity, bone marrow depression, severe hepatic disease, severe renal disease, bacterial infection, pregnancy **D**, viral infection

Precautions: Renal, hepatic disease,
P lactation, children, gout

Ⓝ **Do Not Confuse:**
VePesid/Versed

Pharmacokinetics

Absorption	Variably absorbed
Distribution	Rapidly absorbed, 97% protein binding, crosses placenta
Metabolism	Liver—some
Excretion	Kidneys, unchanged 50%, breast milk
Half-life	3 hr initially, 15 hr terminally

Pharmacodynamics
Unknown

Interactions
Individual drugs
Warfarin: ↑ prothrombin time

NURSING CONSIDERATIONS
Assessment
• Monitor B/P (baseline and q15 min) during administration
• Monitor CBC, differential, platelet count weekly; withhold drug if WBC is <4000/mm^3 or platelet count is <75,000/mm^3; notify prescriber of results; recovery will take 3 wk
• Monitor renal function studies: BUN, urine

CCr before, during therapy; I&O ratio; report fall in urine output of 30 ml/hr; for decreased hyperuricemia
• Monitor for cold, fever, sore throat (may indicate beginning of infection); notify prescriber if these occur
• Assess for bleeding: hematuria, guaiac, bruising or petechiae, mucosa or orifices q8h: no rectal temp; avoid IM inj; use pressure to venipuncture sites
• Identify nutritional status: an antiemetic may need to be prescribed
⬧• Assess for symptoms indicating severe allergic reactions: rash, pruritus, urticaria, itching, flushing, bronchospasm, hypotension; epINEPHrine and crash cart should be nearby

Nursing diagnoses
✓ Injury, risk for (adverse reactions)
✓ Body image, disturbed (adverse reactions)
✓ Infection, risk for (adverse reactions)
✓ Knowledge, deficient (teaching)

Implementation
PO route
• Caps need to be refrigerated
IV route
• Give by intermittent inf
• Sol should be prepared by qualified personnel and only under controlled conditions
• Use Luer-Lok tubing to prevent leakage; do not let sol come in contact with skin; if contact occurs, wash well with soap and water
• Give after diluting 100 mg/250 ml or more D_5W or NaCl to a concentration of 0.2-0.4 mg/ml; infuse over 30-60 min; phosphate may be given over 5 min-3½ hr; may dilute further to 0.1 mg/ml in 0.9% NaCl, D_5W
• Give hyaluronidase 150 units/ml to 1 ml NaCl to infiltration area; ice compress for treatment of vesicant activity

Y-site compatibilities: Allopurinol, amifostine, aztreonam, cladribine, fludarabine, granisetron, melphalan, ondansetron, paclitaxel, piperacillin/tazobactam, sargramostim, sodium bicarbonate, teniposide, thiotepa, vinorelbine

Y-site incompatibility: Idarubicin

Additive compatibilities: Carboplatin, cisplatin, cytarabine, floxuridine, fluorouracil, hydrOXYzine, ifosfamide, ondansetron

Patient/family education
• Teach patient to avoid use of products containing aspirin or ibuprofen, razors, commercial mouthwash because bleeding may occur; to report symptoms of bleeding (hematuria, tarry stools)

• Instruct patient to report signs of anemia (fatigue, headache, irritability, faintness, shortness of breath)
• Teach patient to report any changes in breathing or coughing even several months after treatment
• Advise patient that contraception will be necessary during treatment because teratogenesis may occur
• Caution patient that hair loss may occur during treatment; a wig or hairpiece may make patient feel better; new hair will be different in color, texture
• Advise patient to avoid vaccinations during treatment because serious reactions may occur
• Teach patient to report signs/symptoms of infection; fever, chills, sore throat; patient should avoid crowds and persons with known infections

Evaluation
Positive therapeutic outcome
• Decreased spread of malignant, leukemic cells

---

exemestane (Rx)
(x-ee-mes′-tane)
Aromasin
Func. class.: Antineoplastic
Chem. class.: Aromatase inhibitor
Pregnancy category D

Action: Lowers serum estradiol concentrations; many breast cancers have strong estrogen receptors

Therapeutic Outcome: Prevention of rapidly growing malignant cells

Uses: Advanced breast carcinoma that has not responded to other therapy in estrogen receptor–positive patients (postmenopausal)

Dosage and routes
Adult: PO 25 mg qd pc

Available forms: Tabs 25 mg

Adverse effects
(*italic* = common; **bold** = life-threatening)
CNS: Hot flashes, headache, fatigue, depression, insomnia, anxiety
CV: Hypertension
GI: Vomiting, increased appetite, diarrhea, constipation, abdominal pain
RESP: Cough, dyspnea

Contraindications: Hypersensitivity, premenopausal women, pregnancy **D**

Precautions: Lactation, children, elderly,
 hepatic, renal disease

Pharmacokinetics

Absorption	Rapidly absorbed
Distribution	Unknown
Metabolism	Liver
Excretion	Feces, urine
Half-life	24 hr

Pharmacodynamics
Unknown

NURSING CONSIDERATIONS
Assessment
• Assess B/P, hypertension may occur

Nursing diagnoses
☑ Injury, risk for (adverse reactions)
☑ Knowledge, deficient (teaching)

Implementation
• Give with food or fluids for GI upset
• Store in light-resistant container at room temp

Patient/family education
• Instruct patient to report any complaints, side effects to prescriber; if dose is missed, do not double next dose
• Advise patient that hot flashes can occur, and are reversible after discontinuing treatment
• Inform patient about who should be told about therapy

Evaluation
Positive therapeutic outcome
• Decreased spread of malignant cells in breast cancer

---

ezetimibe (Rx)
(ehz-eh-tim'bee)
Zetia
Func. class.: Antilipemic

Pregnancy category C

Action: Inhibits absorption of cholesterol by the small intestine

⮞ **Therapeutic Outcome:** Decreased cholesterol levels

Uses: Hypercholesterolemia, homozygous familial hypercholesterolemia (HoFH), homozygous sitosterolemia

Dosage and routes
Adult: **PO** 10 mg qd; may be given with

HMG-CoA reductase inhibitor at same time; may be given with bile acid sequestrant; give ezetimibe 2 hr before or 4 hr after the bile acid sequestrant

Available forms: Tabs 10 mg

Adverse effects
(*italic* = common; **bold** = life-threatening)
CNS: Fatigue, dizziness, headache
GI: Diarrhea, abdominal pain
MISC: Chest pain
MS: Myalgias, arthralgias, back pain
RESP: Pharyngitis, sinusitis, cough, URI

Contraindications: Hypersensitivity, severe hepatic disease

Precautions: Pregnancy **C**, lactation,
 children, hepatic disease

Pharmacokinetics

Absorption	Unknown
Distribution	Unknown
Metabolism	Small intestine, liver
Excretion	Urine (11%), feces (78%)
Half-life	Unknown

Pharmacodynamics
Unknown

Interactions
Individual drugs
Cholestyramine, cycloSPORINE: ↓ ezetimibe action
Drug classifications
Antacids, fibric acid derivatives: ↑ ezetimibe action
☑ *Herb/drug*
Glucomannan: ↑ effect
Gotu kola: ↓ effect

NURSING CONSIDERATIONS
Assessment
• Monitor lipid levels, liver function tests baseline and periodically during treatment

Nursing diagnoses
☑ Knowledge, deficient (teaching)
☑ Noncompliance (teaching)

Implementation
• Give without regard to meals

Patient/family education
• Teach patient that compliance is needed
• Advise that risk factors should be decreased: high-fat diet, smoking, alcohol consumption, absence of exercise
• Advise patient to notify prescriber if pregnancy is suspected or planned

---

Evaluation
Positive therapeutic outcome
• Decreased cholesterol

/ **HIGH ALERT**

factor IX complex (human)/ factor IX (Rx)
Benefit, Konyne 80, Proplex T, Proplex SX-T, Alpha Nine, Mononine
Func. class.: Hemostatic
Chem. class.: Factors II, VII, IX, X

Pregnancy category C

Action: Causes an increase in blood levels of clotting factors II, VII, IX, X; factor IX (human) has IX activity only

➡ **Therapeutic Outcome:** Replacement of factors II, VII, IX, X

Uses: Hemophilia B (Christmas disease), factor IX deficiency, anticoagulant reversal, control of bleeding in patients with factor VIII inhibitors; reversal of overdose of anticoagulants in emergencies

Dosage and routes
Bleeding in hemophilia A and inhibitors of factor VIII
P *Adult and child:* 75 units/kg, repeat in 12 hr

Bleeding in hemophilia B
P *Adult and child:* **IV** establish 25% of normal factor IX activity or 60-75 units/kg/day then 10-20 units/kg/day × 1-2 wk

Prophylaxis of bleeding in hemophilia B
P *Adult and child:* 10-20 units/kg/ day × 1 wk

Reversal of oral anticoagulant
P *Adult and child:* 15 units/kg

Factor VII deficiency (use Proplex T only)
P *Adult and child:* 0.5 units/kg × body weight (kg) × desired factor IX increase (in % of normal); repeat q4-6h if needed

Factor IX, Alpha Nine SD (minor to moderate hemorrhage)
P *Adult and child:* **IV** dose to increase plasma factor IX level to 20%-30%

Serious hemorrhage
P *Adult and child:* **IV** dose to increase plasma factor IX level to 30%-50% given as daily inf

Mononine
Minor hemorrhage
P *Adult and child:* **IV** dose to increase plasma factor IX level to 15%-25% (20-30 units/kg), may repeat in 24 hr if needed

Major trauma
P *Adult and child:* **IV** dose to increase plasma factor IX level to 25%-50% (75 units/kg) q18-30h for up to 10 days

Available forms: Inj (number of units noted on label)

Adverse effects
(*italic* = common; **bold** = life-threatening)
CNS: Headache, dizziness, malaise, paresthesia, *lethargy, chills, fever, flushing*
CV: Hypotension, tachycardia, **MI, venous thrombosis, pulmonary embolism**
EENT: Tinnitus, eyelid swelling
GI: Nausea, vomiting, abdominal cramps, jaundice, **viral hepatitis**
HEMA: **Thrombosis, hemolysis, AIDS, disseminated intravascular coagulation (DIC)**
INTEG: Rash, flushing, *urticaria*
RESP: **Bronchospasm**

Contraindications: Hypersensitivity to mouse protein, hepatic disease, DIC, elective surgery, mild factor IX deficiency

P **Precautions:** Neonates/infants, pregnancy **C**

Pharmacokinetics	
Absorption	40% (PO), complete (**IV**)
Distribution	Unknown
Metabolism	Rapidly cleared from plasma, liver 30%
Excretion	Kidneys—70% unchanged
Half-life	24 hr

Pharmacodynamics
Unknown

Interactions
Individual drugs
Aminocaproic acid: ↑ risk of thrombosis; do not use together

NURSING CONSIDERATIONS
Assesment
• Monitor blood studies (coagulation factor assays by % normal: 5% prevents spontaneous hemorrhage, 30%-50% for surgery, 80%-100% for severe hemorrhage); check for bleeding q15-30 min, immobilize and apply ice to affected joints
• Monitor for increased B/P, pulse

- Monitor I&O; if urine becomes orange or red, notify prescriber
- Assess for allergic or pyrogenic reaction: fever, chills, rash, itching; slow inf rate if not severe
- Assess for DIC: bleeding, ecchymosis, hypersensitivity, changes in coagulation tests

Nursing diagnoses
- ✓ Injury, risk for (uses)
- ✓ Tissue perfusion, ineffective (uses)
- ✓ Knowledge, deficient (teaching)

Implementation
IV route
- Give hepatitis B vaccine before administration
- Give **IV** after warming to room temp 3 ml/min or less, with plastic syringe only; do not admix
- Give after dilution with provided diluent, 50 or 25 units/ml; give so as not to exceed 10 ml/min; decrease rate if fever, headache, flushing, tingling occur
- Give after crossmatch is completed if patient has blood type A, B, AB, to determine incompatibility with factor
- Store reconstituted sol for 3 hr at room temp or up to 2 yr if refrigerated (powder); check expiration date
- Incompatible with protein products

Patient/family education
- Advise patient to report any signs of bleeding: gums, under skin, urine, stools, emesis
- Caution patient about risk of viral hepatitis, AIDS; that immunization for hepatitis B may be given first; to be tested q2-3 mo for HIV, even though the risk is low
- Tell patient to carry/wear emergency ID identifying disease and treatment; avoid salicylates, NSAIDs, to inform other health professionals about condition

Evaluation
Positive therapeutic outcome
- Prevention of hemorrhage

---

famciclovir (Rx)
(fam-sye-klo'vir)
Famvir
Func. class.: Antiviral
Chem. class.: Guanosine nucleoside

Pregnancy category B

Action: Inhibits DNA polymerase and viral DNA synthesis by the conversion of this guanosine nucleoside to penciclovir

Therapeutic Outcome: Decreasing size and number of lesions

Uses: Treatment of acute herpes zoster (shingles), genital herpes, recurrent mucocutaneous herpes simplex virus (HSV) in HIV patients

Investigational uses: Initial episodes of herpes genitalis

Dosage and routes
Herpes zoster
Adult: PO 500 mg q8h

Renal dose
Adult: PO CCr ≥ 60 ml/min 500 mg q8h; 40-59 ml/min 500 mg q12h; 20-39 ml/min 500 mg q24h

Recurrent mucocutaneous herpes simplex
Adult: PO 500 mg q12h × 1 wk

Recurrent HSV
Adult: PO 125 mg q12h × 5 days

Suppression of recurrent HSV
Adult: PO 250 mg q12h up to 1 yr

Genital herpes (recurrent)
Adult: PO 125 mg bid × 5 days; begin treatment at first sign of recurrence

Suppression of recurrent genital herpes
Adult: PO 250 mg bid for up to a year

Herpes genitalis
Initial episodes (off-label)
Adult: PO 25 mg tid × 7-10 days

Available forms: Tabs 125, 250, 500 mg

Adverse effects
(*italic* = common; **bold** = life-threatening)
CNS: *Headache, fatigue, dizziness,* paresthesia, somnolence, fever
GI: Nausea, vomiting, diarrhea, constipation, abdominal pain, anorexia
GU: Decreased sperm count
INTEG: *Pruritus*
MS: Back pain, arthralgia
RESP: Pharyngitis, sinusitis

Contraindications: Hypersensitivity to this drug or penciclovir

Precautions: Renal disease, pregnancy **B,** hypersensitivity to acyclovir, ganciclovir, lactation

 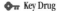

Pharmacokinetics

Absorption	Well absorbed
Distribution	Unknown
Metabolism	Intestinal tissue, blood, liver
Excretion	Breast milk, kidney, bile
Half-life	3 hr

Pharmacodynamics

Onset	Unknown
Peak	1 hr
Duration	8 hr

Interactions
Individual drugs
Cimetidine: ↓ metabolism
Digoxin, probenecid, theophylline: ↓ renal excretion

NURSING CONSIDERATIONS
Assessment
• Assess amount and distribution of lesions; also burning, itching, or pain (early symptoms of herpes infection); neuralgia during and after treatment
• Monitor renal function studies: urine CCr, BUN before and during treatment if patient has decreased renal function; dose may need to be lowered
• Monitor bowel pattern before, during treatment; diarrhea may occur

Nursing diagnoses
✓ Infection, risk for (uses)
✓ Knowledge, deficient (teaching)

Implementation
• Give with or without meals; absorption does not appear to be lowered when taken with food
• Give within 72 hr of the appearance of rash in herpes zoster

Patient/family education
• Teach patient how to recognize signs of beginning of infection
• Teach patient how to prevent the spread of infection to others
• Teach patient reason for medication and expected results
• Advise patient that this medication does not prevent spread of disease to others, that condoms should be used
• Advise women with genital herpes to have yearly Pap smears, cervical cancer is more likely

Evaluation
Positive therapeutic outcome
• Decreased size and spread of lesions

famotidine (Rx, OTC)
(fa-moe′to-deen)
Mylanta AR, Pepcid AC, Pepcid, Pepcid IV, Pepcid RPD ♣
Func. class.: H_2-histamine receptor antagonist, antiulcer agent

Pregnancy category B

Action: Inhibits histamine at H_2-receptor site in gastric parietal cells, which inhibits gastric acid secretion

Therapeutic Outcome: Healing of duodenal ulcers or gastric ulcers; prevention of duodenal ulcers; decreases symptoms of gastroesophageal reflux disease or Zollinger-Ellison syndrome, heartburn

Uses: Short-term treatment of active duodenal ulcer, maintenance therapy for duodenal ulcer, Zollinger-Ellison syndrome, multiple endocrine adenomas, gastric ulcers, heartburn

Investigational uses: GI disorders in those taking NSAIDs, urticaria, prevention of stress ulcers, aspiration pneumonitis, inactivation of oral pancreatic enzymes in pancreatic disorders, prevention of paclitaxel hypersensitivity reactions

Dosage and routes
Active ulcer
Adult: PO 40 mg qd hs × 4-8 wk, then 20 mg qd hs if needed (maintenance); **IV** 20 mg q12h if unable to take PO

Child 1-16 yr: PO 0.5 mg/kg/day hs or divided bid, max 40 mg qd

Hypersecretory conditions
Adult: PO 20 mg q6h; may give 160 mg q6h if needed; **IV** 20 mg q12h if unable to take PO

Child 1-16 yr: PO 1 mg/kg/day divided bid, max 40 mg bid

Paclitaxel hypersensitivity reactions
Adult: **IV** 20 mg ½ hr before inf

Heartburn relief/prevention
Adult: PO 10 mg with water or 1 hr before eating

Renal dose
Adult: PO CCr <10 ml/min 20 mg hs or dose q36-48h

Available forms: Tabs 10 (OTC), 20, 40 mg; powder for oral susp 40 mg/5 ml; inj 10 mg/ml, 20 mg/50 ml 0.9% NaCl; orally disintegrating tabs (RPD) 20, 40 mg; chew tabs 10 mg

F

Adverse effects

(*italic* = common; **bold** = life-threatening)
CNS: *Headache, dizziness,* paresthesia, **seizures,** depression, anxiety, somnolence, insomnia, fever
CV: **Dysrhythmias**
EENT: Taste change, tinnitus, orbital edema
GI: *Constipation,* nausea, vomiting, anorexia, cramps, abnormal liver enzymes, diarrhea
HEMA: **Thrombocytopenia, aplastic anemia**
INTEG: Rash
MS: Myalgia, arthralgia

Contraindications: Hypersensitivity

Precautions: Pregnancy **B**, lactation,
P children <12 yr, severe renal disease, severe
G hepatic disease, elderly

Pharmacokinetics

Absorption	50% absorbed (PO)
Distribution	Plasma, protein binding (15%-20%)
Metabolism	Liver (30% active metabolizing)
Excretion	Kidneys (70%)
Half-life	2½-3½ hr

Pharmacodynamics

	PO	IV
Onset	30-60 min	Immediate
Peak	1-3 hr	½-3 hr
Duration	6-12 hr	8-15 hr

Interactions
Individual drugs
Ketoconazole: ↓ absorption of ketoconazole
Drug classifications
Antacids: ↓ absorption of famotidine

NURSING CONSIDERATIONS
Assessment

• Assess patient with ulcers or suspected ulcers: epigastric, abdominal pain, hematemesis, occult blood in stools, blood in gastric, aspirate before treatment; throughout treatment, monitor gastric pH (5 should be maintained)
• Monitor I&O ratio, BUN, creatinine, CBC with differential monthly

Nursing diagnoses
✓ Pain (uses)
✓ Knowledge, deficient (teaching)

Implementation
PO route
• Give antacids 1 hr before or 2 hr after famotidine; may be given with foods or liq
• Administer oral susp after shaking well; discard unused sol after 1 mo

IV IV route
• Give **IV** direct after diluting 2 ml of drug (10 mg/ml) in 0.9% NaCl to total volume of 5-10 ml; inject over 2 min to prevent hypotension
• Administer **IV** intermittent inf after diluting 20 mg of drug in 100 ml of LR, 0.9% NaCl, D_5W, $D_{10}W$; run over 15-30 min
• Store in cool environment (oral); **IV** solution is stable for 48 hr at room temp; do not use discolored sol

Y-site compatibilities: Acyclovir, allopurinol, amifostine, aminophylline, amphotericin, ampicillin, ampicillin/sulbactam, amrinone, amsacrine, atropine, aztreonam, bretylium, calcium gluconate, cefazolin, cefoperazone, cefotaxime, cefotetan, cefoxitin, ceftazidime, ceftizoxime, ceftriaxone, cefuroxime, cephalothin, cephapirin, chlorproMAZINE, cisplatin, cladribine, cyclophosphamide, cytarabine, dexamethasone, dextran 40, digoxin, diphenhydrAMINE, DOBUTamine, DOPamine, DOXOrubicin, droperidol, enalaprilat, epINEPHrine, erythromycin lactobionate, esmolol, filgrastim, fluconazole, fludarabine, folic acid, gentamicin, granisetron, haloperidol, heparin, hydrocortisone, hydromorphone, hydrOXYzine, imipenem/cilastatin, regular insulin, isoproterenol, labetalol, lidocaine, lorazepam, magnesium sulfate, melphalan, meperidine, methotrexate, methylPREDNISolone, metoclopramide, mezlocillin, midazolam, morphine, nafcillin, nitroglycerin, nitroprusside, norepinephrine, ondansetron, oxacillin, paclitaxel, perphenazine, phenylephrine, phenytoin, phytonadione, piperacillin, potassium chloride, potassium phosphate, procainamide, propofol, sargramostim, sodium bicarbonate, teniposide, theophylline, thiamine, thiotepa, ticarcillin, ticarcillin/clavulanate, verapamil, vinorelbine

Additive compatibilities: Cefazolin, cefmetazole, flumazenil

Patient/family education
• Caution patient to avoid driving, other hazardous activities until stabilized on this medication; dizziness may occur
• Advise patient to avoid black pepper, caffeine, alcohol, harsh spices, extremes in temp of food; tell patient to avoid OTC preparations: aspirin, cough, cold preparations; condition may worsen
• Advise patient to avoid taking the OTC and the prescription preparations of this drug concurrently.

- Tell patient that smoking decreases the effectiveness of the drug; that smoking cessation should be considered
- Instruct patient that drug must be continued for prescribed time to be effective and taken exactly as prescribed; doses are not to be doubled; not to use OTC and prescription products at the same time; to take missed dose when remembered up to 1 hr before next dose
- Tell patient to report bruising, fatigue, malaise; blood dyscrasias may occur
- Tell patient to report diarrhea, black tarry stools, sore throat, rash, dizziness, confusion, or delirium to prescriber immediately

Evaluation
Positive therapeutic outcome
- Decreased pain in abdomen
- Healing of ulcers

---

fat emulsions (Rx)
(fat ee-mul'shuns)
Intralipid 10%, Intralipid 20%, Liposyn II 10%, Liposyn II 20%, Liposyn III 10%, Liposyn III 20%, Soyacal 20%
Func. class.: Caloric
Chem. class.: Fatty acid, long chain
Pregnancy category C

Action: Needed for energy, heat production; consists of neutral triglycerides, primarily unsaturated fatty acids

→**Therapeutic Outcome:** Increased available calories and fatty acids

Uses: Increase calorie intake, prevent fatty acid deficiency

Dosage and routes
Deficiency
P **Adult and child:** IV 8%-10% of required calorie intake (intralipid)

Adjunct to TPN
Adult: IV 1 ml/min over 15-30 min (10%) or 0.5 ml/min over 15-30 min (20%); may increase to 500 ml over 4-8 hr if no adverse reactions occur; not to exceed 2.5 g/kg

P **Child:** IV 0.1 ml/min over 10-15 min (10%) or 0.05 ml/ min over 10-15 min (20%); may increase to 1 g/kg over 4 hr if no adverse reactions occur; not to exceed 4 g/kg

Prevention of deficiency
Adult: IV 500 ml 2 × wk (10%), given 1 ml/min for 30 min, not to exceed 500 ml over 6 hr

P **Child:** IV 5-10 ml/kg/day (10%), given 0.1 ml/min for 30 min, not to exceed 100 ml/hr

Available forms: Inj 10% (50, 100, 200, 250, 500 ml), 20% (50, 100, 200, 250, 500 ml)

Adverse effects
(*italic* = common; **bold** = life-threatening)
CNS: Dizziness, headache, drowsiness, focal seizures
CV: **Shock**
GI: Nausea, vomiting, **hepatomegaly**
HEMA: **Hyperlipemia, hypercoagulation, thrombocytopenia, leukopenia, leukocytosis**
RESP: Dyspnea, **fat in lung tissue**

Contraindications: Hypersensitivity, hyperlipemia, lipid necrosis, acute pancreatitis accompanied by hyperlipemia, hyperbilirubinemia of the newborn

Precautions: Severe liver disease, diabetes mellitus, thrombocytopenia, gastric ulcers, premature, term newborns, pregnancy **C**, sepsis

Pharmacokinetics

Absorption	Completely absorbed
Distribution	Intravascular space
Metabolism	Conversion to triglycerides, to free fatty acids
Excretion	Unknown
Half-life	Unknown

Pharmacodynamics
Unknown

Interactions: None

NURSING CONSIDERATIONS
Assessment
- Monitor triglycerides, free fatty acid levels, platelet counts daily to prevent fat overload, thrombocytopenia
- Monitor liver function studies: AST, ALT, Hct, Hgb; notify prescriber if abnormal
- Assess nutritional status: calorie count by dietitian; monitor weight daily

Nursing diagnoses
✓ Nutrition: less than body requirements, imbalanced (uses)
✓ Knowledge, deficient (teaching)

Implementation
- Administer using infusion pump at prescribed rate; do not use in-line filter sized for lipid emulsion; clogging will occur
- Do not use mixed sol that looks oily or is not separated; discard unused sol
- Change **IV** tubing at each inf: infection may occur with old tubing

- Give by intermittent inf at a rate of 10% sol (1 ml/min); 20% sol (0.5 ml/min) initially for 15-30 min; may be increased to 10% sol (120 ml/hr) or 20% sol (62.5 ml/hr) if no adverse reactions occur; do not give more than 500 ml during the first day; children should be given 10% (0.1 mg/ ml) or 20% (0.05 ml/min) initially for 15-30 min, may be increased 1 g/kg/4 hr, do not give more than 10% (100 ml/hr) or 20% (50 ml/hr)

Y-site compatibilities: Ampicillin, cefamandole, cefazolin, cefoxitin, cephapirin, clindamycin, digoxin, DOPamine, erythromycin, furosemide, gentamicin, IL-2, isoproterenol, lidocaine, kanamycin, norepinephrine, oxacillin, penicillin G potassium, ticarcillin, tobramycin

Y-site incompatibilities: Amikacin, tetracycline

Additive compatibilities: Cefamandole, chloramphenicol, cimetidine, cycloSPORINE, diphenhydrAMINE, famotidine, heparin, hydrocortisone, multivitamins, nizatidine, penicillin G potassium

Patient/family education
- Teach patient reason for use of lipids and expected results

Evaluation
Positive therapeutic outcome
- Increased weight
- Fatty acids at adequate levels

---

felodipine (Rx)
(feh-loh′dih-peen)
Plendil, Renedil ✤
Func. class.: Calcium-channel blocker, antihypertensive, antianginal
Chem. class.: Dihydropyridine

Pregnancy category C

Action: Inhibits calcium ion influx across cell membrane, resulting in inhibition of excitation/contraction

⮕ **Therapeutic Outcome:** Decreased B/P in hypertension

Uses: Essential hypertension, alone or with other antihypertensives, angina pectoris, Prinzmetal's angina (vasospastic)

Dosage and routes
Adult: PO 5 mg qd initially, usual range 5-10 mg qd; max 10 mg qd; do not adjust dosage at intervals of <2 wk

 Elderly: PO 2.5 mg qd

Hepatic dose
PO 2.5-5 mg qd, max 10 mg/day

Available forms: Ext rel tabs 2.5, 5, 10 mg

Adverse effects
(*italic* = common; **bold** = life-threatening)
CNS: Headache, fatigue, drowsiness, dizziness, anxiety, depression, nervousness, insomnia, light-headedness, paresthesia, tinnitus, psychosis, somnolence
CV: **Dysrhythmias,** edema, **CHF,** hypotension, palpitations, **MI, pulmonary edema,** tachycardia, syncope, AV block, angina
GI: Nausea, vomiting, diarrhea, gastric upset, constipation, increased liver function studies, dry mouth
GU: Nocturia, polyuria
HEMA: Anemia
INTEG: Rash, pruritus
MISC: Flushing, sexual difficulties, cough, nasal congestion, shortness of breath, wheezing, epistaxis, respiratory infection, chest pain, **Stevens-Johnson syndrome,** gingival hyperplasia

Contraindications: Hypersensitivity, sick sinus syndrome, 2nd- or 3rd-degree heart block, hypotension <90 mm Hg systolic

Precautions: CHF, hepatic injury, pregnancy **C,** lactation, children, renal disease, elderly

 Do Not Confuse:
Plendil/pindolol, Plendil/Prinivil, Plendil/Prilosec, Plendil/Pletal

Pharmacokinetics	
Absorption	Well absorbed
Distribution	Unknown; protein binding >99%
Metabolism	Liver, extensively
Excretion	Kidneys
Half-life	11-16 hr

Pharmacodynamics	
Onset	2-3 hr
Peak	2½-5 hr
Duration	<24 hr

Interactions
Individual drugs
Alcohol, fentanyl, quinidine: ↑ hypotension
Digoxin: ↑ digoxin levels
Digoxin, disopyramide: ↑ bradycardia, ↑ CHF
Erythromycin, ketoconazole, itraconazole: ↑ toxicity
Phenytoin: ↓ effectiveness

Drug classifications
Antihypertensives, nitrates: ↑ hypotension
β-Adrenergic blockers: ↑ bradycardia, CHF
NSAIDs: ↓ antihypertensive effects
Food/drug
Grapefruit juice: ↑ felodipine level
Herb/drug
Aconite: ↑ toxicity, death
Astragalus, cola tree: ↑ or ↓ antihypertensive effect
Barberry, betony, black catechu, black cohosh, bloodroot, broom, burdock, cat's claw, dandelion, goldenseal, Irish moss, Jamaican dogwood, kelp, khella, mistletoe, parsley: ↑ antihypertensive effect
Coltsfoot, guarana, khat, licorice: ↓ antihypertensive effect

NURSING CONSIDERATIONS
Assessment
• Assess fluid volume status: I&O ratio and record; weight; skin turgor; adequacy of pulses; moist mucous membranes; bilateral lung sounds; peripheral pitting edema; dehydration symptoms of decreasing output, thirst, hypotension, dry mouth, and mucous membranes should be reported; for CHF: weight gain, rales/crackles, dyspnea, edema, jugular venous distention
• Monitor ALT, AST, bilirubin daily if these are elevated
• Monitor cardiac status: B/P, pulse, respiration, ECG, periodically
• Assess for anginal pain: duration, intensity, ameliorating, aggravating factors

Nursing diagnoses
✓ Cardiac output, decreased (uses)
✓ Knowledge, deficient (teaching)

Implementation
• Give once a day, with food for GI symptoms
⊘ • Do not crush, chew tabs, sus rel products

Patient/family education
• Caution patient to avoid hazardous activities until stabilized on drug, and dizziness is no longer a problem
• Instruct patient to limit caffeine consumption; to avoid alcohol and OTC drugs unless directed by prescriber
• Urge patient to comply in all areas of medical regimen: diet, exercise, stress reduction, drug therapy; to notify prescriber of irregular heartbeat, shortness of breath, swelling of feet and hands, pronounced dizziness, constipation, nausea, hypotension
• Advise patient to use protective clothing, sunscreen to prevent photosensitivity

• Teach patient to change positions slowly to prevent orthostatic hypotension
• Advise patient to obtain correct pulse, to contact prescriber if pulse is <50 bpm
• Teach patient to use as directed even if feeling better; may be taken with other CV drugs (nitrates, β-blockers), that capsules may appear in stools, but are insignificant

Evaluation
Positive therapeutic outcome
• Decreased B/P
• Decreased anginal attacks
• Increase in activity tolerance

---

fenofibrate (Rx)
(fen-oh-fee' brate)
Tricor
Func. class.: Antilipemic
Chem. class.: Fibric acid derivative
Pregnancy category C

Action: Increases lipolysis and elimination of triglyceride-rich particles from plasma by activating lipoprotein lipase, resulting in triglyceride change in size and composition of LDL, leading to rapid breakdown of LDL; mobilizes triglycerides from tissue; increases excretion of neutral sterols

⇒ **Therapeutic Outcome:** Decreasing cholesterol levels and low-density lipoproteins, decreased pruritus

Uses: Patients with types IV, V hyperlipidemia who do not respond to other treatment and who are at risk for pancreatitis Fredrickson type IIa, IIb, hypertriglyceridemia

Investigational uses: Polymetabolic syndrome X

Dosage and routes
Hypertriglyceridemia
Adult: PO 54-160 mg/day, may increase q4-8 wk, max 160 mg/day

Primary hypercholesterolemia/ mixed hyperlipidemia
Adult: PO 160 mg/day

Renal dose/elderly
🖸 *Adult:* PO 54 mg/day (CCr <50 ml/min)

Available forms: Tabs 54, 160 mg

Adverse effects
(*italic* = common; **bold** = life-threatening)
CNS: Fatigue, weakness, drowsiness, dizziness, insomnia, depression, vertigo
CV: Angina, **dysrhythmias,** hypertension
GI: Nausea, vomiting, dyspepsia, increased

liver enzymes, flatulence, hepatomegaly, gastritis
GU: Dysuria, proteinuria, oliguria, urinary frequency
HEMA: Anemia, leukopenia, ecchymosis
INTEG: *Rash,* urticaria, pruritus
MISC: Polyphagia, weight gain
MS: Myalgias, arthralgias, myopathy
RESP: Pharyngitis, bronchitis, cough

Contraindications: Hypersensitivity, severe hepatic disease, severe renal disease, primary biliary cirrhosis, preexisting gallbladder disease

Precautions: Peptic ulcer, pregnancy **C,** lactation, pancreatitis, renal, hepatic disease, elderly

Pharmacokinetics

Absorption	Unknown
Distribution	Protein binding 99%
Metabolism	Liver
Excretion	Urine 60%
Half-life	20 hr

Pharmacodynamics

Peak	6-8 hr

Interactions
Drug classifications
Anticoagulants (oral): ↑ effect of anticoagulants
Bile acid sequestrants: ↓ absorption
CycloSPORINE: ↑ nephrotoxicity
HMG-CoA reductase inhibitors: Do not use together, rhabdomyolysis may occur
Immunosuppressants, nephrotoxics: ↓ fenofibrate elimination
Food/drug
↑ Absorption
⊘ *Herb/drug*
Glucomannan: ↑ effect
Gotu kola: ↓ effect

NURSING CONSIDERATIONS
Assessment
• Assess lipid levels, liver function tests, baseline and periodically during treatment; CPK if muscle pain occurs, CBC, Hct, Hgh, Pro-time with anticoagulant therapy
• Assess for pancreatitis, cholelithiasis, renal failure, rhabdomyolysis, (when combined with HMG-CoA reductase inhibitors) myositis, drug should be discontinued
• Assess nutrition: fat, protein, carbohydrates, nutritional analysis should be completed by dietician
• Assess skin integrity after patient has been

receiving drug; itching, pruritus often occur from bile deposits on skin
• Monitor cardiac glycoside level if both drugs are being administered; cardiac glycoside levels will be decreased
• Monitor for signs of vit A, D, K deficiency; serum cholesterol, triglyceride levels, electrolytes if on extended therapy
• Monitor bowel pattern daily; increase bulk, water in diet if constipation develops

Nursing diagnoses
✓ Knowledge, deficient (teaching)
✓ Noncompliance (teaching)

Implementation
• Give with evening meal; if dose is increased, take with breakfast and evening meal
⊘• Do not chew, crush caps
• Store in cool environment in tight, light-resistant container

Patient/family education
• Inform patient that compliance is needed
• Teach patient that risk factors—high-fat diet, smoking, alcohol consumption, absence of exercise—should be decreased
• Caution patient to notify prescriber if pregnancy is planned or suspected
• Teach patient to notify prescriber if the GI symptoms of diarrhea, abdominal or epigastric pain, nausea, or vomiting occur
• Instruct patient to report GU symptoms: dysuria, proteinuria, oliguria, decreased libido, impotence
• Advise patient to notify prescriber of muscle pain, weakness, fever, fatigue, epigastric pain

Evaluation
Positive therapeutic outcome
• Decrease in cholesterol to desired level after 8 wk

---

fenoldopam (Rx)
(fen-nahl'doh-pam)
Corlopam
Func. class.: Antihypertensive, vasodilator
Pregnancy category B

Action: Agonist at D_1-like dopamine receptors; binds to α_2-adrenoceptors; increases renal blood flow

➡ **Therapeutic Outcome:** B/P, decreased

Uses: Hypertensive crisis, malignant hypertension

Dosage and routes
Adult: **IV** 0.01-1.6 mcg/kg/min titrated slowly, result in less reflex tachycardia

Available forms: Inj conc 10 mg/ml in single use ampules

Adverse effects
(*italic* = common; **bold** = life-threatening)
CNS: *Headache,* anxiety, dizziness
CV: *Hypotension,* ST-T-wave changes, angina pectoris, palpitations, **MI, ischemic heart disease,** *flushing*
GI: Nausea, vomiting, constipation, diarrhea
HEMA: **Leukocytosis, bleeding**
META: Increased BUN, glucose, LDH, creatinine, hypokalemia

Contraindications: Hypersensitivity, sulfite sensitivity

Precautions: Tachycardia, pregnancy **B,** lactation, children, intraocular pressure, hypokalemia

Pharmacokinetics

Absorption	Unknown
Distribution	Steady state 20 min
Metabolism	Unknown
Excretion	Unknown
Half-life	5 min (elimination)

Pharmacodynamics

Onset	Unknown
Peak	Unknown
Duration	Unknown

Interactions
Drug classifications
β-Adrenergic blockers: ↑ hypotension
Herb/drug
Aconite: ↑ toxicity, death
Astragalus, cola tree: ↑ or ↓ antihypertensive effect
Barberry, betony, black catechu, black cohosh, bloodroot, broom, burdock, cat's claw, dandelion, goldenseal, Irish moss, Jamaican dogwood, kelp, khella, mistletoe, parsley: ↑ antihypertensive effect
Coltsfoot, guarana, khat, licorice: ↓ antihypertensive effect

NURSING CONSIDERATIONS
Assessment
• Monitor B/P q5 min until stabilized, then q1h × 2 hr, then q4h; pulse, jugular venous distention q4h
• Monitor electrolytes, blood studies: K, Na, Cl, CO_2, CBC, serum glucose
• Assess skin turgor, dryness of mucous membranes for hydration status
• Assess **IV** site for extravasation, rate

Nursing diagnoses
☑ Tissue perfusion, ineffective (uses)
☑ Knowledge, deficient (teaching)
☑ Noncompliance (teaching)

Implementation
IV route
• Administer after diluting contents of ampules in 0.9% NaCl, or 5% dextrose inj (40 mcg/ml); then add 4 ml of conc (40 mg of drug/1000 ml); 2 ml of conc (20 mg of drug/500 ml); 1 ml of conc (10 mg of drug/250 ml); do not admix
• Give to patient in recumbent position; keep in that position for 1 hr after administration
• Diluted sol is stable in normal light/temp for 24 hr

Patient/family education
• Teach patient reason for medication and expected results
• Instruct patient to report dyspnea, chest pain, bleeding

Evaluation
Positive therapeutic outcome
• Decreased B/P

/ HIGH ALERT

fentanyl (Rx)
(fen'ta-nill)
fentanyl, Sublimaze, Fentanyl Oralet, Actiq
Func. class.: Opioid analgesic
Chem. class.: Synthetic phenylpiperidine derivative

Pregnancy category C
Controlled substance schedule II

Action: Inhibits ascending pain pathways in CNS, increases pain threshold, alters pain perception by binding to opiate receptors

Therapeutic Outcome: Relief of pain, supplement to anesthesia

Uses: Preoperatively, postoperatively; adjunct to general anesthetic, adjunct to regional anesthesia; Fentanyl Oralet for anesthesia as premedication, conscious sedation; Actiq for breakthrough cancer pain

Dosage and routes
Anesthetic
Adult: **IV** 25-100 mcg (0.7-2 mcg/kg)

Anesthesia supplement
Adult: **IV** 2-20 mcg/kg **IV** INF 0.025-0.25 mcg/kg/min
Induction and maintenance
Adult: **IV** Bol 5-40 mcg/kg

P *Child 2-12 yr:* **IV** 2-3 mcg/kg

Preoperatively
Adult: IM 0.05-0.1 mg q30-60 min before surgery

Postoperatively
Adult: IM 0.05-0.1 mg q1-2hr prn

P *Child:* IM 0.02-0.03 mg/9 kg

Fentanyl Oralet
Adult: Transmucosal: 5 mcg/kg = fentanyl IM 0.75-1.25 mcg/kg, do not exceed 5 mcg/kg

P *Child:* Transmucosal may need doses of 5-15 mcg/kg; must be watched continuously for hypoventilation

Actiq
Adult: Transmucosal 200 mcg, redose if needed 15 min after completion of 1st dose, do not give more than 2 doses during titration period

Available forms: Inj 0.05 mg/ml; lozenges 100, 200, 300, 400 mcg; lozenges on a stick 200, 400, 600, 800, 1200, 1600 mcg

Adverse effects
(*italic* = common; **bold** = life-threatening)
CNS: Dizziness, delirium, euphoria
CV: **Bradycardia, cardiac arrest,** hypotension or hypertension
EENT: Blurred vision, miosis
GI: Nausea, vomiting
GU: Urinary retention
INTEG: Rash, diaphoresis
MS: Muscle rigidity
RESP: **Respiratory depression, arrest, laryngospasm**

Contraindications: Hypersensitivity to opiates, myasthenia gravis

G **Precautions:** Elderly, respiratory depression, increased ICP, seizure disorders, severe respiratory disorders, cardiac dysrhythmias, pregnancy **C**

N **Do Not Confuse:**
fentanyl/Sufenta

Pharmacokinetics

Absorption	Well absorbed (IM), completely absorbed (**IV**)
Distribution	Unknown, crosses placenta
Metabolism	Extensively—liver, 80% bound to plasma proteins
Excretion	Kidneys—up to 25% unchanged, breast milk
Half-life	1½-6 hr

Pharmacodynamics

	IM	IV
Onset	7-8 min	Rapid
Peak	30 min	3-5 min
Duration	1-2 hr	½-1 hr

Interactions
Individual drugs
Alcohol: ↑ respiratory depression, hypotension, ↑ sedation
Drug classifications
CNS depressants, sedative/hypnotics: ↑ respiratory depression, hypotension
Opioids, skeletal muscle relaxants: effects ↑
Herb/drug
Corkwood: ↑ anticholinergic effect
Jamaican dogwood, kava, lavender, mistletoe, nettle, pokeweed, poppy, senaga, valerian: ↑ fentanyl action
Lab test interferences
↑ Amylase, ↑ lipase

NURSING CONSIDERATIONS
Assessment
• Monitor VS after parenteral route (B/P, pulse, respiration); note muscle rigidity; take drug history before administering drug; check liver, kidney function tests; assess for respiratory dysfunction: respiratory depression, character, rate, rhythm; notify prescriber if respirations are <10/min
• Monitor CNS changes: dizziness, drowsiness, hallucinations, euphoria, LOC, pupil reaction
• Monitor allergic reactions: rash, urticaria; drug should be discontinued
• Assess for pain: intensity, location, duration, type, before and 15 min after IM route or 3-5 min after **IV** route

Nursing diagnoses
☑ Pain (uses)
☑ Sensory-perception disturbed: visual, auditory (adverse reactions)
☑ Breathing pattern, ineffective (adverse reactions)
☑ Knowledge, deficient (teaching)

Implementation
• Give by inj (IM, **IV**), only with resuscitative equipment available; give slowly to prevent rigidity
• Give **IV** undiluted by anesthesiologist or diluted with 5 ml or more sterile water or 0.9% NaCl given through Y-tube or 3-way stopcock given at 0.1 mg or less/1.2 min
• Store in light-resistant area at room temp

Transmucosal route
- Remove foil just before administration, instruct patient to place under tongue and suck, not chew (Oralet); place between cheek and lower gum, moving it back and forth and suck, not chew (Actiq); all products not used or partially used should be flushed down the toilet

Syringe compatibilities: Atracurium, atropine, bupivacaine/ketamine, butorphanol, chlorproMAZINE, cimetidine, clonidine/lidocaine, dimenhyDRINATE, diphenhydrAMINE, droperidol, heparin, hydromorphone, hydrOXYzine, meperidine, metoclopramide, midazolam, morphine, pentazocine, perphenazine, prochlorperazine, promazine, promethazine, ranitidine, scopolamine

Syringe incompatibilities: Pentobarbital

Y-site compatibilities: Amphotericin B cholesteryl, atracurium, cisatracurium, diltiazem, dobutamine, DOPamine, enalaprilat, epINEPHrine, esmolol, etomidate, furosemide, heparin, hydrocortisone, hydromorphone, labetalol, lorazepam, midazolam, milrinone, morphine, nafcillin, niCARdipine, nitroglycerin, norepinephrine, pancuronium, potassium chloride, propofol, ranitidine, remifentanil, sargramostim, thiopental, vecuronium, vit B/C

Additive compatibilities: Bupivacaine, sodium bicarbonate

Additive incompatibilities: Methohexital, pentobarbital, thiopental

Solution compatibilities: D_5W, 0.9% NaCl

Patient/family education
- Advise patient to report any symptoms of CNS changes, allergic reactions
- Instruct patient to avoid CNS depressants: alcohol, sedative/hypnotics for at least 24 hr after taking this drug
- Teach patient that dizziness, drowsiness, confusion are common, and to avoid getting up without assistance
- Discuss in detail with patient all aspects of the drug

Evaluation
Positive therapeutic outcome
- Maintenance of anesthesia
- Decreased pain

Treatment of overdose: Naloxone 0.2-0.8 **IV**, O_2, **IV** fluids, vasopressors

fentanyl transdermal (Rx)
(fen'ta-nill)
Duragesic-25, Duragesic-50, Duragesic-75, Duragesic-100
Func. class.: Opioid, analgesic
Chem. class.: Synthetic phenylpiperidine

Pregnancy category C

Controlled substance schedule II

Action: Inhibits ascending pain pathways in CNS, increases pain threshold, alters pain perception by binding to opiate receptors

→ Therapeutic Outcome: Relief of chronic pain

Uses: Management of chronic pain for those requiring opioid analgesia

Dosage and routes
Adult: TD 25 mcg/hr; may increase until pain relief occurs; apply patch to flat surface on upper torso and wear for 72 hr; apply new patch on different site for continued relief

Available forms: Patches 25, 50, 75, 100 mcg/hr

Adverse effects
(*italic* = common; **bold** = life-threatening)
CNS: Dizziness, delirium, euphoria, lightheadedness, sedation, dysphoria, agitation, anxiety, confusion, headache, depression
CV: Bradycardia, **cardiac arrest,** hypotension or hypertension, facial flushing, chills, chest pain, dysrhythmia
EENT: Blurred vision, miosis
GI: Nausea, vomiting, diarrhea, cramps, anorexia, constipation, dyspepsia
GU: Urinary retention, urgency, dysuria, frequency, oliguria
INTEG: Sweating, pruritus, rash, erythema, papules
MS: Asthenia
RESP: **Respiratory depression, laryngospasm, bronchospasm;** depresses cough; hypoventilation, dyspnea, hiccups, **apnea**

Contraindications: Hypersensitivity to opiates, myasthenia gravis, children <12 yr, patient <18 yr with weight <110 lb

Precautions: Elderly, respiratory depression, increased ICP, seizure disorders, severe respiratory disorders, cardiac dysrhythmias, pregnancy **C,** fever

Pharmacokinetics

Absorption	92% (skin), continuously for 72 hr
Distribution	Crosses placenta
Metabolism	Extensively—liver
Excretion	Up to 25%—kidneys unchanged
Half-life	17 hr after removal of patch

Pharmacodynamics

Onset	6 hr
Peak	12-24 hr
Duration	72 hr

Interactions
Individual drugs
Alcohol: ↑ respiratory depression, hypotension, ↑ sedation
Cimetidine, erythromycin: ↑ recovery
Nalbuphine, pentazocine: ↓ analgesia
Drug classifications
Antihistamines, CNS depressants, phenothiazines, sedative/hypnotics: ↑ respiratory depression, hypotension
MAOIs: Do not use 2 wk before fentanyl
Opioids, skeletal muscle relaxants: effects may be ↑

☑ Herb/drug
Corkwood: ↑ anticholinergic effect
Jamaican dogwood, kava, lavender, mistletoe, nettle, pokeweed, poppy, senega, valerian: ↑ fentanyl level
Lab test interferences
↑ Amylase, ↑ lipase

NURSING CONSIDERATIONS
Assessment
• Assess for respiratory dysfunction: respiratory depression, character, rate, rhythm; notify prescriber if respirations are <10/min
• Monitor CNS changes: dizziness, drowsiness, hallucinations, euphoria, LOC, pupil reaction
• Monitor allergic reactions: rash, urticaria; drug should be discontinued
• Assess for pain: intensity, location, duration, type, before and after administration

Nursing diagnoses
☑ Pain, chronic (uses)
☑ Sensory-perception disturbed: visual, auditory (adverse reactions)
☑ Breathing pattern, ineffective (adverse reactions)
☑ Knowledge, deficient (teaching)

Implementation
• Opioids should be used to control pain until relief is obtained with TD patch; patients may continue to require other opioids for breakthrough pain; if >100 mcg/hr is required, use multiple systems
• Apply patch to chest on a flat area with skin intact; for skin preparation, use clear water with no soap; clip hair, skin should be dry before applying patch; apply immediately after removing from package and press firmly in place with palm of hand; flush old patch down toilet immediately upon removal
Use pain dosing
• Dosage is titrated based on patient's report of pain; dosage is determined by calculating the previous 24-hr requirement and converting to equianalgesic morphine dose
• To convert to another opioid analgesic, remove TD patch and begin treatment with half the equal pain-controlling dose of the new analgesic in 12-18 hr
• Medication should be tapered gradually after long-term use to prevent withdrawal symptoms

Patient/family education
• Advise patient to report any symptoms of CNS changes, allergic reactions
• Instruct patients to avoid CNS depressants: alcohol, sedative/hypnotics for at least 24 hr after this drug
• Discuss with patient that dizziness, drowsiness, and confusion are common and to avoid getting up without assistance
• Discuss with patient that excessive heat may increase absorption; excessive perspiration may alter adhesiveness

Evaluation
Positive therapeutic outcome
• Decreased pain

Treatment of overdose: Naloxone 0.2-0.8 mg **IV**, O_2, **IV** fluids, vasopressors

---

☑ Herb/drug   Ⓢ Do Not Crush   ◈ Alert   ◈_π Key Drug   Ⓖ Geriatric   Ⓟ Pediatric

ferrous fumarate (Rx, OTC)
(fer'us fyu'-muh-rāt)
Femiron, Feostat, Feostat Drops, Hemocyte, Ircon, Nephro-Fer, Novofumar ♣, Palafer ♣, Span-FF

ferrous gluconate (Rx, OTC)
Fergon, Fertinic ♣, Novoferrogluc ♣

ferric gluconate complex (Rx, OTC)
Ferrlecit

ferrous sulfate (Rx, OTC)
Apo-Ferrous Sulfate ♣, ED-INSOL, Feosol, Fer-gen-sol, Fer-Iron Drops, Fero-Grad, Mol-Iron

ferrous sulfate, dried (Rx, OTC)
Fe⁵⁰, Feosol, Feratab, Novoferrosulfa ♣, PMS-Ferrous Sulfate, Slow Fe

iron, carbonyl (OTC)
(kar'boh-nil)
Feosol, Icar

iron polysaccharide (OTC)
(pah-lee-sack'ah-ride)
Hytinic, Niferex, Nu-Iron, Nu-Iron 150
Func. class.: Hematinic
Chem. class.: Iron preparation

Pregnancy category B, C

Action: Replaces iron stores needed for red blood cell development, energy and O_2 transport, utilization; fumarate contains 33% elemental iron; gluconate, 12%; sulfate, 20%; iron, 30%; ferrous sulfate exsiccated

▰ **Therapeutic Outcome:** Prevention and correction of iron deficiency

Uses: Iron deficiency anemia, prophylaxis for iron deficiency in pregnancy

Dosage and routes
Fumarate
Adult: PO 200 mg tid-qid

🄟 *Child 2-12 yr:* PO 3 mg/kg/day (elemental iron) tid-qid

🄟 *Child 6 mo-2 yr:* PO up to 6 mg/kg/day (elemental iron) tid-qid

🄟 *Infants:* PO 10-25 mg/day (elemental iron) in 3-4 divided doses, max 15 mg/day

Gluconate
Adult: PO 200-600 mg tid

🄟 *Child 6-12 yr:* PO 300-900 mg qd

🄟 *Child <6 yr:* PO 100-300 mg qd

Sulfate
Adult: PO 0.750-1.5 g/day in divided doses tid

🄟 *Child 6-12 yr:* 600 mg/day in divided doses

Pregnancy
Adult: PO 300-600 mg/day in divided doses

Complex
Adult: **IV** inf (125 mg) 10 ml/100 ml of NaCl for inj given over 1 hr

Iron polysaccharide
Adult: 100-200 mg tid

🄟 *Child:* PO 4-6 mg/kg/day in 3 divided doses

F

Available forms
Fumarate: Tabs 63, 195, 200, 324, 325 mg; tabs, chewable 100 mg; tabs, controlled-release 300 mg; oral susp 100 mg/5 ml, 45 mg/0.6 ml

Gluconate: Tabs 300, 320, 325, mg; caps 86, 325, 435 mg; tabs, film-coated 300 mg; elix 300 mg/5 ml

Sulfate: Tabs 195, 300, 325, mg; tabs, enteric-coated 325 mg; tabs, ext rel, time-release caps 525 mg

Dried: Tabs, 200 mg; tabs ext rel 160 mg; caplets ext rel 160 mg

Complex: Inj 62.5 mg/5 ml (12.5 mg/ml)

Iron, carboxyl: Tabs 50 mg, susp 15 mg/1.25 ml

Iron polysaccharide: Tabs 50 mg; caps 150 mg; sol 100 mg/5 ml

Adverse effects
(*italic* = common; **bold** = life-threatening)
GI: *Nausea, constipation, epigastric pain, black and red tarry stools,* vomiting, diarrhea
INTEG: Temporarily discolored tooth enamel and eyes

Contraindications: Hypersensitivity, ulcerative colitis/regional enteritis, hemosiderosis/hemochromatosis, peptic ulcer disease, hemolytic anemia, cirrhosis

Precautions: Anemia (long-term), pregnancy **B** (ferric gluconate complex), **C** (iron dextran, oral products)

Pharmacokinetics	
Absorption	Up to 30%
Distribution	Bound to transferrin, crosses placenta
Metabolism	Recycled
Excretion	Feces, urine, skin, breast milk
Half-life	Unknown

Pharmacodynamics
Unknown

Interactions
Individual drugs
Chloramphenicol, vit C: ↑ absorption of iron products

Cholestyramine, cimetidine: ↓ absorption of iron

L-Thyroxine: ↓ L-thyroxine absorption

Levodopa: ↓ absorption of levodopa

Methyldopa: ↓ absorption of methyldopa

Penicillamine: ↓ absorption of penicillamine

Tetracycline: ↓ absorption of tetracycline

Vit E: ↓ absorption of iron preparations

Drug classifications
Antacids: ↓ absorption of iron preparations

Fluoroquinolones: ↓ absorption of fluoroquinolone

Food/drug
Caffeine, dairy products, eggs: ↓ absorption

Herb/drug
Allspice, bilberry, condurango, elderberry, eye bright (PO), gentian, ground ivy, marshmallow, meadowsweet, mistletoe, motherwort, nettle, raspberry, valerian, tea made with artichoke, hawthorn, horse chestnut, lady mantle, lemon balm, oak bark, plantain, poplar, prickly ash, sage: ↓ iron absorption

Anise: ↑ iron effect

Black catechu: Forms insoluble complex

Lab test interferences
False positive: Occult blood

NURSING CONSIDERATIONS
Assessment
- Monitor blood studies: Hct, Hgb, reticulocytes, bilirubin before treatment, at least monthly
- Assess for toxicity: nausea, vomiting, diarrhea (green, then tarry stools,) hematemesis, pallor, cyanosis, shock, coma
- Assess bowel elimination; if constipation occurs, increase water, bulk, activity before laxatives are required
- Assess nutrition: amount of iron in diet (meat, dark green leafy vegetables, dried beans, dried fruits, eggs); provide referral to dietitian if indicated
- Identify cause of iron loss or anemia, including salicylates, sulfonamides, antimalarials, quinidine

Nursing diagnoses
☑ Nutrition, less than body requirements, imbalanced (uses)

☑ Fatigue (uses)

☑ Knowledge, deficient (teaching)

Implementation
- Give between meals for best absorption; may give with juice; do not give with antacids or milk, delay at least 1 hr; if GI symptoms occur, give pc even if absorption is decreased; eggs, milk products, chocolate, caffeine interfere with absorption; ferrous gluconate is less GI irritating than ferrous sulfate
- Do not crush, chew tabs
- Give liq preparations through plastic straw to avoid discoloration of tooth enamel; dilute thoroughly
- Give at least 1 hr before bedtime because corrosion may occur in stomach
- Give for <6 mo for anemia
- Store in airtight, light-resistant container

Patient/family education
- Advise patient that iron will make stools black or dark green; that iron poisoning may occur if increased beyond recommended level
- Tell patient not to crush; swallow tab whole; to keep out of reach of children
- Caution patient not to substitute one iron salt for another; elemental iron content differs (e.g., 300 mg ferrous fumarate contains about 100 mg elemental iron, whereas 300 mg ferrous gluconate contains only about 30 mg elemental iron)
- Caution patient to avoid reclining position for 15-30 min after taking drug to avoid esophageal corrosion; to follow diet high in iron

Evaluation
Positive therapeutic outcome
- Decreased fatigue, weakness
- Improvement in Hct, Hgb, reticulocytes

Treatment of overdose: Induce vomiting; give eggs, milk until lavage can be done

---

fexofenadine (Rx)
(fex-oh-fin′a-deen)

Allegra

Func. class.: H₁-histamine antagonist

Chem. class: Piperidine, peripherally selective

Pregnancy category C

Action: Acts on blood vessels, GI, respiratory system by competing with histamine for H₁-receptor site; decreases allergic response by blocking pharmacologic effects of histamine; less sedation rate than with other antihistamines; causes increased heart rate, vasodilatation, increased secretions

Therapeutic Outcome: Absence of allergy symptoms and rhinitis

---

Uses: Rhinitis, allergy symptoms, chronic idiopathic urticaria

Dosage and routes

P *Adult and child >12 yr:* 60 mg bid

P *Child 6-11 yr:* PO 30 mg bid

Renal dose

Adult: PO CCr <80 ml/min 60 mg qd

Available forms: Caps 60 mg; ext rel tabs 180 mg; tabs 30 mg

Adverse effects

(*italic* = common; **bold** = life-threatening)

CNS: Headache, stimulation, drowsiness, sedation, fatigue, confusion, blurred vision, P tinnitus, restlessness, tremors, paradoxical G excitation in children or elderly

CV: Hypotension, palpitations, bradycardia, tachycardia, **dysrhythmias (rare)**

GI: Nausea, diarrhea, abdominal pain, vomiting, constipation

GU: Frequency, dysuria, urinary retention, impotence

HEMA: **Hemolytic anemia, thrombocytopenia, leukopenia, agranulocytosis, pancytopenia**

INTEG: Rash, eczema, photosensitivity, urticaria

RESP: Thickening of bronchial secretions; dry nose, throat

Contraindications: Hypersensitivity, P newborn or premature infants, lactation, severe hepatic disease

G **Precautions:** Pregnancy **C**, elderly, P children, respiratory disease, narrow-angle glaucoma, prostatic hypertrophy, bladder neck obstruction, asthma

Do Not Confuse:
Allegra/Viagra

Pharmacokinetics

Absorption	Well absorbed
Distribution	Unknown
Metabolism	Liver
Excretion	Kidneys

Pharmacodynamics

Onset	15-30 min
Peak	1-2 hr
Duration	8-12 hr

Interactions
Individual drugs
Alcohol: ↑ sedation

Drug classifications
CNS depressants, opiates, sedative/hypnotics: ↑ sedation

Herb/drug
Corkwood, henbane leaf: ↑ anticholinergic effect

Hops, Jamaican dogwood, khat, senega: ↑ sedation

Lab test interferences
False negative: Skin allergy tests (discontinue antihistamine 3 days before testing)

NURSING CONSIDERATIONS
Assessment
• Assess respiratory status: rate, rhythm, increase in bronchial secretions, wheezing, chest tightness; provide fluids to 2 L/day to decrease secretion thickness
• Monitor I&O ratio: be alert for urinary retention, frequency, dysuria, especially G elderly; drug should be discontinued if these occur

Nursing diagnoses
☑ Airway clearance, ineffective (uses)
☑ Injury, risk for (side effects)
☑ Knowledge, deficient (teaching)
☑ Noncompliance (teaching, overuse)

Implementation
• Give on an empty stomach 1 hr before or 2 hr pc to facilitate absorption
• Store in tight, light-resistant container

Patient/family education
• Teach all aspects of drug uses; to notify prescriber if confusion, sedation, hypotension occur; to avoid driving or other hazardous activity if drowsiness occurs; to avoid alcohol or other CNS depressants that may potentiate effect
• Instruct patient to take 1 hr before or 2 hr pc to facilitate absorption
• Instruct patient not to exceed recommended dose; dysrhythmias may occur
• Teach patient that hard candy, gum, frequent rinsing of mouth may be used for dryness

Evaluation
Positive therapeutic outcome
• Absence of running or congested nose, rashes

Treatment of overdose:
Administer ipecac syrup or lavage, diazepam, vasopressors, barbiturates (short acting)

---

fibrinolysin/ desoxyribonuclease (Rx)
(fye-brin-oe-lye'sin/dez-ox-ee-rye-boe-nuke'lee-ase)
Elase
Func. class.: Enzyme
Chem. class.: Proteolytic, bovine

Pregnancy category C

Action: Dissolves fibrin in clots and fibrinous exudates, attacks DNA in areas of disintegrating cells

Therapeutic Outcome: A clean wound

Uses: Debridement of wounds, vaginitis, cervicitis, ulcerative colitis, 2nd-, 3rd-degree burns; irrigating wounds, topically

Dosage and routes
Debridement/intravaginally
Adult: Oint 5 g × 5 applications

Irrigating
Adult: Irrigating dilution depends on type of wound

Available forms: Fibrinolysin with desoxyribonuclease 666.6 units/g; powder for reconstitution fibrinolysin 25 units/desoxyribonuclease 15,000 units

Adverse effects
(*italic* = common; **bold** = life-threatening)
INTEG: Hyperemia

Contraindications: Hypersensitivity to bovine or mercury products, hematoma

Precautions: Pregnancy **C**

Pharmacokinetics	
Absorption	Not absorbed
Distribution	Unknown
Metabolism	Unknown
Excretion	Unknown
Half-life	Unknown

Pharmacodynamics
Unknown

Interactions: None

NURSING CONSIDERATIONS
Assessment
• Assess for signs of irritation and inflammation around wound; drug should be discontinued
• Assess wound for drainage, color, odor, size, depth before and during therapy

Nursing diagnoses
☑ Skin integrity, impaired (uses)
☑ Knowledge, deficient (teaching)

Implementation
Top route
• Apply after reconstituting top sol with 10-50 ml of sterile NaCl sol; use only fresh sol; reconstituted sol is stable for 24 hr; remove necrotic debris, dry eschar
• Saturate gauze with sol; pack area; remove in 6-8 hr and clean; repeat tid-qid
• Apply top oint after flushing wound with saline, water, or let dry or pat dry, then apply a small amount of oint to area and cover with a nonadhesive dressing; change qd or bid
Vaginal route
• Place 5 ml in applicator, apply with patient recumbent

Patient/family education
• Teach patient reason for treatment and expected results

Evaluation
Positive therapeutic outcome
• Decrease in wound scarring, tissue necrosis

filgrastim (Rx)
(fill-gras'stim)
Neupogen
Func. class.: Biologic modifier
Chem. class.: Granulocyte colony-stimulating factor

Pregnancy category C

Action: Stimulates proliferation and differentiation of neutrophils; a glycoprotein

Therapeutic Outcome: Absence of infection

Uses: To decrease infection in patients receiving antineoplastics that are myelosuppressive; to increase WBC in patients with drug-induced neutropenia

Investigational uses: Neutropenia in HIV infection

Dosage and routes
After myelosuppressive chemotherapy
P *Adult and child:* **IV**/SC 5 mcg/kg/day in a single dose × 14 days; may increase by 5 mcg/kg in each chemotherapy cycle; give qd for up to 2 wk until ANC has reached 10,000/mm³; response to G-CSF is much greater with SC than **IV** therapy

After bone marrow transplantation
Adult: **IV**/SC 10 mcg/kg as an inf (**IV**) over 4 or 24 hr, begin 24 hr after chemotherapy and 24 hr after bone marrow transplantation

Peripheral blood progenitor cell collection/therapy
Adult: 10 mcg/kg/day as a bol or cont inf × 4 days or more before leukapheresis, continue to last leukapheresis, may alter dose if WBC >100,000/mm^3

Severe neutropenia (chronic)
Adult: SC 5 mcg/kg as single SC inj qd

Available forms: Inj 300 mcg/ml

Adverse effects
(*italic* = common; **bold** = life-threatening)
CNS: Fever
GI: Nausea, vomiting, diarrhea, mucositis, anorexia
HEMA: **Thrombocytopenia**
INTEG: Alopecia, exacerbation of skin conditions
MS: Osteoporosis, skeletal pain
RESP: **Respiratory distress syndrome**

Contraindications: Hypersensitivity to proteins of *Escherichia coli*

Precautions: Pregnancy **C,** lactation, cardiac conditions, children, myeloid malignancies

Pharmacokinetics	
Absorption	Well absorbed (SC), completely absorbed (**IV**)
Distribution	Unknown
Metabolism	Unknown
Excretion	Unknown
Half-life	Unknown

Pharmacodynamics		
	IV	SC
Onset	5-60 min	5-60 min
Peak	24 hr	2-8 hr
Duration	up to 1 wk	up to 1 wk

Interactions
Drug classifications
Antineoplastics: ↑ neutrophils, do not use together 24 hr before or after antineoplastics
Lab test interferences
↑ Uric acid, ↑ lactate dehydrogenase, ↑ alkaline phosphatase

NURSING CONSIDERATIONS
Assessment
• Monitor blood studies: CBC, platelet count before treatment and twice weekly; neutrophil counts (ANC) may be increased for 2 days after therapy, but treatment should continue until ANC >10,000/mm^3
• Assess for bone pain: frequency, intensity, duration; analgesics may be given; opiates should not be used
• Check B/P, heart rate, respiration, baseline and during treatment

Nursing diagnoses
☑ Infection, risk for (uses)
☑ Pain, acute (adverse reaction)
☑ Knowledge, deficient (teaching)

Implementation
IV **IV route**
• Give 300 mcg/ml or 480 mcg/1.6 ml; allow to warm to room temp; give single dose over 1 min or less through Y-tube or medport
• Use single-use vials; after dose is withdrawn, do not reenter vial
• Give for 2 wk or until ANC = 10,000/mm^3 after the expected chemotherapy neutrophil nadir
• Store in refrigerator; do not freeze; may store at room temp for up to 6 hr; avoid shaking

Y-site compatibilities: Acyclovir, allopurinol, amikacin, aminophylline, ampicillin, ampicillin/sulbactam, aztreonam, bleomycin, bumetanide, buprenorphine, butorphanol, calcium gluconate, carboplatin, carmustine, cefazolin, cefotetan, ceftazidime, chlorproMAZINE, cimetidine, cisplatin, cyclophosphamide, cytarabine, dacarbazine, DAUNOrubicin, dexamethasone, diphenhydrAMINE, DOXOrubicin, doxycycline, droperidol, enalaprilat, famotidine, floxuridine, fluconazole, fludarabine, gallium, ganciclovir, granisetron, haloperidol, hydrocortisone, hydromorphone, hydrOXYzine, idarubicin, ifosfamide, leucovorin, lorazepam, mechlorethamine, melphalan, meperidine, mesna, methotrexate, metoclopramide, miconazole, minocycline, mitoxantrone, morphine, nalbuphine, netilmicin, ondansetron, plicamycin, potassium chloride, promethazine, ranitidine, sodium bicarbonate, streptozocin, ticarcillin, ticarcillin/clavulanate, tobramycin, trimethoprim-sulfamethoxazole, vancomycin, vinBLAStine, vinCRIStine, vinorelbine, zidovudine

Patient/family education
• Teach patient technique for self-administration: dose, side effects, disposal of containers and needles; provide instruction sheet

Evaluation
Positive therapeutic outcome
- Absence of infection

---

finasteride (Rx)
(fin-ass'te-ride)
Propecia, Proscar
Func. class.: Androgen hormone inhibitor, hair stimulant
Chem. class.: 5-α-Reductase inhibitor

Pregnancy category X

Action: Inhibits 5-α-reductase and reduction in dihydrotestosterone (DHT); DHT induces androgenic effects by binding to androgen receptors in the cell nuclei of the prostate gland, liver, skin; prevents development of benign prostatic hypertrophy (BPH)

Therapeutic Outcome: Reduced prostate size

Uses: Symptomatic BPH; male-pattern baldness (Propecia)

Dosage and routes
BPH
Adult: PO 5 mg qd × 6-12 mo

Male pattern baldness
Adult: PO 1 mg qd

Available forms: Tabs 1, 5 mg

Adverse effects
(*italic* = common; **bold** = life-threatening)
GU: Impotence, decreased libido, decreased volume of ejaculate

Contraindications: Hypersensitivity, pregnancy **X**, children, women who are pregnant or may become pregnant should not handle tabs

Precautions: Large residual urinary volume, severely diminished urinary flow, liver function abnormalities

Do Not Confuse:
Proscar/Prosom, Proscar/Prozac

Pharmacokinetics
Absorption	63%, readily
Distribution	Plasma protein binding, crosses blood-brain barrier
Metabolism	Liver
Excretion	Kidneys—metabolites (39%), feces (57%)
Half-life	6-15 hr

Pharmacodynamics
Onset	Immediate
Peak	1-2 hr
Duration	14 days

Interactions
Drug classifications
Anticholinergics, bronchodilators (adrenergic), theophylline: ↓ effect of finasteride

NURSING CONSIDERATIONS
Assessment
- Assess urinary patterns, residual urinary volume, severely diminished urinary flow; prostate-specific antigen (PSA) levels and digital rectal exam results before initiating therapy and periodically thereafter
- Monitor liver function studies before initiating treatment; extensively metabolized in liver

Nursing diagnoses
✓ Urinary elimination, impaired (uses)
✓ Knowledge, deficient (teaching)

Implementation
- Administer without regard to meals; give for a minimum of 6 mo; not all patients will respond
- Store at temp <86° F (30° C); protect from light; keep container tightly closed

Patient/family education
- Advise patient that pregnant women or women who may become pregnant should not touch crushed tab or come into contact with semen of a patient taking this drug; may adversely affect development of male fetus
- Inform patient that volume of ejaculate may be decreased during treatment; impotence and decreased libido may also occur
- Inform patient that Propecia results may not occur for 3 mo
- Inform patient that Proscar results may not occur for 6-12 mo

Evaluation
Positive therapeutic outcome
- Decreased postvoiding dribbling, frequency, nocturia
- Increased urinary flow
- Hair growth within 3-6 mo

---

flecainide (Rx)
(flek'a-nide)
Tambocor
Func. class.: Antidysrhythmic (Class IC)

Pregnancy category C

Action: Decreases conduction in all parts of the heart, with greatest effect on the His-Purkinje system, which stabilizes the cardiac membrane

➡ **Therapeutic Outcome:** Absence of dysrhythmias

Uses: Life-threatening ventricular dysrhythmias, sustained ventricular tachycardia; supraventricular tachydysrhythmias, paroxysmal atrial fibrillation/flutter associated with disabling symptoms

Dosage and routes
Adult: PO 50-100 mg q12h; may increase every 4 days by 50 mg q12h to desired response, not to exceed 400 mg/day

Renal dose
Adult: PO CCr <35 ml/min dose 50%-75%

Available forms: Tabs 50, 100, 150 mg

Adverse effects
(*italic* = common; **bold** = life-threatening)
CNS: Headache, dizziness, involuntary movement, confusion, psychosis, restlessness, irritability, paresthesias, ataxia, flushing, somnolence, depression, anxiety, malaise, fatigue, asthenia, tremors
CV: Hypotension, **bradycardia,** angina, PVCs, **heart block, cardiovascular collapse, arrest, dysrhythmias, CHF, fatal ventricular tachycardia**
EENT: Tinnitus, *blurred vision,* hearing loss
GI: Nausea, vomiting, anorexia, constipation, abdominal pain, flatulence, change in taste
GU: Impotence, decreased libido, polyuria, urinary retention
HEMA: **Leukopenia, thrombocytopenia**
INTEG: Rash, urticaria, edema, swelling
RESP: Dyspnea, **respiratory depression**

Contraindications: Hypersensitivity, severe heart block, cardiogenic shock, nonsustained ventricular dysrhythmias, frequent PVCs, non–life-threatening dysrhythmias

Precautions: Pregnancy C, lactation,
P children, renal disease, liver disease, CHF, respiratory depression, myasthenia gravis

Pharmacokinetics
Absorption	Well absorbed
Distribution	Widely distributed
Metabolism	Liver
Excretion	30% kidneys, unchanged
Half-life	14 hr

Pharmacodynamics
Onset	Unknown
Peak	3 hr
Duration	Unknown

F

Interactions
Individual drugs
Amiodarone: ↑ blood levels of flecainide
Cimetidine: ↑ level of flecainide
Digoxin: ↑ digoxin levels
Disopyramide, verapamil: ↑ CV depressant action
Drug classifications
Acidifying agents, alkalizing agents: ↑ or ↓ effect
β-Adrenergic blockers: ↑ CV depressant action
▨ *Herb/drug*
Aconite: ↑ toxicity, death
Aloe, broom, buckthorn (chronic use), cascara sagrada (chronic use), Chinese rhubarb, figwort, fumitory, goldenseal, kudzu, licorice: ↑ effect
Coltsfoot: ↓ effect
Horehound: ↑ serotonin effect

NURSING CONSIDERATIONS
Assessment
• Monitor ECG continuously to determine drug effectiveness; measure PR, QRS, QT intervals; check for PVCs, other dysrhythmias; monitor B/P continuously for hypotension, hypertension, and rebound hypertension (after 1-2 hr); check for dehydration or hypovolemia
• Monitor I&O ratio; electrolytes: (K [potassium], Na [sodium]), Cl (chloride); check weight daily and for signs of CHF or pulmonary toxicity: dyspnea, fatigue, cough, fever, chest pain, jugular vein distention, rales, crackles; if these occur, drug should be discontinued
• Monitor liver function studies: AST, ALT, bilirubin, alkaline phosphatase
• Assess patient for CNS symptoms: confusion, psychosis, numbness, depression, involuntary movements; if these occur, drug should be discontinued

• Monitor cardiac rate, respiration: rate, rhythm, character, chest pain; watch for ventricular tachycardia, supraventricular tachycardia, or fibrillation

Nursing diagnoses
☑ Cardiac output, decreased (uses)
☑ Knowledge, deficient (teaching)

Implementation
• Give reduced dosage slowly with ECG monitoring; do not increase dose fewer than 4 days apart
• Give with meals if GI upset occurs

Patient/family education
• Instruct patient to report side effects immediately to prescriber
• Instruct patient to complete follow-up appointment with health care provider including pulmonary function studies, chest x-ray
• Teach patient to change position slowly from lying or sitting to standing to minimize orthostatic hypotension
• Advise patient not to skip or double doses
• Advise patient to carry/wear emergency ID with disorder, medications taken
• Advise patient to avoid hazardous activities that require alertness until response is known

Evaluation
Positive therapeutic outcome
• Absence of dysrhythmias

---

fluconazole (Rx)
(floo-kon'a-zole)
Diflucan
Func. class.: Antifungal
Pregnancy category C

Action: Inhibits ergosterol biosynthesis, causes direct damage to membrane phospholipids in the cell wall of fungi

⮕ **Therapeutic Outcome:** Fungistatic fungicidal against the following susceptible organisms: *Candida, Cryptococcus neoformans*

Uses: Oropharyngeal esophageal candidiasis in AIDS patients, chronic mucocutaneous candidiasis, urinary candidiasis, cryptococcal meningitis, peritonitis

Dosage and routes
Renal dose
Adult: PO CCr 11-50 ml/min dose 50%

Vaginal candidiasis
Adult: PO 150 mg as a single dose

Serious fungal infections
Adult: PO/**IV** 50-400 mg initially, then 200 mg once daily for 4 wk
P *Child:* 6-12 mg/kg/day

Oropharyngeal candidiasis
Adult: PO 200 mg initially, then 100 mg daily for at least 2 wk
P *Child:* 3 mg/kg/day

Available forms: Tabs 50, 100, 150, 200 mg; inj 2 mg/ml; powder for oral susp 50, 200 mg/ml

Adverse effects
(*italic* = common; **bold** = life-threatening)
CNS: Headache
GI: Nausea, vomiting, diarrhea, cramping, flatus, increased AST, ALT, **hepatotoxicity**
INTEG: Stevens-Johnson syndrome

Contraindications: Hypersensitivity

Precautions: Renal disease, pregnancy **C**, lactation

Do Not Confuse:
Diflucan/Diprivan

Pharmacokinetics
Absorption	Well absorbed (PO)
Distribution	Widely distributed (peritoneum, CSF)
Metabolism	<10%—liver
Excretion	80% kidneys (unchanged)
Half-life	30 hr, increased in renal disease

Pharmacodynamics
	PO	IV
Onset	Unknown	Immediate
Peak	2-4 hr	Infusion's end
Duration	Unknown	Unknown

Interactions
Individual drugs
CycloSPORINE, phenytoin, rifabutin, tacrolimus, theophylline: ↑ plasma concentrations
Warfarin: ↑ anticoagulation
Zidovudine: ↑ effect
Drug classification
Oral antidiabetics: hypoglycemia
☑ *Herb/drug*
Gossypol: ↑ nephrotoxicity

NURSING CONSIDERATIONS
Assessment
• Assess for signs and symptoms of infection: clearing of CSF culture during treatment,

---

obtain C&S baseline and during treatment, drug may be started as soon as culture is taken
• Monitor for hepatotoxicity: increased AST, ALT, alkaline phosphatase, bilirubin; drug will be discontinued if hepatotoxicity occurs

Nursing diagnoses
✓ Infection, risk for (uses)
✓ Injury, risk for (adverse reactions)
✓ Knowledge, deficient (teaching)

Implementation
PO route
• Shake oral susp before each use
Ⅳ IV route
• Give after diluting according to package directions; run at 200 mg/hr or less; do not use plastic containers in connections
• Do not admix
• Administer **IV** using an in-line filter, using distal veins; check for extravasation and necrosis q2h
• Give drug only after C&S confirms organism, drug needed to treat condition
• Store protected from moisture and light, diluted sol is stable for 24 hr

Y-site compatibilities: Acyclovir, aldesleukin, allopurinol, amifostine, amikacin, aminophylline, ampicillin/sulbactam, aztreonam, benztropine, cefazolin, cefepime, cefotetan, cefoxitin, chlorproMAZINE, cimetidine, dexamethasone, diphenhydrAMINE, DOBUTamine, DOPamine, droperidol, famotidine, filgrastim, fludarabine, foscarnet, gallium, ganciclovir, gentamicin, granisetron, heparin, hydrocortisone, immune globulin, leucovorin, lorazepam, melphalan, meperidine, meropenem, metoclopramide, metronidazole, midazolam, morphine, nafcillin, nitroglycerin, ondansetron, oxacillin, paclitaxel, pancuronium, penicillin G, potassium, phenytoin, piperacillin/tazobactam, prochlorperazine, promethazine, propofol, ranitidine, sargramostim, sulfamethoxazole, tacrolimus, teniposide, theophylline, thiotepa, ticarcillin/clavulanate, tobramycin, vancomycin, vecuronium, vinorelbine, zidovudine

Y-site incompatibilities: Amphotericin B, ampicillin, calcium gluconate, cefotaxime, ceftriaxone, ceftazidime, cefuroxime, chloramphenicol, clindamycin, diazepam, digoxin, erythromycin lactobionate, furosemide, haloperidol, hydrOXYzine, imipenem/cilastatin, pentamidine, ticarcillin, trimethoprim/sulfamethoxazole

Additive compatibilities: Acyclovir, amikacin, amphotericin B, cefazolin, ceftazidime, clindamycin, gentamicin, heparin, meropenem, metronidazole, morphine, piperacillin, potassium chloride, theophylline

Patient/family education
• Caution patient that long-term therapy may be needed to clear infection; to take entire course of medication; take in equal intervals (PO)
• Teach patient the signs and symptoms of hepatotoxicity: nausea, vomiting, clay-colored stools, dark urine, anorexia, fatigue, jaundice; prescriber should be notified immediately
• Inform patient that medication may be taken with food to reduce GI effects
• Advise patient to consider using alternative contraception if using oral contraceptives

Evaluation
Positive therapeutic outcome
• Decreasing oral candidiasis, fever, malaise, rash
• Negative C&S for infecting organism

---

fludrocortisone (Rx)
(floo-droe-kor′ti-sone)
Florinef
Func. class.: Corticosteroid
Chem. class.: Mineralocorticoid
Pregnancy category C

Action: Promotes increased reabsorption of sodium and loss of potassium, water, hydrogen from the distal renal tubules

➔ **Therapeutic Outcome:** Treatment of adrenal insufficiency symptoms

Uses: Adrenal insufficiency, salt-losing adrenogenital syndrome

Investigational uses: Renal tubular acidosis (type IV), idiopathic orthostatic hypertension

Dosage and routes
Adult: PO 0.1-0.2 mg qd
P *Child:* PO 0.05-0.1 mg/day

Available forms: Tabs 0.1 mg

Adverse effects
(*italic* = common; **bold** = life-threatening)
CNS: Flushing, sweating, headache, paralysis, dizziness
CV: Hypertension, **circulatory collapse, thrombophlebitis, embolism,** tachycardia, **CHF,** edema
ENDO: Weight gain, adrenal suppression
META: Hypokalemia
MISC: Hypersensitivity
MS: Fractures, osteoporosis, weakness

Contraindications: Hypersensitivity, acute glomerulonephritis, amebiasis, psychoses, Cushing's syndrome, fungal infections, P child <2 yr

Precautions: Pregnancy **C**, osteoporosis, P CHF, lactation, child >2 yr, hypertension, diabetes

Pharmacokinetics

Absorption	Well absorbed
Distribution	Widely
Metabolism	Liver
Excretion	Kidneys, breast milk
Half-life	3½ hr

Pharmacodynamics
Unknown

Interactions
Individual drugs
Amphotericin B, mezlocillin, piperacillin: ↑ hypokalemia
Phenytoin: ↓ action of fludrocortisone
Rifampin: ↓ effect of fludrocortisone
Drug classifications
Barbiturates: ↓ action of fludrocortisone
Diuretics (loop): ↑ hypokalemia
Thiazides, potassium-wasting drugs: ↓ potassium levels
Food/drug
↑ Salt/sodium ingestion: ↑ B/P
Herb/drug
Aloe, buckthorn, cascara sagrada, Chinese rhubarb: ↑ hypokalemia
Aloe, licorice, perilla: ↑ corticosteroid effect
Lab test interferences
↑ Potassium, ↑ sodium
↓ Hematocrit

NURSING CONSIDERATIONS
Assessment
• Monitor patient for fluid retention: weigh daily, notify prescriber of weekly gain >5 lb; B/P q4h, pulse; notify prescriber if chest pain occurs; I&O ratio; be alert for decreasing urinary output and increasing edema
• Check for potassium depletion: paresthesias, fatigue, nausea, vomiting, depression, polyuria, dysrhythmias, weakness; also sodium, chloride

Nursing diagnoses
✓ Fluid volume, deficient (uses)
✓ Fluid volume, excess (adverse reactions)
✓ Knowledge, deficient (teaching)

Implementation
• Administer titrated dose; use lowest effective dose; scored tab may be broken if lower dose is necessary
• Give with food or milk to decrease GI symptoms

Patient/family education
• Advise patient to carry/wear emergency ID as steroid user at all times during diagnosis and treatment
• Caution patient not to discontinue this medication abruptly; Addisonian crisis may occur
• Counsel patient to follow dietary regimen recommended by prescriber; should include high potassium and, possibly, low sodium
• Advise patient to report weight gain >5 lb; edema in legs, hands; abdominal cramping; muscle cramps; nausea; vomiting; anorexia; dizziness or weakness, infection, trauma stress
• Advise patient not to breastfeed

Evaluation
Positive therapeutic outcome
• Correction of adrenal insufficiency
• Electrolytes and fluids in normal range

---

flumazenil (Rx)
(flu-maz'e-nil)
Anexate ✦, Romazicon
Func. class.: Benzodiazepine receptor antagonist
Chem. class.: Imidazobenzodiazepine derivative

Pregnancy category C

Action: Antagonizes the actions of benzodiazepines on the CNS, competitively inhibits the activity at the benzodiazepine receptor complex

→ **Therapeutic Outcome:** Reversed benzodiazepine toxic effects

Uses: Reversal of the sedative effects of benzodiazepines

Dosage and routes
Reversal of conscious sedation or in general anesthesia
Adult: **IV** 0.2 mg (2 ml) given over 15 sec; wait 45 sec, then give 0.2 mg (2 ml) if consciousness does not occur; may be repeated at 60-sec intervals as needed (max 3 mg/hr)

P *Child:* **IV** 10 mcg (0.01 mg)/kg; cumulative dose of 1 mg or less

Management of suspected benzodiazepine overdose
Adult: **IV** 0.2 mg (2 ml) given over 30 sec; wait 30 sec, then give 0.3 mg (3 ml) over 30

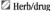 Herb/drug   ⊘ Do Not Crush   ✦ Alert   ✦ᴛ Key Drug   **G** Geriatric   **P** Pediatric

sec if consciousness does not occur; further doses of 0.5 mg (5 ml) can be given over 30 sec at intervals of 1 min up to cumulative dose of 3 mg

P *Child:* **IV** 100 mcg (0.1 mg)/kg; cumulative dose of 1 mg or less

Available forms: Inj 0.1 mg/ml

Adverse effects
(*italic* = common; **bold** = life-threatening)
CNS: Dizziness, agitation, emotional lability, confusion, **seizures,** somnolence
CV: Hypertension, palpitations, cutaneous vasodilatation, **dysrhythmias,** bradycardia, tachycardia, chest pain
EENT: Abnormal vision, blurred vision, tinnitus
GI: Nausea, vomiting, hiccups
SYST: Headache, inj site pain, increased sweating, fatigue, rigors

Contraindications: Hypersensitivity to this drug or benzodiazepines, serous tricyclic antidepressant overdose, patients given benzo-diazepine for control of life-threatening condition

P **Precautions:** Pregnancy **C,** lactation,
G children, elderly, renal disease, seizures, head injury, labor and delivery, hepatic disease, hypoventilation, panic disorder, drug and alcohol dependency, ambulatory patients

N **Do Not Confuse:**
Mazicon/Mivacron

Pharmacokinetics

Absorption	Complete
Distribution	Unknown
Metabolism	Liver
Excretion	Unknown
Half-life	41-79 min

Pharmacodynamics

Onset	1 min
Peak	10 min
Duration	Unknown

Interactions
Toxicity: Mixed drug overdosage

NURSING CONSIDERATIONS
Assessment
• Assess cardiac status using continuous monitoring
• Assess for seizures, protect patient from injury; most likely in those who usually experi-ence withdrawal from sedatives
• Assess for GI symptoms: nausea, vomiting;

place in side-lying position to prevent aspira-tion
• Assess for allergic reactions: flushing, rash, urticaria, pruritus

Nursing diagnoses
✓ Injury, risk for (uses)
✓ Poisoning (uses)

Implementation
• Give directly undiluted or diluted in 0.9% NaCl, D₅W, or LR; give over 15 sec into run-ning **IV**
• Check airway and **IV** access before admin-istration

Additive compatibilities: Aminophylline, cimetidine, DOBUTamine, DOPamine, famoti-dine, heparin, lidocaine, procainamide, ranitidine

Patient/family education
• Caution patient that amnesia may continue
• Instruct patient to avoid any hazardous activities for 18-24 hr after discharge
• Inform patient not to take any alcohol or nonprescription drugs for 18-24 hr; serious reactions may occur

Evaluation
Positive therapeutic outcome
• Decreased sedation, respiratory depression
• Absence of toxicity

⁄ HIGH ALERT

fluorouracil (Rx)
(flure-oh-yoor'a-sil)
Adrucil, Efudex, 5-FU
Func. class.: Antineoplastic, antimetabolite
Chem. class.: Pyrimidine antagonist
Pregnancy category D

Action: Inhibits DNA, RNA synthesis; inter-feres with cell replication by competitively inhibiting thymidylate synthesis, cell cycle–specific (S phase), a vesicant

⊝ Therapeutic Outcome: Prevention of rapidly growing malignant cells

Uses: *Systemic:* cancer of breast, colon, rectum, stomach, pancreas; multiple active keratoses; *Topical:* basal cell carcinoma

Dosage and routes
Adult: **IV** 12 mg/kg/day × 4 days, not to exceed 800 mg/day; may repeat with 6 mg/kg on day 6, 8, 10, 12; maintenance is 10-15 mg/kg/wk as a single dose, not to exceed 1 g/wk

Actinic/solar keratoses
Adult: TOP 1% cream/sol 1-2×/day

Superficial basal cell carcinoma
Adult: TOP 5% sol 2×/day × 3-12 wk

Available forms: Inj 50 mg/ml; cream 1, 5%; sol 1, 2, 5%

Adverse effects
(*italic* = common; **bold** = life-threatening)
Systemic use
CNS: Lethargy, malaise, weakness, acute cerebellar dysfunction
CV: Myocardial ischemia, angina
EENT: Epistaxis
GI: *Anorexia, stomatitis,* diarrhea, nausea, vomiting, **hemorrhage, enteritis glossitis**
HEMA: **Thrombocytopenia, leukopenia, myelosuppression, anemia, agranulocytosis**
INTEG: *Rash,* fever, photosensitivity

Contraindications: Hypersensitivity, myelosuppression, pregnancy **D,** poor nutritional status, serious infections, major surgery within 1 mo

Precautions: Renal disease, hepatic disease, bone marrow depression, angina,
 P lactation, children

 Do Not Confuse:
fluorouracil/flucytosine

Pharmacokinetics	
Absorption	Completely bioavailable (**IV**), minimal (top)
Distribution	Widely distributed, concentration in tumor
Metabolism	Liver—converted to active metabolite
Excretion	Lungs (60%-80%), kidneys (up to 15%)
Half-life	20 hr terminal

Pharmacodynamics
Unknown

Interactions
Individual drugs
Radiation: ↑ toxicity, bone marrow suppression
Drug classifications
Antineoplastics: ↑ toxicity, bone marrow depression
Live virus vaccines: ↓ antibody response
Lab test interferences
↑ Liver function studies, ↑ 6-HIAA
↓ Albumin

NURSING CONSIDERATIONS
Assessment
• Monitor ECG; watch for ST-T wave changes, low QRS and T, possible dysrhythmias (sinus tachycardia, heart block, PVCs)
• Assess buccal cavity q8h for dryness, sores or ulceration, white patches, oral pain, bleeding, dysphagia; obtain prescription for viscous lidocaine (Xylocaine)
• Assess tachypnea, ECG changes, dyspnea, edema, fatigue; identify dyspnea, rales, unproductive cough, chest pain, tachypnea
• Monitor CBC, differential, platelet count qd (**IV**); withhold drug if WBC is <4000/mm³ or platelet count is <100,000/mm³; notify prescriber of results if WBC <20,000/mm³, platelets <50,000/mm³; nadir of leukopenia within 2 wk, recovery 1 mo
• Monitor renal function studies: BUN, creatinine, serum uric acid, urine CCr before and during therapy; I&O ratio; report fall in urine output to <30 ml/hr
• Monitor temp q4h (may indicate beginning of infection)
• Monitor liver function tests before and during therapy (bilirubin, AST, ALT, LDH) as needed or monthly; jaundice of skin, sclera, dark urine, clay-colored stools, itchy skin, abdominal pain, fever, diarrhea
• Assess for bleeding: hematuria, stool guaiac, bruising or petechiae, mucosa or orifices q8h; inflammation of mucosa, breaks in skin

Nursing diagnoses
☑ Injury, risk for (adverse reactions)
☑ Body image, disturbed (adverse reactions)
☑ Infection, risk for (adverse reactions)
☑ Knowledge, deficient (teaching)

Implementation
• Avoid contact with skin (very irritating); wash completely to remove
• Give fluids **IV** or PO before chemotherapy to hydrate patient
• Give antiemetic 30-60 min before giving drug to prevent vomiting, and prn for several days thereafter; antibiotics for prophylaxis of infection
• Provide liq diet: carbonated beverages; gelatin may be added if patient is not nauseated or vomiting
• Provide rinsing of mouth tid-qid with water, club soda; brushing of teeth bid-qid with soft brush or cotton-tipped applicators for stomatitis; use unwaxed dental floss
IV IV route
• Prepare in biologic cabinet using gloves, gown, mask

- **IV** undiluted; may inject through Y-tube or 3-way stopcock; give over 1-3 min
- May be diluted in 0.9% NaCl, D$_5$W, given over 2-8 hr as an **IV** inf

Topical route
- Wear gloves when applying; may use with a loose dressing, use a plastic or wooden applicator

Syringe compatibilities: Bleomycin, cisplatin, cyclophosphamide, furosemide, heparin, leucovorin, methotrexate, metoclopramide, mitomycin, vinBLAStine, vinCRIStine

Syringe incompatibilities: Droperidol

Y-site compatibilities: Allopurinol, amifostine, aztreonam, bleomycin, cefepime, cisplatin, cyclophosphamide, DOXOrubicin, fludarabine, furosemide, granisetron, heparin, hydrocortisone, leucovorin, mannitol, melphalan, methotrexate, metoclopramide, mitomycin, paclitaxel, piperacillin/tazobactam, potassium chloride, propofol, sargramostin, thiotepa, thiposide, vinBLAStine, vinCRIStine, vit B/C

Y-site incompatibilities: Droperidol, vinorelbine

Additive compatibilities: Bleomycin, cephalothin, cyclophosphamide, etoposides, floxuridine, hydromorphone, ifosfamide, leucovorin, methotrexate, mitoxantrone, prednisoLONE, vinCRIStine

Additive incompatibilities: Carboplatin, cisplatin, cytarabine, diazepam, DOXOrubicin

Solution compatibilities: Amino acids 4.25%/D$_{25}$, D$_5$/LR, D$_{3.3}$/0.3% NaCl, D$_5$W, 0.9% NaCl, TPN #23

Patient/family education
- Caution patient that contraceptive measures are recommended during therapy
- Teach patient to avoid using aspirin, NSAIDs, or ibuprofen-containing products, razors, commercial mouthwash because bleeding may occur; to report symptoms of bleeding (hematuria, tarry stools)
- Instruct patient to report signs of anemia (fatigue, headache, irritability, faintness, shortness of breath)
- Instruct patient to report signs of stomatitis (bleeding, white spots, ulcerations in the mouth); tell patient to examine mouth qd, to report symptoms; viscous lidocaine (Xylocaine) may be used
- Teach patient to avoid crowds, persons with known infections

- Advise patient to avoid vaccinations during therapy, to use sunscreen or stay out of the sun to prevent burns; about hair loss, explore use of wigs or other products until hair regrowth occurs

Evaluation
Positive therapeutic outcome
- Prevention of rapid division of malignant cells

---

fluoxetine (Rx) F
(floo-ox'uh-teen)
Prozac, Prozac Weekly, Sarafem
Func. class.: Antidepressant, SSRI (selective serotonin reuptake inhibitor)

Pregnancy category B

Action: Inhibits CNS neuron uptake of serotonin, but not of norepINEPHrine

➔ **Therapeutic Outcome:** Decreased symptoms of depression after 2-3 wk

Uses: Major depressive disorder, obsessive-compulsive disorder (OCD), bulimia nervosa; sarafem: premenstrual dysphoric disorder (PMDD)

Investigational uses: Alcoholism, anorexia nervosa, attention deficit hyperactivity disorder, bipolar II affective disorder, borderline personality disorder, cataplexy, narcolepsy, kleptomania, migraine, obesity, posttraumatic stress disorder, schizophrenia, Gilles de la Tourette's syndrome, trichotillomania, levodopa-induced dyskinesia, social phobia

Dosage and routes
Depression/OCD
Adult: PO 20 mg qd AM; after 4 wk if no clinical improvement is noted, dose may be increased to 20 mg bid in AM, afternoon, not to exceed 80 mg/day; PO weekly

G *Elderly:* PO 5-10 mg/day, increase as needed

P *Child 5-18 yr:* PO 5-10 mg/day, max 20 mg/day

Bulimia nervosa
Adult: PO 60 mg/day in AM

ADHD (unlabeled)
Adult: PO 20-60 mg/day

Alcoholism (unlabeled)
Adult: PO 20-80 mg/day

Anorexia nervosa (unlabeled)
Adult: PO 10 mg qod-20 mg/day

Bipolar II affective disorder (unlabeled)
Adult: PO 10 mg qod-20 mg/day

Borderline personality disorder (unlabeled)
Adult: PO 20 mg/day

Kleptomania (unlabeled)
Adult: PO 60-80 mg/day

Migraine, chronic daily headaches (unlabeled)
Adult: PO 10-80 mg/day

Narcolepsy (unlabeled)
Adult: PO 20-40 mg/day

Posttraumatic stress disorder (unlabeled)
Adult: PO 10-80 mg/day

Premenstrual dysphoric disorder (Sarafem)
Adult: PO 20 mg qd, may be taken qd week before menses

Schizophrenia (unlabeled)
Adult: PO 20-60 mg/day

Available forms: Caps 10, 20, 40 mg; tabs 10, 20 mg; oral sol 20 mg/5 ml; caps, del rel 90 mg

Adverse effects
(*italic* = common; **bold** = life-threatening)
CNS: *Headache, nervousness, insomnia, drowsiness, anxiety, tremor, dizziness, fatigue, sedation, poor concentration, abnormal dreams, agitation,* **seizures,** apathy, euphoria, hallucinations, delusions, psychosis
CV: *Hot flashes, palpitations,* angina pectoris, **hemorrhage,** hypertension, **tachycardia,** 1st-degree AV block, **bradycardia, MI, thrombophlebitis**
EENT: Visual changes, ear/eye pain, photophobia, tinnitus
GI: *Nausea, diarrhea, dry mouth, anorexia, dyspepsia, constipation, cramps, vomiting, taste changes, flatulence, decreased appetite*
GU: *Dysmenorrhea, decreased libido, urinary frequency, urinary tract infection,* amenorrhea, cystitis, impotence, urine retention
INTEG: *Sweating, rash, pruritus,* acne, alopecia, urticaria
MS: *Pain,* arthritis, twitching
RESP: *Infection, pharyngitis, nasal congestion, sinus headache, sinusitis, cough,* *dyspnea, bronchitis,* asthma, hyperventilation, pneumonia
SYST: *Asthenia, viral infection, fever, allergy, chills*

Contraindications: Hypersensitivity

P **Precautions:** Pregnancy **B,** lactation,
G children, elderly, diabetes mellitus

N **Do Not Confuse:**
Prozac/Proscar, Prozac/Prilosec, Prozac/ Prosom
Sarafem/Serophene

Pharmacokinetics

Absorption	Well absorbed
Distribution	Crosses blood-brain barrier
Metabolism	Liver, extensively to norfluoxetine
Excretion	Kidneys, unchanged (12%), metabolite (7%); steady state 28-35 days, protein binding 94%
Half-life	1-3 days metabolite up to 1 wk

Pharmacodynamics

Onset	Unknown
Peak	6-8 hr
Duration	Unknown

Interactions
Individual drugs
Alcohol: ↑ CNS depression
Buspirone: ↑ worsening of OCD
Carbamazepine, digoxin, lithium, warfarin: ↑ toxicity
Cyproheptadine: ↓ fluoxetine effect
Diazepam: ↑ half-life of diazepam
Haloperidol: ↑ haloperidol effect
Phenytoin: ↑ hydantoin levels
Thioridazine: Do not use, or use within 5 wk of discontinuing fluoxetine
Drug classifications
Antidepressants, barbiturates, benzodiazepines, CNS depressants, opioids, sedative/ hypnotics: ↑ CNS depression
Highly protein-bound drugs: ↑ side effects
MAOIs: Hypertensive crisis, seizures; do not use with or 14 days prior to fluoxetine
Oral anticoagulants: ↑ effects
Phenothiazines, tricyclic antidepressants: ↑ levels
Herb/drug
Corkwood, jimsonweed: ↑ anticholinergic effect
Hops, kava, lavender: ↑ CNS effect
St. John's wort, SAM-e: Do not use together; ↑ risk of serotonin syndrome

---

Lab test interferences

↑ Serum bilirubin, ↑ blood glucose, ↑ alkaline phosphatase

↓ VMA, ↓ 5-HIAA

False: ↑ urinary catecholamines

NURSING CONSIDERATIONS
Assessment

• Monitor B/P (lying, standing), pulse q4h; if systolic B/P drops 20 mm hg, hold drug and notify prescriber; take VS q4h in patients with CV disease

• Monitor blood studies: CBC, leukocytes, differential, cardiac enzymes if patient is receiving long-term therapy; check platelets, bleeding can occur

• Monitor hepatic studies: AST, ALT, bilirubin

• Check weight qwk; appetite may increase with drug

• Assess ECG for flattening of T wave, bundle branch block, AV block, dysrhythmias in cardiac patients

• Assess mental status: mood, sensorium, affect, suicidal tendencies; increase in psychiatric symptoms: depression, panic

• Monitor urinary retention, constipation; **P** constipation is more likely to occur in children **G** or elderly

• Identify patient's alcohol consumption; if alcohol is consumed, hold dose until AM

• Assess appetite in bulimia nervosa, weight qd, increase nutritious foods in diet, watch for bingeing and vomiting

• Assess allergic reactions: itching, rash, urticaria, drug should be discontinued; may need to give antihistamine

Nursing diagnoses

✓ Coping, ineffective (uses)

✓ Injury, risk for (side effects)

✓ Knowledge, deficient (teaching)

✓ Noncompliance (teaching)

Implementation

• Give with food or milk for GI symptoms

• Give dosage hs if oversedation occurs **G** during day; may take entire dose hs; elderly may not tolerate once/day dosing, crushed if patient unable to swallow whole (tabs only)

• Prozac weekly: Give on same day each week

• Store at room temp; do not freeze

Patient/family education

• Teach patient that therapeutic effects may take 1-4 wk

• Instruct patient to use caution in driving or other activities requiring alertness because of drowsiness, dizziness, blurred vision; to avoid rising quickly from sitting to standing, espe-**G** cially elderly; to use sunscreen to prevent photosensitivity

• Caution patient to avoid alcohol ingestion, other CNS depressants

• Advise patient not to discontinue medication quickly after long-term use: may cause nausea, headache, malaise

• Instruct patient to increase fluids, bulk in diet if constipation, urinary retention occur, **G** especially elderly

• Advise patient to take gum, hard sugarless candy, or frequent sips of water for dry mouth

• Teach patient to avoid all OTC drugs unless approved by prescriber

• Advise patient to change positions slowly, orthostatic hypotension may occur

Evaluation

Positive therapeutic outcome

• Decrease in depression

• Absence of suicidal thoughts

• Decreased symptoms of OCD

---

fluphenazine decanoate (Rx)
(floo-fen′ah-zeen)

Modecate ✤, Modecate Concentrate, Prolixin Decanoate

fluphenazine enanthate (Rx)

Moditen Enanthate ✤, Prolixin Enanthate

fluphenazine hydrochloride (Rx)

Apo-Fluphenazine ✤, Moditen HCL ✤, Moditen HCl-H.P. ✤, Permitil ✤, Prolixin

Func. class.: Antipsychotic/neuroleptic

Chem. class.: Phenothiazine, piperazine

Pregnancy category C

Action: Depresses cerebral cortex, hypothalamus, limbic system, which control activity and aggression; blocks neurotransmission produced by dopamine at synapse; exhibits strong α-adrenergic and anticholinergic blocking action; mechanism for antipsychotic effects is unclear

→ **Therapeutic Outcome:** Decreased signs and symptoms of psychosis

Uses: Psychotic disorders, schizophrenia

Dosage and routes
Decanoate

P *Adult and child >16 yr:* IM/SC 12.5-25 mg q1-3 wk, may increase slowly

P *Child 12-16 yr:* IM/SC 6.25-18.75 mg, then

repeat q1-3 wk, then increase slowly, max 25 mg

P *Child 5-12 yr:* **IM/SC** 3.125-12.5 mg, then repeat q1-3 wk, increase slowly

HCl
Adult: **PO** 2.5-10 mg, in divided doses q6-8h, not to exceed 20 mg qd; **IM** initially 1.25 mg then 2.5-10 mg in divided doses q6-8h

P *Child:* **PO** 0.25-3.5 mg qd in divided doses q4-6h, max 10 mg/qd

Enanthate
Adult: **IM/SC** 25 mg q1-3 wk, may increase slowly, max 100 mg/dose

Available forms: HCl tabs 1, 2.5, 5, 10 mg; elixir 2.5 mg/5 ml; conc 5 mg/ml; inj 2.5, 10 mg/ml, enanthate, decanoate depot inj 25 mg/ml

Adverse effects
(*italic* = common; **bold** = life-threatening)
CNS: *Extrapyramidal symptoms (EPS), pseudoparkinsonism, akathisia, dystonia, tardive dyskinesia, drowsiness, headache,* **seizures, neuroleptic malignant syndrome**
CV: *Orthostatic hypotension,* hypertension, **cardiac arrest,** ECG changes, **tachycardia**
EENT: Blurred vision, glaucoma, dry eyes
GI: *Dry mouth, nausea, vomiting, anorexia, constipation,* diarrhea, jaundice, weight gain, **paralytic ileus, hepatitis**
GU: Urinary retention, urinary frequency, enuresis, impotence, amenorrhea, gynecomastia
HEMA: Anemia, **leukopenia, leukocytosis, agranulocytosis, aplastic anemia, thrombocytopenia**
INTEG: *Rash,* photosensitivity, dermatitis
RESP: **Laryngospasm,** dyspnea, **respiratory depression**

Contraindications: Hypersensitivity, circulatory collapse, liver damage, cerebral arteriosclerosis, coronary disease, severe hypertension/hypotension, blood dyscrasias, coma, brain damage, bone marrow depression, alcohol and barbiturate withdrawal, narrow-angle glaucoma

Precautions: Pregnancy **C,** lactation,
G seizure disorders, hypertension, hepatic
P disease, cardiac disease, elderly, child <12 yr

N **Do Not Confuse:**
Prolixin/Proloid

Pharmacokinetics
Absorption	Well absorbed (PO, IM)
Distribution	Widely absorbed, crosses blood-brain barrier, placenta
Metabolism	Liver, extensively
Excretion	Kidneys (metabolites)
Half-life	HCl-4.7-15.3 hr, enanthate 3½-4 days, decanoate 6.8-14.3 days

Pharmacodynamics
	PO/IM	IM	IM
	HCl	Enanthate	Decanoate
Onset	1 hr	1-2 days	1-3 days
Peak	1½-2 hr	2-3 days	1-2 days
Duration	6-8 hr	1-3 wk	>4 wk

Interactions
Individual drugs
Alcohol: ↑ effects of both drugs, oversedation
Epinephrine: ↑ toxicity
Levodopa: ↓ antiparkinson activity
Lithium: ↓ effects of lithium
Drug classifications
Anticholinergics: ↑ anticholinergic effects
Barbiturates, general anesthetics, MAOIs, opiates, sedative/hypnotics: ↑ CNS depression
Barbiturates: ↓ effect of fluphenazine
CNS depressants: oversedation
Smoking: ↓ effects of fluphenazine
Ⅾ *Herb/drug*
Betel palm, kava: ↑ EPS
Cola tree, hops, kava, nettle, nutmeg: possible ↑ action
Henbane leaf: ↑ anticholinergic effect
Lab test interferences
↑ Liver function tests, ↑ cardiac enzymes, ↑ cholesterol, ↑ blood glucose, ↑ prolactin, ↑ bilirubin, ↑ PBI, ↑ cholinesterase I
↓ Hormones (blood and urine)
False positive: Pregnancy tests, PKU, urinary steroids, 17-OHCS

NURSING CONSIDERATIONS
Assessment
• Assess mental status: orientation, mood, behavior, presence of hallucinations, and type before initial administration and monthly; this drug should significantly reduce psychotic behavior
• Check for swallowing of PO medication; check for hoarding or giving of medication to other patients
• Monitor I&O ratio, palpate bladder if low
G urinary output occurs, especially in elderly; urinalysis recommended before, during prolonged therapy

---

Ⅾ Herb/drug   **S** Do Not Crush   **◆** Alert   **◆ᴛ** Key Drug   **G** Geriatric   **P** Pediatric

- Monitor bilirubin, CBC, liver function studies monthly
- Assess affect, orientation, LOC, reflexes, gait, coordination, sleep pattern disturbances
- Monitor B/P with patient sitting, standing, and lying down; take pulse and respirations q4h during initial treatment; establish baseline before starting treatment; report drops of 30 mm Hg; obtain baseline ECG, Q-wave and T-wave changes
- Check for dizziness, faintness, palpitations, tachycardia on rising; severe orthostatic hypotension is common
- Assess for neuroleptic malignant syndrome: hyperpyrexia, muscle rigidity, increased CPK, altered mental status; drug should be discontinued
- Assess for EPS including akathisia (inability to sit still, no pattern to movements), tardive dyskinesia (bizarre movements of the jaw, mouth, tongue, extremities), pseudoparkinsonism (rigidity, tremors, pill rolling, shuffling gate), an antiparkinson drug should be prescribed
- Assess for constipation, urinary retention daily; if these occur, increase bulk, water in diet

Nursing diagnoses
✓ Thought processes, disturbed (uses)
✓ Coping, ineffective (uses)
✓ Knowledge, deficient (teaching)
✓ Noncompliance (teaching)

Implementation
PO route
- Give drug in liq form mixed in glass of juice or cola if hoarding is suspected; do not mix in caffeine drinks, tannics, or pectinates; decrease dose in elderly
- Give PO with full glass of water, milk; or give with food to decrease GI upset
- Store in tight, light-resistant container, oral sol in amber bottle
SC route
- May be given by this route; however, it is painful
IM route
- Inject in deep muscle mass, use a 21-G needle into dorsal gluteal site, keep patient recumbent for ½ hr to prevent orthostatic hypotension

Syringe compatibilities: Benztropine, diphenhydrAMINE, hydrOXYzine

Patient/family education
- Teach patient to use good oral hygiene; frequent rinsing of mouth, sugarless gum for dry mouth

- Caution patient to avoid hazardous activities until drug response is determined; dizziness, blurred vision may occur
- Inform patient that orthostatic hypotension occurs often and to rise from sitting or lying position gradually, to remain lying down after IM inj for at least 30 min; tell patient to avoid hot tubs, hot showers, tub baths because hypotension may occur; tell patient that in hot weather, heat stroke may occur; extra precautions are necessary to stay cool
- Instruct patient to avoid abrupt withdrawal of this drug, or EPS may result; drug should be withdrawn slowly
- Teach patient to avoid OTC preparations (cough, hay fever, cold) unless approved by physician because serious drug interactions may occur; avoid use with alcohol, CNS depressants; increased drowsiness may occur
- Instruct patient to use a sunscreen and sunglasses to prevent burns
- Teach patient about EPS and necessity of meticulous oral hygiene because oral candidiasis may occur
- Instruct patient to take antacids 2 hr before or after this drug
- Advise patient to report sore throat, malaise, fever, bleeding, mouth sores; if these occur, CBC should be performed and drug discontinued

Evaluation
Positive therapeutic outcome
- Decrease in emotional excitement, hallucinations, delusions, paranoia
- Reorganization of patterns of thought, speech

Treatment of overdose: Lavage if orally ingested; provide airway; *do not induce vomiting or use epiNEPHrine*

---

flurazepam (Rx)
(flure-az'e-pam)
Apo-flurazepam ✝, Dalmane, flurazepam, Novoflupam ✝, Somnol ✝
Func. class.: Sedative-hypnotic
Chem. class.: Benzodiazepine derivative

Pregnancy category UK

Controlled substance schedule IV (USA), schedule F (Canada)

Action: Produces CNS depression at the limbic, thalamic, hypothalamic levels of CNS; may be mediated by neurotransmitter γ-aminobutyric acid (GABA); results are sedation, hypnosis, skeletal muscle relaxation, anticonvulsant activity, anxiolytic action

➔ **Therapeutic Outcome:** Ability to sleep, relaxation

Uses: Insomnia

Dosage and routes
Adult: PO 15-30 mg hs; may repeat dose once if needed

G *Elderly:* PO 15 mg hs; may increase if needed

Available forms: Caps 15, 30 mg

Adverse effects
(*italic* = common; **bold** = life-threatening)
CNS: Lethargy, drowsiness, daytime sedation, dizziness, confusion, light-headedness, headache, anxiety, irritability
CV: Chest pain, pulse changes, palpitations
GI: Nausea, vomiting, diarrhea, heartburn, abdominal pain, constipation
HEMA: Leukopenia, granulocytopenia (rare)
MISC: Physical, psychologic dependence

Contraindications: Hypersensitivity to benzodiazepines, **pregnancy UK** lactation, intermittent porphyria, uncontrolled pain

Precautions: Anemia, hepatic disease, **G** renal disease, suicidal individuals, drug abuse, **P** elderly, psychosis, child <15 yr

⧄ Do Not Confuse:
flurazepam/temazepam

Pharmacokinetics	
Absorption	Well absorbed
Distribution	Widely absorbed, crosses blood-brain barrier, crosses placenta
Metabolism	Liver to active, inactive metabolites
Excretion	Kidneys, breast milk
Half-life	2½ hr, 30-200 hr active metabolites

Pharmacodynamics	
Onset	15-30 min
Peak	½-1 hr
Duration	7-8 hr

Interactions
Individual drugs
Alcohol: ↑ CNS depression
Cimetidine, disulfiram, fluoxetine, isoniazid, ketoconazole, propranolol, valproic acid: ↑ action of flurazepam
Probenecid: ↑ effects of flurazepam
Rifampin: ↓ action of flurazepam
Theophylline: ↓ effect of flurazepam

Drug classifications
Barbiturates: ↓ effect of flurazepam
CNS depressants: ↑ CNS depression
Oral contraceptives: ↑ effect of flurazepam
⧄ Herb/drug
Black cohosh: ↑ hypotension
Catnip, chamomile, clary, cowslip, kava, lavender, mistletoe, nettle, pokeweed, poppy, Queen Anne's lace, senega, valerian: ↑ effect
Lab test interferences
↑ AST, ↑ ALT, ↑ serum bilirubin
↓ radioactive iodine uptake
False: ↑ urinary 17-OHCS

NURSING CONSIDERATIONS
Assessment
- Assess anxiety reaction: inability to sleep, apprehension, dread, foreboding, or uneasiness related to unidentified source of danger
- Assess for previous drug dependence or tolerance; if drug dependent or tolerant, amount of medication should be restricted
- Monitor B/P (lying, standing), pulse; if systolic B/P drops 20 mm Hg, hold drug, notify prescriber; I&O, may indicate renal dysfunction
- Monitor blood studies: CBC during long-term therapy; blood dyscrasias have occurred rarely
- Monitor hepatic studies: AST, ALT, bilirubin, creatinine, LDH, alkaline phosphatase
- Monitor patient's mental status: mood, sensorium, affect, sleeping patterns, drowsiness, dizziness, suicidal tendencies

Nursing diagnoses
☑ Sleep pattern, disturbed (uses)
☑ Knowledge, deficient (teaching)
☑ Noncompliance (teaching)

Implementation
- Give after removing cigarettes to prevent fires
- Give after trying conservative measures for insomnia
- Give ½-1 hr before hs for sleeplessness; caps may be opened and mixed with food; give pc to decrease GI symptoms if used for sedation
- Provide assistance with ambulation after receiving dose
- Provide safety measures: nightlight, call bell within easy reach
- Check to see if PO medication has been swallowed
- Store in tight container in cool environment

Patient/family education
- Inform patient that drug may be taken with

food; if dose is missed take as soon as remembered; do not double doses
- Advise patient to avoid OTC preparations unless approved by a physician, to avoid alcohol ingestion or other psychotropic medications unless approved by prescriber, that 1-2 wk of therapy may be required before therapeutic effects occur
- Caution patient to avoid driving, activities requiring alertness, drowsiness may occur; until medication response is known, tell patient that drowsiness may worsen at beginning of treatment
- Instruct patient not to discontinue medication abruptly after long-term use
- Caution patient to rise slowly or fainting may occur, especially in elderly
- Inform patient that hangover is common in elderly

Evaluation
Positive therapeutic outcome
- Increased well-being
- Decreased anxiety, restlessness, sleeplessness, dread

Treatment of overdose: Lavage, activated charcoal; monitor electrolytes, VS

---

flutamide (Rx)
(floo'ta-mide)
Eulexin
Func. class.: Antineoplastic hormone
Chem. class.: Antiandrogen
Pregnancy category D

Action: Interferes with testosterone uptake in the nucleus or testosterone activity in target tissues; arrests tumor growth in androgen-sensitive tissue (i.e., prostate gland)

➡ **Therapeutic Outcome:** Prevention of rapidly growing malignant cells

Uses: Metastatic prostatic carcinoma, stage D₂ in combination with LHRH agonistic analogs (leuprolide)

Dosage and routes
Adult: PO 250 mg q8h tid, for a daily dosage of 750 mg

Stage B₂-C prostatic carcinoma
Start 8 wk before radiation therapy and continue during radiation therapy; give with goserelin

Stage D₂ metastatic carcinoma
Adult: Give with LHRH agonist and continue until progression

Available forms: Caps 125 mg
Adverse effects
(*italic* = common; **bold** = life-threatening)
CNS: *Hot flashes,* drowsiness, confusion, depression, anxiety, paresthesia
GI: *Diarrhea, nausea, vomiting,* increased liver function studies, **hepatitis,** anorexia
GU: *Decreased libido, impotence, gynecomastia*
HEMA: Leukopenia, thrombocytopenia, hemolytic anemia
INTEG: Irritation at site, rash, photosensitivity
MISC: Edema, neuromuscular and pulmonary symptoms, hypertension

▧ **Do Not Confuse:**
Eulexin/Edecrin

Contraindications: Hypersensitivity, pregnancy **D**

Pharmacokinetics	
Absorption	Well absorbed
Distribution	Unknown
Metabolism	Liver
Excretion	Unknown
Half-life	6 hr

Pharmacodynamics
Unknown

Interactions
Individual drugs
Leuprolide: ↑ synergistic effect

NURSING CONSIDERATIONS
Assessment
- Monitor CBC, bilirubin, creatinine, AST, ALT, alkaline phosphatase, which may be elevated, drug may need to be discontinued
- Identify CNS symptoms: drowsiness, confusion, depression, anxiety

Nursing diagnoses
✓ Injury, risk for (adverse reactions)
✓ Sexual dysfunction (adverse reactions)
✓ Body image, disturbed (adverse reactions)
✓ Infection, risk for (adverse reactions)
✓ Knowledge, deficient (teaching)

Implementation
- Used in combination with LHRH agonist (leuprolide)
- May be given with food or fluids

Patient/family education
- Tell the patient to report side effects: decreased libido, impotence, breast enlargement, hot flashes, diarrhea, which occur when the two drugs are given together; also nausea,

vomiting; jaundice in eyes, skin; dark urine, clay-colored stools, hepatotoxicity may occur
• Inform patient that this drug is taken with leuprolide for medical castration, do not change dosing

Evaluation
Positive therapeutic outcome
• Prevention of rapid division of malignant cells

---

fluvastatin (Rx)
(flu'vah-stay-tin)
Lescol
Func. class.: Antilipidemic
Chem. class.: HMG-CoA reductase inhibitor

Pregnancy category X

Action: Inhibits HMG-CoA reductase enzyme, which reduces cholesterol synthesis

➔**Therapeutic Outcome:** Decreased cholesterol levels and LDLs, increased HDLs

Uses: As an adjunct in primary hypercholesterolemia (types Ia, Iib), coronary atherosclerosis in CAD

Dosage and routes
Adult: PO 20-40 mg qd in PM initially, usual range 20-80, not to exceed 80 mg; may be given in 2 doses (40 mg AM, 40 mg PM); dosage adjustments may be made in 4-wk intervals or more

Available forms: Caps 20, 40 mg; ext rel tab 80 mg

Adverse effects
(*italic* = common; **bold** = life-threatening)
CNS: Headache, dizziness, insomnia
EENT: Lens opacities
GI: Nausea, constipation, diarrhea, abdominal pain, cramps, dyspepsia, flatus, liver dysfunction, pancreatitis
HEMA: **Thrombocytopenia, hemolytic anemia, leukopenia**
INTEG: Rash, pruritus
MISC: Fatigue, influenza, photosensitivity
MS: Myalgia, *arthritis, arthralgia,* myositis, **rhabdomyolysis**
RESP: Upper respiratory infection, rhinitis, cough, pharyngitis, sinusitis

Contraindications: Hypersensitivity, pregnancy **X,** lactation, active liver disease

Precautions: Past liver disease, alcoholism, severe acute infections, trauma, hypotension, uncontrolled seizure disorders, severe metabolic disorders, electrolyte imbalance

Pharmacokinetics

Absorption	Unknown
Distribution	Unknown
Metabolism	Liver
Excretion	Feces, kidneys
Half-life	14 hr

Pharmacodynamics
Unknown

Interactions
Individual drugs
Alcohol, cimetidine, ranitidine, omeprazole, saquinavir: ↑ fluvastatin effect
Cholestyramine, colestipol, rifampin: ↓ action of fluvastatin
Clofibrate: ↑ myalgia, myositis
CycloSPORINE, erythromycin, gemfibrozil, niacin: ↑ risk of myopathy
Digoxin, warfarin: ↑ action
Drug classifications:
Azole antiinfectives given with clofibrate: ↑ myalgia, ↑ myositis

Drug/food
• Grapefruit juice: Possible increased fluvastatin toxicity
☑ *Herb/drug*
Glucomannan: ↑ effect
Gotu kola: ↓ effect

NURSING CONSIDERATIONS
Assessment
• Assess nutrition: fat, protein, carbohydrates; nutritional analysis should be completed by dietitian before treatment
• Monitor bowel pattern daily; diarrhea may be a problem
• Assess fasting lipid profile (cholesterol, LDL, HDL, triglycerides) q8 wk, then q3-6 mo when stable
• Monitor liver function studies q1-2 mo during the first 1½ yr of treatment; AST, ALT, liver function test results may be increased
• Monitor renal studies in patients with compromised renal system: BUN, I&O ratio, creatinine
• Obtain ophth exam before, 1 mo after treatment begins, annually; lens opacities may occur

Nursing diagnoses
☑ Diarrhea (adverse reactions)
☑ Knowledge, deficient (teaching)
☑ Noncompliance (teaching)

Implementation
• Give with evening meal; if dosage is increased, take with breakfast and evening meal

---

☑ Herb/drug   🚫 Do Not Crush   ◆ Alert   ☙ᵣ Key Drug   🅶 Geriatric   🅿 Pediatric

• Store in cool environment in airtight, light-resistant container

Patient/family education
• Inform patient that compliance is needed for positive results to occur, not to double doses
• Advise patient to notify prescriber if GI symptoms of diarrhea, abdominal or epigastric pain, nausea, vomiting, or if chills, fever, sore throat occur; also muscle pain, weakness, tenderness
• Advise patient that treatment is chronic
• Advise patient that blood studies and eye exam will be necessary during treatment
• Instruct patient to report suspected pregnancy, not to use during pregnancy
• Advise patient that previously prescribed regimen will continue, including diet, exercise, smoking cessation
• Advise patient to use sunscreen or stay out of the sun to prevent burns
• Instruct patient to notify all health care providers of drugs taken

Evaluation
Positive therapeutic outcome
• Decreased LDL, VLDL, total cholesterol levels
• Improved ratio of HDLs

---

folic acid (vitamin B₉) (PO, OTC; IM/IV, Ph)
(foe-lik a'sid)
Apo-Folic ✤, Folate, Folvite, Novofolacid ✤, Vitamin B₉
Func. class.: Vitamin B-complex group
Chem. class.: Supplement

Pregnancy category A

Action: Needed for erythropoiesis; increases RBC, WBC, and platelet formation in megaloblastic anemias

⊅ **Therapeutic Outcome:** Absence of macrocytic, megaloblastic anemias

Uses: Megaloblastic or macrocytic anemia caused by folic acid deficiency; liver disease; alcoholism; hemolysis; intestinal obstruction; pregnancy

Dosage and routes
Therapeutic dose
P **Adult and child:** PO/IM/SC/**IV** up to 1 mg qd

Maintenance dose
P **Adult and child >4 yr:** PO/IM/**IV**/SC 0.4 mg/day

Pregnant and/or lactating: PO/IM/**IV**/SC 0.8 mg/day

P *Child <4 yr:* PO/IM/**IV**/SC up to 0.3 mg/day

P *Infants:* PO/IM/**IV**/SC up to 0.1 mg/day

Available forms: Tabs 0.1, 0.4, 0.8, 1, 5 mg; inj 5, 10 mg/ml

Adverse effects
(*italic* = common; **bold** = life-threatening)
INTEG: Flushing
RESP: **Bronchospasm**

Contraindications: Hypersensitivity, anemias other than megaloblastic/macrocytic anemia, vit B₁₂ deficiency anemia, uncorrected pernicious anemia

Precautions: Pregnancy **A**

Pharmacokinetics
Absorption	Well absorbed
Distribution	Liver, crosses placenta
Metabolism	Liver (converted to active metabolite)
Excretion	Kidneys (unchanged)
Half-life	Unknown

Pharmacodynamics
Onset	Unknown
Peak	½-1 hr
Duration	Unknown

Interactions
Individual drugs
Carbamazepine: ↑ need for folic acid
Fosphenytoin: ↓ fosphenytoin levels
Methotrexate, sulfasalazine: ↓ action of folic acid
Phenytoin: ↓ phenytoin levels
Drug classifications
Estrogens, glucocorticoids, hydantoins: ↑ need for folic acid
Sulfonamides: ↓ action of folic acid

NURSING CONSIDERATIONS
Assessment
• Assess patient for fatigue, dyspnea, weakness, shortness of breath, activity intolerance (signs of megaloblastic anemia)
• Monitor Hgb, Hct, and reticulocyte count; folate levels: 6-15 mcg/ml baseline and throughout treatment
• Assess nutritional status: bran, yeast, dried beans, nuts, fruits, fresh vegetables, asparagus; if high folic acid foods are missing from the diet, a referral to a dietitian may be indicated
• Identify drugs currently taken: alcohol, oral contraceptives, estrogens, glucocorticoids, carbamazepine, hydantoins, trimethoprim;

---

these drugs may cause increased folic acid use by the body and contribute to deficiency

Nursing diagnoses
☑ Nutrition: less than body requirements, imbalanced (uses)
☑ Fatigue (uses)
☑ Activity intolerance (uses)
☑ Knowledge, deficient (teaching)

Implementation
IV IV route
- Give **IV** directly, undiluted 5 mg or less over 1 min or more, or may be added to most **IV** sol or TPN
- Store in light-resistant container

Y-site compatibilities: Famotidine

Solution compatibilities: $D_{20}W$

Solution incompatibilities: $D_{40}W$, $D_{50}W$, calcium gluconate

Patient/family education
- Advise patient to take drug exactly as prescribed; not to double doses, toxicity may occur
- Instruct patient to notify prescriber of side effects; rash or fever may indicate hypersensitivity
- Advise patient that urine may become more yellow
- Instruct patient to increase intake of foods rich in folic acid in diet as recommended by dietitian or health care provider

Evaluation
Positive therapeutic outcome
- Absence of fatigue, weakness, dyspnea
- Absence of symptoms of megaloblastic anemia
- Increase in reticulocyte count within 5 days

---

fondaparinux (Rx)
(fon-dah-pair′ih-nux)
Arixtra
Func. class.: Anticoagulant, antithrombotic
Chem. class.: Synthetic, selective factor Xa inhibitor

Pregnancy category B

Action: Acts by antithrombin III (ATIII)-mediated selective inhibition of factor Xa; neutralization of factor Xa interrupts blood coagulation and inhibits thrombin formation; does not inactivate thrombin (activated factor II) or affect platelets

→ **Therapeutic Outcome:** Prevention of deep vein thrombosis

Uses: Prevention of deep vein thrombosis, pulmonary emboli in hip and knee replacement, hip fracture surgery

Dosage and routes
Adult: SC 2.5 mg qd; after hemostasis established, initial dose is given 6-8 hr after surgery, usual duration 5-9 days

Available forms: Inj 2.5 mg/0.5 ml single-dose syringe

Adverse effects
(*italic* = common; **bold** = life-threatening)
CNS: *Fever,* confusion, headache, dizziness, *insomnia*
GI: *Nausea, vomiting,* diarrhea, dyspepsia, *constipation,* increased AST, ALT
GU: UTI, urinary retention
HEMA: *Anemia,* minor bleeding, purpura, hematoma, **thrombocytopenia, major bleeding (intracranial, cerebral, retroperitoneal hemorrhage), postoperative hemorrhage**
INTEG: Local reaction—*rash,* pruritus, inj site bleeding, increased wound drainage, bullous eruption
META: Hypokalemia
MISC: Hypotension, pain, *edema*

Contraindications: Hypersensitivity to this drug; hemophilia, leukemia with bleeding, peptic ulcer disease, hemorrhagic stroke, surgery, thrombocytopenic purpura, weight <50 kg, severe renal disease (CCr <30 ml/min)

Precautions: Alcoholism, hepatic disease (severe), blood dyscrasias, heparin-induced thrombocytopenia, severe hypertension, subacute bacterial endocarditis, acute nephritis, lactation, pregnancy **B**, elderly, children, mild-moderate renal disease

N Do Not Confuse:
Arixtra/Anti-Xa

Pharmacokinetics	
Absorption	Rapidly, completely absorbed
Distribution	Blood; does not bind to plasma proteins except 94% to ATIII
Metabolism	Unknown
Excretion	Eliminated unchanged in 72 hr in normal renal function
Half-life	17-21 hr

 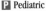

Pharmacodynamics	
Onset	Unknown
Peak	3 hr
Duration	Unknown

Interactions
• Do not mix with other drugs or infusion fluids
• Before starting fondaparinux, discontinue use of other drugs that may increase the risk of hemorrhage; monitor closely if coadministration is essential

🗷 *Herb/drug*
Agrimony, alfalfa, angelica, anise, basil, bay, bilberry, black haw, bogbean, bromelain, buchu, chondroitin, cinchona bark, dong quai, fenugreek, feverfew, garlic, ginger, ginkgo, ginseng, horse chestnut, Irish moss, kelp, kelpware, khella, lovage, lungwort, meadowsweet, motherwort, mugwort, nettle, papaya, parsley (large amounts), pau d'arco, pineapple, poplar, prickly ash, safflower, saw palmetto, tonka bean, turmeric, wintergreen, yarrow: ↑ risk of bleeding
Chamomile, coenzyme Q10, flax, glucomannan, goldenseal, guar gum: ↓ anticoagulant effect

NURSING CONSIDERATIONS
Assessment
• Assess blood studies (Hct, CBC, coagulation studies, platelets, occult blood in stools), anti-Xa; thrombocytopenia may occur
• Assess for bleeding: gums, petechiae, ecchymosis, black tarry stools, hematuria; notify prescriber
• Assess for neurologic symptoms in patients who have received spinal anesthesia

Nursing diagnoses
☑ Injury, risk for (uses, adverse reactions)
☑ Tissue perfusion, ineffective (uses)
☑ Knowledge, deficient (teaching)

Implementation
• Do not mix with other drugs or solutions; cannot be used interchangeably (unit to unit) with other anticoagulants
• Administer for 5-9 days
• Give only after screening patient for bleeding disorders
• Administer SC only; do not give IM
• Store at 77° F (25° C); do not freeze
SC route
• Check for discolored sol or sol with particulate; if present, do not give
• Begin 2 hr prior to surgery
• Administer to recumbent patient, rotate inj sites (left/right anterolateral, left/right posterolateral abdominal wall)
• Wipe surface of inj site with alcohol swab, twist plunger cap and remove, remove rigid needle guard by pulling straight off needle, do not aspirate, do not expel air bubble from surface
• Insert whole length of needle into skin fold held with thumb and forefinger
• When drug is injected, a soft click may be felt or heard
• Give at same time each day to maintain steady blood levels
• Avoid all IM inj that may cause bleeding
◆● Administer only this drug when ordered; not interchangeable with heparin

Patient/family education
• Advise patient to use soft-bristle toothbrush to avoid bleeding gums, to use electric razor
• Advise patient to report any signs of bleeding: gums, under skin, urine, stools
• Caution patient to avoid OTC drugs containing aspirin

Evaluation
Positive therapeutic outcome
• Absence of deep vein thrombosis

---

formoterol fumarate (Rx)
(for-moh'ter-ahl fyoo'mah-rayt)
Foradil Aerolizer
Func. class.: β-Adrenergic agonist
Chem. class.: Sympathomimetic catecholamine

Pregnancy category C

Action: Has β_1 and β_2 action; relaxes bronchial smooth muscle and dilates the trachea and main bronchi by increasing levels of cAMP, which relaxes smooth muscles; causes increased contractility and heart rate by acting on β-receptors in the heart

⊟ **Therapeutic Outcome:** Bronchodilation, increased heart rate and cardiac output from action on β-receptors in heart

Uses: Maintenance, treatment of asthma, COPD, prevention of exercise-induced bronchospasm

Dosage and routes
Maintenance, treatment of asthma
🄿 *Adult/child ≥5 yr:* INH AM and long-term, 1 cap q12h using aerolizer inhaler

Maintenance of COPD
Adult: INH 12 mcg q12h

Prevention of exercise-induced bronchospasm

P *Adult/child ≥12 yr:* prn occasionally 1 cap at least 15 min before exercise

Available forms: INH powder in cap 12 mcg

Adverse effects
(*italic* = common; **bold** = life-threatening)
CNS: Tremors, *anxiety*, insomnia, headache, dizziness, stimulation
CV: Palpitations, tachycardia, hypertension
GI: Nausea, vomiting
RESP: Bronchial irritation, dryness of oropharynx, **bronchospasms** (overuse)

Contraindications: Hypersensitivity to sympathomimetics, narrow-angle glaucoma

Precautions: Pregnancy **C**, cardiac disorders, hyperthyroidism, diabetes mellitus,
G prostatic hypertrophy, elderly

N **Do Not Confuse:**
Foractil/Toradol

Pharmacokinetics
Absorption	Rapid (INH)
Distribution	Plasma protein binding 61%-64% at concentrations of 0.1-100 ng/mL; 31%-38% at concentrations of 5-500 ng/mL
Metabolism	Liver, lungs, GI tract
Excretion	Urine, feces
Half-life	10 hr mean terminal elimination half-life

Pharmacodynamics
Onset	Unknown
Peak	5 min (INH)
Duration	Unknown

Interactions
Drug classifications
β-Blockers: ↓ action of formoterol
Sympathomimetics: ↑ action of both drugs

NURSING CONSIDERATIONS
Assessment
• Assess respiratory function: B/P, pulse, lung sounds
• Assess I&O ratio; check for urinary retention, frequency, hesitancy
• Assess for paresthesias and coldness of extremities; peripheral blood flow may decrease

Nursing diagnoses
☑ Airway clearance, ineffective (uses)
☑ Gas exchange, impaired (uses)
☑ Knowledge, deficient (teaching)

Implementation
• Store at room temp, protect from heat, moisture
• Do not use discolored solution

Patient/family education
• Review package insert with patient and inform about all aspects of drug
• Teach correct use of inhaler
G • Teach use of spacer device in elderly or
P children
• Advise patient to avoid getting aerosol in eyes
• Instruct patient to rinse mouth after use
• Advise patient to wash inhaler in warm water and dry qd
• Advise patient to avoid smoking, smoke-filled rooms, persons with respiratory infections

Evaluation
Positive therapeutic outcome
• Absence of dyspnea, wheezing
• Improved airway exchange
• Improved ABGs

Treatment of overdose: Administer β-blocker

---

foscarnet (Rx)
(foss-kar′net)
Foscavir
Func. class.: Antiviral
Chem. class.: Inorganic pyrophosphate organic analog

Pregnancy category C

Action: Antiviral activity is produced by selective inhibition at the pyrophosphate binding site on virus-specific DNA polymerases and reverse transcriptases at concentrations that do not affect cellular DNA polymerases

⇒ **Therapeutic Outcome:** Virostatic agents against cytomegalovirus (CMV) retinitis

Uses: Treatment of CMV, retinitis, herpes simplex virus (HSV) infections; used with ganciclovir for relapsing patients

Dosage and routes
CMV retinitis
Adult: **IV** inf 60 mg/kg given over at least 1 hr, q8h × 2-3 wk initially, then 90-120 mg/kg/day over 2 hr, usually give with at least 750-1000 ml of 0.9% NaCl qd

HSV
Adult: **IV** 40 mg/kg q8-12h × 2-3 wk

 Herb/drug   Do Not Crush   Alert   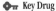 Key Drug   **G** Geriatric   **P** Pediatric

Renal dose
Adult: **IV**
Male:

$$\frac{140 - age}{72 \times serum\ creatinine\ (mg/dl)} = CCr$$

Female: 0.85 × above value; dose based on table provided in package insert

Available forms: Inj 24 mg/ml

Adverse effects
(*italic* = common; **bold** = life-threatening)
CNS: *Fever,* dizziness, *headache,* **seizures,** *fatigue,* neuropathy, tremor, ataxia, dementia, stupor, EEG abnormalities, vertigo, **coma,** abnormal gait, hypertonia, extrapyramidal disorders, hemiparesis, **paralysis,** hyperreflexia, paraplegia, **tetany,** hyporeflexia, neuralgia, neuritis, celebral edema, *paresthesia,* depression, *confusion, anxiety,* insomnia, somnolence, amnesia, hallucinations, agitation
CV: Hypertension, palpitations, ECG abnormalities, 1st-degree AV block, nonspecific ST-T segment changes, hypotension, cerebrovascular disorder, cardiomyopathy, **cardiac arrest,** bradycardia, **dysrhythmias**
EENT: Visual field defects, vocal cord paralysis, speech disorder, taste perversion, eye pain, conjunctivitis, tinnitus, otitis
GI: *Nausea, vomiting, diarrhea, anorexia,* abdominal pain, constipation, dysphagia, rectal hemorrhage, dry mouth, melena, flatulence, ulcerative stomatitis, pancreatitis, enteritis, enterocolitis, glossitis, proctitis, stomatitis, increased amylases, gastroenteritis, **pseudomembranous colitis,** duodenal ulcer, **paralytic ileus, esophageal ulceration,** abnormal A-G ratio, increased AST, ALT, cholecystitis, **hepatitis,** dyspepsia, tenesmus, hepatosplenomegaly, jaundice
GU: **Acute renal failure,** decreased CCr and increased serum creatinine, **glomerulonephritis, toxic nephropathy, nephrosis, renal tubular disorders, pyelonephritis, uremia, hematuria, albuminuria,** dysuria, polyuria
HEMA: Anemia, **granulocytopenia, leukopenia, thrombocytopenia, platelet abnormalities, thrombosis, pulmonary embolism, coagulation disorders, decreased prothrombin, hypochromic anemia, pancytopenia, hemolysis, leukocytosis,** lymphadenopathy, epistaxis, lymphopenia
INTEG: *Rash,* sweating, pruritus, skin ulceration, seborrhea, skin discoloration, alopecia, acne, dermatitis, pain/inflammation at injection site, facial edema, dry skin, urticaria
MS: Arthralgia, myalgia

RESP: *Coughing, dyspnea,* pneumonia, sinusitis, pharyngitis, **pulmonary infiltration,** stridor, **pneumothorax, hemoptysis, bronchospasm,** bronchitis, **respiratory depression, pleural effusion, pulmonary hemorrhage,** rhinitis
SYST: *Hypokalemia, hypocalcemia, hypomagnesemia,* increased alkaline phosphatase, LDH, BUN, acidosis, hypophosphatemia, hyperphosphatemia, dehydration, glycosuria, increased creatine phosphokinase, hypervolemia, infection, **sepsis, death, ascites,** hyponatremia, hypochloremia, hypercalcemia

Contraindications: Hypersensitivity, CCr <0.4 ml/min/kg

P Precautions: Pregnancy **C,** lactation,
G children, elderly, renal disease, seizure disorders, electrolyte/mineral imbalances, severe anemia

Pharmacokinetics	
Absorption	Complete (**IV**)
Distribution	14%-17% plasma protein binding
Metabolism	Not metabolized
Excretion	Kidneys (90%) unchanged, breast milk
Half-life	2-8 hr; ↑ in renal disease

Pharmacodynamics	
Onset	48 hr
Peak	2 wk
Duration	Unknown

Interactions
Individual drugs
Amphotericin B: ↑ nephrotoxicity
Pentamide: ↑ hypocalcemia
Drug classification
Aminoglycosides: ↑ nephrotoxicity

NURSING CONSIDERATIONS
Assessment
• Culture should be done before treatment with foscarnet is begun; cultures of blood, urine, and throat may all be taken; CMV is not confirmed by this method; the diagnosis is made by an ophth exam
• Assess kidney and liver function; increased hemopoietic studies: BUN, serum creatinine, creatinine clearance, if CCr <0.4 ml/min/kg, discontinue drug; AST, ALT, A-G ratio, baseline and during treatment; blood counts should be done q2wk; watch for decreasing granulocytes, Hgb; if low, therapy may have to be discontinued and restarted after hematologic recovery; blood transfusions may be required
• Assess for GI symptoms: severe nausea,

vomiting, diarrhea; severe symptoms may necessitate discontinuing drug
• Monitor electrolytes and minerals: calcium, phosphorous, magnesium, sodium, potassium; watch closely for tetany during first administration
◆• Assess for symptoms of blood dyscrasias (anemia, granulocytopenia); bruising, fatigue, bleeding, poor healing
• Assess for symptoms of allergic reactions: flushing, rash, urticaria, pruritus

Nursing diagnoses
☑ Infection, risk for (uses)
☑ Injury, risk for (adverse reactions)
☑ Knowledge, deficient (teaching)

Implementation
Ⅳ **IV route**
• Administer increased fluids before and during drug administration to induce diuresis and minimize renal toxicity
• Administer via infusion pump, at no more than 1 mg/kg/min; do not give by rapid or bolus **IV**; give by central venous line or peripheral vein; standard 24 mg/ml sol may be used without dilution if using by central line; dilute the 24 mg/ml sol to 12 mg/ml with D₅W or 0.9% NaCl if using peripheral vein
• Monitor patient closely during therapy; if tingling, numbness, paresthesias occur, stop inf and obtain lab sample for electrolytes

Y-site compatibilities: Aldesleukin, aminophylline, amikacin, ampicillin, aztreonam, benzquinamide, cefazolin, cefoperazone, cefoxitin, ceftazidime, ceftizoxime, ceftriaxone, cefuroxime, chloramphenicol, cimetidine, clindamycin, dexamethasone, DOPamine, erythromycin, fluconazole, flucytosine, furosemide, gentamicin, heparin, hydrocortisone, hydromorphone, hydrOXYzine, imipenem-cilastatin, metoclopramide, metronidazole, miconazole, morphine, nafcillin, oxacillin, penicillin G potassium, phenytoin, piperacillin, ranitidine, ticarcillin/clavulanate, tobramycin

Y-site incompatibilities: Acyclovir, amphotericin B, calcium, cotrimoxazole, diazepam, digoxin, ganciclovir, haloperidol, leucovorin, midazolam, pentamidine, phenytoin, prochlorperazine, vancomycin

Patient/family education
• Advise patient to notify prescriber if sore throat, swollen lymph nodes, malaise, fever occur, may indicate presence of other infections
• Advise patient to report perioral tingling, numbness in extremities, and paresthesias; inf

should be stopped and electrolytes should be requested
• Caution patient that serious drug interactions may occur if OTC products are ingested; check first with prescriber
• Inform patient that drug is not a cure, but will control symptoms
• Advise patient that ophth exams must be continued

Evaluation
Positive therapeutic outcome
• Improvement in CMV retinitis

---

fosamprenavir
Lexiva
See Appendix A, Selected New Drugs

---

fosinopril (Rx)
(foss-in-o′pril)
Monopril
Func. class.: Antihypertensive
Chem. class.: Angiotensin-converting enzyme (ACE) inhibitor

Pregnancy category
C (1st trimester),
D (2nd/3rd trimesters)

Action: Selectively suppresses renin-angiotensin-aldosterone system; inhibits ACE; prevents conversion of angiotensin I to angiotensin II; results in dilatation of arterial, venous vessels

▶**Therapeutic Outcome:** Decreased B/P in hypertension

Uses: Hypertension, alone or in combination with thiazide diuretics, systolic CHF

Dosage and routes
Hypertension
Adult: PO 10 mg qd initially, then 20-40 mg/day divided bid or qd, max 80 mg/day

CHF
Adult: PO 10 mg qd, then up to 40 mg/day, increased over several weeks, use lower dose in those undergoing diuresis before fosinopril

Available forms: Tabs 10, 20, 40 mg

Adverse effects
(*italic* = common; **bold** = life-threatening)
CNS: Insomnia, paresthesia, headache, dizziness, fatigue, memory disturbance, tremor, mood change
CV: Hypotension, chest pain, palpitations,

 ☑ Herb/drug   ⑤ Do Not Crush   ◆ Alert   ◆ᴨ Key Drug   ⑥ Geriatric   ⑫ Pediatric

angina, orthostatic hypotension, dysrhythmias, tachycardia

GI: Nausea, constipation, vomiting, diarrhea

GU: **Proteinuria,** increased BUN, creatinine, decreased libido

HEMA: Decreased Hct, Hgb, **eosinophilia, leukopenia, neutropenia**

INTEG: **Angioedema,** rash, flushing, sweating, photosensitivity, pruritus

META: Hyperkalemia

MS: Arthralgia, myalgia

RESP: Cough, sinusitis, dyspnea, **bronchospasm**

Contraindications: Hypersensitivity to ⟨P⟩ ACE inhibitors, lactation, children, pregnancy **D** (2nd/3rd trimesters)

Precautions: Impaired liver function, hypovolemia, blood dyscrasias, CHF, COPD, ⟨G⟩ asthma, elderly, pregnancy **C** (1st trimester)

◣ Do Not Confuse:
Monopril/minoxidil/Accupril/Monoket

Pharmacokinetics

Absorption	30%
Distribution	Crosses placenta
Metabolism	Liver—converted to fosinoprilate
Excretion	50% kidneys (metabolites), 50% feces
Half-life	12 hr—fosinoprilat

Pharmacodynamics

Onset	1 hr
Peak	2-6 hr
Duration	24 hr

Interactions
Individual drugs

Alcohol (acute ingestion): ↑ hypotension (large amounts)

Allopurinol: ↑ hypersensitivity

Digoxin, hydralazine, lithium, prazosin: ↑ toxicity

Indomethacin: ↓ antihypertensive effect

Drug classifications

Adrenergic blockers, antihypertensives, diuretics, ganglionic blockers, nitrates, phenothiazines: ↑ hypotension

Antacids: ↓ absorption

Diuretics (potassium-sparing), sympathomimetics, vasodilators: ↑ toxicity

◪ Herb/drug

Arginine: Fatal hypokalemia

Pill-bearing spurge: ↑ antihypertensive effect

Pineapple, yohimbe: ↓ antihypertensive effect

St. John's wort: Severe photosensitivity

Lab test interferences

↑ AST, ↑ ALT, ↑ alkaline phosphatase, ↑ glucose, ↑ bilirubin, ↑ uric acid

Positive: ANA titer

False positive: Urine acetone

NURSING CONSIDERATIONS
Assessment

• Monitor blood studies: neutrophils, decreased platelets; obtain WBC with differential baseline and qmo × 6 mo, then q2-3 mo × 1 yr; if neutrophils <1000/mm^3, discontinue

• Monitor B/P, check for orthostatic hypotension, syncope; if changes occur, dosage change may be required

• Monitor renal studies: protein, BUN, creatinine; watch for increased levels that may indicate nephrotic syndrome and renal failure; monitor urine daily for protein; monitor renal symptoms: polyuria, oliguria, frequency, dysuria

• Establish baselines in renal, liver function tests before therapy begins

• Check potassium levels throughout treatment although hyperkalemia rarely occurs

• Check for edema in feet, legs daily, monitor weight daily

• Assess for allergic reactions: rash, fever, pruritus, urticaria; drug should be discontinued if antihistamines fail to help

Nursing diagnoses
✓ Cardiac output, decreased (uses)
✓ Injury, risk for (side effects)
✓ Knowledge, deficient (teaching)
✓ Noncompliance (teaching)

Implementation

• Store in airtight container at 86° F (30° C) or less

• Severe hypotension may occur after 1st dose of this medication; hypotension may be prevented by reducing or discontinuing diuretic therapy 3 days before beginning benzapril therapy

Patient/family education

• Advise patient not to discontinue drug abruptly; warn patient to tell all persons associated with his or her care

• Teach patient not to use OTC products (cough, cold, allergy) unless directed by prescriber because serious side effects can occur; xanthines such as coffee, tea, chocolate, cola can prevent action of drug

• Teach patient the importance of complying with dosage schedule, even if feeling better; to continue with medical regimen to decrease B/P: exercise, smoking cessation, decreasing stress, diet modifications

- Emphasize the need to rise slowly to sitting or standing position to minimize orthostatic hypotension; not to exercise in hot weather or increased hypotension can occur
- Teach patient to notify prescriber of mouth sores, sore throat, fever, swelling of hands or feet, irregular heartbeat, chest pain, coughing, shortness of breath
- Instruct patient to report excessive perspiration, dehydration, vomiting, diarrhea; may lead to fall in B/P
- Caution patient that drug may cause dizziness, fainting, light-headedness; may occur during 1st few days of therapy; to avoid activities that may be hazardous
- Teach patient how to take B/P, and normal readings for age-group
- Advise patient to notify prescriber if pregnancy is planned or suspected

Evaluation
Positive therapeutic outcome
- Decreased B/P in hypertension

Treatment of overdose: 0.9% NaCl **IV** inf, hemodialysis

---

fosphenytoin (Rx)
(foss-fen′i-toy-in)
Cerebyx
Func. class.: Anticonvulsant
Chem. class.: Hydantoin
Pregnancy category D

Action: Inhibits spread of seizure activity in motor cortex by altering ion transport; increases AV conduction

→ Therapeutic Outcome: Decreased seizures, absence of dysrhythmias

Uses: Generalized tonic-clonic seizures, status epilepticus

Dosage and routes
PE = Phenytoin equivalent

Status epilepticus
P *Adult and child:* **IV** loading dose 15-20 mg PE/kg given at 100-150 mg PE/min

Nonemergency/maintenance dosing
P *Adult and child:* **IV** loading dose 10-20 mg PE/kg; maintenance dosing 4-6 mg PE/kg/day given at a rate of <150 mg PE/min

Available forms: Inj 150 mg (100 mg PE) 750 mg (500 mg PE)

Adverse effects
(*italic* = common; **bold** = life-threatening)
CNS: Drowsiness, dizziness, insomnia, pares-thesias, depression, suicidal tendencies, aggression, headache, confusion
CV: Hypotension, **ventricular fibrillation**
EENT: Nystagmus, diplopia, blurred vision
GI: Nausea, vomiting, diarrhea, constipation, anorexia, weight loss, hepatitis, jaundice, gingival hyperplasia
***HEMA:* Agranulocytosis, leukopenia, aplastic anemia, thrombocytopenia, megaloblastic anemia**
INTEG: Rash, lupus erythematosus, *Stevens-Johnson syndrome,* hirsutism
SYST: Hyperglycemia

Contraindications: Hypersensitivity, psychiatric conditions, pregnancy **D**, bradycardia, SA and AV block, Stokes-Adams syndrome

Precautions: Allergies, hepatic disease, renal disease, lactation, myocardial insufficiency

Pharmacokinetics
Absorption	Unknown
Distribution	Unknown
Metabolism	Liver
Excretion	Kidneys
Half-life	Unknown

Pharmacodynamics
Unknown

Interactions
Individual drugs
Alcohol: ↑ effects of fosphenytoin (chronic use)
Amiodarone, chloramphenicol, cimetidine, methylphenidate, trazodone: ↑ fosphenytoin level
Carbamazepine: ↓ effectiveness
Folic acid, reserpine, rifampin: ↓ effects of fosphenytoin
Isoniazid: ↓ metabolism, ↑ action
Drug classifications
Antacids, antidepressants (tricyclics), antineoplastics, antihistamines, barbiturates: ↓ effects of fosphenytoin
Azole antiinfectives, benzodiazepines, estrogens, H_2-receptor antagonists, phenothiazines, sulfonamides: ↑ fosphenytoin level
Antihistamines, barbiturates, general anesthetics, hypnotics, opiates, sedatives: ↑ CNS depression
Salicylates: ↑ fosphenytoin level
Food/drug
↓ Folic acid absorption

 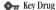

Herb/drug
Ginseng, santonica, valerian: ↓ anticonvulsant effect

Ginkgo: ↑ anticonvulsant effect

Lab test interferences
↓ Dexamethasone, ↓ metyrapone test serum, ↓ PBI, ↓ urinary steroids

↑ Glucose, ↑ alkaline phosphatase

NURSING CONSIDERATIONS
Assessment
• Assess seizure activity including type, location, duration, and character; provide seizure precaution

• Assess renal studies: urinalysis, BUN, urine creatinine

• Monitor hepatic studies: ALT, AST, bilirubin, creatinine

• Assess allergic reaction: red raised rash; if this occurs, drug should be discontinued

• Monitor for toxicity: bone marrow depression, nausea, vomiting, ataxia, diplopia, cardiovascular collapse, slurred speech, confusion

• Assess drug level: toxic level 30-50 mcg/ml

◆ Assess for rash, discontinue as soon as rash develops, serious adverse reactions such as Stevens-Johnson syndrome can occur

• Assess mental status: mood, sensorium, affect, memory (long, short), especially

G elderly

• Assess for blood dyscrasias: fever, sore throat, bruising, rash, jaundice, epistaxis (long-term treatment only)

• Monitor blood studies: RBC, Hct, Hgb, reticulocyte counts weekly for 4 wk then monthly; also check thyroid function tests, serum calcium

Nursing diagnoses
☑ Injury, risk for (uses, adverse reactions)

☑ Knowledge, deficient (teaching)

☑ Noncompliance (teaching)

Implementation
IV IV route

• Administer by direct **IV** after diluting with D_5 or 0.9% NaCl to 1.5-25 mg PE/ml

Solution compatibilities: D_5W, $D_{10}W$, amino acid inj 10%, D_5LR, D_5/0.9% NaCl, Plasmalyte A, LR, per sterile water for inj

Additive compatibilities: Potassium chloride

Patient/family education
• Teach patient the reason for and expected outcome of treatment

• Instruct patient not to use machinery or engage in hazardous activity; drowsiness, dizziness may occur

• Advise patient to carry/wear emergency ID identifying drug used, name of prescriber

• Advise patient to notify prescriber of rash, bleeding, bruising, slurred speech, jaundice of skin or eyes, joint pain, nausea, vomiting, severe headache

• Advise patient to keep all medical appointments, including lab work, physical assessment

• Advise patient to notify prescriber if pregnancy is planned or suspected; to use contraception with this product

Evaluation
Positive therapeutic outcome

• Decreased seizure activity

---

frovatriptan (Rx)
(froh-vah-trip′tan)

Frova

Func. class.: Antimigraine agent

Chem. class.: 5-HT$_1$ receptor agonist

Pregnancy category C

Action: Binds selectively to the vascular 5-HT$_{1B}$, 5-HT$_{1D}$ receptor subtypes, exerts antimigraine effect; binds to benzodiazepine receptor sites

➔ **Therapeutic Outcome:** Absence of migraines

Uses: Acute treatment of migraine with or without aura

Dosage and routes
Adult: PO 2.5 mg, a 2nd dose may be taken after ≥2 hr; max 3 tabs/day (7.5 mg)

Available forms: Tabs 2.5 mg

Adverse effects
(*italic* = common; **bold** = life-threatening)

CNS: Hot sensation, paresthesia, *dizziness,* headache, fatigue, cold sensation

CV: Flushing, **MI,** chest pain

GI: Dry mouth, dyspepsia

INTEG: Photosensitivity

MS: Skeletal pain

Contraindications: Angina pectoris, history of MI, documented silent ischemia, Prinzmetal's angina, ischemic heart disease, concurrent ergotamine-containing preparations, uncontrolled hypertension, hypersensitivity, basilar or hemiplegic migraine; ischemic bowel disease; peripheral vascular disease

Precautions: Postmenopausal women, men >40 yr, risk factors for CAD, hypercholesterolemia, obesity, diabetes, impaired hepatic

P function, pregnancy **C**, lactation, children,
G elderly

Pharmacokinetics

Absorption	Absolute bioavailability of PO dose ~20% in males, 30% in females
Distribution	Protein binding 15%; reversibly bound to blood cells at equilibrium 60%
Metabolism	Liver
Excretion	Urine (32%), feces (62%)
Half-life	25-29 hr

Pharmacodynamics

Onset	10 min-2 hr
Peak	2-4 hr
Duration	Unknown

Interactions
Individual drugs
Ergot: ↑ vasospastic effects
Propranolol: ↑ effects of frovatriptan
Drug classifications
5-HT₁ agonists, ergot derivatives: ↑ vasospastic effects
Oral contraceptives: ↑ effects of frovatriptan
SSRIs: Weakness, incoordination, hyperreflexia
⊘ *Herb/drug*
Butterbur: ↑ effect

NURSING CONSIDERATIONS
Assessment
• Assess B/P; signs/symptoms of coronary vasospasms
• Assess for stress level, activity, recreation, coping mechanisms
• Assess neurologic status: LOC, paresthesia, hot/cold sensations, dizziness, headache, fatigue
• Assess for ingestion of tyramine-containing foods (pickled products, beer, wine, aged cheese), food additives, preservatives, colorings, artificial sweeteners, chocolate, caffeine, which may precipitate these types of headaches

Nursing diagnoses
✓ Pain, acute (uses)
✓ Knowledge, deficient (teaching)

Implementation
• Provide quiet, calm environment with decreased stimulation from noise, bright light, excessive talking
PO route
⊘ • Ensure that tablets are swallowed whole

Patient/family education
• Instruct patient to report any side effects to prescriber

• Advise patient to use contraception while taking drug
• Advise patient that photosensitivity may occur, to use sunscreen and wear protective clothing when outdoors
• Advise patient to have dark, quiet environment available

Evaluation
Positive therapeutic outcome
• Decrease in frequency, severity of migraine

Treatment of overdose: No specific antidote; monitor patient closely for ≥48 hr, treat any symptoms as necessary

---

fulvestrant (Rx)
(full-ves'trant)
Faslodex
Func. class.: Antineoplastic
Pregnancy category D

Action: Inhibits cell division by binding to cytoplasmic estrogen receptors; resembles normal cell complex but inhibits DNA synthesis and estrogen response of target tissue

Therapeutic Outcome: Decreased tumor size, spread of malignancy

Uses: Advanced breast carcinoma in estrogen-receptor–positive patients (usually postmenopausal)

Dosage and routes
Adult: **IM** 250 mg qmo

Available forms: Inj 50 mg/ml

Adverse effects
(*italic* = common; **bold** = life-threatening)
CNS: Headache, depression, dizziness, insomnia, paresthesia, anxiety
GI: Nausea, vomiting, anorexia, constipation, diarrhea, abdominal pain
INTEG: Rash, sweating, hot flashes
MS: Bone pain, arthritis, back pain
RESP: Pharyngitis, dyspnea, cough

Contraindications: Hypersensitivity, pregnancy (D)

P **Precautions:** Lactation, children, hepatic disease

 Herb/drug   Do Not Crush   Alert   Key Drug   Geriatric   P Pediatric

Pharmacokinetics

Absorption	Unknown
Distribution	Unknown
Metabolism	CYP3A4
Excretion	Feces 90%
Half-life	40 days

Pharmacodynamics

Unknown

NURSING CONSIDERATIONS
Assessment
* Monitor for side effects, report to prescriber

Nursing diagnoses
☑ Risk for infection (adverse reactions)
☑ Nutrition: less than body requirements, imbalanced (adverse reactions)
☑ Knowledge, deficient (teaching)

Implementation
IM route
* Give IM 5 ml as a single inj or 2, 2.5 ml inj; give slowly in buttock
* Give antacid before oral agent; give drug after evening meal, before bedtime
* Give antiemetic 30-60 min before giving drug to prevent vomiting
* Provide liquid diet, if needed, including cola, Jell-O; dry toast or crackers may be added if patient is not nauseated or vomiting
* Provide nutritious diet with iron, vitamin supplements as ordered
* Store in refrigerator

Patient/family education
* Advise patient to report any complaints, side effects to prescriber
* Teach patient to increase fluids to 2 L/day unless contraindicated
* Advise patient to report vaginal bleeding immediately
* Teach patient that tumor flare—increase in size of tumor, increased bone pain—may occur and will subside rapidly; may take analgesics for pain
* Teach that premenopausal women must use mechanical birth control because ovulation may be induced

Evaluation
Positive therapeutic outcome
* Decreased tumor size, spread of malignancy

furosemide ⊶ (Rx)
(fur-oh′se-mide)
Apo-Furosemide ✤, Furoside ✤, Lasix,
Lasix Special ✤, Myrosemide,
Novosemide ✤, Uritol ✤
Func. class.: Loop diuretic
Chem. class.: Sulfonamide derivative

Pregnancy category C

Action: Acts on the ascending loop of Henle in the kidney, inhibiting reabsorption of electrolytes sodium and chloride, causing excretion of sodium, calcium, magnesium, chloride, water, and some potassium; decreases reabsorption of sodium and chloride and increases excretion of potassium in the distal tubule of the kidney; responsible for slight antihypertensive effect and peripheral vasodilatation

→ **Therapeutic Outcome:** Decreased edema in lung tissue, peripherally; decreased B/P

Uses: Edema in CHF, nephrotic syndrome, ascites, caused by hepatic disease, hepatic cirrhosis; may be used alone or as adjunct with antihypertensives such as spironolactone, triamterene; should not be used with ethacrynic acid

Investigational uses: Hypercalcemia in malignancy

Dosage and routes
Adult: PO 20-80 mg/day in AM, may give another dose in 6 hr, up to 600 mg/day; IM/**IV** 20-40 mg, increased by 20 mg q2h until desired response

P *Child:* PO/IM/**IV** 2 mg/kg, may increase by 1-2 mg/kg/q6-8h up to 6 mg/kg

Pulmonary edema
Adult: **IV** 40 mg given over several min, repeated in 1 hr; increase to 80 mg if needed

Hypertensive crisis/acute renal failure
Adult: **IV** 100-200 mg over 1-2 min

Antihypercalcemia
Adult: IM/**IV** 80-100 mg q1-4h or PO 120 mg qd or divided bid

P *Child:* IM/**IV** 25-50 mg, repeat q4h if needed

Available forms: Tabs 20, 40, 80 mg; oral sol 10 mg/ml, 40 mg/5 ml; inj IM, **IV** 10 mg/ml

F

Adverse effects

(*italic* = common; **bold** = life-threatening)

CNS: Headache, fatigue, weakness, vertigo, paresthesias

CV: Orthostatic hypotension, chest pain, ECG changes, **circulatory collapse**

EENT: *Loss of hearing,* ear pain, tinnitus, blurred vision

ELECT: *Hypokalemia, hypochloremic alkalosis, hypomagnesemia, hyperuricemia, hypocalcemia, hyponatremia,* metabolic alkalosis

ENDO: *Hyperglycemia*

GI: *Nausea,* diarrhea, dry mouth, vomiting, anorexia, cramps, oral or gastric irritations, pancreatitis

GU: *Polyuria,* **renal failure,** *glycosuria*

HEMA: **Thrombocytopenia, agranulocytosis, leukopenia, neutropenia, anemia**

INTEG: *Rash, pruritus, purpura,* **Stevens-Johnson syndrome,** sweating, photosensitivity, urticaria

MS: Cramps, stiffness

Contraindications: Hypersensitivity to sulfonamides, anuria, hypovolemia, infants, lactation, electrolyte depletion

Precautions: Diabetes mellitus, dehydration, severe renal disease, pregnancy **C,** cirrhosis, ascites

Do Not Confuse:

furosemide/torsemide, Lasix/Lanoxin, Lasix/Lomotil, Lasix/Luvox

Pharmacokinetics

	PO		
Absorption	GI tract (60%-70%)		
	PO/IM/**IV**		
Distribution	Crosses placenta		
Metabolism	Liver (30%-40%)		
Excretion	Breast milk, urine, feces		
Half-life	½-1 hr		

Pharmacodynamics

	PO	IM	IV
Onset	1 hr	½ hr	5 min
Peak	1-2 hrs	Unknown	½ hr
Duration	6-8 hr	4-8 hr	2 hr

Interactions

Individual drugs

Cisplatin, vancomycin: ↑ risk of ototoxicity

Clofibrate: ↑ furosemide effects

Digitalis: ↑ toxicity

Lithium: ↓ renal clearance, causing increased toxicity

Drug classifications

Aminoglycosides: ↑ ototoxicity, nephrotoxicity

Antihypertensives: ↑ antihypertensive effect

Digitalis glycosides: ↑ potassium and magnesium loss with relating dysrhythmias

Nitrates: ↑ hypotensive action

Nondepolarizing skeletal muscle relaxants: ↑ toxicity

Herb/drug

Aloe, cucumber, dandelion, horsetail, khella, pumpkin, Queen Anne's lace, St. John's wort: Severe photosensitivity

Lab test interferences

Interference: GTT

NURSING CONSIDERATIONS

Assessment

• Assess patient for tinnitus, hearing loss, ear pain; periodic testing of hearing is needed when high doses of this drug are given by **IV** route

• Monitor for renal, cardiac, neurologic, GI, pulmonary manifestations of hypokalemia: acidic urine, reduced urine osmolality, nocturia, polyuria and polydipsia; hypotension, broad T-wave, U-wave, ectopy, tachycardia, weak pulse; muscle weakness, altered LOC, drowsiness, apathy, lethargy, confusion, depression; anorexia, nausea, cramps, constipation, distention, paralytic ileus; hypoventilation, respiratory muscle weakness

• Monitor for CNS, GI, cardiovascular, integumentary, neurologic manifestations of hypocalcemia: personality changes, anxiety, disturbances, depression and psychosis; nausea, vomiting, constipation, abdominal pain from muscle spasm; decreased contractility, decreased cardiac output, hypotension, lengthened ST segment, prolonged QT interval; scaling eczema, alopecia, hyperpigmentation; tetany, muscle twitching, cramping grimacing, seizure, altered deep tendon reflexes, spasm

• Monitor for CNS, neuromuscular, GI, cardiac manifestations of hypomagnesemia, agitation; muscle twitching, paresthesias, hyperactive reflexes, positive Babinski reflex, dysphagia, nystagmus seizures, tetnany; nausea, vomiting, diarrhea, anorexia, abdominal distention; ectopy, tachycardia, broad, flat or inverted T-waves, depressed ST segment, prolonged QT, decreased cardiac output, hypotension

• Monitor for CV, GI, neurologic manifestations of hyponatremia: increased B/P, cold, clammy skin, hypovolemia or hypervolemia; anorexia, nausea, vomiting, diarrhea, abdominal cramps; lethargy, increased ICP, confusion, headache, seizures, coma, fatigue, tremors, hyperreflexia

• Monitor for neurologic, respiratory manifestations of hyperchloremia: weakness, lethargy, coma; deep rapid breathing

• Assess fluid volume status: I&O ratios and record, count or weigh diapers as appropriate, weight, distended red veins, crackles in lung, color, quality and sp gr of urine, skin turgor, adequacy of pulses, moist mucous membranes, bilateral lung sounds, peripheral pitting edema; dehydration symptoms of decreasing output, thirst, hypotension, dry mouth and mucous membranes should be reported

• Monitor electrolytes: potassium, sodium, calcium, magnesium; also include BUN, blood pH, ABGs, uric acid, CBC, blood glucose

• Assess B/P before and during therapy lying, standing and sitting as appropriate; orthostatic hypotension can occur rapidly

Nursing diagnoses

✓Fluid volume, deficient (side effects)
✓Fluid volume, excess (uses)
✓Knowledge, deficient (teaching)

Implementation

• Give in AM to avoid interference with sleep
• Potassium replacement if potassium level is <3.0 mg/dl, or use oral sol slightly, drug may be crushed if patient is unable to swallow

PO route

• With food, if nausea occurs, absorption may be reduced

IV IV route

• Do not use sol that is yellow, has a precipitate, or crystals

Implementation

IV Direct IV

• Give undiluted through Y-tube on 3-way stopcock; give 20 mg or less/min

Intermittent Infusion

• May be added to 0.9% NaCl, D_5W, $D_{10}W$, $D_{20}W$; invert sugar 10% in electrolyte #1, LR, use within 24 hr to ensure compatibility; give through Y-tube or 3-way stopcock; give at 4 mg/min or less, use infusion pump

Syringe compatibilities: Bleomycin, cisplatin, cyclophosphamide, fluorouracil, heparin, leucovorin, methotrexate, mitomycin

Syringe incompatibilities: Doxapram, DOXOrubicin, droperidol, metaclopramide, milrinone

Y-site compatibilities: Allopurinol, amifostine, amikacin, aztreonam, bleomycin, cefepime, cefmetazole, cisplatin, cladribine, cyclophosphamide, cytarabine, dexamethasone, epINEPHrine, fentanyl, fludarabine, fluorouracil, foscarnet, gallium, granisetron, heparin, hydrocortisone, hydromorphone, indomethacin, kanamycin, leucovorin, lorazepam, melphalan, meropenem, methotrexate, mitomycin, morphine, nitroglycerin, norepinephrine, paclitaxel, piperacillin/tazobactam, potassium chloride, propofol, ranitidine, sargramostim, tacrolimus, teniposide, thiotepa, tobramycin, tolazoline, vit B complex with C

Y-site incompatibilities: Amsacrine, bleomycin, DOXOrubicin, droperidol, esmolol, fluconazole, gentamicin, idarubicin, metoclopramide, milrinone, netilmicin, ondansetron, quinidine, vinBLAStine, vinCRIStine

Additive compatibilities: Amikacin, aminophylline, ampicillin, atropine, bumetanide, calcium gluconate, cefamandole, cefoperazone, cefuroxime, cimetidine, cloxacillin, dexamethasone, diamorphine, digoxin, epINEPHrine, heparin, isosorbide, kanamycin, lidocaine, meropenem, morphine, nitroglycerin, penicillin G, potassium chloride, ranitidine, scopolamine, sodium bicarbonate, theophylline, tobramycin, verapamil

Additive incompatibilities: Bleomycin, DOBUTamine, gentamicin, chlorproMAZINE, diazepam, erythromycin, isoproterenol, meperidine, metoclopramide, netilmicin, opium alkaloids, prochlorperazine, tetracycline

Patient/family education

General

• Teach patient to take the medication early in the day to prevent nocturia

• Instruct the patient to take with food or milk if GI symptoms of nausea and anorexia occur

• Teach patient to maintain a record of weight on a weekly basis and notify physician of weight loss of >5 lb

• Caution the patient that this drug causes a loss of potassium, that food rich in potassium should be added to the diet; refer to a dietitian for assistance in planning

• Caution the patient not to exercise in hot weather or stand for prolonged periods of time because orthostatic hypotension will be enhanced

• Advise patient to wear protective clothing and sunscreen to prevent photosensitivity

• Teach patient not to use alcohol or any OTC

medications without physician's approval, serious drug reactions may occur

• Emphasize the need to contact physician immediately if muscle cramps, weakness, nausea, dizziness, or numbness occurs

• Teach patient to take and record own B/P and pulse

• Caution the patient that orthostatic hypotension may occur and to rise slowly from sitting or reclining positions and lie down if dizziness occurs

• Teach patient to continue taking medication even if feeling better, this drug controls symptoms but does not cure the condition

• Advise the patient with hypertension to continue other medical treatment (exercise, weight loss, relaxation techniques, cessation of smoking)

Evaluation
Positive therapeutic outcome
• Decreased edema
• Decreased B/P
• Lowered calcium level in malignancy
• Increased diuresis

---

gabapentin (Rx)
(gab'a-pen-tin)
Neurontin
Func. class.: Anticonvulsant

Pregnancy category C

Action: Mechanism unknown; may increase seizure threshold; structurally similar to GABA; gabapentin binding sites in neocortex, hippocampus

➡ **Therapeutic Outcome:** Decreased seizure activity

Uses: Adjunct treatment of partial seizures, with or without generalization in patients >12
🅟 yr; adjunct in partial seizures in children 3-12 yr, postherpetic neuralgia

Investigational uses: Tremors in multiple sclerosis, neuropathic pain, bipolar disorder, migraine prophylaxis, diabetic neuropathy

Dosage and routes
🅟 *Adult and child >12 yr:* PO 900-1800 mg/day in 3 divided doses; may titrate by giving 300 mg on the first day, 300 mg bid on second day, 300 mg tid on third day; may increase to 1800 mg/day by adding 300 mg on subsequent days

🅟 *Child 3-12 yr:* PO 10-15 mg/kg/day in 3 divided doses, initially; titrate dose upward over approximately 3 days; 25-35 mg/kg/day in children ≥5 yr; 40 mg/kg/day in children 3-4 yr; all given in 3 divided doses; rec 200 mg as a single dose

Postherpetic Neuralgia
Adult: PO 300 mg on day 1, 600 mg/day divided bid on day 2, 900 mg/day divided tid, may titrate to 1800 mg divided tid if needed

Renal dose
🅟 *Adult and child >12 yr:* CCr 30-60 ml/min 300 mg bid; CCr 15-30 ml/min 300 mg qd; CCr <15 ml/min 125 mg qd

Available forms: Caps 100, 300, 400 mg; tabs 600, 800 mg; oral sol 250 mg/5 ml

Adverse effects
(*italic* = common; **bold** = life-threatening)
CNS: Dizziness, fatigue, anxiety, somnolence, ataxia, amnesia, abnormal thinking, unsteady
🅟 gait, depression; 3-12 yr old emotional lability, aggression, thought disorder, hyperkinesia
CV: Vasodilatation, peripheral edema
EENT: Dry mouth, blurred vision, diplopia, nystagmus
GI: Constipation, increased appetite, dental abnormalities, nausea, vomiting
GU: Impotence, bleeding, *UTI*
HEMA: **Leukopenia,** decreased WBC
INTEG: Pruritus, abrasion
MS: Myalgia
RESP: Rhinitis, pharyngitis, coughing

Contraindications: Hypersensitivity to this drug

🅟 **Precautions:** Renal disease, pregnancy **C,**
🅖 lactation, child <12 yr, elderly, hemodialysis

🅽 **Do Not Confuse:**
Neurontin/Noroxin/Neoral

Pharmacokinetics	
Absorption	Unknown
Distribution	Unknown
Metabolism	None
Excretion	Urine unchanged
Half-life	5-7 hr

Pharmacodynamics	
Onset	Unknown
Peak	Unknown
Duration	Unknown

Interactions
Individual drugs
Alcohol: ↑ CNS depression

Drug classifications
Antacids: ↓ gabapentin levels
Antihistamines, CNS depressants (other): ↑ CNS depression

Herb/drug
Chamomille, hops, kava, skullcap, valerian: ↑ CNS depression
Ginkgo: ↑ anticonvulsant effect
Ginseng, santonica: ↓ anticonvulsant effect

Lab test interferences
False positive: Urinary protein using Ames N-multistix SG

NURSING CONSIDERATIONS
• Assess seizures: aura, location, duration, activity at onset
• Assess renal studies: urinalysis, BUN, urine creatinine q3 mo
• Assess mental status: mood, sensorium, affect, behavioral changes; if mental status changes, notify prescriber
• Assess eye problems, need for ophth exam before, during, after treatment (slit lamp, fundoscopy, tonometry)

Nursing diagnoses
☑ Knowledge, deficient (teaching)
☑ Noncompliance (teaching)

Implementation
• Give at least 2 hr pc with antacids, give without regard to meals
• Gradually withdraw over 7 days, abrupt withdraw may precipitate seizures
• Store at room temp away from heat and light
• Give hard candy, frequent rinsing of mouth, gum for dry mouth
• Provide assistance with ambulation during early part of treatment; dizziness occurs
• Provide seizure precautions: padded side rails; move objects that may harm patient
• Provide increased fluids, bulk in diet for constipation

Evaluation
Positive therapeutic outcome
• Decreased seizure activity; document on patient's chart

Patient/family education
• Advise patient to carry/wear emergency ID stating patient's name, drugs taken, condition, prescriber's name and phone number
• Teach patient to avoid driving, other activities that require alertness
• Teach patient not to discontinue medication

quickly after long-term use, withdrawal-precipitated seizures may occur, not to double dose; if dose is missed, take if 2 hr or more before next dose
🚫• Teach patient not to break, crush, or chew caps
• Advise patient to notify prescriber if pregnancy is planned or suspected, avoid breast feeding

Treatment of overdose: Lavage, VS

galantamine (Rx)
(gah-lan'tah-meen)
Reminyl
Func. class.: Anti-Alzheimer's agent, cholinesterase inhibitor

Pregnancy category B

Action: May enhance cholinergic functioning by increasing acetylcholine

Therapeutic Outcome: Decreased signs and symptoms of Alzheimer's dementia

Uses: Alzheimer's dementia

Dosage and routes
Adult: PO 4 mg bid; after 4 wk or more may increase to 8 mg bid; after another 4 wk may increase to 12 mg bid

Available forms: Tabs 4, 8, 12 mg; oral sol 4 mg/ml

Adverse effects
(*italic* = common; **bold** = life-threatening)
CNS: Tremors, insomnia, depression, dizziness, headache, somnolence, fatigue
CV: Bradycardia, chest pain
GI: Nausea, vomiting, anorexia, abdominal distress, flatulence, diarrhea
GU: Urinary incontinence, bladder outflow obstruction, hematuria
META: Weight decrease
MISC: Anemia, hematuria
MS: Asthenia, anemia
RESP: URI, rhinitis

Contraindications: Hypersensitivity to this drug

Precautions: Renal disease, hepatic disease, respiratory disease, seizure disorder, peptic ulcer, pregnancy **B**, asthma, lactation, children, peptic ulcer

Pharmacokinetics

Absorption	Rapidly and completely absorbed
Distribution	Unknown
Metabolism	P450 enzyme
Excretion	Kidneys; clearance ↓ in the elderly, hepatic disease, females (20% lower)
Half-life	Unknown

Pharmacodynamics

Onset	Unknown
Peak	Unknown
Duration	Unknown

Interactions
Individual drugs
Amitriptyline, fluvoxamine, quinidine: ↑ galantamine effect
Cimetidine, erythromycin, ketoconazole, paroxetine: ↑ galantamine bioavailability
Drug classifications
Cholinesterase inhibitors, cholinomimetics: Synergistic effect
☑ *Herb/drug*
Jimsonweed, scopolia: cholinergic antagonism
Pill-bearing spurge: ↑ effect

NURSING CONSIDERATIONS
Assessment
• Assess liver function enzymes: AST, ALT, alkaline phosphatase, LDH, bilirubin, CBC
• Assess for severe GI effects: nausea, vomiting, anorexia, weight loss
• Assess B/P, respiration during initial treatment
• Assess mental status: affect, mood, behavioral changes, depression

Nursing diagnoses
✓ Knowledge, deficient (teaching)
✓ Cognitive impairment (uses)

Implementation
• Provide assistance with ambulation during beginning therapy
• Perform complete suicide assessment
PO route
• Give with meals, morning and evening

Patient/family education
• Teach patient or caregiver correct procedure for giving oral solution, using instruction sheet provided
• Instruct patient or caregiver to notify prescriber of severe GI effects
• Instruct patient or caregiver to report hypo/hypertension

Evaluation
Positive therapeutic outcome
• Decreased symptoms of dementia
• Increased coherence
• Improved cognitive performance (memory, orientation, attention, reasoning, language, praxis)

Treatment of overdose: Administer **IV** atropine titrated to effect at an initial dose of 0.5-1.0 mg, with subsequent doses based on clinical response; provide general supportive measures

---

gallium (Rx)
(gal'ee-yum)
Ganite
Func. class.: Electrolyte modifier
Chem. class.: Hypocalcemic drug

Pregnancy category C

Action: Lowers serum calcium levels by inhibiting calcium resorption from bone

➔ **Therapeutic Outcome:** Decrease calcium level to 5-9 mg/dl

Uses: Cancer-related hypercalcemia

Dosage and routes
Adult: IV 100-200 mg/m² qd × 5 days; inf over 24 hr, rest period of 2-4 wk between courses

Available forms: Inj 25 mg/ml

Adverse effects
(*italic* = common; **bold** = life-threatening)
CV: Tachycardia, hypotension
EENT: Blurred vision, optic neuritis, hearing loss
GI: Nausea, vomiting, diarrhea, constipation, mucositis, metallic taste
GU: **Nephrotoxicity**, increased BUN, creatinine
HEMA: **Anemia, leukopenia, thrombocytopenia**
META: *Hypophosphatemia*, hypocalcemia, decreased serum bicarbonate

Contraindications: Hypersensitivity, severe renal disease

Precautions: Pregnancy **C**, lactation, 🅿 children, mild renal disease

Pharmacokinetics

Absorption	Completely absorbed
Distribution	Unknown
Metabolism	Unknown
Excretion	Kidneys (unchanged)
Half-life	Unknown

☑ Herb/drug   🚫 Do Not Crush   ◆ Alert   ◆π Key Drug   🅖 Geriatric   🅿 Pediatric

Pharmacodynamics	
Onset	12-48 hr
Peak	Unknown
Duration	4-14 days

Interactions
Individual drugs
Amphotericin B: ↑ nephrotoxicity
Drug classifications
Aminoglycosides: ↑ nephrotoxicity

NURSING CONSIDERATIONS
Assessment
• Renal status: BUN, creatinine, urine output; if creatinine level is 2.5 mg/dl or more, drug should be discontinued
• Monitor calcium, phosphate, bicarbonate; all levels may be decreased and supplements of phosphate may be needed; calcium daily, phosphate 2-3 ×/wk
• Assess for hypercalcemia: nausea, vomiting, fatigue, weakness, thirst, dehydration, dysrhythmias, headache, confusion, coma, decreased reflexes
• For hypocalcemia: dysrhythmias, hypotension, paresthesia; twitching, colic, laryngospasm; hypercalcemia: poor coordination, myalgia, hypotonia, shortened ST segment and QT interval, prolonged PR interval, cone-shaped T wave, sinus bradycardia; Trousseau's, Chvostek's sign: tremors, tetany, cramping, grimacing, seizures, altered deep tendon reflexes and spasms, personality changes including irritability, depression, psychosis
• Monitor for indications of hypophosphatemia: weakness, malaise, tremors, memory loss, inattention, confusion, decreased reflexes, aching bone pain, joint stiffness, rapid, shallow respiration, decreased tidal volume, nausea, vomiting, anorexia, portal hypertension

Nursing diagnoses
☑ Injury, risk for (uses)
☑ Knowledge, deficient (teaching)

Implementation
• Provide adequate hydration with **IV** saline, 2 L/day during treatment; saline increases the extracellular calcium
• Give by cont **IV** inf after dilution of dose/1 L of 0.9% NaCl or D$_5$W, run over 24 hr, use infusion pump
• Store solution for 48 hr at room temp or 1 wk in refrigerator

Y-site compatibilities: Acyclovir, allopurinol, aminophylline, ampicillin/sulbactam, amifostine, aztreonam, cefazolin, ceftazidime, ceftriaxone, cimetidine, ciprofloxacin, cladribine, cyclophosphamide, dexamethasone, diphenhydrAMINE, filgrastim, fluconazole, furosemide, granisetron, heparin, hydrocortisone, fosfamide, magnesium sulfate, mannitol, melphalan, meperidine, mesna, methotrexate, metoclopramide, ondansetron, piperacillin, piperacillin/tazobactam, potassium chloride, ranitidine, sodium bicarbonate, teniposide, thiotepa, ticarcillin/clavulanate, trimethoprim, sulfamethoxazole, vancomycin, vinorelbine

Patient/family education
• Instruct patient to follow dietary guidelines given by prescriber, including avoiding calcium (dietary products, broccoli) and vit D (fortified milk, grain products, fish oil)
• Explain purpose of drug and expected results

Evaluation
Positive therapeutic outcome
• Decreased serum calcium levels to 5-9 mg/dl

---

ganciclovir (Rx)
(gan-sye'kloe-vir)
Cytovene, Vitrasert
Func. class.: Antiviral
Chem. class.: Synthetic nucleoside analog

Pregnancy category C

Action: Inhibits replication of herpes viruses in vitro, in vivo by selective inhibition of the human cytomegalovirus (CMV) DNA polymerase and by direct incorporation into viral DNA

⇨ **Therapeutic Outcome:** Decreased proliferation of virus responsible for CMV retinitis

Uses: CMV retinitis in immunocompromised persons, including those with AIDS, after indirect ophthalmoscopy confirms diagnosis

Investigational uses: CMV pneumonia in organ transplant patients, CMV gastroenteritis in patients with irritable bowel syndrome, CMV pneumonitis

Dosage and routes
Induction treatment
Adult: **IV** 5 mg/kg given over 1 hr q12h × 2-3 wk

Maintenance treatment
Adult: **IV** inf 5 mg/kg given over 1 hr, qd × 7 days/wk; or 6 mg/kg qd × 5 days/wk; PO 1000

mg tid with food or 500 mg q3h while awake; intravitreal: 4.5-mg implant

Prevention of CMV infection
Adult: IV 5 mg/kg q12h × 1-2 wk, then 5 mg/kg/day × 7 days/wk or 6 mg/kg × 5 days/wk; PO 1000 mg tid

Renal dose
CCr <70 ml/min reduce dose

Available forms: Powder for inj 500 mg/vial, caps 250, 500 mg; implant, intravitreal 4.5 mg

Adverse effects
(*italic* = common; **bold** = life-threatening)
CNS: *Fever,* chills, **coma,** *confusion,* abnormal thoughts, dizziness, bizarre dreams, *headache,* psychosis, tremors, somnolence, *paresthesia, weakness,* **seizures**
CV: Dysrhythmia, hypertension/hypotension
EENT: Retinal detachment in CMV retinitis
GI: *Abnormal liver function tests, nausea, vomiting, anorexia, diarrhea, abdominal pain,* **hemorrhage**
GU: **Hematuria,** increased creatinine, BUN
HEMA: **Granulocytopenia, thrombocytopenia, irreversible neutropenia, anemia, eosinophilia**
INTEG: *Rash,* alopecia, *pruritus,* urticaria, pain at inj site, phlebitis
RESP: Dyspnea

Contraindications: Hypersensitivity to acyclovir or ganciclovir, ANC <500/mm^3, platelet count <25,000/mm^3

Precautions: Preexisting cytopenias, renal **P** function impairment, pregnancy **C**, lactation, **G** children <6 mo, elderly

N Do Not Confuse:
Cytovene/Cytosar

Pharmacokinetics	
Absorption	Completely absorbed
Distribution	Crosses blood-brain barrier, CSF
Metabolism	Not metabolized
Excretion	Kidneys (90%) unchanged, breast milk
Half-life	3 hr

Pharmacodynamics	
Unknown	

Interactions
Individual drugs
Amphotericin B, adriamycin, cycloSPORINE, dapsone, DOXOrubicin, flucytosine, pentamidine, probenecid, trimethoprim/sulfa combinations, vinBLAStine, vinCRIStine: ↑ toxicity

Imipenem with cilastatin: ↑ chance of seizures
Probenecid: ↓ renal clearance of ganciclovir
Radiation, zidovudine: Severe granulocytopenia; do not give together
Drug classifications
Antineoplastics: severe granulocytopenia; do not give together
Nucleoside analogs: ↑ toxicity

NURSING CONSIDERATIONS
Assessment
• Culture should be done before treatment with ganciclovir is initiated; cultures of blood, urine, and throat may all be taken; CMV is not confirmed by this method; the diagnosis is made by an ophth exam
• Assess kidney, liver function; increases in hemopoietic studies: BUN, serum creatinine, AST creatinine clearance, ALT, A-G ratio, baseline, and drip treatment; blood counts should be done q2 wk; watch for decreasing granulocytes, Hgb; if low, therapy may have to be discontinued and restarted after hematologic recovery; blood transfusions may be required
• Assess for GI symptoms: severe nausea, vomiting, diarrhea; severe symptoms may necessitate discontinuing drug
• Monitor electrolytes and minerals: calcium, phosphorus, magnesium, sodium, potassium; watch closely for tetany during 1st administration
• Assess for symptoms of blood dyscrasias (anemia, granulocytopenia); bruising, fatigue, bleeding, poor healing
• Assess for symptoms of allergic reactions: flushing, rash, urticaria, pruritus
• Monitor for leukopenia/neutropenia/thrombocytopenia: WBCs, platelets q2 days during 2 ×/day dosing and q1 wk thereafter; check for leukopenia with qd WBC count in patients with prior leukopenia with other nucleoside analogs or for whom leukopenia counts are <1000 cells/mm^3 at start of treatment
• Monitor serum creatinine or creatinine clearance at least q2 wk

Nursing diagnoses
☑ Infection, risk for (uses)
☑ Injury, risk for (uses, adverse reactions)
☑ Knowledge, deficient (teaching)

Implementation
PO route
• Give with food
IV IV route
• Medicine should be mixed under strict aseptic conditions using gloves, gown, and

mask, and using precautions for antineoplastics

Intermittent Inf Route

- Administer **IV** after diluting 500 mg/10 ml of sterile water for inj (50 mg/ml); shake; further dilute in 100 ml of D_5W, 0.9% NaCl, LR, Ringer's and run over 1 hr; use infusion pump, in-line filter
- Give slowly; do not give by bolus **IV**, IM, SC inj
- Use diluted sol within 12 hr, do not refrigerate or freeze; do not use sol with particulate matter or discoloration, fludarabine, sargramostim

Y-site compatibilities: Allopurinol, cisplatin, cyclophosphamide, enalaprilat, filgrastim, fluconazole, granisetron, melphalan, methotrexate, paclitaxel, propofol, tacrolimus, teniposide, thiotepa

Y-site incompatibilities: Amsacrine, fludarabine, foscarnet, ondansetron, sargramostim, vinorelbine

Patient/family education

- Advise patient to notify prescriber if sore throat, swollen lymph nodes, malaise, fever occur; may indicate other infections
- Advise patient to report perioral tingling, numbness in extremities, and paresthesias
- Caution patient that serious drug interactions may occur if OTC products are ingested; check first with prescriber
- Inform patient that drug is not a cure, but will control symptoms
- Advise patient that regular ophth exams must be continued
- Inform patient that major toxicities may necessitate discontinuing drug
- Instruct patient to use contraception during treatment and that infertility may occur; men should use barrier contraception for 90 days after treatment
- Teach patient to take PO with food
- Teach patient to report infection: fever, chills, sore throat; blood dyscrasias: bruising, bleeding, petechiae
- Tell patient to avoid crowds, persons with respiratory infection
- Advise patient to use sunscreen to prevent burns

Evaluation

Positive therapeutic outcome

- Decreased symptoms of CMV infection

---

ganirelix (Rx)

(gan-i-rell′-ex)

Antagon

Func. class.: Gonadotropin-releasing hormone antagonist

Chem. class.: Synthetic decapeptide

Pregnancy category X

Action: Inhibitor of pituitary gonadotropin secretion; initially increases LH and FSH, induces a rapid suppression of gonadotropin secretion

→ **Therapeutic Outcome:** Pregnancy

G

Uses: For inhibition of premature LH surges in women undergoing controlled ovarian hyperstimulation

Dosage and routes

Adult: SC 250 mcg qd during early to mid follicular phase, continue until day of hCG administration

Available forms: Inj 250 mcg/0.5 ml

Adverse effects

(*italic* = common; **bold** = life-threatening)

CNS: Headache

ENDO: Ovarian hyperstimulation syndrome, abdominal pain (gynecologic)

GI: Nausea

GU: Spotting, breakthrough bleeding

INTEG: Pain on inj

SYST: **Fetal death**

Contraindications: Hypersensitivity, pregnancy **X**, latex allergy, lactation

Pharmacokinetics	
Absorption	Unknown
Distribution	Unknown
Metabolism	To metabolites
Excretion	Unknown
Half-life	13-16 hr

Pharmacodynamics	
Onset	Unknown
Peak	Unknown
Duration	Treatment length

Interactions: None

NURSING CONSIDERATIONS

Assessment

- Assess for suspected pregnancy, drug should not be used
- Assess for latex allergy, drug should not be used

Nursing diagnoses
- ☑ Sexual dysfunction (uses)
- ☑ Knowledge, deficient (teaching)

Implementation
- Administer SC using abdomen, around navel or upper thigh, swab inj area with disinfectant, clean a 2-in circle and allow to dry, pinch up area between thumb and finger, insert needle at 45-90 degrees to surface, if positioned correctly, no blood will be drawn back into syringe, if blood is drawn into syringe, reposition needle without removing it
- Protect from light

Patient/family education
- Teach patient to report abdominal pain, vaginal bleeding

Evaluation
Positive therapeutic outcome
- Pregnancy

---

gatifloxacin (Rx)
(gat-i-floks′-a-sin)
Tequin
Func. class.: Urinary antiinfective
Chem. class.: Fluoroquinolone

Pregnancy category C

Action: Interferes with conversion of intermediate DNA fragments into high-molecular-weight DNA in bacteria; DNA gyrase inhibitor

⇒**Therapeutic Outcome:** Bactericidal action against the following: gram-positive organisms methicillin-resistant strains of *Staphylococcus aureus, Streptococcus pneumoniae;* gram-negative organisms *Escherichia coli, Haemophilus influenzae, Haemophilus parainfluenzae, Klebsiella pneumoniae, Moraxella catarrhalis, Neisseria gonorrhoeae, Proteus mirabilis;* and other microorganisms: *Chlamydia pneumoniae, Legionella pneumophilia, Mycoplasma pneumoniae*

Uses: Adult urinary tract infections (including complicated); lower respiratory, skin, bone, joint infections, acute bacterial exacerbation of chronic bronchitis, acute sinusitis, community-acquired respiratory tract infections, gonorrhea

Investigational uses: Multidrug-resistant *S. pneumoniae;* in children with acute otitis media; sinusitis; *Mycobacterium leprae,* atypical pneumonia, uncomplicated skin, soft tissue infections, chronic prostatitis

Dosage and routes
Renal dose
CCr ≥40 ml/min 400 mg qd; CCr <40 ml/min 200 mg qd after 400 mg initially; hemodialysis 200 mg qd after 400 mg initially

Uncomplicated urinary tract infections
Adult: PO/**IV** 400 mg single dose

Complicated/severe urinary tract infections
Adult: PO/**IV** 400 mg × 7-10 days

Chronic bronchitis
Adult: PO/**IV** 400 mg × 7-10 days

Acute sinusitis
Adult: PO/**IV** 400 mg × 10 days

Community acquired pneumonia
Adult: PO/**IV** 400 mg × 7-14 days

Gonorrhea
Adult: PO/**IV** 400 mg single dose

Available forms: Tabs 200, 400; inj 20 ml (200 mg), 40 ml (400 mg), inj premix 200, 400 mg

Adverse effects
(*italic* = common; **bold** = life-threatening)
CNS: Headache, dizziness, insomnia, paresthesia, tremor, vasodilatation
ENDO: Increased blood glucose
GI: Nausea, increased ALT, AST, diarrhea, **pseudomembranous colitis**
INTEG: Rash, pruritus, urticaria, photosensitivity, flushing, fever, chills
RESP: Dyspnea, pharyngitis
SYST: **Anaphylaxis, Stevens-Johnson syndrome**

Contraindications: Hypersensitivity to quinolones

Precautions: Pregnancy **C**, lactation, ℗ children, renal disease

Pharmacokinetics	
Absorption	Well absorbed (PO); complete (**IV**)
Distribution	Protein binding 20%
Metabolism	Liver
Excretion	Kidneys unchanged (70%)
Half-life	1 hr

Pharmacodynamics		
	PO	IV
Onset	Rapid	Immediate
Peak	1-2 hr	Infusion's end
Duration	24 hr	

Interactions
Individual drugs
Aluminum hydroxide, calcium, sucralfate: ↓ absorption of gatifloxacin

Cimetidine: ↑ serum levels of gatifloxacin

CycloSPORINE: ↑ nephrotoxicity

Probenecid: ↑ blood levels of gatifloxacin

Warfarin: ↑ warfarin level

Drug classifications
Antacids (magnesium): ↓ absorption of gatifloxacin

NURSING CONSIDERATIONS
Assessment
• Assess patient for previous sensitivity reaction

• Assess patient for signs and symptoms of infection including characteristics of wounds, sputum, urine, stool, WBC >10,000/mm³, fever; obtain baseline information before and during treatment

• Obtain C&S before beginning drug therapy to identify if correct treatment has been initiated

• Assess for allergic reactions and anaphylaxis: rash, urticaria, pruritus, chills, fever, joint pain; may occur a few days after therapy begins; epiNEPHrine and resuscitation equipment should be available for anaphylactic reaction

• Identify urine output; if decreasing, notify prescriber (may indicate nephrotoxicity); also check for increased BUN, creatinine

• Monitor blood studies: AST, ALT, CBC, Hct, bilirubin, LDH, alkaline phosphatase, blood glucose, Coombs' test monthly if patient is on long-term therapy

• Monitor electrolytes: potassium, sodium, chloride monthly if patient is on long-term therapy

• Assess bowel pattern qd; if severe diarrhea occurs, drug should be discontinued

• Monitor for bleeding: ecchymosis, bleeding gums, hematuria, stool guaiac daily if on long-term therapy

• Assess for overgrowth of infection: perineal itching, fever, malaise, redness, pain, swelling, drainage, rash, diarrhea, change in cough, sputum

Nursing diagnoses
☑ Infection, risk for (uses)

☑ Diarrhea (side effects)

☑ Injury, risk for (side effects)

☑ Knowledge, deficient (teaching)

☑ Noncompliance (teaching)

Implementation
PO route
• Give 2 hr before or 2 hr after antacids, zinc, iron, calcium

IV IV route
• Check for irritation, extravasation, phlebitis daily

• Do not use flexible containers in series connections; air embolism may occur

• Do not use if particulate matter is present

• Do not admix with other drugs

• Dilute with compatible sol to 2 mg/ml before administration; give over 1 hr; do not give by bolus or rapid IV

Solution compatibilities: D₅, 0.9% NaCl, D₅/0.9% NaCl LR/D₅, water for inj

Patient/family education
• Teach patient to report sore throat, bruising, bleeding, joint pain; may indicate blood dyscrasias (rare)

• Instruct patient to increase fluid intake to 2 L/day to prevent crystalluria

• Advise patient to contact prescriber if vaginal itching, loose, foul-smelling stools, furry tongue occur; may indicate superinfection; report itching, rash, pruritus, urticaria

• Instruct patient to take all medication prescribed for the length of time ordered; drug must be taken around the clock to maintain blood levels: do not give medication to others

• Advise patient to notify prescriber of diarrhea with blood or pus

• Advise patient to notify prescriber if theophylline is also being taken

Evaluation
Positive therapeutic outcome
• Absence of signs/symptoms of infection (WBC <10,000/mm³, temp WNL, absence of pain on urination, urgency)

• Reported improvement in symptoms of infection

gefitinib
(Iressa)
See Appendix A, Selected New Drugs

gemcitabine (Rx)
(gem-sit'a-been)

Gemzar

Func. class.: Antineoplastic—misc.
Chem. class.: Nucleoside analog

Pregnancy category D

Pharmacokinetics

Absorption	Unknown
Distribution	Crosses placenta
Metabolism	Unknown
Excretion	Unknown
Half-life	42-79 min

Pharmacodynamics
Unknown

Action: Exhibits antitumor activity by killing cells undergoing DNA synthesis (S phase) and blocking G_1/S-phase boundary

➡ **Therapeutic Outcome:** Prevention of growth of tumor

Uses: Adenocarcinoma of the pancreas: nonresectable stage II, III, or metastatic stage IV; in combination with cisplatin for inoperable, advanced, or metastatic non–small cell lung cancer

Interactions
Individual drug
Alcohol: ↑ bleeding
Drug classifications
Antineoplastics, radiation: ↑ myelosuppression, diarrhea
Live virus vaccines: ↓ antibody response
NSAIDs, salicylates: ↑ bleeding

Dosage and routes
Pancreatic carcinoma
Adult: IV 1000 mg/m^2 given over ½ hr qwk × 7 wk, then 1 wk rest period; subsequent cycles should be infused once qwk × 3 wk out of every 4 wk

Non–small cell lung cancer
4 wk schedule
Adult: IV 1000 mg/m^2 given over ½ hr on days 1, 8, 15 of each 28-day cycle; give cisplatin **IV** 100 mg/m^2 on day 1 after gemcitabine

3 wk schedule
Adult: IV 1250 mg/m^2 given over ½ hr on days 1, 8 of each 21-day cycle; give cisplatin 100 mg/m^2 after the inf of gemcitabine on day 1

Available forms: Lyophilized powder for inj 20 mg/ml

Adverse effects
(*italic* = common; **bold** = life-threatening)
GI: Diarrhea, nausea, vomiting, anorexia, constipation, stomatitis
GU: Proteinuria, hematuria
***HEMA:* Leukopenia, anemia, neutropenia, thrombocytopenia**
INTEG: Irritation at site, rash, alopecia
MISC: Dyspnea, fever, ***hemorrhage***, infection, flulike syndrome, paresthesia

Contraindications: Hypersensitivity, pregnancy **D**

P **Precautions:** Lactation, children, elderly,
G myelosuppression, irradiation

🗏 **Do Not Confuse:**
Gemzar/Zinecard

NURSING CONSIDERATIONS
Assessment
• Monitor CBC, differential, platelet count before each dose; absolute granulocyte count >1000/mm^3, platelets >100,000/mm^3, give complete dose; absolute granulocyte count 500-1000/mm^3, platelets 50,000-100,000/mm^3, give 75%; absolute granulocyte count <500/mm^3, platelets <50,000/mm^3, do not give
• Assess for blood dyscrasias: bruising, bleeding, petechiae
• Monitor I&O, nutritional intake
• Monitor hepatic/renal studies before and during treatment, may ↑ AST, ALT, alkaline phosphatase, bilirubin, BUN, creatinine
• Assess food preferences: list likes, dislikes
• Assess buccal cavity q8h for dryness, sores or ulceration, white patches, oral pain, bleeding, dysphagia
• Assess GI symptoms: frequency of stools; cramping
• Assess signs of dehydration: rapid respirations, poor skin turgor, decreased urine output, dry skin, restlessness, weakness

Nursing diagnoses
☑ Infection, risk for (adverse reactions)
☑ Nutrition: less than body requirements, imbalanced (adverse reaction)

Implementation
• Provide for rinsing of mouth tid-qid with water, club soda; brushing of teeth bid-tid with soft brush or cotton-tipped applicator for stomatitis; use unwaxed dental floss
• Give nutritious diet with iron, vitamin supplement, low fiber, few dairy products
• Give increased fluid intake to 2-3 L/day to prevent dehydration, unless contraindicated

IV IV route
- Prepare in biologic cabinet using gown, mask, gloves
- After reconstituting with 0.9% NaCl 5 ml/200 mg vial of drug or 25 ml/1 g of drug, shake (40 mg/ml); may be further diluted with 0.9% NaCl to concentrate as low as 0.1 mg/ml; discard unused portion, give over ½ hr, do not admix
- Change **IV** site q48h

Patient/family education
- Advise patient to avoid foods with citric acid or hot or rough texture if stomatitis is present; to drink adequate fluids
- Advise patient to report stomatitis; any bleeding, white spots, ulcerations in mouth; tell patient to examine mouth qd, report symptoms
- Advise patient to report signs of anemia: fatigue, headache, faintness, shortness of breath, irritability; hematuria, dysuria
- Advise patient to use contraception during therapy
- Instruct patient to avoid use with NSAIDs, salicylates, alcohol; not to receive vaccinations during treatment

Evaluation
Positive therapeutic outcome
- Decrease in tumor size, decrease in spread of cancer

Treatment of overdose:
Induce vomiting, provide supportive care

---

gemfibrozil (Rx)
(gem-fye'broe-zil)
gemfibrozil, Lopid
Func. class.: Antilipemic
Chem. class.: Fibric acid derivative

Pregnancy category C

Action: Inhibits biosynthesis of VLDL, decreases triglycerides, increases HDLs

➡ **Therapeutic Outcome:** Decreased hepatic triglyceride production, VLDL; accelerates removal of cholesterol from liver

Uses: Type IIb, IV, V hyperlipidemia as adjunct with diet therapy

Dosage and routes
Adult: PO 1200 mg in divided doses bid 30 min ac

Available forms: Tabs 600 mg

Adverse effects
(*italic* = common; **bold** = life-threatening)
CNS: Fatigue, vertigo, headache, paresthesia, dizziness, somnolence
GI: Nausea, vomiting, *dyspepsia, diarrhea, abdominal pain*
HEMA: **Leukopenia, anemia, eosinophilia, thrombocytopenia**
INTEG: Rash, urticaria, pruritus
MISC: Task perversion

Contraindications: Severe hepatic disease, preexisting gallbladder disease, severe renal disease, primary biliary cirrhosis, hypersensitivity

Precautions: Monitor hematologic and hepatic function, pregnancy **C**, lactation

◼ Do Not Confuse:
Lopid/Levbid/Slo-bid

Pharmacokinetics	
Absorption	Well absorbed
Distribution	Unknown, plasma protein binding >90%
Metabolism	Liver—minimal
Excretion	Kidney—unchanged (70%), feces (6%)
Half-life	1½ hr

Pharmacodynamics	
Onset	1-2 hr
Peak	1-2 hr
Duration	2-4 months

Interactions
Individual drugs
CycloSPORINE: ↓ cycloSPORINE effect
Drug classifications
Anticoagulants (oral): ↑ effect of anticoagulants
HMG-CoA reductase inhibitors: ↑ risk of myositis, myalgia
Sulfonylureas: ↑ hypoglycemic effect
⬚ *Herb/drug*
Glucomannan: ↑ effect
Gotu kola: ↓ effect
Lab test interferences
↑ Liver function studies, ↑ CPK, ↑ BSP, ↑ thymol turbidity, ↑ glucose
↓ Hgb, ↓ Hct, ↓ WBC

NURSING CONSIDERATIONS
Assessment
- Assess nutrition: fat, protein, carbohydrates; nutritional analysis should be performed by dietitian before treatment is initiated
- Assess renal function studies, liver function tests, CBC, blood glucose if patient is on

G

---

long-term therapy; if liver function test results increase, drug should be discontinued
• Monitor bowel pattern daily; diarrhea may be a problem
• Monitor triglycerides, cholesterol, lipids baseline and during treatment; LDL and VLDL should be watched closely and if increased, drug should be discontinued

Nursing diagnoses
☑ Diarrhea (adverse reactions)
☑ Knowledge, deficient (teaching)
☑ Noncompliance (teaching)

Implementation
• Give 30 min before AM and PM meals

Patient/family education
• Inform patient that compliance is needed for positive results to occur; not to double doses; that drug may be discontinued if no improvement in 3 mo
• Caution patient to decrease risk factors: high-fat diet, smoking, alcohol consumption, lack of exercise
• Advise patient to notify prescriber if GI symptoms of diarrhea, abdominal or epigastric pain, nausea, vomiting occur; or if chills, fever, sore throat occur; also occurrence of muscle cramps, abdominal cramps, severe flatulence

Evaluation
Positive therapeutic outcome
• Decreased cholesterol levels, serum triglyceride and improved ratio with HDLs

---

gemifloxacin
(Factive)
See Appendix A, Selected New Drugs

❗ HIGH ALERT

gemtuzumab (Rx)
(gem-tue-zue′mab)
Mylotarg
Func. class.: Antineoplastic—misc.
Chem. class.: Monoclonal antibody

Pregnancy category D

Action: Composed of recombinant humanized IgG_4 κ antibody, binds to CD33 antigen that is released in myeloid cells

➡ **Therapeutic Outcome:** Decreasing signs/symptoms of leukemia

Uses: Acute myeloid leukemia (AML)

Dosage and routes
Adult: **IV** 9 mg/m² as a 2 hr inf; before giving

inf, give diphenhydrAMINE 50 mg PO, acetaminophen 650-1000 mg PO 1 hr before inf; then use acetaminophen 650-1000 mg q1-4h prn

Available forms: Powder for inj, lyophilized 5 mg

Adverse effects
(*italic* = common; **bold** = life-threatening)
CNS: *Dizziness,* insomnia, depression
CV: Hypertension, **hemorrhage,** tachycardia, hypotension
INTEG: *Rash,* herpes simplex, local reaction, petechiae
GI: Anorexia, diarrhea, constipation, nausea, stomatitis, vomiting
GU: Hematuria, **vaginal hemorrhage**
MISC: *Fever, myalgias, headache, chills*
RESP: Cough, pneumonia, epistaxis, rhinitis
META: Hypokalemia, hypomagnesemia

Contraindications: Hypersensitivity, pregnancy **D**, severe myelosuppression

P **Precautions:** Lactation, children, severe renal or hepatic disease

Pharmacokinetics	
Absorption	Unknown
Distribution	Unknown
Metabolism	Unknown
Excretion	Unknown
Half-life	45, 100 hr, respectively

Pharmacodynamics
Unknown

Interactions
None known

NURSING CONSIDERATIONS
Assessment
• Assess for symptoms of infection; chills, fever, headache, may be masked by drug
• Assess CNS reaction: LOC, mental status, dizziness, confusion
• Assess cardiac status: lung sounds; ECG before and during treatment, especially in those with cardiac disease
• Assess bone marrow depression: bruising, bleeding, blood in stools, urine, sputum, emesis

Nursing diagnoses
☑ Infection, risk for (adverse reactions)
☑ Nutrition: less than body requirements, imbalanced (adverse reactions)
☑ Oral mucous membrane, impaired (adverse reactions)

Implementation
- Do not give **IV** push or bolus
- Protect from light, use biologic safety hood, allow to come to room temp
- Reconstitute each vial with 5 ml of sterile water for inj using sterile syringes, swirl each vial, check for discoloration or particulate matter, give over 2 hr, use a separate line with 1.2 micron terminal filter
- Store reconstituted sol for ≤8 hr in refrigerator

Patient/family education
- Advise patient to take acetaminophen for fever
- Instruct patient to avoid hazardous tasks, since confusion, dizziness may occur; avoid prolonged sunlight, use sunscreen
- Instruct patient to report signs of infection: sore throat, fever, diarrhea, vomiting

Evaluation
Positive therapeutic outcome
- Decrease in size, number of lesions

---

gentamicin (Rx)
(jen-ta-mye′sin)
Cidomycin ✤, G-mycin, Garamycin, Gentamicin Sulfate, Jenamicin
Func. class.: Antiinfective
Chem. class.: Aminoglycoside

Pregnancy category C

Action: Interferes with protein synthesis in bacterial cell by binding to ribosomal subunit, causing misreading of genetic code; inaccurate peptide sequence forms in protein chain, causing bacterial death

Therapeutic Outcome: Bactericidal effects for the following organisms: *Pseudomonas aeruginosa, Proteus, Klebsiella, Serratia, Escherichia coli, Enterobacter, Citrobacter, Staphylococcus, Shigella, Salmonella, Acinetobacter*

Uses: Severe systemic infections of CNS; respiratory, GI, and urinary tracts; bone; skin; soft tissues; acute PID caused by susceptible strains

Dosage and routes
Severe systemic infections
Adult: **IV** inf 3-5 mg/kg/day in 3 divided doses q8h; dilute in 50-200 ml 0.9% NaCl or D₅W given over 30 min-1 hr; IM 3 mg/kg/day in divided doses q8h
Child: **IV**/IM 2-2.5 mg/ kg q8h

Neonates and infants: **IV**/IM 2.5 mg/kg q8-12h
Neonates <1 wk: 2.5 mg/kg q12-24h

Once-daily dosing/extended interval dosing (unlabeled)
Adult: **IV** 4-7 mg/kg q24h adjust according to levels
Renal dose
Adult: IM/**IV** 1-1.7 mg/kg initially, then adjust according to CCr levels

Available forms: Inj 10, 40 mg/ml; premixed inj 40, 60, 70, 80, 100 mg/50 ml; 40, 60, 80, 90, 100, 120, 160, 180 mg/ml

Adverse effects
(*italic* = common; **bold** = life-threatening)
CNS: Confusion, depression, numbness, tremors, **seizures,** muscle twitching, **neurotoxicity,** dizziness, vertigo
CV: Hypotension, hypertension, palpitations
EENT: Ototoxicity, deafness, visual disturbances, tinnitus
GI: Nausea, vomiting, anorexia, increased ALT, AST, bilirubin, hepatomegaly, **hepatic necrosis,** splenomegaly
GU: **Oliguria, hematuria, renal damage, azotemia, renal failure, nephrotoxicity**
HEMA: **Agranulocytosis, thrombocytopenia, leukopenia, eosinophilia,** anemia
INTEG: Rash, burning, urticaria, dermatitis, alopecia

Contraindications: Severe renal disease, hypersensitivity

Precautions: Neonates, mild renal disease, pregnancy **C,** hearing deficits, myasthenia gravis, lactation, elderly, Parkinson's disease

Do Not Confuse:
Garamycin/kanamycin

Pharmacokinetics	
Absorption	Well absorbed (IM)
Distribution	Distributed in extracellular fluids, poorly distributed in CSF; crosses placenta
Metabolism	Liver, minimal
Excretion	Mostly unchanged (79%) kidneys
Half-life	1-2 hr, infants 6-7 hr, increased in renal disease

Pharmacodynamics		
	IM	IV
Onset	Rapid	Rapid
Peak	½-1½ hr	Infusion's end

Interactions
Individual drugs
Amphotericin B, cisplatin, ethacrynic acid,

furosemide, mannitol, methoxyflurane, polymyxin, vancomycin: ↑ ototoxicity, neurotoxicity, nephrotoxicity

Drug classifications

Aminoglycosides, cephalosporins, penicillins: ↑ otoxicity, neurotoxicity, nephrotoxicity
Nondepolarizing neuromuscular blockers: ↑ neuromuscular blockade, respiratory depression

NURSING CONSIDERATIONS
Assessment

• Assess patient for previous sensitivity reaction
• Assess patient for signs and symptoms of infection including characteristics of wounds, sputum, urine, stool, WBC >10,000/mm³, fever; obtain baseline information and during treatment
• Complete culture and sensitivity before beginning drug therapy; this will ensure that correct treatment has been initiated
• Assess for allergic reactions: rash, urticaria, pruritus, chills, fever, joint pain may occur a few days after therapy begins
• Identify urine output; if decreasing, notify prescriber (may indicate nephrotoxicity); also, increased BUN, creatinine, urine CCr <80 ml/min
• Monitor blood studies: AST, ALT, CBC, Hct, bilirubin, LDH, alkaline phosphatase, Coombs' test monthly if patient is on long-term therapy
• Monitor electrolytes: potassium, sodium, chloride, magnesium monthly if patient is on long-term therapy
• Monitor for bleeding: ecchymosis, bleeding gums, hematuria; assess stool guaiac daily if on long-term therapy
• Assess for overgrowth of infection: perineal itching, fever, malaise, redness, pain, swelling, drainage, rash, diarrhea, change in cough, sputum
• Obtain weight before treatment; calculation of dosage is usually based on ideal body weight, but may be calculated on actual body weight
• Monitor I&O ratio; urinalysis daily for proteinuria, cells, casts; report sudden change in urine output
• Monitor VS during inf, watch for hypotension, change in pulse
• Assess **IV** site for thrombophlebitis including pain, redness, swelling q30 min, change site if needed; apply warm compresses to discontinue site
• Obtain serum peak, measured at 30-60 min after **IV** inf or 60 min after IM inj, trough level measured just before next dose; blood level should be 2-4 times bacteriostatic level
• Assess urine pH if drug is used for UTI; urine should be kept alkaline
• Assess for deafness by audiometric testing, ringing, roaring in ears, vertigo; assess hearing before, during, after treatment
• Assess for dehydration: high sp gr, decrease in skin turgor, dry mucous membranes, dark urine

Nursing diagnoses

☑ Infection, risk for (uses)
☑ Diarrhea (side effects)
☑ Knowledge, deficient (teaching)
☑ Noncompliance (teaching)
☑ Injury, risk for (side effects)

Implementation
IM route

• Give inj deeply in large muscle mass; rotate sites

Topical route

• Wash hands, wear gloves, clean skin before applying

Ⅳ IV route

• Give in even doses around the clock; drug must be given for 10-14 days to ensure organism death and prevent superimposed infection
• Give by intermittent inf over ½-1 hr, flush with 0.9% NaCl or D₅W after inf
• Separate aminoglycosides and penicillins by ≥1 hr
• Store in tight container

Syringe compatibilities: Clindamycin, methicillin, penicillin G sodium

Y-site compatibilities: Acyclovir, amifostine, amiodarone, amsacrine, atracurium, aztreonam, cefpirome, ciprofloxacin, cyclophosphamide, cytarabine, diltiazem, enalaprilat, esmolol, famotidine, fluconazole, fludarabine, foscarnet, granisetron, hydromorphone, IL-2, insulin, labetalol, lorazepam, magnesium sulfate, melphalan, meperidine, meropenem, midazolam, morphine, multivitamins, ondansetron, paclitaxel, pancuronium, perphenazine, sargramostim, tacrolimus, teniposide, theophylline, thiotepa, tolazine, vecuronium, vinorelbine, vit B with C, zidovudine

Y-site incompatibilities: Idarubicin, indomethacin, zidovudine

Additive compatibilities: Atracurium, aztreonam, bleomycin, cefoxitin, cimetidine, ciprofloxacin, fluconazole, meropenem, methicillin, metronidazole, ofloxacin, penicillin G sodium, ranitidine, verapamil

---

Patient/family education
- Teach patient to report sore throat, bruising, bleeding, joint pain; may indicate blood dyscrasias (rare)
- Advise patient to contact prescriber if vaginal itching, loose foul-smelling stools, furry tongue occur; may indicate superimposed infection

Evaluation
Positive therapeutic outcome
- Absence of signs/symptoms of infection (WBC <10,000/mm³, temp WNL, absence of red, draining wounds)
- Reported improvement in symptoms of infection

Treatment of overdose: Withdraw drug, hemodialysis

---

glatiramer (Rx)
(glah-teer'a-mer)
Copaxone
Func. class.: Multiple sclerosis agent

Pregnancy category B

Action: Unknown; may modify the immune responses responsible for multiple sclerosis

Therapeutic outcome: Decreased symptoms of multiple sclerosis

Uses: Reduction of the frequency of relapses in patients with relapsing-remitting multiple sclerosis

Dosage and routes
Adult: SC 20 mg/day

Available forms: Inj 20 mg/ml

Adverse effects
(*italic* = common; **bold** = life-threatening)
CNS: Anxiety, hypertonia, tremor, vertigo, speech disorder, agitation, confusion
CV: Migraine, palpitations, syncope, tachycardia, vasodilatation
EENT: Ear pain
GI: Nausea, vomiting, diarrhea, anorexia, gastroenteritis
GU: Urgency, dysmenorrhea, vaginal moniliasis
HEMA: Ecchymosis, lymphadenopathy
INTEG: Pruritus, rash, sweating, urticaria, erythema
META: Edema, weight gain
MS: Arthralgia
RESP: Bronchitis, dyspnea

Contraindications: Hypersensitivity to this drug or mannitol

Precautions: Immune disorders, renal disease, pregnancy **B**, lactation

Pharmacokinetics
Absorption	Unknown
Distribution	Unknown
Metabolism	Unknown
Excretion	Unknown
Half-life	Unknown

Pharmacodynamics
Unknown

NURSING CONSIDERATIONS
Assessment
- Monitor blood, renal, hepatic studies; before treatment
- Assess for CNS symptoms: anxiety, confusion, vertigo
- Assess GI status: diarrhea, vomiting, abdominal pain, gastroenteritis
- Assess cardiac status: tachycardia, palpitations, vasodilatation, chest pain

Nursing diagnoses
✓ Knowledge, deficient (teaching)
✓ Noncompliance (teaching)

Implementation
SC route
- Use a sterile syringe/needle to transfer the supplied diluent into the vial, rotate vial gently, do not shake; withdraw medication using a syringe with 27-G needle; administer SC into hip, thigh, arm; discard unused portion
- Use SC route only; do not give IM or **IV**
- Do not use sol that contains precipitate or is discolored

Patient/family education
- Give written, detailed instructions about the drug; provide initial and return demonstrations on inj procedure; give information on use and disposal of drug
- Advise patient that blurred vision, sweating may occur
- Advise patient that irregular menses, dysmenorrhea, or metorrhagia as well as breast pain may occur; use contraception during treatment
- Advise patient that if pregnancy is suspected or if nursing to notify prescriber
- Advise patient not to change dosing or to stop taking drug without advice of prescriber

Evaluation
Positive therapeutic outcome
- Decreased symptoms of multiple sclerosis

glimepiride (Rx)
(gly-meh'pih-ride)
Amaride
***glipiZIDE** (Rx)
(glip-i'zide)
Glucotrol, Glucotrol **XL**
Func. class.: Antidiabetic
Chem. class.: Sulfonylurea (2nd generation)

Pregnancy category C

Action: Causes functioning β-cells in pancreas to release insulin, leading to drop in blood glucose levels; may improve insulin binding to insulin receptors or increase the number of insulin receptors with prolonged administration; may also reduce basal hepatic glucose secretion; not effective if patient lacks functioning β-cells

➔ Therapeutic Outcome: Decrease in polyuria, polydipsia, polyphagia, clear sensorium, absence of dizziness, stable gait

Uses: Stable adult-onset diabetes mellitus (type 2)

Dosage and routes
Glimepiride
Adult: PO 1-2 mg qd, then increase q1-2 wk up to 8 mg/day

Renal dose
Adult: CCr <20 ml/min; PO 1 mg qd with breakfast, may titrate upward as needed

GlipiZIDE
Adult: PO 5 mg initially, then increase to desired response; max 40 mg/day in divided doses or 15 mg/dose

G *Elderly/hepatic dose:* PO 2.5 mg initially, then increase to desired response; max 40 mg/day in divided doses or 15 mg/dose

Available forms: *glimepiride* tabs 1, 2, 4 mg; *glipiZIDE* tabs 5, 10 mg scored; ext rel tab 5, 10 mg

Adverse effects
(*italic* = common; **bold** = life-threatening)
CNS: *Headache, weakness, dizziness, drowsiness,* tinnitus, fatigue, vertigo
ENDO: **Hypoglycemia**
GI: **Hepatotoxicity, cholestatic jaundice,** nausea, vomiting, diarrhea, heartburn
HEMA: **Leukopenia, thrombocytopenia, agranulocytosis, aplastic anemia,** increased AST, ALT, alkaline phosphatase, **pancytopenia, hemolytic anemia**
INTEG: Rash, allergic reactions, pruritus, urticaria, eczema, photosensitivity, erythema

Contraindications: Hypersensitivity to

P sulfonylureas, juvenile or type 1 PM diabetes, diabetic ketoacidosis

G **Precautions:** Pregnancy **C**, elderly, cardiac disease, severe renal disease, severe hepatic disease, thyroid disease

N **Do Not Confuse:**
glipiZIDE/glucotrol/glyBURIDE

Pharmacokinetics	
Absorption	Completely absorbed GI tract
Distribution	Unknown
Metabolism	Liver
Excretion	Via kidneys
Half-life	2-4 hr

Pharmacodynamics	
Onset	1-1½ hr
Peak	1-3 hr
Duration	10-24 hr

Interactions
Individual drugs
Charcoal, cholestyramine, isoniazid, rifampin: possible ↓ action of glipiZIDE
Chloramphenicol, cimetidine, clofibrate, fenfluramine, gemfibrozil, methyldopa, phenylbutazone, probenecid, sulfinpyrizine: ↑ hypoglycemia
Coenzyme Q10: ↑ or ↓ hypoglycemic effect
Diazoxide: Both drugs may have action ↓
Digitalis: ↑ action of digitalis
Digoxin: ↓ action of glipiZIDE
Drug classifications
Androgens, anticoagulants, H₂-antagonists, magnesium salts, MAOIs, NSAIDs, salicylates, sulfonamides, tricyclics, urinary acidifiers: ↑ hypoglycemia
β-Blockers: May mask symptoms of hypoglycemia
Diuretics (thiazide), hydantoins, urinary alkalinizers: Possible ↓ action of glipiZIDE
Glycosides: ↑ action of glycosides
Z *Herb/drug*
Alfalfa, aloe, basil, bay, bilberry, bitter melon, black catechu, buchu, burdock, coriander, dandelion, eyebright (po), fenugreek, garlic, ginseng, glucomannan, glucosamine, goat's rue, gymnema, horehound, horse chestnut, jambul, myrrh, myrtle: ↑ antidiabetic effect
Bee pollen, blue cohosh, broom, chromium, elecampane, eucalyptus, gotu kola: ↓ antidiabetic effect
Glucosamine: ↓ hypoglycemic effect

NURSING CONSIDERATIONS
Assessment
• Assess for hypoglycemic/hyperglycemic reactions that can occur soon pc; hypoglyce-

 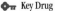

mic reactions (sweating, weakness, dizziness, anxiety, tremors, hunger); hyperglycemic reactions
• Monitor CBC, glycosylated Hgb (baseline, q3 mo) during treatment; check liver function tests periodically: AST, LDH, and renal studies: BUN, creatinine during treatment

Nursing diagnoses
☑ Nutrition: more than body requirements, imbalanced (uses)
☑ Nutrition: less than body requirements, imbalanced (adverse reactions)
☑ Injury, risk for (adverse reactions)
☑ Knowledge, deficient (teaching)
☑ Noncompliance (teaching)

Implementation
• Convert from other oral hypoglycemic agents or insulin dosage of <40 units/day; change may be made without gradual dosage change.
• Patients taking >40 units/day of insulin convert gradually by receiving oral hypoglycemic agents and 50% of previous insulin dosage for 3-5 days
• Monitor serum or urine glucose and ketones 3 ×/day during conversion
• Give drug 30 min before breakfast; if large dose is required, may be divided into 2 doses; give with meals to decrease GI upset and provide best absorption; if patient is NPO, may need to hold dose to prevent hypoglycemia
• Give tab crushed and mixed with meal or fluids for patients with difficulty swallowing; ⊘ do not crush, break, or chew ext rel tabs
• For severe hypoglycemia give **IV** D$_{50}$W, then **IV** dextrose solution
• Store in tight container in cool environment

Patient/family education
• Teach patient to check for symptoms of cholestatic jaundice: dark urine, pruritus, yellow sclera; if these occur, prescriber should be notified
• Teach patient to use capillary blood glucose test or Chemstrip 3 ×/day
• Teach patient symptoms of hypo/hyperglycemia, what to do about each
• Instruct patient that drug must be continued on daily basis; explain consequence of discontinuing drug abruptly
• Teach patient to take drug in AM to prevent hypoglycemic reactions at night
• Caution patient to avoid OTC medications unless approved by a prescriber
• Teach patient that diabetes is a lifelong illness; that this drug is not a cure
• Teach patient to avoid alcohol; inform about

disulfiram reaction (nausea, headache, cramps, flushing, hypoglycemia)
• Instruct patient that all food included in diet plan must be eaten to prevent hypoglycemia
• Advise patient to use sunscreen or stay out of the sun to prevent burns
• Advise patient to carry/wear emergency ID and carry a glucagon emergency kit for emergency purposes; also prescriber name, phone number, and medications taken
• Teach patient ext rel tab may appear in stool

Evaluation
Positive therapeutic outcome
• Decrease in polyuria, polydipsia, polyphagia, clear sensorium, absence of dizziness, stable gait

---

*glyBURIDE (Rx)
(glye′byoor-ide)
Apo-Glyburide ✤, DiaBeta ✤, Euglucon ✤, Gen-Glyben ✤, Glynase PresTab, Micronase, novo-Glyburide ✤, nu-Glyburide ✤
Func. class.: Antidiabetic
Chem. class.: Sulfonylurea (2nd generation)

Pregnancy category C

Action: Causes functioning β-cells in pancreas to release insulin, leading to drop in blood glucose levels; may improve insulin binding to insulin receptors and increase number of insulin receptors with prolonged administration; may also reduce basal hepatic glucose secretion; not effective if patient lacks functioning β-cells

➔**Therapeutic Outcome:** Decrease in polyuria, polydipsia, polyphagia, clear sensorium, absence of dizziness, stable gait

Uses: Stable adult-onset diabetes mellitus (type 2) NIDDM

Dosage and routes
DiaBeta/Micronase
Adult: PO 1.25-5 mg initially, then increased to desired response at weekly intervals up to 20 mg/day

G *Elderly:* PO 1.25 mg initially, then increased to desired response; max 20 mg/day, maintenance 1.25-20 mg/qd

Glynase PresTab (micronized)
Adult: PO 1.5-3 mg/day initially, may increase by 1.5 mg/wk, max 12 mg/day

G *Elderly:* PO 0.75-3 mg/day, may increase by 1.5 mg/wk

Available forms: (Diabeta)Tabs 1.25, 2.5, 5 mg; tabs micronized (Glynase PresTab) 1.5, 3, 6 mg

Adverse effects
(*italic* = common; **bold** = life-threatening)
CNS: *Headache, weakness,* paresthesia, tinnitus, fatigue, vertigo
ENDO: Hypoglycemia
GI: Nausea, fullness, heartburn, **hepatoxicity, cholestatic jaundice,** vomiting, diarrhea
HEMA: **Leukopenia, thrombocytopenia, agranulocytosis, aplastic anemia,** increased AST, ALT, alkaline phosphatase
INTEG: Rash, allergic reactions, pruritus, urticaria, eczema, photosensitivity, erythema
MS: Joint pains

Contraindications: Hypersensitivity to sulfonylureas, juvenile or type 1 diabetes, diabetic ketoacidosis

Precautions: Pregnancy **B,** elderly, cardiac disease, severe renal disease, severe hepatic disease, thyroid disease, severe hypoglycemic reactions

Do Not Confuse:
DiaBeta/Zebeta, glyBURIDE/Glucotrol/glipiZIDE

Pharmacokinetics	
Absorption	Completely absorbed GI tract
Distribution	99% plasma protein binding
Metabolism	Liver
Excretion	Urine, feces (metabolites), crosses placenta
Half-life	10 hr

Pharmacodynamics	
Onset	2-4 hr
Peak	4 hr
Duration	24 hr

Interactions
Individual drugs
Charcoal, cholestyramine, isoniazid, rifampin: ↓ action of glyBURIDE
Chloramphenicol, fenfluramine, fluconazole, gemfibrozil, guanethidine, insulin, methyldopa, phenylbutazone, probenecid, sulfinpyrazone: ↑ hypoglycemia
Coenzyme Q10: ↑ or ↓ hypoglycemic effect
Diazoxide: Both drugs may have action decreased
Digoxin: ↑ level
Drug classifications
Androgens, anticoagulants, antidepressants (tricyclics), H_2-antagonists, magnesium salts, MAOIs, NSAIDs, salicylates, sulfonamides, urinary acidifiers: ↑ hypoglycemia
β-Adrenergic blockers: ↑ masking of symptoms of hypoglycemia
Diuretics (thiazide), hydantoins, urinary alkalinizers: ↓ action of glyBURIDE

Herb/drug
Alfalfa, aloe, basil, bay, bilberry, bitter melon, black catechu, buchu, burdock, coriander, dandelion, eyebright (po), fenugreek, garlic, ginseng, glucomannan, glucosamine, goat's rue, gymnema, horehound, horse chestnut, jambul, myrrh, myrtle: ↑ antidiabetic effect
Bee pollen, blue cohosh, broom, chromium, elecampane, eucalyptus, gotu kola: ↓ antidiabetic effect
Broom, buchu, dandelion, juniper: ↓ hypoglycemic effect
Chromium, fenugreek, ginseng: ↑ or ↓ hypoglycemic effect
Karela: ↑ glucose tolerance

NURSING CONSIDERATIONS
Assessment
• Assess for hypo/hyperglycemic reactions that can occur soon pc; hypoglycemic reactions (sweating, weakness, dizziness, anxiety, tremors, hunger); hyperglycemic reactions
• Monitor CBC, glycosylated Hgb (baseline, q3 mo) during treatment; check liver function tests periodically, AST, LDH, and renal studies: BUN, creatinine during treatment

Nursing diagnoses
☑ Nutrition: more than body requirements, imbalanced (uses)
☑ Nutrition: less than body requirements, imbalanced (adverse reactions)
☑ Injury, risk for (adverse reactions)
☑ Knowledge, deficient (teaching)
☑ Noncompliance (teaching)

Implementation
• Conversion from other oral hypoglycemic agents or insulin dosage of <40 units/day; change may be made without gradual dosage change
• Patients taking >40 units/day of insulin convert gradually by receiving oral hypoglycemic agents and 50% of previous insulin dosage for 3-5 days
• Monitor serum or urine glucose and ketones 3 ×/day during conversion
• Give drug 30 min before breakfast; if large dose is required, may be divided into two; give with meals to decrease GI upset and provide best absorption, if patient is NPO, may need to hold dose to avoid hypoglycemia

 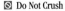

- Give tab crushed and mixed with meal or fluids for patients with difficulty swallowing
- For severe hypoglycemia, give **IV** D$_{50}$W, then **IV** dextrose sol
- Store in tight container in cool environment

Patient/family education

- Teach patient to check for symptoms of cholestatic jaundice: dark urine, pruritus, yellow sclera; if these occur, prescriber should be notified
- Teach patient to use capillary blood glucose test or Chemstrip 3 ×/day
- Teach patient symptoms of hypo/hyperglycemia, what to do about each
- Instruct patient that drug must be continued on daily basis; explain consequence of discontinuing drug abruptly
- Teach patient to take drug in AM to prevent hypoglycemic reactions at night
- Caution patient to avoid OTC medications unless approved by a prescriber
- Teach patient that diabetes is a lifelong illness; that this drug is not a cure
- Instruct patient that all food included in diet plan must be eaten to prevent hypoglycemia
- Advise patient to carry/wear emergency ID and carry a glucagon emergency kit for emergency purposes: have sugar packets available; also prescriber name, phone number, and medications
- Advise patient to use sunscreen or stay out of the sun to prevent burns

Evaluation

Positive therapeutic outcome
- Decrease in polyuria, polydipsia, polyphagia, clear sensorium, absence of dizziness, stable gait

---

glycerin (OTC)
(gli'ser-in)

Fleet Babylax, glycerin USP, Glycerol, Ophthalgan, Sani-Supp

Func. class.: Laxative, hyperosmotic, antiglaucoma agent

Chem. class.: Trihydric alcohol

Pregnancy category C

Action: Increases osmotic pressure by drawing fluid into colon lumen from extravascular spaces to intravascular

➔ **Therapeutic Outcome:** Absence of constipation, intraocular pressure, ICP, absence of edema in the cornea

Uses: Constipation, intraocular pressure in glaucoma; ICP, edema in the superficial layers of the cornea

Dosage and routes

Laxative

P *Adult and child >6 yr:* REC SUPP 3 g; enema 5-15 ml

P *Child <6 yr:* REC SUPP 1-1.5 g; enema 2-5 ml

Intraocular pressure reduction

Adult: PO 1-1.5 g/kg once, then may be given 500 mg/kg q6h

P *Child:* PO 1-1.5 g/kg qd once, then 500 mg/kg 4-8 hr after first dose

Available forms: Rec sol 4 ml/applicator; supp; oral sol 0.6/ml; ophth sol 7.5 ml/container

Adverse effects

(*italic* = common; **bold** = life-threatening)

CNS: Headache, confusion, **seizures**

GI: Nausea, vomiting, diarrhea

META: Dehydration

Contraindications: Hypersensitivity

Precautions: Pregnancy **C**

Pharmacokinetics	
Absorption	Well absorbed (PO), not absorbed (rec)
Distribution	To intravascular space
Metabolism	Liver—80%, kidneys—20%
Excretion	Kidneys
Half-life	30 min

Pharmacodynamics			
	PO	REC	OPHTH
Onset	10-30 min	Unknown	Unknown
Peak	30-120 min	30 min	Unknown
Duration	6-8 hr	Unknown	Up to 4 hr

Interactions

Drug classifications

Diuretics: ↓ effect of glycerin (ophth)

NURSING CONSIDERATIONS

Assessment
- Assess patient for cause of constipation; identify whether fluids, bulk, or exercise is missing from lifestyle; check for distention, bowel sounds
- After administration, check for cramping, rectal bleeding, nausea, vomiting; if these symptoms occur, drug should be discontinued
- Identify stool characteristics: consistency, color, amount, shape, volume

Nursing diagnoses

☑ Constipation (uses)

G

✔ Knowledge, deficient (teaching)

Implementation
Rectal route
- Insert glycerin supp after removing wrapper; may cause evacuation in ½ hr
- For evening use 4-ml applications of fluid, have patient in side-lying position, have patient retain for a few min

Ophthalmic route
- Instill 1-2 gtt in one or both eyes by pulling down on conjunctival sac
- Do not use ophth sol that is discolored, has a precipitate, or is cloudy

PO route
- Pour over cracked ice and sip through a straw
- To prevent severe cerebral dehydration headache have patient recumbent during and after administration
- Give by mixing 50% glycerin sol with 0.9% NaCl with flavoring, or use oral sol that is already flavored; flavoring improves taste and prevents GI symptoms
- Store in cool environment; do not freeze

Patient/family education
- Caution patient not to use laxatives for long-term therapy; normal bowel tone will be lost; that normal bowel movements do not always occur daily
- Advise patient not to use in presence of abdominal pain, nausea, vomiting
- Instruct patient to notify prescriber if constipation is unrelieved or if weakness, dizziness, excessive thirst occur

Evaluation
Positive therapeutic outcome
- Decreased constipation
- Decreased intraocular pressure

---

glycopyrrolate (Rx)
(glye-koe-pye'roe-late)
glycopyrrolate, Robinul, Robinul-Forte
Func. class.: Cholinergic blocker
Chem. class.: Quaternary ammonium compound

Pregnancy category B

Action: Inhibits action of acetylcholine at receptor sites in autonomic nervous system, which controls secretions, free acids in stomach

➡ **Therapeutic Outcome:** Decreased secretions in the respiratory tract, GI system

Uses: Decreased secretions before surgery, reversal of neuromuscular blockade, peptic ulcer disease, irritable bowel syndrome

Investigational uses: Drooling

Dosage and routes
Preoperatively
Adult: IM 4.4 mcg/kg ½-1 hr before surgery, max 0.1 mg

P *Child:* IM 4.4-8.8 mcg/kg ½-1 hr before surgery

Reversal of neuromuscular blockage
P *Adult and child:* IV 200 mcg for each 1 mg of neostigmine or 5 mg IV of pyridostigmine simultaneously

Drooling
Adult: PO doses vary widely

GI disorders
Adult: PO 1-2 mg bid-tid; IM/IV 100-200 mcg tid-qid, titrated to patient response

Antidysrhythmic
Adult: IV 100 mcg, may repeat q2 min

P *Child:* IV 4.4 mcg/kg, may repeat q2 min, max 100 mcg

Available forms: Tabs 1, 2 mg; inj 200 mcg 0.2 mg/ml

Adverse effects
(*italic* = common; **bold** = life-threatening)
CNS: Confusion, anxiety, restlessness, irritability, delusions, hallucinations, headache, sedation, depression, incoherence, dizziness, lethargy, flushing, weakness
CV: Palpitations, tachycardia, postural hypotension, paradoxical bradycardia
EENT: Blurred vision, photophobia, dilated pupils, difficulty swallowing, increased intraocular pressure, mydriasis, cycloplegia
GI: Dryness of mouth, constipation, nausea, vomiting, abdominal distress, paralytic ileus, altered taste perception
GU: Hesitancy, retention, impotence
INTEG: Urticaria, allergic reactions
MISC: Suppression of lactation, nasal congestion, decreased sweating, **anaphylaxis**

Contraindications: Hypersensitivity, narrow-angle glaucoma, myasthenia gravis,
P GI/GU obstruction, child <3 yr, tachycardia, myocardial ischemia, hepatic disease, ulcerative colitis, toxic megacolon

G **Precautions:** Pregnancy **B**, elderly, lactation, prostatic hypertrophy, renal disease, CHF, pulmonary disease, hyperthyroidism

---

 Herb/drug   Do Not Crush   Alert   Key Drug   G Geriatric   P Pediatric

Pharmacokinetics

Absorption	Well absorbed (PO, SC, IM)
Distribution	Unknown
Metabolism	Not metabolized
Excretion	Unchanged feces
Half-life	2 hr

Pharmacodynamics

	PO	IM	IV
Onset	Unknown	15-30 min	Immediate
Peak	1 hr	30-45 min	10-15 min
Duration	8-12 hr	2-7 hr	2-7 hr

Interactions
Individual drugs
Alcohol, amantadine: ↑ anticholinergic effect
Drug classifications
Antacids: ↓ absorption of glycopyrrolate
Antidepressants (tricyclic), antihistamines, phenothiazines: ↑ anticholinergic effect
Antidiarrheals: ↓ absorption of glycopyrrolate

NURSING CONSIDERATIONS
Assessment
• Monitor I&O ratio; retention commonly causes decreased urinary output; check for urinary hesitation; palpate bladder if retention occurs
• Monitor ECG for ectopic ventricular beats, PVC, tachycardia
• Monitor for bowel sounds; check for constipation; increase fluids, bulk, exercise if constipation occurs
• Assess mental status: affect, mood, CNS depression, worsening of psychiatric symptoms during early therapy

Nursing diagnoses
✓ Knowledge, deficient (teaching)

Implementation
IV IV route
• Administer **IV** undiluted, give at a rate of 0.2 mg or less over 5-15 min through Y-tube or 3-way stopcock; do not add to **IV** sol
• Administer parenteral dose with patient recumbent to prevent postural hypotension

Syringe compatibilities: Atropine, benzquinamide, chlorproMAZINE, cimetidine, codeine, diphenhydrAMINE, droperidol, droperidol/fentanyl, hydromorphone, hydrOXYzine, levorphanol, lidocaine, meperidine, meperidine/promethazine, midazolam, morphine, nalbuphine, neostigmine, oxymorphone, procaine, prochlorperazine, promazine, promethazine, pyridostigmine, ranitidine, scopolamine, triflupromazine, trimethobenzamide

Y-site compatibilities: Propofol
Solution compatibilities: D$_5$W, 0.9% NaCl, Ringer's D$_5$/0.45% NaCl
PO route
• Give PO with or after meals to prevent GI upset; may give with fluids other than water
IM route
• Give IM inj deeply in large muscle mass

Patient/family education
• Caution patient not to operate machinery or engage in hazardous activities if drowsiness, blurred vision occurs
• Advise patient not to take OTC products, cough, cold preparations with alcohol, antihistamines without approval of prescriber
• Teach patient to avoid hot temp; since sweating is decreased, heat stroke is possible
• Advise patient to notify prescriber of eye pain, blurred vision, light sensitivity
• Caution patient not to discontinue this drug abruptly; tapering should be done over 1 wk

Evaluation
Positive therapeutic outcome
• Decreased secretions, bronchial, GI
• Decreased pain in GI disorders
• Reversal of neuromuscular blockade

goserelin (Rx)
(goe′se-rel-lin)
Zoladex
Func. class.: Gonadotropin-releasing hormone, antineoplastic
Chem. class.: Synthetic decapeptide analog of LHRH

Pregnancy category X

Action: Inhibitor of pituitary gonadotropin secretion; initially increases LH and FSH, with increases in testosterone, reduction in sex steroid levels (substitute serum testosterone levels)

⟶**Therapeutic Outcome:** Decrease in tumor size and spread of malignant cells

Uses: Advanced prostate cancer (10.8 mg); endometriosis, advanced breast cancer, endometrial thinning (3.6 mg)

Dosage and routes
Adult: SC 3.6 mg q4 wk (implant) or 10.8 mg q12 wk

Endometrial thinning
Adult: SC 1-2 depot inj; usually 1 depot,

surgery performed at 4 wk; if 2 depots, surgery performed 2-4 wk after 2nd depot

Available forms: Depot inj 3.6, 10.8 mg

Adverse effects
(*italic* = common; **bold** = life-threatening)
CNS: Headaches, **spinal cord compression,** anxiety, depression
CV: **Dysrhythmia, cerebrovascular accident,** hypertension, **MI,** chest pain
ENDO: Gynecomastia, breast tenderness, hot flashes
GI: Nausea, vomiting, constipation, diarrhea, ulcer
GU: *Spotting, breakthrough bleeding, decreased libido,* renal insufficiency, urinary obstruction, urinary tract infection, impotence
INTEG: Rash, pain on inj
MS: Osteoneuralgia

Contraindications: Hypersensitivity to LHRH, LHRH-agonist analogs, pregnancy **D** (breast cancer), pregnancy **X** (endometriosis, lactation, nondiagnosed vaginal bleeding)

P Precautions: Children, lactation

Pharmacokinetics	
Absorption	Well absorbed
Distribution	Unknown
Metabolism	Unknown
Excretion	Unknown
Half-life	4½ hr

Pharmacodynamics	
Onset	Unknown
Peak	14-28 days
Duration	Treatment length

Interactions: None
Lab test interferences
↑ Alkaline phosphatase, ↑ estradiol, ↑ FSH, ↑ LH, ↑ testosterone levels
↓ Testosterone levels, ↓ progesterone

NURSING CONSIDERATIONS
Assessment
• Assess for relief of bone pain (back pain), change in motor function
• Monitor I&O ratios, palpate bladder for distention (urinary obstruction) at beginning of treatment; renal insufficiency and obstruction may occur
• Monitor acid phosphatase, PSA baseline and periodically

Nursing diagnoses
☑ Sexual dysfunction (uses)
☑ Knowledge, deficient (teaching)

Implementation
• Administer via implant inserted by qualified persons into upper subcutaneous tissue in abdominal wall q28 days or q12 wk (10.8 mg)

Patient/family education
• Caution patient that gynecomastia and postmenopausal symptoms may occur but will decrease after treatment is discontinued; that bone pain may increase, then decrease
• Teach patient to contact prescriber if difficulty urinating, hot flashes occur during treatment
• Advise patient not to breastfeed while taking drug

Evaluation
Positive therapeutic outcome
• More normal levels of PSA, acid phosphatase, alkaline phosphatase; testosterone level of <25 mg/dl

---

granisetron (Rx)
(grane-iss'e-tron)
Kytril
Func. class.: Antiemetic
Chem. class.: 5-HT₃ receptor antagonist
Pregnancy category C

Action: Prevents nausea, vomiting by blocking serotonin peripherally, centrally, and in the small intestine

⮕ **Therapeutic Outcome:** Absence of nausea and vomiting

Uses: Prevention of nausea, vomiting associated with cancer chemotherapy including high-dose cisplatin

Investigational uses: Acute nausea, vomiting after surgery

Dosage and routes
Nausea, vomiting in chemotherapy
P *Adult and child:* **IV** 10 mcg/kg over 5 min, 30 min before the start of cancer chemotherapy; 1 mg bid, give 1st dose 1 hr before chemotherapy and next dose 12 hr after 1st

Nausea, vomiting in radiation therapy
Adult: PO 2 mg qd 1 hr prior to radiation

Available forms: Inj 1 mg/ml; tabs 1 mg

Adverse effects
(*italic* = common; **bold** = life-threatening)
CNS: *Headache, asthenia,* anxiety, dizziness
CV: Hypertension

GI: Diarrhea, *constipation,* increased AST, ALT, *nausea*
HEMA: **Leukopenia,** anemia, **thrombocytopenia**
MISC: Rash, **bronchospasm**

Contraindications: Hypersensitivity

P Precautions: Pregnancy **B,** lactation,
G children, elderly

Pharmacokinetics

Absorption	Unknown
Distribution	Unknown
Metabolism	Liver
Excretion	Unknown
Half-life	10-12 hr

Pharmacodynamics
Unknown

Interactions: None

NURSING CONSIDERATIONS
Assessment
• Assess patient for absence of nausea, vomiting during chemotherapy
• Assess patient for hypersensitive reaction: rash, bronchospasm

Nursing diagnoses
☑ Fluid volume, deficient (uses)
☑ Knowledge, deficient (teaching)

Implementation
• Administer **IV**
• Dilute in 0.9% NaCl for inj or D_5W (20-50 ml), give over 5-15 min
• Store at room temp for 24-hr dilution

Y-site compatibilities: Acyclovir, allopurinol, amifostine, amikacin, aminophylline, amphotericin B cholesteryl, ampicillin, ampicillin/sulbactam, amsacrine, aztreonam, bleomycin, bumetanide, buprenorphine, butorphanol, calcium gluconate, carboplatin, carmustine, cefazolin, cefepime, cefonicid, cefoperazone, cefotaxime, cefotetan, cefoxitin, ceftazidime, ceftizoxime, ceftriaxone, cefuroxime, chlorproMAZINE, cimetidine, ciprofloxacin, cisplatin, cladribine, clindamycin, cyclophosphamide, cytarabine, dacarbazine, dactinomycin, DAUNOrubicin, dexamethasone, diphenhydrAMINE, DOBUTamine, DOPamine, DOXOrubicin, DOXOrubicin liposome, doxycycline, droperidol, enalaprilat, etoposide, famotidine, filgrastim, floxuridine, fluconazole, fluorouracil, fludarabine, furosemide, gallium, ganciclovir, gentamicin, haloperidol, heparin, hydrocortisone, hydromorphone, hydrOXYzine, idarubicin, ifosfamide, imipenem-cilastatin, leucovorin, lorazepam, magnesium sulfate, melphalan, meperidine, mesna, methotrexate, methylPREDNISolone, metoclopramide, metronidazole, mezlocillin, miconazole, minocycline, mitomycin, mitoxantrone, morphine, nalbuphine, netilmicin, ofloxacin, paclitaxel, piperacillin, piperacillin/tazobactam, plicamycin, potassium chloride, prochlorperazine, promethazine, propofol, ranitidine, sargramostim, sodium bicarbonate, streptozocin, teniposide, thiotepa, ticarcillin, ticarcillin/clavulanate, tobramycin, trimethoprim/sulfamethoxazole, vancomycin, vinBLAStine, vinCRIStine, vinorelbine, zidovudine

Y-site incompatibilities: Fluorouracil, furosemide, sodium bicarbonate

Additive compatibilities: Dexamethasone, methylPREDNISolone

Solution compatibilities: D_5W, 0.9% NaCl

Patient/family education
• Advise patient to report diarrhea, constipation, rash, or changes in respirations

Evaluation
Positive therapeutic outcome
• Absence of nausea, vomiting during cancer chemotherapy

---

guaifenesin (Rx, OTC)
(gwye-fen'e-sin)
Anti-tuss, Benylin-E ✦, Breonesin, Calmylin Expectorant ✦, Diabetic Tussin EX, Duratuss-G, Fenesin, Gee-Gee, Genatuss, GG-Cen, Glyate, Glycotuss, Glytuss, guaifenesin, Guaifenex LA, Guiatuss, Halotussin, Humibid, Humibid L.A., Hytuss, Hytuss 2X, Liquibid, Monafed, Muco-Fen LA, Mytussin, Naldecon Senior EX, Organidin NR, Pneumomist, Respa-GF, Resyl ✦, Robitussin, Scot-Tussin Expectorant, Sinumist-SR, Uni-Tussin
Func. class.: Expectorant

Pregnancy category C

Action: Acts as an expectorant by stimulating a gastric mucosal reflex to increase the production of lung mucus

⇒ Therapeutic Outcome: Decreased cough

Uses: Dry, nonproductive cough

G

Dosage and routes
Adult: PO 200-400 mg q4-6h, or 600-1200 mg q12h (ext rel) not to exceed 2.4 g/day

 Child 6-12 yr: PO 100-200 mg q4h or 600 mg q12h (ext rel); not to exceed 1.2 g/day

 Child 2-6 yr: PO: 50-100 mg q4h; not to exceed 600 mg/day

Available forms: Tabs 100, 200 mg; tabs, ext rel 600, 1200 mg; caps 200 mg; syr 100 mg, 200/5 ml; ext rel caps 300 mg

Adverse effects
(*italic* = common; **bold** = life-threatening)
CNS: Drowsiness
GI: Nausea, anorexia, vomiting

Contraindications: Hypersensitivity, persistent cough

Precautions: Pregnancy **C**

Pharmacokinetics
Absorption	Well absorbed
Distribution	Unknown
Metabolism	Unknown
Excretion	Unknown
Half-life	Unknown

Pharmacodynamics
	PO	PO ER
Onset	½ hr	Unknown
Peak	Unknown	Unknown
Duration	4-6 hr	12 hr

Interactions: None

NURSING CONSIDERATIONS
Assessment
• Assess cough: type, frequency, character, including characteristics of sputum; lung sounds bilaterally; fluids should be increased to 2 L/day to decrease secretion viscosity (thickness)

Nursing diagnoses
☑ Airway clearance, ineffective (uses)
☑ Knowledge, deficient (teaching)

Implementation
• Store at room temp; provide room humidification to assist with liquefying secretions
• Avoid fluids for ½ hr after administration

Patient/family education
• Caution patient to avoid driving, other hazardous activities if drowsiness occurs (rare)
• Advise patient to avoid smoking, smoke-filled rooms, perfumes, dust, environmental pollutants, cleansers

• Instruct patient to notify prescriber if dry, nonproductive cough lasts over 7 days

Evaluation
Positive therapeutic outcome
• Absence of dry cough
• Thinner, more productive cough that raises secretions

---

haloperidol (Rx)
(hal-oh-pehr'ih-dol)
Apo-Haloperidol ✦, Haldol, Novo-Peridol ✦, Peridol ✦
haloperidol decanoate (Rx)
Haldol Decanoate, Haldol LA ✦
haloperidol lactate (Rx)
Haldol, Haloperidol Injection, Haloperidol Intensol
Func. class.: Antipsychotic/neuroleptic
Chem. class.: Butyrophenone

Pregnancy category C

Action: Depresses cerebral cortex, hypothalamus, limbic system, which control activity and aggression; blocks neurotransmission produced by dopamine at synapse; exhibits strong α-adrenergic, anticholinergic blocking action; mechanism for antipsychotic effects unclear

⮞ **Therapeutic Outcome:** Decreased signs and symptoms of psychosis

Uses: Psychotic disorders, control of tics, vocal utterances in Gilles de la Tourette syndrome, short-term treatment of hyperactive children showing excessive motor activity, prolonged parenteral therapy in chronic schizophrenia, control of severe nausea and vomiting in chemotherapy, organic mental syndrome with psychotic features, hiccups (short-term), emergency sedation of severely agitated or delirious patients

Investigational uses: Nausea, vomiting in chemotherapy, surgery

Dosage and routes
Psychosis
Adult: PO 0.5-5 mg bid or tid initially depending on severity of condition; increase to desired dosage, max 100 mg/day; IM (lactate) 2-5 mg q4-8h or bid-tid

G *Elderly:* 0.25-0.5 mg qd-bid, titrate q3-4 days by 0.25-0.5 mg/dose

P *Child 3-12 yr:* PO/IM (lactate) 0.05-0.15 mg/kg/day

Decanoate
Adult: Initial dose IM is 10-15 mg × daily oral dose at 4-wk interval; do not administer **IV**; not to exceed 100 mg

Chronic schizophrenia
Adult: IM 50-100 mg q4 wk (decanoate)

P **Child 3-12 yr:** PO/IM 0.05-0.15 mg/kg/day

Tics/vocal utterances
Adult: PO 0.5-5 mg bid or tid, increased until desired response occurs

P **Child 3-12 yr:** PO 0.05-0.075 mg/kg/day

Hyperactive children
P **Child 3-12 yr:** PO 0.05-0.075 mg/kg/day

Available forms: Tabs 0.5, 1, 2, 5, 10, 20 mg; lactate: conc 2 mg/ml; inj 5 mg/ml; decanoate: 50, 100 mg base/ml

Adverse effects
(*italic* = common; **bold** = life-threatening)
CNS: *Extrapyramidal symptoms (EPS), pseudoparkinsonism, akathisia, dystonia, tardive dyskinesia, drowsiness, headache,* **seizures, neuroleptic malignant syndrome,** confusion
CV: *Orthostatic hypotension,* hypertension, **cardiac arrest,** ECG changes, **tachycardia**
EENT: Blurred vision, glaucoma, dry eyes
GI: *Dry mouth, nausea, vomiting, anorexia, constipation,* diarrhea, jaundice, weight gain, **ileus, hepatitis**
GU: Urinary retention, urinary frequency, dysuria, enuresis, impotence, amenorrhea, gynecomastia
INTEG: *Rash,* photosensitivity, dermatitis
RESP: **Laryngospasm,** dyspnea, **respiratory depression**

Contraindications: Hypersensitivity,
P blood dyscrasias, coma, child <3 yr, brain damage, bone marrow depression, alcohol and barbiturate withdrawal states, Parkinson's disease, angina, epilepsy, urinary retention, narrow-angle glaucoma

Precautions: Pregnancy **C**, lactation, seizure disorders, hypertension, hepatic
G disease, cardiac disease, elderly

N **Do Not Confuse:**
Haldol/Stadol, haloperidol/Halotestin

Pharmacokinetics

Absorption	Well absorbed (PO, IM); decanoate (IM) absorbed slowly
Distribution	High concentrations in liver, crosses placenta
Metabolism	Liver, extensively
Excretion	Kidneys, breast milk
Half-life	21-24 hr

Pharmacodynamics

	PO	IM	IM (decanoate)
Onset	Erratic	½ hr	3-9 days
Peak	2-6 hr	30-45 min	4-11 days
Duration	8-12 hr	4-8 hr	3 wk

H

Interactions
Individual drugs
Alcohol: ↑ effects of both drugs, oversedation
Carbamazepine: ↓ effects of haloperidol
EpINEPHrine: ↑ toxicity
Levodopa: ↓ effects of levodopa
Lithium: ↓ toxicity, ↓ effects of lithium
Phenobarbital: ↓ effectiveness
Drug classifications
Anticholinergics: ↑ anticholinergic effects
Barbiturate anesthetics: oversedation
β-Adrenergic blockers: ↑ effects of both drugs
CNS depressants: oversedation
⊘ *Herb/drug*
Chamomile, cola tree, hops, jimsonweed, kava, nettle, nutmeg, scopolia, skullcap, valerian: ↑ action
Betel palm, kava: ↑ extrapyramidal symptoms
Lab test interferences
↑ Liver function tests, ↑ cardiac enzymes, ↑ cholesterol, ↑ blood glucose, ↑ prolactin, ↑ bilirubin, ↑ PBI, ↑ cholinesterase, ↑ alkaline phosphatase
↓ Hormones (blood and urine), ↓ pro-time
False positive: Pregnancy tests, PKU
False negative: Urinary steroids

NURSING CONSIDERATIONS
Assessment
• Assess mental status: orientation, mood, behavior, presence and type of hallucinations before initial administration and monthly; this drug should significantly reduce psychotic behavior
• Check for swallowing of PO medication; check for hoarding or giving of medication to other patients
• Monitor I&O ratio; palpate bladder if low
G urinary output occurs, especially in elderly; urinalysis is recommended before, during prolonged therapy

- Monitor bilirubin, CBC, liver function studies monthly
- Assess affect, orientation, LOC, reflexes, gait, coordination, sleep pattern disturbances
- Monitor B/P with patient sitting, standing, and lying; take pulse and respirations q4h during initial treatment; establish baseline before starting treatment; report drops of 30 mm Hg; obtain baseline ECG, Q-wave and T-wave changes
- Check for dizziness, faintness, palpitations, tachycardia on rising; severe orthostatic hypotension is common
- Assess for neuroleptic malignant syndrome: hyperpyrexia, muscle rigidity, increased CPK, altered mental status; drug should be discontinued immediately; if seizures, hyper/hypotension, tachycardia occur, notify prescriber immediately
- Assess for EPS including akathisia (inability to sit still, no pattern to movements), tardive dyskinesia (bizarre movements of the jaw, mouth, tongue, extremities), pseudoparkinsonism (ragged tremors, pill rolling, shuffling gate); an antiparkinsonian drug should be prescribed
- Assess for constipation and urinary retention daily; if these occur, increase bulk, water in diet

Nursing diagnoses
☑ Thought processes, disturbed (uses)
☑ Coping, ineffective (uses)
☑ Knowledge, deficient (teaching)
☑ Noncompliance (teaching)

Implementation
PO route
- Give drug in liquid form mixed in glass of juice or caffeine-free cola if hoarding is suspected; do not mix in caffeine drinks, tannics, pectins
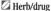 **G** • Give decreased dosage in elderly because of slower metabolism
- Give PO with full glass of water, milk; or give with food to decrease GI upset
- Store in tight, light-resistant container, oral sol in amber bottle

IM route
- Inject in deep muscle mass, do not give SC; use 21-G 2-in needle; do not administer sol with a precipitate; give <3 ml per inj site; give slowly, may be painful

IV **IV route**
- Give undiluted for psychotic episode at 5 mg/min
- Give by intermittent inf after dilution in 30-50 ml of D_5W, run over ½ hr

Syringe compatibilities: Hydromorphone, sufentanil

Y-site compatibilities: Amifostine, amsacrine, aztreonam, cimetidine, cisatracurium, cladribine, DOBUTamine, DOPamine, DOXOrubicin liposome, famotidine, filgrastim, fludarabine, granisetron, lidocaine, lorazepam, melphalan, midazolam, nitroglycerin, norepinephrine, ondansetron, paclitaxel, phenylephrine, propofol, remifentanil, sufentanil, tacrolimus, teniposide, theophylline, thiotepa, vinorelbine

Y-site incompatibilities: Fluconazole, foscarnet, heparin, sargramostim

Patient/family education
- Teach patient to use good oral hygiene; use frequent rinsing of mouth, sugarless gum for dry mouth
- Advise patient to avoid hazardous activities until drug response is determined; dizziness, blurred vision are common
- Inform patient that orthostatic hypotension occurs often and to rise from sitting or lying position gradually; to remain lying down after IM inj for at least 30 min; tell patient to avoid hot tubs, hot showers, tub baths, since hypotension may occur; tell patient that in hot weather heat stroke may occur; take extra precautions to stay cool
- Instruct patient to avoid abrupt withdrawal of this drug, or EPS may result; drug should be withdrawn slowly
- Caution patient to avoid OTC preparations (cough, hay fever, cold) unless approved by prescriber, since serious drug interactions may occur; avoid use with alcohol, CNS depressants since increased drowsiness may occur
- Advise patient to use a sunscreen and sunglasses to prevent burns
- Teach patient about EPS and necessity of meticulous oral hygiene, since oral candidiasis may occur
- Instruct patient to take antacids 2 hr before or after this drug
- Tell patient to report sore throat, malaise, fever, bleeding, mouth sores; if these occur, CBC should be obtained and drug discontinued

Evaluation
Positive therapeutic outcome
- Decrease in emotional excitement, hallucinations, delusions, paranoia, reorganization of patterns of thought, speech; improvement in specific behaviors

Treatment of overdose: Lavage if orally ingested; provide airway; *do not induce vomiting*

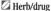

! HIGH ALERT

heparin ⊶ (Rx)
(hep'a-rin)
Calcilean ♣, Calciparine, Hepalean ♣,
Heparin Sodium, Heparin Leo ♣, Heparin
Lock, Hep-Lock, Hep-Lock U/P
Func. class.: Anticoagulant, antithrombotic

Pregnancy category C

Action: Prevents conversion of fibrinogen to
fibrin and prothrombin to thrombin by enhancing inhibitory effects of antithrombin III

➡ **Therapeutic Outcome:** Prevention of
thrombi

Uses: Prevention of deep vein thrombosis
(DVT) and pulmonary emboli (PE) (treatment
and prevention), MI, open heart surgery,
disseminated intravascular clotting syndrome,
atrial fibrillation with embolization, as an
anticoagulant in transfusion and dialysis
procedures, prevention of DVT/PE, to maintain
patency of indwelling venipuncture devices,
diagnosis, treatment of disseminated intravascular coagulation (DIC)

Dosage and routes
DVT/MI
Adult: **IV** push 5000-7000 units q4h then
titrated to PTT or activated coagulation time
(ACT) level; **IV** bol 5000-7500 units, then **IV**
inf; **IV** inf after bol dose, then 1000 units/hr
titrated to PTT or ACT level

P *Child:* **IV** inf 50 units/kg, maintenance 100
units/kg q4h or 20,000 units/m² qd

Anticoagulation
Adult: SC 500 units **IV** then 10,000-20,000
units, then 8,000-10,000 units 8qh or 15,000-
20,000 units q12h

Pulmonary embolism
Adult: **IV** push 7500-10,000 units q4h then
titrated to PTT or ACT level; **IV** bol 7500-
10,000 units, then **IV** inf; **IV** inf after bol dose,
then 1000 units/hr titrated to PTT or ACT level

P *Child:* **IV** inf 50 units/kg; maintenance 100
units/kg q4h or 20,000 units/m² qd

CV surgery
Adult: **IV** inf 150-300 units/kg, prophylaxis
for DVT/PE; SC 5000 units q8-12h

Heparin flush
P *Adult/child:* **IV** 10-100 units

Available forms: Sodium: carpuject 5000
units/ml; disposable inj 1000, 2500, 5000,
7500, 10,000, 15,000, 20,000, 40,000 units/
ml; unit dose 1000, 5000, 10,000, 20,000,
40,000 units/ml; vials 1000, 2000, 2500, 5000,
7500, 10,000, 20,000, 40,000 units/ml; flush,
disposable syringes 10, 100 units/ml; vials, 100
units/ml; ca inj: 5000 units/0.2 ml; ampules
12,500 units/0.5 ml; 20,000 units/0.8 ml

Adverse effects
(*italic* = common; **bold** = life-threatening)
CNS: Fever, chills
GU: **Hematuria**
HEMA: **Hemorrhage, thrombocytopenia,
anemia**
INTEG: Rash, dermatitis, urticaria, pruritus,
delayed transient alopecia, hematoma, cutane-
ous necrosis (SC)
SYST: **Anaphylaxis**

Contraindications: Hypersensitivity,
hemophilia, leukemia with bleeding, peptic
ulcer disease, severe thrombocytopenic
purpura, hepatic disease (severe), renal
disease (severe), blood dyscrasias, severe
hypertension, subacute bacterial endocarditis,
acute nephritis

G **Precautions:** Alcoholism, elderly, preg-
P nancy C, children, hyperlipidemia, diabetes,
renal disease

🖎 **Do Not Confuse:**
heparin/Hespan

Pharmacokinetics
Absorption	Well absorbed (SC)
Distribution	Unknown
Metabolism	Partially in kidney, liver
Excretion	Lymph, spleen, in urine (<50% unchanged)
Half-life	1½ hr

Pharmacodynamics
	SC	IV
Onset	½-1 hr	5 min
Peak	2 hr	10 min
Duration	8-12 hr	2-6 hr

Interactions
Individual drugs
Diazepam, dipyridole, ticlopidine: ↑ action of
diazepam
Digitalis: ↓ action of heparin
Dextran: ↑ action of heparin
Streptokinase: Resistance to heparin
Drug classifications
Anticoagulants (oral), cephalosporins,
NSAIDs, penicillins, platelet inhibitors, salicy-
lates, steroids: ↑ action of heparin
Antihistamines, tetracyclines: ↓ action of
heparin
Corticosteroids: ↓ action of corticosteroids

♣ Canada Only   🖎 Do Not Confuse   * "Tall Man" lettering (See Preface)

☑ *Herb/drug*

Agrimony, alfalfa, angelica, anise, basil, bay, bilberry, black haw, bogbean, bromelain, buchu, chondroitin, cinchona bark, dong quai, fenugreek, feverfew, garlic, ginger, ginkgo, ginseng, horse chestnut, Irish moss, kelp, kelpware, khella, lovage, lungwort, meadow-sweet, motherwort, mugwort, nettle, papaya, parsley (large amounts), pau d'arco, pineapple, poplar, prickly ash, safflower, saw palmetto, tonka bean, turmeric, wintergreen, yarrow: ↑ risk of bleeding

Chamomile, coenzyme Q10, flax, glucomannan, goldenseal, guar gum: ↓ anticoagulant effect

Lab test interferences
↑ ALT, ↑ AST, ↑ INR, ↑ PT, ↑ PTT
↓ Platelets

NURSING CONSIDERATIONS
Assessment
• Assess for blood studies (Hct, occult blood in stools) q3 mo if patient is on long-term therapy
• Monitor PPT, which should be 1½-2 × control, PTT; often done qd, APTT, ACT
• Monitor platelet count q2-3 days; thrombocytopenia may occur on 4th day of treatment and resolve, or continue to 8th day of treatment
◆• Assess for bleeding gums, petechiae, ecchymosis, black tarry stools, hematuria, epistaxis, decrease in Hct, B/P; may indicate bleeding and possible hemorrhage; notify prescriber immediately
• Monitor for hypersensitivity: fever, skin rash, urticaria; notify prescriber immediately

Nursing diagnoses
✓ Injury, risk for (uses, adverse reactions)
✓ Tissue perfusion, ineffective (uses)
✓ Knowledge, deficient (teaching)

Implementation
IV IV route
• Cannot be used interchangeably (unit for unit) with LMWHs or heparinoids
• Give directly; **IV** loading dose over 1 min
• Give **IV** diluted in 0.9% NaCl, dextrose, Ringer's by intermittent or cont inf; inf may run from 4-24 hr; use infusion pump
• When drug is added to inf sol for cont **IV**, invert container at least 6×s to ensure adequate mixing

Syringe compatibilities: Aminophylline, amphotericin B, ampicillin, atropine, azlocillin, bleomycin, cefamandole, cefazolin, cefoperazone, cefotaxime, cefoxitin, chloramphenicol, cimetidine, cisplatin, clindamycin,

cyclophosphamide, diazoxide, digoxin, dimenhyDRINATE, DOBUTamine, DOPamine, epINEPHrine, fentanyl, fluorouracil, furosemide, leucovorin, lidocaine, lincomycin, methotrexate, metoclopramide, mezlocillin, mitomycin, moxalactam, nafcillin, naloxone, neostigmine, nitroglycerin, norepinephrine, pancuronium, penicillin G, phenobarbital, piperacillin, sodium nitroprusside, succinylcholine, trimethoprim-sulfamethoxazole, verapamil, vinCRIStine

Y-site compatibilities: Acyclovir, aldesleukin, allopurinol, amifostine, aminophylline, ampicillin, ampicillin/sulbactam, atracurium, atropine, aztreonam, betamethasone, bleomycin, calcium gluconate, cefazolin, cefotetan, ceftazidime, ceftriaxone, cephalothin, cephapirin, chlordiazepoxide, chlorproMAZINE, cimetidine, cisplatin, cladribine, clindamycin, conjugated estrogens, cyanocobalamin, cyclophosphamide, cytarabine, dexamethasone, digoxin, diphenhydrAMINE, DOPamine, DOXOrubicin liposome, edrophonium, enalaprilat, epINEPHrine, erythromycin, esmolol, ethacrynate, famotidine, fentanyl, fluconazole, fludarabine, fluorouracil, foscarnet, furosemide, gallium, granisetron, hydrALAZINE, hydrocortisone, hydromorphone, regular insulin, isoproterenol, kanamycin, leucovorin, lidocaine, lorazepam, magnesium sulfate, melphalan, menadiol sodium, meperidine, meropenem, methicillin, methotrexate, methoxamine, methyldopate, methylergonovine, metoclopramide, metronidazole, midazolam, milrinone, minocycline, mitomycin, morphine, nafcillin, neostigmine, nitroglycerin, nitroprusside, norepinephrine, ondansetron, oxacillin, oxytocin, paclitaxel, pancuronium, penicillin G potassium, pentazocine, phytonadione, piperacillin, piperacillin/tazobactam, propofol, potassium chloride, prednisoLONE, procainamide, prochlorperazine, propofol, propranolol, pyridostigmine, ranitidine, remifentanil, sargramostim, scopolamine, sodium bicarbonate, streptokinase, succinylcholine, tacrolimus, teniposide, theophylline, thiopental, thiotepa, ticarcillin, ticarcillin/clavulanate, trimethobenzamide, vecuronium, vinBLAStine, vinorelbine, warfarin, zidovudine

Y-site incompatibilities: Alteplase, ciprofloxacin, dacarbazine, diazepam, DOBUTamine, DOXOrubicin, ergotamine, gentamicin, haloperidol, idarubicin, methotrimeprazine, phenytoin, promethazine, tobramycin, triflupromazine

Additive compatibilities: Aminophylline, amphotericin, ascorbic acid, bleomycin, calcium gluconate, cefepime, cephapirin, chloramphenicol, clindamycin, colistimethate, dimenhyDRINATE, doxacillin, DOPamine, enalaprilat, erythromycin, esmolol, floxacillin, fluconazole, flumazenil, furosemide, hydrocortisone, isoproterenol, lidocaine, lincomycin, magnesium sulfate, meropenem, methyldopate, methylPREDNISolone, metronidazole/sodium bicarbonate, nafcillin, norepinephrine, octreotide, penicillin G, potassium chloride, prednisoLONE, promazine, ranitidine, sodium bicarbonate, verapamil, vit B complex, vit B complex with C

Additive incompatibilities: Amikacin, erythromycin lactobionate, gentamicin, kanamycin, meperidine, methadone, morphine, polymyxin B, streptomycin

Heparin lock route
• Inject 10-100 units/0.5-1 ml after each inf or q8-12h

SC route
• Give SC with at least 25-G ⅜-in needle; do not massage area or aspirate fluid when giving SC inj; give in abdomen between pelvic bones, rotate sites; do not pull back on plunger, leave in for 10 sec; apply gentle pressure for 1 min
• Give at same time each day to maintain steady blood levels
• Changing needles is not recommended

Patient/family education
• Advise patient to avoid OTC preparations that may cause serious drug interactions unless directed by prescriber; may contain aspirin or other anticoagulants
• Tell patient that drug may be held during active bleeding (menstruation), depending on condition
• Caution patient to use soft-bristle toothbrush to avoid bleeding gums; avoid contact sports; use electric razor; avoid IM inj
• Instruct patient to carry/wear emergency ID or other identification identifying drug taken and condition treated
• Advise patient to report any signs of bleeding: gums, under skin, urine, stools; or unusual bruising

Evaluation
Positive therapeutic outcome
• Decrease of DVT
• PTT of 1.5-2.5 × control
• Free-flowing **IV**

Treatment of overdose: Withdraw drug, give protamine sulfate 1 mg protamine/100 units heparin

hepatitis B immune globulin (Rx)
(hep-a-tite′iss)
BayHep B, Nabi-HB
Func. class.: Immune globulin
Pregnancy category C

Action: Provides passive immunity to hepatitis B

→ **Therapeutic Outcome:** Passive immunity to hepatitis B

Uses: Prevention of hepatitis B virus in exposed patients, including passive immunity
P in neonates born to HBsAg-positive mothers

Dosage and routes
Acute exposure to blood with HBsAg
Adult: 2 doses, given after exposure and 1 mo later

Perinatal exposure of infants born to HBsAg-positive mothers
P *Infant:* 1 dose at birth, then start hepatitis B vaccine series soon after birth

Sexual exposure to HBsAg
Adult: Administer 1 dose within 2 wk of exposure

Available forms: Bay-Hep B: sol for inj 15%-18% protein; Nabi-HB: sol for inj 5% ± 1% protein

Adverse effects
(*italic* = common; **bold** = life-threatening)
CNS: Headache, dizziness, fever
INTEG: Soreness at inj site, urticaria, erythema, swelling, **anaphylaxis, angioedema**
SYST: Induration

Contraindications: Hypersensitivity to immune globulins, coagulation disorders

G **Precautions:** Pregnancy **C**, elderly,
P lactation, children, active infection, IgA deficiency

Pharmacokinetics
Absorption	Slowly absorbed
Distribution	Unknown
Metabolism	Unknown
Excretion	Unknown
Half-life	3 wk

Pharmacodynamics
Onset	1-7 days
Peak	3-10 days
Duration	2-6 mo

H

NURSING CONSIDERATIONS
Assessment

- Assess for history of allergies, skin conditions (eczema, psoriasis, dermatitis), reactions to vaccinations
- Assess for skin reactions: rash, induration, urticaria
- Assess for sneezing, pruritus, angioedema, dysphagia, vomiting, abdominal pain
- Assess for anaphylaxis: inability to breathe, bronchospasm, hypotension, wheezing, diaphoresis, fever, flushing; epINEPHrine and emergency equipment should be available

Nursing diagnoses
☑ Infection, risk for (uses)
☑ Knowledge, deficient (teaching)

Implementation

- Give after rotating vial; do not shake
- Give in deltoid (adult) or anterolateral thigh for better protection; give 2-ml dose in two different sites; do not give **IV**
- Refrigerate unused portion; sol should be clear, light amber, and thick

Patient/family education

- Teach patient purpose of medication and expected results
- Give patient a list of adverse reactions that need to be reported immediately: wheezing, vomiting, sneezing, abdominal pain, sweating, tightness in chest
- Advise patient that pain, rash, swelling at inj site can be expected
- Give patient written record of immunization

Evaluation
Positive therapeutic outcome

- Prevention of hepatitis B

---

hetastarch (Rx)
(het′a-starch)
Hespan
Func. class.: Plasma expander
Chem. class.: Synthetic polymer

Pregnancy category C

Action: Similar to human albumin, which expands plasma volume by colloidal osmotic pressure

➡ Therapeutic Outcome: Increased plasma volume

Uses: Plasma volume expander for sepsis, trauma, burns, leukapheresis

Dosage and routes
Adult: **IV** inf 500-1000 ml (30-60 g); total dose not to exceed 1500 ml/day, not to exceed 20 ml/kg/hr (hemorrhagic shock)

Leukapheresis
Adult: **IV** inf 250-700 ml infused at 1 : 8 ratio with whole blood; may be repeated twice weekly up to 10 treatments

Available forms: 6% hetastarch/0.9% NaCl (6 g/100 ml)

Adverse effects
(*italic* = common; **bold** = life-threatening)
CNS: Headache
EENT: Periorbital edema
GI: Nausea, vomiting
HEMA: Decreased hematocrit, platelet function, increased bleeding/coagulation times, increased erythrocyte sedimentation rate
INTEG: Rash, urticaria, pruritus, angioedema, chills, fever, flushing, peripheral edema
RESP: Wheezing, dyspnea, **bronchospasm, pulmonary edema**
SYST: **Anaphylaxis**

Contraindications: Hypersensitivity, severe bleeding disorders, renal failure, CHF (severe)

Precautions: Pregnancy **C**, liver disease, pulmonary edema

⚠ Do Not Confuse:
Hespan/heparin

Pharmacokinetics	
Absorption	Completely absorbed
Distribution	Unknown
Metabolism	Degraded
Excretion	Kidneys, unchanged
Half-life	17 days (90%); 48 days (10%)

Pharmacodynamics	
Onset	Immediate
Peak	Infusion's end
Duration	Over 24 hr

Interactions: None
Lab test interferences
False: ↑ Bilirubin

NURSING CONSIDERATIONS
Assessment

- Monitor VS q5 min for 30 min; CVP during inf (5-10 cm H$_2$O normal range); PCWP; urine output q1h: watch for increase, which is common; if output does not increase, inf should be decreased or discontinued
- Monitor CBC with differential, Hgb, Hct, Pro-time, PTT, platelet count, clotting time during treatment; treatment may increase

---

clotting time, PTT, Pro-time, sedimentary rates, Hct may drop due to increased volume and hemodilution; do not allow Hct to be <30% by volume

• Monitor I&O ratio and sp gr, urine osmolarity; if sp gr is very low, renal clearance is low; drug should be discontinued

• Assess for allergy: rash, urticaria, pruritus, wheezing, dyspnea, bronchospasm; drug should be discontinued immediately

◆• Assess for circulatory overload: increased pulse, respirations, dyspnea, wheezing, chest tightness, chest pain, increased CVP, jugular vein distention

• Assess for dehydration after inf; decreased output, increased temp, poor skin turgor, increased sp gr, dry skin

Nursing diagnoses

✓ Fluid volume, deficient (uses)
✓ Tissue perfusion, ineffective (uses)
✓ Fluid volume, excess (adverse reactions)
✓ Knowledge, deficient (teaching)

Implementation

• Give by **IV** cont inf, undiluted, run at 20 ml/kg/hr; reduced rate in septic shock, burns; rate is calculated by blood volume and response of patient

• Give up to 20 ml kg (1.2 g/ kg)/hr

• Store at room temp; discard unused portions; do not freeze; do not use if turbid or deep brown or precipitate forms

Y-site compatibilities: Cimetidine, diltiazem, doxycycline, enalaprilat

Y-site incompatibilities: Amikacin, cefamandole, cefoperazone, cefotaxime, cefoxitin, gentamicin, theophylline, tobramycin

Additive compatibilities: Cloxacillin, fosphenytoin

Patient/family education

• Teach patient the reason for administration and expected results

• Advise patient to notify prescriber if flulike symptoms or allergic symptoms occur

Evaluation

Positive therapeutic outcome
• Increased plasma volume as evidenced by higher B/P, blood volume, output

---

*hydrALAZINE (Rx)
(hye-dral'a-zeen)
Alazine, Apresoline, Novo-Hylazin ✦, hydrALAZINE HCl, Pralzine, Rolzine, Supres ✦
Func. class.: Antihypertensive, direct-acting peripheral vasodilator
Chem. class.: Phthalazine

Pregnancy category C

Action: Vasodilates arterioles in smooth muscle by direct relaxation; reduces B/P with reflex increases in heart rate, stroke volume, cardiac output

Investigational uses: CHF

→**Therapeutic Outcome:** Decreased B/P in hypertension, decreased afterload in CHF

Uses: Essential hypertension, severe essential hypertension, CHF

Dosage and routes
Adult: PO 10 mg qid 2-4 days, then 25 mg for rest of 1st wk, then 50 mg qid individualized to desired response, not to exceed 300 mg qd; **IV**/IM bol 20-40 mg q4-6h; administer PO as soon as possible; IM 20-40 mg q4-6h

P *Child:* PO 0.75-3 mg/kg/day in 4 divided doses; max 7.5 mg/kg/24 hr; **IV** bol 0.1-0.2 mg/kg q4-6h; IM 0.1-0.2 mg/kg q4-6h

Available forms: Inj 20 mg/ml; tabs 10, 25, 50, 100 mg

Adverse effects
(*italic* = common; **bold** = life-threatening)
CNS: Headache, tremors, dizziness, anxiety, peripheral neuritis, depression, fever, chills
CV: Palpitations, reflex tachycardia, angina, **shock,** rebound hypertension
GI: Nausea, vomiting, anorexia, diarrhea, constipation, paralytic ileus
GU: Urinary retention
HEMA: Leukopenia, **agranulocytosis,** anemia, **thrombocytopenia**
INTEG: Rash, pruritus, urticaria
MISC: Nasal congestion, muscle cramps, *lupuslike symptoms,* flushing, edema, dyspnea

Contraindications: Hypersensitivity to hydrALAZINEs, CAD, mitral valvular rheumatic heart disease

Precautions: Pregnancy **C,** CVA, advanced **G** renal disease, elderly, coronary artery disease, lactation

▧ **Do Not Confuse:**
Apresoline/allopurinol
hydrALAZINE/hydrOXYzine

Pharmacokinetics	
Absorption	Rapidly absorbed (PO); well absorbed (IM); completely absorbed (**IV**)
Distribution	Widely distributed; crosses placenta
Metabolism	GI mucosa, liver extensively
Excretion	Kidneys, urine (12%-14%)
Half-life	2-8 hr

Pharmacodynamics			
	PO	IM	IV
Onset	½ hr	10-30 min	5-20 min
Peak	1-2 hr	1 hr	10-80 min
Duration	6-12 hr	4-6 hr	4-6 hr

Interactions
Individual drugs
Indomethacin: ↓ effects of hydrALAZINE
Drug classifications
Antihypertensives, MAOIs: ↑ hypotension
β-Adrenergic blockers: ↑ effects
Sympathomimetics (epinephrine, norepinephrine): ↑ tachycardia, angina
Herb/drug
Aconite: ↑ toxicity, death
Astragalus, cola tree: ↑ or ↓ antihypertensive effect
Barberry, betony, black catechu, black cohosh, bloodroot, broom, burdock, cat's claw, dandelion, goldenseal, Irish moss, Jamaican dogwood, kelp, khella, mistletoe, parsley: ↑ antihypertensive effect
Coltsfoot, guarana, khat, licorice: ↓ antihypertensive effect

NURSING CONSIDERATIONS
Assessment
• Assess B/P q5 min for 2 hr, then q1h for 2 hr, then q4h; pulse, jugular venous distention q4h
• Monitor electrolytes, blood studies: potassium, sodium, chloride, carbon dioxide, CBC, serum glucose; LE prep, ANA titer before starting treatment
• Monitor weight daily, I&O; edema in feet, legs daily; check skin turgor, dryness of mucous membranes for hydration status
• Assess for rales, dyspnea, orthopnea; peripheral edema, fatigue, weight gain, jugular vein distention (CHF)
• For fever, joint pain, rash, sore throat (lupuslike symptoms), notify prescriber
Nursing diagnoses
☑ Cardiac output, decreased (adverse reactions)
☑ Injury, risk for physical (side effects)
☑ Knowledge, deficient (teaching)

Implementation
PO route
• Give with meals to enhance absorption
• Store protected from light and heat
IV IV route
• Give by **IV** undiluted through Y-tube or 3-way stopcock, give ≤10 mg/min
• Administer with patient in recumbent position; keep in that position for 1 hr after administration

Y-site compatibilities: Heparin, hydrocortisone, potassium chloride, verapamil, vit B/C

Y-site incompatibilities: Aminophylline, ampicillin, diazoxide, furosemide, paclitaxel

Additive incompatibilities: Aminophylline, ampicillin, chlorothiazide, edetate calcium disodium, ethacrynate, hydrocortisone, melphalan, mephentermine, methohexital, nitroglycerin, phenobarbital, verapamil, vinorelbine

Additive compatibilities: DOBUTamine
Patient/family education
• Teach patient to take with food to increase bioavailability (PO)
• Teach patient to avoid OTC preparations unless directed by prescriber
• Advise patient to notify prescriber if chest pain, severe fatigue, fever, muscle or joint pain occur
• Advise patient to rise slowly to prevent orthostatic hypertension
• Advise patient to notify prescriber if pregnancy is suspected
Evaluation
Positive therapeutic outcome
• Decreased B/P in hypertension

Treatment of overdose: Administer vasopressors, volume expanders for shock; if PO, lavage or give activated charcoal, digitalization

---

 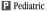

hydrochlorothiazide
⚙️π (Rx)
(hye-droe-klor-oh-thye'a-zide)
Apo-Hydrol ✦, HCTZ, Esidrix, Hydro-Chlor,
hydrochlorothiazide, HydroDIURIL,
Microzide, Neo-Codema ✦,
Novohydrazide ✦, Oretic, Urozide ✦
Func. class: Diuretic, antihypertensive
Chem. class: Thiazide, sulfonamide derivative

Pregnancy category B

Action: Acts on the distal tubule in the kidney, increasing excretion of sodium, water, chloride, magnesium, potassium, and bicarbonate

➡️**Therapeutic Outcome:** Decreased B/P, decreased edema in lung tissues peripherally

Uses: Edema in CHF, nephrotic syndrome; edema in corticosteroid, NSAID therapy; idiopathic lower extremity edema; may be used alone or as adjunct with antihypertensives

Dosage and routes
Adult: PO 25-200 mg/day

🄖 *Elderly:* PO 12.5 mg/day, initially

🄿 *Child >6 mo:* PO 2 mg/kg/day

🄿 *Child <6 mo:* PO up to 4 mg/kg/day in divided doses

Available forms: Tabs 25, 50, 100 mg; caps 12.5 mg; oral sol 10 mg/5 ml, 100 mg/ml

Adverse effects
(*italic* = common; **bold** = life-threatening)
CNS: Drowsiness, paresthesia, anxiety, depression, headache, *dizziness, fatigue, weakness,* fever
CV: Irregular pulse, orthostatic hypotension, palpitations, volume depletion, allergic myocarditis
EENT: Blurred vision
ELECT: *Hypokalemia,* hypercalcemia, hyponatremia, hypochloremia, hypomagnesemia
GI: *Nausea, vomiting, anorexia,* constipation, diarrhea, cramps, pancreatitis, GI irritation, **hepatitis**
GU: *Frequency,* polyuria, **uremia,** glucosuria, hyperuricemia
HEMA: **Aplastic anemia, hemolytic anemia, leukopenia, agranulocytosis, thrombocytopenia, neutropenia**
INTEG: *Rash,* urticaria, purpura, photosensitivity, alopecia, erythema multiform
META: *Hyperglycemia, hyperuricemia,* increased creatinine, BUN

Contraindications: Hypersensitivity to thiazides or sulfonamides, anuria, renal decompensation, hypomagnesemia

Precautions: Hypokalemia, renal disease, hepatic disease, gout, COPD, lupus erythema-🄖tosus, diabetes mellitus, elderly, hyperlipidemia, CCr <25 ml/min, pregnancy **B** lactation

Pharmacokinetics
	PO
Absorption	Variable
Distribution	Extracellular spaces; crosses placenta
Metabolism	Excreted unchanged in urine
Excretion	Breast milk
Half-life	6-15 hr

Pharmacodynamics
Onset	2 hr
Peak	4 hr
Duration	6-12 hr

Interactions
Individual drugs
Amphotericin B: ↑ hypokalemia
Cholestyramine, colestipol: ↓ absorption of hydrochlorothiazide
Diazoxide: ↑ hyperglycemia, hyperuricemia, hypotension
Lithium: ↑ toxicity
Drug classifications
Antidiabetics: ↓ effect of antidiabetic agent
Cardiac glycosides, nondepolarizing skeletal muscle relaxants: ↑ toxicity
Diuretics (loop): ↑ effects of diuretic
Glucocorticoids: ↑ hypokalemia
NSAIDs: ↑ risk of renal failure
Herb/drug
Aloe, buckthorn, cascara sagrada, Chinese rhubarb, gossypol, licorice, nettle, senna: ↑ hypokalemia
Cucumber, dandelion, ginkgo, horsetail, khella, licorice, nettle, pumpkin, Queen Anne's lace: ↑ effect
St. John's wort: severe photosensitivity
Lab test interferences
↑ BSP retention, ↑ amylase, ↑ parathyroid test
↓ PBI, ↓ PSP

NURSING CONSIDERATIONS
Assessment
• Monitor glucose in urine if patient is diabetic
• Assess improvement in CVP q8h
• Check for rashes, temp elevation qd
🄖• Assess for confusion, especially in elderly; take safety precautions if needed
• Monitor manifestations of hypokalemia: acidic urine, reduced urine, osmolality,

nocturia; hypotension, broad T wave, U wave, ectopy, tachycardia, weak pulse; muscle weakness, altered LOC, drowsiness, apathy, lethargy, confusion, depression; anorexia, nausea, cramps, constipation, distention, paralytic ileus; hypoventilation, respiratory muscle weakness

• Monitor for manifestations of hypomagnesemia: agitation, muscle twitching, paresthesias, hyperactive reflexes, positive Babinski reflex, dysphagia, nystagmus seizures, tetany; nausea, vomiting, diarrhea, anorexia, abdominal distention; ectopy, tachycardia, broad, flat, or inverted T waves, depressed ST segment, prolonged QT interval, decreased cardiac output, hypotension

• Monitor for manifestations of hyponatremia: increased B/P, cold, clammy skin, hypovolemia or hypervolemia; anorexia, nausea, vomiting, diarrhea, abdominal cramps; lethargy, increased ICP, confusion, headache, seizures, coma, fatigue, tremors, hyperreflexia

• Monitor for manifestations of hyperchloremia: weakness, lethargy, coma, deep rapid breathing

• Assess fluid volume status: I&O ratios, record, count, or weigh diapers as appropriate, weight, distended red veins, crackles in lungs, color, quality, and sp gr of urine, skin turgor, adequacy of pulses, moist mucous membranes, bilateral lung sounds, peripheral pitting edema; assess for dehydration: symptoms of decreasing output, thirst, hypotension; dry mouth and mucous membranes should be reported

• Monitor electrolytes: potassium, sodium, calcium, magnesium; also include BUN, blood pH, ABGs, uric acid, CBC, blood glucose, renal function

• Assess B/P before and during therapy with patient lying, standing, and sitting as appropriate; orthostatic hypotension can occur rapidly

Nursing diagnoses

☑ Urinary elimination, impaired (side effect)
☑ Fluid volume, deficient (side effects)
☑ Fluid volume, excess (uses)
☑ Knowledge, deficient (teaching)

Implementation

• Give in AM to avoid interference with sleep
• Provide potassium replacement if potassium level is ≤3.0 mg/dl; give whole tab or use oral sol lightly; drug may be crushed if patient is unable to swallow
• Administer with food; if nausea occurs, absorption may be increased

Patient/family education

• Teach patient to take the medication early in the day to prevent nocturia
• Instruct patient to take with food or milk if GI symptoms of nausea and anorexia occur
• Teach patient to maintain a weekly record of weight and notify prescriber of weight loss >5 lb
• Caution patient that this drug causes a loss of potassium and that food rich in potassium should be added to the diet; refer to a dietitian for assistance in planning
• Caution patient not to exercise in hot weather or stand for prolonged periods since orthostatic hypotension will be enhanced
• Teach patient not to use alcohol or any OTC medications without prescriber's approval; serious drug reactions may occur
• Emphasize the need to contact prescriber immediately if muscle cramps, weakness, nausea, dizziness, or numbness occurs
• Teach patient to take own B/P and pulse and record findings
• Caution patient that orthostatic hypotension may occur; patient should rise slowly from sitting or reclining positions and lie down if dizziness occurs
• Teach patient to continue taking medication even if feeling better; this drug controls symptoms but does not cure the condition
• Advise patient with hypertension to continue other medical treatment (exercise, weight loss, relaxation techniques, cessation of smoking)

Evaluation

Positive therapeutic outcome
• Decreased edema
• Decreased B/P
• Increased diuresis

Treatment of overdose: Lavage if taken orally, monitor electrolytes, administer dextrose in saline, monitor hydration, CV, renal status

---

hydrocodone (Rx)
(hye-droe-koe'done)
Hycodan ✸, Robidone ✸, Tussigon
See Combination products section
Func. class.: Antitussive opioid analgesic, nonopioid analgesic

Pregnancy category C
Controlled substance schedule III

Action: Acts directly on cough center in medulla to suppress cough; binds to opiate receptors in the CNS to reduce pain

---

☑ Herb/drug   ⊘ Do Not Crush   ◆ Alert   ⊶ Key Drug   ⑤ Geriatric   ℗ Pediatric

➡️**Therapeutic Outcome:** Pain relief, decreased cough, decreased diarrhea

Uses: Hyperactive and nonproductive cough, mild pain

Dosages and routes
Adult: PO 5-10 mg q4h prn

🅿️ *Child:* PO 1.25-5 mg q4h prn or 0.2 mg/kg q3-4h

Available forms: Syr 5 mg/5 ml; tabs 5 mg (long-acting)

Adverse effects
(*italic* = common; **bold** = life-threatening)
CNS: Drowsiness, dizziness, lightheadedness, confusion, headache, sedation, euphoria, dysphoria, weakness, hallucinations, disorientation, mood changes, dependence, **seizures**
CV: Palpitations, tachycardia, bradycardia, change in B/P, **circulatory depression,** syncope
EENT: Tinnitus, blurred vision, miosis, diplopia
GI: Nausea, vomiting, anorexia, constipation, cramps, dry mouth
GU: Increased urinary output, dysuria, urinary retention
INTEG: Rash, urticaria, flushing, pruritus
RESP: **Respiratory depression**

Contraindications: Hypersensitivity, addiction (opioid)

Precautions: Addictive personality, pregnancy **C,** lactation, increased ICP, MI (acute), severe heart disease, respiratory depression, hepatic disease, renal disease

📵 **Do Not Confuse:**
Hycodan/Vicodin, hydrocodone/hydrocortisone

Pharmacokinetics

Absorption	Well absorbed
Distribution	Unknown; crosses placenta
Metabolism	Liver, extensively
Excretion	Kidneys
Half-life	3½-4½ hr

Pharmacodynamics

	PO (**analgesic**)	PO (**antitussive**)
Onset	10-20 min	Unknown
Peak	30-60 min	Unknown
Duration	4-6 hr	4-6 hr

Interactions
Individual drugs
Alcohol: ↑ respiratory depression, hypotension, sedation

Drug classifications
CNS depressants, phenothiazines, sedative/hypnotics: ↑ respiratory depression, hypotension
General anesthetics, skeletal muscle relaxants: ↑ CNS depression
Tricyclics: ↑ CNS depression
☑️*Herb/drug*
Corkwood: ↑ anticholinergic effect
Jamacian dogwood, lavender, mistletoe, nettle, pokeweed, poppy, senega, valerian: ↑ CNS depression
Lab test interferences
↑ Amylase, ↑ lipase

NURSING CONSIDERATIONS
Assessment
• Assess pain: intensity, type, location, duration, precipitating factor
• Monitor VS after parenteral route; note muscle rigidity, drug history, liver, kidney function tests, cough, and respiratory dysfunction: respiratory depression, character, rate, rhythm; notify prescriber if respirations are <10/min
• Monitor CNS changes: dizziness, drowsiness, hallucinations, euphoria, LOC, pupil reaction
• Monitor allergic reactions: rash, urticaria

Nursing diagnoses
✓Pain, acute (uses)
✓Sensory perception, disturbed: visual, auditory (adverse reactions)
✓Breathing pattern, ineffective (adverse reactions)
✓Knowledge, deficient (teaching)

Implementation
• Give with antiemetic if nausea, vomiting occur
• Give when pain is beginning to return; determine dosage interval by patient response; continuous dosing of medication is more effective given prn
• Medication should be slowly withdrawn after long-term use to prevent withdrawal symptoms
• Store in light-resistant container at room temp
• May be given with food or milk to lessen GI upset
🚫• Do not crush, chew caps

Patient/family education
• Instruct patient to report any symptoms of CNS changes, allergic reactions; to avoid CNS depressants: alcohol, sedative/hypnotics for at least 24 hr after taking this drug
• Teach patient that dizziness, drowsiness, and confusion are common and to avoid getting up

H

without assistance, driving, or other hazardous activities

• Discuss in detail all aspects of the drug

Evaluation
Positive therapeutic outcome
• Decreased pain
• Decreased cough

Treatment of overdose: Naloxone HCl (Narcan) 0.2-0.8 **IV**, O₂, **IV** fluids, vasopressors

---

hydrocortisone (Rx)
(hy-droh-kor'tih-sone)
Cortef, Cortenema, Hydrocortone
hydrocortisone acetate (Rx)
Cortifoam, Hydrocortone Acetate
hydrocortisone cypionate (Rx)
Cortef
hydrocortisone sodium phosphate (Rx)
Hydrocortone Phosphate
hydrocortisone sodium succinate (Rx)
A-hydroCort, Solu-Cortef
Func. class.: Short-acting glucocorticoid
Chem. class.: Natural nonfluorinated, group IV potency (valerate), group VI potency (acetate and plain)

Pregnancy category C

Action: Decreases inflammation by suppressing migration of polymorphonuclear leukocytes and fibroblasts and reversing increased capillary permeability and lysosomal stabilization (systemic); antipruritic, antiinflammatory (top)

⇒ **Therapeutic Outcome:** Decreased inflammation

Uses: Severe inflammation, septic shock, adrenal insufficiency, ulcerative colitis, collagen disorders (systemic), psoriasis, eczema, contact dermatitis, pruritus (top)

Dosage and routes
Adrenal insufficiency/inflammation
Adult: PO 5-30 mg bid-qid; IM/**IV** 100-250 mg (succinate), then 50-100 mg IM as needed; IM/**IV** 15-240 mg q12h (phosphate)

Shock
Adult: 500 mg-2 g q2-6h (succinate)

P *Child:* IM/**IV** 0.186-1 mg/kg bid-tid (succinate)

Colitis
Adult: Enema 100 mg nightly for 21 days

Topical route
P *Adult and child >2 yr:* Apply to affected area qd-qid

Available forms: Tabs 5, 10, 20 mg; inj 25, 50 mg/ml; enema 100 mg/60 ml; acetate-inj 25 ✹, 50 mg/ml ✹, enema 10% aerosol foam, supp 25 mg; cypionate-oral susp 10 mg/5 ml; phosphate-inj 50 mg/ml; succinate inj 100 mg ✹, 250 mg ✹, 500 mg ✹, 1000 mg/vial ✹

Adverse effects
(*italic* = common; **bold** = life-threatening)
CNS: Depression, flushing, sweating, headache, mood changes
CV: Hypertension, **circulatory collapse, thrombophlebitis, embolism,** tachycardia, edema
EENT: Fungal infections, increased intraocular pressure, blurred vision
GI: Diarrhea, nausea, abdominal distention, **GI hemorrhage,** increased appetite, pancreatitis
HEMA: **Thrombocytopenia**
INTEG: Acne, poor wound healing, ecchymosis, petechiae
MS: Fractures, osteoporosis, weakness

Contraindications: Psychosis, hypersensitivity, idiopathic thrombocytopenia (IM), acute glomerulonephritis, amebiasis, fungal
P infections, nonasthmatic bronchial disease, child <2 yr, AIDS, TB

Precautions: Pregnancy **C**, diabetes mellitus, glaucoma, osteoporosis, seizure disorders, ulcerative colitis, CHF, myasthenia gravis, renal disease, esophagitis, peptic ulcer, lactation

▧ **Do Not Confuse:**
hydrocortisone/hydrocodone

Pharmacokinetics	
Absorption	Well absorbed (PO); systemic (top)
Distribution	Crosses placenta
Metabolism	Liver, extensively
Excretion	Kidney
Half-life	3-5 hr, adrenal suppression 3-4 days

Pharmacodynamics				
	PO	IM	IV	TOP
Onset	1-2 hr	20 min	Rapid	Min to hr
Peak	1 hr	4-8 hr	Unkn	Hr to days
Duration	1½ days	1½ days	1½ days	Hr to days

Interactions
Individual drugs
Alcohol, amphotericin B, cycloSPORINE, digitalis: ↑ side effects

Cholestyramine, colestipol, ephedrine, theophylline: ↓ action of hydrocortisone

Phenytoin, rifampin ↓ action

Drug classifications
Anticoagulants, toxoids, vaccines: ↓ action of anticoagulant

Anticonvulsants: ↓ effects of anticonvulsant

Antidiabetics: ↓ effects of antidiabetics

Diuretics: ↑ side effects

Hypoglycemic agents: ↑ need for hypoglycemic agents

NSAIDs, salicylates: ↑ risk of GI bleeding

✓ Herb/drug
Aloe, buckthorn, cascara sagrada, Chinese rhubarb, senna: ↑ hyokalemia

Aloe, licorice, perilla: ↑ corticosteroid effect

Lab test interferences
↑ Cholesterol, ↑ sodium, ↑ blood glucose, ↑ uric acid, ↑ calcium, ↑ urine glucose
↓ Calcium, ↓ potassium, ↓ T_4, ↓ T_3, ↓ thyroid ^{131}I uptake test, ↓ urine 17-OHCS, ↓ 17-KS

False negative: Skin allergy tests

NURSING CONSIDERATIONS
Assessment
• Monitor potassium, blood glucose, urine glucose while patient is on long-term therapy; hypokalemia and hyperglycemia may occur

• Monitor I&O ratio; be alert for decreasing urinary output and increasing edema; weigh daily; notify prescriber of weekly gain >5 lb or edema, hypertension, cardiac symptoms

• Monitor plasma cortisol levels during long-term therapy (normal level is 138-635 nmol/L when obtained at 8 AM); check adrenal function periodically for hypothalamic-pituitary-adrenal axis suppression

• Assess for infection: increased temp, WBC even after withdrawal of medication; drug masks infection symptoms; if fever develops, drug should be discontinued

• Check for potassium depletion: paresthesias, fatigue, nausea, vomiting, depression, polyuria, dysrhythmias, weakness

• Assess mental status: affect, mood, behavioral changes, aggression

• Check nasal passages during long-term treatment for changes in mucus (nasal)

• Assess for systemic absorption: increased temp, inflammation, irritation (top)

Nursing diagnoses
☑ Infection, risk for (adverse reactions)

☑ Knowledge, deficient (teaching)

☑ Noncompliance (teaching) (top/nasal preparation)

Implementation
PO route
• Give with food or milk to decrease GI symptoms

IV IV route
• Give only sodium phosphate product **IV**; reconstitute with sol provided; give 100 mg over >1 min

• May be given by intermittent inf in compatible sol

• Give titrated dose; use lowest effective dosage

Sodium phosphate preparations
Syringe compatibilities: Fluconazole, fludarabine, metoclopramide

Additive compatibilities: Amikacin, amphotericin B, bleomycin, cephapirin, metaraminol, sodium bicarbonate, verapamil

Y-site compatibilities: Allopurinol, amifostine, aztreonam, cefepime, cladribine, famotidine, filgrastim, fluconazole, fludarabine, granisetron, melphalan, ondansetron, paclitaxel, piperacillin/tazobactam, teniposide, thiotepa, vinorelbine

Sodium succinate preparations
Syringe compatibilities: Metoclopramide, thiopental

Y-site compatibilities: Acyclovir, allopurinol, amifostine, aminophylline, ampicillin, amphotericin B cholesteryl, amrinone, amsacrine, atracurium, atropine, aztreonam, betamethasone, calcium gluconate, cefepime, cefmetazole, cephalothin, cephapirin, chlordiazepoxide, chlorproMAZINE, cisatracurium, cladribine, cyanocobalamin, cytarabine, dexamethasone, digoxin, diphenhydramine, DOPamine, DOXOrubicin liposome, droperidol, edrophonium, enalaprilat, epINEPHrine, esmolol, conjugated estrogens, ethacrynate, famotidine, fentanyl, fentanyl/droperidol, filgrastim, fludarabine, fluorouracil, foscarnet, furosemide, gallium, granisetron, heparin, hydrALAZINE, regular insulin, isoproterenol, kanamycin, lidocaine, lorazepam, magnesium sulfate, melphalan, menadiol, meperidine, methicillin, methoxamine, methylergonovine, minocycline, morphine, neostigmine, norepinephrine, ondansetron, oxacillin, oxytocin, paclitaxel, pancuronium, penicillin G potassium, pentazocine, phytonadione, piperacillin/tazobactam, prednisoLONE, procainamide, prochlorperazine, propofol, propranolol, pyridostigmine, remifentanil, scopolamine, sodium bicarbonate, succinylcholine, tacro-

H

limus, teniposide, theophylline, thiotepa, trimethaphan, trimethobenzamide, vecuronium, vinorelbine

Y-site incompatibilities: Diazepam, ergotamine tartrate, idarubicin, phenytoin, sargramostim

Additive compatibilities: Amikacin, aminophylline, amphotericin B, calcium chloride, calcium gluconate, cephalothin, cephapirin, chloramphenicol, clindamycin, cloxacillin, corticotropin, DAUNOrubicin, diphenhydrAMINE, DOPamine, erythromycin, floxacillin, lidocaine, magnesium sulfate, mephentermine, metronidazole/sodium bicarbonate, mitomycin, mitoxantrone, netilmicin, netilmicin/potassium chloride, norepinephrine, penicillin G potassium/sodium, piperacillin, polymyxin B, potassium chloride, sodium bicarbonate, theophylline, thiopental, vancomycin, verapamil, vit B/C

Additive incompatibilities: Bleomycin, DOXOrubicin

Rectal route
• Use applicator provided
• Clean applicator after each use

Topical route
• Apply only to affected areas; do not get in eyes
• Cleanse and dry area before applying medication, then cover with occlusive dressing (only if prescribed); seal to normal skin; change q12h; systemic absorption may occur; use only on dermatoses; do not use on weeping, denuded, or infected area
• Use for a few days after area has cleared
• Store at room temp

Nasal route
• Patient should clear nasal passages before administration; use decongestant if needed; shake inhaler, invert, tilt head backward, insert nozzle into nostril, away from septum; hold other nostril closed and depress activator, inhale through nose, exhale through mouth

Patient/family education
• Teach patient all aspects of drug usage, including cushingoid symptoms
• Advise patient to carry/wear emergency ID as steroid user; not to discontinue abruptly; adrenal crisis can result
• Instruct patient to notify prescriber if therapeutic response decreases; dosage adjustment may be needed
• Instruct patient to notify prescriber of signs of infection
• Caution patient to avoid OTC products

unless directed by perscriber: salicylates, alcohol in cough products, cold preparations
• Teach patient symptoms of adrenal insufficiency: nausea, anorexia, fatigue, dizziness, dyspnea, weakness, joint pain, and when to notify prescriber
• Advise patient that long-term therapy may be needed to resolve infection (1-2 mo depending on type of infection)

Nasal route
• Instruct patient to clear nasal passages if sneezing attack occurs, then repeat dose; to continue using product even if mild nasal bleeding occurs; bleeding is usually transient
• Teach method of instillation after providing written instruction from manufacturer on instillation

Evaluation
Positive therapeutic outcome
• Decrease in runny nose (nasal)
• Ease of respirations, decreased inflammation
• Absence of severe itching, patches on skin, flaking (top)

⚠ HIGH ALERT

hydromorphone (Rx)
(hye-droe-mor'fone)
Dilaudid, Dilaudid-HP, Hydrostat IR, PMS Hydromorphone
Func. class.: Antitussive, opioid analgesic agonist
Chem. class.: Phenanthrene derivative, guaifenesin

Pregnancy category C

Controlled substance schedule II

Action: Depresses pain impulse transmission at the spinal cord level by interacting with opioid receptors; increases respiratory tract fluid by decreasing surface tension and adhesiveness, which increases removal of mucus; analgesic, antitussive

➡ **Therapeutic Outcome:** Decreased cough, decreased pain

Uses: As an antitussive to suppress cough; moderate to severe pain

Dosage and routes
Antitussive
Adult: PO 1 mg q3-4h prn
P *Child 6-12 yr:* PO 0.5 mg q3-4 hr

Analgesic
Adult: PO 1-6 mg q4-6h prn; SC/IM/**IV** 2-4 mg q4-6h prn; rec 3 mg q4-6h prn

G *Geriatric:* PO 1-2 mg q4-6h

Available forms: Inj 1, 2, 3, 4, 10 mg/ml; tabs 1, 2, 3, 4, 8 mg; oral sol 5 mg/5 ml; syr 1 mg/5 ml supp 3 mg

Adverse effects
(*italic* = common; **bold** = life-threatening)
CNS: Dizziness, drowsiness, *sedation, confusion,* headache, euphoria, mood changes, **seizures**
CV: Hypotension, bradycardia, palpitations, change in B/P, tachycardia
EENT: Miosis, diplopia, blurred vision, tinnitus
GI: Nausea, constipation, vomiting, anorexia, dry mouth, cramps
GU: Increased urinary output, dysuria, urinary retention
INTEG: Urticaria, rash, flushing, bruising, diaphoresis, pruritus
RESP: **Respiratory depression**

Contraindications: Hypersensitivity, status asthmaticus, opiate addiction

Precautions: Increased ICP, hypothyroidism, addictive personality, hepatic disease, renal disease, seizure disorders, pregnancy **C**, lactation, MI (acute), severe heart disease, **P** respiratory depression, child <18 yr

N Do Not Confuse:
Dilaudid/Demerol, hydromorphone/meperidine, hydromorphone/morphine

Pharmacokinetics	
Absorption	Well absorbed (PO), complete (**IV**)
Distribution	Unknown; crosses placenta
Metabolism	Liver, extensively
Excretion	Kidneys
Half-life	2-3 hr

Pharmacodynamics			
	PO/IM/SC	IV	REC
Onset	15-30 min	10-15 min	15-30 min
Peak	30-60 min	15-30 min	30-90 min
Duration	4-5 hr	2-3 hr	4-5 hr

Interactions
Individual drugs
Alcohol: ↑ respiratory depression, hypotension, sedation
Nalbuphine, pentazocine: ↓ analgesia

Drug classifications
Antidepressants, antihistamines, CNS depressants, phenothiazines, sedative/hypnotics: ↑ respiratory depression, hypotension
MAOIs: Serious reactions; dosage should be reduced
Opiates, skeletal muscle relaxants: ↑ effects
Z Herb/drug
Chamomile, hops, Jamaican dogwood, lavender, kava, mistletoe, nettle, pokeweed, poppy, senega, skullcap, valerian: ↑ action
Lab test interferences
↑ Amylase

NURSING CONSIDERATIONS
Assessment
• Assess pain control, sedation by scoring on 0-10 scale, around-the-clock dosing is best for pain control
• Monitor VS after parenteral route; note muscle rigidity, drug history, liver, kidney function tests, respiratory dysfunction: respiratory depression, character, rate, rhythm; notify prescriber if respirations are <10/min
• Monitor CNS changes: dizziness, drowsiness, hallucinations, euphoria, LOC, pupil reaction
• Monitor allergic reactions: rash, urticaria; bowel function, constipation

H

Nursing diagnoses
✓ Pain (uses)
✓ Sensory perception, disturbed: visual, auditory (adverse reactions)
✓ Breathing pattern, ineffective (adverse reactions)
✓ Knowledge, deficient (teaching)

Implementation
• Give with antiemetic if nausea, vomiting occur
• Give when pain is beginning to return; determine dosage interval by patient response; continuous dosing of medication is more effective given prn; explain analgesic effect
• Withdraw medication slowly after long-term use to prevent withdrawal symptoms
• Store in light-resistant container at room temp
PO route
• May be given with food or milk to lessen GI upset
IM/SC route
• Do not give if sol is cloudy or a precipitate has formed; rotate inj sites
IV IV route
• Give by direct **IV** after diluting with 5 ml or more of sterile water or 0.9% NaCl for inj
• Give slowly at 2 mg over 3-5 min or less through Y-connector or 3-way stopcock

Syringe compatibilities: Atropine, bupivacaine, ceftazidime, chlorproMAZINE, cimetidine, dimenhyDRINATE, diphenhydrAMINE, fentanyl, glycopyrrolate, haloperidol, hydrOXYzine, lorazepam, midazolam, pentazocaine, pentobarbital, prochlorperazine, promethazine, ranitidine, scopolamine, tetracaine, thiethylperazine, trimethobenzamide

Y-site compatibilities: Acyclovir, allopurinol, amifostine, amikacin, amsacrine, aztreonam, cefamandole, cefepime, cefmetazole, cefoperazone, cefotaxime, cefoxitin, ceftazidime, ceftizoxime, cefuroxime, cephalothin, cephapirin, chloramphenicol, cisplatin, cladribine, clindamycin, cyclophosphamide, cytarabine, diltiazem, DOBUTamine, DOPamine, DOXOrubicin, doxycycline, epINEPHrine, erythromycin lactobionate, famotidine, fentanyl, filgrastim, fludarabine, foscarnet, furosemide, gentamicin, granisetron, heparin, kanamycin, labetalol, lorazepam, magnesium sulfate, melphalan, methotrexate, metronidazole, mezlocillin, midazolam, milrinone, morphine, moxalactam, nafcillin, niCARDipine, nitroglycerin, norepinephrine, ondansetron, oxacillin, paclitaxel, penicillin G potassium, piperacillin, piperacillin/tazobactam, propofol, ranitidine, teniposide, thiotepa, ticarcillin, tobramycin, trimethoprim/sulfamethoxazole, vancomycin, vecuronium, vinorelbine

Y-site incompatibilities: Ampicillin, diazepam, minocycline, phenobarbital, phenytoin, sargramostim

Additive compatibilities: Bupivacaine, fluorouracil, midazolam, ondansetron, promethazine, verapamil

Additive incompatibilities: Sodium bicarbonate, thiopental

Solution compatibilities: D_5W, D_5/0.45% NaCl, D_5/0.9% NaCl, D_5/LR, D_5/Ringer's, 0.45% NaCl, 0.9% NaCl, Ringer's and lactated Ringer's

Patient/family education
- Instruct patient to report any symptoms of CNS changes, allergic reactions; to avoid CNS depressants: alcohol, sedative/hypnotics for at least 24 hr after taking this drug
- Advise patient that dizziness, drowsiness, and confusion are common and to avoid getting up without assistance, driving, or other hazardous activities
- Discuss in detail all aspects of the drug

Evaluation
Positive therapeutic outcome
- Decreased pain
- Decreased cough

Treatment of overdose: Naloxone HCl (Narcan) 0.2-0.8 **IV**, O_2, **IV** fluids, vasopressors

---

hydroxyurea (Rx)
(hye-drox-ee-yoo-ree'ah)
Droxia, Hydrea
Func. class.: Antineoplastic, antimetabolite
Chem. class.: Synthetic urea analog

Pregnancy category D

Action: Acts by inhibiting DNA synthesis without interfering with RNA or protein synthesis; incorporates thymidine into DNA, causing direct damage to DNA strands; cell cycle specific (S phase)

➡ Therapeutic Outcome: Prevention of rapidly growing malignant cells

Uses: Melanoma, chronic myelocytic leukemia, recurrent or metastatic ovarian cancer, squamous cell carcinoma of the head and neck, sickle cell anemia, psoriasis

Dosage and routes
Solid tumors
Adult: PO 80 mg/kg as a single dose q3 days or 20-30 mg/kg as a single dose qd

In combination with radiation
Adult: PO 80 mg/kg as a single dose q3 days; should be started 7 days before irradiation

Resistant chronic myelocytic leukemia
Adult: PO 20-30 mg/kg/day as a single daily dose

Sickle cell anemia
Adult: PO 15 mg/kg/day, may increase by 5 mg/kg/day, max 35 mg/kg/day

Renal dose
Adult: CCr 10-50 ml/min dose 50%; CCr <10 ml/min PO dose 20%

Available forms: Caps 200, 300, 400, 500 mg

Adverse effects
(italic = common; bold = life-threatening)
CNS: Headache, confusion, hallucinations, dizziness, **seizures**
CV: Angina, ischemia
GI: Nausea, vomiting, anorexia, diarrhea, stomatitis, constipation

---

 Herb/drug   Do Not Crush   ◆ Alert   ◆π Key Drug   **G** Geriatric   **P** Pediatric

GU: Increased BUN, uric acid, creatinine, temporary renal function impairment
***HEMA:* Leukopenia, anemia, thrombocytopenia, megaloblastic erythropoiesis**
INTEG: Rash, urticaria, pruritus, dry skin, facial erythema
MISC: Fever, chills, malaise

Contraindications: Hypersensitivity, leukopenia (<2500/mm^3), thrombocytopenia (<100,000/mm^3), anemia (severe), pregnancy **D**, lactation

Precautions: Renal disease (severe)

Pharmacokinetics

Absorption	Well absorbed
Distribution	Crosses blood-brain barrier
Metabolism	Liver (50%)
Excretion	Kidneys, unchanged (50%), eliminated as CO_2
Half-life	4 hr

Pharmacodynamics

Onset	Unknown
Peak	2 hr
Duration	Unknown

Interactions
Individual drugs
Radiation: ↑ toxicity
Drug classifications
Antineoplastics: ↑ toxicity
Lab test interferences
↑ Renal function studies

NURSING CONSIDERATIONS
Assessment
• Assess buccal cavity q8h for dryness, sores or ulceration, white patches, oral pain, bleeding, dysphagia; obtain prescription for viscous lidocaine (Xylocaine)
• Assess symptoms indicating severe allergic reaction: rash, pruritus, urticaria, purpuric skin lesions, itching, flushing
• Monitor CBC, differential, platelet count weekly; withhold drug if WBC is <2500/mm^3 or platelet count is <100,000/mm^3; notify prescriber of results if WBC <20,000/mm^3, platelets <150,000/mm^3
• Assess for increased uric acid levels, swelling, joint pain primarily in extremities; patient should be well hydrated to prevent urate deposits
• Monitor renal function studies: BUN, creatinine, serum uric acid, urine CCr before and during therapy; I&O ratio; report fall in urine output to <30 ml/hr

• Monitor temp q4h (may indicate beginning of infection)
• Monitor liver function tests before and during therapy (bilirubin, AST, ALT, LDH) as needed or monthly
• Assess for bleeding: hematuria, stool guaiac, bruising or petechiae, mucosa or orifices q8h; check for inflammation of mucosa, breaks in skin

Nursing diagnoses
✓ Injury, risk for (adverse reactions)
✓ Body image, disturbed (adverse reactions)
✓ Infection, risk for (adverse reactions)
✓ Knowledge, deficient (teaching)

Implementation
• Avoid contact with skin, very irritating; wash completely to remove
• Give fluids **IV** or PO before chemotherapy to hydrate patient
• Give antiemetic 30-60 min before giving drug and prn to prevent vomiting; antibiotics for prophylaxis of infection
• Provide liq diet: carbonated beverages; gelatin may be added if patient is not nauseated or vomiting
• Provide rinsing of mouth tid-qid with water, club soda; brushing of teeth bid-qid with soft brush or cotton-tipped applicators for stomatitis; use unwaxed dental floss
• For difficulty swallowing, cap contents may be mixed with water
🚫• Do not crush or chew caps

Patient/family education
• Advise patient that contraceptive measures are recommended during therapy
• Teach patient to avoid use of products containing aspirin or ibuprofen, razors, commercial mouthwash, since bleeding may occur; instruct patient to report symptoms of bleeding (hematuria, tarry stools)
• Instruct patient to report signs of anemia (fatigue, headache, irritability, faintness, shortness of breath)
• Advise patient to report any changes in breathing or coughing even several mo after treatment; to avoid crowds and persons with respiratory tract or other infections
• Caution patient not to have any vaccinations without the advice of the prescriber, serious reactions can occur

Evaluation
Positive therapeutic outcome
• Prevention of rapid division of malignant cells

H

*hydrOXYzine (Rx)

(hye-drox'i-zeen)
Apo-hydroxyzine ✤, Atarax, Multipax ✤,
Novohydroxyzine ✤, Vistaril
Func. class.: Antianxiety, sedative, hypnotic,
antihistamine, antiemetic
Chem. class.: Piperazine derivative

Pregnancy category C

Action: Depresses subcortical levels of CNS,
including limbic system, reticular formation;
anticholinergic, antiemetic, antihistaminic
responses; competes with H_1-receptor sites

➥ **Therapeutic Outcome:** Absence of
allergy symptoms, rhinitis, pruritus, absence of
nausea/vomiting, sedation, absence of anxiety

Uses: Anxiety preoperatively, postoperatively
to prevent nausea, vomiting; to potentiate
opioid analgesics; sedation; pruritus; prevention of alcohol, drug withdrawal

Dosage and routes
Adult: PO 25-100 mg tid-qid, max 600
mg/day

G *Elderly:* PO 10 mg tid-qid (pruritus)

P *Child >6 yr:* PO 50-100 mg/day in divided
doses

P *Child <6 yr:* PO 50 mg/day in divided doses

Preoperatively/postoperatively
Adult: IM 25-100 mg q4-6h

P *Child:* IM 0.5-1.1 mg/kg q4-6h

Pruritus
Adult: PO 25 mg tid-qid

Antiemetic
Adult: IM 25-100 mg/dose q4-6h prn

Available forms: Tabs 10, 25, 50, 100
mg; caps 10, 25, 50, 100 mg; oral susp 25
mg/5 ml; inj 25, 50 mg/ml

Adverse effects
(*italic* = common; **bold** = life-threatening)
CNS: Dizziness, drowsiness, confusion,
headache, tremors, fatigue, depression,
seizures
CV: Hypotension
GI: Dry mouth, nausea, diarrhea, increased
appetite, weight gain

Contraindications: Hypersensitivity to
this drug or cetirizine, pregnancy (1st trimester), lactation, acute asthma

G **Precautions:** Elderly, debilitated patients,
hepatic disease, renal disease, pregnancy **C**
(2nd, 3rd trimester), narrow-angle glaucoma,
COPD, prostatic hypertrophy

Do Not Confuse:
Atarax/amoxicillin/Ativan
Vistaril/Versed
hydrOXYzine/hydrALAZINE

Pharmacokinetics

Absorption	Well absorbed
Distribution	Not known
Metabolism	Liver, completely
Excretion	Feces, urine, bile
Half-life	3 hr

Pharmacodynamics

	PO/IM
Onset	15-30 min
Peak	2-4 hr
Duration	4-6 hr

Interactions
Individual drugs
Alcohol, analgesics, barbiturates: ↑ CNS
depression
Atropine, disopyramide, haloperidol,
quinidine: ↑ anticholinergic reactions
Drug classifications
Antidepressants, antihistamines, phenothi-
azines: ↑ anticholinergic reactions
CNS depressants, opiates, sedative/hypnotics:
↑ CNS depression
Herb/drug
Corkwood, henbane leaf, jimsonweed,
scopolia: ↑ anticholinergic effect
Chamomile, cowslip, hops, Jamaican dog-
wood, khat, kava, Queen Anne's lace, senega,
skullcap, valerian: ↑ sedative action
Lab test interferences
False: ↑ 17-OHCS

NURSING CONSIDERATIONS
Assessment
• Assess mental status: mood, sensorium,
affect, behavior, increased sedation
• Assess respiratory status: rate, rhythm,
increase in bronchial secretions, wheezing,
chest tightness; provide fluids to 2 L/day to
decrease secretion thickness
• Monitor I&O ratio: be alert for urinary
retention, frequency, dysuria, especially in the
G elderly; drug should be discontinued if these
occur
• Observe for drowsiness, dizziness
• Assess cough characteristics including type,
frequency, thickness of secretions; evaluate
response to this medication if using for cough

Nursing diagnoses
✓ Injury, risk for (side effects)

✓ Anxiety (uses)
✓ Knowledge, deficient (teaching)

Implementation
PO route
- Give with meals if GI symptoms occur; absorption may be slightly decreased; cap may be opened and drug mixed with food/fluids for patients with swallowing difficulties

IM route
- Give IM inj in large muscle mass; aspirate to prevent **IV** administration; use Z-track method; severe necrosis can result with improper technique; never give **IV**/SC

Syringe compatibilities: Atropine, atropine/meperidine, benzquinamide, bupivacaine, butorphanol, chlorproMAZINE, cimetidine, codeine, diphenhydrAMINE, doxapram, droperidol, fentanyl, fluphenazine, glycopyrrolate, hydromorphone, lidocaine, meperidine, meperidine/atropine, methotrimeprazine, metoclopramide, midazolam, morphine, nalbuphine, oxymorphone, pentazocine, perphenazine, procaine, prochlorperazine, promazine, promethazine, remifentanil, scopolamine, sufentanil, thiothixene

Syringe incompatibilities: Aminophylline, chloramphenicol, dimenhyDRINATE, heparin, penicillin G potassium, pentobarbital, phenobarbital, phenytoin

Additive compatibilities: Cisplatin, cyclophosphamide, cytarabine, dimenhyDRINATE, etoposide, lidocaine, mesna, methotrexate, nafcillin

Patient/family education
- Caution patient to avoid hazardous activities and activities requiring alertness, since dizziness may occur; instruct patient to request assistance with ambulation
- Advise patient to avoid alcohol, other CNS depressants including cough, cold preparations; CNS depression may occur
- Teach all aspects of drug use; to notify prescriber if confusion, sedation, hypotension occur; to avoid driving and other hazardous activity if drowsiness occurs; to avoid alcohol and other CNS depressants that may potentiate effect
- Instruct patient to take 1 hr pc or 2 hr ac to facilitate absorption
- May crush if patient unable to swallow whole
- Caution patient not to exceed recommended dosage; dysrhythmias may occur
- Tell patient hard candy, gum, frequent rinsing of mouth may be used for dryness

Evaluation
Positive therapeutic outcome
- Absence of nausea, vomiting
- Decreased anxiety

Treatment of overdose: Lavage if orally ingested, VS, supportive care, **IV** norepINEPHrine for hypotension

---

ibritumomab tiuxetan (Rx)
(ee-brit-u-moe′mab)
Zevalin
Func. class.: Antineoplastic—misc.

Pregnancy category D

Action: High affinity for indium-111, yttrium-90; induces $CD20^+$ B-cell lines

➡ Therapeutic Outcome: Decrease in tumor size, spread of malignancy

Uses: Non-Hodgkin's lymphoma, B-cell NHL

Dosage and routes
Adult: **IV INF** 250 mg/m^2 at a rate of 50 mg/hr; if hypersensitivity does not occur, increase rate by 50 mg/hr q½h, max 400 mg/hr; slow/interrupt inf if hypersensitivity occurs

Available forms: Inj 3.2 mg/2 ml

Adverse effects
(*italic* = common; **bold** = life-threatening)
CV: **Cardiac dysrhythmias**
GI: Nausea, vomiting, anorexia, abdominal pain, diarrhea
GU: **Renal failure**
HEMA: **Leukopenia, neutropenia, thrombocytopenia,** anemia
INTEG: Irritation at site, rash, **fatal mucocutaneous infections (rare)**
SYST: **Stevens-Johnson syndrome**
OTHER: Fever, chills, asthenia, headache, angioedema, hypotension, myalgia, **bronchospasm, hemorrhage,** infections, cough, dyspnea, dizziness, anxiety

Contraindications: Hypersensitivity to this agent or murine proteins, pregnancy **D**

P Precautions: Lactation, children, elderly,
G cardiac conditions, immunizations after therapy

Pharmacokinetics	
Absorption	Unknown
Distribution	Unknown
Metabolism	Unknown
Excretion	Unknown
Half-life	30 hr

Pharmacodynamics
Unknown

NURSING CONSIDERATIONS
Assessment
◆• Assess for signs of fatal infusion reaction: hypoxia, pulmonary infiltrates, ARDS, MI, ventricular fibrillation, cardiogenic shock; most fatal infusion reactions occur with first infusion; potentially fatal
• Assess biodistribution: 1st image 2-24 hr, 2nd image 48-72 hr, 3rd image 90-120 hr (optimal)
• Assess for signs of severe mucocutaneous reactions: Stevens-Johnson syndrome, lichenoid dermatitis, toxic epidermal lysis; occur 1-13 wk after drug was given
◆• Assess for tumor lysis syndrome: acute renal failure requiring hemodialysis, hyperkalemia, hypocalcemia, hyperuricemia, hyperphosphatemia
• Monitor CBC, differential, platelet count weekly; withhold drug if WBC is <3500/mm³ or platelet count <100,000/mm³; notify prescriber of these results; drug should be discontinued
• Monitor GI symptoms: frequency of stools
• Assess for signs of dehydration: rapid respirations, poor skin turgor, decreased urine output, dry skin, restlessness, weakness

Nursing diagnoses
✓ Infection, risk for (adverse reactions)
✓ Nutrition: less than body requirements, imbalanced (adverse reactions)
✓ Knowledge, deficient (teaching)

Implementation
• Do not use as bolus or **IV** direct
• Provide increased fluid intake to 2-3 L/day to prevent dehydration, unless contraindicated
• Provide nutritious diet with iron, vitamin supplement, low fiber, few dairy products

IV **IV INF route**
• See manufacturer's product labeling for preparation
• Have emergency equipment nearby with epinephrine, antihistamines, corticosteroids
• Change **IV** site q48h
• Store vials at 36°-46° F (2°-7° C), do not freeze

Patient/family education
• To report adverse reactions

Evaluation
Positive therapeutic outcome
• Decrease in tumor size, decrease in spread of cancer

Action: Inhibits prostaglandin synthesis by decreasing enzyme needed for biosynthesis; analgesic, antiinflammatory, antipyretic

⇒**Therapeutic Outcome:** Decreased pain, inflammation, fever

Uses: Rheumatoid arthritis, osteoarthritis, primary dysmenorrhea, gout, dental pain, musculoskeletal disorders, fever

Dosage and routes
Analgesia
Adult: PO 200-400 mg q4-6h, not to exceed 3.2 g/day

P *Child:* PO 4-10 mg/kg/dose q6-8h

Antipyretic
P *Child 6 mo-12 yr:* PO 5 mg/kg (temp <102.5° F or 39.2° C), 10 mg/kg (temp >102.5° F), may repeat q4-6h; max 40 mg/kg/day

Antiinflammatory
Adult: PO 300-800 mg tid-qid; max 3.2 g/day

P *Child:* PO 30-40 mg/kg/day in 3-4 divided doses; max 50 mg/kg/day

Available forms: Tabs 100, 200, 300, 400, 600, 800 mg; Caps, liqui-gel 200 mg; oral susp 100 mg/2.5 ml, 100 mg/5 ml; liq 100 mg/5 ml; tabs, chew 50, 100 mg; drops 50 mg/1.25 ml

Adverse effects
(*italic* = common; **bold** = life-threatening)
CNS: Headache, dizziness, drowsiness, fatigue, tremors, confusion, insomnia, anxiety, depression
CV: Tachycardia, peripheral edema, palpitations, dysrhythmias
EENT: Tinnitus, hearing loss, blurred vision
GI: Nausea, anorexia, vomiting, diarrhea, jaundice, **hepatitis,** constipation, flatulence, cramps, dry mouth, peptic ulcer, **GI bleeding**

GU: **Nephrotoxicity,** dysuria, hematuria, oliguria, azotemia
HEMA: **Blood dyscrasias,** increased bleeding time
INTEG: Purpura, rash, pruritus, sweating
SYST: Anaphylaxis

Contraindications: Hypersensitivity, asthma, severe renal disease, severe hepatic disease, avoid in 2nd/3rd trimester of pregnancy

Precautions: Pregnancy **B** (1st trimester),
P lactation, children, bleeding disorders, GI disorders, cardiac disorders, hypersensitivity
G to other antiinflammatory agents, elderly, CHF, CCr <25 ml/min

◪ **Do Not Confuse:**
Nuprin/Lupron

Pharmacokinetics

Absorption	Well absorbed
Distribution	Not known; crosses placenta
Metabolism	Liver, extensively
Excretion	Kidneys, unchanged (10%)
Half-life	3½ hr

Pharmacodynamics

Onset	½ hr
Peak	1-2 hr
Duration	4-6 hr

Interactions
Individual drugs
Alcohol, aspirin: ↑ GI reactions
Aspirin: ↓ effectiveness
Cefamandole, cefotetan, cefoperazone, valproic acid, warfarin: ↑ risk of bleeding
CycloSPORINE, digoxin, lithium, probenecid: ↑ toxicity
Digoxin: ↑ levels
Furosemide: ↓ effect of furosemide
Insulin: ↑ hypoglycemia
Radiation: ↑ risk of blood dyscrasias
Drug classifications
Anticoagulants, antiplatelet agents, cephalosporins, thrombolytics: ↑ risk of bleeding
Anticoagulants: ↑ toxicity (oral)
Antidiabetics (oral): ↑ hypoglycemia
Antihypertensives: ↓ effect of antihypertensives
Antineoplastics: ↑ risk of blood dyscrasias
Corticosteroids, NSAIDs: ↑ GI reactions
Diuretics: ↓ effectiveness of diuretics (thiazides)
▨ *Herb/drug*
Arginine, gossypol: ↑ gastric irritation
Arnica, bogbean, chamomile, chondroitin, clove, dong quai, fenugreek, feverfew, garlic, ginger, ginkgo, ginseng (panax): ↑ risk of bleeding
Bearberry, bilberry: ↑ NSAIDs effect
Lab test interferences
↑ Bleeding time

NURSING CONSIDERATIONS
Assessment
• Assess pain: location, duration, type, intensity before dose and 1 hr after
• Assess musculoskeletal status: ROM before dose and 1 hr after
• Monitor liver function studies: AST, ALT, bilirubin, creatinine if patient is on long-term therapy
• Monitor renal function studies: BUN, urine creatinine if patient is on long-term therapy
• Assess cardiac status: edema (peripheral), tachycardia, palpitations; monitor B/P, pulse for character, quality, rhythm
• Monitor blood studies: CBC, Hct, Hgb, Pro-time if patient is on long-term therapy
• Check I&O ratio; decreasing output may indicate renal failure if patient is on long-term therapy
• Assess hepatotoxicity: dark urine, clay-colored stools, jaundice of skin and sclera, itching, abdominal pain, fever, diarrhea if patient is on long-term therapy
• Assess for history of peptic ulcer disorder; asthma, aspirin, hypersensitivity, check closely for hypersensitivity reactions
• Assess for allergic reactions: rash, urticaria; if these occur, drug may have to be discontinued
• Assess for ototoxicity: tinnitus, ringing, roaring in ears; audiometric testing needed before, after long-term therapy
• Assess for visual changes: blurring, halos; may indicate corneal, retinal damage
• Identify prior drug history; there are many drug interactions
• Identify fever: length of time in evidence and related symptoms

Nursing diagnoses
☑Pain, acute (uses)
☑Pain, chronic (uses)
☑Mobility, impaired physical (uses)
☑Injury, risk for (side effects)
☑Knowledge, deficient (teaching)

Implementation
• Administer to patient crushed or whole; 800-mg tab may be dissolved in water
• Give with food or milk to decrease gastric symptoms; give 30 min pc or 2 hr ac; absorption may be slowed

Patient/family education

- Teach patient to report any symptoms of hepatotoxicity, renal toxicity, visual changes, ototoxicity, allergic reactions, bleeding if patient is on long-term therapy
- Caution patient not to exceed recommended dosage; acute poisoning may result
- Advise patient to read label on other OTC drugs
- Inform patient that the therapeutic response takes 1 mo (arthritis)
- Caution patient to avoid alcohol ingestion, salicylates, NSAIDs; GI bleeding may occur
- Advise patient with allergies that allergic reactions may develop
- Advise patient to use sunscreen to prevent photosensitivity

Evaluation

Positive therapeutic outcome

- Decreased pain
- Decreased inflammation
- Decreased fever
- Increased mobility

! HIGH ALERT

ibutilide (Rx)

(eye-byoo'te-lide)

Corvert

Func. class.: Antidysrhythmic (Class III)

Pregnancy category C

Action: Prolongs duration of action potential and effective refractory period

Uses: For rapid conversion of atrial fibrillation/flutter occurring within 1 wk of coronary artery bypass or valve surgery

Dosage and routes

Adult: **IV** inf (≥60 kg) 1 vial (1 mg) given over 10 min, may repeat same dose in 10 min; **IV** inf (<60 kg) 0.01 mg/kg given over 10 min, may repeat same dose in 10 min

Available forms: Inj 0.1 mg/ml

Adverse effects

(*italic* = common; **bold** = life-threatening)

CNS: Headache

CV: Hypotension, bradycardia, **sinus arrest, CHF, dysrhythmias,** hypertension, extrasystoles, ventricular tachycardia, bundle branch block, AV block, palpitations, supraventricular extrasystoles, syncope

GI: Nausea

Contraindications: Hypersensitivity

Precautions: Sinus node dysfunction, 2nd- or 3rd-degree AV block, electrolyte imbalances, pregnancy **C,** bradycardia, lactation, children<18 yr, renal/hepatic disease, elderly

Pharmacokinetics

Absorption	Unknown
Distribution	Unknown
Metabolism	Liver
Excretion	Kidney
Half-life	6 hr

Interactions

Individual drugs

Digoxin: masking of cardiotoxicity

Drug classifications

Antidepressants (tricyclic/tetracyclic): Prodysrhythmia

Antihistamines, H₂-receptor antagonists, phenothiazines: ↑ prodysrhythmia

Class Ia antidysrhythmics (disopyramide, quinidine, procainamide), class III agents (amiodarone, sotalol): Do not use within 4 hr of ibutilide

Herb/drug

Aconite: ↑ toxicity, death

Aloe, broom, buckthorn (chronic use), cascara sagrada (chronic use), Chinese rhubarb, figwort, fumitory, goldenseal, kudzu, licorice: ↑ effect

Coltsfoot: ↓ effect

Horehound: ↑ serotonin effect

NURSING CONSIDERATIONS

Assessment

- Monitor I&O ratio; monitor electrolytes: potassium, sodium, chloride
- Monitor liver function studies: AST, ALT, bilirubin, alkaline phosphatase
- Monitor ECG continuously to determine drug effectiveness; measure PR, QRS, QT intervals; check for PVCs, other dysrhythmias; monitor B/P continuously for hypotension, hypertension; check for rebound hypertension after 1-2 hr; discontinue drug when atrial fibrillation/flutter ceases
- Monitor for dehydration or hypovolemia
- Assess for CNS symptoms: confusion, psychosis, numbness, depression, involuntary movements; if these occur drug should be discontinued
- Monitor cardiac rate, respiration; rate, rhythm, character, chest pain, ventricular tachycardia, supraventricular tachycardia or fibrillation

Nursing diagnoses

☑ Cardiac output, decreased (uses)

☑ Gas exchange, impaired (adverse reactions)
☑ Knowledge, deficient (teaching)

Implementation
IV IV route
- Give reduced dosage slowly with ECG monitoring only
- Give undiluted or diluted in 50 ml of 0.9% NaCl or D_5W (0.017 mg/ml), give over 10 min
- Solution is stable for 48 hr refrigerated or 24 hr at room temp
- Do not admix with other solution, drugs

Patient/family education
- Instruct patient to report side effects immediately to prescriber

Evaluation
Positive therapeutic outcome
- Decrease in atrial fibrillation/flutter

⚠ HIGH ALERT

idarubicin (Rx)
(eye-da-roo'bi-sin)
Idamycin, Idamycin PFS
Func. class.: Antineoplastic, antibiotic
Chem. class.: Anthracycline glycoside

Pregnancy category D

Action: Inhibits DNA synthesis derived from DAUNOrubicin by binding to DNA, which causes strand splitting; cell cycle specific (S phase); a vesicant

➡ **Therapeutic Outcome:** Prevention of rapidly growing malignant cells

Uses: Used in combination with other antineoplastics for acute myelocytic leukemia in adults

Investigational uses: Breast cancer, solid tumors

Dosage and routes
Adult: **IV** 12 mg/m^2/day × 3 days in combination with cytosine (induction)

Available forms: Inj 1 mg/ml; powder for inj, lyophilized 5, 10, 20 mg

Adverse effects
(*italic* = common; **bold** = life-threatening)
CNS: Fever, chills, headache
CV: **Dysrhythmias, CHF, pericarditis, myocarditis,** peripheral edema, angina, **MI**
GI: Nausea, vomiting, abdominal pain, mucositis, diarrhea, **hepatotoxicity**
GU: **Nephrotoxicity**
HEMA: **Thrombocytopenia, leukopenia, anemia**

INTEG: Rash, extravasation, dermatitis, reversible alopecia, urticaria, thrombophlebitis, tissue necrosis at inj site

Contraindications: Hypersensitivity, pregnancy **D,** lactation, myelosuppression

Precautions: Renal and hepatic disease,
P gout, bone marrow depression, children

⟩ Do Not Confuse:
Idamycin/Adriamycin, idarubicin/DOXOrubicin

Pharmacokinetics	
Absorption	Complete bioavailability
Distribution	Rapidly distributed; high tissue binding
Metabolism	Liver, extensively
Excretion	Bile
Half-life	22 hr

Pharmacodynamics
Unknown

Interactions
Individual drugs
Radiation: ↑ toxicity
Drug classifications
Antineoplastics: ↑ toxicity
Live virus vaccines: ↓ antibody response
Lab test interferences
↑ Uric acid

NURSING CONSIDERATIONS
Assessment
- Assess symptoms indicating severe allergic reaction: rash, pruritus, urticaria, purpuric skin lesions, itching, flushing; drug should be discontinued
- Assess for tachypnea, ECG changes, dyspnea, edema, fatigue
- Assess for cardiac toxicity: CHF, dysrhythmias, cardiomyopathy; cardiac studies should be done before and periodically during treatment; ECG, chest x-ray
- Monitor CBC, differential, platelet count weekly; withhold drug if WBC is <4000/mm^3 or platelet count is <100,000/mm^3; notify prescriber of results if WBC <20,000/mm^3, platelets <150,000/mm^3
- Monitor renal function studies: BUN, uric acid, urine CCr, electrolytes, before, during therapy
- Monitor temp q4h (may indicate beginning of infection)
- Monitor liver function tests before and during therapy (bilirubin, AST, ALT, LDH) as needed or monthly; note jaundice of skin and sclera, dark urine, clay-colored stools, itchy

- skin, abdominal pain, fever, diarrhea; hepatoxicity can be severe
- Assess for bleeding: hematuria, stool guaiac, bruising or petechiae, mucosa or orifices q8h; assess for inflammation of mucosa, breaks in skin
- Identify effects of alopecia on body image; discuss feelings about body changes

Nursing diagnoses
☑ Injury, risk for (adverse reactions)
☑ Cardiac output, decreased (adverse reactions)
☑ Body image, disturbed (adverse reactions)
☑ Infection, risk for (adverse reactions)
☑ Knowledge, deficient (teaching)

Implementation
- Avoid contact with skin; very irritating; wash completely to remove
- Give fluids **IV** or PO before chemotherapy to hydrate patient
- Administer antiemetic 30-60 min before giving drug and prn to prevent vomiting; administer antibiotics for prophylaxis of infection
- Give a liq diet: carbonated beverages; gelatin may be added if patient is not nauseated or vomiting
- Provide rinsing of mouth tid-qid with water, club soda; brushing of teeth bid-qid with soft brush or cotton-tipped applicators for stomatitis; use unwaxed dental floss
- Drug should be prepared by experienced personnel using proper precautions (biologic cabinet, wearing gown, gloves, mask)
- Give after reconstituting 5-mg vial with 5 ml of 0.9% NaCl (1 mg/1 ml); give over 10-15 min through Y-tube or 3-way stopcock of inf of D_5 or 0.9% NaCl; discard unused portion
- Inject hydrocortisone for extravasation; apply ice compress after stopping inf
- Store at room temp for 3 days after reconstituting or 7 days refrigerated

Y-site compatibilities: Amifostine, amikacin, aztreonam, cimetidine, cladribine, cyclophosphamide, cytarabine, diphenhydrA-MINE, droperidol, erythromycin, filgrastim, granisetron, imipenem/cilastatin, magnesium sulfate, mannitol, melphalan, metoclopramide, potassium chloride, ranitidine, sargramostim, thiotepa, vinorelbine

Y-site incompatibilities: Acyclovir, ampicillin/sulbactam, cefazolin, ceftazidime, clindamycin, dexamethasone, etoposide, furosemide, gentamicin, hydrocortisone, lorazepam, meperidine, methotrexate, mezlocillin, sargramostim, sodium bicarbonate, vancomycin, vinCRIStine

Solution compatibilities: $D_{3.3}$/0.3% NaCl, D_5/0.9% NaCl, D_5W, Ringer's, 0.9% NaCl, LR

Patient/family education
- Teach patient to avoid use of products containing aspirin or ibuprofen, razors, commercial mouthwash, since bleeding may occur; to report symptoms of bleeding (hematuria, tarry stools)
- Instruct patient to report signs of anemia (fatigue, headache, irritability, faintness, shortness of breath)
- Advise patient that hair may be lost during treatment; a wig or hairpiece may make patient feel better; new hair may be different in color, texture
- Tell patient not to have any vaccinations without the advice of the prescriber; serious reactions can occur
- Advise patient that contraception is needed during treatment and for several mo after the completion of therapy

Evaluation
Positive therapeutic outcome
- Prevention of rapid division of malignant cells

❗ HIGH ALERT

ifosfamide ⚬ₓ (Rx)
(i-foss'fa-mide)
Ifex
Func. class.: Antineoplastic alkylating agent
Chem. class.: Nitrogen mustard

Pregnancy category D

Action: Alkylates DNA, RNA; inhibits enzymes that allow synthesis of amino acids in proteins; also responsible for cross-linking DNA strands; activity is not cell cycle stage specific

➔ **Therapeutic Outcome:** Prevention of rapidly growing malignant cells

Uses: Testicular cancer, soft-tissue sarcoma, Ewing's sarcoma, non-Hodgkin's lymphoma, lung, pancreatic cancer, sarcoma

Dosage and routes
Adult: **IV** 1.2 g/m²/day × 5 days; repeat course q3 wk; give with mesna

Available forms: Inj 1, 3 g

Adverse effects
(*italic* = common; **bold** = life-threatening)
CNS: Facial paresthesia, fever, malaise, somnolence, confusion, depression, hallucinations,

---

dizziness, disorientation, **seizures, coma,** cranial nerve dysfunction

GI: Nausea, vomiting, anorexia, **hepatotoxicity,** stomatitis, constipation, diarrhea

GU: **Hematuria, nephrotoxicity, hemorrhagic cystitis,** dysuria, urinary frequency

HEMA: **Thrombocytopenia, leukopenia, anemia**

INTEG: Dermatitis, alopecia, pain at inj site

Contraindications: Hypersensitivity, bone marrow suppression, pregnancy **D**

Precautions: Renal disease, lactation, children

Pharmacokinetics

Absorption	Complete bioavailability
Distribution	Saturation at high dosages
Metabolism	Liver
Excretion	Breast milk
Half-life	15 hr

Pharmacodynamics

Unknown

Interactions

Individual drugs

Allopurinol, radiation: ↑ toxicity

Radiation: ↑ bone marrow suppression

Drug classifications

Antineoplastics, barbiturates: ↑ toxicity

Antineoplastics: ↑ bone marrow suppression

Live virus vaccines: ↓ antibody response

NURSING CONSIDERATIONS

Assessment

• Monitor CBC, differential, platelet count weekly; withhold drug if WBC is <2000 or platelet count is <50,000; notify prescriber of results if WBC <10,000/mm^3, platelets <100,000/mm^3

• Monitor renal function studies: BUN, serum uric acid, urine CCr before, during therapy; I&O ratio; report fall in urine output of 30 ml/hr

• Monitor for cold, fever, sore throat (may indicate beginning of infection); identify edema in feet and joints, stomach pain, shaking; prescriber should be notified

• Assess for bleeding: hematuria, guaiac, bruising or petechiae, mucosa or orifices q8h; no rec temp

• Monitor liver function studies before and during therapy (ALT, AST, LDH); jaundice of skin, sclera, dark urine, clay-colored stools, itching, abdominal pain, fever, diarrhea that may indicate liver involvement

Nursing diagnoses

☑ Injury, risk for (adverse reactions)

☑ Body image, disturbed (adverse reactions)

☑ Infection, risk for (adverse reactions)

☑ Knowledge, deficient (teaching)

Implementation

• Give fluids **IV** or PO before chemotherapy to hydrate patient

• Give antiemetic 30-60 min before giving drug and prn to prevent vomiting

• Provide liq diet: carbonated beverages; gelatin may be added if patient is not nauseated or vomiting

• Give **IV** after diluting 1 g/20 ml of sterile or bacteriostatic water for inj with parabens or benzyl only; shake

• Give by intermittent inf after further diluting with D$_5$W, LR, 0.9% NaCl, sterile water for inj (1 g/20 ml = 50 mg/ml; 1 g/50 ml = 20 mg/ml; 1 g/200 ml = 5 mg/ml); give over ≥30 min; may also give as a cont inf over 72 hr

• Store powder at room temp; always give with mesna, increase fluids to 3 L/day to prevent ifosfamide-induced hemorrhagic cystitis

Syringe compatibilities: Mesna

Y-site compatibilities: Allopurinol, amifostine, aztreonam, filgrastim, fludarabine, gallium, granisetron, melphalan, ondansetron, paclitaxel, piperacillin/tazobactam, propofol, sargramostim, teniposide, thiotepa, vinorelbine

Additive compatibilities: Carboplatin, cisplatin, etoposide, fluorouracil, mesna

Patient/family education

• Teach patient to avoid use of products containing aspirin or NSAIDs, razors, commercial mouthwash, since bleeding may occur; to report symptoms of bleeding (hematuria, tarry stools)

• Instruct patient to report signs of anemia (fatigue, headache, irritability, faintness, shortness of breath)

• Advise patient to report any changes in breathing or coughing even several mo after treatment; to avoid crowds and persons with respiratory tract or other infections

• Teach patient that hair loss is common; discuss the use of wigs or hairpieces; that hair may be a different texture when regrowth occurs

• Caution patient not to have any vaccinations without the advice of the prescriber; serious reactions can occur

- Advise patient that contraception is needed during treatment and for several mo after completion of therapy

Evaluation
Positive therapeutic outcome
- Prevention of rapid division of malignant cells
- Absence of swelling at night
- Increased appetite, increased weight

---

imatinib (Rx)
(im-ah-tin'ib)
Gleevec
Func. class.: Antineoplastic—misc.
Chem. class.: Protein-tyrosine kinase inhibitor

Pregnancy category D

Action: Inhibits Bcr-Abl tyrosine kinase created in chronic myeloid leukemia (CML)

Therapeutic Outcome: Decreased tumor size, prevention of spread of cancer

Uses: Treatment of chronic myeloid leukemia (CML) in blast cell crisis or chronic failure after treatment failure with interferon alfa, gastrointestinal stromal tumors (GIST)

Investigational uses: Polycythemia vera, medullary thyroid carcinoma, recurrent extraabdominal desmoid tumors

Dosage and routes
Adult: PO 400-600 mg/day, may increase to 800 mg qd, give in 2 divided doses; give with meal and large glass of water, continue as long as response is good, may increase by 200 mg/day as needed

Available forms: Cap 100 mg

Adverse effects
(*italic* = common; **bold** = life-threatening)
CV: Hemorrhage
CNS: **CNS hemorrhage,** headache, dizziness, insomnia
GI: *Nausea*, **hepatotoxicity**, *vomiting*, *dyspepsia*, **GI hemorrhage**, *anorexia*, abdominal pain
HEMA: **Neutropenia, thrombocytopenia, bleeding**
INTEG: *Rash, pruritus*
META: Edema, fluid retention, hypokalemia, weight increase
MISC: Fatigue, epistaxis, pyrexia, night sweats, increased weight
MS: Cramps, pain, arthralgia, myalgia
RESP: Cough, dyspnea, nasopharyngitis, pneumonia, URI

Contraindications: Hypersensitivity, pregnancy **D**

P Precautions: Lactation, children, **G** elderly

Pharmacokinetics
Absorption	Well absorbed; bound to plasma protein (98%)
Distribution	Unknown
Metabolism	Liver (metabolites)
Excretion	Feces, primarily (metabolites)
Half-life	18-40 hr

Pharmacodynamics
Onset	Unknown
Peak	2-4 hr
Duration	24 hr (imatinib)
	40 hr (metabolite)

Interactions
Individual drugs
Acetaminophen: ↑ hepatotoxicity
Carbamazepine, dexamethasone, phenobarbital, phenytoin, rifampin: ↓ imatinib concentrations
Clarithromycin, erythromycin, ketoconazole, itraconazole: ↑ imatinib concentrations
Simvastatin: ↑ plasma concentrations
Warfarin: ↑ plasma concentration of warfarin; avoid coadministration; use low molecular weight anticoagulants instead
Herb/drug
St. John's wort: ↓ imatinib concentration

NURSING CONSIDERATIONS
Assessment
- Assess ANC and platelets; in chronic phase if ANC <1 × 10^9/L and/or platelets <50 × 10^9/L, stop until ANC >1.5 × 10^9/L and platelets >75 × 10^9/L; in accelerated phase/blast crisis if ANC <0.5 × 10^9/L and/or platelets <10 × 10^9/L, determine whether cytopenia is related to biopsy/aspirate, if not, reduce dose by 200 mg, if cytopenia continues, reduce dose by another 100 mg; if cytopenia continues for 4 wks, stop drug until ANC ≥1 × 10^9/L
- Assess for hepatotoxicity: monitor liver function tests, before treatment and qmo
- Assess CBC, differential, platelet count weekly; withhold drug if WBC is <3500/mm^3, or platelet count <100,000/mm^3; notify prescriber of these results; drug should be discontinued
- Assess food preferences: list likes, dislikes
- Assess GI symptoms: frequency of stools
- Assess signs of fluid retention, edema:

---

weigh, monitor lung sounds, assess for edema, 50-ml fluid retention is dose dependent

Nursing diagnoses
☑ Injury, risk for (side effects)
☑ Knowledge, deficient (teaching)

Implementation
- Give with meal and large glass of water to decrease GI symptoms
- Provide nutritious diet with iron, vit supplement, low fiber, few dairy products
- Store at 25° C (77° F)

Patient/family education
- Instruct patient to report adverse reactions immediately: shortness of breath, swelling of extremities, bleeding
- Teach patient reason for treatment, expected result

Evaluation
Positive therapeutic outcome
- Decrease in leukemic cells, size of tumors

---

imipenem/ cilastatin (Rx)
(i-me-pen'em sye-la-stat'in)
Primaxin IM, Primaxin IV
Func. class.: Antiinfective—misc. penicillin
Chem. class.: Carbapenem

Pregnancy category C

Action: Interferes with cell wall replication of susceptible organisms; osmotically unstable cell wall swells and bursts from osmotic pressure; addition of cilastatin prevents renal inactivation that occurs with high urinary concentrations of imipenem

➡ **Therapeutic Outcome:** Bactericidal action against the following: *Streptococcus pneumoniae,* group A β-hemolytic streptococci, *Staphylococcus aureus,* enterococcus; gram-negative organisms: *Klebsiella, Proteus, Escherichia coli, Acinetobacter, Serratia, Pseudomonas aeruginosa; Salmonella, Shigella*

Uses: Serious infections caused by gram-positive or gram-negative organisms

Dosage and routes
Adult: **IV** 250-500 mg q8h; severe infections may require 1 g q8h; may give IM q12h (total daily IM dose >1500 mg not recommended); mild to moderate infections

Ⓟ *Child:* **IV** 60-100 mg/kg/day in divided doses max 4 g/day

Renal dose
Adult: **IV** CCr 30-70 ml/min give 50% dose q6-8h; CCr 20-30 ml/min give 40% of dose q8-12h; CCr 5-20 ml/min give 25% of dose q12h

Available forms: IV inj 250, 500; IM inj 500, 750 mg

Adverse effects
(*italic* = common; **bold** = life-threatening)
CNS: Fever, somnolence, **seizures,** confusion, dizziness, weakness, myoclonia
CV: Hypotension, palpitations
GI: Diarrhea, nausea, vomiting, **pseudomembranous colitis, hepatitis,** glossitis
HEMA: **Eosinophilia, neutropenia,** decreased Hgb, Hct
INTEG: Rash, urticaria, pruritus, pain at inj site, phlebitis, erythema at inj site
RESP: Chest discomfort, dyspnea, hyperventilation
SYST: **Anaphylaxis**

Contraindications: Hypersensitivity, IM hypersensitivity to local anesthetics of the amide type

Precautions: Pregnancy **C,** lactation, Ⓖ elderly, hypersensitivity to penicillins, seizure Ⓟ disorders, renal disease, children

◩ **Do Not Confuse:**
imipenem/Omnipen, Primaxin/Premarin

Pharmacokinetics
Absorption	Complete bioavailability (**IV**)
Distribution	Widely distributed; crosses placenta
Metabolism	Liver
Excretion	Kidneys, unchanged (70%-80%); breast milk
Half-life	1 hr; increased in renal disease

Pharmacodynamics
	IV	IM
Onset	Rapid	Unknown
Peak	½-1 hr	Unknown

Interactions
Individual drugs
CycloSPORINE, ganciclovir: ↑ risk of seizures
Probenecid: ↑ imipenem plasma levels
Drug classifications
β-Lactam antibiotics: ↑ toxicity
Lab test interferences
↑ AST, ↑ ALT, ↑ LDH, ↑ BUN, ↑ alkaline phosphatase, ↑ bilirubin, ↑ creatinine
False positive: Direct Coombs' test

NURSING CONSIDERATIONS
Assessment
- Assess patient for previous penicillin sensitivity reaction, may have sensitivity to this drug
- Assess patient for signs and symptoms of infection, including characteristics of wounds, sputum, urine, stool, WBC >10,000/mm³, fever; obtain baseline information before and during treatment
- Complete C&S tests before beginning drug therapy to identify if correct treatment has been initiated
- Assess for allergic reactions, anaphylaxis: rash, urticaria, pruritus, chills, wheezing, laryngeal edema, fever, joint pain; angioedema may occur a few days after therapy begins; epiNEPHrine, resuscitation equipment should be available for anaphylactic reaction
- Identify urine output; if decreasing, notify prescriber (may indicate nephrotoxicity); also check for increased BUN, creatinine
- Monitor blood studies: AST, ALT, CBC, Hct, bilirubin, LDH, alkaline phosphatase, Coombs' test monthly if patient is on long-term therapy
- Monitor electrolytes: potassium, sodium, chloride monthly if patient is on long-term therapy
- Assess bowel pattern qd; if severe diarrhea occurs, drug should be discontinued; may indicate pseudomembranous colitis
- Monitor for bleeding: ecchymosis, bleeding gums, hematuria, stool guaiac daily if patient is on long-term therapy
- Assess for overgrowth of infection: perineal itching, fever, malaise, redness, pain, swelling, drainage, rash, diarrhea, change in cough, sputum

Nursing diagnoses
✓ Infection, risk for (uses)
✓ Diarrhea (adverse reactions)
✓ Injury, risk for (adverse reactions)
✓ Knowledge, deficient (teaching)
✓ Noncompliance (teaching)

Implementation
IM route
- Reconstitute 500 mg/2 ml or 750 mg/3 ml lidocaine without epiNEPHrine; shake well, withdraw and administer entire vial; give inj deep in large muscle mass, massage

IV IV route
- Reconstitute each 250 or 500 mg/10 ml of compatible diluent; shake well; transfer the resulting susp to not less than 100 ml of compatible diluent; add 10 ml to each previously reconstituted vial and shake to ensure all medication is used; transfer the remaining contents of the vial to the infusion container;

do not administer susp by direct inj; reconstitute 120-ml infusion bottles/100 ml of a compatible diluent; shake until clear; may use 0.9% NaCl, D₅W, D₁₀W, D₅/0.2% sodium bicarbonate, D₅/0.9% NaCl, D₅/0.45% NaCl, D₅/0.225% NaCl, mannitol 2.5%, 5%, or 10%
- Give by intermittent inf: each 250- or 500-mg dose over 20-30 min, and each 1-g dose over 40-60 min; administer over 15-20
P min for pediatric patients; do not administer direct **IV**; do not admix with other antibiotics

Y-site compatibilities: Acyclovir, amifostine, aztreonam, cefepime, diltiazem, famotidine, fludarabine, foscarnet, granisetron, idarubicin, regular insulin, melphalan, methotrexate, ondansetron, propofol, tacrolimus, teniposide, thiotepa, vinorelbine, zidovudine

Y-site incompatibilities: Fluconazole, meperidine, sargramostim

Additive incompatibilities: Fluconazole, meperidine, sargramostim

Patient/family education
- Teach patient to report sore throat, bruising, bleeding, joint pain; may indicate blood dyscrasias (rare)
- Advise patient to contact prescriber if vaginal itching, loose foul-smelling stools, furry tongue occur; may indicate superinfection
- Advise patient to notify prescriber of diarrhea with blood or pus; may indicate pseudomembranous colitis

Evaluation
Positive therapeutic outcome
- Absence of signs/symptoms of infection (WBC <10,000/mm³, temp WNL, absence of red, draining wounds)
- Reported improvement in symptoms of infection

Treatment of anaphylaxis: Epinephrine, antihistamines, resuscitate if needed

---

imipramine ⚭π (Rx)
(im-ip′ra-meen)
Apo-Imipramine ♣, Imipramine HCl, Impril ♣, Norfranil, Novo Pramine ♣, Tofranil, Tofranil PM, Tipramine
Func. class.: Antidepressant, tricyclic
Chem. class.: Dibenzazepine, tertiary amine

Pregnancy category C

Action: Blocks reuptake of norepinephrine and serotonin into nerve endings, increasing

---

 Herb/drug   **S** Do Not Crush   ♦ Alert   ⚭π Key Drug   **G** Geriatric   **P** Pediatric

action of norepinephrine and serotonin in nerve cells; has anticholinergic effects

→ **Therapeutic Outcome:** Decreased symptoms of depression after 2-3 wk; decreased bedwetting in children

Uses: Depression, enuresis in children

Investigational uses: Chronic pain, migraine headaches, cluster headaches as adjunct, incontinence

Dosage and routes
Adult: PO/IM 75-100 mg/day in divided doses; may increase by 25-50 mg up to 200 mg, not to exceed 300 mg/day; may give daily dose hs

Elderly: PO 25 mg hs, may increase to 100 mg/day in divided doses

Child: PO 25-75 mg/day

Enuresis

Child 6-12 yr: PO 10 mg at hs, max 50 mg

Available forms: Tabs 10, 25, 50, 75 mg; inj 25 mg/2 ml; caps 75, 100, 125, 150 mg

Adverse effects
(*italic* = common; **bold** = life-threatening)
CV: Orthostatic hypotension, ECG changes, tachycardia, hypertension, palpitations, **dysrhythmias**
CNS: Dizziness, drowsiness, confusion, headache, anxiety, tremors, stimulation, weakness, insomnia, nightmares, extrapyramidal symptoms (EPS) (elderly), increased psychiatric symptoms, paresthesia, seizures
EENT: Blurred vision, tinnitus, mydriasis
GI: Diarrhea, dry mouth, nausea, vomiting, **paralytic ileus,** increased appetite, cramps, epigastric distress, jaundice, **hepatitis,** stomatitis, constipation, taste change
GU: Retention, **acute renal failure**
HEMA: **Agranulocytosis, thrombocytopenia, eosinophilia, leukopenia**
INTEG: Rash, urticaria, sweating, pruritus, photosensitivity

Contraindications: Hypersensitivity to tricyclic antidepressants, recovery phase of MI, seizure disorders, prostatic hypertrophy

Precautions: Suicidal patients, severe depression, increased intraocular pressure, narrow-angle glaucoma, urinary retention, cardiac disease, hepatic disease, hyperthyroidism, electroshock therapy, elective surgery, elderly, pregnancy **C**, lactation

🛇 **Do Not Confuse:**
imipramine/desipramine

Pharmacokinetics
Absorption	Well absorbed
Distribution	Widely distributed; crosses placenta
Metabolism	Liver, extensively
Excretion	Kidneys, breast milk
Half-life	6-20 hr

Pharmacodynamics
	PO	IM
Onset	1 hr	1 hr
Peak	Unknown	Unknown
Duration	Unknown	Unknown

Interactions
Individual drugs
Alcohol: ↑ effects
Clonidine: Severe hypotension; avoid use
Clonidine, guanethidine: ↓ effects
Drug classifications
Barbiturates, benzodiazepines, CNS depressants: ↑ effects
MAOIs: Hypertensive crisis, seizures
Selective serotonin reuptake inhibitors: ↑ toxicity, avoid concurrent use
Sympathomimetics (direct acting): ↑ effects
Sympathomimetics (indirect acting): ↓ effects
🛇 *Herb/drug*
Belladonna, corkwood, henbane, jimsonweed, scopolia: ↑ anticholinergic effect
Chamomile, hops, kava, lavender, skullcap, valerian: ↑ imipramine effect
SAM-e, St. John's wort: serotonin syndrome
Yohimbe: ↑ hypertension
Smoking
↑ Metabolism, ↓ effects
Lab test interferences
↑ Serum bilirubin, ↑ blood glucose, ↑ alkaline phosphatase
↓ VMA, ↓ 5-HIAA, ↓ urinary catecholamines

NURSING CONSIDERATIONS
Assessment
• Monitor B/P (with patient lying, standing), pulse q4h; if systolic B/P drops 20 mm Hg, hold drug, notify prescriber; take vital signs q4h in patients with CV disease
• Monitor blood studies: CBC, leukocytes, differential, cardiac enzymes if patient is receiving long-term therapy
• Monitor hepatic studies: AST, ALT, bilirubin
• Check weight weekly; appetite may increase with drug
• Assess ECG for flattening of T wave, bundle branch block, AV block, dysrhythmias in cardiac patients
• Assess for EPS primarily in elderly: rigidity, dystonia, akathisia

- Assess mental status: mood, sensorium, affect, suicidal tendencies; increase in psychiatric symptoms: depression, panic
- ▣ Monitor urinary retention, constipation; constipation is more likely to occur in children ▣ or elderly
◆▶• Assess for withdrawal symptoms: headache, nausea, vomiting, muscle pain, weakness, diarrhea, insomnia, restlessness; do not usually occur unless drug was discontinued abruptly
- Identify alcohol consumption; if alcohol is consumed, hold dose until AM

Nursing diagnoses
✓ Coping, ineffective (uses)
✓ Injury, risk for (side effects)
✓ Knowledge, deficient (teaching)
✓ Noncompliance (teaching)

Implementation
PO route
- Give with food or milk
⊘• Do not crush, chew caps
- Store at room temp; do not freeze

IM route
- Put ampule under warm running water for 1 min to dissolve crystals; sol may be yellow or red

Syringe compatibilities: Doxapram

Y-site compatibilities: Cladribine

Patient/family education
- Teach patient that therapeutic effects may take 2-3 wk
- Teach patient to use caution in driving and other activities requiring alertness because of drowsiness, dizziness, blurred vision; to avoid rising quickly from sitting position, especially ▣ elderly
- Teach patient to avoid alcohol ingestion, other CNS depressants during treatment
- Teach patient not to discontinue medication quickly after long-term use: may cause nausea, headache, malaise
- Teach patient to wear sunscreen or large hat, since photosensitivity occurs
- Teach patient to increase fluids, bulk in diet if constipation, urinary retention occur, especially ▣ cially elderly
- Teach patient to take gum, hard sugarless candy, or frequent sips of water for dry mouth
- Teach patient to rise slowly, orthostatic hypotension may occur

Evaluation
Positive therapeutic outcome
- Decreased depression

- Absence of suicidal thoughts
▣• Decreased enuresis in children
- Decreased pain

Treatment of overdose: ECG monitoring, induce emesis, lavage, activated charcoal, administer anticonvulsant

---

immune globulin (Rx)
gamma globulin, Gamimune N, Gammagard S/D, Gammar-P IV, Iveegam, polygam, polygam S/D, Sandoglobulin, Venoglobulin-I, Venoglobulin-S, immune serum globulin
Func. class.: Immune serum
Chem. class.: IgG

Pregnancy category C

Action: Provides passive immunity to hepatitis A, measles, varicella, rubella, immune globulin deficiency; contains γ-globulin antibodies (IgG)

➔**Therapeutic Outcome:** Absence of infection

Uses: Immunodeficiency syndrome, B-cell chronic lymphocytic leukemia, Kawasaki syndrome, bone marrow transplantation, ▣ pediatric HIV infection, agammaglobulinemia, hepatitis A, B exposure, measles exposure, measles vaccine complications, purpura, rubella exposure, chickenpox exposure

Dosage and routes
Adult: IM 30-50 ml qmo; **IV** 100 mg/kg qmo, 0.01-0.02 ml/kg/min over 30 min (Gamimune N); **IV** 200 mg/kg qmo, 0.05-1 ml/min over 15-30 min, then increase to 1.5-2.5 ml/min (Sandoglobulin)
▣ *Child:* IM 20-40 ml qmo

Hepatitis A exposure
▣ *Adult and child:* IM 0.02-0.04 ml/kg or 0.1 mg/kg if treatment is delayed

Hepatitis B exposure
▣ *Adult and child:* IM 0.06 ml/kg within 1 wk, qmo

Measles (postexposure)
▣ *Child:* IM 0.25 ml/kg within 6 days

Immunoglobulin deficiency
▣ *Adult and child:* IM 1.3 ml/kg, then 0.66 ml/kg after 2-4 wk and q2-4 wk thereafter

Idiopathic thrombocytopenic purpura
▣ *Adult and child:* **IV** 0.4 g/kg/day × 5 days or 1 g/kg/day × 1-2 days

---

⊘ Herb/drug   ⊘ Do Not Crush   ◆ Alert   ◆⅋ Key Drug   ▣ Geriatric   ▣ Pediatric

Kawasaki syndrome

P *Child:* PO 2 g/kg as a single dose

Available forms: IM inj 2, 10 ml/vial; **IV** inj 5% sol, 0.5, 1, 2.5, 3, 6, 10 g vials

Adverse effects

(*italic* = common; **bold** = life-threatening)

CNS: Headache, fatigue, malaise

GI: Abdominal pain

INTEG: Pain at inj site, rash, pruritus, chills

MS: Arthralgia, chest pain

SYST: Lymphadenopathy, **anaphylaxis**

Contraindications: Hypersensitivity

Precautions: Pregnancy **C**

Pharmacokinetics

Absorption	Well absorbed (IM); completely absorbed (**IV**)
Distribution	Rapidly
Metabolism	Liver, catabolism
Excretion	Kidneys
Half-life	3-4 wk

Pharmacodynamics

	IM	IV
Onset	Unknown	Rapid
Peak	Unknown	Unknown
Duration	Unknown	Unknown

Interactions

Live virus vaccines: Do not give within 3 mo

NURSING CONSIDERATIONS

Assessment

• Assess for exposure date: this drug should be given within 6 days of measles, 1 wk of hepatitis B, 14 days of hepatitis A; if the date of exposure is outside these limits, immune globulin will not be effective

• Monitor blood studies in leukemia, idiopathic thrombocytopenic purpura: WBCs (leukemia), platelets

• Identify the number of inj of this drug patient has received; multiple inj may lead to sensitization (diaphoresis, fever, chills, malaise)

• Assess for anaphylaxis in patient receiving **IV** immune globulin: diaphoresis, flushing, nausea, vomiting, wheezing, difficulty breathing, hypotension, chest tightness, fever, weakness, sneezing, abdominal pain; VS should be monitored during inf and 1 hr after beginning inf; emergency equipment should be available with epINEPHrine and antihistamines to treat anaphylaxis

Nursing diagnoses

✓ Infection, risk for (uses)

✓ Knowledge, deficient (teaching)

Implementation

IM route

• Give IM (IGIM) inj in deltoid or anterolateral thigh in adults or anterolateral thigh in

P young children; if large amounts are given, several inj may be needed

• Do not give the IM preparation **IV**, SC, or intradermally

• Sol should be transparent and clear or slightly colored

IV **IV route**

• Warm to room temp before administration (diluent, powder for inj)

• A transfer device is provided by manufacturer; this drug should not be agitated or shaken

• Do not give the **IV** preparation SC, IM, or intradermally

• Check for adverse reaction during inf; stop inf if adverse reactions are present

Y-site compatibilities: Fluconazole, sargramostim

Gamimune N: Dilute **IV** with D_5; give 0.01 ml/kg/min; may increase to 0.02-0.04 ml/kg/min if no adverse reactions are present; may increase to 0.08 ml/kg/hr; sol should be refrigerated; do not freeze

Gammagard S/D: Reconstitute with sterile water for inj (50 mg protein/ml); give within 2 hr of reconstitution; give 0.5 ml/kg/hr; may increase to 4 ml/kg/hr if no adverse reactions occur; use inf set provided

Gammar-P IV: Give 0.01 ml/kg/min (50 mg/ml sol) over 15-30 min; may increase to 0.02 ml/kg/min; if adverse reactions are not present, may increase to 0.03-0.06 ml/kg/min; do not freeze; store at room temp

Iveegam (5%): Give 1-2 ml/min; refrigerate, do not freeze

Sandoglobulin: **IV** diluted with provided diluent; give 0.5-1 ml/min over 15-30 min; may increase to 1.5-2.5 ml/min; other inf may be given 2-2.5 ml/min; store at room temp

Venoglobulin-I: Give 50 mg/ml sol 0.01-0.02 ml/kg/min over 30 min if no adverse reactions; increase 0.04 ml/kg/min; store at room temp

Patient/family education

• Advise patient that passive immunity is temporary; explain reason for and expected results of this drug

• Advise patient that pain and tenderness may occur at inj site

Evaluation

Positive therapeutic outcome
- Prevention of infection
- Increased platelets

Treatment of anaphylaxis: EpINEPHrine, diphenhydrAMINE, O_2, vasopressors, corticosteroids

---

! HIGH ALERT

inamrinone ⬥π (Rx)

(in-am'rih-nohn)

Inocor

Func. class.: Inotropic agent
Chem. class.: Bipyrimidine derivative

Pregnancy category C

Action: Positive inotropic agent with vasodilator properties; reduces preload and afterload by direct relaxation of vascular smooth muscle; increases myocardial contractility

➲ Therapeutic Outcome: Increased inotropic effect resulting in increased cardiac output

Uses: Short-term management of CHF that has not responded to other medication; can be used with digitalis products

Dosage and routes

P *Adult and child:* **IV** bol 0.75 mg/kg given over 2-3 min; start inf of 5-10 mcg/kg/min; may give another bol 30 min after start of therapy, max 10 mg/kg total daily dose

P *Infants:* **IV** 3-4.5 mg/kg in divided doses, then give by inf 10 mcg/kg/min

P *Neonates:* **IV** 3-4.5 mg/kg in divided doses, then give by inf 3-5 mcg/kg/min

Available forms: Inj 5 mg/ml

Adverse effects

(*italic* = common; **bold** = life-threatening)
CV: Dysrhythmias, hypotension, chest pain
ELECT: Hypokalemia
GI: Nausea, vomiting, anorexia, abdominal pain, **hepatotoxicity (rare), ascites,** jaundice, hiccups
INTEG: Allergic reactions, burning at inj site
RESP: Pleuritis, **pulmonary densities, hypoxemia**

Contraindications: Hypersensitivity to this drug or bisulfites, severe aortic disease, severe pulmonic valvular disease, acute MI

Precautions: Lactation, pregnancy **C**,
P children, renal disease, hepatic disease, atrial
G flutter/fibrillation, elderly, asthma

◣ Do Not Confuse:

inamrinone/amiodarone, Inocor/Cordarone

Pharmacokinetics	
Absorption	Complete bioavailability
Distribution	Unknown
Metabolism	Liver, 50%
Excretion	Kidney, metabolites (60%-90%)
Half-life	4-6 hr, increased in CHF

Pharmacodynamics	
Onset	2-5 min
Peak	10 min
Duration	Variable

Interactions

Individual drugs
Disopyramide: ↑ hypotension
Drug classifications
Antihypertensives: ↑ hypotension
Cardiac glycosides: ↑ inotropic effect
Herb/drug
Aloe, buckthorn, cascara sagrada, senna: ↑ inamrinone action
Lab test interferences
↓ Potassium, ↑ hepatic enzymes

NURSING CONSIDERATIONS
Assessment

- Monitor manifestations of hypokalemia: *RENAL:* acidic urine, reduced urine, osmolality, nocturia; *CV:* hypotension, broad T wave, U wave, ectopy, tachycardia, weak pulse; *NEURO:* muscle weakness, altered LOC, drowsiness, apathy, lethargy, confusion, depression; *GI:* anorexia, nausea, cramps, constipation, distention, paralytic ileus; *RESP:* hypoventilation, respiratory muscle weakness

G • Assess fluid volume status: CVP in elderly, I&O ratio and record, weight, distended red veins, crackles in lung, color, quality, and sp gr of urine, skin turgor, adequacy of pulses, moist mucous membranes, bilateral lung sounds, peripheral pitting edema; dehydration symptoms of decreasing output, thirst, hypotension, dry mouth, and mucous membranes should be reported

- Monitor electrolytes: potassium, sodium, calcium, magnesium; also include BUN, blood pH, ABGs
- Monitor B/P and pulse, PCWP, CVP, index, often during inf; if B/P drops 30 mm Hg, stop infusion and call prescriber
- Monitor ALT, AST, bilirubin daily; if these are elevated, hepatotoxicity is suspected

---

- If platelets are <150,000/mm^3, drug is usually discontinued and another drug started
- Assess for extravasation: change site q48h

Nursing diagnoses
☑ Cardiac output, decreased (uses)
☑ Fluid volume, excess (uses)
☑ Knowledge, deficient (teaching)

Implementation
General
- Patients with low potassium levels (hypokalemia) should receive potassium supplements before inamrinone administration
- Administer potassium supplements if ordered for potassium levels <3.0 mg/dl, correct before using inamrinone

IV IV route
- Do not mix directly with dextrose sol; chemical reaction occurs over 24 hr; precipitate forms if inamrinone and furosemide come in contact

IV Direct IV
- May inject into running dextrose inf through Y-connector or directly into tubing; may give undiluted over 2-3 min or dilute with 0.9%, 0.45% NaCl to concentration of 1-3 mg/ml; run at prescribed rate by cont inf; another loading dose may be given in 30 min

IV Cont IV
- Give after diluting with 0.9% or 0.45% NaCl (1-3 mg/ml); do not dilute with dextrose sol; decomposition of drug will occur; use infusion pump; use sol within 24 hr of dilution; titrate to patient response

Syringe compatibilities: Propranolol, verapamil

Y-site compatibilities: Aminophylline, atropine, bretylium, calcium chloride, cimetidine, cisatracurium, digoxin, DOBUTamine, DOPamine, epINEPHrine, famotidine, hydrocortisone, isoproterenol, lidocaine, metaraminol, methylPREDNISolone, nitroglycerin, nitroprusside, norepinephrine, phenylephrine, potassium chloride, procainamide, propranolol, remifentanil, verapamil

Y-site incompatibilities: Furosemide, inamrinone, sodium bicarbonate

Patient/family education
- Teach patient reason for medication and expected results
- Instruct patient to make position changes slowly; orthostatic hypotension may occur
- Teach patient signs and symptoms of hypersensitivity reactions and hypokalemia
- Advise patient that burning may occur at **IV** site

Evaluation
Positive therapeutic outcome
- Increased cardiac output
- Decreased PCWP, adequate CVP
- Decreased dyspnea, fatigue, edema, ECG

Treatment of overdose: Discontinue drug, support circulation

---

indapamide (Rx)
(in-dap'a-mide)
indapamide, Lozide ✦, Lozol
Func. class.: Diuretic, thiazide-like, antihypertensive
Chem. class.: Thiazide-like sulfonamide derivative

Pregnancy category B

Action: Acts on the distal tubule and thick ascending loop of Henle in the kidney, increasing excretion of sodium, water, chloride, magnesium, potassium, and bicarbonate

➥ **Therapeutic Outcome:** Decreased B/P, decreased edema in lung tissues, peripherally

Uses: May be used alone or as adjunct with antihypertensives (mild to moderate)

Dosage and routes
Edema
Adult: PO 2.5 mg qd in AM; may be increased to 5 mg qd if needed

Antihypertensive
Adult: PO 1.25-5 mg qd; may increase to 5 mg/day over 8 wks

Available forms: Tabs 1.25, 2.5 mg

Adverse effects
(*italic* = common; **bold** = life-threatening)
CNS: Depression, *headache, dizziness, fatigue, weakness, nervousness, agitation,* extremity numbness
CV: Orthostatic hypotension, palpitations, volume depletion, PVCs, dysrhythmias
EENT: Blurred vision, nasal congestion, increased intraocular pressure
ELECT: Hypokalemia, hypercalcemia, hyponatremia, hypochloremic alkalosis, hypomagnesemia, hyperuricemia, hyperglycemia
GI: Nausea, vomiting, anorexia, constipation, diarrhea, cramps, abdominal pain, dry mouth
GU: Frequency, polyuria, nocturia, impotence
INTEG: Rash, *pruritus,*
META: Hyperglycemia, *hyperuricemia,* increased creatinine, BUN
MS: Cramps

Contraindications: Hypersensitivity to thiazides or sulfonamides, anuria, hepatic coma

Precautions: Hypokalemia, renal disease, hepatic disease, gout, diabetes mellitus, **G** elderly, ascites, dehydration, pregnancy **B**, lactation, CCr <25 ml/min (not effective)

Pharmacokinetics

Absorption	Well absorbed
Distribution	Widely distributed
Metabolism	Liver; 7%
Excretion	Unchanged (urine)
Half-life	14-18 hr

Pharmacodynamics

Onset	1-2 hr
Peak	2 hr
Duration	Up to 36 hr

Interactions
Individual drugs
Amphotericin B: ↓ potassium
Cholestyramine, colestipol: ↓ absorption
Diazoxide: hyperglycemia
Digitalis, lithium: ↑ toxicity
Indomethacin: ↓ hypotensive effect
Drug classifications
Anticoagulants, antidiabetics, antigout agents: ↓ effects
Diuretics (other), steroids: ↓ potassium
Muscle relaxants, steroids: ↑ toxicity
NSAIDs: ↓ hypotensive effects
Herb/drug
Aloe, buckthorn, cascara sagrada, licorice, senna: ↑ hypokalemia
Aloe, cucumber, dandelion, horsetail, pumpkin, Queen Anne's lace: ↑ diuretic effect
St. John's wort: severe photosensitivity
Lab test interferences
↑ Calcium, ↑ parathyroid test

NURSING CONSIDERATIONS
Assessment
• Check for rashes, temp elevation qd
• Monitor patients that receive cardiac glycosides for increased hypokalemia, toxicity
• Monitor manifestations of hypokalemia: acidic or reduced urine, osmolality, nocturia; hypotension, broad T-wave, U-wave, ectopy, tachycardia, weak pulse; muscle weakness, altered LOC, drowsiness, apathy, lethargy, confusion, depression; anorexia, nausea, cramps, constipation, distention, paralytic ileus; hypoventilation, respiratory muscle weakness
• Monitor for manifestations of hypomagnese-

mia: agitation, muscle twitching, paresthesias, hyperactive reflexes, positive Babinski reflex, dysphagia, nystagmus, seizures, tetany; nausea, vomiting, diarrhea, anorexia, abdominal distention; ectopy, tachycardia, broad, flat- or inverted T-waves, depressed ST segment, prolonged QT interval, decreased cardiac output, hypotension
• Monitor for manifestations of hyponatremia: increased B/P, cold, clammy skin, hypo/hypervolemia; anorexia, nausea, vomiting, diarrhea, abdominal cramps; lethargy, increased ICP, confusion, headache, seizures, coma, fatigue, tremors, hyperreflexia
• Monitor for manifestations of hyperchloremia: weakness, lethargy, coma, deep rapid breathing
• Assess fluid volume status: I&O ratios and record, weight, distended red veins, crackles in lung, color, quality and sp gr of urine, skin turgor, adequacy of pulses, moist mucous membranes, bilateral lung sounds, peripheral pitting edema; dehydration symptoms of decreasing output, thirst, hypotension, dry mouth and mucous membranes should be reported
• Monitor electrolytes: potassium, sodium, calcium, magnesium; also include BUN, blood pH, ABGs, uric acid, CBC, blood glucose
• Assess B/P before and during therapy with patient lying, standing, and sitting as appropriate; orthostatic hypotension can occur rapidly

Nursing diagnoses
☑ Urinary elimination, impaired (side effect)
☑ Fluid volume, deficient (side effects)
☑ Fluid volume, excess (uses)
☑ Knowledge, deficient (teaching)

Implementation
• Give in AM to avoid interference with sleep
• Provide potassium replacement if potassium level is <3.0 mg/dl; give whole
• Give with food; if nausea occurs, absorption may be increased

Patient/family education
• Teach patient to take the medication early in the day to prevent nocturia
• Instruct the patient to take with food or milk if GI symptoms of nausea and anorexia occur
• Teach patient to maintain weekly record of weight and notify prescriber of weight loss >5 lb
• Caution the patient that this drug causes a loss of potassium, so food rich in potassium should be added to the diet; refer to a dietitian for assistance in planning
• Caution the patient not to exercise in hot

weather or stand for prolonged periods, since orthostatic hypotension will be enhanced
• Teach patient not to use alcohol or any OTC medications without prescriber's approval; serious drug reactions may occur
• Emphasize the need to contact prescriber immediately if muscle cramps, weakness, nausea, dizziness, or numbness occurs
• Teach patient to take own B/P and pulse and record findings
• Caution the patient that orthostatic hypotension may occur and to rise slowly from sitting or reclining positions and lie down if dizziness occurs
• Teach patient to continue taking medication even if feeling better; this drug controls symptoms but does not cure the condition
• Advise the patient with hypertension to continue other medical treatment (exercise, weight loss, relaxation techniques, cessation of smoking)

Evaluation
Positive therapeutic outcome
• Decreased edema
• Decreased B/P
• Increased diuresis

Treatment of overdose: Lavage, monitor electrolytes, administer **IV** fluids, monitor hydration, CV, renal status

---

indinavir (Rx)
(en-den'a-veer)
Crixivan
Func. class.: Antiretroviral
Chem. class.: Protease inhibitor
Pregnancy category C

Action: Inhibits HIV protease; this prevents maturation of the infectious virus

Therapeutic Outcome: Decreased signs/symptoms of HIV infection

Uses: HIV in combination with other antiretrovirals

Investigational uses: Prevention of HIV after exposure

Dosage and routes
Reduce dose in mild/moderate hepatic impairment and ketoconazole coadministration
Adult: PO 800 mg q8h; if given with didanosine, given 1 hr apart on empty stomach
Available forms: Caps 200, 400 mg

Adverse effects
(*italic* = common; **bold** = life-threatening)
CNS: *Headache, insomnia,* dizziness, somnolence
GI: *Diarrhea, abdominal pain, nausea, vomiting,* anorexia, dry mouth
GU: Nephrolithiasis
INTEG: Rash
MISC: Asthenia, **insulin-resistant hyperglycemia,** hyperlipidemia, **ketoacidosis**
MS: Pain

Contraindications: Hypersensitivity

P Precautions: Liver disease, pregnancy **C,** lactation, children, renal disease, history of renal stones

Pharmacokinetics
Absorption	Unknown
Distribution	Unknown
Metabolism	Unknown
Excretion	Unknown
Half-life	Terminal 1-2 hr

Pharmacodynamics
Unknown

Interactions
Individual drugs
Clarithromycin, ketoconazole: ↑ levels of both drugs
Delavirdine, itraconazole: ↑ indinavir level
Efavirenz, fluconazole, nevirapine: ↓ indinavir level
Isoniazid: ↑ isoniazid level
Lovastatin, simvastatin: ↑ myopathy
Midazolam, triazolam: ↑ life-threatening dysrhythmias
Drug classifications
Ergots, rifamycins: ↑ life-threatening dysrhythmias

Food/drug
High fat, high protein, grapefruit juice: ↓ absorption
Herb/drug
St. John's wort: ↓ indinavir level, avoid use

NURSING CONSIDERATIONS
Assessment
• Assess for lower back, flank pain, indicates kidney stones
• Monitor signs of infection, anemia
• Monitor liver studies: ALT, AST; total bilirubin, amylase; all may be elevated
• Determine the presence of other sexually transmitted diseases
• Assess bowel pattern before, during

treatment; if severe abdominal pain with bleeding occurs, drug should be discontinued; monitor hydration
• Assess skin eruptions; rash, urticaria, itching
• Assess allergies before treatment, reaction of each medication; place allergies on chart
• Monitor viral load CD4 during treatment

Nursing diagnoses
☑ Infection, risk for (uses)
☑ Knowledge, deficient (teaching)

Implementation
• Give with water, 1 hr ac or 2 hr pc; may be given with other liquids or small meal; do not give with high-fat, high-protein meals
• Dosage adjustment will need to be considered when given with efavirenz
• Give water to 1.5 L/day minimum, to prevent nephrolithiasis

Patient/family education
• Advise to take as prescribed; if dose is missed, take as soon as remembered up to 1 hr before next dose; do not double dose
🚫• Do not crush, chew caps
• Advise that drug must be taken in equal intervals around the clock to maintain blood levels for duration of therapy
• Instruct patient to increase fluids to prevent kidney stones, if stone formation occurs, treatment may need to be interrupted
• Inform patient that drug does not cure AIDS, controls symptoms only; not to donate blood
• Advise patient that hyperglycemia may occur, watch for symptoms (thirst, hunger, dry, itchy skin); notify prescriber

Evaluation
Positive therapeutic outcome
• Decreased signs/symptoms of infection, HIV

---

indomethacin (Rx)
(in-doe-meth'a-sin)
Apo-Indomethacin ✦, Indameth ✦, Indochron E-R, Indocid ✦, Indocin, Indocin IV, Indocin PDA ✦, Indocin SR, indomethacin, Novomethacin ✦, Nu-Indo ✦
Func. class.: NSAID (nonsteroidal antiinflammatory), antirheumatic
Chem. class.: Propionic acid derivative

Pregnancy category B

Action: Inhibits prostaglandin synthesis by decreasing enzyme needed for biosynthesis; analgesic, antiinflammatory, antipyretic

➡**Therapeutic Outcome:** Decreased pain, inflammation; or closure of patent ductus
Ⓟ arteriosus (premature infants)

Uses: Rheumatoid arthritis, ankylosing rheumatoid spondylitis, acute gouty arthritis, closure of patent ductus arteriosus in
Ⓟ premature infants

Dosage and routes
Arthritis/antiinflammatory
Adult: PO/REC 25-50 mg bid; may increase by 25 mg/day qwk, not to exceed 200 mg/day; sus rel 75 mg qd; may increase to 75 mg bid

Acute arthritis
Adult: PO/REC 50 mg tid; use only for acute attack, then reduce dosage

Patent ductus arteriosus Longer or repeated treatment courses may be necessary
Ⓟ for very premature infants

Ⓟ *Infant<2 days:* IV 0.2 mg/kg, then 0.1 mg/kg × 2 doses after 12, 24 hr

Ⓟ *Infant 2-7 days:* IV 0.2 mg/kg, then 0.2 mg/kg × 2 doses after 12, 24 hr

Ⓟ *Infant >7 days:* IV 0.2 mg/kg, then 0.25 mg/kg × 2 doses after 12, 24 hr

Available forms: Caps 25, 50 mg; sus rel caps 75 mg; oral susp 25 mg/5 ml; rec supp 50, 100 mg; inj 1-mg vials

Adverse effects
(*italic* = common; **bold** = life-threatening)
CNS: Dizziness, drowsiness, fatigue, tremors, confusion, insomnia, anxiety, depression, headache
CV: Tachycardia, peripheral edema, palpitations, dysrhythmias, hypertension
EENT: Tinnitus, hearing loss, blurred vision
GI: *Nausea,* anorexia, *vomiting,* diarrhea, jaundice, **cholestatic hepatitis,** *constipation,* flatulence, cramps, dry mouth, peptic ulcer, **ulceration, perforation, GI bleeding**
GU: **Nephrotoxicity (dysuria, hematuria, oliguria, azotemia)**
HEMA: **Blood dyscrasias,** prolonged bleeding
INTEG: Purpura, rash, pruritus, sweating

Contraindications: Hypersensitivity, asthma, severe renal disease, severe hepatic disease, ulcer disease; avoid in 2nd/3rd trimester of pregnancy

Ⓟ **Precautions:** Lactation, children, bleeding disorders, GI disorders, cardiac disorders, hypersensitivity to other antiinflammatory agents, pregnancy **B** (1st trimester), depression

---

Ⓩ Herb/drug   🚫 Do Not Crush   ✦ Alert   🔑 Key Drug   Ⓖ Geriatric   Ⓟ Pediatric

Pharmacokinetics

Absorption	Well absorbed (PO); erratic (rec); complete (**IV**)
Distribution	Crosses blood-brain barrier; placenta, 99% plasma protein binding
Metabolism	Liver, extensively
Excretion	Breast milk
Half-life	2.6-11 hr

Pharmacodynamics

	IV	PO	PO–EXT REL
Onset	2 day	1-2 hr	½ hr
Peak	Unknown	3 hr	Unknown
Duration	Unknown	4-6 hr	4-6 hr

Interactions
Individual drugs
Acetaminophen (long-term use): ↑ renal reactions
Cyclosporine: ↑ nephrotoxicity
Digoxin, lithium, methotrexate, phenytoin, probenecid, zidovudine: ↑ toxicity
Insulin: ↓ insulin effect
Radiation: ↑ risk of hematologic toxicity
Valproic acid: ↑ bleeding risk
Drug classifications
Aminoglycosides: ↑ effects of aminoglycosides
Anticoagulants, cephalosporins, thrombolytics: ↑ risk of bleeding
Antihypertensives: ↓ effect of antihypertensives
Antineoplastics: ↑ risk of hematologic toxicity
β-Adrenergic blockers: ↑ antihypertension
Diuretics: ↓ effectiveness of diuretics
Diuretics (potassium sparing): ↑ hyperkalemia
Glucocorticoids, NSAIDs: ↑ adverse reactions
Hypoglycemics: ↓ hypoglycemic effect
Potassium supplements: ↑ adverse reactions
Sulfonamides, sulfonylureas: ↑ toxicity
⬜ Herb/drug
Anise, arnica, bogbean, chamomile, chondroitin, clove, dong quai, feverfew, garlic, ginger, ginkgo, ginseng (Panax): ↑ bleeding risk
Arginine, gossypol: ↑ gastric irritation
Bearberry, bilberry: ↑ NSAIDs effect

NURSING CONSIDERATIONS
Assessment
• Assess for patent ductus arteriosus: respiratory rate, character, heart sounds
• Assess for joint pain (duration, intensity, ROM), baseline and during treatment
• Assess for confusion, mood changes,
G hallucinations, especially in elderly
• Assess renal, liver, blood studies: BUN,

creatinine, AST, ALT, Hgb before treatment and periodically thereafter; if renal function decreases, do not give subsequent doses

Nursing diagnoses
☑ Pain, acute (uses)
☑ Pain, chronic (uses)
☑ Mobility impaired (uses)
☑ Knowledge, deficient (teaching)

Implementation
PO route
🚫 • Administer to patient whole; do not crush, chew, or break sus rel cap
• Give with food or milk to decrease gastric symptoms, and prevent ulceration
• Shake susp, do not mix with other liquids
Ⅳ IV route
• Give after diluting 1-2 mg/ml or more normal saline or sterile water for inj without preservative; give over 5-10 sec to avoid dramatic shift in cerebral blood flow; avoid extravasation

Y-site compatibilities: Furosemide, insulin (regular), potassium chloride, sodium bicarbonate, sodium nitroprusside
Rectal route
• Have patient retain rec supp for 1 hr after insertion

Patient/family education
• Advise patient to report change in vision, blurring, rash, tinnitus, black stools
• Tell patient not to use for any other condition than prescribed
• Advise patient to avoid use with OTC medications for pain unless approved by prescriber
• Advise patient to avoid hazardous activities, since dizziness or drowsiness can occur
• Instruct patient to use sunscreen to prevent photosensitivity

Evaluation
Positive therapeutic outcome
• Decreased stiffness
• Increased joint mobility
• Decreased pain

---

infliximab (Rx)
(in-fliks'ih-mab)
Remicade
Func. class.: Monoclonal antibody
Pregnancy category C

Action: Monoclonal antibody that neutralizes the activity of tumor necrosis factor α (TNFα)

that has been found in Crohn's disease; decreased infiltration of inflammatory cells

➡ **Therapeutic Outcome:** Decreased cramping and blood in stools

Uses: Crohn's disease, fistulizing, moderate-severe; rheumatoid arthritis given with methotrexate

Investigational uses: Plaque psoriasis, ankylosing spondylitis, ulcerative colitis, psoriatic arthritis, psoriasis, Behçet syndrome, uveitis, juvenile arthritis

Dosage and routes
Crohn's disease (moderate-severe)
Adult: **IV** inf 5 mg/kg × 1

Crohn's disease (fistulizing)
Adult: **IV** inf 5 mg/kg initially, then repeat dose 2, 6 wk after 1st dose

Rheumatoid arthritis
Adult: **IV** 3 mg/kg initially, and 2, 6 wk and q8 wk thereafter, given with methotrexate

Available forms: Powder for inj 100 mg

Adverse effects
(*italic* = common; **bold** = life-threatening)
CNS: Headache, dizziness, depression, vertigo, fatigue, anxiety, fever, seizures
CV: Chest pain, hypertension and hypotension, tachycardia
GI: Nausea, vomiting, abdominal pain, stomatitis, constipation, dyspepsia, flatulence
GU: Dysuria, frequency
HEMA: **Anemia**
INTEG: Rash, dermatitis, urticaria, dry skin, sweating, flushing, hematoma, pruritus
MS: Myalgia, back pain, arthralgia
RESP: URI, pharyngitis, bronchitis, cough, dyspnea, sinusitis
SYST: **Anaphylaxis, fatal infections, sepsis, malignancies, immunogenicity**

Contraindications: Hypersensitivity to murines, moderate to severe CHF (NYHA class III/IV)

Precautions: Pregnancy **B**, lactation, children, elderly

Pharmacokinetics
Absorption	Unknown
Distribution	Vascular compartment
Metabolism	Unknown
Excretion	Unknown
Half-life	9½ days

Pharmacodynamics
Onset	Unknown
Peak	Unknown
Duration	Unknown

Interactions
Drug classifications
Live virus vaccines: Do not administer live vaccines concurrently

NURSING CONSIDERATIONS
Assessment
• Assess GI symptoms: nausea, vomiting, abdominal pain
• Take periodic blood counts: CBC
• Assess CV status: B/P, pulse, chest pain
• Assess for allergic reaction, anaphylaxis: rash, dermatitis, urticaria, fever, chills, dyspnea, hypotension; discontinue if severe, administer epINEPHrine, corticosteroids; antihistamines; assess for allergy to murine proteins before starting therapy
• Fatal infections: discontinue if infection occurs, do not administer to patients with active infections
• Identify TB before beginning treatment; a TB test should be obtained; if present, TB should be treated prior to receiving infliximab

Nursing diagnoses
☑ Injury, risk for (uses)
☑ Diarrhea (uses)
☑ Knowledge, deficient (teaching)

Implementation
IV infusion route
• Administer immediately after reconstitution; reconstitute each vial with 10 ml of sterile water for inj, further dilute total dose/250 ml of 0.9% NaCl inj to a total conc of between 0.4 and 4 mg/ml; use 21-G or smaller needle for reconstitution, direct sterile water at glass wall of vial, gently swirl
• Give over ≥2 hr, use polyethylene-lined infusion with in-line, sterile, low-protein-bind filter
• Do not admix
• Provide refrigerated storage, do not freeze

Patient/family education
• Teach patient not to breastfeed while taking this drug
• Advise patient to notify prescriber of GI symptoms, hypersensitivity reactions
• Advise patient not to operate machinery or drive if dizziness, vertigo occurs

Evaluation
Positive therapeutic outcome
• Absence of blood in stool

- Reported improvement in comfort
- Weight gain

⚠ HIGH ALERT

insulins

insulin aspart (Rx)
Novolog
insulin glargine
Lantus
insulin, isophane suspension (NPH) ⚷ (Rx)
Humulin N, Iletin NPH, Illetin II NPH ✦, Novolin N
insulin, isophane suspension (NPH), and insulin mixtures (Rx)
Humalin 50/50, Novolin 50/50 ✦,
insulin, isophane suspension, and regular insulin (Rx)
Humilin 70/30, Humalin 30/70 ✦, Novolin 70/30, Novolin 70/30 PenFill, Novolin 70/30 Prefilled, Novolin ge 30/70 ✦
insulin lispro
Humalog
insulin, regular ⚷ (Rx)
Humulin R, Iletin II regular, Novolin ge Toronto ✦, Novolin R, Velosulin BR
insulin, regular concentrated
Regular (concentrated), Iletin II U-500
insulin, zinc suspension extended (ultralente) (Rx)
Humulin U Ultralente, Novolin ge Ultralente ✦, Novolin U, Ultralente U
insulin, zinc suspension (lente) (Rx)
Humulin L, Lente Iletin II, Lente L, Novolin ge Lente ✦, Novolin L
Func. class.: Pancreatic hormone
Chem. class.: Exogenous unmodified insulin

Pregnancy category B

Action: Decreases blood glucose; by transport of glucose into cells and the conversion of glucose to glycogen indirectly increases blood pyruvate and lactate, decreases phosphate and potassium; insulin may be beef, pork, human (processed by recombinant DNA technologies)

➔**Therapeutic Outcome:** Decreased blood glucose levels in diabetes mellitus

P Uses: Adult-onset diabetes, juvenile diabetes, ketoacidosis types 1 and 2, type 2 (non–insulin-dependent) diabetes mellitus, type 1 (insulin-dependent) diabetes mellitus; insulin lispro may be used in combination with
P sulfonylureas in children >3 yr

Dosage and routes
Insulin lispro
Adult: SC 15 min ac

Human regular
Adult: SC ½-1 ac

Insulin, isophane, suspension
Adult: SC dosage individualized by blood, urine glucose; usual dose 7-26 units; may increase by 2-10 units/day if needed

Regular insulin
Ketoacidosis
Adult: **IV** 5-10 units, then 5-10 units/hr until desired response, then switch to SC dose; **IV**/ inf 2-12 units (50 units/500 ml of normal saline)
P *Child:* **IV** 0.1 units/kg

Replacement
P *Adult and child:* SC 0.5-1 units/kg/day qid given 30 min pc

Adolescents: SC 0.8-1.2 mg/kg/day; this dosage is used during rapid growth

Lantus
Adult: SC 10 international units qd, range 2-100 international units/day
P *Child ≥6 yr:* Same as adults

Aspart
P *Adult/child ≥6 yr:* 0.5-1 unit/kg/day divided in treatment, meal-related, highly individualized

Available forms: NPH inj 100 units/ml; regular **IV**/IM/SC inj 100 units/ml; insulin analog inj 100 units/ml; insulin zinc susp, ext (ultralente) 100 units/ml; isophane insulin/ insulin inj 100 units/ml; zinc susp 100 units/ ml; insulin lispro 100 units/ml, 1.5 ml cartridges; Lantus (inj 100 international units); NovoLog (inj 100 units/ml human insulin aspart (rDNA)

Adverse effects
(*italic* = common; **bold** = life-threatening)
EENT: Blurred vision, dry mouth
INTEG: Flushing, rash, urticaria, warmth, *lipodystrophy,* lipohypertrophy, swelling, redness
META: *Hypoglycemia,* rebound hyperglycemia (Somogyi effect 12-72 hr or longer)
SYST: **Anaphylaxis**

Contraindications: Hypersensitivity to protamine

Precautions: Pregnancy **C**, glargine, **B**, all others

I

⬛ Do Not Confuse:
Novolin 70/30 Penfill, Novolin 70/30 Prefilled, Lantus/Lente

Pharmacokinetics	
Absorption	Rapidly absorbed (SC)
Distribution	Widely distributed
Metabolism	Liver, muscle, kidney
Excretion	Kidneys
Half-life	Regular 3-5 min; NPH 10 min

Interactions
Individual drugs
Alcohol: ↑ hypoglycemia
Dobutamine: ↑ insulin need
EpINEPHrine: ↓ hypoglycemia
Fenfluramine, guanethedine, phenylbutazone, sulfinpyrazone, tetracycline: ↓ insulin need
Drug classifications
Anabolic steroids, β-adrenergic blockers, hypoglycemics (oral), salicylates: ↑ hypoglycemia
Contraceptives (oral), corticosteroids, diuretics (thiazide), thyroid hormones: ↓ hypoglycemia
Estrogens: ↑ insulin need
MAOIs: ↓ insulin need
⬚ Herb/drug
Aceitilla, adiantam, agrimony, aloe gel, banana flowers/roots, banyan stem bark, bilberry, bitter melon, broom, bugleweed, burdock, carob, cumin, damiana, dandelion, eucalyptus, fenugreek, fo-ti, garlic, goat's rue, guar gum, horse chestnut, jambul, juniper, konjac, maitake, onion, psyllium, reishi: ↑ hypoglycemia
Alfalfa, aloe, basil, bay, bilberry, bitter melon, black catechu, buchu, burdock, coriander, dandelion, eyebright (po), fenugreek, garlic, ginseng, glucomannan, glucosamine, goat's rue, gymnema, horehound, horse chestnut, jambul, myrrh, myrtle: ↑ antidiabetic effect
Annato, cocoa seeds, coffee beans, cola seeds, guarana, ma huang, maté, rosemary: ↓ hypoglycemic effect

Bee pollen, blue cohosh, broom, chromium, elecampane, eucalyptus, gotu kola: ↓ antidiabetic effect
Chromium: ↑ or ↓ hypoglycemia
Karela: ↑ glucose tolerance
Smoking
↑ Insulin need
Lab test interferences
↑ VMA
↓ Potassium, ↓ calcium
Interference: Liver function studies, thyroid function studies

NURSING CONSIDERATIONS
Assessment
• Monitor fasting blood glucose, 2 hr PC (80-150 mg/dl, normal fasting level; 70-130 mg/dl, normal 2-hr level); also glycosylated Hgb may be measured to identify treatment effectiveness
• Monitor urine ketones during illness; insulin requirements may increase during stress, illness, surgery
• Assess for hypoglycemic reaction that can occur during peak time (sweating, weakness, dizziness, chills, confusion, headache, nausea, rapid weak pulse, fatigue, tachycardia, memory lapses, slurred speech, staggering gait, anxiety, tremors, hunger)
• Assess for hyperglycemia: acetone breath, polyuria, fatigue, polydipsia, flushed, dry skin, lethargy

Nursing diagnoses
☑ Injury, risk for (adverse reactions)
☑ Knowledge, deficient (teaching)
☑ Noncompliance (teaching)

Implementation
SC route
• Give after warming to room temp by rotating in palms to prevent injecting cold insulin; use only insulin syringes with markings or syringe matching units/ml; rotate inj sites within one area: abdomen, upper back, thighs, upper arm, buttocks; keep record of sites

Pharmacodynamics							
	NPH	**INSULIN, REGULAR**		**INSULIN, REGULAR CONC**	**ZINC SUSP**	**ZINC SUSP CONC**	**ZINC SUSP PROMPT**	**LISPRO**
		SC	**IV**				**SC**	
Onset	1-2 hr	½-1 hr	10-30 min	½-1 hr	1-2½ hr	4-8 hr	1-1½ hr	Rapid
Peak	4-12 hr	2-4 hr	30-60 min	2-5 hr	7-15 hr	10-30 hr	5-10 hr	½-1 hr
Duration	18-24 hr	5-7 hr	½-1 hr	5-7 hr	12-24 hr	7-36 hr	12-16 hr	3-4 hr

⬚ Herb/drug   ⬛ Do Not Crush   ◆ Alert   ☗ Key Drug   🄶 Geriatric   🄿 Pediatric

• Give increased dosages if tolerance occurs; give human insulin to those allergic to beef or pork
• Give lispro 15 min ac
• Store at room temp for <1 mo; keep away from heat and sunlight; refrigerate all other supply; do not use if discolored; do not freeze

IV IV route, regular only
• Do not use if cloudy, thick, or discolored
• Give **IV** direct, undiluted via vein, Y-site, 3-way stopcock; give at 50 units/min or less
• Give by cont inf after diluting with **IV** sol and run at prescribed rate; use **IV** infusion pump for correct dosing; give reduced dose at serum glucose level of 250 mg/100 ml

Syringe compatibilities: Metoclopramide

Y-site compatibilities: Amiodarone, ampicillin, ampicillin/sulbactam, aztreonam, cefazolin, cefotetan, DOBUTamine, esmolol, famotidine, gentamicin, heparin, heparin/hydrocortisone, imipenen/cilastatin, indomethacin sodium trihydrate, magnesium sulfate, meperidine, meropenem, midazolam, morphine, nitroglycerin, nitroprusside, oxytocin, pentobarbital, potassium chloride, propofol, ritodrine, sodium bicarbonate, tacrolimus, terbutaline, ticarcillin, ticarcillin/clavulanate, tobramycin, vancomycin, vit B/C

Y-site incompatibilities: Nafcillin

Additive compatibilities: Bretylium, cimetidine, lidocaine, meropenem, ranitidine, verapamil

Additive incompatibilities: Aminophylline, amobarbital, chlorothiazide, cytarabine, DOBUTamine, pentobarbital, phenobarbital, phenytoin, secobarbital, sodium bicarbonate, thiopental

Patient/family education
• Advise patient that blurred vision occurs; not to change corrective lenses until vision is stabilized after 1-2 mo of therapy
• Advise patient to keep insulin and equipment available at all times
• Advise patient to carry/wear emergency ID as diabetic
• Teach patient dosage, route, mixing instructions, disease process; tell patient to continue to use the same brand of insulin and to rotate inj sites
• Instruct patient to carry candy or lump of sugar to treat hypoglycemia; have glucagon emergency kit available; teach how to use these
• Teach patient symptoms of ketoacidosis: nausea, thirst, polyuria, dry mouth, decreased

B/P, dry, flushed skin, acetone breath, drowsiness, Kussmaul respirations; to have insulin available at all times
• Advise patient that a plan is necessary for diet, exercise; all food on diet should be eaten, exercise routine should not vary
• Teach patient to avoid OTC drugs and alcohol unless approved by a prescriber
• Instruct patient to notify prescriber if pregnancy is planned
• Caution patient that treatment is lifelong; insulin does not cure condition

Evaluation
Positive therapeutic outcome
• Decrease in polyuria, polydipsia, polyphagia; clear sensorium, absence of dizziness, stable gait
• Blood glucose level under control

Treatment of overdose: Glucose 25 g **IV**, via dextrose 50% sol, 50 ml or glucagon 1 mg

---

interferon alfa-2a/interferon alfa-2b (Rx)
(in-ter-feer′on)
Roferon-A/Intron-A
Func. class.: Antineoplastic—misc.
Chem. class.: Protein product
Pregnancy category C

Action: Antiviral action inhibits viral replication by reprogramming virus; antitumor action suppresses cell proliferation; immunomodulating action phagocytizes target cells; may also inhibit virus replication

Therapeutic Outcome: Prevention of rapid growth of malignant cells; treatment of hepatitis non-A, non-B (liver function improvement)

Uses: Hairy cell leukemia in persons >18 yr, condylomata acuminata (alfa 2b), malignant melanoma, AIDS-related Kaposi's sarcoma, chronic hepatitis non-A, non-B (alfa 2b), chronic hepatitis B, C (alfa 2b)

Investigational uses: Bladder tumors, carcinoid tumors, non-Hodgkin's lymphoma, essential thrombocytopenia, cytomegaloviruses, herpes simplex, human papilloma virus–associated diseases

Dosage and routes
Hairy cell leukemia (2a)
Adult: SC/IM 3 million international units/day × 16-24 wk, then 3 million international units 3 ×/wk maintenance

Hairy cell leukemia (2b)
2 million international units/m² 3 ×/wk; if severe adverse reactions occur, dose should be skipped or reduced by half

Kaposi's sarcoma (2b)
Adult: SC/IM 30 million international units m² 3 ×/wk

Condylomata acuminata (2a)
1 million international units/lesion 3 ×/wk × 3 wk

Chronic hepatitis B (2b)
Adult: SC/IM 3 million international units 3 ×/wk × 18-24 mo or 5 million international units/day or 10 million international units 3 ×/wk × 16 wk

Chronic hepatitis C
Adult: SC/IM 36 million international units 3 ×/wk

Available forms: Alfa-2a inj 3, 6, 36 million international units/ml; alfa-2b inj 3, 5, 10, 18, 25 million units/vial, powder for inj 5, 10, 18, 25, 50 million units/vial

Adverse effects
(*italic* = common; **bold** = life-threatening)
CNS: *Dizziness, confusion, numbness, paresthesia,* hallucinations, **seizures, coma,** amnesia, anxiety, mood changes, depression, somnolence, paranoia, irritability
CV: *Edema, hypotension,* hypertension, chest pain, palpitations, dysrhythmias, **CHF, MI, CVA,** tachycardia, syncope
GI: *Weight loss, taste changes,* nausea, anorexia, diarrhea, xerostomia
GU: *Impotence*
HEMA: **Neutropenia, thrombocytopenia**
INTEG: *Rash, dry skin, itching, alopecia,* flushing, photosensitivity
MISC: *Flulike syndrome: fever, fatigue, myalgias, headache, chills*

Contraindications: Hypersensitivity

Precautions: Severe hypotension, dysrhythmia, tachycardia, pregnancy **C,** lactation, children, severe renal or hepatic disease, seizure disorder

⊠ Do Not Confuse:
Roferon-A/Imferon

Pharmacokinetics	
Absorption	80%-90% (SC/IM)
Distribution	Unknown
Metabolism	Renal tubular (degraded)
Excretion	Kidneys
Half-life	3.7-8.5 hr (2a); 2-7 hr (2b)

Pharmacodynamics	
Onset	Unknown
Peak	3-8 hr
Duration	Unknown

Interactions
Individual drugs
Aminophylline: ↑ toxicity, blood levels
Zidovudine: ↑ neutropenia
Lab test interferences
Interference: AST, ALT, LDH, alkaline phosphatase, WBC, platelets, granulocytes, creatinine

NURSING CONSIDERATIONS
Assessment
• Assess cardiac status: lung sounds, ECG before and during treatment, especially in those with cardiac disease
• Assess bone marrow depression: bruising, bleeding, blood in stools, urine, sputum, emesis
• Assess mental status: depression, suicidal thoughts, hallucinations, amnesia
• Assess for symptoms of infection; may be masked by drug fever; fever, chills, headache, sore throat may occur 6 hr after dose; give acetaminophen for symptoms
• In AIDS patients with Kaposi's sarcoma, assess characteristics of lesions during therapy; symptoms should decrease
• Assess for bleeding: hematuria, stool guaiac, bruising or petechiae, mucosa or orifices q8h; check for inflammation of mucosa, breaks in skin; avoid IM inj, rec temp, or any other procedures that break the skin
• Assess for CNS reaction: LOC, mental status, dizziness, confusion, poor coordination, difficulty speaking, behavior changes; notify prescriber (alfa-2b)

Nursing diagnoses
☑ Injury, risk for (adverse reactions)
☑ Body image, disturbed (adverse reactions)
☑ Infection, risk for (adverse reactions)
☑ Knowledge, deficient (teaching)

Implementation
• Sol should be prepared by qualified personnel only under controlled conditions in biologic cabinet using gown, gloves, and mask
• Use Luer-Lok tubing to prevent leakage; do not let sol come in contact with skin; if contact occurs, wash well with soap and water
• Give at hs to minimize side effects
• Give acetaminophen as ordered to alleviate fever and headache
• Give by IM/SC after reconstituting 3-5 million international units/1 ml, 10 million

international units/2 ml, 25 million international units/5 ml, of diluent provided; mix gently

Alfa-2a
- SC/IM after reconstituting 18 million units/3 ml of diluent provided (6 million units/ml)
- 36 million units/ml is used for Kaposi's sarcoma only
- Store reconstituted sol; must be used within 30 days

Intralesional route (2b)
- Give by intralesional route after reconstituting 10 million international units/1 ml of bacteriostatic water for inj; no more than 5 lesions can safely be treated at a time; using a 25-G needle inject 0.1 ml into base at center

Patient/family education
- Caution patient to avoid hazardous tasks, since confusion, dizziness may occur; fatigue is common; activity may have to be altered; to take hs to minimize flulike symptoms; to take acetaminophen for fever; avoid prolonged sunlight
- Advise patient that brands of this drug should not be changed; each form is different, with different dosages
- Caution patient not to become pregnant while taking drug; possible mutagenic effects; impotence may occur during treatment but is temporary
- Advise patient to report signs of infection: sore throat, fever, diarrhea, vomiting; sores or white patches in mouth
- Advise patient that emotional lability is common; notify prescriber if severe or incapacitating

Evaluation
Positive therapeutic outcome
- Leukocytes, Hgb, platelets, WNL
- Decreased amount of lesions in AIDS patients with Kaposi's sarcoma
- Decreased amount of genital warts

---

interferon alfa-n 1 lymphoblastoid (Rx)
(in-ter-feer′on)
Wellferon
Func. class.: Recombinant type I interferon
Pregnancy category UK

Action: Induces biologic responses and has antiviral, antiproliferative, and immunomodulatory effects; mixture of α-interferons isolated from human cells after induction with parainfluenza virus

Uses: Chronic hepatitis C infections

Dosage and routes
Adult: SC/IM 3 million units × 3 ×/wk × 6-12 mo

Available forms: Sol 3 million units/ml

Adverse effects
(*italic* = common; **bold** = life-threatening)
CNS: *Headache, fever, insomnia, dizziness, anxiety, hostility, lability, nervousness, depression, confusion, abnormal thinking, amnesia*
GI: *Abdominal pain, nausea, diarrhea, anorexia, vomiting*
HEMA: **Granulocytopenia, thrombocytopenia, leukopenia, ecchymosis**
INTEG: *Alopecia, pruritus, rash, erythema, dry skin*
MS: *Back pain*
PSYCH: *Nervousness, depression, anxiety, lability, abnormal thinking*
RESP: *Pharyngitis, upper respiratory infection, cough, dyspnea, bronchitis, epistaxis*

Contraindications: Hypersensitivity to α interferons, history of anaphylactic reaction to bovine or ovine immunoglobulins, egg protein, polymyxin B, neomycin sulfate

Precautions: Thyroid disorders, myelosuppression, hepatic, cardiac disease, lactation, children <18 yr, depression/suicidal tendencies

Pharmacokinetics	
Peak	24-36 hr

Interactions
Individual drugs
Theophylline: Use cautiously
Drug classifications
Myelosuppressive agents: Use together cautiously

NURSING CONSIDERATIONS
Assessment
- Monitor ALT, hepatitis C viral load, patients who show no reduction in ALT, hepatitis C viral load are unlikely to show benefit from treatment after 6 mo
- Monitor platelet counts, heme concentration, ANC, serum creatinine concentration, albumin, bilirubin, TSH, T_4, AFP
- Monitor for myelosuppression, hold dose if neutrophil count is <500 × 10^6/L or if platelets are <50 × 10^9/L
- Assess for hypersensitivity: discontinue immediately if hypersensitivity occurs

Implementation
• Give the same brand of product during the course of treatment

Patient/family education
• Provide patient or family member with written, detailed information about drug
• Teach patient instructions for home use if appropriate
• Advise patient to take in evening to reduce discomfort, sleep through some side effects

Evaluation
Positive therapeutic outcome
• Decrease chronic hepatitis C signs/ symptoms
• Undetectable viral load

---

interferon alfacon-1 (Rx)
(in-ter-feer'on al'fa-kon)
Infergen
Func. class.: Recombinant type I interferon

Pregnancy category C

Action: Induces biologic responses and has antiviral, antiproliferative, and immunomodulatory effects

Therapeutic Outcome: Decreased signs/symptoms of hepatitis C

Uses: Chronic hepatitis C infections

Investigational uses: Hairy cell leukemia when used with G-CSF

Dosage and routes
Adult: SC 9 mcg as a single inj 3×/wk × 24 wk

Available forms: Inj 9 mg/0.3 ml, 15 mg/0.5 ml

Adverse effects
(*italic* = common; **bold** = life-threatening)
CNS: Headache, fatigue, fever, rigors, insomnia, dizziness
CV: Hypertension, palpitation
EENT: Tinnitus, earache, conjunctivitis, eye pain
GI: Abdominal pain, nausea, diarrhea, anorexia, dyspepsia, vomiting, constipation, flatulence, hemorrhoids, decreased salivation
GU: Dysmenorrhea, vaginitis, menstrual disorders
HEMA: **Granulocytopenia, thrombocytopenia, leukopenia,** ecchymosis
INTEG: Alopecia, pruritus, rash, erythema, dry skin
MS: Back, limb, neck, skeletal pain
PSYCH: Nervousness, depression, anxiety, lability, abnormal thinking
RESP: Pharyngitis, upper respiratory infection, cough, sinusitis, rhinitis, respiratory tract congestion, epistaxis, dyspnea, bronchitis

Contraindications: Hypersensitivity to α-interferons, or products from *Escherichia coli*

Precautions: Thyroid disorders, myelosuppression, hepatic, cardiac disease, lactation, pregnancy **C**, children <18 yr

Pharmacokinetics	
Absorption	Unknown
Distribution	Unknown
Metabolism	Unknown
Excretion	Unknown
Half-life	Unknown

Pharmacodynamics	
Onset	Unknown
Peak	24-36 hr
Duration	Unknown

Interactions: None known

NURSING CONSIDERATIONS
Assessment
• Assess platelet counts, heme concentration, ANC, serum creatinine concentration, albumin, bilirubin, TSH, T_4
• Assess for myelosuppression, low dose if neutrophil count is $<500 \times 10-6/L$ or if platelets are $<50 \times 10-9/L$
• Assess for hypersensitivity; discontinue immediately if hypersensitivity occurs

Nursing diagnoses
☑ Infection, risk for (uses)
☑ Knowledge, deficient (teaching)

Patient/family education
• Provide patient or family member with written, detailed instructions about the drug
• Caution patient to use contraception during treatment

Evaluation
Positive therapeutic outcome
• Decreased hepatitis C signs/symptoms

 Herb/drug   Do Not Crush   Alert   Key Drug   Geriatric   **P** Pediatric

interferon β-1a (Rx)
(in-ter-feer'on)
Avonex
interferon β-1b (Rx)
Betaseron
Func. class.: Multiple sclerosis agent,
immune modifier
Chem. class.: Interferon, *Escherichia coli*
derivative

Pregnancy category C

Action: Antiviral, immunoregulatory; action
not clearly understood; biologic response-
modifying properties mediated through specific receptors on cells, inducing expression of
interferon-induced gene products

➡ **Therapeutic Outcome:** Decreased
symptoms of multiple sclerosis

Uses: Ambulatory patients with relapsing or
remitting multiple sclerosis

Investigational uses: May be useful in
treatment of AIDS, AIDS-related Kaposi's
sarcoma, malignant melanoma, metastatic
renal cell carcinoma, cutaneous T-cell lymphoma, acute non-A, non-B hepatitis

Dosage and routes
Interferon-β-1a
Adult: IM 30 mcg qwk

Interferon-β-1b
Relapsing/remitting multiple
sclerosis
Adult: SC 0.25 mg (8 international units)
qod

Available forms: β-1a 33 mcg (6.6
million international units/vial); β-1b powder
for inj 0.3 mg (9.6 milli-international units)

Adverse effects
(*italic* = common; **bold** = life-threatening)
CNS: Headache, fever, pain, chills, mental
changes, hypertonia, **suicide attempts,**
seizures
CV: Migraine, palpitations, hypertension,
tachycardia, peripheral vascular disorders
EENT: Conjunctivitis, blurred vision
GI: Diarrhea, constipation, vomiting,
abdominal pain
GU: Dysmenorrhea, irregular menses,
metrorrhagia, cystitis, breast pain
HEMA: **Decreased lymphocytes, WBC;**
lymphadenopathy
INTEG: Sweating, inj site reaction, necrosis
MS: Myalgia, **myasthenia**
RESP: Sinusitis, dyspnea

Contraindications: Hypersensitivity to
natural or recombinant interferon-β or human
albumin

Precautions: Pregnancy **C,** lactation,
P children <18 yr, chronic progressive multiple
sclerosis, depression, mental disorders

Pharmacokinetics	
Absorption	50% is absorbed
Distribution	Unknown
Metabolism	Unknown
Excretion	Unknown
Half-life	8 min–4½ hr (β-1b),
	8.6 hr (β-1a)
	β-1a up to 12 hr, 48 hr,
	4 days, β-1b

Pharmacodynamics	
Onset	Rapid
Peak	2-8 hr
Duration	Unknown

Interactions: None

NURSING CONSIDERATIONS
Assessment
• Monitor blood, renal, hepatic studies: CBC,
differential, platelet counts, BUN, creatinine,
ALT, urinalysis; if neutrophil count is <750/
mm³, or if AST, ALT, is 10 × greater than upper
normal limit, or if bilirubin is 5 × greater than
upper normal limit; when neutrophil count
exceeds 750/mm³ and liver function or renal
studies return to normal, treatment may
resume at 50% original dosage
• Assess for CNS symptoms: headache, fatigue,
depression; if depression occurs and is severe,
drug should be discontinued
• Assess for multiple sclerosis symptoms
• Assess mental status: depression, depersonalization, suicidal thoughts, insomnia
• Monitor GI status: diarrhea or constipation,
vomiting, abdominal pain
• Monitor cardiac status: increased B/P,
tachycardia

Nursing diagnoses
☑ Mobility, impaired physical (uses)
☑ Knowledge, deficient (teaching)

Implementation
• Reconstitute 0.3 mg (9.6 million international units)/1.2 ml of supplied diluent
(0.2 mg or 8 million international units
concentration); rotate vial gently, do not shake;
withdraw 1 ml using a syringe with 27-G
needle; administer SC only into hip, thigh, arm;
discard unused portion
• Products are not interchangeable

Interferon β-1a
- Reconstitute with 1.1 ml of diluent, swirl, give within 6 hr

Interferon β-1b
- Reconstitute by injecting diluent provided (1.2 ml) into vial, swirl (8 milli-international units/ml), use 27-G needle for inj
- Give acetaminophen for fever, headache; use SC route only; do not give IM or **IV**
- Store reconstituted sol in refrigerator; do not freeze; do not use sol that contains precipitate or is discolored

Patient/family education
- Provide patient or family member with written, detailed instructions about the drug; provide initial and return demonstrations on inj procedure; give information on use and disposal of drug
- Inform patient that blurred vision, sweating may occur
- Advise women patients that irregular menses, dysmenorrhea, or metorrhagia as well as breast pain may occur; use contraception during treatment; drug may cause spontaneous abortion
- Teach patient to use sunscreen to prevent photosensitivity
- Instruct patient to notify prescriber if pregnancy is suspected
- Teach patient inj technique and care of equipment
- Instruct patient to notify prescriber of increased temp, chills, muscle soreness, fatigue

Evaluation
Positive therapeutic outcome
- Decreased symptoms of multiple sclerosis

---

interferon gamma-1b (Rx)
(in-ter-feer'on)
Actimmune
Func. class.: Biologic response modifier
Chem. class.: Lymphokine, interleukin type

Pregnancy category C

Action: Species-specific protein synthesized in response to viruses; potent phagocyte-activating effects; capable of mediating the killing of *Staphylococcus aureus, Toxoplasma gondii, Leishmania donovani, Listeria monocytogenes, Mycobacterium avium-intracellulare;* enhances oxidative metabolism of macrophages; enhances antibody-dependent cellular cytotoxicity

Therapeutic Outcome: Decreased signs/symptoms of infection (serious) in chronic granulomatous disease

Uses: Serious infections associated with chronic granulomatous disease, osteoporosis

Dosage and routes
Adult: SC 50 mcg/m^2 (1.5 million units/m^2) for patients with a surface area of >0.5 m^2; 1.5 mcg/kg/dose for patient with a surface area of <0.5/m^2; give on Monday, Wednesday, Friday for 3 ×/wk dosing

Available forms: Inj 100 mcg (3 million units)/single-dose vial

Adverse effects
(*italic* = common; **bold** = life-threatening)
CNS: *Headache, fatigue,* depression, fever, chills
GI: *Nausea, anorexia,* abdominal pain, weight loss, diarrhea, vomiting
INTEG: Rash, pain at inj site
MS: Myalgia, arthralgia

Contraindications: Hypersensitivity to interferon γ, *Escherichia coli*–derived products

Precautions: Pregnancy **C**, cardiac disease, seizure disorders, CNS disorders, myelosuppression, lactation, children

Pharmacokinetics	
Absorption	Slowly absorbed; 89%
Distribution	Unknown
Metabolism	Unknown
Excretion	Unknown
Half-life	5.9 hr

Pharmacodynamics	
Onset	Unknown
Peak	7 hr
Duration	Unknown

Interactions
Individual drugs
Radiation: ↑ toxicity, bone marrow suppression
Drug classifications
Antineoplastics: ↑ toxicity, bone marrow suppression

NURSING CONSIDERATIONS
Assessment
- Monitor blood, renal, hepatic studies: CBC with differential, platelet count, BUN, creati-

---

nine, ALT, urinalysis before and q3 mo during treatment

• Assess for infection: headache, fever, chills, fatigue; these are common adverse reactions
• Monitor CNS symptoms: headache, fatigue, depression

Nursing diagnoses
✓ Infection, risk for (uses)
✓ Knowledge, deficient (teaching)

Implementation
• Give at hs to minimize adverse reactions; administer acetaminophen for fever, headache; use 50% of the dosage prescribed if severe reactions occur or discontinue treatment until reactions subside
• Give in right or left deltoid and anterior thigh; warm to room temp before use; do not leave at room temp over 12 hr (unopened vial); does not contain preservatives
• Store in refrigerator upon receipt; do not freeze; do not shake

Patient/family education
• Provide patient or family member with written, detailed instructions about the drug; provide initial and return demonstrations on inj procedure; give information on use and disposal of drug
• Caution patient to use contraception during treatment

Evaluation
Positive therapeutic outcome
• Decreased serious infections
• Improvement in existing infections and inflammatory conditions

ipecac syrup (OTC)
(ip'e-kak)
Func. class.: Emetic
Chem. class.: Cephaelis ipecacuanha derivative

Pregnancy category C

Action: Acts on chemoreceptor trigger zone to induce vomiting; irritates gastric mucosa

➔ **Therapeutic Outcome:** Emesis

Uses: In poisoning from noncaustic substances to induce vomiting

Dosage and routes
Adult: PO 15-30 ml, then 200-300 ml of water; may repeat ×1, if vomiting does not occur within 20 min

P *Child >1 yr:* PO 15 ml, then 200-300 ml of water

P *Child 6-12 mo:* PO 5-10 ml, then 100-200 ml of water; may repeat dose if needed

Available forms: Syr

Adverse effects
(*italic* = common; **bold** = life-threatening)
CNS: Depression, seizures, coma
CV: Circulatory failure, atrial fibrillation, fatal myocarditis, dysrhythmias
GI: Nausea, vomiting, bloody diarrhea

Contraindications: Hypersensitivity, unconscious/semiconscious, depressed gag reflex, poisoning with petroleum products or caustic substances, seizures, shock, alcohol intolerance

P **Precautions:** Lactation, pregnancy **C,** child <6 mo

Pharmacokinetics
Absorption	Not absorbed
Distribution	Unknown
Metabolism	Unknown
Excretion	Unknown
Half-life	Unknown

Pharmacodynamics
Onset	15-30 min
Peak	Unknown
Duration	½ hr

Interactions
Individual drugs
Activated charcoal: ↓ effect; do not use together
Drug classifications
Antiemetics: ↓ effect, do not use together
Food/drug
Dairy products: ↓ effect
Carbonated drinks: ↑ abdominal distention

NURSING CONSIDERATIONS
Assessment
• Assess type of poisoning; do not administer if petroleum products or caustic substances have been ingested: kerosene, gasoline, lye, Drano
• Assess respiratory status before, during, after administration of emetic; check rate, rhythm, character; respiratory depression can occur rapidly with elderly or debilitated patients
• Monitor LOC; do not give to patients who are semiconscious or unconscious or if gag reflex is not present

Nursing diagnoses
✓ Injury, risk for (uses)
✓ Poisoning, risk for (uses)

☑ Knowledge, deficient (teaching)

Implementation
PO route
◆• Give **ipecac *syrup*, not ipecac fluid,** which is 14 times stronger, or death may occur
• Give activated charcoal after the patient has finished vomiting; may begin lavage 10-15 min after 2 doses of ipecac syrup without results
• Give with the patient upright; give water immediately after the ipecac syrup (200-300 P ml for adults; 100-200 ml child <1 yr; 200-300 ml for a child >1 yr)

Patient family education
• Give patient phone number for poison control
• Give patient written guidelines on poisoning and when to induce vomiting; suggest patient P keep ipecac syrup in house if young children are present

Evaluation
Positive therapeutic outcome
• Vomiting within 30 min

---

ipratropium (Rx)
(i-pra-troe′pee-um)
Atrovent
Func. class.: Anticholinergic, bronchodilator
Chem. class.: Synthetic quaternary ammonium compound

Pregnancy category B

Action: Inhibits interaction of acetylcholine at receptor sites on the bronchial smooth muscle, resulting in decreased cyclic guanosine monophosphate (cGMP) and bronchodilatation

⇒**Therapeutic Outcome:** Bronchodilatation

Uses: Bronchodilatation during bronchospasm for patients with COPD; rhinorrhea in P children 6-11 yr (nasal spray)

Dosage and routes
Adult: INH 2 puffs qid, not to exceed 12 puffs/24 hr; sol 500 mcg (1 unit dose) given 3-4 ×1 day

P *Child 6-11 yr:* **Nasal,** 1 spray in each nostril

Available forms: Aerosol 18 mcg/actuation; nasal spray 0.03%, 0.06%; sol for inh 0.02%

Adverse effects
(*italic* = common; **bold** = life-threatening)
CNS: *Anxiety, dizziness, headache,* nervousness
CV: Palpitations
EENT: Dry mouth, blurred vision
GI: *Nausea, vomiting, cramps*
INTEG: Rash
RESP: *Cough, worsening of symptoms,* **bronchospasm**

Contraindications: Hypersensitivity to this drug, atropine, soya lecithin

Precautions: Pregnancy **B**, lactation, P children <12 yr, narrow-angle glaucoma, prostatic hypertrophy, bladder neck obstruction

⊠ **Do Not Confuse:**
Atrovent/Alupent

Pharmacokinetics	
Absorption	Minimal
Distribution	Does not cross blood-brain barrier
Metabolism	Liver, minimal
Excretion	Unknown
Half-life	2 hr

Pharmacodynamics	
Onset	5-15 min
Peak	1-1½ hr
Duration	3-6 hr

Interactions
Drug classifications
Bronchodilators (aerosol): ↑ action of bronchodilator
☑ *Herb/drug*
Black catechu: ↑ constipation
Butterbur, jimsonweed: ↑ anticholinergic effect
Green tea (large amounts), guarana: ↑ bronchodilator effect
Jamborandi tree, pill-bearing spurge: ↓ anticholinergic effect

NURSING CONSIDERATIONS
Assessment
• Monitor respiratory function: vital capacity, FEV, ABGs, lung sounds, heart rate, rhythm (baseline and during treatment); if severe bronchospasm is present, a more rapid medication is required
• Monitor for evidence of allergic reactions, paradoxic bronchospasm; withhold dose and notify prescriber; identify if patient is allergic to belladonna products or atropine; allergy to this drug may occur

---

Nursing diagnoses
☑ Airway clearance, ineffective (uses)
☑ Gas exchange, impaired (uses)
☑ Knowledge, deficient (teaching)

Implementation
• Give after shaking container; have patient exhale, place mouthpiece in mouth, inhale slowly, hold breath, remove, exhale slowly; allow at least 1 min between inhalations

Nebulizer route
• Use solution in nebulizer with a mouthpiece rather than a face mask

Nasal route
• Prime pump, initially requires 7 actuations of the pump, priming again is not necessary if used regularly
• Store in light-resistant container; do not expose to temp over 86° F (30° C)

Patient/family education
• Advise patient not to use OTC medications unless approved by prescriber; extra stimulation may occur; to use this medication before other medications and allow at least 5 min between each to prevent overstimulation
• Teach patient that compliance is necessary with number of inhalations/24 hr, or overdose may occur
• Instruct patient to use spacer device if elderly
• Teach patient the proper use of the inhaler; review package insert with patient; to avoid getting aerosol in eyes; blurring may result; to wash inhaler in warm water qd and dry; to avoid smoking, smoke-filled rooms, persons with respiratory tract infections
• Teach patient if paradoxic bronchospasm occurs to stop drug immediately and notify prescriber; to limit caffeine products such as chocolate, coffee, tea, and colas
• Instruct patient on administration of dose, not to use more than prescribed; serious side effects may occur; if dose is missed, take when remembered; space other doses on new time schedule; do not double doses

Evaluation
Positive therapeutic outcome
• Absence of dyspnea, wheezing after 1 hr
• Improved airway exchange
• Improved ABGs

---

irbesartan (Rx)
(er-be-sar′tan)
Avapro
Func. class.: Antihypertensive
Chem. class.: Angiotensin II receptor (Type AT_1)

Pregnancy category
C (1st trimester);
D (2nd/3rd trimesters)

Action: Blocks the vasoconstrictor and aldosterone-secreting effects of angiotensin II; selectively blocks the binding of angiotensin II to the AT_1 receptor found in tissues

➔**Therapeutic Outcome:** Decreased B/P

Uses: Hypertension, alone or in combination, nephropathy in type 2 diabetic patients

Investigational uses: Heart failure, hypertensive patients with diabetic nephropathy caused by type 2 diabetes

Dosage and routes
Hypertension
Adult: PO 150 mg qd; may be increased to 300 mg qd

Nephropathy in type 2 diabetic patients
Adult: PO maintenance dose 300 mg qd
P *Child 13-16 yr:* PO 150 mg qd, may increase to 300 mg qd
P *Child 6-12 yr:* PO 75 mg qd may increase to 150 mg qd

Volume-depleted patients
Adult: PO 75 mg qd

Available forms: Tabs 75, 150, 300 mg

Adverse effects
(*italic* = common; **bold** = life-threatening)
CNS: Dizziness, anxiety, headache, fatigue
GI: Diarrhea, dyspepsia
RESP: Cough, upper respiratory infection, rhinitis, pharyngitis, sinus disorder
MISC: Edema, chest pain, rash, tachycardia, UTI, **angioedema,** hyperkalemia

Contraindications: Hypersensitivity, pregnancy **D** (2nd/3rd trimesters)

Precautions: Hypersensitivity to ACE
P inhibitors; pregnancy **C** (1st trimester),
G lactation, children, elderly, renal disease

☒ Do Not Confuse:
Avapro/Anaprox

Pharmacokinetics

Absorption	Well
Distribution	Bound to plasma proteins (90%)
Metabolism	Liver (minimal)
Excretion	Feces, urine
Half-life	11-15 hr

Pharmacodynamics

Unknown

Interactions

☑ *Herb/drug*
Aconite: ↑ Toxicity, death
Astragalus, cola tree: ↑ or ↓ antihypertensive effect
Barberry, betony, black catechu, black cohosh, bloodroot, broom, burdock, cat's claw, dandelion, goldenseal, Irish moss, Jamaican dogwood, kelp, khella, mistletoe, parsley: ↑ antihypertensive effect
Coltsfoot, guarana, khat, licorice: ↓ antihypertensive effect

NURSING CONSIDERATIONS
Assessment
- Assess B/P, pulse q4h; note rate, rhythm, quality
- Monitor electrolytes: potassium, sodium, chloride
- Obtain baselines for renal liver function tests before therapy begins
- Monitor for edema in feet, legs daily
- Assess for skin turgor, dryness of mucous membranes for hydration status

Nursing diagnoses
✓ Fluid volume, deficient (side effects)
✓ Noncompliance (teaching)
✓ Knowledge, deficient (teaching)

Implementation
- Administer without regard to meals

Patient/family education
- Advise patient to comply with dosage schedule, even if feeling better
- Inform patient that drug may cause dizziness, fainting; lightheadedness may occur
- Caution patient to rise slowly to sitting or standing position to minimize orthostatic hypotension
- Advise patient to notify prescriber if pregnancy is suspected

Evaluation
Positive therapeutic outcome
- Decreased B/P

! HIGH ALERT

irinotecan (Rx)
(ear-een-oh-tee′kan)
Camptosar
Func. class.: Antineoplastic hormone
Chem. class.: Topoisomerase inhibitor

Pregnancy category D

Action: Cytotoxic by producing damage to double-strand DNA during DNA synthesis

⇒ **Therapeutic Outcome:** Prevention in growth of tumor size

Uses: Metastatic carcinoma of colon or rectum, 1st line treatment in combination with fluorouracil (5-FU) and leucovorin for metastatic carcinoma of colon or rectum

Dosage and routes
Single agent
Adult: **IV** 125 mg/m² given over 1½ hr qwk × 4 wk, then 2 wk rest period, may be repeated; 4 wk or 2 wk off, dosage adjustments may be made to 150 mg/m² (high) or 50 mg/m² (low); adjustments should be made in increments of 25-50 mg/m² depending on patient's tolerance

Combination dosage schedule
Regimen 1: Irinotecan 75-125 mg/m², leucovorin 20 mg/m², 5-FU 300-500 mg/m², depending on dosing levels

Regimen 2: Irinotecan 120-180 mg/m², leucovorin 200 mg/m², 5 FU-BOL 240-400 mg/m², 5 FU infusion 360-600 mg/m²

Hepatic impairment
Adult: 100 mg/m² qwk × 4 wk, then 2 wk rest; may repeat cycle or 300 mg/m² q3wk, dose may be adjusted up or down

Available forms: Inj 20 mg/ml

Adverse effects
(*italic* = common; **bold** = life-threatening)
CNS: Fever, headache, chills, dizziness
CV: Vasodilation
GI: **Severe diarrhea,** nausea, vomiting, anorexia, constipation, cramps, flatus, stomatitis, dyspepsia, **hepatotoxicity**
HEMA: **Leukopenia,** anemia, **neutropenia**
INTEG: Irritation at site, rash, sweating, alopecia
RESP: Dyspnea, increased cough, rhinitis
MISC: Edema, asthenia, weight loss

Contraindications: Hypersensitivity, pregnancy **D**

P Precautions: Lactation, children, elderly, **G** myelosuppression, irradiation

---

 Herb/drug   Do Not Crush   Alert   Key Drug   Geriatric   **P** Pediatric

Pharmacokinetics

Absorption	Complete
Distribution	Widely, 30%-68% bond to plasma proteins
Metabolism	Unknown
Excretion	Urine/bile
Half-life	Unknown

Pharmacodynamics
Unknown

Interactions
Individual drugs
Dexamethasone: ↑ lymphocytopenia
Prochlorperazine: ↑ akathisia
Radiation: ↑ myelosuppression, diarrhea
Drug classifications
Antineoplastics: ↑ myelosuppression, diarrhea
Diuretics: ↑ dehydration

NURSING CONSIDERATIONS
Assessment
- Assess for CNS symptoms: fever, headache, chills, dizziness
- Assess CBC, differential, platelet count weekly; withhold drug if WBC is <2000/mm³, or platelet count is <100,000/mm³, Hgb ≤ g/dl, neutrophils ≤1000/mm³; notify prescriber of these results, drug should be discontinued and colony-stimulating factor given
- Assess buccal cavity q8h for dryness, sores or ulceration, white patches, oral pain, bleeding, dysphagia
- Assess GI symptoms: frequency of stools; cramping; severe life-threatening diarrhea may occur with fluid and electrolyte imbalances
- Assess early diarrhea and other cholinergic symptoms, treat with atropine; late diarrhea must be treated promptly with loperimide, late diarrhea can be life-threatening
- Assess signs of dehydration: rapid respirations, poor skin turgor, decreased urine output; dry skin, restlessness, weakness
- Assess for bone marrow depression: bruising, bleeding, blood in stools, urine, sputum, emesis

Nursing diagnoses
☑ Infection, risk for (adverse reactions)
☑ Knowledge, deficient (teaching)

Implementation
- Give antiemetics and dexamethasone 10 mg at least ½ hr before antineoplastics
- Give after preparing in biologic cabinet using gloves, mask, gown

IV IV route
- Give by intermittent inf after diluting with

0.9% NaCl or D₅W (0.12-1.1 mg/ml); give over 1½ hr
- Do not admix with other solutions or medications
- Provide increased fluid intake to 2-3 L/day to prevent dehydration, unless contraindicated
- Change **IV** site q48h
- Provide rinsing of mouth tid-qid with water, club soda; brushing of teeth bid-tid with soft brush or cotton-tipped applicator for stomatitis; use unwaxed dental floss
- Provide nutritious diet with iron, vitamin supplement, low fiber, few dairy products
- Stable for 24 hr at room temp, 48 hr if refrigerated

Patient/family education
- Advise patient to avoid foods with citric acid or hot or rough texture if stomatitis is present; to drink adequate fluids
- Advise patient to report stomatitis; any bleeding, white spots, ulcerations in mouth; tell patient to examine mouth qd, report symptoms
- Advise patient to report signs of anemia: fatigue, headache, faintness, shortness of breath, irritability
- Advise patient to use contraception during therapy
- Advise patient to avoid vaccinations while taking this drug
- Instruct patient to report diarrhea that occurs 24 hr after administration; severe dehydration can occur rapidly
- Teach patient to avoid salicylates, NSAIDs, alcohol; bleeding may occur

Evaluation
Positive therapeutic outcome
- Decrease in tumor size, decrease in spread of cancer

Treatment of overdose: Induce vomiting, provide supportive care, prevent dehydration

iron, carbonyl
See ferrous fumarate

iron dextran (Rx)

DexFerrum, Imferon, InFed
Func. class.: Hematinic
Chem. class.: Ferric hydroxide complex with dextran

Pregnancy category C

Action: Iron is carried by transferrin to the bone marrow, where it is incorporated into hemoglobin

➡ **Therapeutic Outcome:** Prevention and resolution of iron-deficiency anemia

Uses: Iron-deficiency anemia in patients who cannot take oral preparations

Dosage and routes

P *Adult and child:* IM 0.5 ml as a test dose by Z-track, then no more than the following per day:

Adult <50 kg: IM 100 mg

Adult >50 kg: IM 250 mg

P *Infant <5 kg:* IM 25 mg

P *Child 5-9 kg:* IM 50 mg

Adult: **IV** 0.5 ml (25 mg) test dose, then 100 mg qd after 2-3 days; **IV** 250/1000 ml of NaCl; give 25 mg test dose, wait 5 min, then inf over 6-12 hr or follow equation:

$$\frac{0.3 \times \text{weight (lb)} \times 100 \text{ Hgb (g/dl)} \times 100}{14.8} = \text{mg iron}$$

Patients <30 lb (66 kg) should be given 80% of above formula dose

Available forms: Inj IM/**IV** 50 mg/ml; inj IM only 50 mg/ml (2 ml, 10 ml vials)

Adverse effects

(*italic* = common; **bold** = life-threatening)
CNS: Headache, paresthesia, dizziness, shivering, weakness, **seizures**
CV: Chest pain, **shock,** hypotension, tachycardia
GI: *Nausea,* vomiting, metallic taste, abdominal pain
HEMA: Leukocytosis
INTEG: Rash, pruritus, urticaria, fever, sweating, chills, brown skin discoloration, pain at inj site, necrosis, sterile abscesses, phlebitis
MISC: **Anaphylaxis**
RESP: Dyspnea

Contraindications: Hypersensitivity, all anemias excluding iron-deficiency anemia, hepatic disease

Precautions: Acute renal disease,

P children, asthma, lactation, rheumatoid
P arthritis (**IV**), infants <4 mo, pregnancy **C**

Do Not Confuse:

Imferon/Imuran, Imferon/Roferon-A

Pharmacokinetics

Absorption	Well absorbed; lymphatics over wk or mo
Distribution	Crosses placenta
Metabolism	Slow; blood loss, desquamation
Excretion	Breast milk, feces, urine, bile
Half-life	6 hr

Pharmacodynamics

Unknown

Interactions

Individual drugs
Chloramphenicol, vitamin E: ↓ reticulocyte response
Oral iron: Do not use together, ↑ toxicity
Penicillamine: ↓ absorption of penicillamine
Drug classifications
Fluoroquinolones: ↓ fluoroquinolones absorption

Drug/food
• Iron absorption is ↓ by food
Lab test interferences
False: ↑ Serum bilirubin
False: ↓ Serum calcium
False positive: ^{99m}Tc diphosphate bone scan, iron test (large doses >2 ml)

NURSING CONSIDERATIONS
Assessment

• Monitor blood studies: Hct, Hgb, reticulocytes, transferrin, plasma iron concentrations, ferritin, total iron-binding bilirubin before treatment, at least monthly
• Assess for allergic reaction and anaphylaxis; rash, pruritus, fever, chills, wheezing, notify prescriber immediately, keep emergency equipment available
• Assess cardiac status: anginal pain, hypotension, tachycardia
• Assess for nutrition: amount of iron in diet (meat, dark green leafy vegetables, dried fruits, eggs); cause of iron loss or anemia, including salicylates, sulfonamides
• Monitor pulse, B/P during **IV** administration
• Assess for toxicity: nausea, vomiting, diarrhea, fever, abdominal pain (early symptoms); cyanotic lips, nailbeds, seizures, CV collapse (late symptoms)

 Herb/drug   Do Not Crush   ◆ Alert   Key Drug   **G** Geriatric   **P** Pediatric

Nursing diagnoses
☑ Fatigue (uses)
☑ Activity intolerance (uses)
☑ Knowledge, deficient (teaching)

Implementation
IM route
• Discontinue oral iron before parenteral; give only after test dose of 25 mg by preferred route; wait at least 1 hr before giving remaining portion
• Give IM inj deep in large muscle mass; use Z-track method and 19-, 20-G 2-, 3-inch needle; ensure needle is long enough to place drug deep in muscle; change needles after withdrawing medication and injecting to prevent skin and tissue staining

IV IV route
• Give **IV** after flushing tubing with 10 ml of 0.9% NaCl; give undiluted; give 1 ml (50 mg) or less over 1 min or more; flush line after use with 10 ml of 0.9% NaCl; patient should remain recumbent for 30-60 min to prevent orthostatic hypotension
• **IV** inj requires single-dose vial without preservative; verify on label **IV** use is approved
• Give by cont inf after diluting in 50-250 ml of 0.9% NaCl for inf; administer over 4-5 hr
• Give only with epINEPHrine available in case of anaphylactic reaction during dose
• Store at room temp in cool environment

Additive compatibilities: Netilmicin

Patient/family education
• Caution patient that iron poisoning may occur if increased beyond recommended level; to not take oral iron preparation unless approved by prescriber
• Advise patient that delayed reaction may occur 1-2 days after administration and last 3-4 days (**IV**) or 3-7 days (IM); report fever, chills, malaise, muscle, joint aches, nausea, vomiting, backache

Evaluation
Positive therapeutic outcome
• Increased serum iron levels, Hct, Hgb

Treatment of overdose:
• Discontinue drug, treat allergic reaction, give diphenhydrAMINE or epINEPHrine as needed for anaphylaxis; give iron-chelating drug in acute poisoning

---

iron polysaccharide
See ferrous fumarate

---

iron sucrose (Rx)
Venofer
Func. class.: Hematinic
Chem. class.: Ferric hydroxide complex with dextran

Pregnancy category B

Action: Iron is carried by transferrin to the bone marrow, where it is incorporated into hemoglobin

➡ **Therapeutic Outcome:** Improved signs/symptoms of iron deficiency anemia; iron levels improved

Uses: Iron deficiency anemia

Investigational uses: Dystrophic epidermolysis bullosa (DEB)

Dosage and routes
Adult: **IV** 5 ml (100 mg of elemental iron) given during dialysis, most will need 1000 mg of elemental iron over 10 dialysis sessions

Available forms: Inj 20 mg/ml

Adverse effects
(*italic* = common; **bold** = life-threatening)
CNS: Headache, dizziness
CV: Chest pain, hypo/hypertension, hypervolemia
GI: Nausea, vomiting, abdominal pain
INTEG: Rash, pruritus, urticaria, fever, sweating, chills
MISC: **Anaphylaxis**
RESP: Dyspnea, pneumonia, cough

Contraindications: Hypersensitivity, all anemias excluding iron deficiency anemia, iron overload

G Precautions: Lactation (**IV**), pregnancy **B**,
P elderly, children

Pharmacokinetics	
Absorption	Unknown
Distribution	Unknown
Metabolism	Unknown
Excretion	Urine
Half-life	6 hr

Pharmacodynamics
Unknown

Interactions
Individual drugs
Iron (oral): ↑ toxicity, do not use together

NURSING CONSIDERATIONS
Assessment
- Monitor blood studies: Hct, Hgb, reticulocytes, transferrin, plasma iron concentrations, ferritin, total iron binding, bilirubin before treatment, at least monthly
- Assess for allergy: anaphylaxis, rash, pruritus, fever, chills, wheezing; notify prescriber immediately, keep emergency equipment available
- Assess cardiac status: hypotension, hypertension, hypervolemia
- Assess for toxicity: nausea, vomiting, diarrhea, fever, abdominal pain (early symptoms), cyanotic-looking lips and nailbeds, seizures, CV collapse (late symptoms)

Nursing diagnoses
☑ Nutrition: less than body requirements, imbalanced (uses)
☑ Knowledge, deficient (teaching)

Implementation
◆ Give only with epINEPHrine available in case of anaphylactic reaction during dose

IV **IV route**
- Give directly in dialysis line by slow inj or inf; give by slow inj at 1 ml/min (5 min/vial); inf dilute each vial exclusively in a maximum of 100 ml of 0.9% NaCl, give at rate of 100 mg of iron/15 min, discard unused portions
- Store at room temp in cool environment, do not freeze

Patient/family education
- Teach patient that iron poisoning may occur if increased beyond recommended level; not to take oral iron preparations

Evaluation
Positive therapeutic outcome
- Increased serum iron levels, Hct, Hgb

Treatment of overdose: Discontinue drug, treat allergic reaction, give diphenhydrAMINE or epINEPHrine as needed, give iron-chelating drug in acute poisoning

---

isoniazid ◆π (Rx)
(eye-soe-nye'a-zid)
INH, isoniazid, Isotamine ✦, Laniazid, Nydrazid, PMS-Isoniazid ✦
Func. class.: Antitubercular
Chem. class.: Isonicotinic acid hydrazide

Pregnancy category C

Action: Inhibits RNA synthesis, decreases tubercle bacilli replication

➔ **Therapeutic Outcome:** Resolution of TB infection

Uses: Pulmonary TB as an adjunct; other infections caused by mycobacteria

Dosage and routes
Treatment
Adult: PO/IM 300 mg/day or 15 mg/kg 2-3 ×/wk, max 900 mg 2-3 ×/wk
P *Child and infant:* PO/IM 10-20 mg/kg qd in 1-2 divided doses; max 300 mg/day or 20-40 mg/kg, max 900 mg 2-3 ×/wk

Available forms: Tabs 50, 100, 300 mg; inj 100 mg/ml; powder 50 mg/5 ml; syr 50 mg/5 ml

Adverse effects
(*italic* = common; **bold** = life-threatening)
Hypersensitivity: Fever, skin eruptions, lymphadenopathy, vasculitis
CNS: Peripheral neuropathy, dizziness, memory impairment, **toxic encephalopathy, convulsions,** psychosis, **seizures,** slurred speech
EENT: Blurred vision, optic neuritis
GI: Nausea, vomiting, epigastric distress, jaundice, **fatal hepatitis**
HEMA: **Agranulocytosis, hemolytic anemia, aplastic anemia, thrombocytopenia, eosinophilia, methemoglobinemia**
MISC: Dyspnea, vit B$_6$ deficiency, pellagra, hyperglycemia, metabolic acidosis, gynecomastia, rheumatic syndrome, systemic lupus erythematosus–like syndrome

Contraindications: Hypersensitivity, acute liver disease

Precautions: Pregnancy C, renal disease, diabetic retinopathy, cataracts, ocular defects, **P** hepatic disease, child <13 yr

Pharmacokinetics	
Absorption	Well
Distribution	Widely
Metabolism	Liver
Excretion	Kidneys
Half-life	1-4 hr

Pharmacodynamics		
	PO	IM
Onset	Rapid	Rapid
Peak	1-2 hr	45-60 min
Duration	6-8 hr	6-8 hr

Interactions
Individual drugs
Alcohol, carbamazepine, cycloSERINE, ethion-

 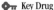

amide, meperidine, phenytoin, rifampin, warfarin: ↑ toxicity

BCG vaccine, ketoconazole: ↓ effectiveness of BCG vaccine

Drug classifications
Antacids, aluminum: ↓ absorption
Benzodiazepines: ↑ toxicity

Food/drug
Tyramine foods: ↑ toxicity

NURSING CONSIDERATIONS
Assessment
• Obtain C&S tests, including sputum tests, before treatment; monitor every mo to detect resistance
• Monitor liver studies weekly: ALT, AST, bilirubin, increased results may indicate hepatitis; renal studies during treatment and monthly: BUN, creatinine, output, sp gr, urinalysis, uric acid
• Assess mental status often: affect, mood, behavioral changes; psychosis may occur with hallucinations, confusion
• Assess hepatic status: decreased appetite, jaundice, dark urine, fatigue
• Assess for visual disturbance that may indicate optic neuritis: blurred vision, change in color perception; may lead to blindness

Nursing diagnoses
☑ Infection, risk for (uses)
☑ Diarrhea (adverse reactions)
☑ Injury, risk for (adverse reactions)
☑ Knowledge, deficient (teaching)
☑ Noncompliance (teaching)

Implementation
• Give antiemetic for vomiting
PO route
• Give with meals to decrease GI symptoms; absorption is better when taken on empty stomach, 1 hr ac or 2 hr pc
IM route
• Give inj deep in large muscle mass, massage; rotate inj sites, warm inj to room temp to dissolve crystals

Patient/family education
• Instruct patient that compliance with dosage schedule for duration is necessary; not to skip or double doses; that scheduled appointments must be kept or relapse may occur
• Caution patient to avoid alcohol while taking drug or hepatoxicity may result; to avoid ingestion of aged cheeses, fish or hypertensive crisis may result; give patient written directions on which foods to avoid while taking this medication
• Tell patient to report peripheral neuritis: weakness, tingling/numbness of hands/feet,

fatigue; hepatoxicity: loss of appetite, nausea, vomiting, jaundice of skin or eyes

Evaluation
Positive therapeutic outcome
• Decreased symptoms of TB
• Culture negative for TB

Treatment of overdose:
Pyridoxine

---

isoproterenol (Rx)
(eye-soe-proe-ter'e-nole)
Aerolone, Dispos-a-Medisoproterenol HCl, Isoproterenol HCl, Isuprel, Isuprel Glossets, Isuprel Mistometer, Medihaler-Iso, Vapo-Iso

Func. class.: β-Adrenergic-agonist, antidysrhythmic, inotropic
Chem. class.: Catecholamine

Pregnancy category C

Action: Has β_1- and β_2-adrenergic action; relaxes bronchial smooth muscle and dilates the trachea and main bronchi by increasing levels of cAMP, which relaxes smooth muscles; causes increased contractility and heart rate by acting on β-receptors in heart

➔**Therapeutic Outcome:** Bronchodilatation, increased heart rate and cardiac output from action on β-receptors in the heart

Uses: Bronchospasm, asthma, heart block, ventricular dysrhythmias, shock

Dosage and routes
Asthma, bronchospasm
Adult: SL tab 10-20 mg q6-8h; inh 1 puff; may repeat in 2-5 min; maintenance 1-2 puffs 4-6 ×/day; **IV** 1020 mg during anesthesia

🄿 *Child:* SL tab 5-10 mg q6-8h; inh 1 puff; may repeat in 2-5 min; maintenance 1-2 puffs 4-6 ×/day

Heart block/ventricular dysrhythmias
Adult: **IV** 0.02-0.06 mg, then 0.01-0.2 mg or 5 mcg/min HCl; 0.2 mg, then 0.02-1 mg as needed

Shock
Adult: **IV** inf 0.5-5 mcg/min (1 mg/500 ml of D₅W) titrate to B/P, CVP, hourly urine output

Available forms: Sol for nebulization 1:400 (0.25%), 1:200 (0.5%), 1:100 (1%); aerosol 0.25%, 0.2%; powder for inh 0.1 mg/cartridge; inj 1:5000 (0.2 mg/ml); glossets (SL) 10, 15 mg

Adverse effects
(*italic* = common; **bold** = life-threatening)
CNS: *Tremors, anxiety,* insomnia, headache, dizziness, stimulation
CV: Palpitations, tachycardia, hypertension, **cardiac arrest**
GI: Nausea, vomiting
META: Hyperglycemia
RESP: Bronchial irritation, edema, dryness of oropharynx, **bronchospasms** (overuse)

Contraindications: Hypersensitivity to sympathomimetics, narrow-angle glaucoma, tachydysrhythmias

Precautions: Pregnancy **C**, cardiac disorders, hyperthyroidism, diabetes mellitus, **G** prostatic hypertrophy, elderly

Pharmacokinetics
Absorption	Erratic (SL, rec), rapid (inh, **IV**)
Distribution	Unknown
Metabolism	Lungs, liver, GI tract
Excretion	Kidneys, unchanged (50%)
Half-life	Unknown

Pharmacodynamics
	SL	INH	IV	REC
Onset	1-2 hr	Rapid	Rapid	2-4 hr
Peak	Unknown	Unknown	Unknown	Unknown
Duration	2 hr	1 hr	10 min	3-4 hr

Interactions
Drug classifications
β-Adrenergic blockers: Block therapeutic effect
MAOIs: ↑ chance of hypertensive crisis
Sympathomimetics: ↑ effects of both drugs

NURSING CONSIDERATIONS
Assessment
• Assess respiratory function: vital capacity, FEV, ABGs, lung sounds, heart rate, rhythm (baseline and during therapy)
• Monitor for evidence of allergic reactions, paradoxic bronchospasm; withhold dose; notify prescriber

Nursing diagnoses
✓ Airway clearance, ineffective (uses)
✓ Gas exchange, impaired (uses)
✓ Knowledge, deficient (teaching)

Implementation
SL route
• Give ≤q3-4h or no more than tid

Inhalation route
• Give after diluting dose in sterile water or 0.9% NaCl, 0.45% NaCl; give over 15-20 min
• Store in light-resistant container; do not expose to temp over 86° F (30° C)
IV IV route
• Give by direct **IV** after diluting 0.2 mg or 1 ml (1:5000 sol)/10 ml of 0.9% NaCl for inj or D₅W (1:50,000 sol); give 1:50,000 sol over 1 min
• Give by cont inf by diluting 2 mg or 10 ml (1:5000 sol)/500 ml of 0.9% NaCl, D₅W, D₁₀W, 0.45% NaCl, Ringer's, LR (1:250,000 sol); give at a rate of 1 ml/min by infusion pump; ratio is adjusted according to patient response

Syringe compatibilities: Ranitidine

Y-site compatibilities: Amiodarone, amrinone, atracurium, bretylium, cisatracurium, famotidine, heparin, hydrocortisone, pancuronium, potassium chloride, propofol, remifentanil, tacrolimus, vecuronium, vit B/C

Additive compatibilities: Atracurium, calcium chloride, calcium gluceptate, cephalothin, cimetidine, DOBUTamine, floxacillin, heparin, magnesium sulfate, multivitamins, netilmicin, potassium chloride, ranitidine, succinylchloride, verapamil, vit B/C

Patient/family education
• Caution patient not to use OTC medications before consulting prescriber; extra stimulation may occur
• Instruct patient to use this medication before other medications and allow at least 5 min between each
• Teach patient use of inhaler; review package insert with patient; advise patient to avoid getting aerosol in eyes, as blurring may result; instruct patient to wash inhaler in warm water qd and dry; to rinse mouth after using; to avoid smoking, smoke-filled rooms, persons with respiratory tract infections
G • Teach elderly patient to use spacer device
• Instruct patient if paradoxic bronchospasm occurs to stop drug immediately and notify prescriber; to limit caffeine products such as chocolate, coffee, tea, and colas
• Instruct patient on administration of dose; not to use more than prescribed; serious side effects may occur; if taking PO regularly and dose is missed, take when remembered; space other doses on new time schedule; do not double dose

---

Evaluation
Positive therapeutic outcome
- Absence of dyspnea, wheezing
- Improved airway exchange
- Improved ABGs

Treatment of overdose: Administer a β_2-adrenergic blocker

---

isosorbide dinitrate (Rx)
(eye-soe-sor'bide)
Apo-ISDN ♣, Cedocard-SR ♣, Coronex ♣, Dilatrate-SR, ISDN, Iso-Bid, Isonate, Isorbid, Isordil, Isosorbide dinitrate, Isotrate, Novasorbide ♣, Sorbitrate
isosorbide mononitrate (Rx)
Imdur, Ismo, Isotrate ER, Monoket
Func. class.: Antianginal, vasodilator
Chem. class.: Nitrate

Pregnancy category C

Action: Relaxation of vascular smooth muscle which leads to decreased preload, afterload, thus decreasing left ventricular end-diastolic pressure, systemic vascular resistance, and reducing cardiac O_2 demand

➡ Therapeutic Outcome: Relief and prevention of angina pectoris

Uses: Treatment, prevention of chronic stable angina pectoris

Dosage and routes
Dinitrate
Adult: PO 5-40 mg qid; SL, buccal tab 2.5-5 mg; may repeat q5-10min × 3 doses; chew tab 5-10 mg prn as prophylaxis; sus rel cap 40-80 mg q8-12h

Mononitrate
Adult: PO (Ismo, Monoket) 10-20 mg bid, 7 hr apart; (Imdur) initiate at 30-60 mg/day as a single dose, increase q3d as needed, may increase to 120 mg qd, max 240 mg/day

Available forms: *dinitrate:* sus rel caps 40 mg; tabs 5, 10, 20, 30, 40 mg; SL tabs 2.5, 5, 10 mg; chew tabs 5, 10 mg; sus rel caps 40 mg; *mononitrate:* tabs 10, 20 mg; (Monoket, Ismo) ext rel tabs 30, 60, 120 mg

Adverse effects
(*italic* = common; **bold** = life-threatening)
CNS: Vascular headache, flushing, dizziness, weakness, faintness
CV: Postural hypotension, tachycardia, **collapse,** syncope, palpitations
GI: Nausea, vomiting, diarrhea

INTEG: Pallor, sweating, rash
MISC: Twitching, hemolytic anemia, **methemoglobinemia**

Contraindications: Hypersensitivity to this drug or nitrates, severe anemia, increased ICP, cerebral hemorrhage, acute MI

Precautions: Postural hypotension, pregnancy **C**, lactation, children, MI, CHF, severe renal, hepatic disease

Do Not Confuse: Monoket/Monopril Imdur/Imuran/Inderal/K-Dur

Pharmacokinetics
Absorption	Well
Distribution	Unknown
Metabolism	Liver
Excretion	Urine, metabolites
Half-life	Dinitrate 1 hr, mononitrate 5 hr

Pharmacodynamics
	SUS REL	SL	PO
Onset	Up to 4 hr	2-5 min	15-30 min
Peak	Unknown	Unknown	Unknown
Duration	6-8 hr	1-4 hr	4-6 hr

Interactions
Individual drugs
Alcohol: ↑ hypotension
Drug classifications
Antihypertensives, β-adrenergic blockers, calcium channel blockers, phenothiazines: ↑ hypotension
Diuretics: ↑ effects
Sildenafil: Fatal hypotension
Herb/drug
Blue cohosh: ↓ antianginal effect

NURSING CONSIDERATIONS
Assessment
- Assess for pain: duration, time started, activity being performed, character, intensity
- Monitor for orthostatic B/P, pulse at baseline and during treatment

Nursing diagnoses
- Cardiac output, decreased (uses)
- Tissue perfusion, ineffective (uses)
- Knowledge, deficient (teaching)

Implementation
SL route
- Hold SL tab under tongue until dissolved (a few min); do not take anything PO when SL tab is in place
PO route
- Give 1 hr ac or 2 hr pc with 8 oz of water
- Sus rel tab should not be chewed, broken,

or crushed; chew tab should be chewed thoroughly

Patient/family education

• Instruct patient to swallow sus rel tab whole, do not chew; SL tab should be dissolved under tongue, do not swallow; chew tab should be chewed thoroughly; do not skip or double doses; if dose is missed take when remembered if 2 hr before next dose (dinitrate), 6 hr before next dose (sus rel), or 8 hr before next dose (mononitrate)

• Caution patient to avoid alcohol and OTC medications unless approved by prescriber

• Inform patient that drug may be taken before stressful activity: exercise, sexual activity

• Advise patient that SL tab may sting mucous membranes

• Caution patient to avoid driving and hazardous activities if dizziness occurs

• Advise patient to comply with complete medical regimen

• Caution patient to make position changes slowly to prevent orthostatic hypotension

Evaluation

Positive therapeutic outcome

• Decrease in, prevention of anginal pain

---

isradipine (Rx)

(is-ra'di-peen)
DynaCirc, DynaCirc CR
Func. class.: Calcium channel blocker, antihypertensive, antianginal
Chem. class.: Dihydropyridine

Pregnancy category C

Action: Inhibits calcium ion influx across cell membrane during cardiac depolarization; produces relaxation of coronary vascular smooth muscle and peripheral vascular smooth muscle; dilates coronary vascular arteries

➡ **Therapeutic Outcome:** Decreased B/P

Uses: Hypertension, pectoris, vasospastic angina

Dosage and routes

Adult: PO 2.5 mg bid; increase at 2-4 wk intervals up to 10 mg bid or 5 mg qd; cont rel, may be increased q2-4wk, max 20 mg/day

Available forms: Caps 2.5, 5 mg; cont rel tabs 5, 10 mg

Adverse effects

(*italic* = common; **bold** = life-threatening)
CNS: Headache, fatigue, dizziness, fainting, sleep disturbances, weakness, depression, drowsiness
CV: Peripheral edema, tachycardia, hypotension, chest pain, **dysrhythmias,** syncope
GI: Nausea, vomiting, diarrhea, gastric upset, constipation, **hepatitis,** abdominal pain, distention, dry mouth
GU: Nocturia, urinary frequency
HEMA: **Leukopenia**
INTEG: Rash, pruritus, urticaria
MISC: Flushing

Contraindications: Sick sinus syndrome, 2nd- or 3rd-degree heart block, hypotension less than 90 mm Hg systolic, hypersensitivity

Precautions: CHF, hypotension, hepatic disease, pregnancy **C,** lactation, children, renal disease, elderly

▶ **Do Not Confuse:**
DynaCirc/Dynabac/Dynacin

Pharmacokinetics	
Absorption	Well absorbed
Distribution	High plasma protein binding (95%)
Metabolism	Liver, extensively and rapidly
Excretion	Kidney
Half-life	8 hr

Pharmacodynamics	
Onset	1-2 hr
Peak	1.5 hr (immediate rel), 7-18 hr (cont rel)
Duration	12 hr

Interactions

Individual drugs
Cimetidine: ↑ effect of isradipine
Disopyramide: ↑ bradycardia, conduction effects
Fentanyl: ↑ hypotension
Flovastatin: ↓ flovastatin concentration
Ranitidine: ↑ or ↓ effect of israpidine
Drug classifications
Antihypertensives, nitrates: ↑ hypotension
β-Adrenergic blockers: ↑ synergistic effect
Herb/drug
Aconite: ↑ toxicity, death
Astragalus, cola tree: ↑ or ↓ antihypertensive effect
Barberry, betony, black catechu, black cohosh, bloodroot, broom, burdock, cat's claw, dandelion, goldenseal, Irish moss, Jamaican dogwood, kelp, khella, mistletoe, parsley: ↑ antihypertensive effect

---

 Herb/drug   ⓢ Do Not Crush   ◆ Alert   ◆☜ Key Drug   Geriatric   Pediatric

Coltsfoot, guarana, khat, licorice: ↓ antihypertensive effect

NURSING CONSIDERATIONS
Assessment
• Assess fluid volume status: I&O ratio and record, weight, distended red veins, crackles in lung, color, quality, and sp gr of urine, skin turgor, adequacy of pulses, moist mucous membranes, peripheral pitting edema; dehydration symptoms of decreasing output, thirst, hypotension, dry mouth and mucous membranes should be reported
• Monitor ALT, AST, bilirubin; if these are elevated, hepatotoxicity is suspected
• Assess renal, hepatic status, electrolytes before and during treatment
• Monitor cardiac status: B/P, pulse, respiration, ECG; assess anginal pain, precipitating, ameliorating factors

Nursing diagnoses
✓ Cardiac output, decreased (uses)
✓ Knowledge, deficient (teaching)

Implementation
• Give once a day, with food for GI symptoms
🚫 • Do not crush, chew caps, cont rel tabs

Patient/family education
• Instruct patient to avoid hazardous activities until stabilized on drug and dizziness is no longer a problem
• Instruct patient to limit caffeine consumption; to avoid alcohol and OTC drugs unless directed by prescriber
• Advise patient to comply in all areas of medical regimen: diet, exercise, stress reduction, drug therapy; to notify prescriber of irregular heartbeat, shortness of breath, swelling of feet and hands, pronounced dizziness, constipation, nausea, hypotension
• Teach patient to use as directed even if feeling better
• Teach patient to take with a full glass of water

Evaluation
Positive therapeutic outcome
• Decreased B/P

Treatment of overdose: Defibrillation, atropine for AV block, vasopressor for hypotension

itraconazole (Rx)
(it-tra-kon′a-zol)
Sporanox
Func. class.: Antifungal (systemic)
Chem. class.: Triazole derivative
Pregnancy category C

Action: Increases cell membrane permeability in susceptible organisms by binding sterols in fungal cell membrane; decreases potassium, sodium, and nutrients in cell

➔ **Therapeutic Outcome:** Fungistatic against *Histoplasma capsulatum, Blastomyces dermatitis, Cryptococcus neoformans, Aspergillus fumigatus, Candida*

Uses: Systemic candidiasis, chronic mucocandidiasis, oral thrush, candiduria, coccidioidomycosis, histoplasmosis, chromomycosis, paracoccidioidomycosis, blastomycosis (pulmonary and extrapulmonary)

Investigational uses: Dermatophytoses, pityriasis versicolor, sebopsoriasis, vaginal candidiasis, cryptococcal, subcutaneous mycoses, dimorphic infections, leishmaniasis, fungal keratitis, alternariosis, zygomycosis

Dosage and routes
Dose varies with type of infection

Adult: PO 200 mg qd with food; may increase to 400 mg qd if needed; life-threatening infections may require a loading dose of 200 mg tid × 3 days; **IV** 200 mg bid × 4 doses, then 200 mg qd; give each dose over 1 hr, maintenance PO 100 mg/day

Child: PO 3-5 mg/kg/day

Available forms: Caps 100 mg; oral sol 10 mg/ml; inj 10 mg/ml

Adverse effects
(*italic* = common; **bold** = life-threatening)
CNS: Headache, dizziness, insomnia, somnolence, depression
GI: Nausea, vomiting, anorexia, diarrhea, cramps, abdominal pain, flatulence, **GI bleeding, hepatotoxicity**
GU: Gynecomastia, impotence, decreased libido
INTEG: Pruritus, fever, rash, **toxic epidermal necrolysis**
MISC: Edema, fatigue, malaise, hypertension, hypokalemia, tinnitus, **rhabdomyolysis**

Contraindications: Hypersensitivity, lactation, fungal meningitis, onychomycosis or dermatomycosis in cardiac dysfunction

Precautions: Hepatic disease, achlorhydria

P or hypochlorhydria (drug-induced), children, pregnancy **C**

Pharmacokinetics

Absorption	Variable
Distribution	Tissue, plasma, CSF, highly protein bound
Metabolism	Liver, extensively, inhibits CYP4503A enzyme
Excretion	Feces, breast milk
Half-life	20-21 hr

Pharmacodynamics

Onset	Unknown
Peak	4 hr
Duration	Unknown

Interactions
Individual drugs
Busulfan, clarithromycin, cycloSPORINE, diazepam, digoxin, felodipine, indinavir, isradipine, niCARdipine, NIFEdipine, nimoldipine, phenytoin, ritonavir, saquinavir, tacrolimus, warfarin: ↑ toxicity
BusPIRone: ↑ busPIRone levels, toxicity
Didanosine: ↓ antifungal action
Dofetilide, pimozide, quinidine: life-threatening CV reaction
Midazolam: ↑ sedation
Quinidine: ↑ tinnitus, hearing loss
Rifamycins: ↓ action of itraconazole
Triazolam: ↑ sedation
Drug classifications
Antacids, H$_2$-receptor antagonists: ↓ action of itraconazole
Calcium channel blockers: ↑ edema
Hepatotoxic drugs: Hepatotoxicity
Oral hypoglycemics: ↑ effects of oral hypoglycemics
Food/drug
↑ Absorption
Herb/drug
Gossypol: Nephrotoxicity

NURSING CONSIDERATIONS
Assessment
• Assess for infection: WBC, sputum baseline and periodically, may start treatment before obtaining results
◆• Monitor for hepatotoxicity: increasing AST, ALT, alkaline phosphatase, bilirubin
• Monitor for allergic reaction: dermatitis, rash; drug should be discontinued, antihistamines (mild reaction) or epINEPHrine (severe reaction) administered; check inj site for thrombophlebitis
• Monitor for hypokalemia, check potassium level: anorexia, drowsiness, weakness, decreased reflexes, dizziness, increased urinary output, increased thirst, paresthesias; if these occur, drug should be decreased or discontinued and potassium administered

Nursing diagnoses
☑ Infection, risk for (uses)
☑ Injury, risk for (adverse reaction)
☑ Knowledge, deficient (teaching)

Implementation
PO route
• Oral sol: patient should swish in mouth vigorously
• Give with food or milk to prevent nausea and vomiting
⊘• Do not crush, chew caps
• Store in tight container at room temp
• Oral sol and caps are not interchangeable on a mg/mg basis
• Give caps after full meal to ensure absorption, swallow whole
IV IV route
• **IV** after adding full contents 25 ml to 50 ml of NaCl, mix gently, use flow control device, give over 1 hr; use separate line, flush after use

Patient/family education
• Advise patient that long-term therapy may be needed to clear infection (1 wk-6 mo depending on type of infection)
• Teach patient side effects and when to notify prescriber
• Instruct patient to avoid hazardous activities if dizziness occurs
• Instruct patient to take 2 hr before administration of other drugs that increase gastric pH (antacids, H$_2$-blockers, omeprazole, sucralfate, anticholinergics)
• Teach patient importance of compliance with drug regimen
• Instruct patient to notify prescriber of GI symptoms, signs of liver dysfunction (fatigue, nausea, anorexia, vomiting, dark urine, pale stools)
⊘• Tell patient not to break, crush, or chew caps

Evaluation
Positive therapeutic outcome
• Decreased fever, malaise, rash
• Negative C&S for infectious organism

kaolin/pectin (OTC)
(kay'-oh-lin pek'tin)
Donnagel-MB ♣, Kao-Spen, Kapectolin, K-P
Func. class.: Antidiarrheal, adsorbent
Chem. class.: Hydrous magnesium aluminum silicate

Pregnancy category C

Action: Decreases gastric motility, water content of stool; adsorbent, demulcent

➡ **Therapeutic Outcome:** Absence of diarrhea

Uses: Diarrhea (cause undetermined)

Dosage and routes
Adult: PO 60-120 ml (45-90 ml conc) after each loose bowel movement

P *Child >12 yr:* PO 60 ml after each loose bowel movement

P *Child 6-12 yr:* PO 30-60 ml (15 ml conc) after each loose bowel movement

P *Child 3-6 yr:* PO 15-30 ml (7.5 ml conc) after each loose bowel movement

Available forms: Susp kaolin 0.87 g/5 ml, pectin 43 mg/5 ml; kaolin 0.98 g/5 ml, pectin 21.7 mg/5 ml

Adverse effects
(*italic* = common; **bold** = life-threatening)
GI: Constipation (chronic use)

P **Contraindications:** Child <3 yr, severe abdominal pain

Precautions: Pregnancy C

Pharmacokinetics

Absorption	Not absorbed
Distribution	Unknown
Metabolism	Unknown
Excretion	Unknown
Half-life	Unknown

Pharmacodynamics

Onset	½ hr
Peak	Unknown
Duration	6 hr

Interactions
All drugs: ↓ action of all other drugs
▨ *Herb/drug*
Nutmeg: ↑ antidiarrheal effect

NURSING CONSIDERATIONS
Assessment
• Assess bowel pattern before, during

treatment; for rebound constipation after termination of medication; check bowel sounds
P • Assess for dehydration in children
• Check response after 48 hr; if no response, drug should be discontinued and other treatment initiated

Nursing diagnoses
✓ Diarrhea (uses)
✓ Constipation (adverse reactions)
✓ Knowledge, deficient (teaching)
✓ Noncompliance (teaching)

Implementation
• Shake susp before use
• Administer for 48 hr only

Patient/family education
• Advise patient not to exceed recommended dosage; to take all other medications ≥2 hr apart

Evaluation
Positive therapeutic outcome
• Decreased diarrhea

ketoconazole (Rx)
(kee-toe-koe'na-zole)
Nizoral
Func. class.: Antifungal
Chem. class.: Imidazole derivative

Pregnancy category C

Action: Alters cell membrane and inhibits several fungal enzymes; prevents production of adrenal sterols; prevents fungal metabolism

➡ **Therapeutic Outcome:** Fungistatic/fungicidal against susceptible organisms: *Blastomycoses, Candida, Coccidioides, Cryptococcus, Histoplasma;* top route: tinea cruris, tinea corporis, tinea versicolor, *Pityrosporum ovale*

Uses: Systemic candidiasis, chronic mucocandidiasis, oral thrush, candiduria, coccidioidomycosis, histoplasmosis, chromomycosis, paracoccidioidomycosis, blastomycosis

Investigational uses: Cushing's syndrome, advanced prostatic cancer

Dosage and routes
Adult: PO 200-400 mg once daily for 1-2 wk (candidiasis), 6 wk (other infections); 400 mg tid (prostate cancer, unlabeled)

P *Children >2 yr:* 3.3-6.6 mg/kg/day as single daily dose; <2 yr daily dose not established

Available forms: Tabs 200 mg; oral

susp 100 mg/5 ml topical (see Appendix D)

Adverse effects

(*italic* = common; **bold** = life-threatening)

CNS: Headache, dizziness, somnolence

GI: Nausea, vomiting, anorexia, diarrhea, abdominal pain, **hepatotoxicity**

GU: Gynecomastia, impotence

HEMA: **Thrombocytopenia, leukopenia, hemolytic anemia**

INTEG: Pruritus, fever, chills, photophobia, rash, dermatitis, purpura, urticaria

SYST: **Anaphylaxis**

Contraindications: Hypersensitivity, lactation, fungal meningitis; coadministration with terfenadine

Precautions: Renal, hepatic disease, achlorhydria (drug induced), pregnancy **C**, children <2 yr, other hepatotoxic agents including terfenadine

Do Not Confuse:

Nizoral/Nasarel/Neoral

Pharmacokinetics

Absorption	pH dependent; ↓ pH ↑ absorption
Distribution	Widely distributed; crosses placenta
Metabolism	Liver, partially
Excretion	Feces, bile, breast milk
Half-life	Biphasic: 2 hr, 8 hr

Pharmacodynamics

Onset	Unknown
Peak	1-3 hr
Duration	Unknown

Interactions

Individual drugs

Alcohol: ↑ hepatotoxicity

Alfentanil, alprazolam, amprenavir, atorvastatin, cerivastatin, clarithromycin, cyclophosphamide, donepezil, erythromycin, fentanyl, ifosfamide, indinavir, lovastatin, midazolam, nelfinavir, nisoldipine, quinidine, ritonavir, saquinavir, sildenafil, simvastatin, sufentanil, tamoxifen, triazolam, vinBLAStine, vinCRIStine, zolpidem: ↑ toxicity

Carbamazepine, isoniazid, phenytoin, rifampin: ↓ effect of ketoconazole

Carbamazepine, phenytoin: ↑ metabolism

Cimetidine, famotidine: ↓ absorption

CycloSPORINE: ↑ toxicity of cycloSPORINE

Didanosine: ↓ action of ketoconazole

Theophylline: ↓ effectiveness

Warfarin: ↑ effects of warfarin

Drug classifications

Anticholinergics, gastric pump inhibitors, H₂-receptor agonists: ↓ ketoconazole action

Anticoagulants (oral): ↑ effects of oral anticoagulants

Calcium channel blockers, corticosteroids, vinca alkaloids: ↑ toxicity

Hepatotoxic agents: ↑ hepatotoxicity

Herb/drug

Gossypol: Nephrotoxicity

Yew: ↓ ketoconazole action

NURSING CONSIDERATIONS

Assessment

• Assess for signs and symptoms of infection: drainage, sore throat, urinary pain, hematuria, fever

• Obtain cultures for C&S before beginning treatment; therapy may be started after culture is taken

• Monitor for hepatotoxicity: increased AST, ALT, alkaline phosphatase, bilirubin; drug is discontinued if hepatotoxicity occurs

Nursing diagnoses

☑ Infection, risk for (uses)

☑ Injury, risk for (adverse reactions)

☑ Knowledge, deficient (teaching)

Implementation

PO route

• Give in the presence of acid products only; do not use alkaline products, proton pump inhibitors, H₂-antagonists, or antacids within 2 hr of drug; may give coffee, tea, acidic fruit juices, cola; give with food to decrease GI symptoms; dissolve tab/4 ml of aqueous sol 0.2 N HCl, use straw to avoid contact with, rinse with water afterward and swallow

• Give with HCl if achlorhydria is present

• Store in tight container at room temp

Topical route

• Use enough medication to cover fungally infected and surrounding area; rub in; do not use occlusive dressing; do not get in eyes

Shampoo

• Hair should be wet; apply shampoo, lather, rub gently into scalp and hair for 1 min; rinse; reapply × 3 min; continue treatment 2 ×/wk for 1 mo, no more than once q3 days

Patient/family education

• Advise patient that long-term therapy may be needed to clear infection (1 wk-6 mo depending on infection)

• Advise patient to avoid hazardous activities if dizziness occurs

• Instruct patient to take 2 hr before adminis-

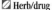

tration of other drugs that increase gastric pH (antacids, H₂-blockers, omeprazole, sucralfate, anticholinergics)
- Stress the importance of compliance with drug regimen
- Advise patient to notify prescriber of GI symptoms, signs of liver dysfunction (fatigue, nausea, anorexia, vomiting, dark urine, pale stools)
- Teach patient proper hygiene: hand washing, nail care, use of concomitant topical agents if prescribed
- Caution patient to avoid alcohol, since nausea, vomiting, hypertension may occur
- Advise patient to use sunscreen or avoid direct sunlight to prevent photosensitivity
- Advise patient to notify prescriber of sore throat, fever, skin rash, which may indicate superinfection
- Advise patient to use sunglasses to prevent photophobia

Evaluation
Positive therapeutic outcome
- Decreased oral candidiasis, fever, malaise, rash
- Negative C&S for infectious organism
- Absence of dandruff, scaling

ketoprofen (OTC, Rx)
(ke-to-proe'fen)
Actron, Apo-Keto ♣, Apo-Keto-E ♣, Ketoprofen, Orudis, Orudis-E ♣, Orudis-KT, Orudis-SR ♣, Oruvail, Rhodis
Func. class.: NSAID; nonopioid analgesic, antirheumatic
Chem. class.: Propionic acid derivative
Pregnancy category B

Action: Inhibits prostaglandin synthesis by decreasing enzyme needed for biosynthesis; analgesic, antiinflammatory

➡ **Therapeutic Outcome:** Decreased pain, inflammation

Uses: Mild to moderate pain, osteoarthritis, rheumatoid arthritis, dysmenorrhea

Dosage and routes
Antiinflammatory
Adult: PO 150-300 mg in divided doses tid-qid, not to exceed 300 mg/day or ext rel 150-200 mg qd

Analgesic
Adult: PO 25-50 mg q6-8h

Available forms: Caps 25, 50, 75 mg; ext rel caps 100, 150, 200 mg; tabs 12.5 mg

Adverse effects
(*italic* = common; **bold** = life-threatening)
CNS: Dizziness, drowsiness, fatigue, tremors, confusion, insomnia, anxiety, depression, headache
CV: Tachycardia, peripheral edema, palpitations, dysrhythmias, hypertension
EENT: Tinnitus, hearing loss, blurred vision
GI: *Nausea, anorexia, vomiting, diarrhea,* jaundice, **hepatitis**, constipation, flatulence, cramps, dry mouth, peptic ulcer, **GI bleeding**
GU: **Nephrotoxicity: dysuria, hematuria, oliguria, azotemia**
HEMA: **Blood dyscrasias**
INTEG: Purpura, rash, pruritus, sweating
SYST: **Anaphylaxis**

Contraindications: Hypersensitivity, asthma, severe renal disease, severe hepatic disease, ulcer disease; avoid in 2nd/3rd trimester of pregnancy

Precautions: Pregnancy **B** (1st trimester), lactation, children, bleeding disorders, GI disorders, cardiac disorders, hypersensitivity to other antiinflammatory agents, elderly

Do Not Confuse:
Oruvail/Clinoril, Oruvail/Elavil

Pharmacokinetics
Absorption	Well absorbed
Distribution	Not known
Metabolism	Liver
Excretion	Kidneys
Half-life	2-4 hr

Pharmacodynamics
Onset	Unknown
Peak	2 hr
Duration	Unknown

Interactions
Individual drugs
Alcohol: ↑ adverse GI reactions, toxicity
Aspirin: ↓ effectiveness, ↑ adverse reactions
Cefamandole, cefaperazone, cefotetan, clopidogrel, eptifibatide, plicamycin, ticlopidine, tirofiban, valproic acid: ↑ risk of bleeding
CycloSPORINE, digoxin, lithium, methotrexate, phenytoin, probenecid, sulfonylurea: ↑ toxicity
Digoxin: ↑ levels
Insulin: ↓ insulin effect
Radiation: ↑ risk of hematologic toxicity
Warfarin: ↑ anticoagulant effect
Drug classifications
Anticoagulants, thrombolytics: ↑ risk of bleeding
Antihypertensives: ↓ effect of antihypertensives

Antineoplastics: ↑ risk of hematologic toxicity
Corticosteroids: ↑ adverse reactions
Diuretics: ↓ effectiveness of diuretics
Hypoglycemics: ↓ hypoglycemic effect
NSAIDs: ↑ adverse GI reactions

⊘ Drug/herb
Anise, arnica, bogbean, chamomile, chondroitin, clove, dong quai, feverfew, garlic, ginger, ginkgo, ginseng (Panax): ↑ risk of bleeding
Arginine, gossypol: ↑ gastric irritation
Bearberry, bilberry: ↑ NSAIDs effect

Lab test interferences
↑ Bleeding time, ↑ potassium, ↑ BUN, ↑ alkaline phosphatase, ↑ AST, ↑ ALT, ↑ creatinine, ↑ LDH, ↓ blood glucose, ↓ Hct, ↓ Hgb, ↓ CCr, ↓ platelets, ↓ leukocytes
Interference: Urine albumin, 17 KS, 17 hydroxycorticosteroids, bilirubin

NURSING CONSIDERATIONS
Assessment
• Assess for pain: type, location, intensity; ROM before and 1-2 hr after treatment
• Monitor liver function, renal function, studies: AST, ALT, bilirubin, creatinine, BUN, urine creatinine, CBC Hct, Hgb, pro-time if patient is on long-term therapy
• Check I&O ratio; decreasing output may indicate renal failure (long-term therapy)
• Assess hepatotoxicity: dark urine, clay-colored stools, jaundice of skin and sclera, itching, abdominal pain, fever, diarrhea if patient is on long-term therapy
• Assess for allergic reactions: rash, urticaria; if these occur, drug may have to be discontinued
• Assess for ototoxicity: tinnitus, ringing, roaring in ears; audiometric testing needed before, after long-term therapy
• Assess for visual changes: blurring, halos; may indicate corneal, retinal damage
• Assess for GI bleeding: blood in sputum, emesis, stools
• Check edema in feet, ankles, legs
• Identify prior drug history; there are many drug interactions
• Monitor pain: location, duration, type, intensity, before dose and 1 hr after; ROM before dose and after

Nursing diagnoses
✓ Pain, acute (uses)
✓ Pain, chronic (uses)
✓ Mobility, impaired physical (uses)
✓ Injury, risk for (adverse reactions)
✓ Knowledge, deficient (teaching)

Implementation
⊘ • Administer to patient whole; do not crush, break, chew, or open cap

• Give with food or milk to decrease gastric symptoms; give 30 min ac or 2 hr pc; absorption may be slowed

Patient/family education
• Teach patient to report any symptoms of hepatotoxicity, renal toxicity, visual changes, ototoxicity, allergic reactions, bleeding (long-term therapy)
• Advise patient to take with 8 oz of water and sit upright for 30 min after dose to prevent ulceration
• Caution patient not to exceed recommended dosage; acute poisoning may result; to take as prescribed; do not double dose
• Advise patient to read label on other OTC drugs; many contain other antiinflammatories
• Advise patient to use sunscreen to prevent photosensitivity
• Inform patient that the therapeutic response takes 2 wk (arthritis)
• Teach patient to report tinnitus, confusion, diarrhea, sweating, hyperventilation, blurred vision, fever, joint aches
• Caution patient to avoid alcohol ingestion; GI bleeding may occur

Evaluation
Positive therapeutic outcome
• Decreased pain
• Decreased inflammation
• Increased mobility
• Decreased fever

ketorolac (Rx)
(kee'toe-role-ak)
Acular, Toradol
Func. class.: NSAID, nonopioid analgesic
Chem. class.: Pyrrolopyrrole

Pregnancy category C

Action: Inhibits prostaglandin synthesis by decreasing an enzyme needed for biosynthesis; analgesic, antiinflammatory, antipyretic effects

Therapeutic Outcome: Decreased pain, inflammation, ocular itching

Uses: Mild to moderate pain (short term); decreased ocular itching in seasonal allergic conjunctivitis

Dosage and routes
Adult <65 yr: PO 20 mg, then 10 mg q4-6h prn, max 40 mg/day; (single dose) IM 60 mg; **IV** 30 mg; (multiple dosing) IM/**IV** 15 mg q6h, max 60 mg/day × 5 days combined either PO/IM/**IV**

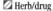

⊿ Herb/drug   ⊘ Do Not Crush   ◆ Alert   ⊙ᴛᴛ Key Drug   🄶 Geriatric   🄿 Pediatric

G *Adult ≥65 yr, renal disease, <50 kg:*
PO 10 mg q4-6h prn, max 40 mg/day; (single dose) IM 30 mg; **IV** 15 mg; (multiple dosing) IM/**IV** 15 mg q6h, max 60 mg/day × 5 days combined either PO/IM/**IV**

Ophthalmic route
See Appendix D

Adult: 1 gtt (0.25 mg) qid × 7 days

P *Child:* **IV** 1 mg/kg then 0.5 mg/kg q6h

Available forms: Inj 15, 30 mg/ml (prefilled syringes); ophth 0.5% sol; tabs 10 mg

Adverse effects
(*italic* = common; **bold** = life-threatening)
CV: Hypertension, flushing, syncope, pallor, edema, vasodilation
CNS: Dizziness, *drowsiness,* tremors
EENT: Tinnitus, hearing loss, blurred vision
GI: Nausea, anorexia, vomiting, diarrhea, constipation, flatulence, cramps, dry mouth, peptic ulcer, **GI bleeding, perforation,** taste change
GU: **Nephrotoxicity: dysuria, hematuria, oliguria, azotemia**
HEMA: **Blood dyscrasias,** prolonged bleeding
INTEG: Purpura, rash, pruritus, sweating

Contraindications: Hypersensitivity, asthma, severe renal disease, severe hepatic disease, peptic ulcer disease, labor and delivery, lactation, CV bleeding

Precautions: Pregnancy **C,** lactation,
P children, bleeding disorders, GI disorders, cardiac disorders, hypersensitivity to other
G antiinflammatory agents, elderly, CCr <25 ml/min

N **Do Not Confuse:**
Toradol/Tegretol/Foradil, Toradol/Inderal, Toradol/Torecan, Toradol/tramadol

Pharmacokinetics	
Absorption	Rapidly, completely absorbed
Distribution	Bound to plasma proteins (99%)
Metabolism	Liver (<50%)
Excretion	Kidney, metabolites (92%); breast milk (6%); feces
Half-life	6 hr (IM); increased in renal disease

Pharmacodynamics		
	IM	OPHTH/PO
Onset	Up to 10 min	Unknown
Peak	50 min IM; 2-3 hr PO	Unknown
Duration	4-6 hr PO	Unknown

Interactions
Individual drugs
Alcohol, aspirin: ↑ GI effects
Aspirin, probenecid: ↑ ketorolac levels
Cefamandole, cefoperazone, cefotetan, clopidogrel, eptifibatide, plicamycin, ticlopidine, tirofiban, valproic acid: ↑ risk of bleeding
Cyclosporine, lithium, methotrexate: ↑ toxicity
Heparin: ↑ bleeding
Drug classifications
ACE inhibitors: ↑ renal impairment
Anticoagulants: ↑ effects
Antihypertensives: ↓ antihypertensive effect
Cephalosporins (some), salicylates, thrombolytics: ↑ risk of bleeding
Corticosteroids, NSAIDs, potassium products, steroids: ↑ GI effects
Diuretics: ↓ antihypertensive effect
Drug/herb
Anise, arnica, bogbean, chamomile, chondroitin, clove, dong quai, feverfew, garlic, ginger, ginkgo, ginseng (Panax): ↑ risk of bleeding
Arginine, gossypol: ↑ gastric irritation
Bearberry, bilberry: ↑ NSAIDs effect
Lab test interferences
↑ Liver function studies, ↑ bleeding time, ↑ BUN, ↑ creatinine, ↑ potassium
↓ Serum potassium, ↓ PBI, ↓ cholesterol
Interference: Urine catecholamines, pregnancy test, urine glucose tests (Clinistix, Tes-Tape)

NURSING CONSIDERATIONS
Assessment
• Monitor blood counts during therapy; watch for decreasing platelets; if low, therapy may need to be discontinued and restarted after hematologic recovery; assess for blood dyscrasia (thrombocytopenia): bruising, fatigue, bleeding, poor healing
• Monitor for aspirin sensitivity, asthma; these patients may be more likely to develop hypersensitivity to NSAIDs
• Assess patient's eyes: redness swelling, tearing, itching
• Monitor for pain: type, location, intensity, ROM before and 1 hr after treatment
• Assess for GI bleeding: blood in sputum, emesis, stools

Nursing diagnoses
✓ Pain, acute (uses)

K

✓ Mobility, impaired physical (uses)
✓ Injury, risk for (adverse reactions)
✓ Knowledge, deficient (teaching)

Implementation
PO route
- Administer to patient crushed or whole
- Give with food or milk to decrease gastric symptoms; give 30 min ac or 2 hr pc; absorption may be slowed

IV IM/IV route
- **IV** give undiluted ≥15 sec
- Give IM/**IV** for 5 days or less, continue with PO

Y-site compatibilities: Cisatracurium, remifentanil, sufentanil

Syringe incompatibilities: Morphine, meperidine, promethazine, hydrOXYzine

Solution compatibilities: D_5W, 0.9% NaCl, LR, D_5, plasmalate

Patient/family education
- Teach patient that drug must be continued for prescribed time to be effective; to avoid aspirin, alcoholic beverages, other NSAIDs, acetaminophen
- Caution patient to report bleeding, bruising, fatigue, malaise, since blood dyscrasias do occur
- Instruct patient to use caution when driving; drowsiness, dizziness may occur
- Ⓢ Teach patient to take with a full glass of water to enhance absorption; do not crush, break, or chew tabs
- Caution patient that this drug may cause eye redness, burning if soft contact lenses are worn

Evaluation
Positive therapeutic outcome
- Decreased pain
- Decreased inflammatory response
- Increased mobility
- Decreased ocular itching

---

labetalol (Rx)
(la-bet'a-lole)
Normodyne, Trandate
Func. class.: Antihypertensive, antianginal
Chem. class.: α- and β-blocker

Pregnancy category C

Action: Competitively blocks stimulation of β-adrenergic receptor within vascular smooth muscle; produces chronotropic, inotropic activity (decreases rate of SA node discharge,

increases recovery time), slows conduction of AV node, decreases heart rate, which decreases O_2 consumption in myocardium; also has α-adrenergic blocking activity

→ **Therapeutic Outcome:** Decreased B/P

Uses: Mild to moderate hypertension; treatment of severe hypertension (**IV**)

Investigational uses: Hypertension in patients with pheochromocytoma, hypertension in clonidine withdrawal

Dosage and routes
Hypertension
Adult: PO 100 mg bid; may be given with a diuretic; may increase to 200 mg bid after 2 days; may continue to increase q1-3 days; max 400 mg bid

Hypertensive crisis
Adult: **IV** inf 200 mg/160 ml D_5W, run at 2 ml/min; stop inf after desired response obtained; repeat q6-8h as needed; **IV** bol 20 mg over 2 min; may repeat 40-80 mg q10 min, not to exceed 300 mg

Available forms: Tabs 100, 200, 300 mg; inj 5 mg/ml in 20-ml ampules

Adverse effects
*(italic = common; **bold** = life-threatening)*
CNS: Dizziness, mental changes, drowsiness, fatigue, headache, catatonia, depression, anxiety, nightmares, paresthesias, lethargy
CV: *Orthostatic hypotension,* **bradycardia, CHF,** chest pain, **ventricular dysrhythmias,** AV block, scalp tingling
EENT: *Tinnitus,* visual changes, sore throat, double vision, dry burning eyes
GI: *Nausea, vomiting, diarrhea,* dyspepsia, taste distortion
GU: Impotence, dysuria, ejaculatory failure
HEMA: **Agranulocytosis, thrombocytopenia, purpura** (rare)
INTEG: Rash, alopecia, urticaria, pruritus, fever
RESP: **Bronchospasm,** dyspnea, wheezing

Contraindications: Hypersensitivity to β-blockers, cardiogenic shock, heart block (2nd or 3rd degree), sinus bradycardia, CHF, bronchial asthma

Precautions: Major surgery, pregnancy **C**, lactation, diabetes mellitus, renal disease, thyroid disease, COPD, well-compensated heart failure, CAD, nonallergic bronchospasm, Ⓖ elderly, hepatic disease

▧ **Do Not Confuse:** Trandate/Tridate

Pharmacokinetics

Absorption	Bioavailability 25% (PO); complete (**IV**)
Distribution	Crosses placenta, CNS
Metabolism	Liver, extensively
Excretion	Breast milk, kidneys, bile
Half-life	6-8 hr

Pharmacodynamics

	PO	IV
Onset	1-2 hr	5 min
Peak	2-4 hr	15 min
Duration	8-12 hr	2-4 hr

Interactions
Individual drugs
Alcohol (large amounts), cimetidine, nitroglycerin: ↑ hypotension
Glutethimide, indomethacin, lidocaine: ↓ effect of each specific drug
Verapamil: ↑ myocardial depression
Drug classifications
Antihypertensives: ↑ hypotension
β-Blockers, bronchodilators, sympathomimetics, xanthines: ↓ effects
Diuretics: ↑ hypotension
General anesthetics, hydantoins: ↑ myocardial depression
Theophyllines: ↓ bronchodilation
⬚ Herb/drug
Aconite: ↑ toxicity, death
Astragalus, cola tree: ↑ or ↓ antihypertensive effect
Barberry, betony, black catechu, black cohosh, bloodroot, broom, burdock, cat's claw, dandelion, goldenseal, Irish moss, Jamaican dogwood, kelp, khella, mistletoe, parsley: ↑ antihypertensive effect
Coltsfoot, guarana, khat, licorice: ↓ antihypertensive effect
Lab test interferences
False: ↑ urinary catecholamines
Increase: ANA titer, blood glucose, alkaline phosphatase, LDH, AST, ALT, BUN, potassium, triglycerides, uric acid

NURSING CONSIDERATIONS
Assessment
• Monitor B/P at beginning of treatment, periodically thereafter; pulse q4h; note rate, rhythm, quality: apical/radial pulse before administration; notify prescriber of any significant changes (pulse <50 bpm)
• Check for baselines in renal, liver function tests before therapy begins
• Assess for edema in feet, legs daily, monitor I&O, daily weight; check for jugular vein distention, rales bilaterally, dyspnea (CHF)
• Monitor skin turgor, dryness of mucous membranes for hydration status, especially Ⓖ elderly

Nursing diagnoses
✓ Cardiac output, decreased (uses)
✓ Injury, risk for (side effects)
✓ Knowledge, deficient (teaching)
✓ Noncompliance (teaching)

Implementation
PO route
• Given ac, hs, tab may be crushed or swallowed whole; give with food to prevent GI upset, increase absorption; reduce dosage in renal dysfunction
• Store protected from light, moisture; place in cool environment
ⅣV IV route
• Give **IV** undiluted 20 mg/2 min; may increase q10 min 40-80 mg until desired effect
• Give **IV** cont inf by diluting in LR, D₅W, D₅ in 0.2%, 0.9%, 0.33% NaCl or Ringer's; inf is titrated to patient response; 200 mg of drug/160 ml sol (1 mg/ml); 300 mg of drug/240 ml sol (1 mg/ml); 200 mg of drug/250 ml sol (2 mg/3ml); use infusion pump
• Keep patient recumbent during and for 3 hr after inf, monitor VS q5-15 min

Y-site compatibilities: Amikacin, aminophylline, amiodarone, ampicillin, butorphanol, calcium gluconate, cefazolin, ceftazidime, ceftizoxime, chloramphenicol, cimetidine, clindamycin, diltiazem, DOBUTamine, DOPamine, enalaprilat, epINEPHrine, erythromycin, esmolol, famotidine, fentanyl, gentamicin, hydromorphone, lidocaine, lorazepam, magnesium sulfate, meperidine, metronidazole, midazolam, milrinone, morphine, niCARdipine, nitroglycerin, nitroprusside, norepinephrine, oxacillin, penicillin G potassium, piperacillin, potassium chloride, potassium phosphate, propofol, ranitidine, sodium acetate, tobramycin, trimethoprim/sulfamethoxazole, vancomycin, vecuronium

Y-site incompatibilities: Cefoperazone, nafcillin

Solution compatibilities: D₅R, D₅LR, D₂½/0.45% NaCl, D₅/0.2% NaCl, D₅/0.33% NaCl, D₅/0.9% NaCl, D₅W, Ringer's, LR

Solution incompatibilities: Sodium bicarbonate 5%

Patient/family education

- Teach patient not to discontinue drug abruptly, or precipitate angina might occur; taper over 2 wk
- Teach patient not to use OTC products containing α-adrenergic stimulants (such as nasal decongestants, cold preparations); to avoid alcohol, smoking and to limit sodium intake as prescribed
- Teach patient how to take pulse and B/P at home; advise when to notify prescriber
- Instruct patient to comply with weight control, dietary adjustments, modified exercise program
- Advise patient to carry/wear emergency ID to identify drugs being taken, allergies; that drug controls symptoms but does not cure the condition
- Caution patient to avoid hazardous activities if dizziness, drowsiness are present
- Teach patient to report symptoms of CHF: difficult breathing, especially on exertion or when lying down, night cough, swelling of extremities, bradycardia, dizziness, confusion, depression, fever
- Teach patient to take drug as prescribed, not to double or skip doses; take any missed doses as soon as remembered if at least 4 hr until next dose

Evaluation

Positive therapeutic outcome

- Decreased B/P in hypertension (after 1-2 wk)
- Absence of dysrhythmias

Treatment of overdose: Lavage, **IV** atropine for bradycardia, **IV** theophylline for bronchospasm, digitalis, O₂, diuretic for cardiac failure, hemodialysis, **IV** glucose for hyperglycemia, **IV** diazepam (or phenytoin) for seizures

---

lactulose (Rx)

(lak'tyoo-lose)
Cephulac, Cholac, Chronulac, Constilac, Constulose, Duphalac, Enulose, Evalose, Heptalac, Kristalose, Lactulax ✤, Lactulose PSE, Portalac
Func. class.: Laxative (hyperosmotic/ammonia detoxicant)
Chem. class.: Lactose synthetic derivative

Pregnancy category B

Action: Increases osmotic pressure; draws fluid into colon; prevents absorption of ammonia in colon; increases water in stool

⮕ **Therapeutic Outcome:** Decreased constipation, decreased blood ammonia level

Uses: Chronic constipation, portal-systemic encephalopathy in patients with hepatic disease

Dosage and routes
Constipation
Adult: PO 15-60 ml qd

P *Child (unlabeled):* PO 7.5 ml qd

Encephalopathy
Adult: PO 30-45 ml tid or qid until stools are soft; **RETENTION ENEMA** 300 ml diluted (unlabeled)

P *Infant (unlabeled):* PO 2.5-10 ml/day in divided doses

P *Child (unlabeled):* PO 40-90 ml/day in divided doses given 2-4 ×/day

Available forms: Syr 10 g/15 ml, single-use packets (Kristalose) 10, 20 g

Adverse effects
(*italic* = common; **bold** = life-threatening)
GI: Nausea, vomiting, anorexia, abdominal cramps, diarrhea, flatulence, *distention, belching*

Contraindications: Hypersensitivity, low-galactose diet

Precautions: Pregnancy **B**, lactation,
G diabetes mellitus, elderly and debilitated patient

Pharmacokinetics	
Absorption	Poorly absorbed
Distribution	Not known
Metabolism	Colonic bacteria to acids
Excretion	Kidneys, unchanged
Half-life	Unknown

Pharmacodynamics
Unknown

Interactions
Individual drugs
Neomycin: ↓ effectiveness (portal-systemic encephalopathy)
Drug classifications
Antiinfectives (oral): ↓ lactulose effect
Laxatives: Do not use together
⬚ *Herb/drug*
Flax, senna: ↑ laxative effect

NURSING CONSIDERATIONS
Assessment

- Monitor glucose levels in diabetic patients (increases)

 Herb/drug   Do Not Crush   ✦ Alert   ✆ Key Drug   **G** Geriatric   **P** Pediatric

• Monitor blood, urine, electrolytes if used often by patient; may cause diarrhea, hypokalemia, hypernatremia; check I&O ratio to identify fluid loss

• Assess cramping, rectal bleeding, nausea, vomiting; if these symptoms occur, drug should be discontinued; identify cause of constipation; identify whether fluids, bulk, or exercise is missing from lifestyle

• Monitor blood ammonia level (30-70 mg/100 ml); monitor for clearing of confusion, lethargy, restlessness, irritability (hepatic encephalopathy); may decrease ammonia level by 50%

Nursing diagnoses

✓ Constipation (uses)
✓ Diarrhea (adverse reactions)
✓ Knowledge, deficient (teaching)
✓ Noncompliance (teaching)

Implementation
PO route

• Give with full glass of fruit juice, water, milk to increase palatability of oral form; increase fluids by 2 L/day; do not give with other laxatives; if diarrhea occurs, reduce dosage

Rectal route

• Administer retention enema by diluting 300 ml of lactulose/700 ml of water or of 0.9% NaCl; administer by rec balloon catheter; retain for 30-60 min; repeat if evacuated too quickly

Patient/family education

• Discuss with patient that adequate fluid consumption is necessary

• Teach patient that normal bowel movements do not always occur daily

• Teach patient not to use in presence of abdominal pain, nausea, vomiting; tell patient to notify prescriber if constipation unrelieved or if symptoms of electrolyte imbalance occur: muscle cramps, pain, weakness, dizziness, excessive thirst

• Teach patient not to use laxatives for longterm therapy; bowel tone will be lost

• Do not give at hs as a laxative; may interfere with sleep

• Notify prescriber if diarrhea occurs; may indicate overdosage

Evaluation
Positive therapeutic outcome

• Decreased constipation
• Decreased blood ammonia level
• Clearing of mental state

---

lamivudine (3TC) (Rx)
(lam-i'vue-dine)
Epivir, Epivir-HBV, 3TC
Func. class.: Antiretroviral
Chem. class.: Nucleoside reverse transcriptase inhibitor

Pregnancy category C

Action: Inhibits replication of HIV virus by incorporating into cellular DNA by viral reverse transcriptase, thereby terminating the cellular DNA chain

➜ **Therapeutic Outcome:** Improved symptoms of HIV infection

Uses: HIV infection in combination with other antiretrovirals; chronic hepatitis B (Epivir-HBV)

Investigational uses: Prophylaxis of HIV postexposure with indinavir and zidovudine

Dosage and routes
HIV infection

🅟 **Adult/child >16 yr:** PO 150 mg bid or 300 mg qd

🅟 **Child 3 mo-16 yr:** PO 4 mg/kg bid; max 150 mg bid

Renal dose

Adult: PO CCr 30-49 ml/min 150 mg qd; CCr 15-29 ml/min 150 mg 1st dose, then 100 mg qd; CCr 5-14 ml/min 150 mg qd, then 50 mg qd; CCr <5 ml/min 50 mg 1st dose, then 25 mg qd

Chronic hepatitis B
Adult: PO 100 mg qd

Renal dose
Adult: PO CCr 30-49 ml/min 100 mg 1st dose, then 50 mg qd; CCr 15-29 ml/min 100 mg 1st dose, then 25 mg qd; CCr 5-14 ml/min 35 mg 1st dose then 15 mg qd; CCr <5 ml/min 35 mg 1st dose, then 10 mg qd

Available forms: Tabs 100, 150, 300 mg; oral sol 10 mg/ml

Adverse effects
(*italic* = common; **bold** = life-threatening)
CNS: *Fever, headache, malaise, dizziness, insomnia, depression, fatigue, chills,* **seizures**
EENT: Taste change, hearing loss, photophobia
GI: *Nausea, vomiting, diarrhea,* anorexia, cramps, dyspepsia, **hepatomegaly with**
🅟 **steatosis, pancreatitis** (pediatric patients)
HEMA: **Neutropenia,** anemia, **thrombocytopenia**

L

INTEG: Rash
MS: Myalgia, arthralgia, pain
RESP: Cough
SYST: **Lactic acidosis, anaphylaxis, Stevens-Johnson syndrome**

Contraindications: Hypersensitivity

Precautions: Granulocyte count <1000/mm^3 or Hgb <9.5 g/dl, pregnancy **C**, lactation, P children, renal disease, severe hepatic dysfunction, G pancreatitis, elderly

⚠ Do Not Confuse:
lamivudine/Lamotrigine

Pharmacokinetics

Absorption	Rapidly absorbed
Distribution	Extravascular space
Metabolism	Unknown
Excretion	Unchanged in urine
Half-life	Unknown

Pharmacodynamics
Unknown

Interactions
Individual drugs
Trimethoprim/sulfamethoxazole: ↑ level of lamivudine

NURSING CONSIDERATIONS
Assessment
• Monitor blood counts q2 wk; watch for neutropenia, thrombocytopenia, Hgb, CD4, viral load, lipase, triglycerides periodically during treatment; if low, therapy may have to be discontinued and restarted after hematologic recovery; blood transfusions may be required
• Monitor liver function studies: AST, ALT, bilirubin; amylase
P • Monitor children for pancreatitis: abdominal pain, nausea, vomiting
• Assess for lactic acidosis, severe hepatomegaly with steatosis: obtain baseline liver function tests; if elevated, discontinue treatment; discontinue even if liver function tests are normal and symptoms of lactic acidosis, severe hepatomegaly develop

Nursing diagnoses
✓ Infection, risk for (uses)
✓ Injury, risk for (adverse reactions)
✓ Knowledge, deficient (teaching)

Implementation
• Administer PO qd, bid without regard to meals
• Give with other antiretrovirals only

• Store in cool environment; protect from light

Patient/family education
• Teach patient that GI complaints and insomnia resolve after 3-4 wk of treatment
• Tell patient that drug is not a cure for AIDS but will control symptoms
• Teach patient to notify prescriber of sore throat, swollen lymph nodes, malaise, fever; other infections may occur
• Teach patient that virus is still infective, may pass AIDS virus to others
• Encourage patient to continue follow-up visits since serious toxicity may occur; blood counts must be done q2 wk
• Teach patient that drug must be taken as prescribed, even if feeling better
• Tell patient that other drugs may be necessary to prevent other infections
• Teach patient that drug may cause fainting or dizziness

Evaluation
Positive therapeutic outcome
• Absence of infection, symptoms of HIV infection

---

lamotrigine (Rx)
(lam-o-trye'geen)
Lamictal, Lamictal Chewable Dispersible
Func. class.: Anticonvulsant—misc.
Chem. class.: Phenyltriazine
Pregnancy category C

Action: Unknown; may inhibit voltage-sensitive sodium channels

➡ **Therapeutic Outcome:** Decrease in intensity and amount of seizures

Uses: Adjunct in the treatment of partial P seizures; children with Lennox-Gastaut syndrome

Investigational uses: Refractory bipolar disorder, generalized tonic-clonic, absence, atypical absence and myoclonic seizures

Dosage and routes
Monotherapy
Adult: PO 50 mg/day for wk 1 and 2, then increase to 100 mg divided bid for wk 3 and 4; maintenance 300-500 mg/day

P *Child:* 2 mg/kg/day in 2 divided doses × 2 wk, then 10 mg/kg/day, max 15 mg/kg/day or 400 mg/day

Multiple therapy
Adult: PO 25 mg every other day, wk 1 through 4, then 150 mg/day in divided doses

---

P *Child:* 0.1-0.2 mg/kg/day initially, then increase q2 wk as needed to 2 mg/kg/day or 150 mg/day

Hepatic dose (Child-Pugh grade B)
Adult: PO: Reduce by 50%; *(Child-Pugh grade C)* reduce by 75%

Available forms: Tabs 25, 100, 150, 200 mg; chew tabs 2, 5, 25 mg

Adverse effects
(*italic* = common; **bold** = life-threatening)
CNS: Fever, insomnia, tremor, depression, anxiety, *dizziness*, ataxia, *headache*
EENT: Nystagmus, **diplopia**, *blurred vision*
GI: *Nausea, vomiting, anorexia*, abdominal pain, **hepatotoxicity**
GU: *Dysmenorrhea*
INTEG: **Rash (potentially life-threatening)**, alopecia, photosensitivity
SYST: **Stevens-Johnson syndrome**

Contraindications: Hypersensitivity

Precautions: Pregnancy **C**, lactation,
P children <16 yr, renal, hepatic disease, elderly,
G cardiac disease

⚠ Do Not Confuse:
Lamictal/Lamisil, Lamictal/Lomotil,
Lamotrigine/Lamivudine

Pharmacokinetics	
Absorption	Well absorbed
Distribution	Unknown
Metabolism	Unknown
Excretion	Unknown
Half-life	Varies, depending on dose

Pharmacodynamics
Unknown

Interactions
Individual drugs
Acetaminophen, contraceptives (oral), rifampin: ↓ lamotrigine serum concentration
Carbamazepine, ethosuximide, oxcarbazepine, phenobarbital, phenytoin, primidone: ↑ metabolic clearance of lamotrigine
Valproic acid: ↓ metabolic clearance of lamotrigine
Herb/drug
Ginkgo: ↑ anticonvulsant effect
Ginseng, santonica: ↓ anticonvulsant effect

NURSING CONSIDERATIONS
Assessment
◆P • Assess for rash (Stevens-Johnson syndrome or toxic epidermal necrolysis) in pediatric

patients, drug should be discontinued at first sign of rash
• Assess for seizure activity: duration, type, intensity, halo before seizure
• Assess for hypersensitive reactions

Nursing diagnoses
☑ Injury, risk for (uses)
☑ Knowledge, deficient (teaching)

Implementation
• May be given with food or fluids
• Dispersible tabs should be swallowed whole, chewed, dispersed in water or diluted fruit juice; if chewed, a small amount of water should be taken

Patient/family education
• Teach patient to take PO in divided doses with or after meals to decrease adverse effects
• Caution patient not to discontinue drug abruptly; seizures may occur
• Caution patient to avoid hazardous activities until stabilized on drug
• Advise patient to notify prescriber of skin rash or increased seizure activity
• Instruct patient to report to prescriber if pregnancy is suspected or planned
• Teach patient to use sunscreen and protective clothing, photosensitivity occurs
• Advise patient to carry/wear emergency ID stating drug use

Evaluation
Positive therapeutic outcome
• Decrease in severity of seizures

lansoprazole (Rx)
(lan-soe'prah-zole)
Prevacid
Func. class.: Anti-ulcer–proton pump inhibitor
Chem. class.: Benzimidazole
Pregnancy category B

Action: Suppresses gastric secretion by inhibiting hydrogen/potassium ATPase enzyme system in gastric parietal cell; characterized as gastric acid pump inhibitor since it blocks final step of acid production

⇒ Therapeutic Outcome: Reduction in gastric pain, swelling, fullness

Uses: Gastroesophageal reflux disease (GERD), severe erosive esophagitis, poorly responsive systemic GERD, pathologic hypersecretory conditions (Zollinger-Ellison syndrome, systemic mastocytosis, multiple endocrine adenomas); possibly effective for treatment of duodenal, gastric ulcers, maintenance of healed duodenal ulcers

Dosage and routes
NG tube
Adult: Use intact granules mixed in 40 ml of apple juice injected through NG tube, then flush with apple juice

Duodenal ulcer
Adult: PO 15 mg qd ac for 4 wk, then 15 mg qd to maintain healing of ulcers; ulcers associated with *Helicobacter:* 30 mg lansoprazole, 500 mg clarithromycin, 1 g amoxicillin bid × 14 days or 30 mg lansoprazole, 1 g amoxicillin tid × 14 days

Erosive esophagitis
Adult: PO 30 mg qd ac for up to 8 wk, may use another 8-wk course if needed

Pathologic hypersecretory conditions
Adult: PO 60 mg qd, may give up to 90 mg bid

Available forms: Caps delayed rel 15, 30 mg

Adverse effects
(*italic* = common; **bold** = life-threatening)
CNS: Headache, dizziness, confusion, agitation, amnesia, depression
CV: Chest pain, angina, tachycardia, bradycardia, palpitations, **CVA,** hypertension/hypotension, **MI,** shock, vasodilation
EENT: Tinnitus, taste perversion, deafness, eye pain, otitis media
GI: Diarrhea, abdominal pain, vomiting, nausea, constipation, flatulence, acid regurgitation, anorexia, irritable colon
GU: Hematuria, glycosuria, impotence, kidney calculus, breast enlargement
HEMA: **Hemolysis,** anemia
INTEG: Rash, urticaria, pruritus, alopecia
META: Weight gain/loss, gout
RESP: Upper respiratory infections, cough, epistaxis, asthma, bronchitis, dyspnea

Contraindications: Hypersensitivity

Precautions: Pregnancy **B,** lactation, P children

⊠ Do Not Confuse:
Prevacid/Pravachol/Prinivil

Pharmacokinetics
Absorption	Rapid after granules leave stomach
Distribution	Protein binding 97%
Metabolism	Liver extensively
Excretion	Urine, feces; clearance decreased **G** in elderly, renal, hepatic disease
Half-life	Plasma 1.5 hr

Pharmacodynamics
Unknown

Interactions
Individual drugs
Ampicillin, digoxin, iron, itraconazole, ketoconazole: ↓ absorption of each specific drug
Sucralfate: Delayed absorption of lansoprazole

NURSING CONSIDERATIONS
Assessment
• Assess GI system; bowel sounds q8h, abdomen for pain, swelling, anorexia
• Monitor hepatic enzymes (AST, ALT, alkaline phosphatase) during treatment

Nursing diagnoses
☑ Pain, chronic (uses)
☑ Knowledge, deficient (teaching)

Implementation
• Administer before eating; swallow capsule whole
⊘ • Do not open, chew, crush

Patient/family education
• Instruct patient to report severe diarrhea; drug may have to be discontinued
• Inform diabetic patient that hypoglycemia may occur
• Encourage patient to avoid hazardous activities; dizziness may occur
• Tell patient to avoid alcohol, salicylates, ibuprofen; may cause GI irritation

Evaluation
Positive therapeutic outcome
• Absence of gastric pain, swelling, fullness

---

laronidase
Aldurazyme
See Appendix A, Selected New Drugs

---

leflunomide (Rx)
(leh-floo'noh-mide)
Arava
Func. class.: Antirheumatic (DMARDs)
Chem. class.: Immune modulator, pyrimidine synthesis inhibitor

Pregnancy category X

Action: Inhibits an enzyme involved in pyrimidine synthesis and has antiproliferative, antiinflammatory effect

---

☑ Herb/drug   ⊘ Do Not Crush   ◆ Alert   ◔ᴛᴛ Key Drug   **G** Geriatric   **P** Pediatric

→ **Therapeutic Outcome:** Decreased pain, joint swelling, increased mobility

Uses: Rheumatoid arthritis, to reduce disease process as well as symptoms

Dosage and routes
Adult: **PO** loading dose 100 mg/day × 3 days maintenance 20 mg/day, may be decreased to 10 mg/day if not well tolerated

Available forms: Tabs 10, 20, 100 mg

Adverse effects
(*italic* = common; **bold** = life-threatening)
CNS: Dizziness, insomnia, depression, paresthesia, anxiety, migraine, neuralgia, headache
CV: Palpitations, hypertension, chest pain, angina pectoris, migraine, peripheral edema
EENT: Pharyngitis, oral candidiasis, stomatitis, dry mouth, blurred vision
HEMA: Anemia, ecchymosis, hyperlipidemia
GI: *Nausea, anorexia, vomiting, constipation, flatulence, diarrhea,* ↑ *liver function tests*
INTEG: Rash, pruritus, alopecia, acne, hematoma, herpes infections
RESP: Pharyngitis, rhinitis, bronchitis, cough, respiratory infection, pneumonia, sinusitis

Contraindications: Hypersensitivity, pregnancy **X,** lactation

Precautions: Hepatic, renal disorders

Pharmacokinetics
Absorption	Unknown
Distribution	Unknown
Metabolism	Liver
Excretion	Kidneys
Half-life	Unknown

Pharmacodynamics
Onset	Unknown
Peak	Unknown
Duration	Unknown

Interactions
Individual drugs
Activated charcoal, cholestyramine: ↓ effect of leflunomide
Methotrexate: ↑ leflunomide side effects
Rifampin: ↑ rifampin levels
Drug classifications
Live virus vaccines: ↓ antibody reaction
NSAIDs: ↑ NSAID effect
Hepatotoxic agents: ↑ side effects of leflunomide

NURSING CONSIDERATIONS
Assessment
• Monitor liver function studies: if ALT elevations are >2 times baseline, reduce dose to 10 mg/day
• Assess arthritic symptoms: ROM, mobility, swelling of joints, baseline and during treatment

Nursing diagnoses
☑ Mobility, impaired (uses)
☑ Pain, chronic (uses)
☑ Knowledge, deficient (teaching)

Implementation
PO route
• Give PO with food for GI upset
• To eliminate drug give cholestyramine 8 g tid × 11 days, check levels

Patient/family education
• Teach patient that drug must be continued for prescribed time to be effective
• Instruct patient to take with food, milk, or antacids to avoid GI upset
• Advise patient to use caution when driving; drowsiness, dizziness may occur
• Advise patient to take with a full glass of water to enhance absorption
• Advise patient to avoid pregnancy while taking this drug
• Inform patient that hair may be lost, review alternatives
• Advise patient to avoid live virus vaccinations during treatment

Evaluation
Positive therapeutic outcome
• Increased joint mobility without pain
• Decreased joint swelling

L

⚠ HIGH ALERT

lepirudin ⊶ (Rx)
(lep-ih-roo'din)
Refludan
Func. class.: Anticoagulant
Chem. class.: Thrombin inhibitor, hirudin

Pregnancy category B

Action Direct inhibitor of thrombin that is highly specific

→ **Therapeutic Outcome:** Absence of thrombocytopenia, stroke, MI, or other thromboembolic conditions

Uses: Heparin-induced thrombocytopenia and other thromboembolic conditions

Investigational uses: Adjunct therapy in unstable angina, acute MI without ST elevation, prevention of deep vein thrombosis, percutaneous coronary intervention

Dosage and routes
Adult: **IV** 0.4 mg/kg (≤110 kg) over 15-20 sec; then 0.15 mg/kg (≤110 kg/hr) as a cont inf for 2-10 days or longer

Renal dose
Adult: **IV** BOL 0.2 mg/kg over 15-20 sec; CCr 45-60 ml/min 0.075 mg/kg/hr; CCr 30-44 ml/min 0.045 mg/kg/hr; CCr 15-29 ml/min 0.0225 mg/kg/hr

Concomitant use with thrombolytic therapy
Adult: **IV** BOL 0.2 mg/kg initially
Adult: Cont **IV** INF 0.1 mg/kg/hr

Available forms: Powder for inj 50 mg

Adverse effects
(*italic* = common; **bold** = life-threatening)
CNS: Fever, **intracranial bleeding**
CV: **Heart failure, pericardial effusion, ventricular fibrillation**
GI: GI bleeding, abnormal liver function tests
GU: **Hematuria,** abnormal kidney function, vaginal bleeding
HEMA: **Hemorrhage, thrombocytopenia**
INTEG: Allergic skin reactions
RESP: Pneumonia
SYST: **Multiorgan failure, sepsis, anaphylaxis**

Contraindications: Hypersensitivity to hirudins

Precautions: Intracranial bleeding, lactation, children, hepatic disease, pregnancy **B,** recent major surgery, hemorrhagic diathesis, bacterial endocarditis, severe uncontrolled hypertension, advanced renal disease, recent active peptic ulcer, recent CVA, stroke, intracerebral surgery, elderly, women

Pharmacokinetics	
Absorption	Unknown
Distribution	Unknown
Metabolism	Possibly by the release of amino acids during catabolism
Excretion	50% unchanged in urine
Half-life	Unknown

Pharmacodynamics	
Onset	Unknown
Peak	Unknown
Duration	Unknown

Interactions
Individual drugs
Aspirin, cefamandole, cefoperazone, cefotetan, clopidogrel, dipyridamole, eptifibatide, plicamycin, ticlopidine, tirofiban, valproic acid: ↑ bleeding risk
Drug classifications
NSAIDs, warfarin derivatives: ↑ bleeding risk
Thrombolytics: ↑ action of lepirudin
Herb/drug
Agrimony, alfalfa, angelica, anise, basil, bay, bilberry, black haw, bogbean, bromelain, buchu, chondroitin, cinchona bark, dong quai, fenugreek, feverfew, garlic, ginger, ginkgo, ginseng, horse chestnut, Irish moss, kelp, kelpware, khella, lovage, lungwort, meadowsweet, motherwort, mugwort, nettle, papaya, parsley (large amounts), pau d'arco, pineapple, poplar, prickly ash, safflower, saw palmetto, tonka bean, turmeric, wintergreen, yarrow: ↑ risk of bleeding
Chamomile, coenzyme Q10, flax, glucomannan, goldenseal, guar gum: ↓ anticoagulant effect

NURSING CONSIDERATIONS
Assessment
- Obtain baseline APTT before treatment; do not start treatment if APTT ratio is ≥2.5, then APTT 4 hr after initiation of treatment and at least qd thereafter; if APTT is above target, stop infusion for 2 hr, then restart at 50%, take APTT in 4 hr; if below target, increase inf rate by 20%, take APTT in 4 hr, do not exceed inf rate of 0.21 mg/kg/hr without checking for coagulation abnormalities
- Monitor APTT, which should be 1.5-2.5 × control
- Assess bleeding gums, petechiae, ecchymosis, black tarry stools, hematuria/epistaxis, B/P, vaginal bleeding, puncture sites; may indicate bleeding and possible hemorrhage
- Assess fever, skin rash, urticaria

Nursing diagnoses
☑ Tissue perfusion, ineffective (uses)
☑ Injury, risk for (side effects)
☑ Knowledge, deficient (teaching)

Implementation
- Administer after reconstitution and further dilution under sterile conditions; use water for inj or 0.9% NaCl; for further dilution 0.9% NaCl or D$_5$; for rapid and complete reconstitution, inject 1 ml of diluent into vial and shake gently, use immediately, warm to room temp before use
- Avoid all IM inj that may cause bleeding

 Herb/drug   Do Not Crush   Alert   Key Drug   Geriatric   Pediatric

IV route

- Administer **IV** bol: use sol with conc of 5 mg/ml, reconstitute 5 mg (1 vial)/1 ml of water for inj or 0.9% NaCl, use body weight for correct weight calculation
- Administer **IV** inf: use sol with a conc of 0.2 or 0.4 mg/ml; reconstitute 100 mg (2 vials) with 1 ml each (2 ml) water for inj or 0.9% NaCl, transfer to infusion bag with either 500 or 250 ml of 0.9% NaCl or D$_5$W

Patient/family education

- Teach patient to use soft bristle toothbrush to avoid bleeding gums, avoid contact sports, use electric razor, avoid IM inj
- Teach patient to report any signs of bleeding: gums, under skin, urine, stools

Evaluation

Positive therapeutic outcome

- Absence of thrombocytopenia without significant bleeding

---

letrozole (Rx)

(let'tro-zohl)

Femara

Func. class.: Antineoplastic, nonsteroidal aromatase inhibitor

Pregnancy category D

Action: Binds to the heme group of aromatase; inhibits conversion of androgens to estrogens to reduce plasma estrogen levels; 30% of breast cancers decrease in size when deprived of estrogen

→ **Therapeutic Outcome:** Decreased spread of malignancy

Uses: Metastatic breast cancer in postmenopausal women

Dosage and routes

Adult: PO 2.5 mg qd

Available forms: Tabs 2.5 mg

Adverse effects

(*italic* = common; **bold** = life-threatening)

CNS: Somnolence, dizziness, depression, anxiety, *headache, lethargy*

CV: Hypertension

GI: *Nausea, vomiting, anorexia,* **hepatotoxicity,** constipation, heartburn, diarrhea

INTEG: *Rash, pruritus,* alopecia, sweating, hot flashes

RESP: Dyspnea, cough

Contraindications: Hypersensitivity, pregnancy **D**

Precautions: Hepatic disease, respiratory disease

Pharmacokinetics

Absorption	Well absorbed
Distribution	Widely
Metabolism	Liver
Excretion	Kidneys
Half-life	Unknown

Pharmacodynamics

Unknown

NURSING CONSIDERATIONS

Assessment

- Monitor temperature q4h; may indicate beginning of infection
- Monitor liver function tests before, during therapy (bilirubin, AST, ALT, LDH) as needed or monthly
- Monitor inflammation of mucosa, breaks in skin, yellowing of skin and sclera, dark urine, clay-colored stools, itchy skin, abdominal pain, fever, diarrhea

Nursing diagnoses

- ☑ Injury, risk for (adverse reactions)
- ☑ Body image, disturbed (adverse reactions)
- ☑ Infection, risk for (adverse reactions)
- ☑ Knowledge, deficient (teaching)

Implementation

- Give with food or fluids for GI upset
- Give in equal intervals q6h

Patient/family education

- Instruct patient to report side effects
- Advise patient to avoid use of alcohol, which potentiates this drug
- Tell patient that drug may be taken without regard to meals

Evaluation

Positive therapeutic outcome

- Prevention of rapid division of malignant cells, postmenopausal cancer, prostate cancer

Treatment of overdose:

Induce vomiting, provide supportive care

leucovorin (Rx)

(loo-koe-vor'in)

Citrovorum Factor, Folinic Acid, leucovorin calcium, Wellcovorin

Func. class.: Vitamin/folic acid antagonist antidote

Chem. class.: Tetrahydrofolic acid derivative

Pregnancy category C

Action: Needed for normal growth patterns; prevents toxicity during antineoplastic therapy by protecting normal cells

➔ **Therapeutic Outcome:** Reversal of severe toxic effects of folic acid antagonists

Uses: Megaloblastic or macrocytic anemia caused by folic acid deficiency, overdose of folic acid antagonist, methotrexate toxicity, toxicity caused by pyrimethamine or trimethoprim, pneumocystosis, toxoplasmosis

Dosage and routes
Megaloblastic anemia caused by enzyme deficiency

P *Adult and child:* PO/IM/**IV** up to 6 mg/day

Megaloblastic anemia caused by deficiency of folate

P *Adult and child:* IM 1 mg or less qd until adequate response

Advanced colorectal cancer

Adult: **IV** 200 mg/m^2, then 5-fluorouracil 370 mg/m^2; or leucovorin 20 mg/m^2, then 5-fluorouracil 425 mg/m^2; give qd × 5 days q4-5 wk

Methotrexate toxicity

P *Adult and child:* PO/IM/**IV** (normal elimination) given 6-36 hr after dose of methotrexate 10 mg/m^2 until methotrexate is <10^{-8} M, CCr has increased 50% above prior level or methotrexate level is 5 × 10 at 24 hr, or at 48 hr level is >9 × 10 M, give leucovorin 100 mg/m^2 q3h until level drops to <10 M

Pyrimethamine toxicity

P *Adult and child:* PO/IM 5-15 mg qd

Trimethoprim toxicity

P *Adult and child:* PO/IM 400 mcg qd

Available forms: Tabs 5, 10, 15, 25 mg; inj 3, 5 mg/ml; powder for inj 10 mg/ml

Adverse effects
(*italic* = common; **bold** = life-threatening)

HEMA: Thrombocytosis (intraarterial)

INTEG: Rash, pruritus, erythema, thrombocytosis, urticaria

RESP: Wheezing

Contraindications: Hypersensitivity, anemias other than megaloblastic not associated with vit B$_{12}$ deficiency

Precautions: Pregnancy **C**

◪ **Do Not Confuse:**

leucovorin/Leukeran, leucovorin/Leukine

Pharmacokinetics

Absorption	Rapidly absorbed (PO); completely absorbed (**IV**)
Distribution	Widely distributed
Metabolism	Liver
Excretion	Kidney
Half-life	3½ hr

Pharmacodynamics

	PO/IM/IV
Onset	Up to 5 min
Peak	Unknown
Duration	4-6 hr

Interactions
Individual drugs

Chloramphenicol: ↓ folate levels

Phenobarbital: ↑ metabolism of phenobarbital

Drug classifications

Hydantoins: ↑ metabolism of hydantoins

NURSING CONSIDERATIONS
Assessment

• Obtain CCr before leucovorin rescue and qd to detect nephrotoxicity, methotrexate level

• Monitor I&O; watch for nausea and vomiting; if vomiting occurs IM or **IV** route may be necessary

• Assess drugs currently taken: alcohol, hydantoins, trimethoprim may cause increased folic acid use by body

• Assess for allergic reactions: rash, dyspnea, wheezing

Nursing diagnoses

☑ Injury, risk for (uses)

☑ Nutrition: less than body requirements, imbalanced (uses)

☑ Knowledge, deficient (teaching)

Implementation
PO route

• Use PO route only if patient is not vomiting

IM route

• Treatment of megaloblastic anemia uses IM dosing

• Give within 1 hr of folic acid antagonist, no reconstitution needed

• Give increased fluid intake if used to treat folic acid inhibitor overdose

• Provide protection from light and heat when storing ampules

---

☑ Herb/drug   ◩ Do Not Crush   ◆ Alert   ◑π Key Drug   ℍ Geriatric   **P** Pediatric

IV IV route

- Reconstitute 50 mg/5 ml of bacteriostatic water or sterile water for inj (10 mg/ml) or 100 mg/10 ml; use immediately if sterile water for inj is used to reconstitute
- Give by direct **IV** over 160 mg/min or less (16 ml of 10 mg/ml sol/min)
- Give by intermittent inf after diluting in 100-500 ml of 0.9% NaCl, D_5W, $D_{10}W$, LR, Ringer's

Syringe compatibilities: Bleomycin, cisplatin, cyclophosphamide, DOXOrubicin, fluorouracil, furosemide, heparin, methotrexate, metoclopramide, mitomycin, vinBLAStine, vinCRIStine

Y-site compatibilities: Amifostine, aztreonam, bleomycin, cefepime, cisplatin, cladribine, cyclophosphamide, DOXOrubicin, filgrastim, fluconazole, fluorouracil, furosemide, granisetron, heparin, methotrexate, metoclopramide, mitomycin, piperacillin/tazobactam, tacrolimus, teniposide, thiotepa, vinBLAStine, vinCRIStine

Additive compatibilities: Cisplatin, cisplatin/floxuridine, floxuridine

Patient/family education

- Advise patient to take drug exactly as prescribed; to notify prescriber of side effects immediately
- Advise patient to report signs of hypersensitivity reaction immediately
- Instruct patient about leucovorin rescue; have patient drink 3 L of fluid each day of rescue
- Advise patient with folic acid deficiency to eat folic acid–rich foods: bran, yeast, dried beans, nuts, fruits, fresh green leafy vegetables, asparagus

Evaluation

Positive therapeutic outcome
- Increased weight
- Improved orientation, well-being
- Absence of fatigue
- Reversal of toxicity: methotrexate, folic acid antagonist overdose

---

⚠ HIGH ALERT

leuprolide (Rx)
(loo-proe′lide)
Leupron Depo PED, Lupron Depot, Lupron, Lupron Depot-3 month, Viadur
Func. class.: Antineoplastic hormone
Chem. class.: Gonadotropin-releasing hormone

Pregnancy category X (depot)

Action: Causes initial increase in circulating levels of LH, FSH; continuous administration results in decreased LH, FSH; in men testosterone is reduced to castration levels; in premenopausal women estrogen is reduced to menopausal levels

➡ **Therapeutic Outcome:** Prevention of rapidly growing malignant cells in prostate cancer, decreased pain in endometriosis, resolution of central precocious puberty (CPP)

Uses: Metastatic prostate cancer, management of endometriosis (depot), CPP

Dosage and routes
Prostate cancer
Adult: SC 1 mg/day; Depot IM 7.5 mg/dose qmo; or IM 22.5 mg q3 mo; or implant 1 implant q12 mo Viadur implant 72 mg qyr

Endometriosis/fibroids
Adult: IM 3.75 mg once a month or 11.25 mg q3 mo; or IM 30 mg q4 mo

Central precocious puberty
P *Child:* SC 50 mcg/kg/day; increase as needed by 10 mcg/kg/day

P *Child:* >37.5 kg: IM 15 mg q4 wk
25-37.5 kg: IM 11.25 mg q4 wk
≤25 kg: 7.5 mg q4 wk

Available forms: Inj (depot) 3.75, 7.5 mg single-dose, multiple-dose vials (5 mg/ml); single-use kit 11.25 mg vial; pediatric depot 7.5, 11.25, 15 mg; 3 mo depot 22.5 mg single use; Viadur once/yr implant

Adverse effects
(*italic* = common; **bold** = life-threatening)
CV: **MI, pulmonary emboli, dysrhythmias**
GI: Anorexia, diarrhea, **GI bleeding**
GU: Edema, hot flashes, impotence, decreased libido, amenorrhea, vaginal dryness, gynecomastia

Contraindications: Hypersensitivity to GnRH or analogs, thromboembolic disorders, pregnancy **X**, lactation, undiagnosed vaginal bleeding

L

Precautions: Edema, hepatic disease, CVA, MI, seizures, hypertension, diabetes mellitus

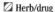 Do Not Confuse:
Lupron/Lopurin, Lupron/Nuprin

Pharmacokinetics

Absorption	Rapidly absorbed (SC); slowly absorbed (IM depot)
Distribution	Unknown
Metabolism	Unknown
Excretion	Unknown
Half-life	3-4 hr

Pharmacodynamics
Unknown

Interactions
Individual drugs
Flutamide, megestrol: ↑ antineoplastic action

NURSING CONSIDERATIONS
Assessment
• Assess for symptoms of endometriosis/fibroids including lower abdominal pain, excessive vaginal bleeding, bloating if drug is given for the diagnosis of endometriosis
• If giving this drug for CPP, the diagnosis should have been confirmed by development of secondary sex characteristics in child <9 yr; also included to confirm the diagnosis of CPP is estradiol/testosterone, GnRH test, tomography of head, adrenal steroid, chorionic gonadotropin, wrist x-ray, height, weight; patients diagnosed with CPP display the signs of testicular growth, facial, body hair (males), breast development, menses (females)
• Monitor liver function tests before, during therapy (bilirubin, AST, ALT, LDH) as needed or monthly; prostate-specific antigen in prostate cancer
• Monitor pituitary gonadotropic and gonadal function during therapy and 4-8 wk after therapy is decreased; check LH, FSH, acid phosphatase at beginning of treatment
• Monitor worsening of signs and symptoms (normal during beginning therapy): fatigue, increased pulse, pallor, lethargy, edema in feet, joints, stomach pain, shaking
• Monitor renal status: I&O ratio, check for bladder distention daily during beginning therapy (renal obstruction)

Nursing diagnoses
☑ Sexual dysfunction (adverse reactions)
☑ Injury, risk for (adverse reactions)
☑ Knowledge, deficient (teaching)

Implementation
• Use syringe and drug packaged together; give deep in large muscle mass; rotate sites
• Use depot only IM; never give SC
• Unused vials may be stored at room temp
• Give monthly: reconstitute single use vial with 1 ml of diluent, if multiple vials are used, withdraw 0.5 ml and inject into each vial (1 ml) withdraw all and inject
• Give 3 month: reconstitute microspheres using 1.5 ml of diluent and inject in vial, shake, withdraw and inject; 12-month: inserted into upper arm at the end of 12 months, implant must be removed

Patient/family education
• Advise patient to notify prescriber if menstruation continues; menstruation should stop; to use a nonhormonal method of contraception during therapy
• Instruct patient to report any complaints, side effects to nurse or prescriber; hot flashes may occur; record weight, report gain of 2 lb/day
• Teach patient how to prepare, administer; to rotate sites for SC inj; to keep accurate records of dosing (prostate cancer)
• Instruct patient that tumor flare may occur: increase in size of tumor, increased bone pain; tell patient that bone pain disappears after 1 wk; may take analgesics for pain; premenopausal women must use mechanical birth control; ovulation may be induced
• Advise the patient not to breastfeed while taking this drug
• Inform patient that voiding problems may increase in beginning of therapy, but will decrease in several weeks

Evaluation
Positive therapeutic outcome
• Decreased size, spread of malignancy
• Decreased pain in endometriosis, fibroids
• Decreased signs of CPP

levalbuterol (Rx)
(lev-al-bute′er-ole)
Xopenex
Func. class.: Bronchodilator
Chem. class.: Adrenergic β₂-agonist

Pregnancy category C

Action: Causes bronchodilatation by action on β_2 (pulmonary) receptors by increasing levels of cyclic adenosine monophosphate (cAMP), which relaxes smooth muscle; produces bronchodilatation; CNS, cardiac stimulation, increased diuresis, and increased gastric acid secretion; longer acting than isoproterenol

➡ **Therapeutic Outcome:** Increased ability to breathe because of bronchodilatation

Uses: Treatment or prevention of bronchospasm (reversible obstructive airway disease)

Dosage and routes
🅿 *Adult and child ≥12 yr:* INH 0.63 mg tid, q6-8h by nebulization; may increase to 1.25 mg q8h

🅿 *Child 6-11 yr:* INH 0.31 mg tid via neb, max 0.63 mg tid

Available forms: Sol, inh 0.63, 1.25 mg/3 ml

Adverse effects
(*italic* = common; **bold** = life-threatening)
CNS: Tremors, anxiety, insomnia, headache, dizziness, stimulation, ***restlessness,*** hallucinations, flushing, irritability
CV: Palpitations, tachycardia, hypertension, angina, hypotension, dysrhythmias
EENT: Dry nose, irritation of nose and throat
GI: Heartburn, nausea, vomiting
MS: Muscle cramps

Contraindications: Hypersensitivity to sympathomimetics, tachydysrhythmias, severe cardiac disease

Precautions: Lactation, pregnancy **C**, cardiac disorders, hyperthyroidism, diabetes mellitus, hypertension, prostatic hypertrophy, narrow-angle glaucoma, seizures

Pharmacokinetics

Absorption	Unknown
Distribution	Unknown
Metabolism	Liver extensively, tissues
Excretion	Unknown, breast milk
Half-life	Unknown

Pharmacodynamics

	INH
Onset	5-15 min
Peak	1-1½ hr
Duration	6-8 hr

Interactions
Drug classifications
Adrenergics: ↑ levalbuterol action
Antidepressants (tricyclics): ↑ levalbuterol action
β-Adrenergic blockers: Block therapeutic effect

Bronchodilators (aerosol): ↑ action of bronchodilator
MAOIs: ↑ chance of hypertensive crisis
Sympathomimetics: ↑ adrenergic side effects
🗹 *Herb/drug*
Cola nut, guarana, tea (black/green), yerba maté: ↑ stimulation

NURSING CONSIDERATIONS
Assessment
• Assess respiratory function: vital capacity, forced expiratory volume, ABGs, lung sounds, heart rate, rhythm (baseline and during therapy); character of sputum: color, consistency, amount
• Determine that patient has not received theophylline therapy before giving dose, to prevent additive effect; client's ability to self-medicate
• Monitor for evidence of allergic reactions; paradoxic bronchospasm; withhold dose; notify prescriber

Nursing diagnoses
☑ Airway clearance, ineffective (uses)
☑ Gas exchange, impaired (uses)
☑ Knowledge, deficient (teaching)

Implementation
• Give by nebulization q6-8h; wait at least 1 min between inhalation of aerosols

Patient/family education
• Tell patient not to use OTC medications before consulting prescriber; extra stimulation may occur; instruct patient to use this medication before other medications and allow at least 5 min between each to prevent overstimulation; to limit caffeine products such as chocolate, coffee, tea, and cola or herbs such as cola nut, guarana, yerba maté
◆• Teach patient that if paradoxic bronchospasm occurs to stop drug immediately and notify prescriber

Evaluation
Positive therapeutic outcome
• Absence of dyspnea and wheezing after 1 hr
• Improved airway exchange
• Improved ABGs

Treatment of overdose: Administer a β₁-adrenergic blocker

levetiracetam (Rx)

(lev-ee-tye'ra-see-tam)
Keppra
Func. class.: Anticonvulsant

Pregnancy category C

Action: Unknown; may inhibit nerve impulses by limiting influx of sodium ions across cell membrane in motor cortex

➡ **Therapeutic Outcome:** Absence of seizures

Uses: Adjunctive therapy in partial onset seizures

Dosage and routes
Adult: PO 500 mg bid, may increase by 1000 mg/day q2 wk, max 3000 mg/day

Available forms: Tabs 250, 500, 750 mg

Adverse effects
(*italic* = common; **bold** = life-threatening)
MISC: Abdominal pain, pharyngitis, infection
CNS: Dizziness, somnolence, asthenia
HEMA: Decreased Hct, Hgb, RBC, infection

Contraindications: Hypersensitivity

Precautions: Renal disease, cardiac
Ⓟ disease, pregnancy C, lactation, children

Pharmacokinetics	
Absorption	Rapidly absorbed
Distribution	Widely distributed, not protein bound
Metabolism	Small amount liver
Excretion	Kidneys (66%) unchanged
Ⓖ **Half-life**	6-8 hr or more in elderly

Pharmacodynamics	
Unknown	

Interactions
None known

NURSING CONSIDERATIONS
Assessment
• Monitor urine function tests (BUN, urine protein) periodically during treatments
• Assess seizure activity including type, location, duration, and character; provide seizure precautions

Nursing diagnoses
☑ Injury, risk for (side effects)
☑ Knowledge, deficient (teaching)

Implementation
• Give with food, milk to decrease GI symptoms (rare)

Patient/family education
• Teach patient to carry/wear emergency ID stating patient's name, drugs taken, condition, prescriber's name, phone number
• Caution patient to avoid driving, other activities that require alertness until stabilized on medication
• Teach patient not to discontinue medication quickly after long-term use
• Teach patient to use a nonhormonal type of contraception to prevent harm to the fetus
• Teach patient to take exactly as prescribed, do not double or omit doses

Evaluation
Positive therapeutic outcome
• Decreased seizure activity

levodopa ✚ℼ (Rx)

(lee'voe-doe-pa)
Dopar, Larodopa, L-Dopa
Func. class.: Antiparkinsonian agent
Chem. class.: Catecholamine, dopamine agonist

Pregnancy category C

Action: Decarboxylation to dopamine, which increases dopamine levels in brain

➡ **Therapeutic Outcome:** Decreased symptoms of Parkinson's disease (involuntary movements)

Uses: Parkinsonism

Dosage and routes
Adult: PO 0.5-1 g qd divided bid-qid with meals; may increase by up to 0.75 g q3-7 days, max 8 g/day unless closely supervised

Available forms: Caps 100, 250, 500 mg; tabs 100, 250, 500 mg

Adverse effects
(*italic* = common; **bold** = life-threatening)
CNS: *Involuntary choreiform movements, hand tremors, fatigue, headache, anxiety, twitching, numbness, weakness, confusion, agitation, insomnia, nightmares,* psychosis, hallucinations, hypomania, severe depression, dizziness
CV: *Orthostatic hypotension,* tachycardia, hypertension, palpitations
EENT: Blurred vision, diplopia, dilated pupils
GI: *Nausea, vomiting, anorexia, abdominal distress, dry mouth, flatulence, dysphagia,* bitter taste, diarrhea, constipation
HEMA: **Hemolytic anemia, leukopenia, agranulocytosis**
INTEG: Rash, sweating, alopecia

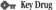
�herb/drug   🚫 Do Not Crush   ◆ Alert   ✚ℼ Key Drug   Ⓖ Geriatric   Ⓟ Pediatric

MISC: Urinary retention, incontinence, weight change, dark urine

Contraindications: Hypersensitivity, narrow-angle glaucoma, undiagnosed skin lesions

Precautions: Renal disease, cardiac disease, hepatic disease, respiratory disease, MI with dysrhythmias, seizures, peptic ulcer, pregnancy **C**, asthma, endocrine disease, affective disorders, psychosis, lactation, ⟨P⟩ children <12 yr peptic ulcer

⬛ Do Not Confuse:
L-dopa/methyldopa

Pharmacokinetics

Absorption	Well absorbed
Distribution	Widely distributed
Metabolism	Liver, GI tract, extensively
Excretion	Kidneys to metabolites; breast milk
Half-life	1 hr

Pharmacodynamics

Onset	10-15 min
Peak	1-3 hr
Duration	Up to 24 hr

Interactions
Individual drugs
Papaverine, phenytoin, pyridoxine, reserpine: ↓ effects of levodopa
Drug classifications
Antacids: ↓ absorption
Anticholinergics, hydantoins: ↓ effects of levodopa
MAOIs: Hypertensive crisis
⊘ Herb/drug
Kava: ↑ Parkinson's symptoms
Indian snakeroot: ↑ extrapyramidal symptoms (EPS), ↓ levodopa effect
Food/drug
↑ Pyridoxine will ↓ levodopa effect, ↑ protein food will ↓ absorption
Lab test interferences
↓ VMA
False positive: Urine ketones, urine glucose, Coombs' test
False negative: Urine glucose (glucose oxidase)
False: ↑ uric acid, ↑ urine protein
↓ VMA

NURSING CONSIDERATIONS
Assessment
• Monitor B/P, respiration during initial treatment; hypotension or hypertension should be reported
• Assess mental status: affect, mood, behav-

ioral changes, depression; complete suicide assessment
• Monitor liver function, renal function studies: AST, ALT, alkaline phosphatase; also check LDH, bilirubin, CBC, BUN, PBI
• Assess for involuntary movements in parkinsonism: akinesia, tremors, staggering gait, muscle rigidity, drooling; these symptoms should improve with levodopa therapy
◆• Assess for levodopa toxicity: mental, personality changes, increased twitching, grimacing, tongue protrusion; these should be reported to prescriber

Nursing diagnoses
☑ Mobility, impaired (uses)
☑ Injury, risk for (uses)
☑ Knowledge, deficient (teaching)
☑ Noncompliance (teaching)

Implementation
• Levodopa/carbidopa should not be started until levodopa is withheld for 8 hr; toxicity may result if the two drugs are taken close together
• Give levodopa until NPO before surgery
• Adjust dosage to patient response
• Give with meals to decrease GI upset; limit protein taken with drug
• Give only after MAOIs have been discontinued for 2 wk

Patient/family education
• Advise patient that therapeutic effects may take several wk to a few months
• Caution to change positions slowly to prevent orthostatic hypotension
• Instruct patient to report side effects: twitching, eye spasms; indicate overdose
• Instruct patient to use drug exactly as prescribed; if drug is discontinued abruptly, parkinsonian crisis may occur
• Inform patient that urine, sweat may darken
• Advise patient to avoid vit B_6 preparations, vitamin-fortified foods containing B_6; these foods can reverse effects of levodopa; also OTC preparations should be avoided unless approved by prescriber

Evaluation
Positive therapeutic outcome
• Decreased akathisia, other involuntary movements
• Improved mood

levofloxacin (Rx)
(lev-o-floks'a-sin)
Levaquin
Func. class.: Antiinfective
Chem. class.: Fluoroquinolone antibacterial

Pregnancy category C

Action: Interferes with conversion of intermediate DNA fragments into high molecular weight DNA in bacteria; DNA gyrase inhibitor

→**Therapeutic Outcome:** Bacterial action against the following: *Streptococcus pneumoniae, Haemophilus influenzae, Haemophilus parainfluenzae, Moraxella catarrhalis, Staphylococcus aureus, Klebsiella pneumoniae, Mycoplasma pneumoniae*

Uses: Adult urinary tract infections (including complicated); lower respiratory, skin infection

Dosage and routes
Adult: **IV** inf 500 mg by slow inf over 1 hr q24h × 7-14 days depending on infection; PO 500 mg q24h × 7 days depending on infection

Renal dose
Adult: PO/**IV** CCr 20-49 ml/min initial 500 mg, then 250 mg q24h; CCr 10-19 ml/min 250 or 500 mg, depending on condition, then 250 mg q48h

Available forms: Single-use vials (500 mg), 25 mg/ml 20-ml vials, premixed flexible container; tabs 250, 500, 750 mg

Adverse effects:
(*italic* = common; **bold** = life-threatening)
CNS: Headache, dizziness, *insomnia,* anxiety, **seizures,** encephalopathy, paresthesia
CV: Chest pain, palpitations, vasodilatation
EENT: Dry mouth
GI: Nausea, flatulence, *vomiting,* diarrhea, abdominal pain, **pseudomembranous colitis**
GU: Vaginitis, crystalluria
HEMA: Eosinophilia, **hemolytic anemia,** lymphophemia
INTEG: Rash, pruritus, urticaria, photosensitivity, **Stevens-Johnson syndrome**
MISC: Hypoglycemia, hypersensitivity
RESP: Pneumonitis
SYST: **Anaphylaxis, multisystem organ failure**

Contraindications: Hypersensitivity to quinolones

Precautions: Pregnancy **C**, lactation, **P** children

Pharmacokinetics
Absorption	Unknown
Distribution	Unknown
Metabolism	Liver
Excretion	Kidneys unchanged
Half-life	6-8 hr

Pharmacodynamics
Onset	Immediate
Peak	Infusion's end

Interactions
Individual drugs
Calcium, iron, sucralfate, zinc: ↓ absorption of levofloxacin
Cimetidine, digoxin, theophylline, warfarin: ↑ toxicity
Cyclosporine: ↑ nephrotoxicity
Foscarnet: ↑ CNS stimulation, seizures
Magnesium: ↓ levofloxacin absorption; do not use in same **IV** line
Theophylline: ↓ theophylline clearance
Warfarin: ↑ bleeding
Drug classifications
Antacids: ↓ absorption of levofloxacin
Antidiabetics: Altered blood glucose levels
NSAIDs: ↑ CNS stimulation, seizures
Herb/drug
Cola tree: ↑ antiinfective effect
Lab test interferences
↓ Glucose, ↓ lymphocytes

NURSING CONSIDERATIONS
Assessment
• Assess patient for previous sensitivity reaction
• Assess patient for signs and symptoms of infection including characteristics of wounds, sputum, urine, stool, WBC >10,000/mm³, fever; baseline and during treatment
• Obtain C&S before beginning drug therapy to identify if correct treatment has been initiated
• Assess for allergic reactions and anaphylaxis: rash, urticaria, pruritus, chills, fever, joint pain; may occur a few days after therapy begins; epINEPHrine and resuscitation equipment should be available for anaphylactic reaction
• Determine urine output; if decreasing, notify prescriber (may indicate nephrotoxicity); also check for increased BUN, creatinine
• Monitor blood studies: AST, ALT, CBC, Hct, bilirubin, LDH, alkaline phosphatase, Coombs' test monthly if patient is on long-term therapy
• Monitor electrolytes: potassium, sodium,

chloride monthly if patient is on long-term therapy

• Assess bowel pattern qd; if severe diarrhea occurs, drug should be discontinued

• Monitor for bleeding: ecchymosis, bleeding gums, hematuria, stool guaiac daily if on long-term therapy

• Assess for overgrowth of infection: perineal itching, fever, malaise, redness, pain, swelling, drainage, rash, diarrhea, change in cough, sputum

Nursing diagnoses
✓ Infection, risk for (uses)
✓ Diarrhea (side effects)
✓ Injury, risk for (side effects)
✓ Knowledge, deficient (teaching)
✓ Noncompliance (teaching)

Implementation
• Give PO 4 hr before or 2 hr after antacids, iron, calcium, zinc

• Check for irritation, extravasation, phlebitis daily

Patient/family education
• Teach patient to report sore throat, bruising, bleeding, joint pain; may indicate blood dyscrasias (rare)

• Advise patient to contact prescriber if vaginal itching, loose foul-smelling stools, furry tongue occur, may indicate superinfection; report itching, rash, pruritus, urticaria

• Instruct patient to take all medication prescribed for the length of time ordered; drug must be taken around the clock to maintain blood levels; do not give medication to others

• Advise patient to notify prescriber of diarrhea with blood or pus

• Instruct patient to take 4 hr before antacids, iron, calcium, zinc products

• Tell patient to complete full course of therapy; to increase fluid intake to 2 L/day to prevent crystalluria

• Advise patient to avoid hazardous activities until response to drug is known

• Instruct patient to rinse mouth frequently and use sugarless candy or gum for dry mouth

• Instruct patient to avoid taking other medications unless approved by prescriber

• Advise patient not to use theophylline with this product, as toxicity may result; to contact prescriber if taking theophylline

• Advise patient to avoid sun exposure or use sunscreen to prevent phototoxicity

Evaluation
Positive therapeutic outcome
• Absence of signs/symptoms of infection (WBC <10,000/mm^3, temp WNL)

• Reported improvement in symptoms of infection

---

levothyroxine ⚷ (Rx)
(lee-voe-thye-rox'een)
Eltroxin ✤, Levo-T, Levothroid, levothyroxine sodium, Levoxyl, PMS-Levothyroxine Sodium ✤, Synthroid, T_4
Func. class.: Thyroid hormone
Chem. class.: Levoisomer of thyroxine
Pregnancy category A

Action: Controls protein synthesis; increases metabolic rate, cardiac output, renal blood flow, O_2 consumption, body temp, blood volume, growth, development at cellular level, exact mechanism unknown

⇥ **Therapeutic Outcome:** Correction of lack of thyroid hormone

Uses: Hypothyroidism, myxedema coma, thyroid hormone replacement, cretinism, thyrotoxicosis, congenital hypothyroidism, some types of thyroid cancer

Dosage and routes
Severe hypothyroidism
Adult: PO 50 mcg qd, increase by 0.05-0.1 mg q1-4 wk until desired response; maintenance dosage 75-125 mcg qd, IM/**IV** 50-100 mcg/day as a single dose or 50% of usual oral dosage

P *Child >12 yr:* PO 2-3 mcg/kg/day given as a single dose AM

P *Child 6-12 yr:* PO 4-5 mcg/kg/day given as a single dose AM

P *Child 1-5 yr:* PO 5-6 mcg/kg/day given as a single dose AM

P *Child 6-12 mo:* PO 6-8 mcg/kg/day given as a single dose AM

P *Child to 6 mo:* PO 8-10 mcg/kg/day given as a single dose AM

Myxedema coma
Adult: **IV** 200-500 mcg; may increase by 100-300 mcg after 24 hr; give oral medication as soon as possible

Available forms: Powder for inj 50, 200, 500 mcg/vial; tabs 0.025, 0.05, 0.075, 0.088, 0.1, 0.112, 0.125, 0.137, 0.15, 0.175, 0.2, 0.3 mg

Adverse effects

(*italic* = common; **bold** = life-threatening)
CNS: *Anxiety, insomnia, tremors,* headache, **thyroid storm**
CV: *Tachycardia, palpitations, angina, dysrhythmias,* hypertension, **cardiac arrest**
GI: Nausea, diarrhea, increased or decreased appetite, cramps
MISC: Menstrual irregularities, weight loss, sweating, heat intolerance, fever, alopecia

Contraindications: Adrenal insufficiency, recent MI, thyrotoxicosis, hypersensitivity to beef, alcohol intolerance (inj only)

G **Precautions:** Elderly, angina pectoris, hypertension, ischemia, cardiac disease, pregnancy **A**, lactation, diabetes

N **Do Not Confuse:**
Synthroid/Symmetrel

Pharmacokinetics	
Absorption	Erratic (PO); complete (**IV**)
Distribution	Widely distributed
Metabolism	Liver; enterohepatic recirculation
Excretion	Feces via bile; breast milk (small amounts)
Half-life	6-7 days

Pharmacodynamics		
	PO	IV
Onset	3-5 days	6-8 hr
Peak	12-48 hr	12-48 hr
Duration	Unknown	Unknown

Interactions
Individual drugs
Cholestyramine: ↓ absorption of thyroid hormone
Colestipol, ferrous sulfate: ↓ absorption of levothyroxine
Digitalis: ↓ effect of digitalis
Insulin: ↑ requirement for insulin
Phenytoin (**IV**): ↑ release of thyroid hormone
Drug classifications
Amphetamines, decongestants, vasopressors: ↑ CNS, cardiac stimulation
Anticoagulants (oral): ↑ requirements for anticoagulants
Antidepressants (tricyclics): ↑ tricyclic effect
β-Adrenergic blockers: ↓ effect of β-blockers
Estrogens: ↓ thyroid hormone effects
Hypoglycemics: ↓ hypoglycemic effect
Sympathomimetics: ↑ sympathomimetic effect
Z Herb/drug
Agar, bugleweed, carnitine, kelpware, soy, spirulina: ↓ thyroid hormone effect

Lab test interferences
↑ CPK, ↑ LDH, ↑ AST, ↑ PBI, ↑ blood glucose
↓ Thyroid function tests

NURSING CONSIDERATIONS
Assessment
• Determine if the patient is taking anticoagulants, antidiabetic agents; document on chart
• Take B/P, pulse before each dose; monitor I&O ratio and weight every day in same clothing, using same scale, at same time of day
• Monitor height, weight, psychomotor development and growth rate if given to a **P** child
• Monitor T_3, T_4, which are decreased; radioimmunoassay of TSH, which is increased; radioactive iodine uptake (RAIU), which is increased if patient is on too low a dosage of medication
• Monitor Pro-time (may require decreased anticoagulant); check for bleeding, bruising
• Assess for increased nervousness, excitability, irritability, which may indicate too high a dosage of medication, usually after 1-3 wk of treatment
• Assess cardiac status: angina, palpitations, **G** chest pain, change in VS; the elderly patient may have undetected cardiac problems and baseline ECG should be completed before treatment

Nursing diagnoses
☑ Knowledge, deficient (teaching)
☑ Noncompliance (teaching)

Implementation
PO route
• Give in AM if possible as a single dose to decrease sleeplessness; give at same time each day to maintain drug level
• Give crushed and mixed with water, non-soy **P** formula, or breast milk for infants/children
• Give only for hormone imbalances; not to be used for obesity, male infertility, menstrual conditions, lethargy; give lowest dosage that relieves symptoms; lower dosage for the **G** elderly and in cardiac diseases
• Store in tight, light-resistant container
• Remove medication 4 wk before RAIU test
IV IV route
• Give **IV** after diluting with provided diluent (0.9% NaCl), 0.5 mg/5 ml; shake well; give through Y-tube or 3-way stopcock; give 0.1 mg or less over 1 min; do not add to **IV** inf; 0.1 mg = 1 ml; discard any unused portion

Patient/family education
• Teach patient that drug is not a cure but controls symptoms and treatment is long term
• Instruct patient to report excitability, irrita-

---

bility, anxiety, sweating, heat intolerance, chest pain, palpitations, which indicate overdose
• Advise patient not to switch brands unless approved by prescriber; bioavailability may differ; do not take with food; absorption will be decreased
• Teach patient that drug may be discontinued after giving birth; thyroid panel will be evaluated after 1-2 mo
• Teach patient or parent that hyperthyroid **P** child will show almost immediate behavior/personality change; that hair loss will occur in child but is temporary
• Caution patient that drug is not to be taken to reduce weight
• Caution patient to avoid OTC preparations with iodine; read labels; other medications should not be used unless approved by prescriber
• Teach patient to avoid iodine-rich food: iodized salt, soybeans, tofu, turnips, high iodine seafood, some bread

Evaluation
Positive therapeutic outcome
• Absence of depression
• Weight loss, increased diuresis, pulse, appetite
• Absence of constipation, peripheral edema, cold intolerance, pale, cool dry skin, brittle nails, alopecia, coarse hair, menorrhagia, night blindness, paresthesias, syncope, stupor, coma, rosy cheeks
• Improved levels of T_3, T_4 by laboratory tests
P • Child: age-appropriate weight, height and psychomotor development

Treatment of overdose: Withhold dose for up to 1 wk: acute overdose: gastric lavage or induced emesis, activated charcoal; provide supportive treatment to control symptoms

---

❗HIGH ALERT

lidocaine, parenteral
☙ₙ (Rx)
(lye'doe-kane)
Lidopen Auto-Injector, Xylocard ✦, Xylocaine
Func. class.: Antidysrhthmic (class IB)
Chem. class.: Aminoacyl amide

Pregnancy category B
See also, topical products

Action: Increases electrical stimulation threshold of ventricle and His-Purkinje system, which stabilizes cardiac membrane and decreases automaticity; locally produces anesthesia by preventing initiation and conduction of nerve impulses

➡ **Therapeutic Outcome:** Decreased ventricular dysrhythmia; produces anesthesia locally

Uses: Ventricular tachycardia, ventricular dysrhythmias during cardiac surgery, MI, digitalis toxicity, cardiac catheterization; anesthesia locally

Dosage and routes
Adult: **IV** bol 50-100 mg (1 mg/kg) over 2-3 min; repeat q3-5 min, max 300 mg in 1 hr; begin **IV** inf 20-50 mcg/kg/min; IM 200-300 mg (4.3 mg/kg) in deltoid muscle, may repeat in 1-1½ hr if needed

G *Elderly with CHF, reduced liver function:* **IV** bol ½ adult dose

P *Child:* **IV** bol 1 mg/kg, then **IV** inf 30 mcg/kg/min

Available forms: **IV** inf 0.2% (2 mg/ml), 0.4% (4 mg/ml), 0.8% (8 mg/ml); **IV** admixture 4% (40 mg/ml), 10% (100 mg/ml), 20% (200 mg/ml); **IV** direct 1% (10 mg/ml), 2% (20 mg/ml); IM 300 mg/3 ml

Adverse effects
(*italic* = common; **bold** = life-threatening)
CNS: *Headache, dizziness,* involuntary movement, confusion, tremor, *drowsiness,* euphoria, **seizures**
CV: *Hypotension, bradycardia,* **heart block, cardiovascular collapse, arrest**
EENT: Tinnitus, blurred vision
GI: Nausea, vomiting, anorexia
INTEG: Rash, urticaria, edema, swelling
MISC: Febrile response, phlebitis at inj site
RESP: Dyspnea, **respiratory depression**

Contraindications: Hypersensitivity to amides, severe heart block, supraventricular dysrhythmias, Adams-Stokes syndrome, Wolff-Parkinson-White syndrome

Precautions: Pregnancy **B**, lactation, **P** children, renal disease, liver disease, CHF, respiratory depression, malignant hyperthermia

Pharmacokinetics	
Absorption	Complete bioavailability (**IV**)
Distribution	Erythrocytes, cardiovascular endothelium
Metabolism	Liver
Excretion	Kidneys
Half-life	Biphasic 8 min, 1-2 hr

Pharmacodynamics

	IV	IM	TOP
Onset	2 min	5-15 min	Unknown
Peak	Unknown	½ hr	5 min
Duration	20 min	1½ hr	½-1 hr

Interactions
Individual drugs
Cimetidine, metoprolol, phenytoin: ↑ lidocaine effects
Propranolol: ↑ toxicity
Drug classifications
Barbiturates: ↓ lidocaine effects
β-Adrenergic blockers: ↑ toxicity
Neuromuscular blockers: ↑ neuromuscular blockade
☑ Herb/drug
Aconite: ↑ toxicity, death
Aloe, broom, buckthorn (chronic use), cascara sagrada (chronic use), Chinese rhubarb, figwort, fumitory, goldenseal, kudzu, licorice: ↑ effect
Aloe, buckthorn, cascara sagrada, senna: ↑ action of lidocaine
Coltsfoot: ↓ effect
Horehound: ↑ serotonin effect
Lab test interferences
↑ CPR

NURSING CONSIDERATIONS
Assessment
• Assess for oxygenation or perfusion deficit: decreased B/P, chest pain, dizziness, loss of consciousness
• Assess respiratory status: auscultate lung fields for bibasilar crackles in patients with advanced CHF
• Assess for urinary retention: check for pain, abdominal absorption, palpate bladder; check males with benign prostatic hypertrophy; anticholinergic reaction may cause retention
• Monitor I&O ratio, electrolytes (potassium, sodium, chloride); watch for decreasing urinary output, possible retention
• Monitor liver function studies: AST, ALT, bilirubin, alkaline phosphatase
• Monitor ECG continuously to determine drug effectiveness, measure PR, QRS, QT intervals, check for PVCs, other dysrhythmias; monitor B/P continuously for hypotension, hypertension; check for rebound hypertension after 1-2 hr, prolonged PR/QT intervals, QRS complex; if QT or QRS increases by 50% or more, withhold next dose, notify prescriber
• Monitor for CNS symptoms: confusion, numbness, depression, involuntary movements; if these occur, drug should be discontinued

• Monitor blood levels (therapeutic level 1.5-5 mcg/ml), notify prescriber of abnormal results

Nursing diagnoses
☑ Cardiac output, decreased (uses)
☑ Gas exchange, impaired (adverse reactions)
☑ Knowledge, deficient (teaching)

Implementation
IM route
• Administer in deltoid, aspirate to prevent **IV** administration
• Check site daily for extravasation
IV IV route
• Give **IV** bolus undiluted (1%, 2% only); give 6 mg or less over 1 min; if using an **IV** line, use port near insertion site, flush with 0.9% NaCl (50 ml)
• Store at room temp; sol should be clear
• Give by cont inf after adding 1 g/250-1000 ml of D₅W; give 1-4 mg/min; use infusion
P pump for correct dosage; pediatric inf is 120 mg of lidocaine/100 ml of D₅W; 1-2.5 ml/kg/hr = 20-50 mcg/kg/min; use only 1%, 2% sol

Solution compatibilities: D₅W, D₅/0.9% NaCl, D₅/0.45% NaCl, D₅/LR, LR, 0.9% NaCl, 0.45% NaCl

Syringe compatibilities: Cloxacillin, glycopyrrolate, heparin, hydrOXYzine, methicillin, metoclopramide, milrinone, moxalactam, nalbuphine

Syringe incompatibilities: Cefazolin

Y-site compatibilities: Alteplase, amiodarone, amrinone, cefazolin, ciprofloxacin, diltiazem, DOBUTamine, DOPamine, enalaprilat, etomidate, famotidine, haloperidol, heparin, heparin with hydrocortisone, labetalol, meperidine, morphine, nitroglycerin, nitroprusside, potassium chloride, propofol, streptokinase, theophylline, vit B/C, warfarin

Additive compatibilities: Alteplase, aminophylline, amiodarone, atracurium, bretylium, calcium chloride, calcium gluceptate, calcium gluconate, chloramphenicol, chlorothiazide, cimetidine, dexamethasone, digoxin, diphenhydrAMINE, DOBUTamine, DOPamine, epHEDrine, erythromycin, floxacillin, flumazenil, furosemide, heparin, hydrocortisone, nafcillin, hydrOXYzine, regular insulin, mephentermine, metaraminol, nafcillin, nitroglycerin, penicillin G potassium, pentobarbital, phenylephrine, potassium chloride, procainamide, prochlorperazine, promazine, ranitidine, sodium bicarbonate, sodium lactate, theophylline, verapamil, vit B/C

Additive incompatibilities: Methohexital, phenytoin; do not admix with blood transfusions

Infiltration

Physician may order lidocaine with epINEPHrine to minimize systemic absorption and prolong local anesthesia

Patient/family education
• Teach patient or family reason for use of medication and expected results
• Instruct patient in at-home use of Lidopen Auto-Injector; patient should call prescriber before use if heart attack is imminent

Evaluation
Positive therapeutic outcome
• Decreased B/P, dysrhythmias
• Decreased heart rate
• Normal sinus rhythm

Treatment of overdose: Oxygen, artificial ventilation, ECG, administer DOPamine for circulatory depression, diazepam or thiopental for seizures, decreased drug or discontinuation may be required

---

lindane (OTC)
(lin-dane)
GBH ✚, G-Well, Hexit ✚, Kwell, lindane, PMS Lindane ✚, Scabene
Func. class.: Scabicide/pediculicide
Chem. class.: Chlorinated hydrocarbon (synthetic)

Pregnancy category B

Action: Stimulates nervous system of arthropods, resulting in seizures, death of organism

⮕ **Therapeutic Outcome:** Resolution of infestation

Uses: Scabies, lice (head/pubic/body), nits

Dosage and routes
Lice
P *Adult and child:* Top/cream/lotion: wash area with soap and water 8-12 hr after application; may reapply in 1 wk if needed; shampoo using 30 ml: work into lather, rub for 5 min, rinse, dry with towel; use fine-toothed comb to remove nits

Scabies
P *Adult and child:* Top apply 1% cream/lotion to skin from neck to bottom of feet, toes; repeat in 1 wk if necessary

Available forms: Lotion, shampoo, cream (1%)

Adverse effects
(*italic* = common; **bold** = life-threatening)
CNS: Tremors, **seizures,** stimulation, dizziness (chronic inhalation of vapors), **CNS toxicity**
CV: **Ventricular fibrillation** (chronic inhalation of vapors)
GI: *Nausea, vomiting, diarrhea,* liver damage (inhalation of vapors)
HEMA: **Aplastic anemia** (chronic inhalation of vapors)
INTEG: *Pruritus, rash, irritation, contact dermatitis*
GU: **Kidney damage** (chronic inhalation of vapors)

Contraindications: Hypersensitivity, **P** premature neonate, patients with known seizure disorders, inflammation of skin, abrasions, or breaks in skin

P Precautions: Pregnancy **B,** children <10 yr, infants, lactation; avoid contact with eyes

Pharmacokinetics	
Absorption	20%
Distribution	Fat
Metabolism	Liver
Excretion	Kidneys
Half-life	18 hr

Pharmacodynamics	
Onset	Rapid
Peak	Rapid
Duration	3 hr

Interactions
Oil-based hair dressing: ↑ absorption; wash, rinse, and dry hair before using lindane

NURSING CONSIDERATIONS
Assessment
• Assess head, hair for lice and nits before and after treatment; if scabies are present, check all skin surfaces
• Identify source of infection: school, family members, sexual contacts

Nursing diagnoses
✓ Skin integrity, impaired (uses)
✓ Knowledge, deficient (teaching)

Implementation
• Apply to body areas, scalp only; do not apply to face, lips, mouth, eyes, any mucous membrane, anus, or meatus
• Give top corticosteroids as ordered to

decrease contact dermatitis; provide antihistamines
- Apply menthol or phenol lotions to control itching
- Give top antibiotics for infection
- Provide isolation until areas on skin, scalp have cleared and treatment is completed
- Remove nits by using a fine-toothed comb rinsed in vinegar after treatment; use gloves

Patient/family education
- Advise patient to wash all inhabitants' clothing, using insecticide; preventive treatment may be required for all persons living in same house, using lotion or shampoo to decrease spread of infection; use rubber gloves when applying drug
- Instruct patient that itching may continue for 4-6 wk; that drug must be reapplied if accidently washed off, or treatment will be ineffective; remove after specified time to prevent toxicity
- Advise patient not to apply to face; if accidental contact with eyes occurs, flush with water
- Advise patient that sexual contacts should be treated simultaneously
- Inform the patient of CNS toxicity: dizziness, cramps, anxiety, nausea, vomiting, seizures

Evaluation
Positive therapeutic outcome
- Decreased crusts, nits, brownish trails on skin, itching papules in skinfolds
- Decreased itching after several wk

Treatment of ingestion: Gastric lavage, saline laxatives, **IV** diazepam (Valium) for seizures (if taken orally)

---

linezolid (Rx)
(lih-nee′zoh-lid)
Zyvox
Func. class.: Broad-spectrum antiinfective
Chem. class.: Oxazolidinone

Pregnancy category C

Action: Binds to bacterial 23S ribosomal RNA of the 50S subunit preventing formation of the bacterial translation process

Therapeutic Outcome: Negative blood cultures, absence of signs/symptoms of infection

Uses: Vancomycin-resistant *Enterococcus faecium* infections, nosocomial pneumonia, uncomplicated or complicated skin and skin structure infections, community-acquired pneumonia

Dosage and routes
Vancomycin-resistant E. faecium *infections*
Adult: **IV** 600 mg q12h × 14-28 days PO

Nosocomial pneumonia/complicated skin infections/community-acquired pneumonia/concurrent bacterial infection
Adult: **IV**/PO 600 mg q12h × 10-14 days

Uncomplicated skin infections
Adult: **IV**/PO 400 mg q12h × 10-14 days

Available forms: Tabs 400, 600 mg; oral susp 100 mg/5 ml; inj 2 mg/ml

Adverse effects
(*italic* = common; **bold** = life-threatening)
CNS: Headache, dizziness, confusion
GI: Nausea, diarrhea, increased ALT, AST, *vomiting,* taste change, tongue color change
HEMA: Myelosuppression
MISC: Vaginal moniliasis, fungal infection, oral moniliasis

Contraindications: Hypersensitivity

Precautions: Pregnancy **C**, lactation, children, thrombocytopenia

Do Not Confuse:
Zyvox/Vioxx

Pharmacokinetics	
Absorption	Rapidly, excessively
Distribution	Protein binding 31%
Metabolism	Oxidation of the morpholine ring
Excretion	Unknown
Half-life	Unknown

Pharmacodynamics
Unknown

Interactions
Drug classifications
Adrenergic blockers: ↑effects of adrenergics
MAOIs: ↓ effects of MAOIs
Serotonergic agents: ↑ effect

NURSING CONSIDERATIONS
Assessment
- Assess CNS symptoms: headache, dizziness
- Monitor liver function studies: AST, ALT
- Monitor allergic reactions: fever, flushing, rash, urticaria, pruritus
- Assess for pseudomembranous colitis: severe diarrhea, cramping
- Monitor CBC weekly, assess for myelosup-

---

pression (anemia, leukopenia, pancytopenia, thrombocytopenia)

Nursing diagnoses

☑ Infection, risk for (uses)
☑ Knowledge, deficient (teaching)

Implementation

PO route

- Store reconstituted oral suspension at room temperature, use within 3 wk

Ⅳ IV route

- Give over 30-120 min; do not use **IV** infusion bag in series connections, do not use with additives in sol, do not use with another drug, administer separately

Y-site compatibilities: Acyclovir, alfentanil, amikacin, aminophylline, ampicillin, aztreonam, bretylium, buprenorphine, butorphanol, calcium gluconate, carboplatin, cefazolin, cefoperazone, cefotetan, cefoxitin, ceftazidine, ceftizoxime, ceftriaxone, cefuroxime, cimetidine, ciprofloxacin, cisatracurium, cisplatin, clindamycin, cyclophosphamide, cycloSPORINE, cytarabine, hydromorphone, ifosfamide, labetalol, leucovorin, levofloxacin, lidocaine, lorazepam, magnesium sulfate, mannitol, meperidine, meropenem, mesna, methotrexate, methylPREDNISolone, metoclopramide, metronidazole, midazolam, minocycline, mitoxantrone, morphine, nalbuphine, naloxone, nitroglycerin, ofloxacin, ondansetron, paclitaxel, pentobarbital, piperacillin, potassium chloride, prochlorperazine, promethazine, propranolol, ranitidine, remifentanil, theophylline, ticarcillin, tobramycin, vancomycin, vecuronium, verapamil, vinCRIStine, zidovudine

Solution compatibilities: D₅, 0.9% NaCl, LR

Patient/family education

- Advise patient if dizziness occurs, to ambulate, perform activities with assistance
- Advise patient to complete full course of drug therapy
- Advise patient to contact prescriber if adverse reaction occurs
- Advise patient to avoid large amounts of tyramine-containing foods (give list)

Evaluation

Positive therapeutic outcome

- Decreased symptoms of infection, blood cultures negative

---

liothyronine (T₃) (Rx)

(lye-oh-thye'roe-neen)
Cytomel, l-Triiodothyronine, liothyronine sodium, Triostat, T₃
Func. class.: Thyroid hormone
Chem. class.: Synthetic T₃

Pregnancy category A

Action: Controls protein synthesis; increases metabolic rates, cardiac output, renal blood flow, O₂ consumption, body temp, blood volume, growth, development at cellular level, exact mechanism unknown

➡ **Therapeutic Outcome:** Correction of lack of thyroid hormone

Uses: Hypothyroidism, myxedema coma, thyroid hormone replacement, nontoxic goiter, T₃ suppression test, congenital hypothyroidism

Dosage and routes

Adult: PO 25 mcg qd, increased by 12.5-25 mcg q1-2 wk until desired response, maintenance dosage 25-75 mcg qd

G *Elderly:* PO 5 mcg/day, increase by 5 mcg/day q1-2 wk

Congenital hypothyroidism
P *Child >3 yr:* PO 50-100 mcg qd
P *Child <3 yr:* PO 5 mcg qd, increased by 5 mcg q3-4 days titrated to response

Myxedema, severe hypothyroidism
Adult: PO 25-50 mcg then may increase by 5-10 mcg q1-2 wk; maintenance dosage 50-100 mcg qd

Myxedema coma/precoma
Adult: **IV** 25-50 mcg initially; 5 mcg in
G elderly; 10-20 mcg in cardiac disease; give doses q4-12h

Nontoxic goiter
Adult: PO 5 mcg qd, increased by 12.5-25 mcg q1-2 wk; maintenance dosage 75 mcg qd

Suppression test (T₃)
Adult: PO 75-100 mcg qd × 1 wk; ¹³¹I is given before and after 1st wk dose

Available forms: Tabs 5, 25, 50 mcg; inj 10 mcg/ml

Adverse effects

(*italic* = common; **bold** = life-threatening)
CNS: Insomnia, tremors, headache, **thyroid storm**
CV: Tachycardia, palpitations, angina, dysrhythmias, hypertension, cardiac arrest
GI: Nausea, diarrhea, increased or decreased appetite, cramps

MISC: Menstrual irregularities, weight loss, sweating, heat intolerance, fever, alopecia

Contraindications: Adrenal insufficiency, MI, thyrotoxicosis

G Precautions: Elderly, angina pectoris, hypertension, ischemia, cardiac disease, pregnancy **A,** lactation, diabetes

Pharmacokinetics

Absorption	Well (PO); complete (**IV**)
Distribution	Widely distributed; does not cross placenta
Metabolism	Liver
Excretion	Feces via bile, breast milk
Half-life	1-2 days

Pharmacodynamics

	PO/IV
Onset	Unknown
Peak	12-24 hr
Duration	72 hr

Interactions
Individual drugs
Cholestyramine, colestipol: ↓ absorption of thyroid hormone
Digitalis: ↓ effect of digitalis
Insulin: ↑ requirement for insulin
Phenytoin (**IV**): ↑ release of thyroid hormone
Drug classifications
Amphetamines, decongestants, vasopressors: ↑ CNS, cardiac stimulation
Anticoagulants (oral): ↑ requirements for anticoagulants
Antidepressants (tricyclics), sympathomimetics, tricyclics: ↑ effect of each specific drug
β-Adrenergic blockers, hypoglycemics: ↓ effect of each specific drug
☑ Herb/drug
Agar, bugleweed, carnitine, kelpware, soy, spirulina: ↓ thyroid hormone effect
Lab test interferences
↑ CPK, ↑ LDH, ↑ AST, ↑ PBI, ↑ blood glucose
↓ Thyroid function tests

NURSING CONSIDERATIONS
Assessment
• Determine if the patient is taking anticoagulants, antidiabetic agents; document on patient record
• Take B/P, pulse before each dose; monitor I&O ratio and weight every day in same clothing, using same scale, at same time of day
• Monitor height, weight, psychomotor development, and growth rate if given to a
P child

• Monitor T$_3$, T$_4$, FTIs, which are decreased; radioimmunoassay of TSH, which is increased; radioactive iodine uptake, which is increased if medication dose is too low
• Monitor Pro-time; may require decreased anticoagulant; check for bleeding, bruising
• Assess for increased nervousness, excitability, irritability, which may indicate too high a dose, usually after 1-3 wk of treatment
• Assess cardiac status: angina, palpitations,
G chest pain, change in VS; elderly patients may have undetected cardiac problems, and baseline ECG should be completed before treatment

Nursing diagnoses
✓ Knowledge, deficient (teaching)
✓ Noncompliance (teaching)

Implementation
PO route
• Give in AM if possible as a single dose to decrease sleeplessness; give at same time each day to maintain drug level
• Give only for hormone imbalances; not to be used for obesity, male infertility, menstrual conditions, lethargy; give lowest dose that relieves symptoms; give lower dose to the
G elderly and those with cardiac diseases
• Store in airtight, light-resistant container
IV IV route
• Administer **IV** for myxedema coma and precoma; do not give IM or SC; give q4-12h; use PO dose as soon as feasible

Patient/family education
• Teach patient that drug is not a cure but controls symptoms, and treatment is long term
• Instruct patient to report excitability, irritability, anxiety, sweating, heat intolerance, chest pain, palpitations, which indicate overdose
• Advise patient not to switch brands unless approved by prescriber; bioavailability may differ; do not take with food or absorption will be decreased
• Teach patient that drug may be discontinued after giving birth; thyroid panel will be evaluated after 1-2 mo
P • Teach patient that hyperthyroid child will show almost immediate behavior/personality change; that hair loss will occur in child but is temporary
• Caution patient that drug is not to be taken to reduce weight
• Caution patient to avoid OTC preparations with iodine; read labels; other medications should not be used unless approved by prescriber
• Teach patient to avoid iodine-rich food:

☑ Herb/drug　　Ⓢ Do Not Crush　　◆ Alert　　◆$_{\text{m}}$ Key Drug　　**G** Geriatric　　**P** Pediatric iodized salt, soybeans, tofu, turnips, high iodine seafood, some bread

Evaluation

Positive therapeutic outcome

- Absence of depression
- Weight loss
- Increased diuresis, pulse, appetite
- Absence of constipation, peripheral edema, cold intolerance, pale, cool dry skin, brittle nails, alopecia, coarse hair, menorrhagia, night blindness, paresthesias, syncope, stupor, coma, rosy cheeks
- Improved levels of T_3, T_4 by laboratory tests
- **P** Child: age-appropriate weight, height, and psychomotor development

Treatment of overdose: Withhold dose for up to 1 wk; for acute overdose: gastric lavage or induce emesis, then activated charcoal; provide supportive treatment to control symptoms

liotrix (Rx)

(lye'oh-trix)
T_3/T_4, Thyrolar
Func. class.: Thyroid hormone
Chem. class.: Levothyroxine/liothyronine (synthetic T_4, T_3)

Pregnancy category A

Action: Controls protein synthesis; increases metabolic rates, cardiac output, renal blood flow, O_2 consumption, body temp, blood volume, growth, development at cellular level, exact mechanism unknown

➡ **Therapeutic Outcome:** Correction of lack of thyroid hormone

Uses: Hypothyroidism, thyroid hormone replacement

Dosage and routes

P *Adult and child:* PO 50 mcg levothyroxine/12.5 mcg liothyronine qd, increased by 50 mcg levothyroxine/12.5 mcg liothyronine q2-3 wk until desired response; may increase by 15-30 mg q2 wk in child

G *Elderly:* PO 12.5-25 mcg levothyroxine/3.1-6.2 mcg liothyronine, may increase by 12.5-25 mcg levothyroxine/3.1-6.2 mcg liothyronine q6-8 wk until adequate response

Available forms: Tabs 12.5/3.1, 25/6.25, 50/12.5, 100/25, 150 mcg levothyroxine/37.5 mcg liothyronine

Adverse effects

(*italic* = common; **bold** = life-threatening)
CNS: *Insomnia, tremors,* headache, **thyroid storm**
CV: *Tachycardia, palpitations, angina, dysrhythmias,* hypertension, cardiac arrest
GI: Nausea, diarrhea, increased or decreased appetite, cramps
MISC: Menstrual irregularities, weight loss, sweating, heat intolerance, fever

Contraindications: Adrenal insufficiency, MI, thyrotoxicosis

G **Precautions:** Elderly, angina pectoris, hypertension, ischemia, cardiac disease, pregnancy **A,** lactation, diabetes

N **Do Not Confuse:**
Thyrolar/Thyrar

Pharmacokinetics

Absorption	50%-80% (T_4); 95% (T_3)
Distribution	Widely distributed; does not cross placenta
Metabolism	Liver, tissues
Excretion	Feces via bile; breast milk
Half-life	6-7 days (T_4); 2 days (T_3)

Pharmacodynamics

	PO (T_4)	PO (T_3)
Onset	Unknown	Unknown
Peak	Unknown	24-72 hr
Duration	Unknown	72 hr

Interactions

Individual drugs
Cholestyramine: ↓ absorption of thyroid hormone
Colestipol: ↓ absorption of liotrix
Digitalis: ↓ effect of digitalis
Insulin: ↑ requirement for insulin
Phenytoin (**IV**): ↑ release of thyroid hormone
Drug classifications
Amphetamines, decongestants, vasopressors: ↑ CNS, cardiac stimulation
Anticoagulants (oral): ↑ requirements for anticoagulants
Antidepressants (tricyclics): ↑ tricyclic effect
β-Adrenergic blockers: ↓ effect of β-blockers
Catecholamines: ↑ catecholamine effect
Estrogens: ↓ liotrix effect
Hypoglycemics: ↓ hypoglycemic effect
Sympathomimetics: ↑ sympathomimetic effect
⚋ *Herb/drug*
Agar, bugleweed, carnitine, kelpware, soy, spirulina: ↓ thyroid hormone effect

L

Lab test interferences
↑ CPK, ↑ LDH, ↑ AST, ↑ PBI, ↑ blood glucose
↓ Thyroid function tests

NURSING CONSIDERATIONS
Assessment
• Determine if the patient is taking anticoagulants, antidiabetic agents; document on chart
• Take B/P, pulse before each dose; monitor I&O ratio and weight every day in same clothing, using same scale, at same time of day
• Monitor height, weight, psychomotor development, and growth rate if given to a **P** child
• Monitor T_3, T_4, FTIs, which are decreased; radioimmunoassay of TSH, which is increased; radioactive iodine uptake (RAinternational units), which is increased if medication dose is too low
• Monitor Pro-time; may require decreased anticoagulant; check for bleeding, bruising
• Assess for increased nervousness, excitability, irritability, which may indicate too high a dose of medication, usually after 1-3 wk of treatment
• Assess cardiac status: angina, palpitations, **G** chest pain, change in VS; the elderly patient may have undetected cardiac problems, and baseline ECG should be completed before treatment

Nursing diagnoses
✓ Knowledge, deficient (teaching)
✓ Noncompliance (teaching)

Implementation
• Give in AM if possible as a single dose to decrease sleeplessness; give at same time each day to maintain drug level
• Give only for hormone imbalances; not to be used for obesity, male infertility, menstrual conditions, lethargy; give lowest dose that relieves symptoms; give lower dose to the **G** elderly and those with cardiac diseases
• Store in airtight, light-resistant container
• Remove medication 4 wk before RAIU test

Patient/family education
• Teach patient that drug is not a cure but controls symptoms, and treatment is long term
• Instruct patient to report excitability, irritability, anxiety, sweating, heat intolerance, chest pain, palpitations, which indicate overdose
• Advise patient not to switch brands unless approved by prescriber; bioavailability may differ; do not take with food or absorption will be decreased
• Teach patient that drug may be discontinued after giving birth; thyroid panel will be evaluated after 1-2 mo

P • Teach patient that hyperthyroid child will show almost immediate behavior/personality change; that hair loss will occur in child but is temporary
• Caution patient that drug is not to be taken to reduce weight
• Caution patient to avoid OTC preparations with iodine; read labels; other medications should not be used unless approved by prescriber
• Teach patient to avoid iodine-rich food: iodized salt, soybeans, tofu, turnips, high iodine seafood, some bread

Evaluation
Positive therapeutic outcome
• Absence of depression
• Weight loss
• Increased diuresis, pulse, appetite
• Absence of constipation, peripheral edema, cold intolerance, pale, cool dry skin, brittle nails, alopecia, coarse hair, menorrhagia, night blindness, paresthesias, syncope, stupor, coma, rosy cheeks
• Improved levels of T_3, T_4 by laboratory tests
P • Child: age-appropriate weight, height, and psychomotor development

Treatment of overdose: Withhold dose for up to 1 wk; acute overdose: gastric lavage or induce emesis, then activated charcoal; provide supportive treatment to control symptoms

lisinopril (Rx)
(lyse-in'oh-pril)
Prinivil, Zestril
Func. class.: Antihypertensive, angiotensin converting enzyme (ACE) inhibitor
Chem. class.: Enalaprilat lysine analog

Pregnancy category
C (1st trimester),
D (2nd/3rd trimesters)

Action: Selectively suppresses renin-angiotensin-aldosterone system; inhibits ACE; prevents conversion of angiotensin I to angiotensin II; results in dilatation of arterial, venous vessels

⇒**Therapeutic Outcome:** Decreased B/P in hypertension, decreased preload, afterload in CHF

Uses: Mild to moderate hypertension, adjunctive therapy of systolic CHF, acute MI

Dosage and routes
Hypertension
Adult: PO 10-40 mg qd; may increase to 80 mg qd if required

G **Elderly:** PO 2.5-5 mg/day, increase q7 days

CHF
Adult: PO 5 mg initially with diuretics/digitalis, range 5-20 mg

Available forms: Tabs 2.5, 5, 10, 20, 40 mg

Adverse effects
(*italic* = common; **bold** = life-threatening)
CNS: *Vertigo,* depression, stroke, insomnia, paresthesias, *headache,* fatigue, asthenia, dizziness
CV: Chest pain, hypotension
EENT: Blurred vision, nasal congestion
GI: Nausea, vomiting, anorexia, constipation, flatulence, GI irritation, diarrhea
GU: Proteinuria, renal insufficiency, sexual dysfunction, impotence
INTEG: Rash, pruritus
MISC: Muscle cramps
RESP: Dry cough, dyspnea
SYST: Angioedema

Contraindications: Hypersensitivity, pregnancy **D** (2nd/3rd trimesters)

Precautions: Pregnancy **C** (1st trimester), lactation, renal disease, hyperkalemia, renal artery stenosis

Do Not Confuse:
Prinivil/Plendil, Prinivil/Prilosec, Prinivil/Proventil
lisinopril/Risperdal

Pharmacokinetics	
Absorption	Variable
Distribution	Unknown
Metabolism	Not metabolized
Excretion	Kidneys, unchanged
Half-life	12 hr

Pharmacodynamics	
Onset	1 hr
Peak	6-8 hr
Duration	24 hr

Interactions
Individual drugs
Alcohol (large amounts), probenecid: ↑ hypotension
Allopurinol: ↑ hypersensitivity
CycloSPORINE: ↑ hyperkalemia
Digoxin: ↑ serum levels, toxicity

Indomethacin: ↓ antihypertensive effect
Lithium: ↑ levels of lithium, toxicity
Drug classifications
Antihypertensives, diuretics, nitrates, phenothiazines: ↑ hypotension
Diuretics, potassium-sparing, potassium supplements: ↑ hyperkalemia
NSAIDs: ↓ lisinopril effect
Food/drug
High-potassium diet (bananas, orange juice, avocados, broccoli, nuts, spinach) should be avoided; hyperkalemia may occur
Herb/drug
Aconite: ↑ toxicity, death
Astragalus, cola tree: ↑ or ↓ antihypertensive effect
Barberry, betony, black catechu, black cohosh, bloodroot, broom, burdock, cat's claw, dandelion, goldenseal, Irish moss, Jamaican dogwood, kelp, khella, mistletoe, parsley: ↑ antihypertensive effect
Coltsfoot, guarana, khat, licorice: ↓ antihypertensive effect
Lab test interferences
Interference: Glucose/insulin tolerance tests, ANA titer

NURSING CONSIDERATIONS
Assessment
- Assess blood studies: platelets, WBC with differential, baseline and periodically q3 mo; if neutrophils <1000/mm^3, discontinue treatment
- Monitor B/P, check for orthostatic hypotension, syncope; if changes occur, dosage change may be required
- Establish baselines in renal, liver function tests before therapy begins
- Monitor renal, liver studies: protein, BUN, creatinine; watch for increased levels that may indicate nephrotic syndrome and renal failure; monitor renal symptoms: polyuria, oliguria, frequency, dysuria; liver function tests
- Check potassium levels throughout treatment, although hyperkalemia rarely occurs
- Check for edema in feet, legs daily
- Assess for allergic reactions: rash, fever, pruritus, urticaria; drug should be discontinued if antihistamines fail to help

Nursing diagnoses
☑ Cardiac output, decreased (uses)
☑ Injury, risk for (side effects)
☑ Knowledge, deficient (teaching)
☑ Noncompliance (teaching)

Implementation
- Store in airtight container at 86° F (30° C) or less

- Severe hypotension may occur after 1st dose of this medication; may be prevented by reducing or discontinuing diuretic therapy 3 days before beginning lisinopril therapy

Patient/family education
- Caution patient not to discontinue drug abruptly; advise patient to inform all health care providers about taking this drug
- Teach patient not to use OTC products (cough, cold, allergy) unless directed by prescriber; serious side effects can occur
- Teach patient the importance of complying with dosage schedule, even if feeling better; to continue with medical regimen to decrease B/P: exercise, cessation of smoking, decreasing stress, diet modifications
- Teach patient to notify prescriber of mouth sores, sore throat, fever, swelling of hands or feet, irregular heartbeat, chest pain, coughing, shortness of breath
- Caution patient to report excessive perspiration, dehydration, vomiting, diarrhea; may lead to fall in B/P
- Emphasize the need to rise slowly to sitting or standing position to minimize orthostatic hypotension; not to exercise in hot weather or increased hypotension can occur
- Caution patient that drug may cause dizziness, fainting, light-headedness; may occur during 1st few days of therapy; to avoid activities that may be hazardous
- Teach patient how to take B/P, and normal readings for age group; advise patient to take B/P regularly
- Instruct patient to avoid increasing potassium in the diet

Evaluation
Positive therapeutic outcome
- Decreased B/P in hypertension
- Decreased CHF symptoms

Treatment of overdose: 0.9% NaCl **IV** inf, hemodialysis

---

lithium (Rx)
(li'thee-um)
Carbolith ✤, Duralith ✤, Eskalith, Eskalith CR, lithium carbonate, Lithizine ✤, Lithonate, Lithotabs
Func. class.: Antimanic, antipsychotic
Chem. class.: Alkali metal ion salt

Pregnancy category D

Action: May alter sodium, potassium ion transport across cell membrane in nerve, muscle cells; may balance biogenic amines of norepinephrine, serotonin in CNS areas involved in emotional responses

➤**Therapeutic Outcome:** Stable mood

Uses: Bipolar disorders (manic phase), prevention of bipolar manic-depressive psychosis

Dosage and routes
Adult: PO 300-600 mg tid; maintenance 300 mg tid or qid; slow rel tab 300 mg bid; dosage should be individualized to maintain blood levels at 0.5-1.5 mEq/L

G *Elderly:* PO 300 mg bid, increase q7 days by 300 mg to desired dose

P *Child:* PO 15-20 mg (0.4-0.5 mEq)/kg/day in 2-3 divided doses, increase as needed, do not exceed adult doses

Renal dose
Adult: PO CCr 10-50 ml/min 50-75% of dose; CCr <10 ml/min 25%-50% of dose

Available forms: Caps 150, 300, 600 mg; tabs 300 mg; ext rel tabs 300, 450 mg; syr 300 mg/5 ml (8 mEq/5 ml); slow rel caps 150, 300 mg ✤

Adverse effects
(*italic* = common; **bold** = life-threatening)
CNS: *Headache, drowsiness, dizziness, tremors,* twitching, ataxia, **seizures,** slurred speech, restlessness, *confusion,* stupor, memory loss, clonic movements, *fatigue*
CV: *Hypotension,* ECG changes, **dysrhythmias, circulatory collapse, edema**
EENT: Tinnitus, blurred vision
ENDO: Hypothyroidism, goiter, hyperglycemia, hyperthyroidism
GI: *Dry mouth, anorexia, nausea, vomiting, diarrhea,* incontinence, abdominal pain, metallic taste
GU: **Polyuria, glycosuria, proteinuria, albuminuria,** urinary incontinence, polydipsia, edema, **renal toxicity**
HEMA: **Leukocytosis**
INTEG: Drying of hair, alopecia, rash, pruritus, hyperkeratosis, *acneiform rash, folliculitis*
MS: *Muscle weakness,* rigidity
SYST: Hyponatremia

Contraindications: Hepatic disease, renal disease, brain trauma, OBS, pregnancy **D,** lactation, schizophrenia, severe cardiac disease, severe renal disease, severe
P dehydration, children <12 yr

G **Precautions:** Elderly, thyroid disease, seizure disorders, diabetes mellitus, systemic infection, urinary retention

---

▨ Herb/drug   ⓢ Do Not Crush   ◆ Alert   ◆☜ Key Drug   **G** Geriatric   **P** Pediatric

Pharmacokinetics

Absorption	Completely absorbed
Distribution	Reabsorbed by renal tubules (80%); crosses blood-brain barrier; crosses placenta
Metabolism	Unknown
Excretion	Urine, unchanged
Half-life	18-36 hr depending on age

Pharmacodynamics

Onset	Rapid
Peak	½-4 hr
Duration	Unknown

Interactions
Individual drugs
Acetazolamide, aminophylline, mannitol, sodium bicarbonate: ↑ renal clearance
Calcium iodide, iodinated glycerol, potassium: ↑ hypothyroid effect
Carbamazepine, fluoxetine, methyldopa, probenecid: ↑ lithium toxicity
Haloperidol: ↑ neurotoxicity
Indomethacin, losartan, urea: ↑ toxicity
Thioridazine: Brain damage

Drug classifications
Antithyroid agents: ↑ hypothyroid effects
Neuromuscular blocking agents: ↑ neuromuscular blocking effects
NSAIDs, thiazides: ↑ lithium toxicity
Phenothiazines: ↑ effect of phenothiazines
Theophyllines: ↓ effect of lithium

☑ Herb/drug
Broom, buchu, dandelion, goldenrod, horsetail, juniper, nettle, parsley: ↑ lithium effect
Cola nut, guarana, plantain, tea (black/green), yerba maté: ↓ lithium effect

Food/drug
Significant changes in sodium intake will alter lithium excretion

Lab test interferences
↑ Potassium excretion, ↑ urine glucose, ↑ blood glucose, ↑ protein, ↑ BUN
↓ VMA, ↓ T$_3$, ↓ T$_4$, ↓ PBI, ↓ ^{131}I

NURSING CONSIDERATIONS
Assessment
• Assess for minor lithium toxicity: vomiting, diarrhea, poor coordination, fine motor tremors, weakness, lassitude; major toxicity: coarse tremors, severe thirst, tinnitus, dilute urine
• Assess weight daily; check for edema in legs, ankles, wrists; report if present; check skin turgor at least daily
• Monitor sodium intake; decreased sodium intake with decreased fluid intake may lead to lithium retention; increased sodium and fluids may decrease lithium retention
• Monitor urine for albuminuria, glycosuria, uric acid during beginning treatment, q2 mo thereafter
• Assess neurologic status: LOC, gait, motor reflexes, hand tremors
• Monitor serum lithium levels weekly initially, then q2 mo (therapeutic level: 0.5-1.5 mEq/L); toxicity and therapeutic levels are very close; toxicity may occur rapidly; blood levels are measured before the AM dose

Nursing diagnoses
☑ Coping, ineffective (uses)
☑ Thought processes, disturbed (uses)
☑ Knowledge, deficient (teaching)
☑ Noncompliance (teaching)

Implementation
G • Administer reduced dosage to elderly; give with meals to avoid GI upset
• Provide adequate fluids (2-3 L/day) to prevent dehydration during initial treatment, 1-2 L/day during maintenance

Patient/family education
• Provide patient with written information on symptoms of minor toxicity: vomiting, diarrhea, poor coordination, fine motor tremors, weakness, lassitude; major toxicity: coarse tremors, severe thirst, tinnitus, dilute urine
• Advise patient to monitor urine sp gr; emphasize need for follow-up care to determine lithium effects
• Advise patient that contraception is necessary, since lithium may harm fetus
• Caution patient not to operate machinery until lithium levels are stable and response determined; that beneficial effects may take 1-3 wk
• Provide to the patient a list of drugs that interact with lithium and discuss need for adequate, stable intake of salt and fluid
Ⓢ • Advise patient not to crush, chew caps

Evaluation
Positive therapeutic outcome
• Decrease in excitement, poor judgment, insomnia (manic phase)
• Decreased mood swings and lability

Treatment of overdose: Induce emesis or lavage, maintain airway, respiratory function; dialysis for severe intoxication

L

lomefloxacin (Rx)
(lome-flocks'a-sin)
Maxaquin
Func. class.: Antiinfective
Chem. class.: Fluoroquinolone

Pregnancy category C

Action: Interferes with conversion of intermediate DNA fragments into high molecular weight DNA in bacteria; DNA gyrase inhibitor

➡ **Therapeutic Outcome:** Bactericidal for gram-negative organisms *Aeromonas, Citrobacter, Enterobacter, Escherichia coli, Haemophilus influenzae, Klebsiella, Legionella, Moraxella catarrhalis, Morganella morganii, Proteus vulgaris, Proteus mirabilis, Providencia alcalifaciens, Providencia rettgeri, Pseudomonas aeruginosa, Serratia;* gram-positive organisms *Staphylococcus aureus, Staphylococcus epidermidis, Staphylococcus saprophyticus* (methicillin-resistant strains also)

Uses: Treatment of lower respiratory tract infections (pneumonia, bronchitis), genitourinary tract infections (prostatitis, UTIs), preoperatively to reduce UTIs in transurethral surgical procedures

Dosage and routes
Lower respiratory tract infection/uncomplicated cystitis
Adult: PO 400 mg × 10 days

Complicated UTI
Adult: PO 400 mg × 14 days

Renal dose
Adult: PO CCr ≤40 ml/min 400 mg, then 200 mg/day

Surgical prophylaxis of UTI
Adult: PO 400 mg 2-6 hr before surgery

Available forms: Tabs 400 mg

Adverse effects
(*italic* = common; **bold** = life-threatening)
CNS: Dizziness, headache, somnolence, depression, insomnia, nervousness, confusion, agitation, **seizures**
EENT: Visual disturbances
GI: Diarrhea, *nausea,* vomiting, anorexia, flatulence, heartburn, dry mouth, increased AST, ALT, constipation, abdominal pain, oral thrush, glossitis, stomatitis, **pseudomembranous colitis**
INTEG: Rash, pruritus, urticaria, *photosensitivity*
SYST: **Anaphylaxis, Stevens-Johnson syndrome**

Contraindications: Hypersensitivity to quinolones

🅟 **Precautions:** Pregnancy **C,** lactation, 🅖 children, elderly, renal disease, seizure disorders, excessive exposure to sunlight, psychosis, ICP

Pharmacokinetics
Absorption	Well absorbed
Distribution	Widely distributed
Metabolism	Unknown
Excretion	Kidney, unchanged
Half-life	6-8 hr; increased in renal disease

Pharmacodynamics
Onset	Unknown
Peak	1-2 hr

Interactions
Individual drugs
Caffeine: ↑ levels
Calcium: ↓ effects of lomefloxacin
Cimetidine, probenecid: ↑ lomefloxacin levels, toxicity
CycloSPORINE: ↑ levels of cycloSPORINE, toxicity
Nitrofurantoin, sucralfate: ↓ lomefloxacin levels
Theophylline: ↓ clearance, ↑ toxicity
Warfarin: ↑ levels of warfarin, toxicity
Drug classifications
Antacids (aluminum, magnesium), iron sulfate, zinc sulfate: ↓ levels of lomefloxacin
NSAIDs: ↑ CNS stimulation, seizures
⊘ *Herb/drug*
Cola tree: ↑ antiinfective effect

NURSING CONSIDERATIONS
Assessment
• Assess patient for previous sensitivity reaction
• Assess patient for signs and symptoms of infection: characteristics of wounds, sputum, urine, stool, WBC >10,000/mm³, fever; baseline and during treatment
• Obtain C&S before beginning drug therapy to identify if correct treatment has been initiated
• Assess for allergic reactions and anaphylaxis: rash, urticaria, pruritus, chills, fever, joint pain; may occur a few days after therapy begins; epINEPHrine and resuscitation equipment should be available for anaphylactic reaction
• Monitor blood studies: AST, ALT, CBC, Hct,

bilirubin, LDH, alkaline phosphatase, Coombs' test monthly if patient is on long-term therapy

• Assess bowel pattern qd; if severe diarrhea occurs, drug should be discontinued

• Assess for overgrowth of infection: perineal itching, fever, malaise, redness, pain, swelling, drainage, rash, diarrhea, change in cough, sputum

• Assess for CNS symptoms: insomnia, vertigo, headaches, agitation, confusion

Nursing diagnoses
☑ Infection, risk for (uses)
☑ Diarrhea (adverse reactions)
☑ Injury, risk for (adverse reactions)
☑ Knowledge, deficient (teaching)
☑ Noncompliance (teaching)

Implementation
• Give with food for GI symptoms; give with 8 oz of water

• Give 2 hr before or 2 hr after iron, calcium, zinc, magnesium products, or antacids, which decrease absorption

Patient/family education
• Instruct patient to take all medication prescribed for the length of time ordered; drug must be taken around the clock to maintain blood levels; do not give medication to others

• Teach patient to use sunscreen when outdoors to decrease phototoxicity

• Advise patient to increase fluids to 2 L/day to prevent crystalluria

• Caution patient to avoid driving and other hazardous activities until response is known; dizziness, confusion, drowsiness may occur

• Advise patient to rinse mouth frequently, use sugarless candy or gum for dry mouth

• Instruct patient to avoid other medications unless approved by prescriber

Evaluation
Positive therapeutic outcome
• Negative C&S, absence of signs/symptoms of infection (WBC <10,000/mm³, temp WNL)

• Reported improvement in symptoms of infection

---

lomustine (Rx)
(loe-mus´teen)
CCNU, CeeNU
Func. class.: Antineoplastic alkylating agent
Chem. class.: Nitrosourea

Pregnancy category D

Action: Changes essential cellular ions to covalent bonding with resultant alkylation; this interferes with normal biologic function of DNA; activity is not phase specific; action is due to myelosuppression

→ **Therapeutic Outcome:** Prevention of rapid growth of malignant cells in chronic myelocytic leukemia

Uses: Hodgkin's disease, lymphomas, multiple myeloma

Investigational uses: Brain, breast, renal, GI tract, bronchogenic carcinoma; melanomas

Dosage and routes
Adult: PO 100, 130 mg/m² as a single dose q6 wk; titrate dosage to WBC level; do not give repeat dose unless WBCs are >4000/mm³, platelet count >100,000/mm³

Available forms: Caps 10, 40, 100 mg

Adverse effects
(*italic* = common; **bold** = life-threatening)
GI: Nausea, vomiting, anorexia, stomatitis, **hepatotoxicity**
GU: **Azotemia, renal failure**
HEMA: **Thrombocytopenia, leukopenia, myelosuppression, anemia**
INTEG: Burning at inj site
RESP: **Fibrosis, pulmonary infiltrate**

Contraindications: Lactation, pregnancy **D** (3rd trimester), "blastic" phase of chronic myelocytic leukemia, hypersensitivity, leukopenia, thrombocytopenia

Precautions: Radiation therapy

Pharmacokinetics	
Absorption	Rapidly absorbed
Distribution	Widely
Metabolism	Liver
Excretion	Kidneys, breast milk
Half-life	16-48 hr

Pharmacodynamics
Unknown

Interactions
Individual drugs
Allopurinol, radiation: ↑ bone marrow suppression
Chloral hydrate, phenytoin, radiation: ↑ toxicity
Phenobarbital: ↑ lomustine metabolism
Succinylcholine: ↑ lomustine effect
Drug classifications
Anticoagulants: ↑ bleeding
Antineoplastics: ↑ toxicity, bone marrow suppression

L

Lab test interferences
False positive: Cytology tests for breast, bladder, cervix, lung

NURSING CONSIDERATIONS
Assessment
◆● Monitor CBC, differential, platelet count weekly; withhold drug if WBC is <4000/mm³ or platelet count is <100,000/mm³; notify prescriber of results if WBC <20,000/mm³, platelets <150,000/mm³
● Monitor pulmonary function tests, chest x-ray films before, during therapy; chest film should be obtained q2 wk during treatment; assess for dyspnea, rales, unproductive cough, chest pain, tachypnea
● Monitor renal function studies: BUN, serum uric acid, urine CCr before, during therapy; I&O ratio; report fall in urine output of 30 ml/hr; check for decreased hyperuricemia
● Monitor for cold, fever, sore throat (may indicate beginning of infection); identify edema in feet, joint and stomach pain, shaking; prescriber should be notified
● Assess for bleeding: hematuria, guaiac, bruising or petechiae, mucosa or orifices q8h, no rec temp

Nursing diagnoses
☑ Injury, risk for (adverse reactions)
☑ Body image, disturbed (adverse reactions)
☑ Infection, risk for (adverse reactions)
☑ Knowledge, deficient (teaching)

Implementation
● Give drug after evening meal, before hs; administer antiemetic 30-60 min before giving drug to prevent vomiting
● Antiinfectives for prophylaxis of infection may be prescribed since infection potential is high
● Store in tight container

Patient/family education
● Teach patient to avoid use of products containing aspirin or ibuprofen, razors, commercial mouthwash, since bleeding may occur; to report symptoms of bleeding (hematuria, tarry stools)
● Advise patient to report signs of anemia (fatigue, headache, irritability, faintness, shortness of breath)
● Caution patient to report any changes in breathing or coughing even several mo after treatment; to avoid crowds and persons with respiratory tract or other infections
● Caution patient not to have any vaccinations without the advice of prescriber; serious reactions can occur
● Tell patient contraception is needed during treatment and for several mo after the completion of therapy

Evaluation
Positive therapeutic outcome
● Decreased tumor sizes
● Decreased spread of malignancy

loperamide (OTC, Rx)
(loe-per´a-mide)
loperamide solution, Imodium, Imodium A-D, Imodium A-D Caplet, Loperamide, Kaopectate II Caplets, Maalox Antidiarrheal Caplets, Neo-Diaral, Pepto Diarrhea Control
Func. class.: Antidiarrheal
Chem. class.: Piperidine derivative

Pregnancy category B

Action: Direct action on intestinal muscles to decrease GI peristalsis; reduces volume, increases bulk; electrolytes are not lost

➔**Therapeutic Outcome:** Absence of diarrhea

Uses: Diarrhea (cause undetermined), chronic diarrhea, to decrease amount of ileostomy discharge

Dosage and routes
Adult: PO 4 mg, then 2 mg after each loose stool, max 16 mg/day

P *Child 9-11 yr:* PO 2 mg, then 1 mg after each loose stool, max 6 mg/24 hr

P *Child 2-5 yr:* PO 1 mg on day 1, then 0.1 mg/kg after each loose stool, max 4 mg/24 hr

Available forms: Caps 2 mg; liq 1 mg/5 ml; tabs 2 mg

Adverse effects
(*italic* = common; **bold** = life-threatening)
CNS: Dizziness, drowsiness, fatigue, fever
GI: Nausea, dry mouth, vomiting, constipation, abdominal pain, anorexia, **toxic megacolon**
INTEG: Rash

Contraindications: Hypersensitivity, severe ulcerative colitis, pseudomembranous colitis, acute diarrhea associated with *Escherichia coli*

Precautions: Pregnancy **B**, lactation,
P children <2 yr, liver disease, dehydration, bacterial disease

Pharmacokinetics

Absorption	Poor
Distribution	Unknown
Metabolism	Liver
Excretion	Feces, unchanged; small amount in urine
Half-life	7-14 hr

Pharmacodynamics

Onset	½-1 hr
Peak	Unknown
Duration	4-5 hr

Interaction
Individual drugs
Alcohol: ↑ CNS depression
Drug classifications
Antihistamines, analgesics (opioids), sedative/hypnotics: ↑ CNS depression
Solutions: Do not mix with other oral sol
⚠ *Herb/drug*
Chamomile, hops, kava, skullcap, valerian: ↑ CNS depression
Nutmeg: ↑ antidiarrheal effect

NURSING CONSIDERATIONS
Assessment
• Monitor electrolytes (potassium, sodium, chloride) if patient is on long-term therapy; check fluid status, skin turgor
• Assess bowel pattern before, during treatment; check for rebound constipation after termination of medication; check bowel sounds
• Check response after 48 hr; if no response, drug should be discontinued and other treatment initiated
• Assess for abdominal distention, toxic megacolon, which may occur in ulcerative colitis
• Assess for dehydration, CNS symptoms in
P children

Nursing diagnoses
✓ Diarrhea (uses)
✓ Constipation (adverse reactions)
✓ Knowledge, deficient (teaching)
✓ Noncompliance (teaching)

Implementation
🚫 • Do not chew, crush caps
• Store in airtight containers

Patient/family education
• Caution patient to avoid alcohol and OTC products unless directed by prescriber; may cause increased CNS depression
• Advise patient not to exceed recommended dosage; drug may be habit forming; ileostomy patient may take this drug for extended time
• Advise patient that drug may cause drowsiness and to avoid hazardous activities until response to drug is determined
• Teach patient that dry mouth can be decreased by frequent sips of water, hard candy, sugarless gum

Evaluation
Positive therapeutic outcome
• Decreased diarrhea

loracarbef
See cephalosporins—2nd generation

loratadine (Rx, OTC)
(lor-a'ti-deen)
Alavert, Claritin, Claritin Non-Drowsy Allergy, Claritin Reditabs, Tavist ND
Func. class.: Antihistamine (2nd generation)
Chem. class.: Selective histamine (H₁) receptor antagonist

Pregnancy category B

Action: Binds to peripheral histamine receptors, which provides antihistamine action without sedation

➔ **Therapeutic Outcome:** Decreased nasal stuffiness, itching, swollen eyes

Uses: Seasonal rhinitis

Investigational uses: Chronic idiopathic urticaria for those ≥2 yr

Dosage and routes
P *Adult and child ≥6 yr:* PO 10 mg qd
P *Child 2-5 yr:* PO 5 mg qd

Available forms: Tabs 10 mg; tab rapid-disintegrating 10 mg; tabs, orally disintegrating 10 mg; syr 1 mg/ml

Adverse effects
(*italic* = common; **bold** = life-threatening)
CNS: Sedation (more common with increased dosages), headache

Contraindications: Hypersensitivity, acute asthma attacks, lower respiratory tract disease

Precautions: Pregnancy **B**, increased intraocular pressure, bronchial asthma

L

Pharmacokinetics

Absorption	Well absorbed
Distribution	Unknown
Metabolism	Liver, extensively, to active metabolites
Excretion	Kidneys
Half-life	8½-28 hr

Pharmacodynamics

Onset	Unknown
Peak	1½ hr
Duration	Unknown

Interactions

Individual drugs
Alcohol: ↑ CNS depression
Drug classifications
CNS depressants, antihistamines (other), opiates, sedative/hypnotics: ↑ CNS depression
MAOIs: ↑ antihistamine effects
Food/drug
↑ Absorption
☑ *Herb/drug*
Chamomile, hops, Jamaican dogwood, kava, khat, senega, skullcap, valerian: ↑ CNS depression
Corkwood, henbane: ↑ anticholinergic effect
Lab test interferences
False negative: Skin allergy tests (discontinue antihistamine 3 days before testing)

NURSING CONSIDERATIONS
Assessment
- Assess allergy: hives, rash, rhinitis
- Assess respiratory status: rate, rhythm, increase in bronchial secretions, wheezing, chest tightness; provide fluids to 2 L/day to decrease secretion thickness

Nursing diagnoses
✓ Airway clearance, ineffective (uses)
✓ Knowledge, deficient (teaching)
✓ Noncompliance (teaching, overuse)

Implementation
- Give on an empty stomach, 1 hr ac or 2 hr pc to facilitate absorption
- Place rapidly disintegrating tabs on tongue, then swallow after disintegrated with or without water
- Store in airtight, light-resistant container

Patient/family education
- Teach all aspects of drug uses; to notify prescriber if confusion, sedation, hypotension occur; to avoid driving and other hazardous activity if drowsiness occurs; to avoid alcohol and other CNS depressants that may potentiate effect

- Teach patient to take 1 hr ac or 2 hr pc to facilitate absorption
- Advise patient to use sunscreen or stay out of the sun to prevent burns
- Caution patient not to exceed recommended dosage; dysrhythmias may occur
- Teach patient hard candy, gum, frequent rinsing of mouth may be used for dryness

Evaluation
Positive therapeutic outcome
- Absence of runny or congested nose, other allergy symptoms

lorazepam (Rx)
(lor-az'e-pam)
Apo-Lorazepam ✦, Ativan, lorazepam, Novo-Lorazem ✦, Nu-Loraz ✦
Func. class.: Sedative/hypnotic, antianxiety agent
Chem. class.: Benzodiazepine

Pregnancy category D
Controlled substance schedule IV

Action: Potentiates the actions of GABA, an inhibitory neurotransmitter, especially in the limbic system and reticular formation, which depresses the CNS

➡ **Therapeutic Outcome:** Decreased anxiety, relaxation

Uses: Anxiety, irritability in psychiatric or organic disorders, preoperatively, insomnia

Investigational uses: Antiemetic before chemotherapy, status epilepticus, rectal use

Dosage and routes
Anxiety
Adult: PO 2-6 mg/day in divided doses, not to exceed 10 mg/day
G *Elderly:* PO 0.5-1 mg/day in divided doses; or 0.5-1 mg hs
P *Child:* PO 0.05 mg/kg/dose, q4-8 hr

Insomnia
Adult: PO 2-4 mg hs; only minimally effective after 2 wk continuous therapy
G *Elderly:* PO 1-2 mg initially

Preoperatively
Adult: IM 50 mcg/kg 2 hr before surgery; **IV** 44 mcg/kg 15-20 min before surgery
P *Child:* 0.05 mg/kg

Status epilepticus
P *Neonate:* 0.05 mg/kg

P *Child:* 0.1 mg/kg up to 4 mg/dose; rec (off label) 0.05-0.1 mg × 2; wait 7 min before giving 2nd dose

Available forms: Tabs 0.5, 1, 2 mg; inj 2, 4 mg/ml; conc sol 2 mg/ml

Adverse effects
(*italic* = common; **bold** = life-threatening)
CNS: Dizziness, drowsiness, confusion, headache, anxiety, tremors, stimulation, fatigue, depression, insomnia, hallucinations, weakness, unsteadiness
CV: Orthostatic hypotension, **ECG changes, tachycardia,** hypotension; **apnea, cardiac arrest (IV, rapid)**
EENT: Blurred vision, tinnitus, mydriasis
GI: Constipation, dry mouth, nausea, vomiting, anorexia, diarrhea
INTEG: Rash, dermatitis, itching

Contraindications: Hypersensitivity to benzodiazepines, narrow-angle glaucoma, **P** psychosis, pregnancy **D**, lactation, child <12 yr, history of drug abuse, COPD

G **Precautions:** Elderly, debilitated patients, hepatic disease, renal disease

N **Do Not Confuse:**
lorazepam/alprazolam/clonazepam

Pharmacokinetics	
Absorption	Well absorbed (PO); completely absorbed (IM)
Distribution	Widely distributed; crosses placenta, blood-brain barrier
Metabolism	Liver, extensively
Excretion	Kidneys, breast milk
Half-life	14 hr

Pharmacodynamics			
	PO	IM	IV
Onset	½ hr	15-30 min	5-15 min
Peak	1-3 hr	1-1½ hr	Unknown
Duration	3-6 hr	3-6 hr	3-6 hr

Interactions
Individual drugs
Alcohol: ↑ CNS depression
Cimetidine, disulfiram, fluoxetine: ↑ action
Levodopa: ↓ action of levodopa
Drug classifications
Antidepressants, antihistamines, opiates: ↑ CNS depression
Smoking
↑ Metabolism, ↓ effect
Herb/drug
Black cohosh: ↑ hypotension
Catnip, chamomile, clary, cowslip, hops, lavender, mistletoe, nettle, pokeweed, poppy, Queen Anne's lace, senega, skullcap, valerian: ↑ CNS depression
Kava: ↑ action
Lab test interferences
↑ AST, ↑ ALT, ↑ serum bilirubin
False: ↑ 17-OHCS
↓ Radioactive iodine uptake

NURSING CONSIDERATIONS
Assessment
• Assess degree of anxiety; what precipitates anxiety and whether drug controls symptoms; other signs of anxiety: dilated pupils, inability to sleep, restlessness, inability to focus
• Assess for alcohol withdrawal symptoms, including hallucinations (visual, auditory), delirium, irritability, agitation, fine to coarse tremors
• Monitor B/P (with patient lying/standing), pulse, check respiratory rate; if systolic B/P drops 20 mm Hg, hold drug, notify prescriber; respirations q5-15 min if given **IV**
• Monitor CBC during long-term therapy; blood dyscrasias have occurred (rarely)
• Monitor for seizure control; type, duration, and intensity of seizures; what precipitates seizures
• Monitor hepatic studies: AST, ALT, bilirubin, creatinine, LDH, alkaline phosphatase
• Assess mental status: mood, sensorium, affect, sleeping pattern, drowsiness, dizziness, suicidal tendencies, and ability of drug to control these symptoms; check for tolerance, withdrawal symptoms: headache, nausea, vomiting, muscle pain, weakness after long-term use

Nursing diagnoses
✓ Sleep pattern, disturbed (uses)
✓ Coping, ineffective (uses)
✓ Knowledge, deficient (teaching)
✓ Noncompliance (teaching)

Implementation
PO route
• Give with food or milk for GI symptoms; crush tab if patient is unable to swallow medication whole; provide sugarless gum, hard candy, frequent sips of water for dry mouth
• Use by SL route for rapid response (investigational use)
IM route
• Give deep in muscle mass; if using for preoperative sedation, give 2 hr or more before surgical procedure
IV **IV route**
• Dilute with sterile water for inj, 0.9% NaCl, or D₅W just before using; give by Y-site or 3-way stopcock at 2 mg/min

• Do not use sol that is discolored or contains a precipitate

Syringe compatibilities: Cimetidine, hydromorphone

Y-site compatibilities: Acyclovir, albumin, allopurinol, amifostine, amikacin, amoxicillin, amoxicillin/clavulanate, amsacrine, atracurium, bumetanide, cefepime, cefmetazole, cefotaxime, ciprofloxacin, cisatracurium, cisplatin, cladribine, clonidine, cyclophosphamide, cytarabine, dexamethasone, diltiazem, DOBUTamine, DOPamine, DOXOrubicin, epINEPHrine, erythromycin, etomidate, famotidine, fentanyl, filgrastim, fluconazole, fludarabine, furosemide, gentamicin, granisetron, haloperidol, heparin, hydrocortisone, hydromorphone, ketanserin, labetalol, melphalan, methotrexate, metronidazole, midazolam, milrinone, morphine, niCARdipine, nitroglycerin, norepinephrine, paclitaxel, pancuronium, piperacillin, piperacillin/tazobactam, potassium chloride, propofol, ranitidine, tacrolimus, teniposide, thiotepa, trimethoprim/sulfamethoxazole, vancomycin, vecuronium, vinorelbine, zidovudine

Y-site incompatibilities: Idarubicin, ondansetron, sargramostim

Patient/family education

• Advise patient that drug may be taken with food; that drug is not to be used for everyday stress or used longer than 4 mo unless directed by a prescriber; to take no more than prescribed amount; may be habit forming
• Caution patient to avoid OTC preparations unless approved by prescriber; to avoid alcohol, other psychotropic medications unless prescribed by physician; not to discontinue medication abruptly after long-term use
• Inform patient to avoid driving and activities that require alertness; drowsiness may occur; to rise slowly or fainting may occur, especially in elderly
• Inform patient that drowsiness may worsen at beginning of treatment

Evaluation

Positive therapeutic outcome
• Decreased anxiety, restlessness, insomnia

Treatment of overdose: Lavage, VS, supportive care

losartan (Rx)

(low-sar'tan)
Cozaar
Func. class.: Antihypertensive
Chem. class.: Angiotensin II receptor (type AT$_1$)

Pregnancy category
C (1st trimester);
D (2nd/3rd trimesters)

Action: Blocks the vasoconstrictor and aldosterone-secreting effects of angiotensin II; selectively blocks the binding of angiotensin II to the AT$_1$ receptor found in tissues

Therapeutic Outcome: Decreased B/P

Uses: Hypertension, alone or in combination; nephropathy in type 2 diabetes, hypertension with left ventricular hypertrophy

Dosage and routes
Hypertension
Adult: PO 50 mg qd alone or 25 mg qd when used in combination with diuretic

Nephropathy in type 2 diabetes
Adult: PO 50 mg qd, may increase to 100 mg qd

Hepatic dose
Adult: PO 25 mg qd as starting dose

Hypertension with left ventricular hypertrophy
Adult: PO 50 mg qd, add hydrochlorothiazide 12.5 mg/day and/or increase losartan to 100 mg qd, then increase hydrochlorothiazide to 25 mg qd

Available forms: Tabs 25, 50, 100 mg

Adverse effects
(*italic* = common; **bold** = life-threatening)
CNS: Dizziness, insomnia, anxiety, confusion, abnormal dreams, migraine, tremor, vertigo, headache
CV: Angina pectoris, 2nd- degree AV block, **CVA,** hypotension, **MI, dysrhythmias**
EENT: Blurred vision, burning eyes, conjunctivitis
GI: Diarrhea, dyspepsia, anorexia, constipation, dry mouth, flatulence, gastritis, vomiting
GU: Impotence, nocturia, urinary frequency, urinary tract infection, **renal failure**
HEMA: Anemia
INTEG: Alopecia, dermatitis, dry skin, flushing, photosensitivity, rash, pruritus, sweating
META: Gout
MS: Cramps, myalgia, pain, stiffness
RESP: Cough, upper respiratory infection, congestion, dyspnea, bronchitis

---

Contraindications: Hypersensitivity, pregnancy **D** (2nd/3rd trimesters)

Precautions: Hypersensitivity to ACE
P inhibitors; pregnancy **C** (1st trimester);
G lactation, children, elderly

🔌 **Do Not Confuse:**
Cozaar/Zocor
losartan/valsartan

Pharmacokinetics

Absorption	Well
Distribution	Bound to plasma proteins
Metabolism	Extensive
Excretion	Feces, urine
Half-life	Biphasic, 2 hr, 6-9 hr

Pharmacodynamics
Unknown

Interactions
Individual drugs
Fluconazole: ↑ antihypertensive effect
Lithium: ↑ toxicity
Phenobarbital, rifamycin: ↓ antihypertensive effect
🖉 *Herb/drug*
Aconite: ↑ toxicity, death
Astragalus, cola tree: ↑ or ↓ antihypertensive effect
Barberry, betony, black catechu, black cohosh, bloodroot, broom, burdock, cat's claw, dandelion, goldenseal, Irish moss, Jamaican dogwood, kelp, khella, mistletoe, parsley: ↑ antihypertensive effect
Coltsfoot, guarana, khat, licorice: ↑ antihypertensive effect

NURSING CONSIDERATIONS
Assessment
• Assess B/P with position changes, pulse q4h; note rate, rhythm, quality
• Monitor electrolytes: potassium, sodium, chloride
• Obtain baselines for renal, liver function tests before therapy begins
• Monitor for edema in feet, legs daily
• Assess for skin turgor, dryness of mucous membranes for hydration status

Nursing diagnoses
✓ Fluid volume, deficient (side effects)
✓ Noncompliance (teaching)
✓ Knowledge, deficient (teaching)

Implementation
• Administer without regard to meals

Patient/family education
• Teach patient to avoid sunlight or wear sunscreen if in sunlight; photosensitivity may occur
• Advise patient to comply with dosage schedule, even if feeling better
• Teach patient to notify prescriber of mouth sores, fever, swelling of hands or feet, irregular heartbeat, chest pain
• Advise patient that excessive perspiration, dehydration, vomiting, diarrhea may lead to fall in blood pressure, consult prescriber if these occur
• Inform patient that drug may cause dizziness, fainting; light-headedness may occur
• Caution patient to rise slowly to sitting or standing position to minimize orthostatic hypotension
• Advise patient to use contraception while taking this product

Evaluation
Positive therapeutic outcome
• Decreased B/P

---

lovastatin ⊕π (Rx)
(loe′va-sta-tin)
Altocor, Mevacor
Func. class.: Antilipemic
Chem. class.: HMG-CoA reductase inhibitor

Pregnancy category X

Action: By inhibiting HMG-CoA reductase, inhibits biosynthesis of VLDL and LDL, which are responsible for cholesterol development

➔ **Therapeutic Outcome:** Decreased cholesterol levels and LDLs, increased HDLs

Uses: As an adjunct in primary hypercholesterolemia (types IIa, IIb), atherosclerosis, primary and secondary prevention of coronary events

Dosage and routes
(Patient should first be consuming a cholesterol-lowering diet)

Adult: PO 20 mg qd with evening meal; may increase to 20-80 mg/day in single or divided doses; not to exceed 80 mg/day; dosage adjustments should be made monthly; reduce dose in renal disease

Available forms: Tabs 10, 20, 40 mg; ext rel tab 10, 20, 40, 60 mg

Adverse effects
(*italic* = common; **bold** = life-threatening)
CNS: Dizziness, headache, tremor, insomnia, paresthesia
EENT: Blurred vision, dysgeusia, lens opacities
GI: Nausea, constipation, diarrhea, dyspepsia,

flatus, abdominal pain, heartburn, **liver dysfunction,** vomiting, acid regurgitation, dry mouth, dysgeusia
***HEMA:* Thrombocytopenia, hemolytic anemia, leukopenia**
INTEG: Rash, pruritus, photosensitivity
MS: Muscle cramps, myalgia, **myositis, rhabdomyolysis,** leg, shoulder or localized pain

Contraindications: Hypersensitivity, pregnancy **X,** lactation, active liver disease

Precautions: Past liver disease, alcoholism, severe acute infections, trauma, hypotension, uncontrolled seizure disorders, severe metabolic disorders, electrolyte imbalances, visual **P** condition, children

🔌 Do Not Confuse:
lovastatin/Lotensin

Pharmacokinetics

Absorption	Poorly absorbed, erratic
Distribution	Crosses placenta, blood-brain barrier
Metabolism	Liver, extensively
Excretion	Feces (83%); kidneys, urine (10%)
Half-life	3-4 hr

Pharmacodynamics

Onset	Unknown
Peak	2-4 hr
Duration	Unknown

Interactions
Individual drugs
Cholestyramine: ↓ action of lovastatin
Clofibrate, cycloSPORINE, erythromycin, gemfibrozil, niacin: ↑ myopathy risk
Digoxin: ↑ digoxin effect
Propranolol: ↓ antihyperlipidemic effect
Warfarin: ↑ bleeding

Drug classifications
Azole antifungals: ↑ myositis, myalgia
Bile acid sequestrants: ↑ lovastatin effects
Food/drug
↑ Levels of lovastatin with food, must be taken with food
Grapefruit juice: ↑ toxicity
🖊 *Herb/drug*
Glucomannan: ↑ effect
Gotu kola: ↓ effect
Lab test interferences
↑ CPK, ↑ liver function tests

NURSING CONSIDERATIONS
Assessment
• Assess nutrition: fat, protein, carbohydrates; nutritional analysis should be completed by dietitian before treatment

• Monitor bowel pattern daily; diarrhea may be a problem
• Monitor triglycerides, fasting cholesterol LDL, HDL at baseline and throughout treatment; watch LDL and VLDL closely; if increased, drug should be discontinued
• Assess for muscle pain, tenderness, obtain CPK; if these occur, drug may need to be discontinued

Nursing diagnoses
☑ Diarrhea (adverse reactions)
☑ Knowledge, deficient (teaching)
☑ Noncompliance (teaching)

Implementation
• Give with evening meal; if dosage is increased, take with breakfast and evening meal
• Store in cool environment in airtight, light-resistant container

Patient/family education
• Inform patient that compliance is needed for positive results to occur; not to double doses
• Inform patient that blood work and ophthalmic exam will be necessary during treatment
• Teach patient that risk factors should be decreased: high-fat diet, smoking, alcohol consumption, absence of exercise
• Advise patient to report if pregnancy is suspected
• Advise patient to notify prescriber if the GI symptoms of diarrhea, abdominal or epigastric pain, nausea, vomiting occur; or if chills, fever, sore throat, blurred vision, dizziness, headache, muscle pain, weakness occur
• Advise patient to stay out of the sun or use sunscreen to prevent burns

Evaluation
Positive therapeutic outcome
• Decreased cholesterol, serum triglyceride levels
• Improved ratio of HDLs

---

loxapine (Rx)
(lox'a-peen)
Loxapac ✦, loxapine succinate, Loxitane IM, Loxitane, Loxitane-C
Func. class.: Antipsychotic/neuroleptic
Chem. class.: Dibenzoxazepine
Pregnancy category C

Action: Depresses cerebral cortex, hypothalamus, limbic system, which control activity and aggression; blocks neurotransmission produced by DOPamine at synapse; exhibits strong

 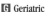

α-adrenergic, anticholinergic blocking action; mechanism for antipsychotic effects is unclear

→**Therapeutic Outcome:** Decreased psychotic behavior

Uses: Psychotic disorders, nonpsychotic symptoms associated with dementia

Investigational uses: Depression, anxiety

Dosage and routes
Adult: PO 10 mg bid-qid initially; may be rapidly increased depending on severity of condition; maintenance 60-100 mg/day; IM 12.5-50 mg q4-6h or more until desired response, then start PO form

G *Elderly:* PO 5-10 mg qd bid, increase q4-7 days by 5-10 mg, max 125 mg

Available forms: Caps 5, 10, 25, 50 mg; conc 25 mg/ml; inj 50 mg/ml; tabs 5, 10, 25, 50 mg

Adverse effects
(*italic* = common; **bold** = life-threatening)
CNS: Extrapyramidal symptoms (EPS): pseudoparkinsonism, akathisia, dystonia, tardive dyskinesia, drowsiness, headache, **seizures,** confusion, **neuroleptic malignant syndrome**
CV: Orthostatic hypotension, **cardiac arrest,** ECG changes, tachycardia
EENT: Blurred vision, glaucoma
GI: Dry mouth, nausea, vomiting, anorexia, constipation, diarrhea, jaundice, weight gain
GU: Urinary retention, urinary frequency, enuresis, impotence, amenorrhea, gynecomastia
HEMA: **Anemia, leukopenia, leukocytosis, agranulocytosis**
INTEG: Rash, photosensitivity, dermatitis
RESP: **Laryngospasm,** dyspnea, **respiratory depression**

Contraindications: Hypersensitivity, blood dyscrasias, coma, severe CNS depression, brain damage, bone marrow depression, alcohol and barbiturate withdrawal states, narrow-angle glaucoma

Precautions: Pregnancy **C,** lactation, seizure disorders, hepatic disease, cardiac **P** disease, prostatic hypertrophy, cardiac condi-**G** tions, child <16 yr, elderly

N **Do Not Confuse:**
Loxitane/Soriatane

♣ Canada Only   **N** Do Not Confuse   * "Tall Man" lettering (See Preface)

Pharmacokinetics

Absorption	Well absorbed (PO)
Distribution	Unknown
Metabolism	Liver, extensively
Excretion	Kidneys
Half-life	Biphasic 5 hr, 19 hr

Pharmacodynamics

	PO	IM
Onset	½ hr	15-30 min
Peak	2-4 hr	15-20 min
Duration	12 hr	12 hr

Interactions
Individual drugs
Alcohol: ↑ effects of both drugs, oversedation
Aluminum hydroxide: ↓ absorption
EpINEPHrine: ↑ toxicity
Drug classifications
Anticholinergics: ↑ anticholinergic effects
Antidepressants, antihistamines, barbiturates, MAOIs, opiates, sedative/hypnotics: ↑ CNS depression
Antipsychotics: ↑ EPS
☑ *Herb/drug*
Betel palm, kava: ↑ EPS
Chamomile, cola tree, hops, nettle, nutmeg, skullcap, valerian: ↑ CNS depression

NURSING CONSIDERATIONS
Assessment
• Assess mental status: orientation, mood, behavior, presence and type of hallucinations before initial administration and monthly; this drug should significantly reduce psychotic behavior
• Check for swallowing of PO medication; check for hoarding or giving of medication to other patients
• Monitor I&O ratio; palpate bladder if low
G urinary output occurs, especially in elderly; urinalysis recommended before, during prolonged therapy, urinary retention may be cause
• Monitor bilirubin, CBC, liver function studies monthly
• Assess affect, orientation, LOC, reflexes, gait, coordination, sleep pattern disturbances
• Monitor B/P with patient sitting, standing, and lying; take pulse and respirations q4h during initial treatment; establish baseline before starting treatment; report drops of 30 mm Hg
• Check for dizziness, faintness, palpitations, tachycardia on rising; severe orthostatic hypotension is common
◆ • Identify for neuroleptic malignant

L

syndrome: hyperpyrexia, muscle rigidity, increased CPK, altered mental status; drug should be discontinued
• Assess for EPS including akathisia (inability to sit still, no pattern to movements), tardive dyskinesia (bizarre movements of the jaw, mouth, tongue, extremities), pseudoparkinsonism (ragged tremors, pill rolling, shuffling gait); an antiparkinsonian drug should be prescribed
• Assess for constipation, urinary retention daily; if these occur, increase bulk, water in diet

Nursing diagnoses
☑ Thought processes, disturbed (uses)
☑ Coping, ineffective (uses)
☑ Knowledge, deficient (teaching)
☑ Noncompliance (teaching)

Implementation
PO route
• Administer drug in liq form mixed in glass of juice or cola if hoarding is suspected; do not mix in caffeine drinks, tannics, pectins
G • Administer lowered dose in elderly, since metabolism is slowed
• Administer with full glass of water or milk; or give with food to decrease GI upset
• Store in airtight, light-resistant container, oral sol in amber bottle

IM route
• Inject deep in muscle mass; do not give SC; do not administer sol with a precipitate; amber-colored sol can be used

Patient/family education
• Teach patient to use good oral hygiene; suggest frequent rinsing of mouth, sugarless gum for dry mouth
• Caution patient to avoid hazardous activities until drug response is determined; dizziness, blurred vision may occur
• Inform patient that orthostatic hypotension occurs often and to rise from sitting or lying position gradually; to remain lying down after IM inj for at least 30 min; caution patient to avoid hot tubs, hot showers, tub baths, since hypotension may occur; tell patient that in hot weather heat stroke may occur; take extra precautions to stay cool
• Advise patient to avoid abrupt withdrawal of this drug, or EPS may result; drug should be withdrawn slowly
• Advise patient to avoid use with alcohol, CNS depressants; increased drowsiness may occur
• Advise patient to use a sunscreen and sunglasses to prevent burns

• Teach patient about EPS and necessity of meticulous oral hygiene, since oral candidiasis may occur
• Suggest patient take antacids 2 hr before or after taking this drug
• Instruct patient to report sore throat, malaise, fever, bleeding, mouth sores; if these occur, CBC should be performed and drug discontinued

Evaluation
Positive therapeutic outcome
• Decrease in emotional excitement, hallucinations, delusions, paranoia
• Reorganization of patterns of thought, speech

Treatment of overdose: Lavage if orally ingested; barbiturates; provide airway, **IV** fluids; do not use epINEPHrine, which may increase hypotension

lymphocyte immune globulin (anti-thymocyte) (Rx)
Atgam
Func. class.: Immune globulin immunosuppressant

Pregnancy category C

Action: Produces immunosuppression by inhibiting the function of T-lymphocytes

➡ **Therapeutic Outcome:** Absence of transplant rejection; hematologic remission (aplastic anemia)

Uses: Organ transplants to prevent rejection, aplastic anemia

Investigational uses: Multiple sclerosis, myasthenia gravis, immunosuppressant in liver, bone marrow, heart and other organ transplants, pure red cell aplasia, scleroderma

Dosage and routes
Renal allograft
Adult: **IV** 10-30 mg/kg/day
P *Child:* **IV** 5-25 mg/kg/day

Delay of renal allograft rejection
Adult: **IV** 15 mg/kg/day × 14 days, then qod × 14 days for a total of 21 doses in 28 days

Aplastic anemia
Adult: **IV** 10-20 mg/kg/day × 8-14 days

Available forms: Inj 50 mg horse gamma globulin/ml

☑ Herb/drug   ⊗ Do Not Crush   ◆ Alert   ✦☐ Key Drug   **G** Geriatric   **P** Pediatric

Adverse effects
(*italic* = common; **bold** = life-threatening)
Renal transplant
CNS: Fever, chills, headache, dizziness, weakness, faintness, seizures
CV: Chest pain, hypertension, tachycardia
GI: Diarrhea, nausea, vomiting, epigastric pain
INTEG: Rash, pruritus, urticaria, wheal
SYST: **Anaphylaxis**

Aplastic anemia
CNS: Fever, chills, headache, seizures, lightheadedness, encephalitis, postviral encephalopathy
CV: Bradycardia, myocarditis, irregularity
GI: Nausea, liver function test abnormality

Contraindications: Hypersensitivity

Precautions: Severe renal disease, severe hepatic disease, pregnancy **C**, lactation, children

Pharmacokinetics
Absorption	Unknown
Distribution	Unknown
Metabolism	Unknown
Excretion	Unknown
Half-life	5.7 days

Pharmacodynamics
Onset	Rapid
Peak	Unknown
Duration	Unknown

Interactions
None known

NURSING CONSIDERATIONS
Assessment
• Assess for infection, if infection occurs evaluation will be needed to continue treatment
• Monitor renal studies: BUN, creatinine at least monthly during treatment, 3 mo after treatment
• Monitor liver function studies: alkaline phosphatase, AST, ALT, bilirubin

Nursing diagnoses
☑ Mobility, impaired (uses)
☑ Infection, risk for (uses)
☑ Knowledge, deficient (teaching)

Implementation
IV route
• Do not infuse <4 hr

Delay of renal allograft rejection
Adult: **IV** 15 mg/kg/day × 14 days, then qod × 14 days for a total of 21 doses in 28 days

Aplastic anemia
Adult: **IV** 10-20 mg/kg/day × 8-14 days
• Keep emergency equipment nearby for severe allergic reactions
• Skin testing must be completed before treatment; use intradermal inj of 0.1 ml of a 1:1000 dilution (5 mcg of horse IgG) in 0.9% NaCl, if a wheal or rash >10 mm or both, use caution during inf
• Dilute in saline sol before inf; invert **IV** bag, so undiluted drug does not contact the air inside, concentration should not be >1 mg/ml

Patient/family education
• Advise patient to report fever, rash, chills, sore throat, fatigue, since serious infections may occur
• Caution patient to use contraceptive measures during treatment and for 12 wk after ending therapy; drug is teratogenic
• Caution patient to avoid crowds and persons with known infections to reduce risk of infection

Evaluation
Positive therapeutic outcome
• Absence of graft rejection
• Hematologic recovery (aplastic anemia)

M

magaldrate (OTC)
(mag'al-drate)
Losapan ✚, Lowsium, Riopan, Riopan Extra Strength ✚
Func. class.: Antacid
Chem. class.: Aluminum/magnesium hydroxide

Pregnancy category C

Action: Neutralizes gastric acidity; drug is dissolved in gastric contents; this drug is a combination of aluminum and magnesium

Therapeutic Outcome: Decreased pain of ulcers

Uses: Antacid, peptic ulcer disease (adjunct), indigestion/heartburn, duodenal and gastric ulcers, reflux esophagitis, hyperacidity

Dosage and routes
Adult: SUSP 5-10 ml (400-800 mg) with water between meals, hs, not to exceed 100 ml/day

Available forms: Susp 540 mg/5 ml; liq 540 mg/5 ml

Adverse effects
(*italic* = common; **bold** = life-threatening)
GI: Constipation, diarrhea
META: Hypermagnesemia, hypophosphatemia

Contraindications: Hypersensitivity to this drug or aluminum products

G Precautions: Elderly, fluid restriction, decreased GI motility, GI obstruction, dehydration, renal disease, sodium-restricted diets, pregnancy **C**

Pharmacokinetics
Absorption	Not absorbed
Distribution	Not distributed
Metabolism	Not metabolized
Excretion	Kidneys
Half-life	Unknown

Pharmacodynamics
Onset	Unknown
Peak	½ hr
Duration	1 hr

Interactions
Individual drugs
Chlordiazepoxide, cimetidine, phenytoin: ↓ absorption of each specific drug
Ketoconazole, tetracycline: ↓ effect of each specific drug
Drug classifications
Anticholinergics, iron salts, phenothiazines, salicylates: ↓ absorption of each specific drug

NURSING CONSIDERATIONS
Assessment
• Assess GI status: location of pain, intensity, characteristics, what aggravates, ameliorates pain; heartburn/indigestion; hematemesis
• Monitor serum magnesium, calcium, phosphate, potassium if using long term or with impaired renal function
• Assess for constipation: increase bulk in diet if needed or obtain order for stool softener

Nursing diagnoses
✓ Pain (uses)
✓ Knowledge, deficient (teaching)

Implementation
• Give laxatives or stool softeners if constipation occurs
• Give susp after shaking; give between meals and hs
• Give when stomach is empty pc and hs

Patient/family education
• Advise patient to separate ingestion of enteric-coated drugs and antacid by 2 hr
• Advise patient to use 2 wk or less; drug should not be used for long periods
• Teach patient to notify prescriber immediately if coffee-ground emesis, emesis with frank blood, or black tarry stools occur

Evaluation
Positive therapeutic outcome
• Absence of abdominal pain
• Decreased acidity

magnesium salts (OTC)
(mag-neez′ee-um)
magnesium chloride (OTC)
Chloromag, Slo-Mag
magnesium citrate (OTC)
Citrate of Magnesia, Citroma, Citromag ✦, Evac-Q-Mag
magnesium gluconate magtrate (OTC)
Mag-G
magnesium hydroxide (OTC)
Phillips Magnesium Tablets, Phillips Milk of Magnesia, MOM
magnesium oxide (OTC)
Mag-Ox 400, Maox, Uro-Mag
magnesium sulfate (OTC, Rx)
Epsom Salt
Func. class.: Electrolyte; anticonvulsant, laxative, saline; antacid

Pregnancy category A, B (magnesium sulfate)

Action: Increases osmotic pressure, draws fluid into colon, neutralizes HCl

⊃ **Therapeutic Outcome:** Magnesium levels WNL, absence of constipation

Uses: Constipation, bowel preparation before surgery or exam, electrolyte, anticonvulsant, in preeclampsia, eclampsia (magnesium sulfate)

Dosage and routes
Laxative
Adult: PO 30-60 ml hs (Milk of Magnesia), 300 mg

P *Adult and child >6 yr:* PO 15 g in 8 oz of H_2O (magnesium sulfate); PO 10-20 ml (Concentrated Milk of Magnesia); PO 5-10 oz hs (magnesium citrate)

P *Child 2-6 yr:* 5-15 ml/day (Milk of Magnesia)

Prevention of magnesium deficiency

P *Adult and child ≥10 yr:* PO male: 350-400 mg/day; female: 280-300 mg/day; lactation: 335-350 mg/day; pregnancy 320 mg/day

P *Child 8-10 yr:* PO 170 mg/day

P *Child 4-7 yr:* PO 120 mg/day

P *Infant to 4 yr:* 40-80 mg/day

Magnesium sulfate deficiency
Adult: PO 200-400 mg in divided doses tid-qid; IM 1 g q6h × 4 doses; **IV** 5 g (severe)

P *Child 6-12 yr:* 3-6 mg/kg/day in divided doses tid-qid

Preeclampsia/eclampsia magnesium sulfate
Adult: IM/**IV** 4-5 g **IV** inf; with 5 g IM in each gluteus, then 5 g q4h or 4 g **IV** inf then 1-2 g/hr cont inf

Available forms: *Chloride:* sus rel tabs 535 mg (64 mg Mg); enteric tabs 833 mg (100 mg Mg) *Hydroxide:* liq 400 mg/5 ml (164 mg Mg/5 ml); conc liq 800 mg/5 ml (328 mg Mg/5 ml); chew tabs 300, 600 mg *Oxide:* tabs 200, 400 mg (241.3 mg Mg); caps 140 mg (84.5 mg Mg) *Sulfate:* powder for oral; bulk packages; Epsom salts, bulk packages; inj 10, 12.5, 25, 50%

Adverse effects
(*italic* = common; **bold** = life-threatening)
CNS: Muscle weakness, flushing, sweating, confusion, sedation, depressed reflexes, **flaccid paralysis, hypothermia**
CV: Hypotension, heart block, **circulatory collapse**
GI: Nausea, vomiting, anorexia, cramps
META: Electrolyte, fluid imbalances
RESP: Respiratory depression

Contraindications: Hypersensitivity, abdominal pain, nausea/vomiting, obstruction, acute surgical abdomen, rectal bleeding

Precautions: Pregnancy **A; B** (magnesium sulfate) renal disease, cardiac disease

Pharmacokinetics
PO	Onset 3-6 hr
IM	Onset 1 hr, duration 4 hr
IV	Duration ½ hr

Pharmacodynamics
Onset	Unknown
Distribution	Unknown
Metabolized	Unknown
Excreted	Kidneys
Half-life	Unknown
	effective anticonvulsant levels 2.5-7.5 mEq/L.

Interactions
Drug classifications
Antiinfectives (aminoquinolones), tetracyclines: ↓ absorption
Neuromuscular blockers: ↑ effect

NURSING CONSIDERATIONS
Assessment
- Assess I&O ratio; check for decrease in urinary output
- Assess cause of constipation; lack of fluids, bulk, exercise
- Assess cramping, rectal bleeding, nausea, vomiting; drug should be discontinued
- Assess Mg toxicity: thirst, confusion, decrease in reflexes
- Assess visual changes: blurring, halos, corneal and retinal damage
- Assess edema in feet, ankles, legs
- Assess prior drug history; there are many drug interactions

Implementation
PO route
- Administer with 8 oz of H_2O
- Refrigerate magnesium citrate before administration
- Shake susp before using
- Give as antacid at least 2 hr pc
- Administer to patient crushed or whole; chewable tablets may be chewed
- Administer with food or milk to decrease gastric symptoms; give 30 min before or 2 hr after antacids

IV route
- Administer only when calcium gluconate available for magnesium toxicity
- Administer **IV** undiluted 1.5 ml of 10% sol over 1 min; may dilute to 20% sol, infuse over 3 hr
- Administer **IV** at less than 150 mg/min; circulatory collapse may occur

Y-site compatibilities: Acyclovir, aldesleukin, amifostine, amikacin, ampicillin,

M

aztreonam, cefamandole, cefazolin, cefmetazole, cefoperazone, cefotaxime, cefoxitin, cephalothin, cephapirin, chloramphenicol, cisatracurium, DOBUTamine, doxycycline, DOXOrubicin liposome, enalaprilat, erythromycin, esmolol, famotidine, fludarabine, gallium, gentamicin, granisetron, heparin, hydromorphone, idarubicin, insulin, kanamycin, labetalol, meperidine, metronidazole, minocycline, morphine, moxalactam, nafcillin, ondansetron, oxacillin, paclitaxel, penicillin G potassium, piperacillin, piperacillin/tazobactam, potassium chloride, propofol, remifentanil, sargramostim, thiotepa, ticarcillin, tobramycin, trimethoprim/sulfamethoxazole, vancomycin, vit B complex/C

Additive compatibilities: Cephalothin, chloramphenicol, cisplatin, heparin, hydrocortisone, isoproterenol, meropenem, methyldopate, norepinephrine, penicillin G potassium, potassium phosphate, verapamil

Patient/family education
• Inform patient to report any symptoms of hepatotoxicity, renal toxicity, visual changes, ototoxicity, allergic reactions, bleeding (long-term therapy)
• Inform patient not to exceed recommended dosage; acute poisoning may result
• Inform patient to read label on other OTC drugs; many contain aspirin
• Inform patient that therapeutic response takes 2 wk (arthritis)
• Inform patient to avoid alcohol ingestion; GI bleeding may occur
• Inform patient that if anticoagulants are given with this drug, both should be discontinued 2 wk before surgery

Evaluation
Positive therapeutic outcomes
• Decreased pain, fever

Treatment of overdose: Lavage, activated charcoal, monitor electrolytes, VS

---

mannitol (Rx)
(man'i-tole)
mannitol, Osmitrol, Resectisol
Func. class.: Diuretic-osmotic
Chem. class.: Hexahydric alcohol

Pregnancy category C

Action: Increases osmolarity of glomerular filtrate, which raises osmotic pressure of fluid in renal tubules; there is a decrease in reabsorption of water, electrolytes; increases in urinary output, sodium, chloride, potassium, calcium, phosphorus, uric acid, urea, magnesium

Uses: Edema; promote systemic diuresis in cerebral edema, decrease intraocular pressure, improve renal function in acute renal failure, chemical poisoning

Dosage and routes
Oliguria, prevention
Adult: **IV** 50-100 g of a 5%-25% sol, may use test dose 0.2 g/kg over 3-5 min

Oliguria, treatment
Adult: **IV** 300-400 mg/kg of a 20%-25% sol up to 100 g of a 15%-20% sol over 30-60 min

P *Child:* **IV** 0.25-2 g/kg as a 15%-20% sol, run over 2-6 hr

Intraocular pressure/ICP
Adult: **IV** 1.5-2 g/kg of a 15%-25% sol over 30-60 min

P *Child:* **IV** 1-2 g/kg (30-60 g/m^2) as a 15%-20% sol run over 30-60 min

Renal failure
Adult: **IV** 50-200 g/24 hr, adjusting to maintain output of 30-50 mg/hr

Diuresis in drug intoxication
P *Adult and child >12 yr:* 5%-10% sol continuously up to 200 g **IV**, while maintaining 100-500 ml urine output/hr

Available forms: Inj 5%, 10%, 15%, 20%, 25%; GU irrigation 5%

Adverse effects
(*italic* = common; **bold** = life-threatening)
CNS: Dizziness, headache, *seizures,* **rebound increased ICP,** confusion
CV: Edema, hypotension, hypertension, **tachycardia, CHF,** thrombophlebitis, angina-like chest pains, fever, chills
EENT: Loss of hearing, blurred vision, nasal congestion, decreased intraocular pressure
ELECT: Fluid, electrolyte imbalances, **acidosis,** electrolyte loss, dehydration
GI: *Nausea, vomiting,* dry mouth, diarrhea
GU: Marked diuresis, urinary retention, thirst
RESP: Pulmonary congestion

Contraindications: Active intracranial bleeding, hypersensitivity, anuria, severe pulmonary congestion, edema, severe dehydration, progressive heart disease, renal failure

Precautions: Dehydration, pregnancy **C,** severe renal disease, CHF, lactation

---

Pharmacokinetics

Absorption	Complete
Distribution	Extracellular spaces
Metabolism	Minimal
Excretion	Renal
Half-life	100 min

Pharmacodynamics

Onset	½-1 hr
Peak	1 hr
Duration	6-8 hr

Interactions
Individual drugs
Lithium: ↓ action, ↑ excretion
Food/drug
Potassium foods: ↑ hyperkalemia
Lab test interferences
Interference: Inorganic phosphorus, ethylene glycol

NURSING CONSIDERATIONS
Assessment
• Assess neurologic status: LOC, ICP reading, pupil size and reaction when drug is given for increased ICP
• Assess for visual changes or eye discomfort or pain before and during treatment; (increases intraocular pressure); neurologic checks, ICP during treatment (increased ICP)
• Assess patient for tinnitus, hearing loss, ear pain; periodic testing of hearing is needed when high doses of this drug are given by **IV** route
• Monitor manifestations of hypokalemia: acidic urine, reduced urine osmolality, nocturia, polyuria, polydipsia; hypotension, broad T wave, U wave, ectopy, tachycardia, weak pulse; muscle weakness, altered LOC, drowsiness, apathy, lethargy, confusion, depression; anorexia, nausea, cramps, constipation, distention, paralytic ileus; hypoventilation, respiratory muscle weakness
• Monitor for manifestations of hyponatremia: increased B/P, cold, clammy skin, hypovolemia or hypervolemia; anorexia, nausea, vomiting, diarrhea, abdominal cramps; lethargy, increased ICP, confusion, headache, seizures, coma, fatigue, tremors, hyperreflexia
• Assess fluid volume status: check I&O ratios and record hourly urine values, CVP, breath sounds, weight, distended red veins, crackles in lung, color, quality and sp gr of urine, skin turgor, adequacy of pulses, moist mucous membranes, bilateral lung sounds, peripheral pitting edema
• Assess for dehydration; symptoms of decreasing output, thirst, hypotension, dry mouth and mucous membranes should be reported
• Monitor electrolytes: potassium, sodium, calcium, magnesium; also include BUN, ABGs, CVP, PAP, CBC; regularly monitor serum and urine levels of sodium and potassium
• Assess B/P before and during therapy with patient lying, standing, and sitting as appropriate; orthostatic hypotension can occur rapidly
• Monitor for rebound ICP: headache, confusion

Nursing diagnoses
☑ Urinary elimination, impaired (adverse reactions)
☑ Fluid volume, deficient (adverse reactions)
☑ Fluid volume, excess (uses)
☑ Knowledge, deficient (teaching)

Implementation
• Administer potassium replacement if potassium level is less than 3 mg/ml
• Use an in-line filter for 15%, 20%, 25% give with infusion pump; check **IV** patency at infusion site before and during administration; do not use sol that is yellow or has a precipitate or crystals; to redissolve, run bottle under hot water and shake vigorously; cool to body temp before giving
• Run at 30-50 ml/hr in oliguria
• Run over 30-60 min in increased ICP
• Run over 30 min for intraocular pressure; 60-90 min after surgery

Irrigation
• Use 100 ml of 25%/900 ml of sterile water for inj (2.5% sol)

Y-site compatibilities: Allopurinol, amifostine, aztreonam, cladribine, fludarabine, fluorouracil, gallium, idarubicin, melphalan, ondansetron, paclitaxel, piperacillin, propofol, sargramostim, teniposide, thiotepa, vinorelbine

Y-site incompatibilities: Amsacrine, bleomycin, DOXOrubicin, fluconazole, gentamicin, quinidine, vinBLAStine, vinCRIStine

Additive compatibilities: Amikacin, bretylium, cefamandole, cefoxitin, cimetidine, cisplatin, DOPamine, fosphenytoin, furosemide, gentamicin, metoclopramide, netilmicin, nizatidine, ofloxacin, ondansetron, sodium bicarbonate, tobramycin, verapamil

Additive incompatibilities: Blood, blood products, imipenem-cilastatin, potassium chloride, sodium chloride

M

Patient/family education
- Teach patient reason for and method of treatment

Evaluation
Positive therapeutic outcome
- Decreased intraocular pressure
- Prevention of hypokalemia (diuretic use)
- Decreased edema
- Decreased ICP
- Increased diuresis of >30 ml/hr
- Increased excretion of toxic substances

Treatment of overdose: Discontinue inf, correct fluid, electrolyte imbalances, hemodialysis, monitor hydration, CV, renal function

---

mebendazole (Rx)
(me-ben'da-zole)
Vermox
Func. class.: Anthelmintic
Chem. class.: Carbamate

Pregnancy category C

Action: Inhibits glucose uptake, degeneration of cytoplasmic microtubules in the cell; interferes with absorption, secretory function

➡ **Therapeutic Outcome:** Parasite, cyst, egg death

Uses: Infestation with pinworms, roundworms, hookworms, whipworms, threadworms, pork tapeworms, dwarf tapeworms, beef tapeworms; hydatid cyst

Dosage and routes
P *Adult and child >2 yr:* PO 100 mg as a single dose (pinworms) or bid × 3 days (whip-, round-, or hookworms); course may be repeated in 3 wk if needed

Available forms: Chew tab 100 mg

Adverse effects
(*italic* = common; **bold** = life-threatening)
CNS: Dizziness, fever, headache
GI: Transient diarrhea, abdominal pain, nausea, vomiting

Contraindication: Hypersensitivity

P **Precautions:** Child <2 yr, lactation, pregnancy C (1st trimester)

Pharmacokinetics
Absorption	Minimal
Distribution	Highly bound to plasma proteins
Metabolism	Liver
Excretion	Feces in metabolites (>95%); urine, unchanged
Half-life	2½-9 hr; increased in hepatic disease

Pharmacodynamics
Onset	Unknown
Peak	½-7 hr
Duration	Unknown

Interactions
Individual drugs
Carbamazepine: ↓ effect of mebendazole
Drug classifications
Hydantoins: ↓ effect of mebendazole
Food/drug
High-fat foods: ↑ absorption

NURSING CONSIDERATIONS
Assessment
- Assess stools during entire treatment, also 1-3 wk after treatment is completed; specimens must be sent to lab while still warm; monitor for diarrhea during expulsion of worms; avoid self-contamination with patient's feces
- Assess for allergic reaction: rash (rare)
- Identify infestation in other family members, since transmission from person to person is common
- If pinworms are suspected, place a piece of cellophane tape over the anal area at night for 1 wk after treatment at night to identify ova; negative perianal swabs taken every ᴀᴍ for 3 days confirm that the patient is no longer infested
- Monitor blood studies: AST, ALT, alkaline phosphatase, BUN, CBC during treatment

Nursing diagnoses
☑ Infection, risk for (uses)
☑ Knowledge, deficient (teaching)

Implementation
- Tabs may be chewed or crushed and mixed with food if patient is unable to swallow whole
- Give PO after meals to avoid GI symptoms, since absorption is not decreased by food
- Give second course after 3 wk if needed; usually recommended (pinworms)
- Store in airtight container

Patient/family education
- Teach patient proper hygiene after bowel movements, including hand-washing tech-

---

nique; tell patient to avoid putting fingers in mouth; clean fingernails

• Advise patient that infested person should sleep alone; do not shake bed linen; wash bed linen daily in hot water; change and wash undergarments daily; that all members of the family should be treated (pinworms)

• Advise patient to clean toilet daily with disinfectant (green soap sol)

• Inform patient that compliance is needed with dosage schedule, duration of treatment

• Tell patient to wear shoes, wash all fruits and vegetables well before eating, use commercial fruit and vegetable cleaner solution

Evaluation
Positive therapeutic outcome
• Expulsion of worms
• Three negative stool cultures after completion of treatment

---

mechlorethamine (Rx)
(me-klor-eth′a-meen)
Mustargen, nitrogen mustard
Func. class.: Antineoplastic alkylating agent
Chem. class.: Nitrogen mustard
Pregnancy category D

Action: Alkylates DNA, RNA; inhibits enzymes that allow synthesis of amino acids in proteins; activity is not cell cycle phase specific; a vesicant

➔ **Therapeutic Outcome:** Prevention of rapidly growing malignant cells

Uses: Hodgkin's disease, lymphomas, leukemias, lymphosarcoma; ovarian, breast, lung carcinoma; neoplastic effusions

Dosage and routes
Adult: **IV** 0.4 mg/kg or 10 mg/m² as 1 dose or 2-4 divided doses over 2-4 days; second course after 3 wk depending on blood cell count

Neoplastic effusions
Adult: Intracavity 0.4 mg/kg, may be 200-400 mcg/kg

Available forms: Inj 10 mg/vial

Adverse effects
(*italic* = common; **bold** = life-threatening)
CNS: *Headache, dizziness, drowsiness, paresthesia,* peripheral neuropathy, **coma**
EENT: Tinnitus, hearing loss
GI: *Nausea, vomiting, diarrhea, stomatitis, weight loss,* colitis, **hepatotoxicity**
HEMA: **Thrombocytopenia, leukopenia, agranulocytosis,** anemia

INTEG: *Alopecia,* pruritus, herpes zoster, extravasation

Contraindications: Lactation, pregnancy **D,** myelosuppression, acute herpes zoster

Precautions: Radiation therapy, chronic lymphocytic leukemia

Pharmacokinetics
Absorption	Complete (**IV**)
Distribution	Unknown
Metabolism	Tissues/fluids
Excretion	Kidneys
Half-life	Unknown

Pharmacodynamics
	IV
Onset	1 day
Peak	1-2 wk
Duration	1-3 wk

Interactions
Individual drugs
Amphotericin B: ↑ blood dyscrasia
Radiation: ↑ toxicity, bone marrow suppression
Drug classifications
Antineoplastics: ↑ toxicity
Antineoplastics, bone marrow–suppressing drugs: ↑ bone marrow suppression
Live virus vaccines: ↓ antibody reaction
Lab test interferences
↑ Uric acid

NURSING CONSIDERATIONS
Assessment
• Monitor CBC, differential, platelet count weekly; withhold drug if WBC is <1000/mm³ or platelet count is <75,000/mm³; notify prescriber of results if WBC <20,000/mm³, platelets <150,000/mm³; recovery of WBC platelets within 20 days

• Monitor pulmonary function tests, chest x-ray films before, during therapy; chest film should be obtained q2 wk during treatment; assess for dyspnea, rales, unproductive cough, chest pain, tachypnea

• Assess for increased uric acid levels, swelling, joint pain primarily in extremities; patient should be well hydrated to prevent urate deposits

• Monitor renal function studies: BUN, serum uric acid, urine CCr before, during therapy; I&O ratio; report fall in urine output of 30 ml/hr; for decreased hyperuricemia

• Monitor for cold, fever, sore throat (may indicate beginning of infection); identify

---

M

edema in feet, joint and stomach pain, shaking; prescriber should be notified
• Assess for bleeding: hematuria, guaiac, bruising or petechiae, mucosa or orifices q8h; no rec temp

Nursing diagnoses
☑ Injury, risk for (adverse reactions)
☑ Body image, disturbed (adverse reactions)
☑ Infection, risk for (adverse reactions)
☑ Knowledge, deficient (teaching)

Implementation
• Give fluids **IV** or PO before chemotherapy to hydrate patient
• Give antacid before oral agent; give drug after evening meal, before hs; administer antiemetic 30-60 min before giving drug and prn to prevent vomiting; give antibiotics for prophylaxis of infection
• Give top or systemic analgesics for pain
• Give in AM so drug can be eliminated before hs
• Use a liq diet: carbonated beverages; gelatin may be added if patient is not nauseated or vomiting

IV IV route
• Give **IV** after diluting 10 mg/10 ml sterile water or 0.9% NaCl; leave needle in vial, shake, withdraw dose, give through Y-tube or 3-way stopcock or directly over 3-5 min into running **IV** of 0.9% NaCl

Y-site compatibilities: Amifostine, aztreonam, filgrastim, fludarabine, granisetron, melphalan, ondansetron, sargramostim, teniposide, vinorelbine

Additive incompatibilities: Methohexital

Solution incompatibilities: D$_5$W, 0.9% NaCl (**IV** only)

Intracavity route
• Further dilute in 100 ml of 0.9% NaCl; administration is completed by prescriber
• Watch for infiltration; if infiltration occurs, infiltrate area with isotonic sodium thiosulfate or 1% lidocaine; apply ice for 6-12 hr

Patient/family education
• Teach patient to avoid use of products containing aspirin or ibuprofen, razors, commercial mouthwash, since bleeding may occur; to report symptoms of bleeding (hematuria, tarry stools)
• Teach patient to report signs of anemia (fatigue, headache, irritability, faintness, shortness of breath)
• Advise patient to report any changes in breathing or coughing even several mo after treatment; to avoid crowds and persons with respiratory tract or other infections
• Tell patient hair loss is common; discuss the use of wigs or hairpieces
• Caution patient not to have any vaccinations without the advice of the prescriber, serious reactions can occur
• Advise patient that contraception is needed during treatment and for several mo after the completion of therapy
• Have patient rinse mouth tid-qid with water, club soda; brush teeth bid-qid with soft brush or cotton-tipped applicators for stomatitis; use unwaxed dental floss

Evaluation
Positive therapeutic outcome
• Decreased size of tumor
• Decreased spread of malignancy
• Improved blood values
• Absence of sweating at night
• Increased appetite, increased weight

---

*medroxyPROGESTERone (Rx)
(me-drox-ee-proe-jess'te-rone)
Amen, Curretab, Cycrin, Depo-Provera, medroxyPROGESTERone, Provera
Func. class.: Hormone—progestogen; contraceptive; antineoplastic
Chem. class.: Progesterone derivative

Pregnancy category X

Action: Inhibits secretion of pituitary gonadotropins, which prevents follicular maturation and ovulation; stimulates growth of mammary tissue; antineoplastic action against endometrial cancer

→ **Therapeutic Outcome:** Decreased abnormal uterine bleeding, absence of amenorrhea

Uses: Uterine bleeding (abnormal), secondary amenorrhea, endometrial cancer, renal cancer, contraceptive, prevention of endometrial changes associated with estrogen replacement therapy (ERT)

Investigational uses: Pickwickian syndrome, sleep apnea, hypersomnolence

Dosage and routes
Secondary amenorrhea
Adult: PO 5-10 mg qd × 5-10 days

Endometrial/renal cancer
Adult: IM 400-1000 mg/wk; may repeat qwk, dose may be decreased after adequate response

---

Uterine bleeding
Adult: PO 5-10 mg qd × 5-10 days starting on 16th or 21st day of menstrual cycle

Contraceptive
Adult: IM 150 mg q3 mo

With ERT
Adult: PO monophasic 2.5 mg qd; biphasic 5 mg days 15-28 of cycle

Available forms: Tabs 2.5, 5, 10 mg; inj susp 50, 100, 150, 400 mg/ml

Adverse effects
(*italic* = common; **bold** = life-threatening)
CNS: Dizziness, headache, migraines, depression, fatigue

CV: Hypotension, thrombophlebitis, edema, **thromboembolism, stroke, pulmonary embolism, MI**

EENT: Diplopia

GI: *Nausea,* vomiting, anorexia, cramps, increased weight, **cholestatic jaundice**

GU: Amenorrhea, cervical erosion, breakthrough bleeding, dysmenorrhea, vaginal candidiasis, breast changes, *gynecomastia, testicular atrophy, impotence,* endometriosis, **spontaneous abortion**

INTEG: Rash, urticaria, acne, hirsutism, alopecia, oily skin, seborrhea, purpura, melasma, photosensitivity

META: Hyperglycemia

SYST: **Angioedema, anaphylaxis**

Contraindications: Breast cancer, hypersensitivity, thromboembolic disorders, reproductive cancer, genital bleeding (abnormal, undiagnosed), pregnancy **X**

Precautions: Lactation, hypertension, asthma, blood dyscrasias, gallbladder disease, CHF, diabetes mellitus, bone disease, depression, migraine headache, seizure disorders, hepatic disease, renal disease, family history of cancer of breast or reproductive tract

◤ Do Not Confuse:
Amen/Ambien, medroxyPROGESTERone/methylPREDNISolone, Provera/Premarin

Pharmacokinetics	
Absorption	Unknown
Distribution	Unknown
Metabolism	Unknown
Excretion	Unknown
Half-life	Unknown

Pharmacodynamics		
	PO	IM
Onset	Unknown	Unknown
Peak	Unknown	Unknown
Duration	2-4 hr	Unknown

Interactions
Individual drugs
Aminoglutethimide: ↓ contraceptive effect
Bromocriptine: ↓ effectiveness
Lab test interferences
↑ Alkaline phosphatase, ↑ pregnanediol, ↑ amino acids, ↑ sodium
↓ GTT, ↓ HDL

NURSING CONSIDERATIONS
Assessment
• Assess for symptoms indicating severe allergic reaction, angioedema; have epINEPHrine and resuscitative equipment available
• Monitor B/P at beginning of treatment and periodically; check weight daily; notify prescriber of weekly weight gain >5 lb
• Monitor I&O ratio: be alert for decreasing urinary output, increasing edema, hypertension
• Assess liver function studies: ALT, AST, bilirubin, periodically during long-term therapy
• Assess for edema, hypertension, cardiac symptoms, jaundice
• Assess mental status: affect, mood, behavioral changes, depression

Nursing diagnoses
☑ Sexual dysfunction (uses)
☑ Tissue perfusion, ineffective (adverse reactions)
☑ Injury, risk for (adverse reactions)
☑ Knowledge, deficient (teaching)

Implementation
PO route
• Give with food or milk to decrease GI symptoms
IM route
• Store in dark area
• Give titrated dosage; use lowest effective dosage; give oil sol deep in large muscle mass (IM); rotate sites; use after warming to dissolve crystals

Patient/family education
• Advise patients to avoid sunlight or use sunscreen; photosensitivity and melasma (brown patches on the face) can occur
• Teach patient about cushingoid symptoms
• Teach women patients to report breast lumps, vaginal bleeding, edema, jaundice,

M

dark urine, clay-colored stools, dyspnea, headache, blurred vision, abdominal pain, numbness or stiffness in legs, chest pain; men to report impotence or gynecomastia
• Teach patient to report suspected pregnancy immediately

Evaluation
Positive therapeutic outcome
• Decreased abnormal uterine bleeding
• Absence of amenorrhea
• Prevention of pregnancy
• Arrested spread of malignant cells

---

megestrol (Rx)
(me-jess'trole)
Megace, megestrol
Func. class.: Antineoplastic hormone
Chem. class.: Progestin

Pregnancy category D (tabs), X (susp)

Action: Affects endometrium by antiluteinizing effect; this is thought to bring about cell death

⮞ Therapeutic Outcome: Prevention of rapidly growing malignant cells; weight gain, increased appetite in AIDS

Uses: Breast, endometrial, renal cell cancer; increase weight, decrease cachexia and anorexia associated with AIDS

Investigational uses: Hot flashes

Dosage and routes
Endometrial/ovarian carcinoma
Adult: PO 40-320 mg/day in divided doses

Breast carcinoma
Adult: PO 40 mg qid or 160 mg qd

Anorexia (AIDS)
Adult: PO 800 mg qd (oral susp)

Hot flashes (off-label)
Adult: PO 20 mg qd

Available forms: Tabs 20, 40 mg; oral susp 40 mg/ml

Adverse effects
(*italic* = common; **bold** = life-threatening)
CNS: Mood swings
CV: **Thrombophlebitis, thrombembolism**
GI: Nausea, vomiting, diarrhea, abdominal cramps, weight gain
GU: Gynecomastia, fluid retention, hypercalcemia, vaginal bleeding, discharge, impotence, decreased libido
INTEG: Alopecia, rash, pruritus, purpura, itching

Contraindications: Hypersensitivity, pregnancy X (susp), D (tabs)

◪ Do Not Confuse:
Megace/Reglan

Pharmacokinetics	
Absorption	Well absorbed
Distribution	Unknown
Metabolism	Liver, completely
Excretion	Unknown
Half-life	1 hr

Pharmacodynamics	
Onset	Several wk-mo
Peak	Unknown
Duration	1-3 days

Interactions: None
Lab test interferences
↑ Alkaline phosphatase, ↑ urinary pregnanediol, ↑ plasma amino acids, ↑ urinary sodium
↓ HDL, ↓ GTT
False positive: Urine glucose

NURSING CONSIDERATIONS
Assessment
• Monitor effects of alopecia on body image; discuss feelings about body changes
• In AIDS patients monitor calorie counts, weight, appetite
• Assess for thrombophlebitis: pain, redness, swelling in legs; notify prescriber immediately if these occur

Nursing diagnoses
☑ Knowledge, deficient (teaching)

Implementation
• Administer with meals for GI symptoms
• Oral susp is usually used for AIDS patients, shake well
• Give tablets for carcinoma

Patient/family education
• Teach patient to report any complaints or side effects to prescriber
• Advise patient that contraceptive measures must be used during and several mo after treatment; drug is teratogenic
• Explore with patient the need for wig or a hairpiece for hair loss
• Caution patient to report vaginal bleeding to prescriber
• Review with patient the need to comply with dosage schedule, not to miss or double doses; missed doses may be taken up to 1 hr before next dose
• Teach patient how to recognize signs of fluid

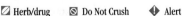

retention, thromboembolism and report immediately

Evaluation
Positive therapeutic outcome
- Decreased spread of malignant cells
- Weight gain, increased appetite in AIDS patients

---

meloxicam (Rx)
(mel-ox'i-kam)
Mobic
Func. class.: Nonsteroidal antiinflammatory/nonopioid analgesic (NSAIDs)
Chem. class.: Oxicam

Pregnancy category C

Action: Inhibits prostaglandin synthesis by decreasing an enzyme needed for biosynthesis; analgesic, antiinflammatory, antipyretic effects

Therapeutic Outcome: Decreased pain, swelling of joints; improved mobility

Uses: Osteoarthritis

Dosage and routes
Adult: PO 7.5 mg qd, may increase to 15 mg qd

Available forms: Tabs 7.5 mg

Adverse effects
(*italic* = common; **bold** = life-threatening)
CV: Hypertension, angina, **cardiac failure, MI,** hypotension, palpitations, **dysrhythmias,** tachycardia
CNS: Dizziness, drowsiness, tremors, headache, nervousness, malaise, fatigue, insomnia, depression, **seizures**
EENT: Tinnitus, hearing loss
GI: Pancreatitis, nausea, colitis, GERD, vomiting, diarrhea, constipation, flatulence, cramps, dry mouth, peptic ulcer, **GI bleeding, perforation**
GU: Nephrotoxicity: **dysuria, hematuria, oliguria, azotemia**
HEMA: **Blood dyscrasias,** anemia, prolonged bleeding
INTEG: Rash, urticaria, photosensitivity
SYST: **Angioedema, anaphylaxis**

Contraindications: Hypersensitivity, asthma, severe renal disease, severe hepatic disease, peptic ulcer disease, labor and delivery, lactation, CV bleeding, avoid in 2nd/3rd trimester

Precautions: Pregnancy **C,** children, bleeding disorders, GI disorders, cardiac disorders, hypersensitivity to other antiinflammatory agents, elderly, CCr <25 ml/min

Pharmacokinetics
Absorption	Unknown
Distribution	Unknown
Metabolism	Liver <50%
Excretion	Breast milk, kidneys
Half-life	6 hr

Pharmacodynamics
	PO	IM
Onset	Unknown	Unknown
Peak	4-5 hr	50 min
Duration	Unknown	Unknown

Interactions
Individual drugs
Cholestyramine: ↓ action of meloxicam
Cyclosporine: ↑ nephrotoxicity
Phenytoin: ↑ action of meloxicam
Drug classifications
Aminoglycosides, anticoagulants, diuretics, hydantoins, salicylates, sulfonamides: ↑ action of each specific drug
β-Adrenergic blockers: ↓ action of β-blockers
Herb/drug
Arginine, gossypol: ↑ gastric irritation
Bearberry, bilberry: ↑ NSAIDs effect
Bogbean, chondroitin: ↑ bleeding risk

NURSING CONSIDERATIONS
Assessment
- Monitor renal, liver, blood studies: BUN, creatinine, AST, ALT, Hgb before treatment, periodically thereafter
- Assess for bleeding times; check for bruising, bleeding; test for occult blood in urine
- Assess for anaphylaxis and angioedema; emergency equipment should be nearby
- Assess for hepatic dysfunction: jaundice, yellow sclera and skin, clay-colored stools
- Assess for audiometric, ophth exam before, during, after treatment
- Assess for GI condition, hypertension, cardiac conditions

Nursing diagnoses
✓ Mobility, impaired (uses)
✓ Pain, chronic (uses)
✓ Knowledge, deficient (teaching)

Implementation
- May take without regard to meals, take with food for GI upset

M

- Take with full glass of water and sit upright for ½ hr
- Store at room temp

Patient/family education
- Advise patient to report blurred vision or ringing, roaring in ears (may indicate toxicity)
- Advise patient to avoid driving, other hazardous activities if dizziness or drowsiness occurs
- Teach patient to report change in urine pattern, weight increase, edema, pain increase in joints, fever, blood in urine (indicates nephrotoxicity); to report rash, black stools, or continuing headache
- Teach patient to avoid alcohol, aspirin, acetaminophen without consulting prescriber

Evaluation
Positive therapeutic outcome
- Decreased pain, stiffness, swelling in joints, able to move more easily

---

! HIGH ALERT

melphalan (Rx)
(mel′fa-lan)
Alkeran, ʟ-Pam, phenylalanine mustard
Func. class.: Antineoplastic, alkylating agent
Chem. class.: Nitrogen mustard

Pregnancy category D

Action: Alkylates DNA, RNA; inhibits enzymes that allow synthesis of amino acids in proteins; activity is not cell cycle phase specific

➔ **Therapeutic Outcome:** Prevention of rapidly growing malignant cells

Uses: Multiple myeloma, malignant melanoma, advanced ovarian cancer

Investigational uses: Breast, testicular, prostate carcinoma; osteogenic sarcoma, chronic myelogenous leukemia

Dosage and routes
Multiple myeloma
Adult: PO 150 mcg/kg/day × 1 wk, then 21 days off, then 50 mcg/kg/day or 100-150 mcg/kg/day or 250 mcg/kg/day × 4 days for 2-3 wk, then 2-4 wk off, then 2-4 mg/day or 7 mg/m² × 5 days q5-6 wk

Adult: **IV** inf 16 mg/m²; reduce in renal insufficiency; give over 15-20 min; give at 2-wk intervals × 4 doses, then at 4-wk intervals

Ovarian carcinoma
Adult: PO 200 mcg/kg/day × 5 days q4-5 wk

Available forms: Tabs 2 mg; inj 50 mg

Adverse effects
(*italic* = common; **bold** = life-threatening)
GI: *Nausea, vomiting,* stomatitis, diarrhea
GU: Amenorrhea, hyperuricemia, gonadal suppression
HEMA: **Thrombocytopenia, neutropenia, leukopenia,** anemia
INTEG: Rash, urticaria, alopecia, pruritus
RESP: **Fibrosis, dysplasia**
SYST: **Anaphylaxis,** allergic reaction

Contraindications: Lactation, pregnancy **D,** hypersensitivity to this drug or other nitrogen mustards

Precautions: Radiation therapy, bone marrow depression, infection, renal disease, ▣ children

▨ Do Not Confuse:
melphalan/myleran

Pharmacokinetics
Absorption	Variable; incompletely absorbed
Distribution	Rapidly distributed
Metabolism	Bloodstream
Excretion	Kidneys, unchanged (10%)
Half-life	1½ hr

Pharmacodynamics
Unknown

Interactions
Individual drugs
Carmustine: ↑ pulmonary toxicity
CycloSPORINE: ↑ renal failure risk
Nalidixic acid: ↑ enterocolitis risk
Radiation: ↑ toxicity, bone marrow suppression
Drug classifications
Antineoplastics: ↑ toxicity
Antineoplastics, bone marrow–suppressing drugs: ↑ bone marrow suppression
Live virus vaccines: ↑ adverse reactions, ↓ antibody reaction

Lab test interferences
↑ Uric acid

NURSING CONSIDERATIONS
Assessment
- Monitor CBC, differential, platelet count weekly; withhold drug if WBC is <3000/mm³ or platelet count is <100,000/mm³; notify prescriber of results if WBC <20,000/mm³, platelets <100,000/mm³; recovery usually occurs in 6 wk
- Monitor pulmonary function tests, chest x-ray films before, during therapy; chest film should be obtained q2 wk during treatment;

check for dyspnea, rales, unproductive cough, chest pain, tachypnea

• Assess for increased uric acid levels, swelling, joint pain primarily in extremities; patient should be well hydrated to prevent urate deposits

• Monitor renal function studies: BUN, serum uric acid, urine CCr before, during therapy; check I&O ratio; report fall in urine output of 30 ml/hr; check for decreased hyperuricemia; monitor AST, ALT

• Monitor for cold, fever, sore throat (may indicate beginning of infection); identify edema in feet, joint and stomach pain, shaking; prescriber should be notified

• Assess for bleeding: hematuria, guaiac, bruising or petechiae, from mucosa or orifices q8h; no rec temp

• Assess for symptoms indicating severe allergic reaction: rash, pruritus, urticaria, purpuric skin lesions, itching, flushing; assess allergy to chlorambucil, cross-sensitivity may occur

Nursing diagnoses
✓ Injury, risk for (adverse reactions)
✓ Body image, disturbed (adverse reactions)
✓ Infection, risk for (adverse reactions)
✓ Knowledge, deficient (teaching)

Implementation
• Give fluids **IV** or PO before chemotherapy to hydrate patient

• Give antacid before oral agent; give drug after evening meal, before hs; provide antiemetic 30-60 min before giving drug and prn to prevent vomiting; give antibiotics for prophylaxis of infection

• Give in AM so drug can be eliminated before hs

• Use a liq diet: carbonated beverages; gelatin may be added if patient is not nauseated or vomiting

PO route
• Give 1 hr ac or 2 hr pc to prevent nausea/vomiting

IV IV route
• Give as intermittent inf: reconstitute with provided diluent (10 ml) to 5 mg/ml; shake until clear; further dilute with 0.9% NaCl to <0.45 mg/ml; give over 15 min, give within 1 hr

Y-site compatibilities: Acyclovir, amikacin, aminophylline, ampicillin, aztreonam, bleomycin, bumetanide, buprenorphine, butorphanol, calcium gluconate, carboplatin, carmustine, cefazolin, cefepime, cefoperazone, cefotaxime, cefotetan, ceftazidime, ceftizoxime, ceftriaxone, cefuroxime, cimetidine, cisplatin,

clindamycin, cyclophosphamide, cytarabine, dacarbazine, dactinomycin, DAUNOrubicin, dexamethasone, diphenhydrAMINE, DOXOrubicin, doxycycline, droperidol, enalaprilat, etoposide, famotidine, floxuridine, fluconazole, fludarabine, fluorouracil, furosemide, gallium, ganciclovir, gentamicin, granisetron, haloperidol, heparin, hydrocortisone sodium phosphate, hydromorphone, hydrOXYzine, idarubicin, ifosfamide, imipenem-cilastatin, lorazepam, mannitol, mechlorethamine, meperidine, mesna, methylPREDNISolone, metoclopramide, methotrexate, metronidazole, miconazole, minocycline, mitomycin, mitoxantrone, morphine, nalbuphine, netilmicin, ondansetron, pentostatin, piperacillin, plicamycin, potassium chloride, prochlorperazine, promethazine, ranitidine, sodium bicarbonate, streptozocin, teniposide, thiotepa, ticarcillin, ticarcillin/clavulanate, tobramycin, trimethoprim/sulfamethoxazole, vancomycin, vinBLAStine, vinCRIStine, vinorelbine, zidovudine

Patient/family education
• Teach patient to avoid use of products containing aspirin or ibuprofen, razors, commercial mouthwash, since bleeding may occur; to report symptoms of bleeding (hematuria, tarry stools)

• Instruct patient to report signs of anemia (fatigue, headache, irritability, faintness, shortness of breath)

• Instruct patient to report any changes in breathing or coughing even several mo after treatment; to avoid crowds and persons with respiratory tract or other infections

• Tell patient hair loss is common; discuss the use of wigs or hairpieces

• Caution patient not to have any vaccinations without the advice of the prescriber, serious reactions can occur

• Advise patient that contraception is needed during treatment and for several mo after the completion of therapy

• Teach patient to rinse mouth tid-qid with water, club soda; brush teeth bid-qid with soft brush or cotton-tipped applicators for stomatitis; use unwaxed dental floss

Evaluation
Positive therapeutic outcome
• Decreased size of tumor
• Decreased spread of malignancy

M

memantine
Namenda
See Appendix A, Selected New Drugs

---

menotropins (Rx)
(men-oh-troe′pinz)
Humegon, Pergonal, Repronex
Func. class.: Gonadotropin
Chem. class.: Exogenous gonadotropin
Pregnancy category X

Action: In women, increases follicular growth, maturation; in men, when given with hCG, stimulates spermatogenesis; contains FSH and LH

➡ **Therapeutic Outcome:** Pregnancy, ovulation

Uses: Infertility, anovulation in women; stimulates spermatogenesis in men; usually used with hCG

Dosage and routes
Infertility
Adult (men): IM 1 ampule 3 times a wk with hCG 2000 units 2 times a wk × 4 mo

Anovulation
Adult (women): IM 75 international units of FSH, LH qd × 9-12 days, then 10,000 units of hCG 1 day after these drugs; repeat × 2 menstrual cycles, then increase to 150 international units of FSH, LH qd × 9-12 days, then 10,000 units of hCG 1 day after these drugs × 2 menstrual cycles

Available forms: Powder for inj lyophilized 75, 150 international units FSH, LH activity

Adverse effects
(*italic* = common; **bold** = life-threatening)
CNS: Fever
CV: **Hypovolemia**, thrombophlebitis, **pulmonary embolism, thromboembolism**
GI: *Nausea*, vomiting, diarrhea, anorexia, abdominal distention/pain
GU: **Ovarian enlargement**, multiple births, ovarian hyperstimulation, sudden ovarian enlargement, ascites with or without pain, gynecomastia in men
HEMA: **Hemoperitoneum, arterial thromboembolism**
RESP: **ARDS, pulmonary embolism, pulmonary infarction, pleural effusion**
OTHER: Anaphylaxis

Contraindications: Primary ovarian failure, abnormal bleeding, thyroid/adrenal dys-

function, organic intracranial lesion, ovarian cysts, primary testicular failure, pregnancy **X**

Pharmacokinetics
Absorption	Well absorbed
Distribution	Unknown
Metabolism	Unknown
Excretion	Kidneys, unchanged (8%)
Half-life	70 hr (FSH); 4 hr (LH)

Pharmacodynamics
Unknown

Interactions: None

NURSING CONSIDERATIONS
Assessment
• Monitor weight qd; notify prescriber if weight gain increases rapidly
• Monitor estrogen excretion level; if >100 mcg/24 hr, drug is withheld; hyperstimulation syndrome may occur
• Monitor I&O ratio; be alert for decreasing urinary output
• Assess for ovarian enlargement, abdominal distention/pain; report symptoms immediately

Nursing diagnoses
☑ Sexual dysfunction (uses)
☑ Knowledge, deficient (teaching)

Implementation
• Give after reconstituting with 1-2 ml of sterile saline inj; use immediately

Patient/family education
• Advise patient that multiple births are possible; if pregnancy occurs, it is usually 4-6 wk after start of treatment
• Instruct patient to keep daily appointment for 2 wk during treatment

Evaluation
Positive therapeutic outcome
• Pregnancy

⚠ HIGH ALERT

meperidine ⊙π (Rx)
(me-per′i-deen)
Demerol, meperidine HCl, Pethandol, Pethidine
Func. class.: Opioid analgesic
Chem. class.: Phenylpiperidine derivative

Pregnancy category B
Controlled substance schedule II

Action: Depresses pain impulse transmission at the spinal cord level by interacting with opioid receptors; produces CNS depression

---

 Herb/drug   Do Not Crush   Alert   Key Drug   Geriatric   Pediatric

→ **Therapeutic Outcome:** Relief of pain

Uses: Moderate to severe pain, preoperatively, during labor

Investigational uses: Rigors

Dosage and routes
Pain
Adult: PO/SC/IM 50-150 mg q3-4h prn; **IV** 15-35 mg/hr as a cont inf; PCA 10 mg, then 1-5 mg incremental dose; lockout interval 6-10 min

P *Child:* PO/SC/IM 1 mg/kg q3-4h prn, not to exceed 100 mg q4h

Preoperatively
Adult: IM/SC 50-100 mg q30-90 min before surgery; dosage should be reduced if given **IV**

P *Child:* IM/SC 1-2.2 mg/kg 30-90 min before surgery

Renal dose
Adult: CCr 10-50 ml/min 75% of dose; CCr <10 ml/min 50% of dose

Labor analgesia
Adult: SC/IM 50-100 mg given when contractions are regulary spaced, repeat q1-3h prn

Available forms: Inj 10, 25, 50, 75, 100 mg/ml; tabs 50, 100 mg; syr 50 mg/5 ml

Adverse effects
(*italic* = common; **bold** = life-threatening)
CNS: Drowsiness, dizziness, confusion, headache, sedation, euphoria, **increased ICP, seizures**
CV: Palpitations, bradycardia, change in B/P, tachycardia (**IV**)
EENT: Tinnitus, blurred vision, miosis, diplopia, depressed corneal reflex
GI: Nausea, vomiting, anorexia, constipation, cramps
GU: Urinary retention, dysuria
INTEG: Rash, urticaria, bruising, flushing, diaphoresis, pruritus
RESP: **Respiratory depression**

Contraindications: Hypersensitivity, addiction (opiate)

Precautions: Addictive personality, pregnancy **B**, lactation, increased ICP, MI (acute), severe heart disease, respiratory depression, **P** hepatic disease, renal disease, child <18 yr, **G** elderly

◩ **Do Not Confuse:**
Demerol/Dilaudid, meperidine/
hydromorphone
meprobamate/morphine

Pharmacokinetics

Absorption	Well absorbed (IM, SC); 50% (PO)
Distribution	Widely distributed; crosses placenta
Metabolism	Liver, extensively
Excretion	Kidneys; breast milk
Half-life	3-4 hr

Pharmacodynamics

	PO	IM/SC	IV
Onset	15 min	10 min	Rapid
Peak	½-1 hr	½-1 hr	5-7 min
Duration	2-4 hr	2-4 hr	2-4 hr

Interactions
Individual drugs
Alcohol: ↑ respiratory depression, hypotension, sedation
Phenytoin: ↓ meperidine effect
Procarbazine: Fatal reaction, do not use together
Drug classifications
Antihistamines, barbiturates, CNS depressants, phenothiazines, sedative/hypnotics: ↑ respiratory depression
Antihistamines, CNS depressants, phenothiazines, sedative/hypnotics: ↑ hypotension
MAOIs: Do not use for 2 wk before taking meperidine
Protease inhibitor antiretrovirals: ↑ adverse reactions
◩ *Herb/drug*
Chamomile, hops, Jamaican dogwood, kava, mistletoe, nettle, pokeweed, poppy, senega, skullcap, valerian: ↑ CNS depression
Parsley: May promote serotonin syndrome, avoid concurrent medicinal use
Lab test interferences
↑ Amylase

NURSING CONSIDERATIONS
Assessment
● Assess pain: location, duration, intensity before and 1 hr (IM, SC, PO) and 5-10 min (**IV**) after administration
● Assess renal function before initiating therapy; poor renal function can lead to accumulation of toxic metabolite and seizures
● Monitor VS after parenteral route; note muscle rigidity, drug history, liver, kidney function tests, respiratory dysfunction: respiratory depression, character, rate, rhythm; notify prescriber if respirations are <10/min
● Monitor CNS changes: dizziness, drowsiness, hallucinations, euphoria, LOC, pupil reaction; these are due to metabolite produced, CNS stimulation occurs with chronic or high doses
● Monitor allergic reactions: rash, urticaria

M

Nursing diagnoses

☑ Pain, acute (uses)
☑ Sensory perception, disturbed: visual, auditory (adverse reactions)
☑ Breathing pattern, ineffective (adverse reactions)
☑ Injury, risk for (adverse reactions)
☑ Knowledge, deficient (teaching)

Implementation

• Give with antiemetic if nausea, vomiting occur
• Administer when pain is beginning to return; determine dosage interval by patient response; continuous dosing of medication is more effective given prn
• Medication should be slowly withdrawn after long-term use to prevent withdrawal symptoms
• Store in light-resistant container at room temp

PO route
• May be given with food or milk to lessen GI upset
• Syr should be mixed with 4 oz of water

IM/SC route
• Do not give if cloudy or a precipitate has formed
• Patient should remain recumbent for 1 hr after administration

Ⅳ IV route
• Give by direct **IV** after diluting to 10 mg/ml with sterile water, 0.9% NaCl for inj; give slowly at 25 mg/1 min; rapid administration may cause respiratory depression, hypotension, circulatory collapse
• Give cont inf after diluting to 1 mg/ml with D_5W, $D_{10}W$, dextrose/saline combinations, dextrose/Ringer's, inj combinations, 0.45% NaCl, 0.9% NaCl, Ringer's, LR; give by infusion pump; titrate according to response

Syringe compatibilities: Atropine, benzquinamide, butorphanol, chlorproMAZINE, cimetidine, dimenhyDRINATE, diphenhydrAMINE, droperidol, fentanyl, glycopyrrolate, hydrOXYzine, ketamine, metoclopramide, midazolam, pentazocine, perphenazine, prochlorperazine, promazine, promethazine, ranitidine, scopolamine

Syringe incompatibilities: Heparin, morphine, pentobarbital

Y-site compatibilities: Amifostine, amikacin, ampicillin, atenolol, aztreonam, bumetanide, cefamandole, cefazolin, cefmetazole, cefotaxime, cefotetan, cefoxitin, ceftazidime, ceftizoxime, ceftriaxone, cefuroxime, cephalothin, cephapirin, chloram-

phenicol, cladribine, clindamycin, dexamethasone, diltiazem, diphenhydrAMINE, DOBUTamine, DOPamine, doxycycline, droperidol, erythromycin lactobionate, famotidine, filgrastim, fluconazole, fludarabine, gallium, gentamicin, granisetron, heparin, hydrocortisone, regular insulin, kanamycin, labetalol, lidocaine, magnesium sulfate, melphalan, methyldopate, methylPREDNISolone, metoclopramide, metoprolol, metronidazole, moxalactam, ondansetron, oxacillin, oxytocin, paclitaxel, penicillin G potassium, piperacillin, potassium chloride, propofol, propranolol, ranitidine, sargramostim, teniposide, thiotepa, ticarcillin, ticarcillin/clavulanate, tobramycin, trimethoprim/sulfamethoxazole, vancomycin, verapamil, vinorelbine

Y-site incompatibilities: Cefoperazone, idarubicin, imipenem/cilastatin, mezlocillin, minocycline

Additive compatibilities: Cefazolin, DOBUTamine, ondansetron, scopolamine, succinylcholine, triflupromazine, verapamil

Patient/family education

• Advise patients to avoid CNS depressants (alcohol, sedative/hypnotics) for at least 24 hr after taking this drug
• Discuss with patient that dizziness, drowsiness, and confusion are common; to avoid getting up without assistance
• Discuss in detail with patient all aspects of the drug, including its purpose and what to expect
• Caution patient to make position changes carefully to lessen orthostatic hypotension

Evaluation

Positive therapeutic outcome
• Decreased pain

Treatment of overdose: Naloxone 0.2-0.8 mg **IV**, O_2, **IV** fluids, vasopressors

---

mercaptopurine (Rx)
(mer-kap-toe-pyoor′een)
6-MP, Purinethol
Func. class.: Antineoplastic, antimetabolite
Chem. class.: Purine analog

Pregnancy category D

Action: Inhibits purine metabolism at multiple sites, which inhibits DNA and RNA synthesis S phase of cell cycle

⇥ **Therapeutic Outcome:** Prevention of rapidly growing malignant cells

Uses: Chronic myelocytic leukemia, acute

P lymphoblastic leukemia in children, acute
myelogenous leukemia

Investigational uses: Polycythemia
vera, psoriatic arthritis, colitis, lymphoma

Dosage and routes
Adult: PO 80-100 mg/m² qd, max 5 mg/kg/
day; maintenance 1.5-2.5 mg/kg/day
P *Child:* 75 mg/m²/day (2.5 mg/kg/day);
maintenance 1.5-2.5 mg/kg/day

Available forms: Tabs 50 mg

Adverse effects
(*italic* = common; **bold** = life-threatening)
CNS: Fever, headache, weakness
*GI: Nausea, vomiting, anorexia, diarrhea,
stomatitis,* **hepatotoxicity** (with high doses),
jaundice, gastritis
GU: **Renal failure,** hyperuricemia, **oliguria,**
crystalluria, **hematuria**
HEMA: **Thrombocytopenia, leukopenia,
myelosuppression, anemia**
INTEG: Rash, dry skin, urticaria

Contraindications: Patients with prior
drug resistance, leukopenia (<2500/mm³),
thrombocytopenia (<100,000/mm³), anemia,
pregnancy **D,** lactation

Precautions: Renal disease

Pharmacokinetics

Absorption	Variable
Distribution	Widely—body water
Metabolism	Liver—extensively
Excretion	Kidneys unchanged (small amounts)
Half-life	Unknown

Pharmacodynamics
Unknown

Interactions
Individual drugs
Allopurinol, cotrimoxazole, radiation: ↑ bone
marrow depression
Cyclophosphamide: ↑ cardiotoxicity, CHF
Radiation: ↑ toxicity
Warfarin: ↑ or ↓ effect of warfarin
Drug classifications
Antineoplastics: ↑ toxicity, bone marrow
suppression
Hepatotoxic agents: ↑ hepatotoxicity
Live virus vaccines: ↓ antibodies
Nondepolarizing muscle relaxants: Reversal of
neuromuscular blockade

NURSING CONSIDERATIONS
Assessment
• Assess buccal cavity q8h for dryness, sores
or ulceration, white patches, oral pain, bleeding, dysphagia; obtain prescription for viscous
lidocaine (Xylocaine)
◆• Assess symptoms indicating severe allergic
reaction: rash, pruritus, urticaria, purpuric
skin lesions, itching, flushing
• Monitor CBC, differential, platelet count
weekly; withhold drug if WBC is <4000/mm³
or platelet count is <100,000/mm³; notify
prescriber of results if WBC <20,000/mm³,
platelets <150,000/mm³
• Assess for increased uric acid levels, swelling, joint pain primarily in extremities; patient
should be well hydrated to prevent urate
deposits
• Monitor renal function studies: BUN, creatinine, serum uric acid, urine CCr before and
during therapy; check I&O ratio; report fall in
urine output to <30 ml/hr
• Monitor temp q4h (may indicate beginning
of infection)
• Monitor liver function tests before and
during therapy (bilirubin, AST, ALT, LDH) as
needed or monthly; check for yellowing of skin
or sclera, dark urine, clay-colored stools, itchy
skin, abdominal pain, fever, diarrhea
• Assess for bleeding: hematuria, stool guaiac,
bruising or petechiae, mucosa or orifices q8h;
check for inflammation of mucosa, breaks in
skin

Nursing diagnoses
☑ Injury, risk for (adverse reactions)
☑ Body image, disturbed (adverse reactions)
☑ Infection, risk for (adverse reactions)
☑ Knowledge, deficient (teaching)

Implementation
• Give fluids **IV** or PO before chemotherapy
to hydrate patient
• Give antiemetic 30-60 min before giving
drug and prn to prevent vomiting; give antibiotics for prophylaxis of infection
• Give in AM so drug can be eliminated before hs
• Provide liq diet: carbonated beverages;
gelatin may be added if patient is not nauseated or vomiting
• Encourage patient to rinse mouth tid-qid
with water, club soda; brush teeth bid-qid with
soft brush or cotton-tipped applicators for
stomatitis; use unwaxed dental floss
• Tab may be crushed and added to fluids or
food to facilitate swallowing

Patient/family education
• Advise patient that contraceptive measures

M

are recommended during therapy; serious teratogenic effects may occur, to avoid breast-feeding
• Teach patient to avoid use of products containing aspirin or NSAIDs, razors, commercial mouthwash, since bleeding may occur; to report symptoms of bleeding (hematuria, tarry stools)
• Instruct patient to report signs of anemia (fatigue, headache, irritability, faintness, shortness of breath)
• Instruct patient to report any changes in breathing or coughing even several mo after treatment; to avoid crowds and persons with respiratory tract or other infections
• Caution patient not to have any vaccinations without the advice of the prescriber; serious reactions can occur

Evaluation
Positive therapeutic outcome
• Prevention of rapid division of malignant cells

---

meropenem (Rx)
(mer-oh-pen'em)
Merrem **IV**
Func. class.: Antiinfective—misc.

Pregnancy category B

Action: Interferes with cell wall replication of susceptible organisms; osmotically unstable cell wall swells and bursts from osmotic pressure

➡ **Therapeutic Outcome:** Bactericidal action against the following: *Streptococcus pneumoniae,* group A β-hemolytic streptococci, *viridans* group streptococci, enterococcus; gram-negative organisms *Klebsiella, Proteus, Escherichia coli, Pseudomonas aeruginosa, Bacteroides fragilis, Bacteroides thetaiotamicron,* bacterial
P meningitis (>3 mo old)

Uses: Serious infections caused by gram-positive or gram-negative organisms (appendicitis, peritonitis)

Dosage and routes
Adult: **IV** 1 g q8h, given over 15-30 min or as an **IV** bolus 5-20 ml given over 3-5 min

Renal dose
Adult: **IV** CCr 26-50 ml/min 1 g q12h; CCr 10-25 ml/min 500 mg q12h; CCr <10 ml/min 500 mg q24h

P *Child ≥ 3 mo:* **IV** 20-40 mg/kg q8h (max 2 g q8h meningitis)

P *Child >50 kg:* **IV** 1 g q8h (intraabdominal infection) or 2 g q8h (meningitis) given over 15-30 min or as an **IV** bolus 5-20 ml over 3-5 min

Available forms: Inj 500 mg, 1 g

Adverse effects
(*italic* = common; **bold** = life-threatening)
CNS: Fever, somnolence, *seizures,* dizziness, weakness, *headache*
CV: Hypotension, palpitations
GI: Diarrhea, nausea, vomiting, **pseudomembranous colitis, hepatitis,** glossitis
HEMA: **Eosinophilia, neutropenia,** decreased Hgb, Hct
INTEG: Rash, urticaria, *pruritus,* pain at inj site, phlebitis, erythema at inj site
RESP: Chest discomfort, dyspnea, hyperventilation
SYST: **Anaphylaxis**

Contraindications: Hypersensitivity to meropenem or imipenem

Precautions: Pregnancy **B,** lactation, **G** elderly, renal disease

Pharmacokinetics	
Absorption	Complete bioavailability
Distribution	Widely distributed
Metabolism	Liver
Excretion	Kidneys
Half-life	1 hr; increased in renal disease

Pharmacodynamics	
Onset	Rapid
Peak	Dose dependent

Interactions
Individual drugs
Probenecid: ↑ meropenem levels
Lab test interferences
False positive: Direct Coombs' test
↑ AST, ↑ ALT, ↑ LDH, ↑ BUN, ↑ alkaline phosphatase, ↑ bilirubin, ↑ creatinine

NURSING CONSIDERATIONS
Assessment
• Assess patient for previous sensitivity reaction to carbapenem antiinfectives, penicillins
• Assess patient for signs and symptoms of infection, including characteristics of wounds, sputum, urine, stool, WBC >10,000/100 mm^3, fever; obtain baseline information before and during treatment
• Complete C&S tests before beginning drug therapy to identify if correct treatment has been initiated
• Assess for allergic reactions, anaphylaxis:

---

rash, urticaria, pruritus, chills, fever, joint pain; angioedema may occur a few days after therapy begins; epINEPHrine and resuscitation equipment should be available for anaphylactic reaction

• Identify urine output; if decreasing, notify prescriber (may indicate nephrotoxicity); also check for increased BUN, creatinine

• Monitor blood studies: AST, ALT, CBC, Hct, bilirubin, LDH, alkaline phosphatase, Coombs' test monthly if patient is on long-term therapy

• Monitor electrolytes: potassium, sodium, chloride monthly if patient is on long-term therapy

• Assess bowel pattern qd; if severe diarrhea occurs, drug should be discontinued; may indicate pseudomembranous colitis

• Monitor for bleeding: ecchymosis, bleeding gums, hematuria, stool guaiac daily on long-term therapy

• Assess for overgrowth of infection: perineal itching, fever, malaise, redness, pain, swelling, drainage, rash, diarrhea, change in cough, sputum

Nursing diagnoses
☑ Infection, risk for (uses)
☑ Diarrhea (adverse reactions)
☑ Injury, risk for (adverse reactions)
☑ Knowledge, deficient (teaching)
☑ Noncompliance (teaching)

Implementation
IV IV route
• Reconstitute with 0.9% NaCl, D_5W, LR, dilute in 5-20 ml of compatible sol; give by direct **IV** over 3-5 min
• Give by intermittent inf, dilute in 5-20 ml of compatible sol, give over 15-30 min

Y-site compatibilities: Aminophylline, atenolol, atropine, cimetidine, dexamethasone, digoxin, diphenhydrAMINE, enalaprilat, fluconazole, furosemide, gentamicin, heparin, insulin (regular), metoclopramide, morphine, norepinephrine, phenobarbital, vancomycin

Additive compatibilities: Aminophylline, atropine, cimetidine, dexamethasone, DOBUTamine, DOPamine, enalaprilat, fluconazole, furosemide, gentamicin, heparin, insulin (regular), magnesium sulfate, metoclopramide, morphine, norepinephrine, phenobarbital, ranitidine, vancomycin

Patient/family education
• Teach patient to report sore throat, bruising, bleeding, joint pain; may indicate blood dyscrasias (rare)
• Advise patient to contact prescriber if vaginal itching, loose foul-smelling stools,

furry tongue occur; may indicate superinfection
• Advise patient to avoid breastfeeding, drug is excreted in breast milk
• Advise patient to notify prescriber of diarrhea with blood or pus, may indicate pseudomembranous colitis

Evaluation
Positive therapeutic outcome
• Absence of signs/symptoms of infection (WBC <10,000/mm³, temp WNL, absence of red draining wounds)
• Reported improvement in symptoms of infection

Treatment of anaphylaxis:
EpINEPHrine, antihistamines, resuscitate if needed

---

mesalamine (Rx)
(mez-al'a-meen)
Asacol, Canasa, Mesasal, Pentasa, Rowasa, Salofulk ✦
Func class.: GI antiinflammatory
Chem class.: 5-Aminosalicylic acid
Pregnancy category B

Action: May diminish inflammation by blocking cyclooxygenase, inhibiting prostaglandin production in colon, local action only

➔**Therapeutic Outcome:** Decreased cramping, pain in GI conditions

Uses: Mild to moderate active distal ulcerative colitis, proctosigmoiditis, proctitis

Dosage and routes
Adult: Rec 60 ml (4 g) hs, retained for 8 hr × 3-6 wk; PO 800 mg tid for 6 wk; supp 500 mg bid for 3-6 wk

Available forms: Rec susp 4 g/60 ml; supp 500 mg; delayed rel tabs 400 mg; caps cont rel 250 mg (Pentasa)

Adverse effects
(*italic* = common; **bold** = life-threatening)
CNS: Headache, fever, dizziness, insomnia, asthenia, weakness, fatigue
CV: Pericarditis, myocarditis
EENT: Sore throat, cough, pharyngitis, rhinitis
GI: Cramps, gas, nausea, diarrhea, rectal pain, constipation
INTEG: Rash, itching, acne
SYST: Flu, malaise, back pain, peripheral edema, leg and joint pain, arthralgia, dysmenorrhea, **anaphylaxis,** acute intolerance syndrome

M

Contraindications: Hypersensitivity to this drug or salicylates

Precautions: Renal disease, pregnancy **B**, **P** lactation, children, sulfite sensitivity

N Do Not Confuse:
Asacol/Ansaid

Pharmacokinetics	
Absorption	20%-30% (PO), 10%-25% (rec)
Distribution	Unknown
Metabolism	Unknown
Excretion	Feces
Half-life	1 hr; metabolite 5-10 hr

Pharmacodynamics	
Unknown	

Interactions
Individual drugs
Omeprazole: ↑ mesalamine absorption
Lab test interferences
↑ AST, ↑ ALT, ↑ alkaline phosphatase, ↑ LDH, ↑ GGTP, ↑ amylase, ↑ lipase

NURSING CONSIDERATIONS
Assessment
• Assess for GI symptoms: cramping, gas, nausea, diarrhea, rectal pain, abdominal pain; if severe, the drug should be discontinued
• Assess for allergy to salicylates, sulfonamides; if allergic reactions occur, discontinue drug
• Assess renal function before and during treatment: BUN, creatinine
• Monitor I & O ratios, increase fluids to 1500 ml qd to prevent crystalluria

Nursing diagnoses
☑ Pain, chronic (uses)
☑ Diarrhea (uses)
☑ Knowledge, deficient (teaching)

Implementation
PO route
◎• Do not crush, chew tabs
• May give orally
Rectal route (susp)
• Give hs, retained until AM; empty bowel before insertion
• Store at room temp
• Usual course of therapy is 3-6 wk
• Give after shaking bottle well

Patient/family education
• Advise patient to notify prescriber if abdominal pain, cramping, diarrhea with blood, headache, fever, rash, chest pain occur; drug should be discontinued

• Teach correct administration for PO, or enema

Evaluation
Positive therapeutic outcome
• Absence of pain, bleeding from GI tract

---

metaproterenol (Rx)
(met-a-proe-ter'e-nole)
Alupent
Func. class.: Selective β₂-agonist, bronchodilator

Pregnancy category C

Action: Relaxes bronchial smooth muscle by direct action on β₂-adrenergic receptors, with increased levels of cAMP and increased bronchodilatation, diuresis, and cardiac and CNS stimulation

⇒**Therapeutic Outcome:** Bronchodilatation with ease of breathing

Uses: Bronchial asthma, bronchospasm

Dosage and routes
P *Adult and child >12 yr:* INH 2-3 puffs; may repeat q3-4h, not to exceed 12 puffs/day

Asthma/bronchospasm
Adult: PO 20 mg q6-8h

G *Elderly:* PO 10 mg tid-qid, initially

P *Child >9 yr or >27 kg:* PO 20 mg q6-8h or 0.4-0.9 mg/kg tid

P *Child 6-9 yr or <27 kg:* PO 10 mg q6-8h or 0.4-0.9 mg/kg tid

P *Child 2-6 yr:* PO 1.3-2.6 mg/kg divided q6-8h

Available forms: Tabs 10, 20 mg; aerosol 0.65 mg/dose; syr 10 mg/5 ml; sol for inh 0.4%, 0.6%, 5%

Adverse effects
(*italic* = common; **bold** = life-threatening)
CNS: Tremors, anxiety, insomnia, headache, dizziness, stimulation
CV: Palpitations, tachycardia, hypertension, **dysrhythmias, cardiac arrest** (high dose)
GI: Nausea, vomiting, dry mouth
RESP: **Paradoxical bronchospasm**

Contraindications: Hypersensitivity to sympathomimetics, narrow-angle glaucoma, cardiac dysrhythmias with tachycardia

Precautions: Pregnancy **C**, cardiac disorders, hyperthyroidism, diabetes mellitus, **G** prostatic hypertrophy, seizure disorder, elderly, **P** child <6 yr (PO)

◪ Do Not Confuse:
Alupent/Atrovent

Pharmacokinetics

Absorption	Well absorbed (PO)
Distribution	Unknown
Metabolism	Liver, tissues
Excretion	Unknown
Half-life	2-4 hr

Pharmacodynamics

	PO	INH
Onset	15 min	5 min
Peak	1 hr	1 hr
Duration	4 hr	1-6 hr

Interactions
Drug classifications
β-Adrenergic blockers: Block therapeutic effect
Bronchodilators, aerosol: ↑ action of bronchodilator
MAOIs: ↑ chance of hypertensive crisis
Sympathomimetics: ↑ effects of both drugs
◪ Herb/drug
Coffee, cola nut, guarana, tea (black/green): ↑ effect

NURSING CONSIDERATIONS
Assessment
• Monitor respiratory function: vital capacity, FEV, ABGs, lung sounds, heart rate, rhythm (baseline)
• Determine that patient has not received theophylline therapy before giving dose; identify client's ability to self-medicate
• Monitor for evidence of allergic reactions; paradoxic bronchospasm; withhold dose; notify prescriber

Nursing diagnoses
☑ Airway clearance, ineffective (uses)
☑ Gas exchange, impaired (uses)
☑ Knowledge, deficient (teaching)

Implementation
Aerosol route
• Give after shaking, exhale, place mouthpiece in mouth, inhale slowly, hold breath, remove, exhale slowly; allow at least 1 min between inhalations
• Store in light-resistant container, do not expose to temp over 86° F (30° C)
◪ • Provide spacer device for elderly
PO route
• Give PO with meals to decrease gastric
◪ irritation; syr to children (no alcohol, sugar)

Patient/family education
• Advise patient not to use OTC medications; excess stimulation may occur; to use this medication before other medications and allow at least 5 min between each to prevent overstimulation
• Teach patient use of inhaler; review package insert with patient; teach patient to avoid getting aerosol in eyes, since blurring may result; to wash inhaler in warm water qd and dry; to avoid smoking, smoke-filled rooms, persons with respiratory tract infections
• Advise patient that paradoxic bronchospasm may occur and to stop drug immediately and notify prescriber; to limit caffeine products such as chocolate, coffee, tea, and colas
• Instruct patient on administration of dose; not to use more than prescribed; serious side effects may occur

Evaluation
Positive therapeutic outcome
• Absence of dyspnea, wheezing after 1 hr
• Improved airway exchange
• Improved ABGs

Treatment of overdose: Administer a β₁-adrenergic blocker

M

metformin (Rx)
(met-for′min)
Glucophage, Glucophage XR, Novo-Metformin ✦
Func. class.: Antidiabetic, oral
Chem. class.: Biguanide
Pregnancy category B

Action: Inhibits hepatic glucose production and increases sensitivity of peripheral tissue to insulin

⇒ Therapeutic Outcome: Blood glucose at normal levels

Uses: Stable adult-onset diabetes mellitus, type 2

Dosage and routes
Adult: PO 500 mg bid initially, then increase to desired response 1-3 g; dosage adjustment q2-3 wk or 850 mg qd with morning meal with dosage increased every other week, max 2500 mg/day; ext rel max 2000 mg/day

◪ *Elderly:* PO use lowest effective dose

Available forms: Tabs 500, 850, 1000 mg; ext rel tab 500 mg

Adverse effects:
(*italic* = common; **bold** = life-threatening)
CNS: Headache, weakness, dizziness, drowsiness, tinnitus, fatigue, vertigo, *agitation*
ENDO: **Lactic acidosis,** hypoglycemia
GI: Nausea, vomiting, diarrhea, heartburn, anorexia, metallic taste
HEMA: **Thrombocytopenia,** decreased vit B_{12} concentration
INTEG: Rash

Contraindications:
Hypersensitivity, hepatic disease, creatinine >1.5 mg/ml (males) ≥1.4 (females), CHF, alcoholism, cardiopulmonary disease, history of lactic acidosis

G **Precautions:** Pregnancy **B,** elderly, thyroid disease, previous hypersensitivity

Pharmacokinetics	
Absorption	Unknown
Distribution	Unknown
Metabolism	Unknown
Excretion	Kidneys, unchanged (35%-50%)
Half-life	1½-5, Terminal 6-20 hr

Pharmacodynamics	
Onset	Unknown
Peak	1-3 hr
Duration	Unknown

Interactions
Individual drugs
Acetazolamide: ↑ blood glucose levels
Cimetidine, digoxin, morphine, procainamide, ranitidine, triamterone, vancomycin: ↑ hypoglycemia
Ethanol: ↑ risk of lactic acidosis
Radiologic contrast media: Do not give together, may cause renal failure
Drug classifications
Calcium channel blockers, contraceptives (oral), diuretics, estrogens, phenothiazines, thyroid agents, sympathomimetics: ↑ hypoglycemia
Glucocorticoids: ↑ risk of lactic acidosis
Herb/drug
Alfalfa, aloe, basil, bay, bilberry, bitter melon, black catechu, buchu, burdock, coriander, dandelion, eyebright (po), fenugreek, garlic, ginseng, glucomannan, glucosamine, goat's, rue, gymnema, horehound, horse chestnut, jambul, myrrh, myrtle: ↑ antidiabetic effect
Bee pollen, blue cohosh, broom, chromium, elecampane, eucalyptus, gotu kola: ↓ antidiabetic effect

Chromium, coenzyme Q10, fenugreek, glucosamine: ↑ hyperglycemia
Quinine: ↑ metformin level

NURSING CONSIDERATIONS
Assessment
• Assess for hypoglycemic reactions (sweating, weakness, dizziness, anxiety, tremors, hunger), hyperglycemic reactions soon after meals
• Monitor CBC (baseline, q3 mo) during treatment; check liver function tests (AST, LDH) and renal studies (BUN, creatinine) periodically during treatment; glucose, glycosylated Hgb
⊕• Monitor for lactic acidosis: malaise, myalgia, abdominal distress; risk increases with age, poor renal function; monitor electrolytes, lactate, pyruvate, blood pH, ketones, glucose

Nursing diagnoses
☑ Knowledge, deficient (teaching)

Implementation
• Conversion from other oral hypoglycemic agents; change may be made without gradual dosage change; monitor serum or urine glucose and ketones tid during conversion
• Give twice a day with meals to decrease GI upset and provide best absorption, may also be taken as a single dose
⊘• Give tabs crushed and mixed with meal or fluids for patients with difficulty swallowing; do not crush, chew, break ext rel tab
• Store in tight container in cool environment

Patient/family education
• Teach patient to use capillary blood glucose test or Chemstrip tid
• Teach patient symptoms of hypo/hyperglycemia, what to do about each
• Advise patient that drug must be continued on daily basis; explain consequence of discontinuing drug abruptly
• Advise patient to take drug in morning to prevent hypoglycemic reactions at night
• Advise patient to avoid OTC medications unless approved by the prescriber
• Teach patient that diabetes is a lifelong illness; that this drug controls symptoms, but does not cure the condition
• Teach patient symptoms of lactic acidosis: hyperventilation, fatigue, malaise, myalgia, chills, somnolence to notify prescriber immediately
• Teach patient that all food included in diet plan must be eaten to prevent hypoglycemia
• Teach patient to carry/wear emergency ID and glucagon emergency kit for emergencies
• Advise patient that glucophage XR tab may appear in stool

Evaluation
• Therapeutic response: decrease in polyuria, polydipsia, polyphagia; clear sensorium; absence of dizziness; stable gait, blood glucose at normal level

Treatment of overdose: Glucose 25 g **IV** via dextrose 50% sol, 50 ml or 1 mg glucagon

---

⚠ HIGH ALERT

methadone (Rx)
(meth′a-done)
Dolophine, methadone HCl, Methadose
Func. class.: Opioid analgesic
Chem. class.: Synthetic diphenylheptane derivative

Pregnancy category C
Controlled substance schedule II

Action: Depresses pain impulse transmission at the spinal cord level by interacting with opioid receptors; produces CNS depression

➡ **Therapeutic Outcome:** Relief of pain; successful opioid withdrawal

Uses: Severe pain, opiate withdrawal

Dosage and routes
Severe pain
Adult: PO/SC/IM 2.5-10 mg q3-4h prn

Opiate withdrawal
Adult: PO 15-40 mg/day individualized initially, then 20-120 mg/day titrated to patient response

🄟 **Child:** 0.05-0.1 mg/kg/dose q6-12h

Renal dose
Adult: PO CCr 10-50 ml/min dose q8h; CCr <10 ml/min dose q8-12h

Available forms: Inj 10 mg/ml; tabs 5, 10 mg; oral sol 5, 10 mg/5 ml; dispersible tabs 40 mg; oral conc 10 mg/ml; oral sol 5, 10 mg/5 ml, 10 mg/10 ml

Adverse effects
(*italic* = common; **bold** = life-threatening)
CNS: Drowsiness, dizziness, confusion, headache, sedation, euphoria, **seizures**
CV: Palpitations, bradycardia, change in B/P, **cardiac arrest, shock**
EENT: Tinnitus, blurred vision, miosis, diplopia
GI: Nausea, vomiting, anorexia, constipation, cramps, biliary tract spasm
GU: Increased urinary output, dysuria, urinary retention

INTEG: Rash, urticaria, bruising, flushing, diaphoresis, pruritus
RESP: **Respiratory depression, respiratory arrest**

Contraindications: Hypersensitivity to this drug, or hypersensitivity to chlorobutanol (inj route), addiction (opiate)

Precautions: Addictive personality, pregnancy **C**, lactation, increased ICP, MI (acute), severe heart disease, respiratory depression, 🄟 hepatic disease, renal disease, child <18 yr, 🄖 elderly

🄝 **Do Not Confuse:**
methadone/methylphenidate

Pharmacokinetics
Absorption	Well absorbed (PO, SC, IM)
Distribution	Widely distributed; crosses placenta
Metabolism	Liver, extensively
Excretion	Kidneys, breast milk
Half-life	15-30 hr; extended interval with continued dosing

Pharmacodynamics
	PO	IM/SC
Onset	½-1hr	20 min
Peak	1½-2 hr	1½-2 hr
Duration	4-12 hr	4-6 hr

Interactions
Individual drugs
Alcohol: ↑ respiratory depression, hypotension, sedation
Nalbuphine, pentazocine, phenytoin, rifampin: ↓ analgesia
Drug classifications
Antihistamines, CNS depressants, phenothiazines, sedative/hypnotics: ↑ respiratory depression, hypotension
MAOIs: Do not use for 2 wk before taking methadone
🖊 *Herb/drug*
Chamomile, hops, Jamaican dogwood, kava, lavender, mistletoe, nettle, pokeweed, poppy, senega, skullcap, valerian: ↑ CNS depression
Corkwood: ↑ anticholinergic effect
Lab test interferences
↑ amylase, ↑ lipase

NURSING CONSIDERATIONS
Assessment
• Assess for pain: type, location, intensity, grimacing before and 1½-2 hr after administration; use pain scoring
• Monitor VS after parenteral route; note muscle rigidity, drug history, liver, kidney function tests, respiratory dysfunction: respira-

tory depression, character, rate, rhythm; notify prescriber if respirations are <10/min
• Monitor CNS changes: dizziness, drowsiness, hallucinations, euphoria, LOC, pupil reaction
• Monitor allergic reactions: rash, urticaria
• Monitor opioid detoxification: no analgesia occurs, only prevention of withdrawal symptoms
• Monitor B/P, pulse
• Monitor bowel changes, bulk, fluids, laxatives should be used for constipation

Nursing diagnoses
☑ Pain (uses)
☑ Sensory perception, disturbed: visual, auditory (adverse reactions)
☑ Breathing pattern, ineffective (adverse reactions)
☑ Knowledge, deficient (teaching)

Implementation
• Medication should be slowly withdrawn after long-term use to prevent withdrawal symptoms
PO route
• May be given with food or milk to lessen GI upset
• Store in light-resistant container at room temp
IM/SC route
• Do not give if cloudy or a precipitate has formed
• Give deeply in large muscle mass; rotate inj sites

Patient/family education
• Instruct patient to report any symptoms of CNS changes, allergic reactions; to avoid CNS depressants: alcohol, sedative/hypnotics for at least 24 hr after taking this drug
• Discuss with patient that dizziness, drowsiness, and confusion are common; to avoid getting up without assistance
• Discuss in detail with patient all aspects of the drug
• Caution patient to make position changes slowly to prevent orthostatic hypotension

Evaluation
Positive therapeutic outcome
• Decreased pain
• Successful opioid withdrawal

Treatment of overdose: Naloxone (Narcan) 0.2-0.8 mg **IV**, O$_2$, **IV** fluids, vasopressors

methimazole (Rx)
(meth-im′a-zole)
Tapazole
Func. class.: Thyroid hormone antagonist (antithyroid)
Chem. class.: Thioamide

Pregnancy category D

Action: Inhibits synthesis of thyroid hormones by decreasing iodine use in the manufacture of thyroglobin and iodothyronine; does not affect already formed hormones

→**Therapeutic Outcome:** Decreased T$_4$ levels, hyperthyroid symptoms

Uses: Hyperthyroidism, preparation for thyroidectomy, thyrotoxic crisis, thyroid storm

Dosage and routes
Hyperthyroidism
Adult: PO 5-20 mg tid depending on severity of condition; continue until euthyroid; maintenance dosage 5-15 mg qd-tid; max dosage 150 mg qd

P *Child:* PO 0.4 mg/kg/day in divided doses q8h; continue until euthyroid; maintenance dosage 0.2 mg/kg/day in divided doses q8h

Preparation for thyroidectomy
P *Adult and child:* PO same as above; iodine may be added for 10 days before surgery

Thyrotoxic crisis
P *Adult and child:* PO same as hyperthyroidism with iodine and propranolol

Available forms: Tabs 5, 10 mg

Adverse effects
(*italic* = common; **bold** = life-threatening)
CNS: Drowsiness, headache, vertigo, fever, paresthesias, neuritis
ENDO: Enlarged thyroid
GI: Nausea, diarrhea, vomiting, jaundice, **hepatitis,** loss of taste
GU: **Nephritis**
HEMA: **Agranulocytosis, leukopenia, thrombocytopenia, hypothrombinemia, lymphadenopathy,** bleeding, vasculitis
INTEG: Rash, urticaria, pruritus, alopecia, hyperpigmentation, lupus-like syndrome
MS: Myalgia, arthralgia, nocturnal muscle cramps

Contraindications: Hypersensitivity, pregnancy **D,** lactation

Precautions: Infection, bone marrow depression, hepatic disease, patient >40 yr

---

☑ Herb/drug   🚫 Do Not Crush   ◆ Alert   ◆☎ Key Drug   **G** Geriatric   **P** Pediatric

Pharmacokinetics

Absorption	Rapidly absorbed
Distribution	Crosses placenta
Metabolism	Liver, extensively
Excretion	Kidneys, unchanged; breast milk
Half-life	5-13 hr

Pharmacodynamics

Onset	½ hr
Peak	Unknown
Duration	2-4 hr

Interactions
Individual drugs
Amiodarone, potassium iodide: ↓ effectiveness
Digitalis, warfarin: ↑ response
Potassium iodide: ↑ antithyroid effect
Radiation: ↑ bone marrow depression
Drug classifications
Antineoplastics: ↑ bone marrow depression
Phenothiazines: ↑ granulocytosis
Lab test interferences
↑ Pro-time, ↑ AST, ↑ ALT, ↑ alkaline phosphatase

NURSING CONSIDERATIONS
Assessment
• Monitor pulse, B/P, temp; check I&O ratio; check for edema (puffy hands, feet, periorbititis); indicates hypothyroidism
• Check weight qd; same clothing, scale, time of day
• Monitor T₃, T₄, which are increased; serum TSH, which is decreased; free thyroxine index, which is increased if dosage is too low; discontinue drug 3-4 wk before radioactive iodine uptake
◆• Monitor blood studies: CBC for blood dyscrasias (leukopenia, thrombocytopenia, agranulocytosis), if these occur, drug should be discontinued and other treatment initiated; liver function tests
• Assess for hypersensitivity (rash, enlarged cervical lymph nodes); drug may have to be discontinued
• Assess for hypoprothrombinemia (bleeding, petechiae, ecchymosis)
• Monitor clinical response: after 3 wk should include increased weight, pulse, decreased T₄
◆• Assess for bone marrow depression: sore throat, fever, fatigue

Nursing diagnoses
✓ Knowledge, deficient (teaching)
✓ Noncompliance (teaching)

Implementation
• Give with meals to decrease GI upset; give at same time each day to maintain drug level
• Give lowest dosage that relieves symptoms
• Store in light-resistant container
• Increase fluids to 3-4 L/day, unless contraindicated

Patient/family education
• Advise patient to abstain from breast-feeding after delivery; drug appears in breast milk
• Instruct patient to take pulse daily; to keep graph of weight, pulse, mood
• Advise patient to report redness, swelling, sore throat, mouth lesions, which indicate blood dyscrasias
• Caution patient to avoid OTC products that contain iodine; that seafood and other iodine-containing products may be restricted by prescriber
• Caution patient not to discontinue this medication abruptly; thyroid crisis may occur; stress patient compliance
• Advise patient that response may take several mo if thyroid is large
• Teach patient symptoms/signs of overdose: periorbital edema, cold intolerance, mental depression; notify prescriber at once
• Teach patient symptoms of inadequate dosage: tachycardia, diarrhea, fever, irritability; prescriber should be notified to adjust
• Teach patient to take medication exactly as prescribed, not to skip or double doses; missed doses should be taken when remembered up to 1 hr before next dose
• Instruct patient to carry ID describing medication taken and condition being treated

Evaluation
Positive therapeutic outcome
• Decreased weight gain
• Decreased pulse
• Decreased T₄
• Decreased B/P

M

---

methocarbamol (Rx)
(meth-oh-kar′ba-mole)
Carbacot, methocarbamol, Robaxin
Func. class.: Skeletal muscle relaxant, central acting
Chem. class.: Carbamate derivative

Pregnancy category C

Action: Depresses multisynaptic pathways in the spinal cord, causing skeletal muscle relaxation

⮑ **Therapeutic Outcome:** Decreased pain, spasm

Uses: Adjunct for relief of spasm and pain in musculoskeletal conditions

Dosage and routes
Pain of muscle spasm
Adult: PO 1.5 g × 2-3 days, then 1 g qid; IM 500 mg in each gluteal region; may repeat q8h; **IV** bol 1-3 g/day at 3 ml/min; **IV** inf 1 g/250 ml D₅W or 0.9% NaCl, not to exceed 3 g/day

G *Elderly:* PO 500 mg qid, titrate to needed dose

Available forms: Tabs 500, 750 mg; inj 100 mg/ml

Adverse effects
(*italic* = common; **bold** = life-threatening)
CNS: Dizziness, weakness, drowsiness, headache, tremor, depression, insomnia; **seizures** (**IV**, IM only)
CV: Postural hypotension, *bradycardia*
EENT: Diplopia, temporary loss of vision, blurred vision, nystagmus
GI: Nausea, vomiting, hiccups, anorexia, metallic taste
GU: Brown, black, green urine
HEMA: Hemolysis, increased hemoglobin (**IV** only)
INTEG: Rash, pruritus, fever, facial flushing, urticaria
MISC: **Anaphylaxis** (IM, **IV**)

Contraindications: Hypersensitivity, **P** child <12 yr, intermittent porphyria

Precautions: Renal disease, hepatic disease, addictive personalities, pregnancy **C**, myasthenia gravis, epilepsy

Pharmacokinetics
Absorption	Rapidly absorbed (PO)
Distribution	Widely distributed; crosses placenta
Metabolism	Liver, partially
Excretion	Kidney, unchanged
Half-life	1-2 hr

Pharmacodynamics
	PO	IM	IV
Onset	½ hr	Rapid	Rapid
Peak	1-2 hr	Unknown	Inf end
Duration	>8 hr	Unknown	Unknown

Interactions
Individual drugs
Alcohol: ↑ CNS depression
Drug classifications
Antidepressants, barbiturates, opioids, sedative/hypnotics, tricyclic: ↑ CNS depression

Herb/drug
Chamomile, hops, kava, skullcap, valerian: ↑ CNS depression
Lab test interferences
False: ↑ VMA, ↑ urinary 5-HIAA

NURSING CONSIDERATIONS
Assessment
• Assess for pain and spasm: location, duration, intensity, range of motion
• Monitor during and after inj: CNS effects, rash, conjunctivitis, and nasal congestion may occur
• Monitor ECG in epileptic patients; poor seizure control has occurred in patients taking this drug
• Assess allergic reactions: rash, fever, respiratory distress; check for severe weakness, numbness in extremities
• Assess for tolerance: increased need for medication, more frequent requests for medication, increased pain
• Assess for CNS depression: dizziness, drowsiness, psychiatric symptoms

Nursing diagnoses
✓ Mobility, impaired physical (uses)
✓ Injury, risk for (adverse reactions)
✓ Knowledge, deficient (teaching)

Implementation
PO route
• Give with meals if GI symptoms occur
• Store in airtight container at room temp
IM route
• Give inj deep in large muscle mass; rotate sites
• Do not give SC
IV **IV route**
• Give **IV** undiluted over 1 min or more; give 300 mg or less/1 min or longer; may be diluted in 250 ml or less D₅ or isotonic NaCl sol
• Give by slow **IV** to prevent phlebitis; keep recumbent for 15 min to prevent orthostatic hypotension; check for extravasation

Patient/family education
• Advise patient not to discontinue medication quickly; insomnia, nausea, headache, spasticity, tachycardia will occur; drug should be tapered off over 1-2 wk
• Inform patient that urine may turn green, black, or brown
• Caution patient not to take with alcohol, other CNS depressants; increased CNS depression can occur
• Advise patient to avoid altering activities while taking this drug
• Caution patient to avoid hazardous activities

if drowsiness, dizziness occur; driving should be avoided until drug response is known

• Advise patient to avoid using OTC medications that are CNS depressants (cough preparations, antihistamines) unless directed by prescriber; CNS depression can occur

Evaluation
Positive therapeutic outcome
• Decreased pain, spasticity

Treatment of overdose: Induce emesis in conscious patient; lavage, dialysis; have epINEPHrine, antihistamines, and corticosteroids available

---

! HIGH ALERT

methotrexate ⊖π (Rx)
(meth-oh-trex'ate)
Amethopterin, Folex, Folex PFS, methotrexate, Rheumatrex
Func. class.: Antineoplastic, antimetabolite
Chem. class.: Folic acid antagonist

Pregnancy category X

Action: Inhibits an enzyme that reduces folic acid, which is needed for nucleic acid synthesis in all cells; cell cycle specific (S phase); immunosuppressive

➔ **Therapeutic Outcome:** Prevention of rapidly growing malignant cells; immunosuppression

Uses: Acute lymphocytic leukemia, in combination for breast, lung, head, neck carcinoma, lymphosarcoma, gestational choriocarcinoma, hydatidiform mole, psoriasis, rheumatoid arthritis, mycosis fungoides

Dosage and routes
Acute lymphocytic leukemia
P *Adult and child:* PO/IM/**IV** 3.3 mg/m²/day × 4-6 wk until remission, then 20-30 mg/m² PO/IM qwk in 2 divided doses or 2.5 mg/kg **IV** × 2 wk

Burkitt's lymphoma (stages I, II, III)
Adult: PO 10-25 mg qd × 4-8 days with 7-day rest period

Lymphosarcoma (stage III)
Adult: PO/IM/IV, 0.625-2.5 mg/kg/day

Meningeal leukemia
P *Adult and child:* 12 mg/m² IT q2-5 days until CSF is normal, then one additional dose, max 15 mg

Choriocarcinoma
P *Adult and child:* PO/IM 15-30 mg/m² qd × 5 days, then off 1 wk; may repeat

Breast cancer
Adult: **IV** 40 mg/m² on days 1 and 8 with other antineoplastics

Rheumatoid arthritis
Adult: PO 7.5 mg/wk or divided doses of 2.5 mg q12h × 3 given qwk, max 20 mg/wk

Polyarticular-course juvenile RA
Child: PO 10 mg/m² qwk

Osteosarcoma
P *Adult and child:* **IV** 12 g/m² given over 4 hr, then leucovorin rescue is given

Mycosis fungoides
Adult: PO 2.5-10 mg/day until cleared (may be many mo); IM 50 mg qwk or 25 mg 2 ×/wk

Psoriasis
Adult: PO/IM/**IV** 10-25 mg qwk or 2.5 mg PO q12hr × 3 doses; may increase to 25 mg qwk

Available forms: Tabs 2.5, 5, 7.5, 10, 15 mg; inj 25 mg/ml; powder for inj 20, 25, 50, 100, 250 mg, 1 g

Adverse effects
(*italic* = common; **bold** = life-threatening)
CNS: Dizziness, **seizures**, headache, confusion, hemiparesis, malaise, fatigue, chills, fever, **leukoencephalopathy; arachnoiditis** (intrathecal)
GI: Nausea, vomiting, anorexia, diarrhea, stomatitis, **hepatotoxicity,** cramps, ulcerative ulcer, gastritis, **GI hemorrhage,** abdominal pain, hematemesis, **hepatic fibrosis, acute toxicity**
GU: Urinary retention, **renal failure,** menstrual irregularities, defective spermatogenesis, **hematuria, azotemia, uric acid nephropathy**
HEMA: **Leukopenia, thrombocytopenia, myelosuppression, anemia**
INTEG: Rash, alopecia, dry skin, urticaria, photosensitivity, folliculitis, vasculitis, petechiae, ecchymosis, acne, alopecia, **severe fatal skin reactions**
RESP: **Methotrexate-induced lung disease**
SYST: **Sudden death,** *pneumocystis carinii* pneumonia

Contraindications: Hypersensitivity, leukopenia (<3500/mm³), thrombocytopenia (<100,000/mm³), anemia, psoriatic patients with severe renal/hepatic disease, pregnancy X, alcoholism, HIV infection

Precautions: Renal disease, lactation, P children

🔳 **Do Not Confuse:**
methotrexate/metolazone

M

Pharmacokinetics

Absorption	Well absorbed (GI)
Distribution	Widely distributed; crosses placenta
Metabolism	Not metabolized
Excretion	Kidneys, unchanged; breast milk (minimal)
Half-life	2-4 hr; increased in renal disease

Pharmacodynamics

	PO	IM/IV	IT
Onset	Unknown	Unknown	Unknown
Peak	1-4 hr	½-2 hr	Unknown
Duration	Unknown	Unknown	Unknown

Interactions
Individual drugs
Alcohol, phenylbutazone, probenecid, radiation, theophylline : ↑ toxicity
Digoxin (PO), fosphenytoin: ↓ effect
Folic acid: ↓ effect of methotrexate
Fosphenytoin, phenytoin: ↓ effect of each specific drug
Radiation: ↑ bone marrow suppression
Drug classifications
Antineoplastics: ↑ bone marrow suppression
Antineoplastics, NSAIDs, penicillins, salicylates, sulfonylureas: ↑ toxicity
Hepatotoxic agents: ↑ hepatotoxicity
Live virus vaccines: ↓ antibodies

NURSING CONSIDERATIONS
Assessment
• Assess buccal cavity q8h for dryness, sores or ulceration, white patches, oral pain, bleeding, dysphagia; obtain prescription for viscous lidocaine (Xylocaine)
• Assess symptoms indicating severe allergic reaction: rash, pruritus, urticaria, purpuric skin lesions, itching, flushing
• Assess tachypnea, ECG changes, dyspnea, edema, fatigue; identify dyspnea, rales, unproductive cough, chest pain, tachypnea
• Monitor CBC, differential, platelet count weekly; withhold drug if WBC is <3500/mm³ or platelet count is <100,000/mm³; notify prescriber of results if WBC <20,000/mm³, platelets <150,000/mm³; WBC, platelet nadirs occur on day 7
• Assess for increased uric acid levels, swelling, joint pain primarily in extremities; patient should be well hydrated to prevent urate deposits
• Monitor renal function studies: BUN, creatinine, serum uric acid, urine CCr before and during therapy; check I&O ratio; report fall in urine output to <30 ml/hr

• Monitor temp q4h (may indicate beginning of infection)
• Monitor liver function tests before and during therapy (bilirubin, AST, ALT, LDH) as needed or monthly; check for jaundice of skin and sclera, dark urine, clay-colored stools, itchy skin, abdominal pain, fever, diarrhea (hepatotoxicity)
• Assess for bleeding: hematuria, stool guaiac, bruising or petechiae, mucosa or orifices q8h; check for inflammation of mucosa, breaks in skin
• Identify effects of alopecia on body image; discuss feelings about body changes
• Identify edema in feet, joint and stomach pain, shaking; prescriber should be notified
• Monitor methotrexate levels, adjust leucovorin dose based on the level

Nursing diagnoses
☑ Injury, risk for (adverse reactions)
☑ Body image, disturbed (adverse reactions)
☑ Infection, risk for (adverse reactions)
☑ Knowledge, deficient (teaching)

Implementation
• Avoid contact with skin, since drug is very irritating; wash completely to remove
◆• Administer leucovorin calcium within 24 hr of giving this drug to prevent tissue damage; check agency policy; continue until methotrexate level <10⁻⁸m
• Give fluids **IV** or PO before chemotherapy to hydrate patient
• Give antacid before oral agent; give drug after evening meal, before hs; give antiemetic 30-60 min before giving drug and prn to prevent vomiting; administer antibiotics for infection prophylaxis
• Give in AM so drug can be eliminated before hs
• Provide liq diet: carbonated beverages; gelatin may be added if patient is not nauseated or vomiting
• Encourage patient to rinse mouth tid-qid with water, club soda; brush teeth bid-qid with soft brush or cotton-tipped applicators for stomatitis; use unwaxed dental floss
PO route
• Give 1 hr ac or 2 hr pc to prevent vomiting
• Make sure drug is taken weekly in RA, JRA
IM route
• Give deeply in large muscle mass
IV route
• Give **IV** after diluting 5 mg/2 ml of sterile water for inj; give through Y-tube or 3-way stopcock at 10 mg or less/min
• Give **IV** inf after diluting in 0.9% NaCl, D₅W, D₅/0.9% NaCl and give as prescribed

• Give sodium bicarbonate tabs or **IV** fluids to prevent precipitation of drug at high doses, urine pH should be >7; may need to reduce dose if BUN is 20-30 mg/dl or creatinine is 1.2-2 mg/dl; stop drug if BUN >30 mg/dl or creatitine is >2 mg/dl

Syringe compatibilities: Bleomycin, cisplatin, cyclophosphamide, doxapram, DOXOrubicin, fluorouracil, furosemide, heparin, leucovorin, mitomycin, vinBLAStine, vinCRIStine

Syringe incompatibilities: Droperidol, ranitidine

Y-site compatibilities: Allopurinol, amifostine, asparaginase, aztreonam, bleomycin, cefepime, ceftriaxone, cimetidine, cisplatin, cyclophosphamide, cytarabine, DAUNOrubicin, dexchlorpheniramine, diphenhydrAMINE, DOXOrubicin, etoposide, famotidine, filgrastim, fludarabine, fluorouracil, furosemide, gallium, ganciclovir, granisetron, heparin, hydromorphone, imipenem-cilastatin, leucovorin, lorazepam, melphalan, mesna, methylPREDNISolone, metoclopramide, mitomycin, morphine, ondansetron, oxacillin, paclitaxel, piperacillin/tazobactam, prochlorperazine, ranitidine, sargramostim, teniposide, thiotepa, vinBLAStine, vinCRIStine, vinorelbine

Y-site incompatibilities: Droperidol, idarubicin

Additive compatibilities: Cephalothin, cyclophosphamide, cytarabine, fluorouracil, hydrOXYzine, mercaptopurine, ondansetron, sodium bicarbonate, vinCRIStine

Additive incompatibilities: Bleomycin, prednisoLONE

Solution compatibilities: Amino acids, 4.25%/D_{25}, D_5W, sodium bicarbonate 0.05 mol/L, sodium chloride 0.9%

Patient/family education
• Advise patient that contraceptive measures are recommended during therapy; drug is teratogenic; contraception should be used for 3 mo (male) and 4-6 wk (female); to discontinue breastfeeding; toxicity to infant may occur
• Teach patient to avoid use of products containing aspirin or NSAIDs, razors, commercial mouthwash, since bleeding may occur; to report symptoms of bleeding (hematuria, tarry stools)
• Caution patient to report signs of anemia (fatigue, headache, irritability, faintness, shortness of breath)

• Advise patient to report any changes in breathing or coughing even several mo after treatment; to avoid crowds and persons with respiratory tract or other infections
• Advise patient to report stomatitis: any bleeding, white spots, ulcerations in mouth to prescriber; tell patient to examine mouth qd, report symptoms, use good oral hygiene
• Teach patient that hair may be lost during treatment; a wig or hairpiece may make patient feel better; new hair may be different in color, texture
• Caution patient not to have any vaccinations without the advice of the prescriber; serious reactions can occur
• Advise patient to use sunblock or protective clothing to prevent burns

Evaluation
Positive therapeutic outcome
• Prevention of rapid division of malignant cells

methyldopa/methyldopate (Rx)
(meth-ill-doe′pa)
Aldomet, Apo-methyldopa ✤, Dopamet ✤, methyldopa/methyldopate HCl, Novamedopa, Nu-Medopa ✤
Func. class.: Antihypertensive
Chem. class.: Centrally acting α-adrenergic inhibitor

Pregnancy category C

Action: Stimulates central α_2-adrenergic receptors in the CNS, resulting in decreased sympathetic outflow from the brain with decreased peripheral resistance

Therapeutic Outcome: Decreased B/P in hypertension

Uses: Hypertension, hypertensive crisis

Dosage and routes
Adult: PO 250-500 mg bid or tid, then adjusted q2 days prn, 0.5-2 g qd in 2-4 divided doses (maintenance), max 3 g/day; **IV** 250-500 mg in 100 ml D_5W q6h, run over 30-60 min, not to exceed 1 g q6h, switch to PO as soon as possible

G *Elderly:* PO 125 mg bid tid, increase q2 days as needed, max 3 g/day

P *Child:* PO 10 mg/kg/day in 2-4 divided doses, max 65 mg/kg or 3 g/day, whichever is less; **IV** 20-40 mg/kg/day in 4 divided doses, max 65 mg/kg or 3 g, whichever is less

M

Available forms: Methyldopa tabs 125, 250, 500 mg; oral susp 50 mg/ml; methyldopate inj 50 mg/ml (250 mg/5 ml)

Adverse effects

(*italic* = common; **bold** = life-threatening)

CNS: *Drowsiness, weakness, dizziness, sedation, headache,* depression, psychosis, paresthesias, parkinsonism, Bell's palsy, nightmares

CV: Bradycardia, **myocarditis,** orthostatic hypotension, angina, edema, weight gain, **CHF,** paradoxical pressor response (**IV** use)

EENT: Nasal congestion, eczema

ENDO: Breast enlargement, gynecomastia, lactation, amenorrhea

GI: Nausea, vomiting, diarrhea, constipation, **hepatic dysfunction,** sore or "black" tongue, **pancreatitis,** colitis, flatulence

GU: Impotence, failure to ejaculate

HEMA: Leukopenia, thrombocytopenia, hemolytic anemia, granulocytopenia, positive Coombs' test

INTEG: Lupus-like syndrome, rash, toxic epidural necrolysis

Contraindications: Active hepatic disease, hypersensitivity

Precautions: Pregnancy **B** (PO), **C** (**IV**) liver disease, eclampsia, severe cardiac disease, renal disease

 Do Not Confuse:
methyldopa/ʟ-dopa (levodopa)

Pharmacokinetics

Absorption	50% (PO)
Distribution	Crosses placenta, blood-brain barrier
Metabolism	Liver, moderately
Excretion	Kidneys, unchanged (partially)
Half-life	1½ hr

Pharmacodynamics

	PO	IV
Onset	Unknown	Unknown
Peak	2-4 hr	2 hr
Duration	12-24 hr	10-16 hr

Interactions

Individual drugs

Alcohol: CNS depression

Alcohol, levodopa: ↑ hypotension

Haloperidol: ↑ psychosis

Levodopa: ↑ CNS toxicity

Lithium: ↑ lithium toxicity

Tolbutamide: ↑ hypoglycemia

Drug classifications

Amphetamines, NSAIDs, phenothiazines: ↓ antihypertensive effect

Analgesics, antihistamines, sedative/hypnotics: ↑ CNS depression

Antidepressants (tricyclic), barbiturates: ↓ effects of methyldopa

Antihypertensives, nitrates: ↑ hypotension

β-Adrenergic blockers: ↑ B/P

MAOIs: ↑ pressor effect

Herb/drug

Aconite: ↑ toxicity, death

Astragalus, cola tree: ↑ or ↓ antihypertensive effect

Barberry, betony, black catechu, black cohosh, bloodroot, broom, burdock, cat's claw, dandelion, goldenseal, Irish moss, Jamaican dogwood, kelp, khella, mistletoe, parsley: ↑ antihypertensive effect

Capsicum, Indian snakeroot: ↓ methyldopa effect

Coltsfoot, guarana, khat, licorice: ↓ antihypertensive effect

Lab test interferences

Interference: Urinary uric acid, serum creatinine, AST

False: ↑ Urinary catecholamines

NURSING CONSIDERATIONS

Assessment

• Monitor blood studies: neutrophils, decreased platelets; direct Coombs' test before and after 6, 12 mo of therapy

• Monitor renal studies: protein, BUN, creatinine; watch for increased levels that may indicate nephrotic syndrome: polyuria, oliguria, frequency; report weight gain >5 lb

• Obtain baselines in renal, liver function tests before therapy begins; check potassium levels, although hyperkalemia rarely occurs

• Monitor B/P, pulse if the drug is being used for hypertension; notify prescriber of changes

• Monitor edema in feet, legs daily; monitor I&O; check weight for decreasing output

• Assess for allergic reaction: rash, fever, pruritus, urticaria; drug should be discontinued if antihistamines fail to help

• Monitor CNS symptoms, especially in the elderly, depression, change in mental status

Nursing diagnoses

☑ Cardiac output, decreased (uses)

☑ Injury, risk for (side effects)

☑ Knowledge, deficient (teaching)

☑ Noncompliance (teaching)

Implementation

PO route

• Give ac

- Shake susp before using
- Store in airtight container at room temp

IV route
- Give by intermittent inf after diluting in 100 ml of 0.9% NaCl, D$_5$W, D$_5$/0.9% NaCl, 5% sodium bicarbonate, Ringer's; administer over 30-60 min

Y-site compatibilities: Esmolol, heparin, meperidine, morphine, theophylline

Additive compatibilities: Aminophylline, ascorbic acid, chloramphenicol, diphenhydrA-MINE, heparin, magnesium sulfate, multivitamins, netilmicin, potassium chloride, promazine, sodium bicarbonate, succinylcholine, verapamil, vit B/C

Additive incompatibilities: Amphotericin B, barbiturates, methohexital, sulfonamides

Solution compatibilities: D$_5$W, D$_5$/0.9% NaCl, Ringer's, sodium bicarbonate 5%, 0.9% NaCl, amino acids 4.25%/D$_{25}$, Dextran$_6$/0.9% NaCl, Normosol R, Normosol M/D$_5$W

Patient/family education
- Instruct patient not to discontinue drug abruptly, or withdrawal symptoms may occur: anxiety, increased B/P, headache, insomnia, increased pulse, tremors, nausea, sweating
- Caution patient not to use OTC (cough, cold, or allergy) products unless directed by prescriber
- Teach patient to comply with dosage schedule even if feeling better; drug controls symptoms, does not cure
- Caution patient to change position slowly, to rise slowly to sitting or standing position to minimize orthostatic hypotension, especially elderly
- Teach patient about excessive perspiration, dehydration, vomiting, diarrhea, may lead to fall in B/P; consult prescriber if these occur
- Advise patient that drug may cause dizziness, fainting; lightheadedness may occur during 1st few days of therapy; that drug may cause dry mouth; use hard candy, saliva product, or frequent rinsing of mouth
- Caution patient that compliance is necessary; not to skip or stop drug unless directed by prescriber
- Teach patient that drug may cause skin rash
- Teach patient to avoid hazardous activities, since drug may cause drowsiness, dizziness
- Teach patient to take ac

Evaluation
Positive therapeutic outcome
- Decreased B/P

Treatment of overdose: Gastric evacuation, sympathomimetics, may be indicated if severe; hemodialysis

methylergonovine (Rx)
(meth-ill-er-goe-noe'veen)
Methergine, methylergonovine
Func. class.: Oxytocic
Chem. class.: Ergot alkaloid
Pregnancy category C

Action: Stimulates uterine and vascular smooth muscle, causing contractions, decreased bleeding

Therapeutic Outcome: Absence of hemorrhage

Uses: Treatment of hemorrhage postpartum or after abortion

Dosage and routes
Adult: PO 200-400 mcg q6-12h × 2-7 days
IM/**IV** 200 mcg q2-4hr for 1-5 doses

Available forms: Inj 200 mcg/ml; tabs 200 mcg

Adverse effects
(*italic* = common; **bold** = life-threatening)
CNS: Headache, dizziness, **seizures**
CV: **Hypotension,** chest pain, palpitations, *hypertension,* **dysrhythmias; CVA (IV)**
EENT: Tinnitus
GI: Nausea, vomiting
GU: Cramping
INTEG: Sweating, rash, allergic reactions
RESP: Dyspnea

Contraindications: Hypersensitivity to ergot preparations, indication of labor, before delivery of placenta, hypertension, pelvic inflammatory disease, respiratory disease, cardiac disease, peripheral vascular disease

Precautions: Pregnancy **C,** severe hepatic disease, severe renal disease, jaundice, diabetes mellitus, convulsive disorders, sepsis

Pharmacokinetics	
Absorption	Well absorbed (PO, IM)
Distribution	Unknown
Metabolism	Liver, possibly
Excretion	Unknown
Half-life	½-2 hr

M

Pharmacodynamics			
	PO	**IM**	**IV**
Onset	5-15 min	5 min	Immediate
Peak	Unknown	Unknown	Unknown
Duration	3 hr	3 hr	Unknown

Interactions
Individual drugs
Cyclopropane anesthesia: ↑ hypotension
Drug classifications
Vasopressors: ↑ hypertension
Smoking
↑ Vasoconstriction

NURSING CONSIDERATIONS
Assessment
• Monitor B/P, pulse; watch for change that may indicate hemorrhage; check respiratory rate, rhythm, depth; notify prescriber of abnormalities
• Assess fundal tone, nonphasic contractions; check for relaxation or severe cramping
• Assess for ergotism or overdose: nausea, vomiting, weakness, muscular pain, insensitivity to cold, paresthesia of extremities; drug should be decreased or inf discontinued
• Before administering ergonovine, check calcium levels; if hypocalcemia is present, correction should be made to increase effectiveness of this drug
• Monitor prolactin levels and for decreased breast milk production

Nursing diagnoses
☑ Tissue perfusion, ineffective (uses)
☑ Injury, risk for (adverse reactions)
☑ Knowledge, deficient (teaching)

Implementation
PO route
• PO is the preferred route
IM route
• Give inj deeply in large muscle mass
Ⅳ IV route
• Give by this route for severe, life-threatening hemorrhage
• Give directly undiluted or diluted with 5 ml of 0.9% NaCl given through Y-site or 3-way stopcock; give 0.2 mg/min; use clear, colorless sol
• Store up to 2 mo if unused

Y-site compatibilities: Heparin, hydrocortisone sodium succinate, potassium chloride, vit B/C

Patient/family education
• Advise patient to stop smoking, since increased vasoconstriction will result

• Inform patient that abdominal cramps are a side effect of this medication
• Instruct patient to notify prescriber if chest pain, nausea, vomiting, headache, muscle pain, weakness or cold, numb extremities occur

Evaluation
Positive therapeutic outcome
• Prevention of hemorrhage

---

methylphenidate ⬥ₙ (Rx)
(meth-ill-fen'i-date)
Concerta, Metadate CD, Metadate ER, Methidate, Methylin, Methylin SR, PMS-Methylphenidate, Riphenidate ✦, Ritalin, Ritalin SR
Func. class.: Cerebral stimulant
Chem. class.: Piperidine derivative

Pregnancy category C

Controlled substance schedule II

Action: Increases release of norepinephrine and dopamine in cerebral cortex to reticular activating system; exact action not known

⇒ **Therapeutic Outcome:** Increased alertness, decreased fatigue, ability to stay awake (narcolepsy), increased attention span, decreased hyperactivity (ADHD)

Uses: Attention deficit disorder with hyperactivity (ADHD), narcolepsy

Investigational uses: Depression in the
Ⓖ elderly, cancer, poststroke, HIV, brain injury, anesthesia-related hiccups

Dosage and routes
ADHD
Adult: PO 5-20 bid-tid

Ⓟ *Child >6 yr:* PO 5 mg before breakfast and lunch, increasing by 5-10 mg/wk, not to exceed 60 mg/day; sus rel 20 mg qd-tid

Narcolepsy
Adult: PO 10 mg bid-tid, 30-45 min ac; may increase up to 40-60 mg/day

Depression
Ⓖ *Elderly:* PO 2.5 mg q AM, increase q 3rd day by 2.5 mg to desired dose, max 20 mg/day

Available forms: Tabs 5, 10, 20 mg; ext rel caps 20 mg; ext rel tabs 10, 20 mg; ext rel tabs (concerta) 18, 36, 54 mg

Adverse effects
(*italic* = common; **bold** = life-threatening)
CNS: Hyperactivity, insomnia, restlessness, talkativeness, dizziness, headache, akathisia,

---

dyskinesia, masking or worsening of Gilles de la Tourette's syndrome, **seizures,** drowsiness, toxic psychosis
CV: Palpitations, tachycardia, B/P changes, angina, **dysrhythmias**
ENDO: Growth retardation
GI: Nausea, anorexia, dry mouth, weight loss, abdominal pain
HEMA: **Leukopenia,** anemia, **thrombocyto-penic purpura**
INTEG: **Exfoliative dermatitis,** urticaria, rash, erythema multiforme
MISC: Fever, arthralgia, scalp hair loss

Contraindications: Hypersensitivity, anxiety, history of Gilles de la Tourette's P syndrome; children <6 yr, glaucoma

Precautions: Hypertension, depression, pregnancy **C,** seizures, lactation, drug abuse

🔃 **Do Not Confuse:**
methylphenidate/methadone

Pharmacokinetics

Absorption	Well absorbed (PO); delayed (sus rel)
Distribution	Widely distributed; crosses placenta
Metabolism	Liver
Excretion	Kidneys
Half-life	1-3 hr

Pharmacodynamics

	PO	PO–SUS REL
Onset	½-1 hr	2 hr
Peak	1-3 hr	4 hr
Duration	4-6 hr	6-8 hr

Interactions
Drug classifications
Anticonvulsants, antidepressants (tricyclics), selective serotonin reuptake inhibitors: ↑ effects
MAOIs, vasopressors: Hypertensive crisis
Food/drug
Caffeine: ↑ stimulation
🔃 *Herb/drug*
Cola nut, guarana, horsetail, yerba maté, yohimbe: ↑ CNS stimulation
Melatonin: Synergistic effect

NURSING CONSIDERATIONS
Assessment
• Monitor VS, B/P, since this drug may reverse antihypertensives; check patients with cardiac disease more often for increased B/P
• Perform CBC, urinalysis; for diabetic patients monitor blood glucose, urine glucose;

insulin changes may be required, since eating will decrease
• Monitor height and weight q3 mo since P growth rate in children may be decreased; appetite is suppressed, weight loss is common during the first few mo of treatment
• Monitor mental status: mood sensorium, affect, stimulation, insomnia; aggressiveness may occur; depression with crying spells may occur after drug has worn off
• Assess for tolerance; should not be used for extended time except in ADHD; dosage should be discontinued gradually to prevent with-drawal symptoms
• Assess for narcoleptic symptoms before medication and after; ability to stay awake should increase significantly
P • In children or adults with ADHD, monitor for improved organizational skills, attention span, attending to tasks, impulse control, socialization, and ability to get along better with others
🔃 • Assess for withdrawal symptoms: headache, nausea, vomiting, muscle pain, weakness; drug tolerance will develop after long-term use; dosage should not be increased if tolerance develops
• Assess appetite, sleep, speech patterns

Nursing diagnoses   **M**
☑ Thought processes, disturbed (uses, adverse reactions)
☑ Coping, ineffective (uses)
☑ Knowledge, deficient (teaching)
☑ Coping, compromised family (uses)

Implementation
• Give at least 6 hr before hs (regular release); at least 10 hr (sus rel, ext rel) to avoid sleeplessness; titrate to patient's response; lowest dosage should be used to control symptoms
🚫 • Do not chew, crush time rel tabs
• Give gum, hard candy, frequent sips of water for dry mouth at beginning of treatment; these symptoms tend to lessen with time

Patient/family education
• Teach patient to decrease caffeine consump-tion (coffee, tea, cola, chocolate); not to use guarana, cola nut, yerba maté; which may increase irritability and stimulation; to avoid OTC preparations unless approved by prescriber; to avoid alcohol ingestion; these may cause serious drug interactions
• Advise patient to taper off drug over several wk, or depression, increased sleeping, lethargy may occur
• Caution patient to avoid hazardous activities until stabilized on medication

• Instruct patient not to double doses if medication is missed; prescriber may suggest drug holidays (ADHD) during the school year to assess progress and determine continued drug necessity

• Instruct patient/family to notify presciber if significant side effects occur: tremors, insomnia, palpitations, restlessness; drug changes may be needed

• Inform patient that if dry mouth occurs to use frequent sips of water, sugarless gum, hard candy during beginning therapy; dry mouth lessens with continued treatment

• Encourage patient to get needed rest; patient will feel more tired at end of day; to take last dose at least 6 hr before hs to avoid insomnia

• Advise patient that shell of Concerta tab may appear in stools

Evaluation
Positive therapeutic outcome
• Decreased hyperactivity in ADHD
• Improved attention span in ADHD
• Absence of sleeping during day in narcolepsy

Treatment of overdose: Administer fluids, hemodialysis, peritoneal dialysis, antihypertensives for increased B/P

---

*methylPREDNISolone (Rx)
(meth-ill-pred-niss'oh-lone)
A-Methapred, dep Medalone, Depoject, Depo-Medrol, Depopred, Depo-Predate, Duralone, Medralone, Medrol, Rep-Pred, Solu-Medrol
Func. class.: Corticosteroid
Chem. class.: Glucocorticoid, immediate acting

Pregnancy category C

Action: Decreases inflammation by suppression of migration of polymorphonuclear leukocytes, fibroblasts; reverses increased capillary permeability and lysosomal stabilization; antipruritic, antiinflammatory (top)

⮊**Therapeutic Outcome:** Decreased inflammation

Uses: Severe inflammation, shock, adrenal insufficiency, collagen disorders, management of acute spinal cord injury

Dosage and routes
Adrenal insufficiency/inflammation
Adult: PO 2-60 mg in 4 divided doses; IM 10-80 mg (acetate); IM/**IV** 10-250 mg (succinate); intraarticular 4-30 mg (acetate); Rec 40 mg 3-7 × wk for ≥2 wk

P Child: IV 117 mcg-1.66 mg/kg in 3-4 divided doses (succinate); Rec 0.5-1 mg/kg (15-30 mg/m²) qd or qod × 1 wk or more

Shock
Adult: IV 100-250 mg q2-6h or 30 mg/kg, then q4-6h prn × 2-3 days (succinate)

Multiple sclerosis
Adult: PO 160 mg/day × 1 wk, then 64 mg qod × 30 days

Available forms: Tabs 2, 4, 6, 8, 16, 24, 32 mg; inj 20, 40, 80 mg/ml acetate; inj 40, 125, 500, 1000, 2000 mg/vial succinate; 1%; dose pack 4 mg tabs; susp for inj 20, 40, 80 mg/ml; enema 40 mg

Adverse effects
(*italic* = common; **bold** = life-threatening)
CNS: Depression, flushing, sweating, headache, mood changes
CV: Hypertension, **circulatory collapse, thrombophlebitis, embolism,** tachycardia
EENT: Fungal infections, increased intraocular pressure, blurred vision, cataracts
GI: Diarrhea, nausea, abdominal distention, **GI hemorrhage,** increased appetite, **pancreatitis**
HEMA: Thrombocytopenia
INTEG: Acne, poor wound healing, ecchymosis, petechiae
MS: Fractures, osteoporosis, weakness

Contraindications: Hypersensitivity to corticosteroids, fungal infections, psychosis, idiopathic thrombocytopenia, acute glomerulonephritis, amebiasis, nonasthmatic bronchial **P** disease, child <2 yr, AIDS, TB

Precautions: Pregnancy **C**, lactation, diabetes mellitus, glaucoma, osteoporosis, seizure disorders, ulcerative colitis, CHF, myasthenia gravis, renal disease, esophagitis, peptic ulcer

📎 **Do Not Confuse:**
methylPREDNISolone/
medroxyPROGESTERone,
methylPREDNISolone/predniSONE,
methylPREDNISolone/methylTESTOSTERone

Pharmacokinetics	
Absorption	Well absorbed (PO); systemic (top)
Distribution	Crosses placenta
Metabolism	Liver, extensively
Excretion	Kidney
Half-life	3-5 hr; adrenal suppression 3-4 days

Pharmacodynamics				
	PO	IM	IV	TOP
Onset	Unknown	Unknown	Rapid	Min to hr
Peak	2 hr	4-8 days	Unknown	Hr to days
Dura-tion	1½ days	1-4 wk	Unknown	Hr to days

Interactions
Individual drugs
Amphotericin B, mezlocillin, piperacillin, ticarcillin: ↑ hypokalemia
Insulin: ↑ need for insulin
Phenytoin, rifampin: ↓ action, ↑ metabolism
Drug classifications
Barbiturates: ↓ action, ↑ metabolism
Contraceptives, oral: ↓ effect
Diuretics: ↑ hypokalemia
Hypoglycemic agents: ↑ need for hypoglycemic agents
NSAIDs: ↑ GI reactions
Food/drug
Grapefruit juice: ↑ methylPREDNISolone level, do not use concurrently
☑ Herb/drug
Aloe, buckthorn, cascara sagrada, Chinese rhubarb, rhubarb root, senna: ↑ hypokalemia
Aloe, licorice, perilla: ↑ corticosteroid effect
Lab test interferences
↑ Cholesterol, ↑ sodium, ↑ blood glucose, ↑ uric acid, ↑ calcium, ↑ urine glucose
↓ Calcium, ↓ potassium, ↓ T₄, ↓ T₃, ↓ thyroid radioactive iodine uptake test, ↓ urine 17-OHCS, ↓ 17-KS, ↓ PBI
False negative: Skin allergy tests

NURSING CONSIDERATIONS
Assessment
• Monitor potassium, blood glucose, urine glucose while patient is on long-term therapy; hypokalemia and hyperglycemia
• Monitor weight daily; notify prescriber of weekly gain >5 lb
• Monitor B/P q4h, pulse; notify prescriber if chest pain occurs
• Monitor I&O ratio; be alert for decreasing urinary output and increasing edema
• Monitor plasma cortisol levels during long-term therapy (normal level 138-635 nmol/L when drawn at 8 AM)
• Monitor adrenal function periodically for hypothalamic-pituitary-adrenal axis suppression
• Assess for infection: increased temp, WBC even after withdrawal of medication; drug masks infection symptoms
• Assess for potassium depletion: paresthe-sias, fatigue, nausea, vomiting, depression, polyuria, dysrhythmias, weakness
• Assess for edema, hypertension, cardiac symptoms
• Assess mental status: affect, mood, behavioral changes, aggression
• Check temp; if fever develops, drug should be discontinued
• Assess for systemic absorption: increased temp, inflammation, irritation (top)

Nursing diagnoses
☑ Infection, risk for (adverse reactions)
☑ Knowledge, deficient (teaching)
☑ Noncompliance (teaching)

Implementation
IV IV route
• Give **IV**, use only sodium phosphate product; give >1 min; may be given by **IV** inf in compatible sol
• Give after shaking susp (parenteral)
• Give titrated dosage; use lowest effective dosage

Syringe compatibilities: Granisetron, metoclopramide

Y-site compatibilities: Acyclovir, amifostine, amrinone, aztreonam, cefepime, cisplatin, cladribine, cyclophosphamide, cytarabine, DOPamine, DOXOrubicin, enalaprilat, famotidine, fludarabine, granisetron, heparin, melphalan, meperidine, methotrexate, metronidazole, midazolam, morphine, piperacillin/tazobactam, sodium bicarbonate, tacrolimus, teniposide, theophylline, thiotepa, vit B with C

Y-site incompatibilities: Ondansetron, paclitaxel, sargramostim, vinorelbine

Additive compatibilities: Chloramphenicol, cimetidine, clindamycin, DOPamine, granisetron, heparin, norepinephrine, penicillin G potassium, ranitidine, theophylline, verapamil
PO route
• Give with food or milk to decrease GI symptoms
IM route
• Give IM inj deep in large muscle mass; rotate sites; avoid deltoid; use 21-G needle
• Give in one dose in AM to prevent adrenal suppression; avoid SC administration; may damage tissue
Inhalation route
• Give inh with water to decrease possibility of fungal infections
• Give titrated dosage; use lowest effective dosage

M

- Clean aerosol top daily with warm water; dry thoroughly
- Store in cool environment; do not puncture or incinerate container

Topical route
- Cleanse area before applying drug
- Apply only to affected areas; do not get in eyes
- Apply medication, then cover with occlusive dressing (only if prescribed); seal to normal skin; change q12h; systemic absorption may occur
- Apply only to dermatoses; do not use on weeping, denuded, or infected area
- Apply treatment for a few days after area has cleared
- Store at room temp

Patient/family education
- Teach patient that emergency ID as steroid user should be carried/worn
- Advise patient to notify prescriber if therapeutic response decreases; dosage adjustment may be needed
- Caution patient not to discontinue abruptly; adrenal crisis can result
- Caution patient to avoid OTC products: salicylates, alcohol in cough products, cold preparations unless directed by prescriber
- Teach patient all aspects of drug usage including cushingoid symptoms
- Teach patient symptoms of adrenal insufficiency: nausea, anorexia, fatigue, dizziness, dyspnea, weakness, joint pain
- Inform patient that long-term therapy may be needed to clear infection (1-2 mo depending on type of infection)

Nasal route
- Advise patient to clear nasal passages if sneezing attack occurs; repeat dose
- Advise patient to continue using product even if mild nasal bleeding occurs; is usually transient
- Teach patient method of instillation after providing written instructions from manufacturer

Topical route
- Advise patient to avoid sunlight on affected area; burns may occur

Evaluation
Positive therapeutic outcome
- Ease of respirations, decreased inflammation
- Absence of severe itching, patches on skin, flaking (top)

methysergide (Rx)
(meth-i-ser′jide)
Sansert
Func. class.: Adrenergic blocker, serotonin antagonist
Chem. class.: Ergot derivative

Pregnancy category X

Action: Competitively blocks serotonin (hydroxytryptamine) receptors in CNS and periphery; potent vasoconstrictor

Therapeutic Outcome: Absence of migraines and other vascular headaches

Uses: Prophylaxis for migraine and other vascular headaches; if no improvement is noted in 3 wk, drug is unlikely to be beneficial

Dosage and routes
Adult: PO 2-4 mg bid with meals; 3-4 wk rest period after each 6-mo treatment

Available forms: Tabs 2 mg

Adverse effects
(*italic* = common; **bold** = life-threatening)
CNS: Tremors, anxiety, insomnia, headache, dizziness, euphoria, confusion, depersonalization, hallucinations, paresthesias, drowsiness
CV: **Retroperitoneal fibrosis,** valvular thickening, palpitations, tachycardia, postural hypertension, angina, thrombophlebitis, ECG changes, **cardiac fibrosis**
GI: Nausea, vomiting, weight gain
HEMA: **Blood dyscrasias**
INTEG: Flushing, rash, alopecia
MS: Arthralgia, myalgia

Contraindications: Hypersensitivity to ergot, tartrazine, peripheral vascular occlusion, CAD, hepatic disease, renal disease, peptic ulcer, hypertension, connective tissue disease, fibrotic pulmonary disease, pregnancy **X**

Precautions: Lactation, children

Pharmacokinetics	
Absorption	Rapidly absorbed
Distribution	Widely distributed
Metabolism	Liver
Excretion	Kidneys, breast milk
Half-life	10 hr

Pharmacodynamics
Unknown

Interactions
Drug classifications
β-Adrenergic blockers: ↑ vasoconstriction
Opiates: ↓ effect of opiates
Smoking
↑ Vasoconstriction

NURSING CONSIDERATIONS
Assessment
• Monitor stress level, activity, reaction, coping mechanisms of patient
• Assess neurologic status: LOC, blurring vision, nausea, vomiting, tingling in extremities preceding headache
• Assess for ingestion of tyramine-containing foods (pickled products, beer, wine, aged cheese), food additives, preservatives, colorings, artificial sweeteners, chocolate, caffeine, which may precipitate these types of headaches

Nursing diagnoses
☑ Pain, chronic (uses)
☑ Injury, risk for (adverse reactions)
☑ Knowledge, deficient (teaching)

Implementation
• Provide quiet, calm environment with decreased stimulation; no noise, bright lights, or excessive talking
• Give with or pc to avoid GI symptoms
• Store in dark area

Patient/family education
• Caution patient to avoid OTC medications and alcohol; serious drug interactions may occur
• Caution patient to maintain dosage at approved level; not to increase even if drug does not relieve headache
• Advise patient that an increase in headaches may occur when this drug is discontinued after long-term use
• Caution patient to keep drug out of the ℗ reach of children; death may occur
• Caution patient to use drug for less than 6 mo continuously; a 3-4 wk drug-free period must follow each 6-mo period

Evaluation
Positive therapeutic outcome
• Decrease in frequency, severity of headache

---

metoclopramide (Rx)
(met-oh-kloe-pra′mide)
Apo-Metoclop ♣, Clopra, Emex ♣, Maxeran ♣, metoclopramide, Octamide-PFS, Reclomide, Reglan
Func. class.: Cholinergic, antiemetic
Chem. class.: Central dopamine receptor antagonist

Pregnancy category B

Action: Enhances response to acetylcholine of tissue in upper GI tract, which causes contraction of gastric muscle, relaxes pyloric, duodenal segments, increases peristalsis without stimulating secretions, blocks dopamine in chemoreceptor trigger zone of CNS

→ **Therapeutic Outcome:** Decreased symptoms of delayed gastric emptying, decreased nausea, vomiting

Uses: Prevention of nausea, vomiting induced by chemotherapy, radiation; delayed gastric emptying, gastroesophageal reflux

Investigational uses: Hiccups, migraines

Dosage and routes
Nausea/vomiting
Adult: **IV** 1-2 mg/kg 30 min before administration of chemotherapy, then q2h × 2 doses, then q3h × 3 doses

℗ *Child:* **IV** 0.1-0.2 mg/kg/dose

Facilitation of small bowel intubation in radiologic exams
℗ *Adult and child >14 yr:* **IV** 10 mg over 1-2 min

℗ *Child <6 yr:* **IV** 0.1 mg/kg
℗ *Child 6-14 yr:* **IV** 2.5-5 mg

Diabetic gastroparesis
Adult: PO 10 mg 30 min ac, hs × 2-8 wk

Ⓖ *Elderly:* PO 5 mg ½ hr ac hs, increase to 10 mg if needed

Hiccups
Adult: PO/IM 10-20 mg qid (PO); may give 10 mg IM

Gastroesophageal reflux
Adult: PO 10-15 mg qid 30 min ac

℗ *Child:* PO 0.4-0.8 mg/kg/day divided in 4 doses

Renal dose
Adult: **IV** CCr <40 ml/min 50% of dose

Available forms: Tabs 5, 10 mg; syr 5 mg/5 ml; inj 5 mg/ml, conc sol 10 mg/ml

M

Adverse effects
(*italic* = common; **bold** = life-threatening)
CNS: *Sedation, fatigue, restlessness, headache, sleeplessness, dystonia,* dizziness, drowsiness, suicide ideation, **seizures,** extrapyramidal symptoms (EPS)
CV: Hypotension, **supraventricular tachycardia**
GI: Dry mouth, constipation, nausea, anorexia, vomiting, diarrhea
GU: Decreased libido, prolactin secretion, amenorrhea, galactorrhea
HEMA: **Neutropenia, leukopenia, agranulocytosis**
INTEG: Urticaria, rash

Contraindications: Hypersensitivity to this drug or procaine or procainamide, seizure disorder, pheochromocytoma, breast cancer (prolactin dependent), GI obstruction

Precautions: Pregnancy **B,** lactation, GI hemorrhage, CHF, Parkinson's disease

Do Not Confuse:
metoclopramide/metolazone, Reglan/Megace

Pharmacokinetics
Absorption	Well absorbed (PO)
Distribution	Widely distributed; crosses blood-brain barrier, placenta
Metabolism	Liver, minimally
Excretion	Kidneys, breast milk
Half-life	4 hr

Pharmacodynamics
	PO	IM	IV
Onset	½-1 hr	10-15 min	1-3 min
Peak	Unknown	Unknown	Unknown
Duration	1-2 hr	1-2 hr	1-2 hr

Interactions
Individual drugs
Alcohol: ↑ sedation
Digoxin: ↓ action
Haloperidol: ↑ extrapyramidal reaction
Drug classifications
Anticholinergics, opiates: ↓ action of metoclopramide
Antidepressants, antihistamines, sedative/hypnotics: ↑ CNS depression
CNS depressants: ↑ sedation
MAOIs: Avoid use
Phenothiazines: ↑ extrapyramidal reaction
Lab test interferences
↑ Prolactin, ↑ aldosterone, ↑ thyrotropin

NURSING CONSIDERATIONS
Assessment
• Assess GI complaints: nausea, vomiting, anorexia, constipation, abdominal distention before and after administration
• Assess for extrapyramidal symptoms and tardive dyskinesia, more likely to occur in
G elderly patient: rigidity, grimacing, shuffling gait, tremors, rhythmic involuntary movements of tongue, mouth, jaw, feet, hands; these side effects should be reported to prescriber immediately; some effects may be irreversible
• Assess mental status: depression, anxiety, irritability during treatment

Nursing diagnoses
☑ Injury, risk for (adverse reactions)
☑ Knowledge, deficient (teaching)

Implementation
PO route
• Give ½-1 hr before meals for better absorption
IV **IV route**
• Give **IV** undiluted if dose is ≤10 mg; give over 2 min
• Dilute more than 10 mg in 50 ml or more D$_5$W, NaCl, Ringer's, LR and give over 15 min or more
• Give diphenhydrAMINE **IV** for EPS
• Discard open ampules

Syringe compatibilities: Aminophylline, ascorbic acid, atropine, benztropine, bleomycin, butorphanol, chlorproMAZINE, cisplatin, cyclophosphamide, cytarabine, dexamethasone, dimenhyDRINATE, diphenhydrAMINE, DOXOrubicin, droperidol, fentanyl, fluorouracil, heparin, hydrocortisone, hydrOXYzine, regular insulin, leucovorin, lidocaine, magnesium sulfate, meperidine, methotrimeprazine, methylPREDNISolone, midazolam, mitomycin, morphine, pentazocine, perphenazine, prochlorperazine, promazine, promethazine, ranitidine, scopolamine, sufentanil, vinBLAStine, vinCRIStine, vit B/C

Syringe incompatibilities: Ampicillin, calcium gluconate, cephalothin, chloramphenicol, furosemide, penicillin G potassium, sodium bicarbonate

Y-site compatibilities: Acyclovir, aldesleukin, amifostine, aztreonam, bleomycin, ciprofloxacin, cisplatin, cladribine, cyclophosphamide, cytarabine, diltiazem, DOXOrubicin, droperidol, famotidine, filgrastim, fluconazole, fludarabine, fluorouracil, foscarnet, gallium, granisetron, heparin, idarubicin, leucovorin, melphalan, meperidine, meropenem, methotrexate, mitomycin, morphine, ondansetron, paclitaxel, piperacillin/tazobactam, propofol, sargramostim, sufentanil, tacrolimus, teniposide, thiotepa, vinBLAStine, vinCRIStine, vinorelbine, zidovudine

Y-site incompatibilities: Furosemide

Additive compatibilities: Clindamycin, meropenem, morphine, multivitamins, potassium acetate/chloride/phosphate, verapamil

Additive incompatibilities: Cisplatin, erythromycin, tetracycline

PO route
• Give 30-60 min ac for better absorption and at hs
• Use gum, hard candy, frequent rinsing of mouth for dryness of oral cavity

Patient/family education
• Instruct patient to avoid driving, other hazardous activities until stabilized on this medication
• Advise patient to avoid alcohol and other CNS depressants that enhance sedating properties of this drug
• Advise patient to notify prescriber if involuntary movements occur

Evaluation
Positive therapeutic outcome
• Absence of nausea, vomiting, anorexia, fullness

---

metolazone (Rx)
(me-tole′a-zone)
MyKrox, Zaroxolyn
Func. class.: Diuretic, antihypertensive
Chem. class.: Thiazide-like quinazoline derivative

Pregnancy category B

Action: Acts on the distal tubule and cortical thick ascending limb of the loop of Henle in the kidney, increasing excretion of sodium, water, chloride, magnesium, potassium, and bicarbonate

Therapeutic Outcome: Decreased B/P, decreased edema in lung tissue and peripherally

Uses: Edema in CHF, nephrotic syndrome; may be used alone or as adjunct with antihypertensives for mild to moderate hypertension

Dosage and routes
Edema
Adult: PO 5-20 mg/day

Hypertension
Adult: PO 2.5-5 mg/day (Zaroxolyn)
P *Child:* PO 0.2-0.4 mg/kg/day divided q12-24h
Adult: PO 0.5 mg (MyKrox) qd in AM: may increase to 1 mg

Available forms: MyKrox tabs 0.5; Zaroxolyn tabs 2.5, 5, 10 mg

Adverse effects
(*italic* = common; **bold** = life-threatening)
CNS: Drowsiness, paresthesia, anxiety, depression, headache, *dizziness, fatigue, weakness*
CV: Irregular pulse, orthostatic hypotension, palpitations, volume depletion, chest pain
EENT: Blurred vision
ELECT: Hypokalemia, hypercalcemia, hyponatremia, hypochloremia, hypomagnesemia, hypophosphatemia
GI: Nausea, vomiting, anorexia, constipation, diarrhea, cramps, **pancreatitis,** GI irritation, **hepatitis**
GU: Frequency, polyuria, **uremia,** glucosuria
HEMA: **Aplastic anemia, hemolytic anemia, leukopenia, agranulocytosis, neutropenia**
INTEG: Rash, urticaria, purpura, photosensitivity, fever
META: Hyperglycemia, increased creatinine, BUN

Contraindications: Hypersensitivity to thiazides or sulfonamides, anuria, lactation

Precautions: Hypokalemia, renal disease, hepatic disease, gout, COPD, lupus erythematosus, diabetes mellitus, elderly, pregnancy **B,** lactation

Do Not Confuse:
metolazone/methotrexate, metolazone/metoclopramide

Pharmacokinetics	
Absorption	GI tract (10%-20%)
Distribution	Crosses placenta
Metabolism	Urine, unchanged
Excretion	Breast milk
Half-life	8 hr (extended); 14 hr (prompt)

Pharmacodynamics	
Onset	1 hr
Peak	2 hr
Duration	12-24 hr

Interactions
Individual drugs
Alcohol: ↑ hypotension (large amounts)

Amphotericin B, digoxin, mezlocillin, piper-
acillin, ticarcillin: ↑ hypokalemia
Lithium: ↑ toxicity
Drug classifications
Antihypertensives: ↑ antihypertensive effect
Barbiturates, nitrates, opioids: ↑ hypotension
Glucocorticoids, laxatives (stimulant): ↑
hypokalemia
NSAIDs: ↓ action of metolazone
🖉 *Herb/drug*
Aconite: ↑ toxicity, death
Astragalus, cola tree: ↑ or ↓ antihypertensive
effect
Barberry, betony, black catechu, black cohosh,
bloodroot, broom, burdock, cat's claw, dande-
lion, goldenseal, Irish moss, Jamaican dog-
wood, kelp, khella, mistletoe, parsley: ↑
antihypertensive effect
Coltsfoot, guarana, khat, licorice: ↓ antihyper-
tensive effect
Lab test interferences
↑ BSP retention, ↑ calcium, ↑ amylase, ↑
parathyroid test
↓ PBI, ↓ PSP

NURSING CONSIDERATIONS
Assessment
- Monitor blood glucose if patient is diabetic
- Check for rashes, temp elevation qd
- Monitor patients receiving cardiac glycosides for increased hypokalemia
- Monitor manifestations of hypokalemia;
acidic urine, reduced urine, osmolality,
nocturia; hypotension, broad T wave, U wave,
ectopy, tachycardia, weak pulse; muscle
weakness, altered LOC, drowsiness, apathy,
lethargy, confusion, depression; anorexia,
nausea, cramps, constipation, distention,
paralytic ileus; hypoventilation, respiratory
muscle weakness
- Monitor for manifestations of hypomagnesemia: agitation, muscle twitching, paresthesias, hyperactive reflexes, positive Babinski
reflex, dysphagia, nystagmus seizures, tetany;
nausea, vomiting, diarrhea, anorexia, abdominal distention; ectopy, tachycardia, broad, flat,
or inverted T-waves, depressed ST segment,
prolonged QT interval, decreased cardiac
output, hypotension
- Monitor for manifestations of hyponatremia;
increased B/P, cold, clammy skin, hypovolemia
or hypervolemia; anorexia, nausea, vomiting,
diarrhea, abdominal cramps; lethargy, increased ICP, confusion, headache, seizures,
coma, fatigue, tremors, hyperreflexia
- Monitor for manifestations of hyperchloremia: weakness, lethargy, coma, deep
rapid breathing

- Assess and record fluid volume status: I&O
ratios; monitor weight, distended red veins,
crackles in lung, color, quality and sp gr of
urine, skin turgor, adequacy of pulses, moist
mucous membranes, bilateral lung sounds,
peripheral pitting edema; dehydration symptoms of decreasing output, thirst, hypotension,
dry mouth and mucous membranes should be
reported
- Monitor electrolytes: potassium, sodium,
calcium, magnesium; also include BUN, blood
pH, ABGs, uric acid, CBC, blood glucose
- Assess B/P before and during therapy with
patient lying, standing, and sitting as appropriate; orthostatic hypotension can occur
rapidly

Nursing diagnoses
☑ Urinary elimination, impaired (adverse reac-
tions)
☑ Fluid volume, deficient (adverse reactions)
☑ Fluid volume, excess (uses)
☑ Knowledge, deficient (teaching)

Implementation
- Give in AM to avoid interference with sleep
- Provide potassium replacement if potassium
level is 3.0; drug may be crushed if patient is
unable to swallow
- Give with food; if nausea occurs, absorption
may be increased; extended release product is
Zaroxolyn; prompt action product is MyKrox;
the two formulations are not equivalent

Patient/family education
- Teach patient to take the medication early in
the day to prevent nocturia
- Instruct patient to take with food or milk if
GI symptoms of nausea and anorexia occur
- Teach patient to maintain a weekly record
of weight and notify prescriber of weight loss
>5 lb
- Caution patient that this drug causes a loss
of potassium, so foods rich in potassium
should be added to the diet; refer to a dietitian
for assistance in planning
- Caution the patient not to exercise in hot
weather or stand for prolonged periods, since
orthostatic hypotension will be enhanced
- Teach patient not to use alcohol or any OTC
medications without prescriber's approval;
serious drug reactions may occur
- Emphasize the need to contact prescriber
immediately if muscle cramps, weakness,
nausea, dizziness, or numbness occurs
- Teach patient to take own B/P and pulse and
record
- Advise patient to use sunscreen to prevent
burns
- Caution the patient that orthostatic hypoten-

🖉 Herb/drug   🚫 Do Not Crush   ✦ Alert   ☞ Key Drug   G Geriatric   P Pediatric sion may occur and to rise slowly from sitting or reclining positions, lie down if dizziness occurs

• Teach patient to continue taking medication even if feeling better; this drug controls symptoms but does not cure the condition

• Advise patient with hypertension to continue other medical regimen (exercise, weight loss, relaxation techniques, cessation of smoking)

Evaluation
Positive therapeutic outcome
• Decreased edema
• Decreased B/P

Treatment of overdose:
Lavage if taken orally, monitor electrolytes; administer dextrose in saline; monitor hydration, CV, renal status

---

metoprolol (Rx)
(met-oh-proe'lole)
Betaloc ✦, Betaloc Durules ✦, Lopressor ✦, Lopressor SR ✦, Novometoprol ✦, Toprol XL
Func. class.: Antihypertensive, antianginal
Chem. class.: β₁-Adrenergic blocker

Pregnancy category C

Action: Competitively blocks stimulation of β₁-adrenergic receptor within vascular smooth muscle; produces chronotropic, inotropic activity (decreases rate of SA node discharge, increases recovery time), slows conduction of AV node, decreases heart rate, which decreases O_2 consumption in myocardium; also decreases renin-aldosterone-angiotensin system at high doses

➡ **Therapeutic Outcome:** Decreased B/P, heart rate, AV conduction

Uses: Mild to moderate hypertension, acute MI to reduce cardiovascular mortality, angina pectoris, New York Heart Association class II, III heart failure

Investigational uses: Atrial ectopy, antipsychotic-induced akathisia, rapid heart rate control, unstable angina, variceal bleeding in portal hypertension

Dosage and routes
Hypertension
Adult: PO 50 mg bid, or 100 mg qd; may give 200-450 mg in divided doses; ext rel tabs give qd

🄶 *Elderly:* PO 25 mg/day initially, increase weekly as needed

MI
Adult: Early treatment, **IV** bol 5 mg q2 min × 3 doses, then 50 mg PO 15 min after last dose and q6h × 48 hr; late treatment, PO maintenance 100 mg bid for 3 mo

Angina
Adult: PO 100 mg qd, increase qwk as needed or 100 mg ext rel tab qd

Available forms: Tabs 50, 100 mg; inj 1 mg/ml; ext rel tabs 25, 50, 100, 200 mg

Adverse effects
(*italic* = common; **bold** = life-threatening)
CNS: Insomnia, dizziness, mental changes, hallucinations, **depression,** anxiety, headaches, nightmares, confusion, fatigue
CV: **CHF,** *palpitations,* dysrhythmias, **cardiac arrest, AV block,** hypotension, **bradycardia, pulmonary edema, chest pain**
EENT: Sore throat, dry burning eyes
GI: *Nausea, vomiting,* colitis, cramps, *diarrhea,* constipation, flatulence, dry mouth, *hiccups*
GU: Impotence
HEMA: **Agranulocytosis, eosinophilia, thrombocytopenic purpura**
INTEG: Rash, purpura, alopecia, dry skin, urticaria, pruritus
RESP: **Bronchospasm,** dyspnea, wheezing

Contraindications: Hypersensitivity to β-blockers, cardiogenic shock, heart block (2nd- and 3rd-degree), sinus bradycardia, CHF, bronchial asthma

Precautions: Major surgery, pregnancy C, lactation, diabetes mellitus, renal disease, thyroid disease, COPD, CAD, nonallergic bronchospasm, hepatic disease

🚫 **Do Not Confuse:**
metoprolol/misoprostol

Pharmacokinetics
Absorption	Well absorbed (PO); completely absorbed (**IV**)
Distribution	Crosses blood-brain barrier, placenta
Metabolism	Liver, extensively
Excretion	Kidneys, breast milk
Half-life	3-4 hr

Pharmacodynamics
	PO	IV
Onset	15 min	Immediate
Peak	2-4 hr	20 min
Duration	6-19 hr	5-8 hr

M

Interactions
Individual drugs
DOBUTamine: ↓ effect of DOBUTamine

DOPamine: ↓ DOPamine

EpINEPHrine, hydrALAZINE, methyldopa prazosin, reserpine: ↑ hypotension, bradycardia

Indomethacin: ↓ antihypertensive effect

Insulin: ↑ hypoglycemia

Drug classifications
Amphetamines: ↑ hypertension

Amphetamines, cardiac glycosides, histamine H_2 antagonists: ↑ bradycardia

Antidiabetics: ↑ hypoglycemia

Antihypertensive, calcium channel blockers, histamine H_2 antagonists, nitrates: ↑ hypotension

Benzodiazepines: ↑ effect of benzodiazepines

β_2-Adrenergic agonists, theophyllines: ↓ bronchodilatation

MAOIs: Do not use together

NSAIDs, salicylates: ↓ antihypertensive effect

Sulfonylureas: ↓ hypoglycemic effect

Food/drug
↑ Absorption with food

Herb/drug
Aconite: ↑ toxicity, death

Astragalus, cola tree: ↑ or ↓ antihypertensive effect

Barberry, betony, black catechu, black cohosh, bloodroot, broom, burdock, cat's claw, dandelion, goldenseal, Irish moss, Jamaican dogwood, kelp, khella, mistletoe, parsley: ↑ antihypertensive effect

Coltsfoot, guarana, khat, licorice: ↑ antihypertensive effect

Lab test interferences
↑ liver function tests

↑ renal function tests

NURSING CONSIDERATIONS
Assessment
• Monitor B/P during beginning treatment, periodically thereafter; pulse q4h; note rate, rhythm, quality; check apical/radial pulse before administration; notify prescriber of any significant changes (pulse <50 bpm)

• Check for baselines in renal, liver function tests before therapy begins and periodically thereafter

• Assess for edema in feet, legs daily; monitor I&O, daily weight; check for jugular vein distention, rales bilaterally, dyspnea (CHF)

• Monitor skin turgor, dryness of mucous membranes for hydration status, especially

G elderly

Nursing diagnoses
☑ Cardiac output, decreased (uses)

☑ Injury, risk for (adverse reactions)

☑ Knowledge, deficient (teaching)

☑ Noncompliance (teaching)

Implementation
PO route
• Given ac, hs; tab may be crushed or swallowed whole; give with food to prevent GI upset; reduced dosage in renal dysfunction

🚫 • Do not crush or chew ext rel tabs

• Store protected from light, moisture; place in cool environment

IV IV route
• Give by direct **IV** 5 mg/2 min or more × 3 doses at 2 min intervals, start PO 15 min after last **IV** dose

Y-site compatibilities:
Alteplase, meperidine, morphine

Patient/family education
• Teach patient not to discontinue drug abruptly; taper over 2 wk; may cause precipitate angina if stopped abruptly

• Teach patient not to use OTC products containing α-adrenergic stimulants (such as nasal decongestants, cold preparations); to avoid alcohol, smoking and to limit sodium intake as prescribed

• Teach patient how to take pulse and B/P at home; advise when to notify prescriber

• Instruct patient to comply with weight control, dietary adjustments, modified exercise program

• Tell patient to carry/wear emergency ID to identify drug being taken, allergies; tell patient drug controls symptoms but does not cure

• Caution patient to avoid hazardous activities if dizziness, drowsiness is present, to avoid driving until drug response is known

• Teach patient to report symptoms of CHF; difficult breathing, especially with exertion or when lying down, night cough, swelling of extremities or bradycardia, dizziness, confusion, depression, fever

• Teach patient to take drug as prescribed, not to double doses or skip doses; take any missed doses as soon as remembered if at least 4 hr until next dose

Evaluation
Positive therapeutic outcome
• Decreased B/P in hypertension (after 1-2 wk)

• Absence of dysrhythmias

Treatment of overdose: Lavage, **IV** atropine for bradycardia, **IV** theophylline for bronchospasm, digitalis, O_2, diuretic for cardiac failure, hemodialysis, **IV** glucose for

 Herb/drug   🚫 Do Not Crush   ✦ Alert   ☎ Key Drug   **G** Geriatric   **P** Pediatric

hyperglycemia, **IV** diazepam (or phenytoin) for seizures

---

metronidazole (Rx)
(me-troe-ni'da-zole)
Apo-Metronidazole ♣, Flagyl, Flagyl ER, Flagyl IV, Flagyl IV RTU, Metronidazole, Novonidazole ♣, Protostat, Trikacide ♣
Func. class.: Trichomonacide, amebicide, antiinfective
Chem. class.: Nitroimidazole derivative

Pregnancy category B (2nd, 3rd trimesters)

Action: Direct-acting amebicide/trichomonacide; binds, degrades DNA in organism

Therapeutic Outcome: Trichomonacidal, amebicidal, bactericidal for the following susceptible organisms: *Bacteroides, Clostridium, Trichomonas vaginalis, Giardia lamblia, Entamoeba histolytica*

Uses: Intestinal amebiasis, amebic abscess, trichomoniasis, refractory trichomoniasis, bacterial anaerobic infections, giardiasis; septicemia, endocarditis, bone, joint, and lower respiratory tract infections

Dosage and routes
Trichomoniasis
Adult: PO 250 mg tid × 7 days or 2 g in single dose; do not repeat treatment for 4-6 wk
P Child: PO 5 mg/kg/day in divided doses × 7-10 days

Refractory trichomoniasis
Adult: PO 250 mg bid × 10 days

Amebic hepatic abscess
Adult: PO 500-750 mg tid × 5-10 days
P Child: PO 35-50 mg/kg/day in 3 divided doses × 10 days

Intestinal amebiasis
Adult: PO 750 mg tid × 5-10 days
P Child: PO 35-50 mg/kg/day in 3 divided doses × 10 days; then oral iodoquinol

Anaerobic bacterial infections
Adult: IV inf 15 mg/kg/over 1 hr, then 7.5 mg/kg **IV** or PO q6h, max 4 g/day; first maintenance dose should be administered 6 hr after loading dose

Giardiasis
Adult: PO 250 mg tid × 5 days
P Child: PO 5 mg/kg tid × 5 days

Antibiotic-associated pseudomembranous colitis
Adult: PO 250-500 mg 3-4 ×/day × 10-14 days
P Child: PO 20 mg/kg/day (max 2 g) divided q6h

Available forms: Tabs 250, 375, 500 mg; ext rel tabs 750 mg; inj 500 mg/100 ml; powder for inj 500 mg single dose

Adverse effects
(*italic* = common; **bold** = life-threatening)
CNS: Headache, dizziness, confusion, irritability, restlessness, ataxia, depression, fatigue, drowsiness, insomnia, paresthesia, peripheral neuropathy, **seizures,** incoordination, depression
CV: Flat T-waves
EENT: Blurred vision, sore throat, retinal edema, dry mouth, metallic taste, furry tongue, glossitis, stomatitis
GI: Nausea, vomiting, diarrhea, epigastric distress, *anorexia,* constipation, *abdominal cramps,* metallic taste, **pseudomembranous colitis**
GU: Darkened urine, vaginal dryness, polyuria, **albuminuria,** dysuria, cystitis, decreased libido, **nephrotoxicity,** incontinence, dyspareunia
HEMA: Leukopenia, bone marrow depression, aplasia
INTEG: Rash, pruritus, urticaria, flushing

Contraindications: Hypersensitivity to this drug, renal disease, hepatic disease, contracted visual or color fields, blood dyscrasias, lactation, CNS disorders, pregnancy (1st trimester)

Precautions: Candidal infections, pregnancy **B** (2nd, 3rd trimesters)

Pharmacokinetics
Absorption	80% (PO)
Distribution	Widely distributed, crosses placenta
Metabolism	Liver
Excretion	Urine, unchanged; feces
Half-life	6-11 hr

Pharmacodynamics
	PO	IV
Onset	Rapid	Immediate
Peak	1-2 hr	Infusion's end

Interactions
Individual drugs
Alcohol: ↑ disulfiram-like reaction
Cimetidine, lithium: ↑ toxicity

M

Phenobarbital, phenytoin: ↓ effect of metronidazole

Drug classifications
Anticoagulants (oral): ↑ risk of bleeding

Lab test interferences
↓ AST, ↓ ALT

NURSING CONSIDERATIONS
Assessment
• Assess patient for signs and symptoms of infection including characteristics of wounds, WBC >10,000/mm^3, vaginal secretions, fever; obtain baseline information and during treatment
• Obtain C&S before beginning drug therapy to identify if correct treatment has been initiated
• Assess for allergic reactions: rash, urticaria, pruritus
• Identify urine output; if decreasing, notify prescriber (may indicate nephrotoxicity); also check for increased BUN, creatinine
• Assess bowel pattern qd; if severe diarrhea occurs, drug should be discontinued
• Assess for overgrowth of infection: perineal itching, fever, malaise, redness, pain, swelling, drainage, rash, diarrhea, change in cough, sputum

Nursing diagnoses
☑ Infection, risk for (uses)
☑ Diarrhea (adverse reactions)
☑ Injury, risk for (adverse reactions)
☑ Knowledge, deficient (teaching)
☑ Noncompliance (teaching)

Implementation
IV **IV route**
• Give intermittent **IV** prediluted; for Flagyl **IV** dilute with 4.4 ml of sterile water or 0.9% NaCl; must be diluted further with 8 mg/ml or more 0.9% NaCl, D$_5$W, or LR; must neutralize with 5 mEq of NaCO$_3$/500 mg; CO$_2$ gas will be generated and may require venting; run over 1 hr or more; primary **IV** must be discontinued; may be given as cont inf; do not use aluminum products; **IV** may require venting

Y-site compatibilities: Acyclovir, allopurinol, amifostine, amiodarone, cefepime, cyclophosphamide, diltiazem, DOPamine, enalaprilat, esmolol, fluconazole, foscarnet, granisetron, heparin, hydromorphone, labetalol, lorazepam, magnesium sulfate, melphalan, meperidine, methylPREDNISolone, midazolam, morphine, perphenazine, piperacillin/tazobactam, sargramostim, tacrolimus, teniposide, theophylline, thiotepa, vinorelbine

Additive compatibilities: Amikacin, aminophylline, cefazolin, cefotaxime, ceftazidime, ceftizoxime, ceftriaxone, cefuroxime, chloramphenicol, ciprofloxacin, clindamycin, disopyramide, floxacillin, fluconazole, gentamicin, heparin, moxalactam, multielectrolyte concentrate, multivitamins, netilmicin, penicillin G potassium, tobramycin

Topical route
• A thin coating should be applied to affected area after cleaning with soap and water and patting dry

PO route
• Give with or after a meal to avoid GI symptoms, metallic taste; crush tab if needed
• Store in light-resistant container; do not refrigerate

Patient/family education
• Teach patient to report sore throat, bruising, bleeding, joint pain; may indicate blood dyscrasias (rare)
• Advise patient to contact prescriber if vaginal itching, loose foul-smelling stools, furry tongue occur; may indicate superinfection
• Advise patient to notify physician of numbness or tingling of extremities
• Teach trichomoniasis patient that both partners need to be treated; condoms should be used during intercourse to prevent reinfection
• Advise patient of disulfiram-like reaction to alcohol ingestion; alcohol should not be used within 48 hr of this drug
• Inform patient drug has a metallic taste and urine may turn dark
• Advise patient to contact prescriber if pregnancy is suspected
• Advise patient to use sips of water, sugarless gum, candy for dry mouth

Evaluation
Positive therapeutic outcome
• Decreased symptoms of infection

---

mexiletine (Rx)
(mex-il'e-teen)
Mexitil
Func. class.: Antidysrhythmic (class IB)
Chem. class.: Lidocaine analog

Pregnancy category C

Action: Increases electrical stimulation threshold of ventricle and His-Purkinje system, which stabilizes cardiac membrane and decreases automaticity

---

 Herb/drug   Do Not Crush   Alert   Key Drug   Geriatric   **P** Pediatric

→ **Therapeutic Outcome:** Decreased ventricular dysrhythmia

Uses: Life-threatening ventricular tachycardia; because of proarrhythmic effects, use with lesser dysrhythmias is not recommended

Investigational uses: Diabetic neuropathy

Dosage and routes
Adult: PO 200-400 mg (loading dose), then 200 mg q8h, then 200-400 mg q8h

Diabetic neuropathy (off-label)
Adult: PO 150 mg/day for 3 days, then 300 mg/day for 3 days followed by 10 mg/kg/day

Available forms: Caps 100 ♣, 150, 200, 250 mg

Adverse effects
(*italic* = common; **bold** = life-threatening)
CNS: Headache, dizziness, confusion, **seizures,** tremors, psychosis, nervousness, paresthesias, weakness, fatigue, coordination difficulties, change in sleep habits
CV: Hypotension, bradycardia, angina, PVCs, **heart block, cardiovascular collapse, arrest,** sinus node slowing, **left ventricular failure,** syncope, **cardiogenic shock, AV conduction disturbances, CHF, atrial dysrhythmias, palpitations, ventricular dysrhythmias,** ventricular tachycardia, other ventricular arrhythmias in acute phase of MI
EENT: Blurred vision, hearing loss, tinnitus
GI: Nausea, vomiting, anorexia, diarrhea, abdominal pain, **hepatitis,** dry mouth, peptic ulcer, altered taste, **GI bleeding,** constipation
GU: Urinary hesitancy, decreased libido
HEMA: **Thrombocytopenia, leukopenia, agranulocytosis**
INTEG: Rash, alopecia, dry skin
MISC: Edema, arthralgia, fever, systemic lupus erythematosus syndrome
RESP: Dyspnea

Contraindications: Hypersensitivity, cardiogenic shock, severe heart block

Precautions: Pregnancy **C**, lactation, ℗ children, liver disease, CHF, seizure disorders, hypotension

Pharmacokinetics	
Absorption	Well absorbed
Distribution	Body tissues
Metabolism	Liver, extensively
Excretion	Kidneys, unchanged (10%)
Half-life	12 hr

Pharmacodynamics	
Onset	½-2 hr
Peak	2-3 hr
Duration	8-12 hr

Interactions
Individual drugs
Atropine: ↓ mexiletine levels
Cimetidine: ↑ toxicity
Metoclopramide: ↑ effects of mexiletine
Phenobarbital, rifampin: ↓ effect
Phenytoin: ↑ effect
Drug classifications
Acidifers (urinary): ↓ mexiletine levels
Alkalinizers (urinary): ↑ mexiletine levels
Analgesics (opioid), antacids: ↓ absorption
⧄ *Herb/drug*
Aconite: ↑ toxicity, death
Aloe, broom, buckthorn (chronic use), cascara sagrada (chronic use), Chinese rhubarb, figwort, fumitory, goldenseal, kudzu, licorice: ↑ effect
Aloe, buckthorn, cascara sagrada, rhubarb, senna: ↑ hypokalemia, ↑ antidysrhythmic action
Coltsfoot: ↓ effect
Horehound: ↑ serotonin effect
Lab test interferences
↑ CPK

NURSING CONSIDERATIONS
Assessment
• Assess for oxygenation or perfusion deficit: decreased B/P, chest pain, dizziness, loss of consciousness
• Assess respiratory status: auscultate lung fields for bibasilar crackles in patients with advanced CHF
• Assess for urinary retention: check for pain, abdominal absorption, palpate bladder; check males with benign prostatic hypertrophy; anticholinergic reaction may cause retention
• Monitor I&O ratio; electrolytes potassium, sodium, chloride; watch for decreasing urinary output, possible retention
• Monitor liver function studies: AST, ALT, bilirubin, alkaline phosphatase
• Monitor ECG periodically to determine drug effectiveness; measure PR, QRS, QT intervals; check for PVCs, other dysrhythmias; assess B/P for hypotension, hypertension, for rebound hypertension after 1-2 hr; for prolonged PR/QT intervals, QRS complex, if QT or QRS increase by 50% or more, withhold next dose, notify prescriber
• Monitor for dehydration and hypovolemia
• Monitor blood levels (therapeutic level

M

0.5-2 mcg/ml), notify prescriber of abnormal results
- Assess pulmonary toxicity: dyspnea, fatigue, cough, fever, chest pain; drug should be discontinued
- Assess cardiac rate, respiration: rate, rhythm, character, chest pain, ventricular tachycardia, supraventricular tachycardia, fibrillation

Nursing diagnoses
✓ Cardiac output, decreased (uses)
✓ Gas exchange, impaired (adverse reactions)
✓ Knowledge, deficient (teaching)

Implementation
- Give with meals for GI upset

Patient/family education
- Teach patient to report side effects immediately to prescriber; to take exactly as prescribed; if dose is missed, take when remembered if within 3-4 hr of next dose; do not double doses
- Caution patient to avoid temp extremes; impairment of heat-regulating mechanism can occur
- Encourage patient to complete follow-up appointment with health care provider, including pulmonary function studies, chest x-ray
- Instruct patient that dry mouth may be relieved by frequent sips of water, hard candy, sugarless gum
- Caution patient to make position changes from lying to standing slowly to prevent orthostatic hypotension

Evaluation
Positive therapeutic outcome
- Decreased B/P, dysrhythmias
- Decreased heart rate
- Normal sinus rhythm

Treatment of overdose: O_2, artificial ventilation, ECG monitoring, administer DOPamine for circulatory depression, administer diazepam or thiopental for convulsions, isoproterenol

---

mezlocillin (Rx)
(mez-loe-sill'in)
Mezlin
Func. class.: Antiinfective—broad-spectrum
Chem. class.: Extended-spectrum penicillin

Pregnancy category B

Action: Interferes with cell wall replication of susceptible organisms; osmotically unstable cell wall swells, bursts from osmotic pressure

Uses: Infection due to penicillinase-producing staphylococci, streptococci; respiratory tract, skin, skin structure, urinary tract, bone, joint infections; sinusitis, endocarditis, septicemia, meningitis; may be combined with an aminoglycoside for *Pseudomonas* infection

➔ **Therapeutic Outcome:** Bactericidal effects on the following: gram-positive cocci *Staphylococcus aureus, Streptococcus viridans, Streptococcus faecalis, Streptococcus pneumoniae;* gram-negative coccus *Neisseria gonorrhoeae;* gram-positive bacilli *Clostridium perfringens, Clostridium tetani;* gram-negative bacilli *Bacteroides, Escherichia coli, Haemophilus influenzae, Klebsiella, Morganella morganii, Enterobacter, Serratia, Pseudomonas, Proteus mirabilis, Proteus vulgaris, Proteus rettgeri, Shigella, Citrobacter, Veillonella;* and *Peptococcus, Peptostreptococcus*

Dosage and routes
Adult: IM/**IV** 200-300 mg/kg/day (serious infections) q4-6h or **IV** 500 mg q8h; may give up to 24 g/day for severe infections

P *Child:* IM/**IV** 50 mg/kg q4-6h

P *Infants >8 days:* (>2000 g) 75 mg/kg q6h; <2000 g, 75 mg/kg q8h

P *Infants <8 days:* 75 mg/kg q12h

Renal dose
Adult: IM/**IV** dose reduction indicated if CCr <30 ml/min

Hepatic dose
Adult: Give 50% of dose

Available forms: Powder for inj 1, 2, 3, 4 g; **IV** inf 2, 3, 4 g

Adverse effects
(*italic* = common; **bold** = life-threatening)
CNS: Lethargy, hallucinations, anxiety, depression, twitching, **coma, seizures**
GI: Nausea, vomiting, diarrhea, increased AST, ALT, abdominal pain, glossitis, colitis, abnormal taste
GU: Oliguria, proteinuria, hematuria vaginitis, moniliasis, **glomerulonephritis**, increased BUN, creatinine
HEMA: Anemia, increased bleeding time, **bone marrow depression, granulocytopenia**
META: Hyperkalemia, hypokalemia, alkalosis, hypernatremia

Contraindications: Hypersensitivity to penicillins

Precautions: Pregnancy **B**, hypersensitivity
P to cephalosporins, neonates, renal disease

 Herb/drug   Do Not Crush   ◆ Alert   ☚ Key Drug   G Geriatric   P Pediatric

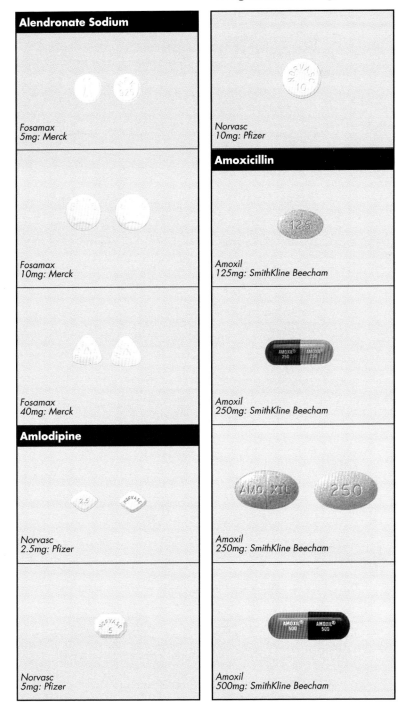

Alendronate Sodium

Fosamax
5mg: Merck

Fosamax
10mg: Merck

Fosamax
40mg: Merck

Amlodipine

Norvasc
2.5mg: Pfizer

Norvasc
5mg: Pfizer

Norvasc
10mg: Pfizer

Amoxicillin

Amoxil
125mg: SmithKline Beecham

Amoxil
250mg: SmithKline Beecham

Amoxil
250mg: SmithKline Beecham

Amoxil
500mg: SmithKline Beecham

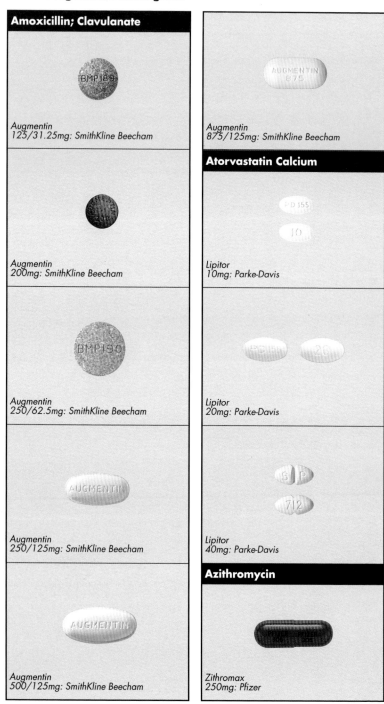

Amoxicillin; Clavulanate

Augmentin
125/31.25mg: SmithKline Beecham

Augmentin
200mg: SmithKline Beecham

Augmentin
250/62.5mg: SmithKline Beecham

Augmentin
250/125mg: SmithKline Beecham

Augmentin
500/125mg: SmithKline Beecham

Augmentin
875/125mg: SmithKline Beecham

Atorvastatin Calcium

Lipitor
10mg: Parke-Davis

Lipitor
20mg: Parke-Davis

Lipitor
40mg: Parke-Davis

Azithromycin

Zithromax
250mg: Pfizer

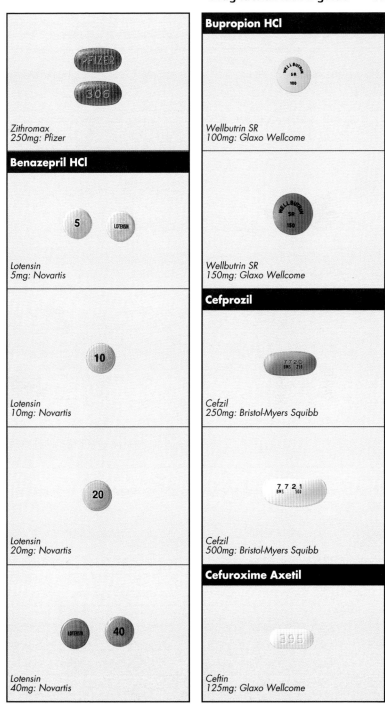

Zithromax
250mg: Pfizer

Benazepril HCl

Lotensin
5mg: Novartis

Lotensin
10mg: Novartis

Lotensin
20mg: Novartis

Lotensin
40mg: Novartis

Bupropion HCl

Wellbutrin SR
100mg: Glaxo Wellcome

Wellbutrin SR
150mg: Glaxo Wellcome

Cefprozil

Cefzil
250mg: Bristol-Myers Squibb

Cefzil
500mg: Bristol-Myers Squibb

Cefuroxime Axetil

Ceftin
125mg: Glaxo Wellcome

Ceftin
250mg: Glaxo Wellcome

Ceftin
500mg: Glaxo Wellcome

Celecoxib

Celebrex
100mg: Searle

Celebrex
200mg: Searle

Cetirizine

Zyrtec
10mg: Pfizer

Ciprofloxacin HCl

Cipro
250mg: Miles

Cipro
500mg: Miles

Cipro
750mg: Miles

Clarithromycin

Biaxin
250mg: Abbott

Biaxin
500mg: Abbott

Biaxin XL
500mg: Abbott

Cardizem CD
300mg: Hoechst Marion Roussel

Digoxin

Divalproex

Lanoxicaps
0.1mg: Glaxo Wellcome

Depakote
125mg: Abbott

Diltiazem HCl

Cardizem CD
120mg: Hoechst Marion Roussel

Depakote
250mg: Abbott

Cardizem CD
180mg: Hoechst Marion Roussel

Depakote
500mg: Abbott

Doxazosin

Cardizem CD
240mg: Hoechst Marion Roussel

Cardura
1mg: Roerig

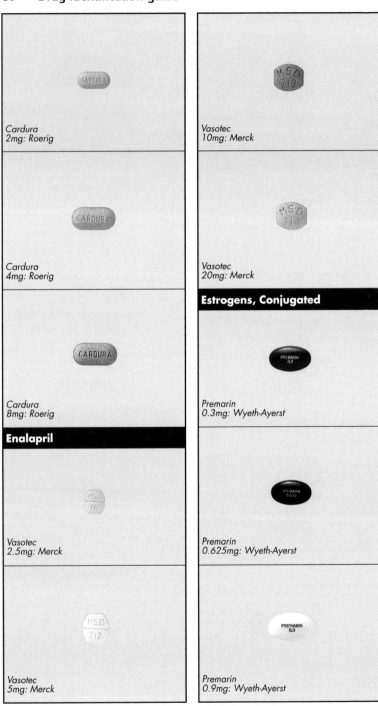

Cardura
2mg: Roerig

Cardura
4mg: Roerig

Cardura
8mg: Roerig

Enalapril

Vasotec
2.5mg: Merck

Vasotec
5mg: Merck

Vasotec
10mg: Merck

Vasotec
20mg: Merck

Estrogens, Conjugated

Premarin
0.3mg: Wyeth-Ayerst

Premarin
0.625mg: Wyeth-Ayerst

Premarin
0.9mg: Wyeth-Ayerst

Premarin
1.25mg: Wyeth-Ayerst

Premarin
2.5mg: Wyeth-Ayerst

Estrogens, Conjugated, Medroxyprogesterone

Prempro
0.625/2.5mg: Wyeth-Ayerst

Premphase
0.625/5mg: Wyeth-Ayerst

Ethinyl Estradiol; Levonorgestrel

Triphasil Inert/ 0.03/0.125/0.03/0.05/
0.04/0.075mg: Wyeth-Ayerst

Famotidine

Pepcid
20mg: Merck

Pepcid
40mg: Merck

Fexofenadine HCl

Allegra
180mg: Aventis

Allegra
60mg: Hoechst Marion Roussel

Fluconazole

Diflucan
50mg: Roerig

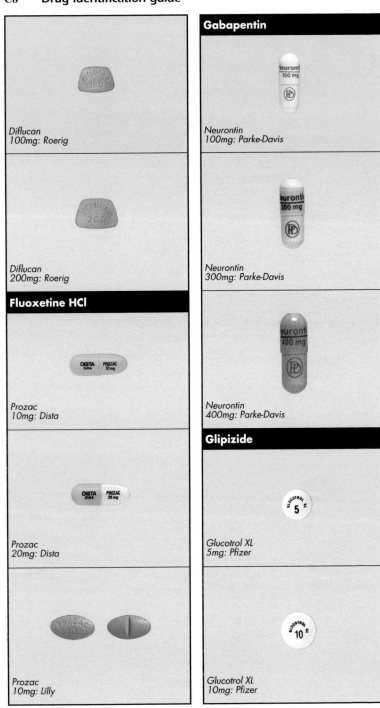

Diflucan
100mg: Roerig

Diflucan
200mg: Roerig

Fluoxetine HCl

Prozac
10mg: Dista

Prozac
20mg: Dista

Prozac
10mg: Lilly

Gabapentin

Neurontin
100mg: Parke-Davis

Neurontin
300mg: Parke-Davis

Neurontin
400mg: Parke-Davis

Glipizide

Glucotrol XL
5mg: Pfizer

Glucotrol XL
10mg: Pfizer

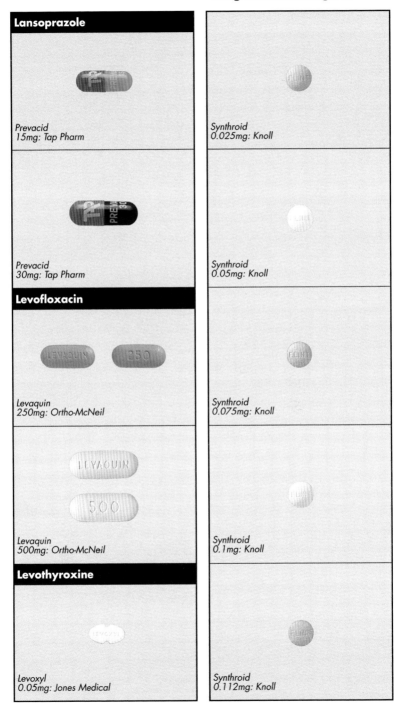

Lansoprazole

Prevacid
15mg: Tap Pharm

Prevacid
30mg: Tap Pharm

Levofloxacin

Levaquin
250mg: Ortho-McNeil

Levaquin
500mg: Ortho-McNeil

Levothyroxine

Levoxyl
0.05mg: Jones Medical

Synthroid
0.025mg: Knoll

Synthroid
0.05mg: Knoll

Synthroid
0.075mg: Knoll

Synthroid
0.1mg: Knoll

Synthroid
0.112mg: Knoll

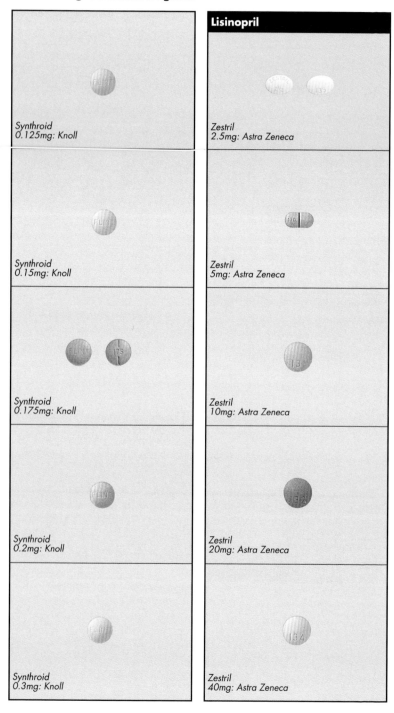

Synthroid
0.125mg: Knoll

Lisinopril

Zestril
2.5mg: Astra Zeneca

Synthroid
0.15mg: Knoll

Zestril
5mg: Astra Zeneca

Synthroid
0.175mg: Knoll

Zestril
10mg: Astra Zeneca

Synthroid
0.2mg: Knoll

Zestril
20mg: Astra Zeneca

Synthroid
0.3mg: Knoll

Zestril
40mg: Astra Zeneca

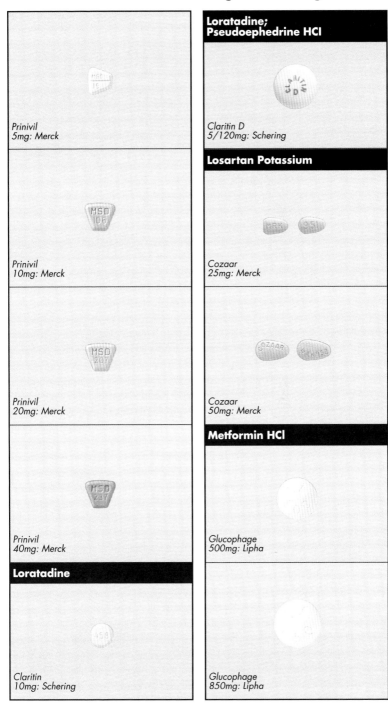

Prinivil
5mg: Merck

Prinivil
10mg: Merck

Prinivil
20mg: Merck

Prinivil
40mg: Merck

Loratadine

Claritin
10mg: Schering

Loratadine;
Pseudoephedrine HCl

Claritin D
5/120mg: Schering

Losartan Potassium

Cozaar
25mg: Merck

Cozaar
50mg: Merck

Metformin HCl

Glucophage
500mg: Lipha

Glucophage
850mg: Lipha

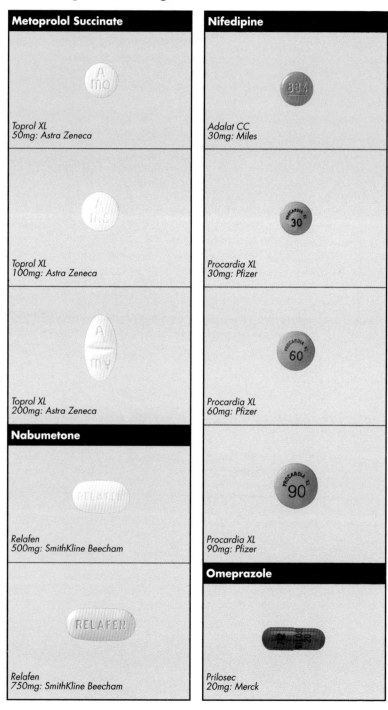

Metoprolol Succinate

Toprol XL
50mg: Astra Zeneca

Toprol XL
100mg: Astra Zeneca

Toprol XL
200mg: Astra Zeneca

Nabumetone

Relafen
500mg: SmithKline Beecham

Relafen
750mg: SmithKline Beecham

Nifedipine

Adalat CC
30mg: Miles

Procardia XL
30mg: Pfizer

Procardia XL
60mg: Pfizer

Procardia XL
90mg: Pfizer

Omeprazole

Prilosec
20mg: Merck

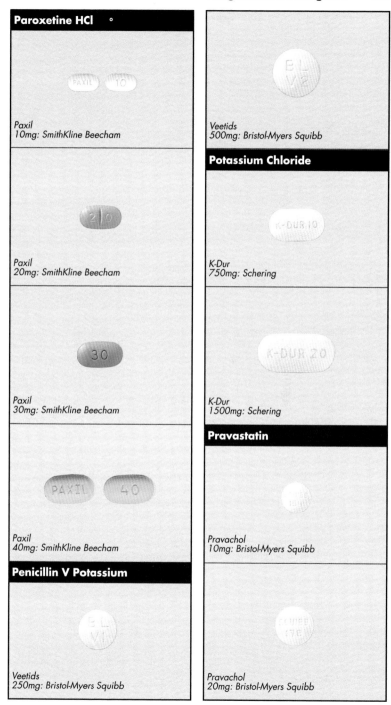

Paroxetine HCl °

Paxil
10mg: SmithKline Beecham

Paxil
20mg: SmithKline Beecham

Paxil
30mg: SmithKline Beecham

Paxil
40mg: SmithKline Beecham

Penicillin V Potassium

Veetids
250mg: Bristol-Myers Squibb

Veetids
500mg: Bristol-Myers Squibb

Potassium Chloride

K-Dur
750mg: Schering

K-Dur
1500mg: Schering

Pravastatin

Pravachol
10mg: Bristol-Myers Squibb

Pravachol
20mg: Bristol-Myers Squibb

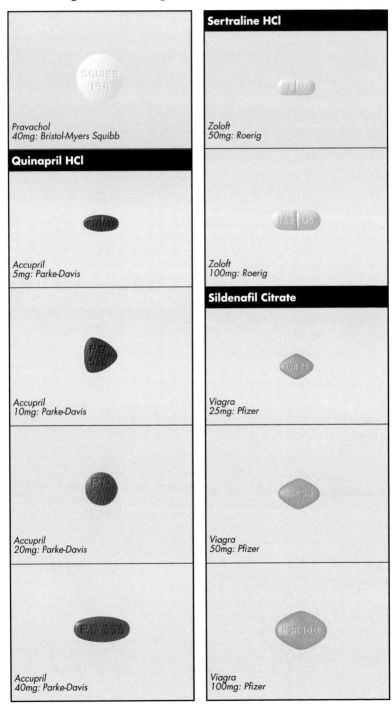

Pravachol
40mg: Bristol-Myers Squibb

Quinapril HCl

Accupril
5mg: Parke-Davis

Accupril
10mg: Parke-Davis

Accupril
20mg: Parke-Davis

Accupril
40mg: Parke-Davis

Sertraline HCl

Zoloft
50mg: Roerig

Zoloft
100mg: Roerig

Sildenafil Citrate

Viagra
25mg: Pfizer

Viagra
50mg: Pfizer

Viagra
100mg: Pfizer

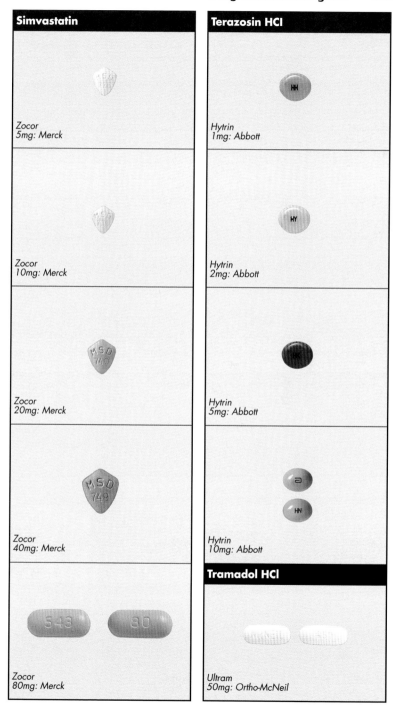

Simvastatin

Zocor
5mg: Merck

Zocor
10mg: Merck

Zocor
20mg: Merck

Zocor
40mg: Merck

Zocor
80mg: Merck

Terazosin HCl

Hytrin
1mg: Abbott

Hytrin
2mg: Abbott

Hytrin
5mg: Abbott

Hytrin
10mg: Abbott

Tramadol HCl

Ultram
50mg: Ortho-McNeil

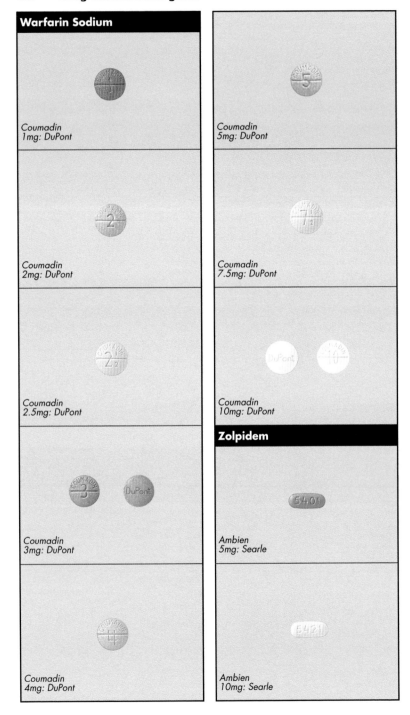

Warfarin Sodium

Coumadin
1mg: DuPont

Coumadin
2mg: DuPont

Coumadin
2.5mg: DuPont

Coumadin
3mg: DuPont

Coumadin
4mg: DuPont

Coumadin
5mg: DuPont

Coumadin
7.5mg: DuPont

Coumadin
10mg: DuPont

Zolpidem

Ambien
5mg: Searle

Ambien
10mg: Searle

*All color plates are from Potter PA and Perry AG: *Fundamentals of Nursing,* ed. 6, St. Louis, 2004, Mosby (except where noted).

Standard Precautions

The following precautions are used in the care of all patients regardless of their diagnosis or disease. They are also applied when handling or cleaning equipment or supplies that are potentially contaminated.

1. Wear gloves any time that you may contact blood, any moist body fluid (except sweat), secretions, excretions, nonintact skin, or mucous membranes.

2. Remove your gloves, wash your hands, and reapply clean gloves if your gloves become soiled with infective material.

3. Even if you are wearing gloves, remove them, wash your hands, and apply clean gloves *immediately before* contact with mucous membranes or nonintact skin.

4. Wear a protective cover gown of waterproof material if your clothing is likely to have substantial contact with infective material or if splashing of body fluids is likely.

5. Wear a face shield or goggles to protect your eyes if splashing of secretions is likely.

6. Any time a face shield or goggles is worn, wear a surgical mask to protect the mucous membranes of your nose and mouth. A surgical mask may be worn during certain sterile procedures without protective eyewear. However, protective eyewear is *never* worn without a surgical mask.

7. Handle needles, razors, broken glass, and other sharp objects with care. Needles should never be recapped. All sharps should be disposed of in a puncture-resistant sharps container.

8. Wash your hands before and after each patient contact.

9. Wash your hands before you apply and after you remove gloves. Do not assume that handwashing is unnecessary because gloves were worn. Do not wash your hands with gloves on them.

10. Gloves are used for the care of one patient only, then discarded.

11. Follow your facility policy for disposal of gloves and other contaminated items. These items are generally not disposed of in open trash containers. Facilities have designated disposal sites for these biohazardous waste materials.

12. Use resuscitation barrier devices as an alternative to mouth-to-mouth resuscitation.

13. Linen should be handled in a manner that prevents contamination of the outside of the container. Linen from isolation rooms was previously double bagged. Double bagging is no longer recommended, since all linen is handled as potentially infectious. Double bag linen only if the outside of the bag becomes contaminated during the bagging process.

Plate 1 Needles. Top to bottom: 19 gauge, 1½-inch length; 20 gauge, 1-inch length; 21 gauge, 1-inch length; 23 gauge, 1-inch length; and 25 gauge, ⅝-inch length.

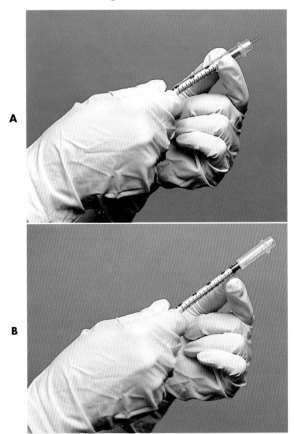

Plate 2 Needle with plastic guard to prevent needle sticks. **A,** Position of guard before injection. **B,** After injection, the guard locks in place, covering the needle.

Plate 3 Preparing an injection from a vial. Remove needle cap from syringe. Pull back on the plunger to draw amount of air into syringe equivalent to volume of medication to be aspirated from vial. **A,** Insert tip of needle, with bevel pointing up, through center of rubber seal. Apply pressure on tip of needle during insertion. **B,** Allow air pressure to fill syringe gradually with medication. Pull back slightly on plunger if necessary.   *Continued*

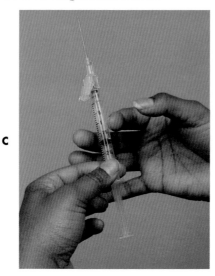

C

Plate 3, cont'd C, Remove remaining air from syringe by holding it and needle upright. Tap barrel to dislodge air bubbles. Draw back slightly on plunger and then push plunger upward to eject air. Do not eject fluid.

Plate 4 Administering an injection. Cleanse site with antiseptic swab. Apply swab at center of site and rotate outward in circular direction for about 5 cm (2 inches).

A

Plate 5 A, For a subcutaneous injection, hold the syringe between the thumb and forefinger of the dominant hand as a dart, with the palm down.   *Continued*

B

Plate 5, cont'd **B,** After injecting the needle at a 45- to 90-degree angle, grasp lower end of syringe barrel with nondominant hand to end of plunger. Avoid moving syringe while slowly pulling back on plunger to aspirate drug. If blood appears in syringe, remove needle, discard medication and syringe, and repeat procedure. *Exception:* Do not aspirate when giving heparin.

Plate 6 For an intradermal injection, note formation of small bleb approximately 6 mm (¼ inch) in diameter at injection site.

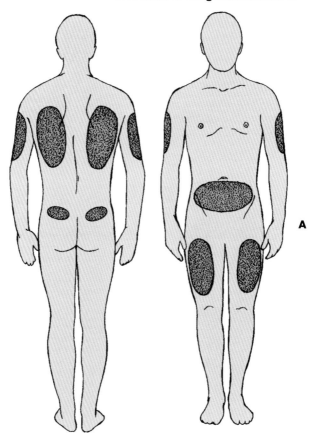

A

Plate 7 A, Sites recommended for subcutaneous injections.

Continued

B

Plate 7, cont'd B, Giving SQ injection in the abdomen.

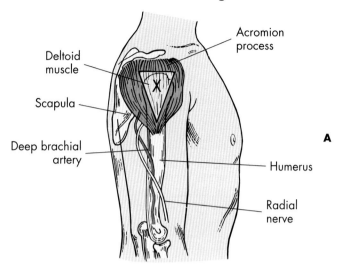

A

Plate 8 A, Landmarks for IM injection into the deltoid muscle.
Continued

Plate 8, cont'd B, Giving IM injection in deltoid muscle.

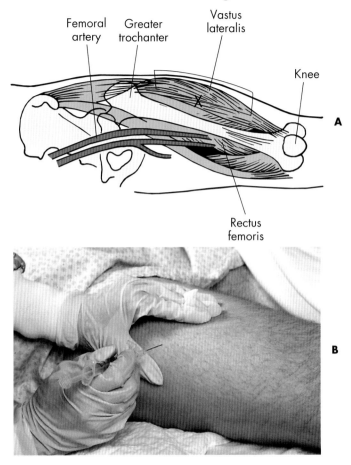

Plate 9 A, Landmarks for IM injection in vastus lateralis. **B,** Giving IM injection in vastus lateralis site.

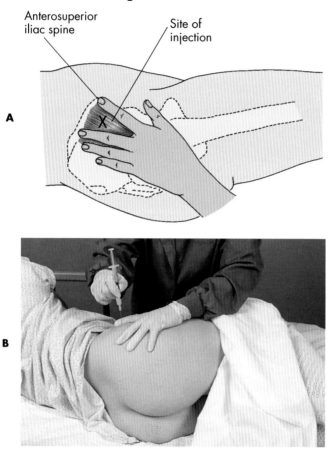

Plate 10 **A,** Anatomical view of ventrogluteal site. **B,** Giving IM injection into ventrogluteal muscle to avoid major nerves and blood vessels.

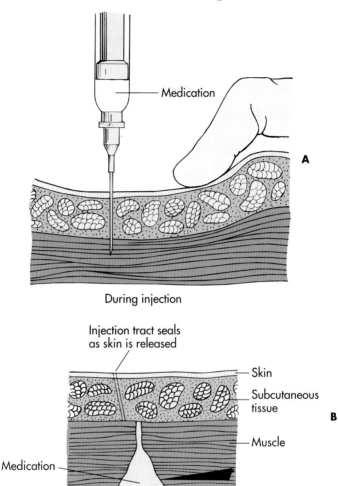

Medication

During injection

Injection tract seals
as skin is released

Skin

Subcutaneous
tissue

Muscle

Medication

After release

Plate 11 Z-track method of injection. **A,** Pulling on overlying skin
during IM injection moves tissues to prevent later tracking. **B,** The
Z-track left after injection prevents the deposit of medication through
sensitive tissue.

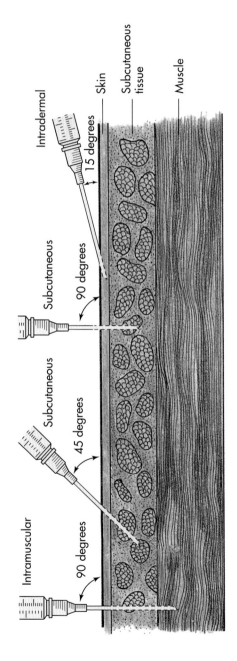

Plate 12 Comparison of angles of insertion for IM (90 degrees), SQ (45 degrees and 90 degrees), and ID (15 degrees) injections.

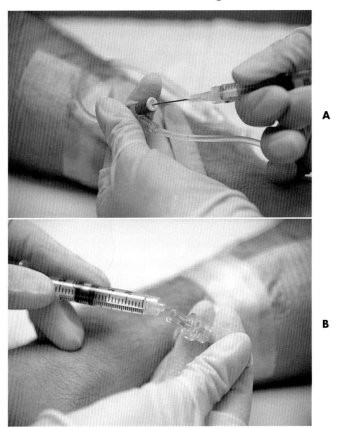

Plate 13 Administering medication by IV bolus (push). **A,** Needle system: Insert small-gauge needle of syringe containing prepared drug through center of injection port. **B,** Needleless system: Remove cap of needleless injection port. Connect tip of syringe directly. (From Potter PA and Perry AG: *Fundamentals of Nursing,* ed 5, St. Louis, 2001, Mosby.)   *Continued*

Plate 13, cont'd C, Occlude IV line by pinching tubing just above injection port. Pull back gently on syringe's plunger to aspirate blood return. **D,** After noting blood return, continue to occlude tubing and inject medication slowly over several minutes (read directions on drug package). Use watch to time administration.

E

Plate 13, cont'd **E,** IV lock: Insert needle of syringe containing prepared drug through center of diaphragm.

Plate 14 Administering IV medication by piggyback, volume administration sets or miniinfusors (syringe pump). Use needle-lock device to secure needle of secondary piggyback line through injection port of main line.

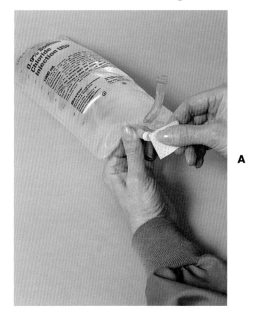

A

Plate 15 Adding medications to IV fluid containers. **A,** Wipe off port or injection site with alcohol or antiseptic swab.   *Continued*

Plate 15, cont'd B, Remove needle cap from syringe and insert needle of syringe through center of injection port or site, and inject medication.

◼ Do Not Confuse:
methicillin/mezlocillin

Pharmacokinetics

Absorption	Well absorbed
Distribution	Widely distributed; crosses placenta
Metabolism	Liver, small amounts
Excretion	Kidneys, unchanged (40%-70%); breast milk, bile (15%-30%)
Half-life	50-55 min; increased in renal disease

Pharmacodynamics

	IM	IV
Onset	Rapid	Rapid
Peak	5 min	Inf end

Interactions
Individual drugs
Probenecid: ↑ mezlocillin levels, ↓ renal excretion
Vecuronium: ↑ effect
Drug classifications
Aminoglycosides: ↓ effectiveness of aminoglycosides if mixed together
Oral contraceptives: ↓ contraceptive effectiveness
Food/drug
Food, carbonated drinks, citrus fruit juices: ↓ absorption
◰ *Herb/drug*
Khat: ↓ absorption, separate by ≥2 hr
Lab test interferences
False positive: Urine glucose, urine protein

NURSING CONSIDERATIONS
Assessment
• Assess patient for previous sensitivity reaction to penicillins or other cephalosporins; cross-sensitivity between penicillins and cephalosporins is common
• Assess patient for signs and symptoms of infection including characteristics of wounds, sputum, urine, stool, WBC >10,000/mm³, fever; obtain baseline information and during treatment
• Obtain C&S before beginning drug therapy to identify if correct treatment has been initiated
• Assess for allergic reactions: rash, urticaria, pruritus, chills, fever, joint pain; angioedema may occur a few days after therapy begins; epINEPHrine, resuscitation equipment should be available for anaphylactic reaction
• Identify urine output; if decreasing, notify prescriber (may indicate nephrotoxicity); also check for increased BUN, creatinine
• Monitor blood studies: AST, ALT, CBC, Hct,
bilirubin, LDH, alkaline phosphatase, Coombs' test monthly if patient is on long-term therapy
• Monitor electrolytes: potassium, sodium, chloride monthly if patient is on long-term therapy
• Assess bowel pattern qd; if severe diarrhea occurs, drug should be discontinued; may indicate pseudomembranous colitis
• Assess for symptoms of vaginitis during therapy
• Monitor for bleeding: ecchymosis, bleeding gums, hematuria, stool guaiac daily if on long-term therapy
• Assess for overgrowth of infection: perineal itching, fever, malaise, redness, pain, swelling, drainage, rash, diarrhea, change in cough, sputum
• Assess for possible seizures; use seizure precautions in those receiving high doses

Nursing diagnoses
☑ Infection, risk for (uses)
☑ Diarrhea (adverse reactions)
☑ Injury, risk for (adverse reactions)
☑ Knowledge, deficient (teaching)
☑ Noncompliance (teaching)

Implementation
◻ **IV route**
• Dilute 1 g or less/10 ml of sterile water, for inj; D₅, 0.9% NaCl, for inj; shake, dilute further with D₅W or 0.45 NaCl, give over 3-5 min, change site q48h

Syringe compatibilities: Heparin

Y-site compatibilities: Amifostine, aztreonam, cyclophosphamide, famotidine, fludarabine, granisetron, hydromorphone, morphine, perphenazine, sargramostim, tacrolimus, teniposide, thiotepa

Patient/family education
• Teach patient to report sore throat, bruising, bleeding, joint pain; may indicate blood dyscrasias (rare)
• Advise patient to contact prescriber if vaginal itching, loose foul-smelling stools, furry tongue occur; may indicate superinfection
• Advise patient to notify prescriber of diarrhea with blood or pus, which may indicate pseudomembranous colitis

Evaluation
Positive therapeutic outcome
• Absence of signs/symptoms of infection (WBC <10,000/mm³, temp WNL, absence of red, draining wounds)
• Reported improvement in symptoms of infection

M

Treatment of anaphylaxis: Withdraw drug, maintain airway, administer epINEPHrine, aminophylline, O_2, **IV** corticosteroids

---

mibefradil (Rx)
(mi-be-fray′dill)
Posicor
Func. class.: Calcium channel blocker; antihypertensive; antianginal
Chem. class.: Benzimidazole-substituted tetraline derivative

Pregnancy category C

Action: Inhibits calcium ion influx across cell membrane during cardiac depolarization; produces relaxation of coronary vascular smooth muscle; peripheral vascular smooth muscle; dilates coronary vascular arteries; increases myocardial oxygen delivery in patients with vasospastic angina; only calcium channel blocker that blocks both T-type and L-type channels

⇒ Therapeutic Outcome: Decreased angina pectoris

Uses: Chronic stable angina pectoris

Dosage and routes
Adult: PO 50-100 mg qd

Available forms: Tabs 50, 100 mg

Adverse effects
(*italic* = common; **bold** = life-threatening)
CNS: Headache, dizziness
CV: Bradycardia, hypotension, palpitation, AV block, Wenckebach episodes
GI: Gastric upset, heartburn
***HEMA:* Intravascular hemolysis**

Contraindications: Sick sinus syndrome, 2nd- or 3rd-degree heart block, hypotension less than 90 mm Hg systolic, cardiogenic shock, severe CHF

Precautions: CHF, hypotension, hepatic injury, pregnancy **C**, lactation, children, renal disease, concomitant β-blocker therapy, elderly

---

Pharmacokinetics

Absorption	Unknown
Distribution	Unknown
Metabolism	Liver
Excretion	Kidneys
Half-life	27 hr

Pharmacodynamics

Onset	Unknown
Peak	2 hr
Duration	24 hr

Interactions
Drug classifications
β-Adrenergic blockers: ↑ depressant effects on myocardial contractility

NURSING CONSIDERATIONS
Assessment
• Assess fluid volume status: I&O ratio and record; weight; distended red veins; crackles in lung; color, quality, and sp gr of urine; skin turgor; adequacy of pulses; moist mucous membranes; bilateral lung sounds; peripheral pitting edema; dehydration symptoms of decreasing output, thirst, hypotension, dry mouth, and mucous membranes should be reported
• Monitor if platelets are <150,000/mm³; if so, drug is usually discontinued and another drug started
• Assess for extravasation: change site q48h
• Monitor cardiac status: B/P, pulse, respiration, ECG

Nursing diagnoses
☑ Cardiac output, decreased (uses)
☑ Knowledge, deficient (teaching)

Implementation
• Give once a day, with food for GI symptoms

Patient/family education
• Caution patient to avoid hazardous activities until stabilized on drug, dizziness is no longer a problem
• Instruct patient to limit caffeine consumption; to avoid alcohol and OTC drugs unless directed by prescriber
• Advise patient to comply with medical regimen: diet, exercise, stress reduction, drug therapy; to notify prescriber of irregular heartbeat, shortness of breath, swelling of feet and hands, pronounced dizziness, constipation, nausea, hypotension
• Teach patient to use as directed even if feeling better; may be taken with other cardiovascular drugs (nitrates, β-blockers)

Evaluation
Positive therapeutic outcome
• Decreased anginal pain

Treatment of overdose: Defibrillation, atropine for AV block, vasopressor for hypotension

---

miconazole ⊶ (OTC)
(mi-kon'a-zole)
Monistat, Monistat I.V.; topical: Micatin, Micatin Liquid, miconazole nitrate, Monistat-Derm, Monistat 3, Monistat 7, Monistat Dual-Pak
Func. class.: Antifungal
Chem. class.: Imidazole

Pregnancy category C

Action: Alters cell membranes, inhibits fungal enzymes, inhibits sterols so intracellular contents are lost, prevents biosynthesis of phospholipids/triglycerides

⇥ Therapeutic Outcome: Fungistatic/fungicidal against *Aspergillus, Coccidioides, Cryptococcus, Candida, Dermatophytes, Histoplasma*

Uses: Coccidioidomycosis, candidiasis, cryptococcosis, paracoccidioidomycosis, chronic mucocutaneous candidiasis, fungal meningitis; **IV** used for severe infections only; (top) tinea pedis, tinea cruris, tinea corporis, tinea versicolor, vaginal or vulva candidal infections

Dosage and routes
Adult: **IV** inf 200-3600 mg/day; may be divided in 3 inf at 200-1200 mg/inf; may have to repeat course; IT 20 mg given simultaneously with **IV** for fungal meningitis q1-2 days

P *Child:* **IV** 20-40 mg/kg/day, max 15 mg/kg/day

P *Adult and child:* Top apply to affected area bid × 2-4 wk

Adult: Intravaginal give 1 applicator or supp × 7 days hs

Available forms: Inj 10 mg/ml; aerosol 2%; cream 2%; lotion 2%; powder 2%; spray 2%; vag cream 2%; vag supp 100, 200 mg

Adverse effects
(*italic* = common; **bold** = life-threatening)
CNS: Drowsiness, headache, lethargy
CV: Tachycardia, **dysrhythmias** (rapid **IV**)
GI: Nausea, vomiting, anorexia, diarrhea, cramps
GU: Vulvovaginal burning, itching, hyponatremia, pelvic cramps (topical forms)
HEMA: Decreased Hct, thrombocytopenia, hyperlipidemia
INTEG: Pruritus, rash, fever, flushing, hives
SYST: Anaphylaxis

Contraindications: Hypersensitivity

Precautions: Renal disease, hepatic disease, pregnancy **C**

Pharmacokinetics
Absorption	Poorly absorbed (PO)
Distribution	Widely distributed (**IV**); bound to serum proteins (90%)
Metabolism	Liver, extensively
Excretion	Unknown
Half-life	Triphasic: 0.4, 2.1, 24 hr

Pharmacodynamics
	IV	TOP	VAG
Onset	Rapid	Unknown	Unknown
Peak	Infusion's end	Unknown	Unknown

Interactions
Individual drugs
Amphotericin B, isoniazid, rifampin: ↓ effect of miconazole
Amphotericin B: ↓ effect of amphotericin B
Phenytoin: ↑ effect
Warfarin: ↑ anticoagulant effect
Drug classifications
Sulfonylureas: ↑ effect
Lab test interferences
False positive: Urine glucose, urine protein

M

NURSING CONSIDERATIONS
Assessment
• Assess for signs and symptoms of infection: drainage, sore throat, urinary pain, hematuria, fever
• Obtain C&S before beginning treatment; therapy may be started after culture is taken; monitor signs of infection before and throughout treatment
• Monitor bowel pattern before and during treatment; diarrhea may occur
• Monitor cardiac system: B/P, pulse; watch for increasing pulse, cardiac dysrhythmias; drug should be discontinued
• Monitor blood studies: WBC, RBC, Hgb, Hct, bleeding time; patients taking anticoagulants may need a decreased dosage; monitor liver and renal studies periodically for patients on long-term therapy
• Monitor I&O ratio; watch for decreasing urinary output, change in sp gr; discontinue drug to prevent renal damage; patients with renal disease may require lowered dose
• Monitor **IV** site for thrombophlebitis; site should be changed q48-72h
• Monitor for allergies before initiation of treatment and reaction to each medication; highlight allergies on chart; check for allergic reaction: burning, stinging, swelling, redness

(top); observe for skin eruptions after administration of drug to 1 wk after discontinuing drug

Nursing diagnoses

☑ Skin integrity, impaired (uses)
☑ Infection, risk for (uses)
☑ Injury, risk for (adverse reactions)
☑ Knowledge, deficient (teaching)

Implementation

• Have adrenalin, suction, tracheostomy set, endotracheal intubation equipment available

IV IV route

• Give 200 mg initially to prevent severe hypersensitive reaction
• Give **IV** after diluting ≤1 g/10 ml of sterile water, D₅W, or 0.45% NaCl over 3-5 min
• Give by intermittent **IV** after diluting in 200 ml or more, D₅W or 0.9% NaCl; give over 30-60 min
• Store at room temp; reconstituted sol is stable for 24 hr refrigerated

Y-site compatibilities: Allopurinol, filgrastim, foscarnet, granisetron, melphalan, ondansetron, propofol, sargramostim, teniposide, thiotepa, vinorelbine

Y-site incompatibilities: Fludarabine

Topical route

• Apply after cleansing area with soap and water before each application; use enough medication to cover lesions completely; dry well
• Store at room temp in dry place

Vaginal route

• Administer 1 applicator full every night high into the vagina
• Store at room temp in dry place

Patient/family education

• Inform patient that culture may be performed after completed course of medication
• Advise patient to notify nurse of diarrhea, symptoms of candidal vaginitis

Topical route

• Teach patient to use medical asepsis (hand washing) before, after each application; to apply with glove to prevent further infection; to avoid contact with eyes; not to use occlusive dressings
• Caution patient to avoid use of OTC creams, ointments, lotions unless directed by prescriber
• Instruct patient to notify prescriber if no improvement in condition in 4 wk or if symptoms return in 2 mo; pregnancy or a serious medical condition may be the cause

• Teach patient to use for full prescribed treatment time, or reinfection may occur

Vaginal route

• Instruct patient in asepsis (hand washing) before, after each application
• Teach patient to apply with applicator only; to avoid use of any other vaginal product unless directed by prescriber; sanitary napkin may prevent soiling of undergarments; to abstain from sexual intercourse until treatment is completed; reinfection and irritation may occur
• Instruct patient to notify prescriber if symptoms persist

Evaluation

Positive therapeutic outcome

• Decreasing oral candidiasis, fever, malaise, rash
• Negative C&S for infectious organism
• Decrease in size, number of lesions
• Decrease in itching or white discharge (vaginal)

Treatment of overdose: Withdraw drug; maintain airway; administer epINEPHrine, aminophylline, O₂, **IV** corticosteroids for anaphylaxis

---

midazolam (Rx)

(mid′ay-zoe-lam)
Versed
Func. class.: Sedative/hypnotic, antianxiety
Chem. class.: Benzodiazepine, short-acting

Pregnancy category D

Controlled substance schedule IV

Action: Depresses subcortical levels in CNS; may act on limbic system, reticular formation; may potentiate GABA by binding to specific benzodiazepine receptors

▶ **Therapeutic Outcome:** Sedation for anesthesia induction and procedures

Uses: Preoperative sedation, general anesthesia induction, sedation for diagnostic endoscopic procedures, intubation

Investigational uses: Epileptic seizures, refractory status epilepticus

Dosage and routes
Preoperative sedation
Adult: IM 0.07-0.08 mg/kg 30-60 min before general anesthesia

P *Child <6 mo:* IM 0.1-0.15 mg/kg, may give up to 0.5 mg/kg if needed

---

P *Child 6 mo-5 yr:* PO 0.25-1 mg/kg, max 20 mg as a single dose

P *Child 6 yr-16 yr:* PO 0.25-0.5 mg/kg, max 20 mg as a single dose

Induction of general anesthesia

P *Adult and child 12-16 yr:* Unpremedicated patients, **IV** 0.3-0.35 mg/kg over 30 sec, wait 2 min, follow with 25% of initial dose if needed; premedicated patients, 0.15-0.35 mg/kg over 20-30 sec, allow 2 min for effect

P *Child 6-12 yr:* **IV** 0.025-0.05 mg/kg, total dose up to 0.4 mg/kg if needed

P *Child 6 mo-5 yr:* **IV** 0.05-0.1 mg/kg, total dose up to 0.6 mg/kg may be needed

P *Child <6 mo:* Titrate with small increments

Continuous infusion for intubation (critical care)

Adult: **IV** 0.01-0.05 mg/kg over several min; repeat at 10-15 min intervals, until adequate sedation; then 0.02-0.10 mg/kg/hr maintenance

Child: **IV** 0.05-0.2 mg/kg over 2-3 min then 0.06-0.12 mg/kg/hr by cont inf; adjust as needed

Available forms: Inj 1, 5 mg/ml; syr 2 mg/ml

Adverse effects

(*italic* = common; **bold** = life-threatening)

CNS: Retrograde amnesia, euphoria, confusion, headache, anxiety, insomnia, slurred speech, paresthesia, tremors, weakness, chills

CV: Hypotension, PVCs, tachycardia, bigeminy, nodal rhythm, **cardiac arrest**

EENT: Blurred vision, nystagmus, diplopia, blocked ears, loss of balance

GI: *Nausea, vomiting,* increased salivation, hiccups

INTEG: Urticaria, pain, swelling at inj site, rash, pruritus

RESP: Coughing, **apnea, bronchospasm, laryngospasm,** dyspnea, **respiratory depression**

Contraindications: Pregnancy **D**, hypersensitivity to benzodiazepines, shock, coma, alcohol intoxication, acute narrow-angle glaucoma

G **Precautions:** COPD, CHF, chronic renal **P** failure, chills, debilitated, elderly, children, lactation

N **Do Not Confuse:**
Versed/Vepesid, Versed/Vistaril

Pharmacokinetics

Absorption	Well absorbed
Distribution	Crosses placenta, blood-brain barrier
Metabolism	Liver
Excretion	Kidneys, breast milk
Half-life	1-12 hr

Pharmacodynamics

	IM	IV
Onset	15 min	3-5 min
Peak	½-1 hr	Unknown
Duration	2-6 hr	2-6 hr

Interactions

Individual drugs

Alcohol: ↑ CNS depression

Cimetidine: ↑ levels of midazolam

Erythromycin, theophylline: May alter midazolam metabolism

Fluvoxamine, indinavir, ritonavir, verapamil: ↑ respiratory depression

Drug classifications

Antifungals, azole: ↑ levels of midalozam

Antihistamines, opiates, sedative/hypnotics: ↑ CNS depression

Antihypertensives, nitrates: ↑ hypotension

Oral contraceptives: ↑ half-life of midazolam

Theophyllines: ↓ effect of midazolam

Food/drug

Grapefruit juice: ↑ midazolam effect

Herb/drug

Black cohosh: ↑ hypotension

Catnip, chamomile, clary, cowslip, hops, kava, lavender, mistletoe, nettle, pokeweed, poppy, Queen Anne's lace, senega, skullcap, valerian: ↑ CNS depression

NURSING CONSIDERATIONS
Assessment

• Monitor B/P, pulse, respiration during **IV**; O₂ and emergency equipment should be nearby

• Monitor inj site for redness, pain, swelling

G • Assess degree of amnesia in elderly; may be increased

• Assess anterograde amnesia

• Assess vital signs for recovery period in obese patient, since half-life may be extended

• Assess for apnea, respiratory depression, **G** which may be increased in the elderly

Nursing diagnoses

✓ Knowledge, deficient (teaching)

Implementation
PO route

• Remove cap of press-in bottle adaptor and

M

push adaptor into neck of bottle, close with cap, remove cap and insert tip of dispenser and insert into adaptor, turn upside-down and withdraw correct dose, place in mouth

IM route
• Give inj deep into large muscle mass

IV IV route
• Give **IV** undiluted or after diluting with D_5W or 0.9% NaCl to a conc of 0.25 mg/ml; give over 2 min (conscious sedation) or over 30 sec (anesthesia induction)
• Ensure immediate availability of resuscitation equipment, O_2 to support airway; do not give by rapid bol

Syringe compatibilities: Atracurium, atropine, benzquinamide, buprenorphine, butorphanol, chlorproMAZINE, cimetadine, diphenhydrAMINE, droperidol, fentanyl, glycopyrrolate, hydromorphine, hydrOXYzine, meperidine, metoclopramide, morphine, nalbuphine, promazine, promethazine, scopolamine, sufentanil, thiethylperazine, trimethobenzamide

Syringe incompatibilities: Dimenhydrinate, pentobarbital, perphenazine, prochlorperazine, ranitidine

Y-site compatibilities: Amikacin, amiodarone, atracurium, calcium gluconate, cefazolin, cefmetazole, cefotaxime, cimetidine, ciprofloxacin, clindamycin, digoxin, diltiazem, DOPamine, epINEPHrine, erythromycin, esmolol, etomidate, famotidine, fentanyl, fluconazole, gentamicin, haloperidol, heparin, hydromorphone, insulin (regular), labetalol, lorazepam, methylPREDNISolone, metronidazole, milrinone, morphine, niCARdipine, nitroglycerin, norepinephrine, pancuronium, piperacillin, potassium chloride, ranitidine, sodium nitroprusside, sufentanil, theophylline, tobramycin, vancomycin, vecuronium

Y-site incompatibilities: Foscarnet
IM route
• Give IM inj deep in large muscle mass
• Store at room temp

Patient/family education
• Inform patient that amnesia occurs; events may not be remembered
• Caution patient to avoid CNS depressants including alcohol for 24 hr after taking this drug

Evaluation
Positive therapeutic outcome
• Induction of sedation, amnesia

Treatment of overdose: O_2, vasopressors, physostigmine, resuscitation; flumazenil will reverse effects

---

midodrine (Rx)
(mye'doh-dreen)
ProAmatine
Func. class.: Prodrug

Pregnancy category C

Action: Activates α-adrenergic receptors of arteriolar, venous vasculature; increases vascular tone

➡ Therapeutic Outcome: Decreased feeling of faintness upon rising, absence of significant change in B/P

Uses: Orthostatic hypotension

Dosage and routes
Adult: PO 10 mg tid

Renal dose
Adult: PO 2.5 mg tid

Available forms: Tabs 2.5, 5 mg

Adverse effects
(*italic* = common; **bold** = life-threatening)
CNS: Drowsiness, restlessness, headache, paresthesia, pain, chills, confusion
CV: **Supine hypertension,** vasodilatation, flushing face
EENT: Dry mouth, blurred vision
GI: Nausea, anorexia
GU: Dysuria
INTEG: Pruritus, piloerection, rash

Contraindications: Hypersensitivity, severe organic heart disease, acute renal disease, urinary retention, pheochromocytoma, thyrotoxicosis, persistent/excessive supine hypertension

P Precautions: Children, urinary retention, lactation, prostatic hypertrophy, pregnancy **C**, hepatic function impairment, orthostatic diabetic patients

N Do Not Confuse:
ProAmatine/Protamine

Pharmacokinetics	
Absorption	Unknown
Distribution	Unknown
Metabolism	Unknown
Excretion	Unknown
Half-life	3-4 hr

Pharmacodynamics

Onset	Unknown
Peak	1-2 hr
Duration	Unknown

Interactions
Individual drugs:
Fludrocortisone: ↑ supine hypertension
Drug classifications
α-Adrenergic agonists: ↑ pressor effects
β-Adrenergic blockers, cardiac glycosides, psychotropics: ↑ bradycardia
Steroids: ↑ intraocular pressure

NURSING CONSIDERATIONS
Assessment
• Monitor VS, B/P (standing, supine); notify prescriber if B/P supine is increased
• Observe for drowsiness, dizziness, LOC

Implementation
• Tablets may be swallowed whole, chewed, or allowed to dissolve
• Administer upon arising, at midday, and in late afternoon (no later than 6 PM)
• Avoid administering if patient is to be supine during day

Nursing diagnoses
☑ Knowledge, deficient (teaching)

Patient/family education
• Advise to avoid hazardous activities; activities requiring alertness; dizziness may occur; instruct patient to request assistance with ambulation
• Advise to avoid alcohol, other depressants

Evaluation
Positive therapeutic outcome
• Decreased orthostatic hypotension

mifepristone (Rx)
(mif-ee-press'tone)
Mifeprex
Func. class.: Abortifacient
Chem. class.: Antiprogestational
Pregnancy category C

Action: Stimulates uterine contractions, causing complete abortion

⮞ **Therapeutic Outcome:** Termination of pregnancy

Uses: Abortion through 49 days gestation

Investigational uses: Postcoital contraception/contragestation, intrauterine fetal death, endometriosis, Cushing's syndrome, unresectable meningioma

Dosage and routes
Coadministration of mifepristone/ misoprostol
• Day 1: PO single dose 600 mg mifepristone
• Day 3: 400 mcg misoprostol

Available forms: Tabs 200 mg

Adverse effects
(*italic* = common; **bold** = life-threatening)
CNS: Dizziness, insomnia, anxiety, syncope, fainting, headache
GI: Nausea, vomiting, diarrhea, dyspepsia
GU: Uterine cramping, uterine hemorrhage, vaginitis, pelvic pain
MISC: Fatigue, back pain, fever, viral infections, chills, sinusitis

Contraindications: Hypersensitivity, severe hepatic disease, severe renal disease, PID, respiratory disease, cardiac disease, IUD, ectopic pregnancy, chronic adrenal failure, bleeding disorder, inherited porphyrias

Precautions: Asthma, anemia, jaundice, diabetes mellitus, seizure disorders, women >35 yr/smoking ≥10 cigarettes/day, past uterine surgery, pregnancy **C**

Pharmacokinetics

Absorption	Rapidly
Distribution	98% protein binding, albumin, glycoprotein
Metabolism	Unknown
Excretion	Feces, urine
Half-life	Unknown

Pharmacodynamics

Onset	Unknown
Peak	90 min
Duration	Unknown

Interactions
Individual drugs
Erythromycin, itraconazole, ketoconazole: ↓ metabolism of each specific drug
Food/drug
Grapefruit juice: ↓ metabolism of mifepristone
☑ *Herb/drug*
St. John's wort: ↓ mifepristone action

NURSING CONSIDERATIONS
Assessment
• Monitor B/P, pulse; watch for change that may indicate hemorrhage
• Monitor respiratory rate, rhythm, depth; notify prescriber of abnormalities
• Assess for length, duration of contraction;

M

notify prescriber of contractions lasting over 1 min or absence of contractions
• Assess for incomplete abortion, pregnancy must be terminated by another method; drug is teratogenic

Nursing diagnoses
☑ Pain, acute (adverse reactions)
☑ Knowledge, deficient (teaching)

Implementation
• Provide emotional support before and after abortion

Patient/family education
• Advise patient to report increased blood loss, abdominal cramps, increased temperature, foul-smelling lochia
• Teach patient some methods of comfort control and pain control
• Advise patient to continue with follow-up
• Advise patient that cramping and vaginal bleeding will occur

Evaluation
Positive therapeutic outcome
• Expulsion of fetus

---

miglitol (Rx)
(mig'le-tol)
Glyset
Func. class.: Oral hypoglycemic
Chem. class.: α-Glucosidase inhibitor

Pregnancy category B

Action: Delays the digestion of ingested carbohydrates, results in a smaller rise in blood glucose after meals; does not increase insulin production

⇨ **Therapeutic Outcome:** Decreased blood glucose levels in diabetes mellitus

Uses: Stable adult-onset diabetes mellitus, (type 2)

Dosage and routes
Initial dose
Adult: PO 25 mg tid with first bite of meal

Maintenance dose
Adult: PO may be increased to 50 mg tid; may increase to 100 mg tid if needed only in patients >60 kg; dosage adjustment at 4-8 wk intervals

Available forms: Tabs 25, 50, 100 mg

Adverse effects
(*italic* = common; **bold** = life-threatening)
GI: *Abdominal pain, diarrhea, flatulence,* **hepatotoxicity**

HEMA: Low iron
INTEG: Rash

Contraindications: Hypersensitivity, diabetic ketoacidosis, cirrhosis, inflammatory bowel disease, colonic ulceration, partial intestinal obstruction, chronic intestinal disease

Precautions: Pregnancy **B,** renal disease, ☑ lactation, children, hepatic disease

Pharmacokinetics	
Absorption	Unknown
Distribution	Unknown
Metabolism	Not metabolized
Excretion	Kidneys, unchanged drug
Half-life	2 hr

Pharmacodynamics	
Onset	Unknown
Peak	2-3 hr
Duration	Unknown

Interactions
Individual drugs
Digoxin: ↓ levels of digoxin
Propranolol: ↓ levels of propranolol
Ranitidine: ↓ levels of ranitidine
Drug classifications
Adsorbents (intestinal), enzymes (digestive): ↓ miglitol levels; do not use together

Food/drug
Carbohydrates: ↑ diarrhea
☑ *Herb/drug*
Broom, buchu, dandelion, juniper: ↓ hypoglycemia
Chromium, fenugreek, ginseng: ↑ or ↓ hypoglycemic effect
Karela: Improved glucose tolerance

NURSING CONSIDERATIONS
Assessment
• Assess for hypoglycemia, hyperglycemia; even though this drug does not cause hypoglycemia, if taking a sulfonylurea or insulin, hypoglycemia may be additive
• Monitor blood glucose levels, glycosylated hemoglobin, liver function tests

Nursing diagnoses
☑ Nutrition: more than body requirements, imbalanced (uses)
☑ Nutrition: less than body requirements, imbalanced (adverse reactions)
☑ Knowledge, deficient (teaching)
☑ Noncompliance (teaching)

Implementation
• Give tid with first bite of each meal

☑ Herb/drug   🚫 Do Not Crush   ◆ Alert   ◆☊ Key Drug   🅖 Geriatric   🅿 Pediatric

- Provide storage in airtight container in cool environment

Patient/family education
- Teach patient the symptoms of hypoglycemia, hyperglycemia and what to do about each
- Instruct that medication must be taken as prescribed; explain consequences of discontinuing the medication abruptly; that during periods of stress, infection, surgery, insulin may be required
- Tell patient to avoid OTC medications unless approved by prescriber
- Teach patient that diabetes is a lifelong illness; drug will not cure condition
- Instruct patient to carry/wear emergency ID as diabetic
- Teach patient that diet and exercise regimen must be followed

Evaluation
Positive therapeutic outcome
- Decreased signs, symptoms of diabetes mellitus (polyuria, polydipsia, polyphagia, clear sensorium, absence of dizziness, stable gait)

miglustat
Zavesa
See Appendix A, Selected New Drugs

! HIGH ALERT

milrinone (Rx)
(mill-re′none)
Primacor
Func. class.: Inotropic/vasodilator agent with phosphodiesterase activity
Chem. class.: Bipyridine derivative

Pregnancy category C

Action: Positive inotropic agent with vasodilator properties; increases contractility of cardiac muscle; reduces preload and afterload by direct relaxation of vascular smooth muscle; increases myocardial contractility

Therapeutic Outcome: Increased inotropic effect resulting in increased cardiac output

Uses: Short-term management of advanced CHF that has not responded to other medication; can be used with digitalis products

Dosage and routes
Adult: **IV** bol 50 mcg/kg given over 10 min; start inf of 0.375-0.75 mcg/kg/min; reduce dosage in renal impairment

Available forms: Inj 1 mg/ml; premixed inj 200 mcg/ml in D^{5}W

Adverse effects
(*italic* = common; **bold** = life-threatening)
CV: Dysrhythmias, hypotension, chest pain
GI: Nausea, vomiting, anorexia, abdominal pain, **hepatotoxicity,** jaundice
HEMA: **Thrombocytopenia**
MISC: Headache, hypokalemia, tremor

Contraindications: Hypersensitivity to this drug, severe aortic disease, severe pulmonic valvular disease, acute MI

Precautions: Lactation, pregnancy **C,** children, renal disease, hepatic disease, atrial flutter/fibrillation, elderly

Pharmacokinetics
Absorption	Completely absorbed
Distribution	Unknown
Metabolism	Liver (50%)
Excretion	Kidney, unchanged (83%), metabolites (12%)
Half-life	2.4 hr; increased in CHF

Pharmacodynamics
Onset	2-5 min
Peak	10 min
Duration	Variable

Interactions: None

NURSING CONSIDERATIONS
Assessment
- Monitor manifestations of hypokalemia: acidic urine, reduced urine, osmolality, nocturia; hypotension, broad T-wave, U-wave, ectopy, tachycardia, weak pulse; muscle weakness, altered LOC, drowsiness, apathy, lethargy, confusion, depression; anorexia, nausea, cramps, constipation, distention, paralytic ileus; hypoventilation, respiratory muscle weakness
- Assess fluid volume status: complete I&O ratio and record; note weight, distended red veins, crackles in lung, color, quality, and sp gr of urine, skin turgor, adequacy of pulses, moist mucous membranes, bilateral lung sounds, peripheral pitting edema; dehydration symptoms of decreasing output, thirst, hypotension, dry mouth and mucous membranes should be reported
- Monitor electrolytes: potassium, sodium, calcium, magnesium; also include BUN, blood pH, ABGs
- Monitor B/P and pulse, ECG continuously during **IV**, ventricular dysrhythmia can occur,

PCWP, CVP, index often during inf; if B/P drops 30 mm Hg, stop inf and call prescriber
• Monitor ALT, AST, bilirubin daily; if these are elevated, hepatoxicity is suspected
• Monitor platelets; if <150,000/mm³, drug is usually discontinued and another drug started
• Assess for extravasation: change site q48h

Nursing diagnoses
☑ Cardiac output, decreased (uses)
☑ Fluid volume, excess (uses)
☑ Knowledge, deficient (teaching)

Implementation
IV IV route
• Give **IV** loading dose undiluted over 10 min
• Do not mix directly with glucose sol; chemical reaction occurs over 24 hr; precipitate forms if milrinone and furosemide come in contact
• Administer by direct **IV** into inf through Y-connector or directly into tubing; may give undiluted over 2-3 min
• Give by cont inf diluted with 0.9% NaCl to conc of 1-3 mg/ml, run at prescribed rate; give by infusion pump for doses other than bol
• Administer potassium supplements if ordered for potassium levels <3.0 mg/dl

Syringe compatibilities: Atropine, calcium chloride, digoxin, epINEPHrine, lidocaine, morphine, propranolol, sodium bicarbonate, verapamil

Y-site compatibilities: Digoxin, diltiazem, DOBUTamine, DOPamine, epINEPHrine, fentanyl, heparin, hydromorphone, labetalol, lorazepam, midazolam, morphine, niCARdipine, nitroglycerin, norepinephrine, propranolol, quinidine, ranitidine, thiopental, vecuronium

Additive compatibilities: Quinidine

Patient/family education
• Teach patient reason for medication and expected results
• Instruct patient to make position changes slowly; orthostatic hypotension may occur
• Teach patient signs and symptoms of hypersensitivity reactions and hypokalemia

Evaluation
Positive therapeutic outcome
• Increased cardiac output
• Decreased PCWP, adequate CVP
• Decreased dyspnea, fatigue, edema, ECG

Treatment of overdose: Discontinue drug, support circulation

---

minocycline (Rx)
(min-oh-sye'kleen)
Dynacin, Minocin
Func. class.: Antiinfective
Chem. class.: Tetracycline

Pregnancy category D

Action: Inhibits protein synthesis and phosphorylation in microorganisms by binding to 30S ribosomal subunits and reversibly binding to 50S ribosomal subunits; bacteriostatic

➡ **Therapeutic Outcome:** Bactericidal action against susceptible organisms, including *Neisseria meningitidis, Neisseria gonorrhoeae, Treponema pallidum, Chlamydia trachomatis, Ureaplasma urealyticum, Mycoplasma pneumoniae, Nocardia, Rickettsia*

Uses: Syphilis, chlamydial infection, gonorrhea, lymphogranuloma venereum, rickettsial infections, inflammatory acne, meningitis carriers, periodontitis

Investigational uses: Rheumatoid arthritis

Dosage and routes
Adult: PO/**IV** 200 mg, then 100 mg q12h or 50 mg q6h, max 400 mg/24 hr **IV**; subgingival insert into periodontal pocket

P *Child >8 yr:* PO/**IV** 4 mg/kg then 4 mg/kg/day PO in divided doses q12h

Gonorrhea
Adult: PO 200 mg, then 100 mg q12h × 4 days

C. trachomatis infection
Adult: PO 100 mg bid × 7 days

Syphilis
Adult: PO 200 mg, then 100 mg q12h × 10-15 days

Uncomplicated gonococcal urethritis in men
Adult: PO 100 mg q12h × 5 days

Rheumatoid arthritis (off-label)
Adult: PO 100 mg bid for ≤48 wk

Available forms: Caps 50, 75, 100 mg; oral susp 50 mg/5 ml; powder for inj 100 mg; caps, pellet filled 50, 100 mg

Adverse effects
(*italic* = common; **bold** = life-threatening)
CNS: Dizziness, fever, lightheadedness, vertigo
CV: Pericarditis
EENT: Dysphagia, glossitis, decreased calcifi-

---

cation, permanent discoloration of teeth, oral candidiasis
GI: Nausea, abdominal pain, *vomiting, diarrhea,* anorexia, enterocolitis, **hepatotoxicity,** flatulence, abdominal cramps, epigastric burning, stomatitis
GU: Increased BUN, polyuria, polydipsia, **renal failure, nephrotoxicity**
HEMA: **Eosinophilia, neutropenia, thrombocytopenia, hemolytic anemia**
INTEG: Rash, urticaria, photosensitivity, increased pigmentation, **exfoliative dermatitis,** pruritus, angioedema, blue-gray color of skin and mucous membranes

Contraindications: Hypersensitivity to ☐ tetracyclines, children <8 yr, pregnancy **D**

Precautions: Hepatic disease, lactation

Pharmacokinetics	
Absorption	Well absorbed (PO)
Distribution	Widely distributed (70%-75% protein bound); some distribution in CSF, crosses placenta
Metabolism	Liver, some
Excretion	Kidneys, unchanged (20%), bile, feces
Half-life	11-17 hr

Pharmacodynamics		
	PO	IV
Onset	Rapid	Rapid
Peak	2-3 hr	Infusion's end

Interactions
Individual drugs
Calcium, iron, magnesium: Forms chelates, ↓ absorption
Carbamazepine, phenytoin: ↓ effect
Kaolin/pectin, sodium bicarbonate: ↓ minocycline effect
Warfarin: ↑ effect
Drug classifications
Antacids, alkali products: ↓ minocycline effect
Antidiarrheals (adsorbent): ↓ absorption
Barbiturates, penicillins: ↓ effect
Oral contraceptives: ↓ effect of oral contraception
Lab test interferences
False negative: Urine glucose with Clinistix, Tes-Tape

NURSING CONSIDERATIONS
Assessment
• Assess patient for previous sensitivity reaction
• Assess patient for signs and symptoms of infection including characteristics of wounds, sputum, urine, stool, WBC >10,000/mm³,

fever; obtain baseline information, before and during treatment
• Obtain C&S before beginning drug therapy to identify if correct treatment has been initiated
• Assess for allergic reactions: rash, urticaria, pruritus
• Monitor blood studies: AST, ALT, CBC, Hct, bilirubin, alkaline phosphatase, amylase monthly if patient is on long-term therapy
• Assess bowel pattern qd; if severe diarrhea occurs, drug should be discontinued
• Monitor for bleeding: ecchymosis, bleeding gums, hematuria, stool guaiac daily if on long-term therapy; blood dyscrasias may occur
• Assess for overgrowth of infection: perineal itching, fever, malaise, redness, pain, swelling, drainage, rash, diarrhea, change in cough, sputum; black, furry tongue

Nursing diagnoses
☑ Infection, risk for (uses)
☑ Diarrhea (adverse reactions)
☑ Knowledge, deficient (teaching)
☑ Noncompliance (teaching)

Implementation
PO route
• Give around the clock to maintain proper blood levels; give with food to increase absorption of drug; do not give within 3 hr of other agents; drug interactions may occur
• Give with 8 oz of water 1 hr before hs to prevent ulceration
• Shake liq preparation well before giving; use calibrated device for proper dosing
• Do not give with iron, calcium, magnesium products, or antacids, which decrease absorption and form insoluble chelate
☑ **IV route**
• Check for irritation, extravasation, phlebitis daily; change site q72h
• For intermittent inf, dilute each 100 mg/10 ml of 0.9% NaCl, sterile water for inj; further dilute in 500-1000 ml of 0.9% NaCl, D₅W, Ringer's, LR, D₅/LR; give over 6 hr

Y-site compatibilities: Cyclophosphamide, fludarabine, granisetron, heparin, hydrocortisone, magnesium sulfate, melphalan, perphenazine, potassium chloride, sargramostim, sodium succinate, vinorelbine, vit B/C

Y-site incompatibilities: Aztreonam, filgrastim, hydromorphone, meperidine, morphine, teniposide

Patient/family education
• Teach patient to use sunscreen when outdoors to decrease photosensitivity reaction

M

- Teach patient to report sore throat, bruising, bleeding, joint pain; may indicate blood dyscrasias (rare)
- Advise patient to contact prescriber if vaginal itching, loose foul-smelling stools, furry tongue occur; may indicate superinfection; report itching, rash, pruritus, urticaria
- Instruct patient to take all medication prescribed for the length of time ordered; drug must be taken around the clock to maintain blood levels; do not give medication to others; take with a full glass of water; may take with food; not to use outdated product, Fanconi's syndrome may occur
- Advise patient to use a form of contraception other than hormonal

Evaluation
Positive therapeutic outcome
- Absence of signs/symptoms of infection (WBC <10,000/mm^3, temp WNL, absence of red, draining wounds)
- Reported improvement in symptoms of infection

---

minoxidil (Rx, OTC)
(mi-nox'i-dill)
Loniten, minoxidil, Rogaine (top)
Func. class.: Antihypertensive, hair growth stimulant
Chem. class.: Vasodilator, peripheral

Pregnancy category C

Action: Directly relaxes arteriolar smooth muscle, causing vasodilatation; increased cutaneous blood flow; stimulation of hair follicles

Therapeutic Outcome: Decreased B/P in hypertension; hair growth

Uses: Severe hypertension unresponsive to other therapy (use with diuretic); topically to treat alopecia

Dosage and routes
Severe hypertension
Adult: PO 2.5-5 mg/day max 100 mg daily; usual range 10-40 mg/day in single doses

Elderly: PO 2.5 mg qd, may be increased gradually

Child <12 yr: Initial, 0.2 mg/kg/day; effective range, 0.25-1 mg/kg/day; max, 50 mg/day

Alopecia
Adult: Top 1 ml bid rub into scalp daily, max 2 ml/day

Available forms: Tabs 2.5, 10 mg; top 2% sol

Adverse effects
(*italic* = common; **bold** = life-threatening)
CNS: Headache, fatigue
CV: Severe rebound hypertension (withdrawal in children), tachycardia, angina, increased T-wave, **CHF, pulmonary edema, pericardial effusion,** edema, sodium retention, water retention
GI: Nausea, vomiting
GU: Breast tenderness
HEMA: Hct, Hgb, erythrocyte count may decrease initially
INTEG: Pruritus, **Stevens-Johnson syndrome,** rash, hirsutism

Contraindications: Acute MI, dissecting aortic aneurysm, hypersensitivity, pheochromocytoma

Precautions: Pregnancy **C**, lactation, children, renal disease, CAD, CHF, elderly

Do Not Confuse:
Loniten/Lotensin, minoxidil/Monopril

Pharmacokinetics	
Absorption	Well absorbed (PO); minimally absorbed (top)
Distribution	Widely distributed
Metabolism	Liver
Excretion	Kidneys, breast milk
Half-life	4.2 hr

Pharmacodynamics		
	PO	TOP
Onset	½ hr	4 mo
Peak	2-3 hr	Unknown
Duration	75 hr	4 mo

Interactions
Drug classifications
Antihypertensives: ↑ orthostatic hypotension

Lab test interferences
↑ Renal function studies
↓ Hgb, ↓ Hct, ↓ RBC

NURSING CONSIDERATIONS
Assessment
- Monitor closely, usually given with β-blocker to prevent tachycardia and increased myocardial workload, usually given with diuretic to prevent serious fluid accumulation, patient should be hospitalized during beginning treatment
- Monitor B/P, pulse, jugular venous distention periodically throughout treatment

---

 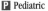

- Monitor electrolytes, blood studies: potassium, sodium, chloride, carbon dioxide, CBC, serum glucose
- Monitor weight daily, I&O; assess edema in feet, legs daily; check skin turgor, dryness of mucous membranes for hydration status
- Assess for rales, dyspnea, orthopnea, peripheral edema, fatigue, weight gain, jugular vein distention (CHF)
- Assess for signs of hyperglycemia: acetone breath, increased urinary output, severe thirst, lethargy, dizziness

Nursing diagnoses
✓ Cardiac output, decreased (adverse reactions)
✓ Injury, risk for (side effects)
✓ Knowledge, deficient (teaching)

Implementation
PO route
- Give with meals to decrease GI symptoms
- Give with β-blockers and/or diuretic for hypertension
- Store protected from light and heat

Topical route
- Administer 1 ml dose no matter how much balding has occurred; increasing dose does not speed hair growth
- Treatment must continue long term or new hair will be lost again

Patient/family education
Topical route
- Teach patient that new hair will be soft and hardly visible
- Caution patient not to use on other parts of the body; drug is to be used on the scalp only
- Instruct patient that hair should be clean before applying medication; do not get on clothing
- Caution patient not to get medication near mucous membranes (mouth, nose, eyes) and to contact prescriber if burning, stinging, or rash occurs

Evaluation
Positive therapeutic outcome
- Decreased B/P in hypertension
- Hair growth (Top)

---

mirtazapine (Rx)
(mer-ta′za-peen)
Remeron, Remeron Soltab
Func. class.: Antidepressant
Chem. class.: Tetracyclic

Pregnancy category C

Action: Blocks reuptake of norepinephrine, serotonin into nerve endings, increasing action of norepinephrine, serotonin in nerve cells; has anticholinergic action

Therapeutic Outcome: Decreased symptoms of depression after 2-3 wk

Uses: Depression, dysthymic disorder, bipolar disorder: depression, agitated depression

Dosage and routes
Adult: PO 15 mg/day at hs, maintenance to continue for 6 mo, titrate up to 45 mg/day; orally disintegrating tabs, open blister pack, place tab on tongue, allow to disintegrate, swallow

Elderly: PO 7.5 mg qhs, increase by 7.5 mg q1-2 wk to desired dose, max 45 mg/day

Available forms: Tabs 15, 30 mg; orally disintegrating tabs 15, 30, 45 mg

Adverse effects
(*italic* = common; **bold** = life-threatening)
CNS: Dizziness, drowsiness, confusion, headache, anxiety, tremors, stimulation, weakness, insomnia, nightmares, extrapyramidal symptoms (EPS) (elderly), increased psychiatric symptoms, *seizures*
CV: Orthostatic hypotension, ECG changes, tachycardia, hypertension, palpitations
EENT: Blurred vision, tinnitus, mydriasis
GI: Diarrhea, dry mouth, nausea, vomiting, **paralytic ileus,** increased appetite; cramps, epigastric distress, **jaundice, hepatitis,** stomatitis, constipation
GU: Retention, **acute renal failure**
HEMA: **Agranulocytosis, thrombocytopenia, eosinophilia, leukopenia**
INTEG: Rash, urticaria, sweating, pruritus, photosensitivity
SYST: Flulike symptoms

Contraindications: Hypersensitivity to tricyclic antidepressants, recovery phase of MI, seizure disorders, prostatic hypertrophy

Precautions: Suicidal patients, severe depression, increased intraocular pressure, narrow-angle glaucoma, urinary retention, cardiac disease, hepatic disease, renal disease, hypothyroidism, hyperthyroidism, electroshock therapy, elective surgery, elderly, pregnancy **C**

Pharmacokinetics	
Absorption	Slow, complete
Distribution	Widely distributed; crosses placenta
Metabolism	Liver, extensively
Excretion	Feces; breast milk
Half-life	20-40 hr

M

Pharmacodynamics	
Onset	Unknown
Peak	2 hr
Duration	Unknown

Interactions
Individual drugs
Alcohol: ↑ CNS depression
Cimetidine, fluoxetine: ↑ levels, ↑ toxicity
Clonidine: Severe hypotension; avoid use
Disulfiram: Organic brain syndrome
Drug classifications
Analgesics, antihistamines, sedative/hypnotics: ↑ CNS depression
Anticholinergics: ↑ side effects
Antihypertensives: May block antihypertensive effect
Barbiturates, CNS depressants (other), contraceptives (oral): ↑ effects
MAOIs: Hypertensive crisis, seizures
Phenothiazines, oral contraceptives: ↑ toxicity
Smoking
↑ Metabolism, ↓ effects

☑ Herb/drug
Belladonna, henbane: ↑ anticholinergic effect
Chamomile, hops, kava, skullcap, valerian: ↑ CNS depression
St. John's wort, SAM-e: serotonin syndrome
Scopolia: ↑ antidepressant effect
Lab test interferences
↑ Serum bilirubin, ↑ blood glucose, ↑ alkaline phosphatase
↓ VMA, ↓ 5-HIAA
False: ↑ Urinary catecholamines

NURSING CONSIDERATIONS
Assessment
• Monitor B/P (with patient lying, standing), pulse q4h during beginning treatment; if systolic B/P drops 20 mm Hg, hold drug, notify prescriber; take VS q4h in patients with CV disease
• Monitor blood studies: CBC, leukocytes, differential, cardiac enzymes if patient is receiving long-term therapy
• Monitor hepatic studies: AST, ALT, bilirubin
• Check weight weekly, drug may increase appetite
• Assess ECG for flattening of T-wave, bundle branch block, AV block, dysrhythmias in cardiac patients
G • Assess for EPS primarily in elderly: rigidity, dystonia, akathisia
• Assess mental status: mood, sensorium, affect, suicidal tendencies; assess increase in psychiatric symptoms: depression, panic

• Identify alcohol consumption; if alcohol is consumed, hold dose until AM

Nursing diagnoses
☑ Coping, ineffective (uses)
☑ Injury, risk for (side effects)
☑ Knowledge, deficient (teaching)
☑ Noncompliance (teaching)

Implementation
• Give with food or milk for GI symptoms; crush if patient is unable to swallow medication whole
S • Give dose hs if oversedation occurs during day; may take entire dose hs; elderly may not tolerate once/day dosing
• Store at room temp; do not freeze
Orally disintegrating tablets
• No water needed, allow to dissolve on tongue

Patient/family education
• Inform patient that therapeutic effects may take 2-3 wk
G • Advise patient to use caution in driving and other activities requiring alertness because of drowsiness, dizziness, blurred vision; to avoid rising quickly from sitting to standing, especially elderly
• Caution patient to avoid alcohol ingestion, other CNS depressants
G • Teach patient to increase fluids, bulk in diet if constipation, urinary retention occur, especially elderly
• Teach patient to use gum, hard sugarless candy, or frequent sips of water for dry mouth
• To report immediately urinary retention

Evaluation
Positive therapeutic outcome
• Decrease in depression
• Absence of suicidal thoughts

Treatment of overdose: ECG monitoring, induce emesis, lavage, activated charcoal, administer anticonvulsant

---

misoprostol (Rx)
(mye-soe-prost'ole)
Cytotec
Func. class.: Gastric mucosa protectant; antiulcer
Chem. class.: Prostaglandin E_1 analog

Pregnancy category X

Action: Inhibits gastric acid secretion; may protect gastric mucosa; can increase bicarbonate, mucus production

⇒ **Therapeutic Outcome:** Prevention of gastric ulcers

Uses: Prevention of NSAID-induced gastric ulcers

Dosage and routes
Adult: PO 200 mcg qid with food for duration of NSAID therapy; if 200 mcg is not tolerated, 100 mcg may be given

Available forms: Tabs 100, 200 mcg

Adverse effects
(*italic* = common; **bold** = life-threatening)
GI: Diarrhea, nausea, vomiting, flatulence, constipation, dyspepsia, abdominal pain
GU: Spotting, cramps, hypermenorrhea, menstrual disorders

Contraindications: Hypersensitivity, pregnancy **X**

P Precautions: Lactation, children, elderly,
G renal disease

N Do Not Confuse:
Cytotec/Cytoxan, misoprostol/metoprolol

Pharmacokinetics	
Absorption	Well absorbed
Distribution	Unknown
Metabolism	Liver
Excretion	Kidneys
Half-life	½-1 hr

Pharmacodynamics	
Onset	½ hr
Peak	Unknown
Duration	3 hr

Interactions
Drug classifications
Antacids (magnesium): ↑ diarrhea
Food/drug
↓ Absorption with food

NURSING CONSIDERATIONS
Assessment
• Assess patient for GI symptoms: hematemesis, occult or frank blood in stools, also severe abdominal pain, cramping, severe diarrhea
• Obtain a negative pregnancy test in women of childbearing age before starting medication; miscarriages are common

Nursing diagnoses
✓ Pain, chronic (uses)
✓ Knowledge, deficient (teaching)

Implementation
• Give with meals for prolonged drug effect; avoid use of magnesium antacids

Patient/family education
• Advise patient to avoid black pepper, caffeine, alcohol, harsh spices, extremes in temp of food, which may aggravate condition
• Caution patient to avoid OTC preparations: aspirin, cough, cold preparations; condition may worsen
• Teach patient that drug must be continued for prescribed time to be effective and taken exactly as prescribed; doses are not to be doubled
• Instruct patient to report to prescriber diarrhea, black tarry stools, abdominal pain, cramping, menstrual disorders
• Caution patient to prevent pregnancy while taking this drug; spontaneous abortion may occur

Evaluation
Positive therapeutic outcome
• Prevention of ulcers

! HIGH ALERT

mitomycin (Rx)
(mye-toe-mye′sin)
mitomycin, Mutamycin
Func. class.: Antineoplastic, antibiotic

Pregnancy category D

Action: Inhibits DNA synthesis, primarily; derived from *Streptomyces caespitosus;* appears to cause cross-linking of DNA, a vesicant

→ Therapeutic Outcome: Prevention of rapidly growing malignant cells

Uses: Pancreas, stomach, head and neck, breast cancer

Investigational uses: Palliative treatment of head, neck, colon, breast, biliary, cervical, lung malignancies

Dosage and routes
Adult: **IV** 10-20 mg/m² q6-8 wk

Available forms: Inj 5, 20, 40 mg/vial

Adverse effects
(*italic* = common; **bold** = life-threatening)
CNS: Fever, headache, confusion, drowsiness, syncope, fatigue
EENT: Blurred vision, drowsiness, syncope
GI: Nausea, vomiting, anorexia, stomatitis, **hepatotoxicity,** diarrhea
GU: Urinary retention, **renal failure,** edema
HEMA: **Thrombocytopenia, leukopenia, anemia**
INTEG: Rash, alopecia, ***extravasation***
RESP: **Fibrosis, pulmonary infiltrate,** dyspnea
MISC: **Hemolytic uremic syndrome**

M

Contraindications: Hypersensitivity, pregnancy **D** (1st trimester), as a single agent, thrombocytopenia, coagulation disorders, lactation

Precautions: Renal disease, bone marrow depression

Pharmacokinetics

Absorption	Complete bioavailability
Distribution	Widely distributed; concentrates in tumor
Metabolism	Liver, extensively
Excretion	Kidneys, unchanged
Half-life	1 hr

Pharmacodynamics
Unknown

Interactions
Individual drugs
Radiation: ↑ toxicity, bone marrow suppression
Drug classifications
Antineoplastics: ↑ toxicity, bone marrow suppression

NURSING CONSIDERATIONS
Assessment
◆• Assess for fatal hemolytic uremic syndrome: hypertension, thrombocytopenia, microangiopathic hemolytic anemia, occurs during long-term therapy
• Assess buccal cavity q8h for dryness, sores or ulceration, white patches, oral pain, bleeding, dysphagia; obtain prescription for viscous lidocaine (Xylocaine)
• Assess symptoms indicating severe allergic reaction: rash, pruritus, urticaria, purpuric skin lesions, itching, flushing
• Monitor CBC, differential, platelet count weekly; withhold drug if WBC is <2000/mm^3 or platelet count is <100,000/mm^3 or granulocyte count is <1000/mm^3, notify prescriber of results if WBC <20,000/mm^3, platelets <150,000/mm^3
• Monitor renal function studies: BUN, creatinine, serum uric acid, urine CCr before and during therapy; check I&O ratio; report fall in urine output to <30 ml/hr
◆• Assess for pulmonary fibrosis, bronchospasm, dyspnea, rales, unproductive cough, chest pain, tachypnea, fatigue, increased pulse, pallor, lethargy
• Monitor temp q4h (may indicate beginning of infection)
• Monitor liver function tests before and during therapy (bilirubin, AST, ALT, LDH) as

needed or monthly; check for jaundiced skin and sclera, dark urine, clay-colored stools, itchy skin, abdominal pain, fever, diarrhea
• Assess for bleeding: hematuria, stool guaiac, bruising or petechiae, mucosa or orifices q8h; inflammation of mucosa, breaks in skin
• Identify effects of alopecia on body image; discuss feelings about body changes
• Identify edema in feet, joint pain, stomach pain, shaking; check for inflammation of mucosa, breaks in skin

Nursing diagnoses
☑ Injury, risk for (adverse reactions)
☑ Body image, disturbed (adverse reactions)
☑ Infection, risk for (adverse reactions)
☑ Knowledge, deficient (teaching)

Implementation
IV route
• Avoid contact with skin, since medication is very irritating; wash completely to remove
• Give fluids **IV** or PO before chemotherapy to hydrate patient
• Provide antacid before oral agent; give drug after evening meal, before hs; administer antiemetic 30-60 min before giving drug and prn to prevent vomiting; use antibiotics for prophylaxis of infection
• Give top or syst analgesics for pain
• Give in AM so drug can be eliminated before hs
• Provide a liq diet: carbonated beverages; gelatin may be added if patient is not nauseated or vomiting
• Encourage patient to rinse mouth tid-qid with water, club soda, brush teeth bid-qid with soft brush or cotton-tipped applicators for stomatitis, use unwaxed dental floss
• Drug should be prepared by experienced personnel using proper precautions in a biologic cabinet using gown, gloves, mask
• Give by direct **IV** after diluting 5 mg/10, or 10 mg/40 ml sterile water for inj; shake, allow to stand, give through Y-tube or 3 way stopcock; give over 5-10 min through running D$_5$W, 0.9% NaCl **IV**, color of reconstituted sol is gray
• Apply ice compress for extravasation

Syringe compatibilities: Bleomycin, cisplatin, cyclophosphamide, DOXOrubicin, droperidol, fluorouracil, furosemide, heparin, leucovorin, methotrexate, metoclopramide, vinBLAStine, vinCRIStine

Y-site compatibilities: Allopurinol, amifostine, bleomycin, cisplatin, cyclophosphamide, DOXOrubicin, droperidol, fluorouracil, furosemide, granisetron, heparin, leucovorin, melphalan, methotrexate, metoclopramide, ondansetron, teniposide, thiotepa, vinBLAStine, vinCRIStine

Y-site incompatibilities: Sargramostim, vinorelbine

Additive compatibilities: Dexamethasone, hydrocortisone

Additive incompatibilities: Bleomycin

Solution compatibilities: LR, 0.3% NaCl, 0.5% NaCl

Patient/family education
• Teach patient to avoid use of products containing aspirin or ibuprofen, razors, commercial mouthwash, since bleeding may occur; to report symptoms of bleeding (hematuria, tarry stools)
• Caution patient to report signs of anemia (fatigue, headache, irritability, faintness, shortness of breath)
• Advise patient to report any changes in breathing or coughing even several mo after treatment; to avoid crowds and persons with respiratory tract or other infections
• Inform patient that hair may be lost during treatment; a wig or hairpiece may make patient feel better; new hair may be different in color, texture
• Advise patient not to have any vaccinations without the advice of the prescriber, serious reactions can occur
• Teach patient that contraception is needed during treatment and for several mo after completion of therapy

Evaluation
Positive therapeutic outcome
• Prevention of rapid division of malignant cells

⚠ HIGH ALERT

mitoxantrone (Rx)
(mye-toe-zan'trone)
Novantrone
Func. class.: Antineoplastic-antibiotic, immunomodulator
Chem. class.: Synthetic anthraquinone

Pregnancy category D

Action: DNA reactive agent; cytocidal effect on both proliferating and nonproliferating cells, suggesting lack of cell cycle phase specificity; a vesicant

➡ **Therapeutic Outcome:** Prevention of rapidly growing malignant cells

Uses: Acute nonlymphocytic leukemia (adult), relapsed leukemia, breast cancer, multiple sclerosis

Investigational uses: Breast and liver malignancies, non-Hodgkin's lymphoma

Dosage and routes
Induction
Adult: **IV** inf 12 mg/m² /day on days 1-3, and 100 mg/m² cytosine arabinoside × 7 days as a cont 24-hr inf

Consolidation
Adult: **IV** inf 12 mg/m² given as a short 5-15 min inf

Multiple sclerosis
Adult: **IV** inf 12 mg/m² as a 5-15 min infusion q3 mo

Available forms: Inj 2 mg/ml

Adverse effects
*(italic = common; **bold** = life-threatening)*
CNS: Headache, **seizures**
CV: **CHF, cardiomyopathy, dysrhythmias,** ECG changes
EENT: Conjunctivitis, blue-green sclera
GI: *Nausea, vomiting, diarrhea, anorexia, mucositis,* **hepatotoxicity**
HEMA: **Thrombocytopenia, leukopenia, myelosuppression, anemia**
INTEG: *Rash, necrosis at inj site,* alopecia, dermatitis, thrombophlebitis at inj site
MISC: Fever
RESP: Cough, dyspnea

Contraindications: Hypersensitivity, pregnancy **D**

Precautions: Myelosuppression, lactation, cardiac disease, children, renal, hepatic disease, gout

Pharmacokinetics	
Absorption	Completely absorbed
Distribution	Widely distributed
Metabolism	Liver
Excretion	Bile; kidneys, unchanged (<10%)
Half-life	24-72 hr

Pharmacodynamics
Unknown

Interactions
Individual drugs
Radiation: ↑ toxicity, bone marrow suppression

Drug classifications
Antineoplastics: ↑ toxicity, bone marrow suppression
Live virus vaccines: ↑ adverse reactions

NURSING CONSIDERATIONS
Assessment
• Multiple sclerosis: obtain baseline multi-gated angiogram, left ventricular ejection fraction (LVEF) if symptoms of CHF occur, repeat LVEF or if cumulative dose is >100 mg/m^2; do not administer to patients who have received a lifetime dose of ≥140 mg/m^2 or if LVEF <50% or significant decrease in LVEF
• Do not administer in multiple sclerosis if neutrophils <1500/mm^3
• Obtain pregnancy test in all women of childbearing age
◆• Monitor ECG; watch for ST-T wave changes, low QRS and T, possible dysrhythmias (sinus tachycardia, heart block, PVCs); also monitor ECHO, chest x-ray, RAI angiography to assess ejection fraction before and during treatment, drug is cardiotoxic, may develop during treatment or months to years after treatment
• Assess buccal cavity q8h for dryness, sores or ulceration, white patches, oral pain, bleeding, dysphagia; obtain prescription for viscous lidocaine (Xylocaine)
• Assess symptoms indicating severe allergic reaction: rash, pruritus, urticaria, purpuric skin lesions, itching, flushing
• Assess tachypnea, ECG changes, dyspnea, edema, fatigue
• Monitor CBC, differential, platelet count weekly; withhold drug if WBC is <4000/mm^3 or platelet count is <100,000/mm^3, notify prescriber of results if WBC <20,000/mm^3, platelets <150,000/mm^3
• Assess for increased uric acid levels, swelling, joint pain primarily in extremities; patient should be well hydrated to prevent urate deposits
• Monitor renal function studies: BUN, creatinine, urine CCr before and during therapy; determine I&O ratio
• Monitor temp q4h (may indicate beginning of infection)
• Monitor liver function tests before and during therapy (bilirubin, AST, ALT, LDH) as needed or monthly; check for jaundiced skin and sclera, dark urine, clay-colored stools, itchy skin, abdominal pain, fever, diarrhea
• Assess for bleeding: hematuria, stool guaiac, bruising or petechiae, mucosa or orifices q8h; check for inflammation of mucosa, breaks in skin

• Identify effects of alopecia on body image; discuss feelings about body changes
◆• Assess for MS: obtain MUGA, LVEF baselines; repeat LVEF if symptoms of CHF occur or if cumulative dose is >100 mg/m^2; do not give to patients who have received a lifetime dose of ≥140 mg/m^2 or if LVEF <50% or significant LVEF
◆• Assess for secondary acute myelogenous leukemia (AML) that can develop after taking this drug

Nursing diagnoses
☑ Injury, risk for (adverse reactions)
☑ Body image, disturbed (adverse reactions)
☑ Infection, risk for (adverse reactions)
☑ Knowledge, deficient (teaching)

Implementation
• Avoid contact with skin, since medication is very irritating; wash completely to remove
• Give fluids **IV** or PO before chemotherapy to hydrate patient
• Give antacid before oral agent; give drug after evening meal, before hs; provide antiemetic 30-60 min before giving drug and prn to prevent vomiting; administer antibiotics for prophylaxis of infection
• Give top or systemic analgesics for pain
• Liq diet: carbonated beverages; gelatin may be added if patient is not nauseated or vomiting
• Encourage patient to rinse mouth tid-qid with water, club soda, brush teeth bid-qid with soft brush or cotton-tipped applicators for stomatitis, use unwaxed dental floss
• Sol should be prepared by qualified personnel only under controlled conditions in a biologic cabinet using mask, gloves, gown
• Use Luer-Lok tubing to prevent leakage; do not let sol come in contact with skin; if contact occurs wash well with soap and water
• Give by direct **IV** after diluting with 50 ml or more of 0.9% NaCl or D$_5$W; give over 3-5 min, running **IV** of D$_5$W or 0.9% NaCl
• Intermittent inf may be diluted further in D$_5$W, 0.9% NaCl and run over 15-30 min; check for extravasation

Y-site compatibilities: Allopurinol, amifostine, cladribine, filgrastim, fludarabine, granisetron, melphalan, ondansetron, sargramostim, teniposide, thiotepa, vinorelbine

Y-site incompatibilities: Paclitaxel

Additive compatibilities: Cyclophosphamide, cytarabine, fluorouracil, hydrocortisone, potassium chloride

---

🖉 Herb/drug   🚫 Do Not Crush   ◆ Alert   ◆ℼ Key Drug   🄶 Geriatric   🄿 Pediatric

Additive incompatibilities: Heparin

Solution compatibilities: D$_5$/0.9 NaCl, D$_5$W, 0.9% NaCl

Patient/family education
• Teach patient to avoid use of products containing aspirin or NSAIDs, razors, commercial mouthwash, since bleeding may occur; to report symptoms of bleeding (hematuria, tarry stools)
• Caution patient to report signs of anemia (fatigue, headache, irritability, faintness, shortness of breath)
• Inform patient that hair may be lost during treatment; a wig or hairpiece may make patient feel better; new hair may be different in color, texture
• Caution patient not to have any vaccinations without the advice of the prescriber; serious reactions can occur
• Advise patient that contraception is needed during treatment and for several mo after completion of therapy
• Advise patient that sclera, urine may turn blue or green

Evaluation
Positive therapeutic outcome
• Prevention of rapid division of malignant cells

! HIGH ALERT

mivacurium (Rx)
(mi-va-kure'ee-um)
Mivacron
Func. class.: Nondepolarizing neuromuscular blocker

Pregnancy category C

Action: Inhibits transmission of nerve impulses by binding with cholinergic receptor sites, antagonizing action of acetylcholine; no analgesic response

➡ Therapeutic Outcome: Paralysis of all skeletal muscles

Uses: Facilitation of endotracheal intubation; skeletal muscle relaxation during mechanical ventilation, surgery, or general anesthesia; reduction of fractures/dislocations

Dosage and routes
Adult: **IV** 0.15 mg/kg; maintenance q15 min
P *Child 2-12:* **IV** 0.2 mg/kg for a 10-min block

Available forms: 5, 10 ml single-use vial

(2 mg/ml); premixed inf in D$_5$W 50 ml flexible container

Adverse effects
(*italic* = common; **bold** = life-threatening)
CV: Decreased B/P, bradycardia, tachycardia
EENT: Diplopia
INTEG: Rash, urticaria
MS: Weakness, prolonged skeletal muscle relaxation, **paralysis**
RESP: **Prolonged apnea, bronchospasm, wheezing, respiratory depression**

Contraindications: Hypersensitivity

Precautions: Pregnancy **C**, renal or hepatic **P** disease, lactation, children <3 mo, fluid and electrolyte imbalances, neuromuscular dis-**G** ease, respiratory disease, obesity, elderly

▣ Do Not Confuse:
Mivacron/Mazicon

Pharmacokinetics	
Absorption	Completely absorbed
Distribution	Extracellular spaces; crosses placenta
Metabolism	Plasma
Excretion	Kidneys
Half-life	2 hr

Pharmacodynamics	
Onset	2-2½ min
Peak	2-3 min
Duration	20-30 min

Interactions
Individual drugs
Clindamycin, colistin, lidocaine, lithium, magnesium, polymyxin B, procainamide, quinidine, succinylcholine: ↑ paralysis length and intensity
Drug classifications
Anesthetics (general), antibiotics, aminoglycosides, β-adrenergic blockers, diuretics (potassium-losing): ↑ paralysis length and intensity

NURSING CONSIDERATIONS
Assessment
• Monitor VS (B/P, pulse, respirations, airway) until fully recovered; rate, depth, pattern of respirations, strength of hand grip; patient should be intubated before use
• Monitor for electrolyte imbalances (potassium, magnesium) before drug is used; electrolyte imbalances may lead to increased action of this drug
• Monitor for recovery: decreased paralysis of face, diaphragm, leg, arm, rest of body;

residual weakness and respiratory problems may occur during recovery period
• Assess for hypersensitive reactions: rash, fever, respiratory distress, pruritus; drug should be discontinued

Nursing diagnoses
☑ Breathing pattern, ineffective (uses)
☑ Communication, impaired verbal (adverse reactions)
☑ Fear (adverse reactions)
☑ Knowledge, deficient (teaching)

Implementation
• Use peripheral nerve stimulator (anesthesiologist) to determine neuromuscular blockade; deep tendon reflexes should be monitored during extended periods
• Give direct **IV** undiluted over 5-15 min
• Give cont **IV** diluted to 0.5 mg ml in D_5W, 0.9% NaCl, D_5/0.9% NaCl, LR, D_5/LR and give as an inf at prescribed rate (only by qualified person, usually an anesthesiologist); do not administer IM
• Store in light-resistant container
• Give anticholinesterase to reverse neuromuscular blockade

Y-site compatibilities: Etomidate, thiopental

Y-site incompatibilities: Barbiturates

Patient/family education
• Provide reassurance if communication is difficult during recovery from neuromuscular blockade
• Provide explanation to patients regarding all procedures or treatments; patient will remain conscious if anesthesia is not given also

Evaluation
Positive therapeutic outcome
• Paralysis of jaw, eyelid, head, neck, rest of body as evaluated by peripheral nerve stimulator

Treatment of overdose: Edrophonium or neostigmine, atropine; monitor VS; may require mechanical ventilation

---

moexipril (Rx)
(moe-ex'i-pril)
Univasc
Func. class.: Antihypertensive
Chem. class.: Angiotensin-converting enzyme (ACE) inhibitor

Pregnancy category
C (1st trimester),
D (2nd/3rd trimesters)

Action: Selectively suppresses renin-angiotensin-aldosterone system; inhibits ACE; prevents conversion of angiotensin I to angiotensin II; results in dilatation of arterial, venous vessels

➔ **Therapeutic Outcome:** Decreased B/P in hypertension

Uses: Hypertension, alone or in combination with thiazide diuretics

Dosage and routes
Initial treatment
Adult: PO 7.5 mg 1 hr ac, may be increased or divided depending on B/P response

Maintenance
Adult: PO 7.5-30 mg qd in 1-2 divided doses 1 hr ac

Renal dose
Adult: PO CCr <40 ml/min 3.75 mg/day titrate to desired dose

Available forms: Tabs 7.5, 15 mg

Adverse effects
(*italic* = common; **bold** = life-threatening)
CNS: Fever, chills
CV: Hypotension, postural hypotension
GI: Loss of taste
GU: Impotence, dysuria, nocturia, proteinura, nephrotic syndrome, acute reversible renal failure, polyuria, oliguria, frequency
HEMA: **Neutropenia**
INTEG: Rash
META: Hypokalemia
RESP: **Bronchospasm,** dyspnea, dry cough
SYST: **Angioedema,** anaphylaxis

Contraindications: Hypersensitivity, children, lactation, heart block, bilateral renal stenosis, potassium-sparing diuretics, pregnancy **D** (2nd/3rd trimesters)

Precautions: Dialysis patients, hypovolemia, leukemia, scleroderma, lupus erythematosus, blood dyscrasias, CHF, diabetes mellitus, renal disease, thyroid disease, COPD, asthma, pregnancy **C** (1st trimester)

Pharmacokinetics	
Absorption	Unknown
Distribution	Unknown
Metabolism	Liver to metabolites
Excretion	Via kidneys, crosses placenta, excreted in breast milk
Half-life	Unknown

Pharmacodynamics
Unknown

Interactions
Individual drugs
Allopurinol: ↑ hypersensitivity
CycloSPORINE: ↑ hyperkalemia
Digoxin, lithium: ↑ toxicity
Drug classification
Antihypertensives, diuretics, ganglionic blockers, phenothiazines: ↑ hypotension
Diuretics (potassium-sparing), potassium supplements, sympathomimetics: Do not use together
NSAIDs: ↓ antihypertensive effect
Lab test interferences
False positive: Urine acetone

NURSING CONSIDERATIONS
Assessment
• Monitor blood studies: neutrophils, decreased platelets
• Monitor B/P
• Monitor renal studies: protein, BUN, creatinine; watch for increased levels that may indicate nephrotic syndrome
• Monitor baselines in renal, liver function tests before therapy begins
• Monitor potassium levels, although hyperkalemia rarely occurs
• Assess edema in feet, legs daily
• Assess allergic reaction: rash, fever, pruritus, urticaria; drug should be discontinued if antihistamines fail to help
• Assess for symptoms of CHF: edema, dyspnea, wet rales, B/P
• Monitor for renal symptoms: polyuria, oliguria, frequency

Implementation
• Give PO 1 hr ac
• Store in airtight container at 86° F or less

Nursing diagnoses
✓ Knowledge, deficient (teaching)

Patient/family education
• Teach patient to take 1 hr ac
• Instruct patient not to discontinue drug abruptly

• Tell patient not to use OTC (cough, cold, allergy) products unless directed by prescriber
• Teach patient to comply with dosage schedule, even if feeling better
• Encourage patient to rise slowly to sitting or standing position to minimize orthostatic hypotension
• Teach patient to notify prescriber of mouth sores, sore throat, fever, swelling of hands or feet, irregular heartbeat, chest pain, signs of angioedema
• Tell patient that excessive perspiration, dehydration, vomiting, diarrhea may lead to fall in B/P; consult prescriber if this occurs
• Teach patient that dizziness, fainting, lightheadedness may occur during first few days of therapy
• Tell patient that skin rash or impaired perspiration may occur
• Teach patient how to take B/P

Evaluation
Positive therapeutic outcome
• Decreased B/P in hypertension

Treatment of overdose: 0.9% NaCl **IV** inf, hemodialysis

---

montelukast (Rx) M
(mon-teh-loo'kast)
Singulair
Func. class.: Bronchodilator
Chem. class.: Leukotriene antagonist, cysteinyl
Pregnancy category B

Action: Inhibits leukotriene (LTD$_4$) formation; leukotrienes exert their effects by increasing neutrophil, eosinophil migration; aggregation of neutrophils, monocytes; smooth muscle contraction, capillary permeability; these actions further lead to bronchoconstriction, inflammation, edema

⇒**Therapeutic Outcome:** Ability to breathe with ease

Uses: Chronic asthma

Investigational uses: Chronic urticaria

Dosage and routes
Asthma
P *Adult and child ≥15 yr:* PO 10 mg qd PM
P *Child 6-14 yr:* PO 5 mg chew tabs qd PM
P *Child 2-5 yr:* PO chew tabs 4 mg qd
P *Child 12-23 mo:* PO 1 packet of granules taken PM

Available forms: Tabs 10 mg; chewable tabs 4, 5 mg; oral granules 4 mg/packet

Adverse effects
(*italic* = common; **bold** = life-threatening)
CNS: Dizziness, fatigue, headache
GI: Abdominal pain, dyspepsia
INTEG: Rash
MS: Asthenia
RESP: Influenza, cough, nasal congestion

Contraindications: Hypersensitivity

Precautions: Acute attacks of asthma, alcohol consumption, pregnancy **B,** lactation, ▣ child <6 yr, aspirin sensitivity

Pharmacokinetics	
Absorption	Rapidly
Distribution	Protein binding 99%
Metabolism	Liver
Excretion	Bile
Half-life	2.7-5.5 hr

Pharmacodynamics	
Onset	Unknown
Peak	3-4 hr
Duration	Unknown

Interactions
Individual drugs
Phenobarbitol, rifampin: ↓ montelukast levels
▣ *Herb/drug*
Tea (green, black), guarana: ↑ stimulation

Lab test interferences
↑ ALT, ↑ AST

NURSING CONSIDERATIONS
Assessment
◆● Assess adult patients carefully for symptoms of Churg-Strauss syndrome (rare), including eosinophilia, vasculitic rash, worsening pulmonary symptoms, cardiac complications and/or neuropathy
● Monitor CBC, blood chemistry during treatment
● Assess respiratory rate, rhythm, depth; auscultate lung fields bilaterally; notify prescriber of abnormalities
● Assess allergic reactions: rash, urticaria; drug should be discontinued

Nursing diagnoses
☑ Airway clearance, ineffective (uses)
☑ Activity intolerance (uses)
☑ Knowledge, deficient (teaching)

Implementation
PO route
● Give PO in PM qd

● Do not open packet until ready to use, mix whole dose, give within 15 min
Granules
● May give directly in mouth or mixed with a spoonful of soft food (carrots, applesauce, ice cream, rice)

Patient/family education
● Instruct patient to check OTC and current prescription medications for epHEDrine, which will increase stimulation; to avoid alcohol
● Advise patient to avoid hazardous activities; dizziness may occur
● Teach patient that drug is not to be used for acute asthma attacks
● Advise patient to avoid NSAIDs if sensitive to aspirin
● Advise patient to continue to use inhaled β-agonists if exercise-induced asthma occurs

Evaluation
Positive therapeutic outcome
● Increased ease of breathing
● Decreased bronchospasm

moricizine (Rx)
(more-i'siz-een)
Ethmozine
Func. class.: Antidysrhythmic, group 1A
Chem. class.: Phenothiazine

Pregnancy category B

Action: Decreased rate of rise of action potential, prolonging refractory period and shortening the action potential duration; depression of inward influx if sodium mediates the effects; may slow atrial and AV nodal conduction

⇥**Therapeutic Outcome:** Resolution of life-threatening dysrhythmias

Uses: Life-threatening ventricular dysrhythmias

Dosage and routes
Hospitalization is required when initiating therapy

Adult: PO 10-15 mg/kg/day in 2-3 divided doses or 600-900 mg/day given in 2-3 divided doses

Hepatic dose
Adult: PO 600 mg or less qd

Available forms: Film-coated tabs 200, 250, 300 mg

 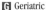

Adverse effects
(*italic* = common; **bold** = life-threatening)
CNS: *Dizziness, headache, fatigue, perioral numbness, euphoria,* nervousness, sleep disorders, depression, tinnitus, fatigue, anxiety
CV: Palpitations, chest pain, CHF, hypertension, syncope, **dysrhythmias,** bradycardia, **MI, thrombophlebitis,** ECG abnormalities, **cardiac arrest**
GI: Nausea, abdominal pain, vomiting, diarrhea
GU: Sexual dysfunction, difficult urination, dysuria, incontinence, urinary retention
MISC: Sweating, musculoskeletal pain, drug fever, blurred vision, dry mouth
RESP: Dyspnea, hyperventilation, **apnea,** asthma, pharyngitis, cough

Contraindications: 2nd- to 3rd-degree AV block, right bundle branch block, cardiogenic shock, hypersensitivity

Precautions: CHF, hypokalemia, hyperkalemia, sick sinus syndrome, pregnancy **B,** lactation, children, impaired hepatic and renal function, cardiac dysfunction

Pharmacokinetics
Absorption	Well absorbed
Distribution	Plasma protein binding (95%)
Metabolism	Liver, extensively
Excretion	Kidneys, breast milk
Half-life	1½-3½ hr

Pharmacodynamics
Onset	Unknown
Peak	½-2 hr
Duration	8-12 hr

Interactions
Individual drugs
Cimetidine: ↑ effect of moricizine
Theophylline: ↓ effect of theophylline

Herb/drug
Aconite: ↑ toxicity, death
Aloe, broom, buckthorn (chronic use), cascara sagrada (chronic use), Chinese rhubarb, figwort, fumitory, goldenseal, kudzu, licorice: ↑ effect
Aloe, buckthorn, cascara sagrada, rhubarb, senna: ↑ hypokalemia, ↑ antidysrhythmic effect
Coltsfoot: ↓ effect
Henbane: ↑ anticholinergic effect
Horehound: ↑ serotonin effect

Lab test interferences
↑ CPK

NURSING CONSIDERATIONS
Assessment
• Monitor ECG at baseline and periodically to determine drug effectiveness; measure PR, QRS, QT intervals, check for PVCs, other dysrhythmias; check B/P for hypotension, hypertension and for rebound hypertension after 1-2 hr; check for dehydration or hypovolemia

• Monitor I&O ratio and electrolytes: potassium, sodium, chloride; check weight daily and for signs of CHF or pulmonary toxicity: dyspnea, fatigue, cough, fever, chest pain; drug should be discontinued

• Monitor liver function studies: AST, ALT, bilirubin, alkaline phosphatase

• Monitor cardiac rate; monitor respiration rate, rhythm, character, and chest pain; watch for ventricular tachycardia, supraventricular tachycardia, or fibrillation

• Monitor for toxicity: fine tremors, dizziness, emesis, lethargy, coma, syncope, hypotension conduction disturbances

Nursing diagnoses
✓ Cardiac output, decreased (uses)
✓ Gas exchange, impaired (adverse reactions)
✓ Knowledge, deficient (teaching)

Implementation
• Give with meals for GI upset; may be given in 2 divided doses if adverse reactions are minimal
• Make dosage adjustment q3 days or more
• Initiate therapy in hospital

Patient/family education
• Instruct patient to report side effects to prescriber immediately
• Instruct patient to complete follow-up appointment with health care provider including pulmonary function studies, chest x-ray, ophth and otoscopic examinations
• Advise patient to carry/wear emergency ID indicating condition and treatment
• Caution patient to avoid driving and other hazardous activities until drug response is determined
• Instruct patient to take medication as prescribed, not to double doses; missed doses may be taken up to 6 hr after previous dose

Treatment of overdose: O₂, artificial ventilation, ECG, administer DOPamine for circulatory depression, administer diazepam or thiopental for seizures, isoproterenol

M

! HIGH ALERT

morphine ⊶ (Rx)
(mor'feen)

Astramorph, Astramorph PF, Duramorph, Epimorph �, Infumorph, Morphine H.P. �, morphine sulfate, Morphitec �, M.O.S. �, M.O.S.-S.R. �, MS Contin, MSIR, MSIR, OMS Concentrate, Oramorph SR, RMS, Roxanol, Roxanol Rescudose, Roxanol-T, Statex �

Func. class.: Opioid analgesic

Pregnancy category C

Controlled substance schedule II

Action: Depresses pain impulse transmission at the spinal cord level by interacting with opioid receptors, produces CNS depression

➡ **Therapeutic Outcome:** Decreased pain

Uses: Severe pain; often given after or during an MI

Dosage and routes
Adult: SC/IM 5-20 mg q4h prn; PO 10-30 mg q4h prn; ext rel 70 kg patient q8-12h; rec 10-30 mg q4h prn; **IV** 4-10 mg diluted in 4-5 ml of water for inj, over 5 min

P *Child:* SC/**IV** 0.1-0.2 mg/kg, max 15 mg; PO 0.2-0.5 mg/kg q4-6h (regular rel), q12h (sus rel)

Available forms: Inj 0.5, 1, 2, 3, 4, 5, 8, 10, 15, 25, 50 mg/ml; sol tabs 10, 15, 30 mg; oral sol 10, 20 mg/5 ml, 20 mg/10 ml, 20 mg/ml; oral tabs 15, 30 mg; rec supp 5, 10, 20, 30 mg; ext rel tabs 15, 30, 60, 100, 200 mg; caps 15, 30 mg; syr 1, 5 mg/ml

Adverse effects
(*italic* = common; **bold** = life-threatening)
CNS: Drowsiness, dizziness, *confusion,* headache, *sedation,* euphoria
CV: Palpitations, **bradycardia,** change in B/P, **shock, cardiac arrest**
EENT: Tinnitus, blurred vision, miosis, diplopia
GI: Nausea, vomiting, anorexia, *constipation,* cramps, biliary tract pressure
GU: Urinary retention
HEMA: **Thrombocytopenia**

INTEG: Rash, urticaria, bruising, flushing, diaphoresis, pruritus
RESP: **Respiratory depression, respiratory arrest, apnea**

Contraindications: Hypersensitivity, addiction (opioid), hemorrhage, bronchial asthma, increased intracranial pressure

Precautions: Addictive personality, pregnancy **C**, lactation, acute MI, severe heart **G** disease, elderly, respiratory depression, **P** hepatic disease, renal disease, child <18 yr

▧ Do Not Confuse:
morphine/hydromorphone, Roxanol/Roxicet

Pharmacokinetics	
Absorption	Variably absorbed (PO); well absorbed (IM, SC, rec); completely absorbed (**IV**)
Distribution	Widely distributed; crosses placenta
Metabolism	Liver, extensively
Excretion	Kidneys
Half-life	1½-2 hr

Interactions
Individual drugs
Alcohol: ↑ respiratory depression, hypotension, sedation
Rifampin: ↓ analgesic action
Drug classifications
Antihistamines, CNS depressants, sedative/hypnotics: ↑ respiratory depression, hypotension
Antipsychotics, opiates, skeletal muscle relaxants: ↑ effects
MAOIs: Unpredictable reaction may occur, avoid use

Food/drug
Cranberry juice, oats: ↓ morphine effect (excessive amounts)
▧ Herb/drug
Chamomile, hops, Jamaican dogwood, kava, lavender, mistletoe, nettle, pokeweed, poppy, senega, skullcap, valerian: ↑ CNS depression
Lab test interferences
↑ Amylase

Pharmacodynamics							
	PO	PO–EXT REL	IM	SC	REC	IV	IT
Onset	Variable	Unknown	10-30 min	20 min	Unknown	Rapid	Rapid
Peak	1 hr	Unknown	½-1 hr	1-1½ hr	½-1 hr	20 min	Unknown
Duration	4-5 hr	8-12 hr	3-7 hr	4-5 hr	4-5 hr	4-5 hr	Ext

 Herb/drug   Do Not Crush   Alert   Key Drug   Geriatric   Pediatric

NURSING CONSIDERATIONS
Assessment
- Assess pain: location, type, character, intensity; give dose before pain becomes extreme
- Monitor I&O ratio; check for decreasing output; may indicate urinary retention; check for constipation; increase fluids, bulk in diet if needed or stool softeners may be prescribed
- Monitor CNS changes: dizziness, drowsiness, hallucinations, euphoria, LOC, pupil reactions
- Monitor allergic reactions: rash, urticaria
- Assess respiratory dysfunction: depression, character, rate, rhythm; notify prescriber if respirations are <10/min

Nursing diagnoses
☑ Pain, acute (uses)
☑ Sensory perception, disturbed: visual, auditory (adverse reactions)
☑ Breathing pattern, ineffective (adverse reactions)
☑ Knowledge, deficient (teaching)

Implementation
- Give with antiemetic if nausea, vomiting occur
- Administer when pain is beginning to return; determine dosage interval by patient response; continuous dosing of medication is more effective than giving prn
- Withdraw medication slowly after long-term use to prevent withdrawal symptoms
- Store in light-resistant container at room temp

PO route
- May be given with food or milk to lessen GI upset; may be crushed and mixed with food or fluids; ext rel tabs should be swallowed whole

IM/SC route
- Do not give if cloudy or a precipitate has formed

IV IV route
- Give direct **IV** by diluting with ≥5 ml of sterile water or 0.9% NaCl for inj; give 2.5-15 mg/4-5 min; rapid administration may lead to increased respiratory depression, death
- Give cont inf by adding to D_5W, $D_{10}W$, 0.9% NaCl, 0.45% NaCl, Ringer's, LR, any dextrose/saline sol, or any dextrose/Ringer's, 0.1-1 mg/ml
- Give by infusion pump to deliver correct dosage; titrate to provide adequate pain relief without serious sedation, respiratory depression, hypotension
- May be given by patient-controlled analgesia (PCA) pump in terminal illnesses; patient is able to control amount of morphine

- Administer epidurally with caution in the elderly

Syringe compatibilities: Atropine, benzquinamide, bupivacaine, butorphanol, cimetidine, dimenhyDRINATE, diphenhydrAMINE, droperidol, fentanyl, glycopyrrolate, hydrOXYzine, ketamine, metoclopramide, midazolam, milrinone, pentazocine, perphenazine, promazine, ranitidine, scopolamine

Syringe incompatibilities: Meperidine, thiopental

Y-site compatibilities: Allopurinol, amifostine, amikacin, aminophylline, amiodarone, ampicillin, ampicillin/sulbactam, amsacrine, atenolol, atracurium, aztreonam, bumetanide, calcium chloride, cefamandole, cefazolin, cefmetazole, cefoperazone, cefotaxime, cefotetan, cefoxitin, ceftazidime, ceftizoxime, ceftriaxone, cefuroxime, cephalothin, cephapirin, chloramphenicol, cisplatin, cladribine, clindamycin, cyclophosphamide, cytarabine, dexamethasone, digoxin, diltiazem, dobutamine, DOPamine, doxycycline, enalaprilat, epINEPHrine, erythromycin, esmolol, etomidate, famotidine, fentanyl, filgrastim, fluconazole, fludarabine, foscarnet, gentamicin, granisetron, heparin, hydrocortisone, hydromorphone, IL-2, insulin (regular), kanamycin, labetalol, lidocaine, lorazepam, magnesium sulfate, melphalan, meropenem, methotrexate, methyldopate, methylPREDNISolone, metoclopramide, metoprolol, metronidazole, mezlocillin, midazolam, milrinone, moxalactam, nafcillin, niCARdipine, nitroglycerin, norepinephrine, ondansetron, oxacillin, oxytocin, paclitaxel, pancuronium, penicillin G potassium, piperacillin, piperacillin/tazobactam, potassium chloride, propofol, propranolol, ranitidine, sodium bicarbonate, sodium nitroprusside, teniposide, thiotepa, ticarcillin, ticarcillin/clavulanate, tobramycin, trimethoprim/sulfamethoxazole, vancomycin, vecuronium, vinorelbine, vit B/C, warfarin, zidovudine

Y-site incompatibilities: Furosemide, minocycline, tetracycline

Additive compatibilities: Alteplase, atracurium, baclofen, bupivacaine, DOBUTamine, fluconazole, furosemide, meropenem, metoclopramide, ondansetron, succinylcholine, verapamil

Additive incompatibilities: Aminophylline

M

Patient/family education

- Advise patient to report any symptoms of CNS changes, allergic reactions
- Caution patients to avoid CNS depressants (alcohol, sedative/hypnotics) for at least 24 hr after taking this drug
- Discuss with patient that dizziness, drowsiness, and confusion are common; to avoid getting up without assistance
- Discuss in detail all aspects of the drug and expected response

Evaluation

Positive therapeutic outcome
- Decreased pain

Treatment of overdose: Naloxone (Narcan) 0.2-0.8 **IV**, O₂, **IV** fluids, vasopressors

---

moxifloxacin (Rx)

(mox-i-floks′a-sin)
Avelox, Avelox IV
Func. class.: Antiinfective
Chem. class.: Fluoroquinolone

Pregnancy category C

Action: Interferes with conversion of intermediate DNA fragments into high molecular weight DNA in bacteria; DNA gyrase inhibitor

➤ Therapeutic Outcome: Bactericidal action against the following: *Staphylococcus aureus, Streptococcus pneumoniae, Haemophilus influenzae, Haemophilus parainfluenzae, Moraxella catarrhalis, Klebsiella pneumoniae, Mycoplasma pneumoniae, Chlamydia pneumoniae;* uncomplicated skin/skin structure infections: *Staphylococcus aureus, Streptococcus pyogenes*

Uses: Acute bacterial sinusitis, acute bacterial exacerbation of chronic bronchitis, community-acquired pneumonia (mild to moderate)

Dosage and routes
Acute bacterial sinusitis
Adult: PO/**IV** 400 mg q24h × 10 days

Acute bacterial exacerbation of chronic bronchitis
Adult: PO/**IV** 400 mg q24h × 5 days

Community acquired pneumonia
Adult: PO/**IV** 400 mg q24h × 7-14 days

Uncomplicated skin/skin structure infections
Adult: PO/**IV** 400 mg q24h × 7 days

Available forms: Tabs 400 mg; inj premix 400 mg

Adverse effects
(*italic* = common; **bold** = life-threatening)
CNS: Headache, dizziness, fatigue, insomnia, depression, restlessness, **seizures,** confusion
CV: Prolonged QT interval, ***dysrhythmias***
GI: Nausea, constipation, increased ALT, AST, flatulence, insomnia, heartburn, vomiting, diarrhea, oral candidiasis, dysphagia, **pseudomembranous colitis**
INTEG: Rash, pruritus, urticaria, photosensitivity, flushing, fever, chills
EENT: Blurred vision, tinnitus
SYST: **Anaphylaxis, Stevens-Johnson syndrome**
MS: Tremor, arthralgia, tendon rupture

Contraindications: Hypersensitivity to quinolones

Precautions: Pregnancy C, lactation, **P** children, renal disease, uncorrected hypokalemia, prolonged QT interval, patients receiving class IA, III antidysrhythmics

Pharmacokinetics

Absorption	Well absorbed (75%) (PO)
Distribution	Widely distributed
Metabolism	Liver
Excretion	Kidneys
Half-life	Increased in renal disease

Pharmacodynamics

	PO
Onset	Rapid
Peak	1 hr

Interactions
Individual drugs
Aluminum hydroxide, calcium, didanosine, iron, sucralfate, zinc sulfate: ↓ absorption of moxifloxacin
Caffeine: ↓ effect of moxifloxacin
CycloSPORINE: ↑ nephrotoxicity
Probenecid: ↑ blood levels
Theophylline: ↑ toxicity
Warfarin: ↑ warfarin effect
Drug classifications
Antacids, iron salts: ↓ absorption of moxifloxacin
Antidysrhythmics IA, III: Prolonged QT interval
Food/drug
Enteral feeding: ↓ absorption of moxifloxacin
Herb/drug
Cola tree: ↑ antiinfective effect

 Herb/drug   Do Not Crush   Alert   Key Drug   Geriatric   Pediatric

Lab test interferences
↑ AST, ↑ ALT, ↑ BUN, ↑ creatinine, ↑ alkaline phosphatase

NURSING CONSIDERATIONS
Assessment
• Assess patient for previous sensitivity reaction
• Assess patient for signs and symptoms of infection including characteristics of wounds, sputum, urine, stool, WBC >10,000/mm³, fever; baseline and during treatment
• Obtain C&S before beginning drug therapy to identify if correct treatment has been initiated
• Assess for allergic reactions and anaphylaxis: rash, urticaria, pruritus, chills, fever, joint pain; may occur a few days after therapy begins; epINEPHrine and resuscitation equipment should be available for anaphylactic reaction
• Assess for CNS symptoms: headache, dizziness, fatigue, insomnia, depression, **seizures**
• Identify urine output; if decreasing, notify prescriber (may indicate nephrotoxicity); also check for increased BUN, creatinine
• Monitor blood studies: AST, ALT, CBC, Hct, bilirubin, LDH, alkaline phosphatase, Coombs' test monthly if patient is on long-term therapy
• Monitor electrolytes: potassium, sodium chloride monthly if patient is on long-term therapy
• Assess bowel pattern qd; if severe diarrhea occurs, drug should be discontinued
• Monitor for bleeding: ecchymosis, bleeding gums, hematuria, stool guaiac daily if on long-term therapy
• Assess for overgrowth of infection: perineal itching, fever, malaise, redness, pain, swelling, drainage, rash, diarrhea, change in cough, sputum

Nursing diagnoses
☑ Infection, risk for (uses)
☑ Diarrhea (side effects)
☑ Injury, risk for (side effects)
☑ Knowledge, deficient (teaching)
☑ Noncompliance (teaching)

Implementation
PO route
• Give once a day for 5-10 days depending on condition

Ⅳ IV route
• Discontinue primary **IV** while administering moxifloxacin
• Do not give SC, IM

Solution compatibilities: 0.9% NaCl, D₅, D₁₀, LR, sterile water for inj

Patient/family education
• Teach patient to report sore throat, bruising, bleeding, joint pain; may indicate blood dyscrasias (rare)
• Advise patient to contact prescriber if vaginal itching, loose foul-smelling stools, furry tongue occur; may indicate superinfection; report itching, rash, pruritus, urticaria
• Instruct patient to take all medication prescribed for the length of time ordered; do not give medication to others
• Advise patient to notify prescriber of diarrhea with blood or pus
• Advise patient to rinse mouth frequently, use sugarless candy or gum for dry mouth
• Advise patient to take as prescribed, not to double or miss doses
• Instruct patient not to use theophylline with this product, may cause toxicity; contact prescriber if taking theophylline

Evaluation
Positive therapeutic outcome
• Absence of signs/symptoms of infection (WBC <10,000/mm³, temp WNL)
• Reported improvement in symptoms of infection

M

multivitamins
(PO, OTC, **IV**, Rx)
Adavite, Dayalets, LKV Drops, Multi-75, Multi-Day, One-A-Day, Optilets, Poly-Vi-Sol, Quintabs, Rulets, Sesame Street Vitamins, Tab-A-Vite, Therabid, Theragran, Unicaps, Vita-Bob, Vita-Kid, many other brands; Berocca Parenteral, M.V.C. 9+3, M.V.I. Pediatric
Func. class.: Vitamins, multiple

Pregnancy category A

Action: Needed for adequate metabolism

➔**Therapeutic Outcome:** Prevention and treatment of vitamin deficiencies

Uses: Prevention and treatment of vitamin deficiencies

Dosage and routes
P *Adult and child:* PO depends on brand

Available forms: Many forms available

Adverse effects
Rare at recommended dosage

Precautions: Pregnancy **A**

Ⓝ Do Not Confuse:
Theragran/Phenergan

Pharmacokinetics	
Absorption	Well absorbed (PO)
Distribution	Widely distributed; crosses placenta
Metabolism	Widely metabolized
Excretion	Kidney, unchanged (water soluble)
Half-life	Unknown

Pharmacodynamics
Unknown

NURSING CONSIDERATIONS
Assessment
• Assess patient for vitamin deficiency; usually more than one vitamin deficiency is present

Nursing diagnoses
☑ Nutrition: less than body requirements, imbalanced (uses)
☑ Knowledge, deficient (teaching)

Implementation
PO route
• Liq multivitamins can be diluted or dropped into patients' mouth using dropper provided with some brands
• Chew tabs should be chewed and not swallowed whole

IV IV route
• Give by cont inf only after diluting 5-10 ml (multivitamins)/500-1000 ml of D_5W, $D_{10}W$, $D_{20}W$, LR, D_5/LR, D_5/0.9% NaCl, 0.9% NaCl, 3% NaCl
• Do not use sol with crystals, precipitate, or color other than bright yellow

Y-site compatibilities: Acyclovir, ampicillin, cefazolin, cephalothin, cephapirin, diltiazem, erythromycin, fludarabine, gentamicin, tacrolimus, tetracycline

Additive compatibilities: Cefoxitin, isoproterenol, methyldopa, metoclopramide, metronidazole, netilmicin, norepinephrine, sodium bicarbonate, verapamil

Additive incompatibilities: Penicillin G, erythromycin, tetracycline, kanamycin, streptomycin, doxycycline, lincomycin should not be admixed

Patient/family education
• Advise patient that adequate nutrition must be maintained to prevent further deficiencies; to comply with treatment regimen
• Advise patient to avoid treating flavored
P multivitamins as candy; child may overdose
• Caution patient to store vitamins out of
P children's reach

Evaluation
Positive therapeutic outcome
• Check each individual vitamin for guidelines
• Absence of vitamin deficiencies

---

muromonab-CD3 (Rx)
(mur-oe-mone'ab)
Orthoclone OKT3
Func. class.: Immunosuppressive
Chem. class.: Murine monoclonal antibody

Pregnancy category C

Action: Reverses graft rejection by blocking T-cell function

➡ Therapeutic Outcome: Prevention of graft rejection

Uses: Acute allograft rejection in renal, cardiac, hepatic transplant patients

Dosage and routes
Adult: **IV** bol 5 mg/day × 10-14 days; usually methylPREDNISolone sodium succinate, 1 mg/kg **IV**, is given before muromonab-CD3, 100 mg **IV** hydrocortisone sodium succinate is given 30 min after muromonab-CD3

P *Child:* **IV** 100 mcg/kg/day × 10-14 day

Cardiac/hepatic allograft rejection, steroid resistant
Adult: **IV** bol 5 mg/day × 10-14 days; begin when it is known that rejection has not been reversed by steroids

Available forms: Inj 5 mg/5 ml

Adverse effects
(*italic* = common; **bold** = life-threatening)
CNS: Pyrexia, chills, tremors, **aseptic meningitis**
CV: Chest pain
GI: Vomiting, nausea, diarrhea
MISC: Infection, cytokine release syndrome, **anaphylaxis**
RESP: Dyspnea, wheezing, **pulmonary edema**

Contraindications: Hypersensitivity to murine origin, fluid overload

P Precautions: Pregnancy **C**, child <2 yr, fever

Pharmacokinetics	
Absorption	Completely absorbed
Distribution	Unknown
Metabolism	Unknown
Excretion	Unknown
Half-life	Unknown

 Herb/drug   🚫 Do Not Crush   ◆ Alert   ✪☞ Key Drug   **G** Geriatric   **P** Pediatric

Pharmacodynamics
Unknown

Interactions
Individual drugs
Azathioprine, cycloSPORINE: ↑ risk of infection
Indomethacin: ↑ CNS symptoms
Drug classifications
Antineoplastics: ↑ myelosuppression
Corticosteroids: ↑ risk of infection
Immunosuppressants: ↑ immunosuppression
Live virus vaccines: ↓ antibody response
Herb/drug
Astragalus, echinacea, melatonin: immunosuppression
Ginseng, maitake, mistletoe, schisandra, St. John's wort, turmeric: ↓ effect

NURSING CONSIDERATIONS
Assessment
• Assess for cytosine release syndrome (CRS): nausea, vomiting, chills, fever, joint pain, weakness, dizziness, diarrhea, tremors, abdominal pain; occurs 30-60 min after first dose; methylPREDNISolone sodium succinate may be prescribed to lessen this reaction
• Assess for hypersensitivity reaction, anaphylaxis: dyspnea, bronchospasm, urticaria, tachycardia, hypotension, angioedema; discontinue drug; emergency equipment must be nearby
• Assess for headache, photophobia, fever, rigidity; indicate aseptic meningitis has developed
• Assess for sore throat, fever, chills, rash, dysuria, which may indicate infection; therapy may be discontinued
• Assess for fluid overload: edema, pulmonary edema, increasing weight
• Monitor blood studies: CBC with differential, platelets, BUN, creatinine, alkaline phosphatase, bilirubin during treatment monthly
• Monitor AST, ALT, BUN, creatinine, alkaline phosphatase, bilirubin
• Obtain human-mouse antibody; if titer is >1:1000, this drug should not be used
• Monitor T-cells with CD3, CD4, CD8 antigen qd; report should be CD3 positive and T-cells <25/mm³

Nursing diagnoses
Infection, risk for (uses)
Knowledge, deficient (teaching)

Implementation
• Give by direct IV undiluted; withdraw with a 0.2-0.22 low–protein binding μm filter; discard and use new needle for administration; give over 1 min
• Give for several days before transplant surgery

Patient/family education
• Instruct patient to report fever, chills, sore throat, fatigue, since serious infections may occur; rash, rapid heartbeat
• Advise patient to use contraceptive measures during treatment and for 12 wk after ending therapy; drug is mutagenic
• Advise patient to avoid crowds and persons with known infections to reduce risk of infection
• Advise patient to report symptoms of cytokine release syndrome, aseptic meningitis, give list of symptoms
• Instruct patient to avoid vaccinations during treatment

Evaluation
Positive therapeutic outcome
• Absence of graft rejection

mycophenolate mofetil (Rx)
(mie-koe-feen'oh-late moe-feh-til)
CellCept
Func. class.: Immunosuppressant
Pregnancy category C

Action: Inhibits inflammatory responses that are mediated by the immune system; prolongs survival of allogenic transplants

Therapeutic Outcome: Absence of graft rejection

Uses: Organ transplants to prevent rejection (renal); prophylaxis of rejection in allogenic cardiac, hepatic, renal transplants

Investigational uses: Refractory uveitis, 2nd-line therapy for Churg-Strauss syndrome, diffuse proliferative lupus nephritis (in combination)

Dosage and routes
Renal transplant
Adult: PO/IV give initial dose 72 hr before transplantation; 1 g bid given to renal transplant patients in combination with corticosteroids and cycloSPORINE

Renal dose
Adult: PO/IV GFR <25 ml/min, max 2 g/day

Cardiac transplant
Adult: PO/IV 1.5 g bid, IV can be started ≤24 hr after transplant, switch to PO when able

Hepatic transplant
Adult: PO/**IV** 1.5 g bid, give **IV** over ≥2 hr

Available forms: Caps 250 mg; tabs 250, 500 mg; inj (powder) 500 mg/20 ml vial; powder for oral susp 200 mg/ml

Adverse effects
(*italic* = common; **bold** = life-threatening)

CNS: *Tremor, dizziness, insomnia, headache, fever*

CV: *Hypertension, chest pain*

GI: *Nausea, vomiting,* stomatitis, *diarrhea, constipation,* GI bleeding

GU: *UTI, hematuria,* **renal tubular necrosis**

HEMA: **Leukopenia, thrombocytopenia, anemia, pancytopenia**

INTEG: *Rash*

META: *Peripheral edema, hypercholesterolemia, hypophosphatemia, edema, hyperkalemia, hypokalemia, hyperglycemia*

MS: *Arthralgia, muscle wasting*

RESP: *Dyspnea, respiratory infection, increased cough, pharyngitis, bronchitis, pneumonia*

SYST: **Lymphoma, nonmelanoma skin carcinoma**

Contraindications: Hypersensitivity to this drug or mycophenolic acid

Precautions: Lymphomas, malignancies, neutropenia, renal disease, pregnancy **C**, lactation

Pharmacokinetics	
Absorption	Rapidly and completely absorbed
Distribution	Unknown
Metabolism	To active metabolite (MPA)
Excretion	Urine, feces
Half-life	Unknown

Pharmacodynamics
Unknown

Interactions
Individual drugs

Acyclovir, ganciclovir: ↑ concentration of both drugs

Azathioprine: Avoid use

Cholestyramine: ↓ levels of mycophenolate

Phenytoin: ↓ protein binding of phenytoin

Probenecid: ↑ levels of mycophenolate

Theophylline: ↓ protein binding of theophylline

Drug classifications

Antacids: ↓ levels of mycophenolate

Salicylates: ↑ levels of mycophenolate

Food/drug

Decreased absorption if taken with food

Herb/drug

Astragalus, echinacea, melatonin: Interferes with immunosuppression

NURSING CONSIDERATIONS
Assessment
• Monitor blood studies: CBC monthly during treatment

• Monitor liver function studies: alkaline phosphatase, AST, ALT, bilirubin

Nursing diagnoses
☑ Infection, risk for (uses)

☑ Knowledge, deficient (teaching)

Implementation
• Give 72 hr before transplantation; may be given in combination with corticosteroids and cycloSPORINE

PO route
• Give alone for better absorption

⃠ • Do not crush, chew tabs, do not open caps

IV IV route
• Do not give by rapid or bolus inj: reconstitute and dilute to 6 mg/ml with D$_5$, give over ≥2 hr

• Do not admix with mycophenolate **IV** in infusion catheter or with other **IV** drug or infusion admixtures

Patient/family education
• Teach patient to report fever, rash, severe diarrhea, chills, sore throat, fatigue, since serious infections may occur

• Instruct patient to avoid crowds to reduce risk of infection

• Advise patient that repeated lab tests are necessary

• Advise patient to limit exposure to sunlight/UV light

• Instruct patient to use contraception before, during, and 6 wk after therapy

Evaluation
Positive therapeutic outcome
• Absence of graft rejection

 Herb/drug   Do Not Crush   Alert   Key Drug   Geriatric   **P** Pediatric

nabumetone (Rx)

(na-byoo'me-tone)

Relafen

Func. class.: Nonsteroidal antiinflammatory
Chem. class.: Acetic acid derivative

Pregnancy category
C (1st trimester),
B (2nd trimester)

Action: Inhibits prostaglandin synthesis by decreasing an enzyme needed for biosynthesis; analgesic, antiinflammatory

➡ **Therapeutic Outcome:** Decreased pain, swelling of joints

Uses: Osteoarthritis, rheumatoid arthritis, acute or chronic treatment

Dosage and routes

Adult: PO 1 g as a single dose; may increase to 1.5-2 g/day if needed; may give qd or bid (as a divided dose)

Available forms: Tabs 500, 750 mg

Adverse effects

(*italic* = common; **bold** = life-threatening)

CNS: Dizziness, headache, drowsiness, fatigue, tremors, confusion, insomnia, anxiety, depression, nervousness

CV: Tachycardia, peripheral edema, palpitations, **dysrhythmias, CHF**

EENT: Tinnitus, hearing loss, blurred vision

GI: Nausea, anorexia, vomiting, diarrhea, jaundice, cholestatic hepatitis, constipation, flatulence, cramps, dry mouth, peptic ulcer, gastritis, **ulceration, perforation**

GU: **Nephrotoxicity, dysuria, hematuria, oliguria, azotemia,** cystitis

HEMA: **Blood dyscrasias**

INTEG: Purpura, rash, pruritus, sweating, photosensitivity

RESP: Dyspnea, pharyngitis, **bronchospasm**

SYST: **Anaphylaxis, angioneurotic edema**

Contraindications: Hypersensitivity to this drug or aspirin, iodides, NSAIDs, asthma, severe renal disease, severe hepatic disease, avoid in late pregnancy

Precautions: Pregnancy **C** (1st trimester), **P** lactation, children, bleeding disorders, GI disorders, cardiac disorders, renal disorders, **G** hepatic dysfunction, elderly

Pharmacokinetics

Absorption	Well absorbed
Distribution	Unknown
Metabolism	Liver, extensively, to inactive metabolite
Excretion	Unknown
Half-life	22-30 hr

Pharmacodynamics

Onset	Unknown
Peak	2½-4 hr
Duration	Unknown

Interactions

Individual drugs

Alcohol: ↑ GI reactions
Cefamandole, cefoperazone, cefotetan, clopidogrel, eptifibatide, plicamycin, ticlopidine, valproic acid: ↑ risk of bleeding
Radiation: ↑ risk of hematologic reactions

Drug classifications

Anticoagulants, thrombolytics: ↑ risk of bleeding
Antihypertensives: ↓ effect of antihypertensives
Antineoplastics: ↑ risk of hematologic reactions
Corticosteroids, NSAIDs, potassium supplements, salicylates: ↑ GI reactions
Diuretics: ↓ effectiveness of diuretics

🗌 *Herb/drug*

Arginine, gossypol: ↑ gastric irritation
Bearberry, bilberry: ↑ NSAIDs effect
Bogbean, chondroitin: ↑ bleeding risk

N

NURSING CONSIDERATIONS

Assessment

• Assess for pain: frequency, characteristics, location, duration, intensity, relief of pain after medication; and for inflammation of joints, ROM

• Monitor blood counts during therapy; watch for decreasing platelets; if low, therapy may need to be discontinued, restarted after hematologic recovery; check for blood dyscrasias (thrombocytopenia): bruising, fatigue, bleeding, poor healing; monitor liver function tests: AST, ALT, alkaline phosphatase; LDH, blood glucose, WBC, CCr

• Assess for asthma, aspirin sensitivity, nasal polyps; increased hypersensitivity reactions

Nursing diagnoses

☑ Pain, acute (uses)
☑ Pain, chronic
☑ Mobility, impaired (uses)
☑ Injury, risk for (adverse reactions)
☑ Knowledge, deficient (teaching)

Implementation
- Administer tab to patient crushed or whole
- Give with food or milk to decrease gastric symptoms

Patient/family education
- Tell patient that drug must be continued for prescribed time to be effective; to avoid aspirin, alcoholic beverages, NSAIDs, and OTC medications unless approved by prescriber
- Caution patient to report bleeding, bruising, fatigue, malaise, since blood dyscrasias do occur
- Instruct patient to use caution when driving; drowsiness, dizziness may occur
- Advise patient to use sunscreen, hat, and other protective clothing to prevent burns
- Instruct patient to take with a full glass of water and sit upright
- Advise patient to report dark stools, a change in urine pattern, increased weight, edema, increased pain in joints, fever, blood in urine, blurred vision, ringing or roaring in ears

Evaluation
Positive therapeutic outcome
- Decreased pain
- Decreased inflammation
- Increased mobility

---

nadolol (Rx)

(nay-doe′lole)

Corgard, Syn-Nadolol

Func. class.: Antihypertensive, antianginal

Chem. class.: β-Adrenergic receptor blocker

Pregnancy category C

Action: Competitively blocks stimulation of β-adrenergic receptor within vascular smooth muscle; produces chronotropic, inotropic activity (decreases rate of SA node discharge, increases recovery time), slows conduction of AV node, decreases heart rate, which decreases O_2 consumption in myocardium; also decreases renin-aldosterone-angiotensin system at high doses, inhibits $β_2$-receptors in bronchial system

▶ **Therapeutic Outcome:** Decreased B/P, heart rate

Uses: Chronic stable angina pectoris, mild to moderate hypertension

Investigational uses: Tachydysrhythmias, aggression, anxiety, tremors, esophageal varices (rebleeding only), prophylaxis of migraine headaches, hyperthyroidism adjunctive therapy

Dosage and routes
Adult: PO 40 mg qd; increase by 40-80 mg q3-7 days; maintenance 40-240 mg/day for angina, 40-320 mg/day for hypertension

G *Elderly:* PO 20 mg/day, may increase by 20 mg until desired dose

Renal dose
Adult: PO CCr 31-50 ml/min give q24-36h; CCr 10-30 ml/min give q24-48h; CCr <10 ml/min give q40-60h

Available forms: Tabs 20, 40, 80, 120, 160 mg

Adverse effects
(*italic* = common; **bold** = life-threatening)

CNS: Depression, hallucinations, dizziness, fatigue, lethargy, paresthesia, headache

CV: **Bradycardia,** *hypotension,* **CHF,** palpitations, AV block, chest pain, peripheral ischemia, flushing, edema, vasodilatation, conduction disturbances, **pulmonary edema**

EENT: Sore throat

GI: Nausea, vomiting, diarrhea, colitis, constipation, cramps, dry mouth, flatulence, hepatomegaly, **pancreatitis,** taste distortion

GU: *Impotence*

HEMA: **Agranulocytosis, thrombocytopenia**

INTEG: Rash, pruritus, fever, alopecia

RESP: Dyspnea, respiratory dysfunction, **bronchospasm,** cough, wheezing, nasal stuffiness, pharyngitis, **laryngospasm**

Contraindications: Hypersensitivity to this drug, cardiac failure, cardiogenic shock, 2nd- or 3rd-degree heart block, bronchospastic disease, sinus bradycardia, CHF, COPD

Precautions: Diabetes mellitus, pregnancy C, renal disease, lactation, hyperthyroidism, peripheral vascular disease, myasthenia gravis, major surgery, nonallergic bronchospasm

◥ **Do Not Confuse:**
Corgard/Cognex

Pharmacokinetics	
Absorption	Variably absorbed
Distribution	Crosses placenta; minimal concentration in CNS, protein binding 30%
Excretion	Kidneys, unchanged
Half-life	10-24 hr; increased in renal disease

Pharmacodynamics	
Onset	Variable
Peak	3-4 hr
Duration	20-24 hr

Interactions
Individual drugs
Clonidine, epinephrine, prazosin: ↑ hypotension, bradycardia

Thyroid: ↓ β-blocking effect
Drug classifications
Antihypertensives: ↑ hypotension

Contraceptives (oral): ↓ β-blocking effect

Diuretics, phenothiazines: ↑ hypotensive effects

Ergots: Peripheral ischemia

MAOIs: ↑ bradycardia; do not use together

NSAIDs: ↓ antihypertensive effect
Herb/drug
Aconite: ↑ toxicity, death

Astragalus, cola tree: ↑ or ↓ antihypertensive effect

Barberry, betony, black catechu, black cohosh, bloodroot, broom, burdock, cat's claw, dandelion, goldenseal, Irish moss, Jamaican dogwood, kelp, khella, mistletoe, parsley: ↑ antihypertensive effect

Coltsfoot, guarana, khat, licorice: ↓ antihypertensive effect
Lab test interferences
↑ Serum potassium, ↑ serum uric acid, ↑ ALT, ↑ AST, ↑ alkaline phosphatase, ↑ LDH, ↑ blood glucose, ↑ cholesterol

NURSING CONSIDERATIONS
Assessment
- Monitor B/P at beginning of treatment, periodically thereafter; note rate, rhythm, quality of apical/radial pulse before administration; notify prescriber of any significant changes (pulse <55 bpm), orthostatic hypotension
- Check for baselines in renal, liver function tests before therapy begins
- Assess for edema in feet, legs daily; monitor I&O, daily weight; check for jugular vein distention and rales bilaterally, dyspnea (CHF)
- Monitor skin turgor, dryness of mucous membranes for hydration status, especially elderly

Nursing diagnoses
✓ Cardiac output, decreased (uses)
✓ Injury, risk for (adverse reactions)
✓ Knowledge, deficient (teaching)
✓ Noncompliance (teaching)

Implementation
- Given ac, hs, tab may be crushed or swallowed whole; give with food to prevent GI upset; give reduced dosage in renal dysfunction
- Store protected from light, moisture; place in cool environment

Patient/family education
- Teach patient not to discontinue drug abruptly; taper over 2 wk; may cause precipitate angina, serious dysrhythmias if stopped abruptly
- Teach patient not to use OTC products containing α-adrenergic stimulants (such as nasal decongestants, cold preparations); to avoid alcohol, smoking and to limit sodium intake as prescribed
- Teach patient how to take pulse and B/P at home; advise when to notify prescriber
- Instruct patient to comply with weight control, dietary adjustments, modified exercise program
- Advise patient to carry/wear emergency ID to identify drug being taken, allergies; teach patient drug controls symptoms but does not cure condition
- Caution patient to avoid hazardous activities if dizziness, drowsiness present; to rise slowly to prevent orthostatic hypotension
- Teach patient to report symptoms of CHF: difficult breathing, especially on exertion or when lying down, night cough, swelling of extremities or bradycardia, dizziness, confusion, depression, fever
- Teach patient to take drug as prescribed, not to double doses, skip doses; take any missed doses as soon as remembered if at least 4 hr until next dose

Evaluation
Positive therapeutic outcome
- Decreased B/P in hypertension

nafcillin (Rx)
(naf-sill'in)

Nafcillin sodium, Nallpen, Unipen

Func. class.: Antiinfective—broad-spectrum

Chem. class.: Penicillinase-resistant penicillin

Pregnancy category B

Action: Interferes with cell wall replication of susceptible organisms; osmotically unstable cell wall swells, bursts from osmotic pressure

Therapeutic Outcome: Bactericidal effects for gram-positive cocci *Staphylococcus*

aureus, Streptococcus viridans, Streptococcus pneumoniae and infections caused by penicillinase-producing *Staphylococcus*

Uses: Infections caused by penicillinase-producing staphylococci, streptococci; respiratory tract, skin, skin structure, urinary tract, bone, joint infections, sinusitis, endocarditis, septicemia, meningitis

Dosage and routes
Adult: PO 250-1000 mg q4-6h; IM 500 mg q4-6h; **IV** 500-1500 mg q4-6h

P *Child and infants, most infections:* PO 6.25-12.5 mg/kg q6h; pharyngitis PO 250 mg q8h; IM 25 mg/kg q12h; **IV** most infections 10-20 mg/kg q4h or 20-40 mg/kg q8h, max 200 mg/kg/day

P *Neonates:* PO 10 mg/kg q6-8h; IM 10 mg/kg q12h; **IV:** most infections 10-20 mg/kg q4h or 20-40 mg/kg q8h, max 200 mg/kg/day

Meningitis

P *Neonates ≥2 kg:* 50 mg/kg q8h × 1 wk of life, then 50 mg/kg q6h

P *Neonates <2 kg:* 25-50 mg/kg q12h × 1 wk of life, then 50 mg/kg q8h

Available forms: Caps 250 mg; tabs 500 mg; powder for inj 1, 2, 10 g

Adverse effects
(*italic* = common; **bold** = life-threatening)
CNS: Lethargy, hallucinations, anxiety, depression, muscle twitching, **coma, seizures**
GI: *Nausea, vomiting, diarrhea,* increased AST, ALT, abdominal pain, glossitis, **pseudomembranous colitis**
GU: Oliguria, **proteinuria, hematuria, vaginitis, moniliasis, glomerulonephritis,** interstitial nephritis
HEMA: Anemia, increased bleeding time, **bone marrow depression, granulocytopenia**
SYST: **Anaphylaxis, serum sickness**

Contraindications: Hypersensitivity to penicillins

Precautions: Pregnancy **B**, hypersensitivity
P to cephalosporins, neonates

Pharmacokinetics
Absorption	Well absorbed (IM); erratic (PO)
Distribution	Widely distributed; crosses placenta
Metabolism	Not metabolized
Excretion	Kidneys, unchanged; breast milk
Half-life	1 hr; increased in renal disease

Pharmacodynamics
	PO	IM	IV
Onset	½ hr	½ hr	Immediate
Peak	1-2 hr	1-2 hr	Inf end

Interactions
Individual drugs
Aspirin, probenecid: ↑ nafcillin levels, ↓ renal excretion
Dilsulfiram: ↑ nafcillin concentrations
Drug classifications
Anticoagulants (oral): ↓ anticoagulant effects
Contraceptives (oral): ↓ contraceptive effectiveness
Food/drug
Food, carbonated drinks, citrus fruit juices: ↓ absorption
Herb/drug
Acidophilus: Do not use with antiinfectives
Khat: ↓ absorption
Lab test interferences
False positive: Urine glucose, urine protein

NURSING CONSIDERATIONS
Assessment
• Assess patient for previous sensitivity reaction to penicillins or other cephalosporins; cross-sensitivity between penicillins and cephalosporins is common
• Assess patient for signs and symptoms of infection including characteristics of wounds, sputum, urine, stool, WBC >10,000/mm³, earache, fever; obtain baseline information and during treatment
• Obtain C&S before beginning drug therapy to identify if correct treatment has been initiated
• Assess for allergic reactions, anaphylaxis: rash, urticaria, pruritus, chills, fever, dyspnea, laryngeal edema, joint pain; angioedema may occur a few days after therapy begins; epiNEPHrine, resuscitation equipment should be available for anaphylactic reaction
• Assess renal studies: urinalysis, protein, blood, BUN, creatinine
• Identify urine output; if decreasing, notify prescriber (may indicate nephrotoxicity)
• Monitor blood studies: AST, ALT, CBC, Hct, bilirubin, LDH, alkaline phosphatase, Coombs' test monthly if patient is on long-term therapy
• Monitor electrolytes: potassium, sodium, chloride monthly if patient is on long-term therapy
• Assess bowel pattern qd; if severe diarrhea occurs, drug should be discontinued; may indicate pseudomembranous colitis
• Monitor for bleeding: ecchymosis, bleeding

gums, hematuria, stool guaiac daily if on long-term therapy
• Assess for overgrowth of infection: perineal itching, fever, malaise, redness, pain, swelling, drainage, rash, diarrhea, change in cough, sputum

Nursing diagnoses
✓ Infection, risk for (uses)
✓ Diarrhea (adverse reactions)
✓ Injury, risk for (adverse reactions)
✓ Knowledge, deficient (teaching)
✓ Noncompliance (teaching)

Implementation
PO route
• Give in even doses around the clock; if GI upset occurs, give with food; drug must be given for 10-14 days to ensure organism death and prevent superinfection; store in tight container.
🚫 • Do not crush, chew caps
• Shake susp; store in refrigerator for 2 wk, 1 wk at room temp
IM route
• Reconstitute 500 mg/1.7-1.8 ml; 1 g/3.4 ml; 2 g/6.6-6.8 ml with sterile water or bacteriostatic water for a conc of 250 mg/ml; store unused portion in refrigerator for up to 7 days
• Give deep in large muscle mass
IV route
• Reconstitute 1 g/3.4 ml, 2 g/6.6-6.8 ml with sterile water or bacteriostatic water for a conc of 250 mg/ml; store unused portion in refrigerator for up to 7 days
• Give by direct **IV** by diluting reconstituted sol with 15-30 ml of sterile water or 0.9% NaCl; give over 5-10 min
• Give by intermittent inf by diluting to a conc of 2-40 mg/ml with 0.9% NaCl, D_5W, D_{10}W, D_5/0.9% NaCl, D_5/LR, LR, Ringer's; store in refrigerator for up to 96 hr or 24 hr room temp; run over 30-60 min

Syringe compatibilities: Cimetidine, heparin

Y-site compatibilities: Acyclovir, atropine, cyclophosphamide, diazepam, enalaprilat, esmolol, famotidine, fentanyl, fluconazole, foscarnet, hydromorphone, magnesium sulfate, morphine, perphenazine, propofol, theophylline, zidovudine

Y-site incompatibilities: Droperidol, fentanyl/droperidol, labetalol, nalbuphine, pentazocine, regular insulin, verapamil

Additive compatibilities: Chloramphenicol, chlorothiazide, dexamethasone, diphenhy-

drAMINE, epHEDrine, heparin, hydrOXYzine, lidocaine, potassium chloride, prochlorperazine, sodium bicarbonate, sodium lactate

Additive incompatibilities: Ascorbic acid, aztreonam, bleomycin, cytarabine, gentamicin, hydrocortisone sodium succinate, methylPREDNISolone sodium succinate, promazine

Patient/family education
• Teach patient to report sore throat, bruising, bleeding, joint pain; may indicate blood dyscrasias (rare)
• Advise patient to contact prescriber if vaginal itching, loose foul-smelling stools, furry tongue occur; may indicate superinfection
• Instruct patient to take all medication prescribed for the length of time ordered
• Advise patient to notify prescriber of diarrhea with blood or pus, which may indicate pseudomembranous colitis
• Advise patient to carry/wear emergency ID if allergic to penicillins

Evaluation
Positive therapeutic outcome
• Absence of signs/symptoms of infection (WBC <10,000/mm³, temp WNL, absence of red, draining wounds, earache)
• Reported improvement in symptoms of infection

Treatment of anaphylaxis: Withdraw drug, maintain airway, administer epINEPHrine, aminophylline, O_2, **IV** corticosteroids

---

❗HIGH ALERT

nalbuphine (Rx)
(nal′byoo-feen)
Nubain, nalbuphine HCl
Func. class.: Opioid analgesic
Chem. class.: Synthetic opioid agonist/antagonist

Pregnancy category C

Action: Inhibits ascending pain pathways in limbic system, thalamus, midbrain, hypothalamus by binding to opiate receptor sites, thus altering pain perception and response

Therapeutic Outcome: Relief of pain

Uses: Moderate to severe pain, labor analgesia, balanced anesthesia (adjunct)

Dosage and routes
Analgesic
Adult: SC/IM/**IV** 10-20 mg q3-6h prn, not to exceed 160 mg/day

Balanced anesthesia supplement
Adult: IV 0.3-3 mg/kg given over 10-15 min; may give 0.25-0.5 mg/kg as needed (maintenance)

Available forms: Inj 10, 20 mg/ml

Adverse effects
(*italic* = common; **bold** = life-threatening)
CNS: *Drowsiness, dizziness, confusion, headache, sedation, euphoria,* dysphoria (high doses), hallucinations, increased dreaming, tolerance, physical and psychologic dependency
CV: Palpitations, bradycardia, change in B/P, orthostatic hypotension
EENT: Tinnitus, blurred vision, miosis (high doses), diplopia
GI: *Nausea, vomiting, anorexia, constipation, cramps*
GU: Increased urinary output, dysuria, urinary retention, urgency
INTEG: *Rash,* urticaria, bruising, flushing, *diaphoresis,* pruritus
RESP: **Respiratory depression,** pulmonary edema

Contraindications: Hypersensitivity, addiction (opioid)

Precautions: Addictive personality, pregnancy **C**, lactation, increased intracranial pressure, MI (acute), severe heart disease, respiratory depression, hepatic disease, renal disease

Pharmacokinetics
Absorption	Well absorbed (SC, IM); completely absorbed (**IV**)
Distribution	Crosses placenta
Metabolism	Liver, extensively
Excretion	Feces, kidneys, unchanged (small amounts); breast milk
Half-life	5 hr

Pharmacodynamics
	IM	SC	IV
Onset	Up to 15 min	Up to 15 min	Rapid
Peak	1 hr	Unknown	½ hr
Duration	3-6 hr	3-6 hr	3-6 hr

Interactions
Individual drugs
Alcohol: ↑ respiratory depression, hypotension, sedation

Drug classifications
Antihistamines, CNS depressants, phenothiazines, sedative/hypnotics: ↑ respiratory depression, hypotension
MAOIs: Use cautiously, results are unpredictable
Opiates: ↑ opioid withdrawals (dependency)
⬚ Herb/drug
Chamomile, hops, Jamaican dogwood, kava, lavender, mistletoe, nettle, pokeweed, poppy, senega, skullcap, valerian: ↑ CNS depression
Corkwood: ↑ anticholinergic effect
Lab test interferences
↑ amylase, ↑ lipase

NURSING CONSIDERATIONS
Assessment
- Assess pain characteristics (location, intensity, type) before medication administration and after treatment
- Monitor VS after parenteral route; note muscle rigidity, drug history, liver, kidney function tests; respiratory dysfunction: respiratory depression, character, rate, rhythm; notify prescriber if respirations are <10/min
- Monitor CNS changes: dizziness, drowsiness, hallucinations, euphoria, LOC, pupil reaction
- Monitor allergic reactions: rash, urticaria

Nursing diagnoses
☑ Pain, acute (uses)
☑ Sensory perception, disturbed: visual, auditory (adverse reactions)
☑ Breathing pattern, ineffective (adverse reactions)
☑ Knowledge, deficient (teaching)

Implementation
- Give by inj (IM, **IV**), only with resuscitative equipment available; give slowly to prevent rigidity
- Store in light-resistant area at room temp
IM route
- Give inj deeply in large muscle mass; rotate inj sites
IV IV route
- Give direct **IV** undiluted 10 mg or less over 3-5 min or more

Syringe compatibilities: Atropine, cimetidine, diphenhydrAMINE, droperidol, glycopyrrolate, hydrOXYzine, lidocaine, midazolam, prochlorperazine, promethazine, ranitidine, scopolamine, trimethobenzamide

Syringe incompatibilities: Diazepam, pentobarbital

Y-site compatibilities: Amifostine, aztreonam, cefmetazole, cladribine, filgrastim,

⬚ Herb/drug   ⓢ Do Not Crush   ◆ Alert   ◆⚏ Key Drug   ⒼGeriatric   ⓅPediatric

fludarabine, granisetron, melphalan, paclitaxel, propofol, teniposide, thiotepa, vinorelbine

Y-site incompatibilities: Nafcillin,
sargramostim

Patient/family education
• Instruct patient to report any symptoms of
CNS changes, allergic reactions
• Caution patients to avoid CNS depressants:
alcohol, sedative/hypnotics for at least 24 hr
after taking this drug
• Discuss with patient that dizziness, drowsiness, confusion are common; to avoid getting
up without assistance
• Discuss in detail all aspects of the drug:
reason for taking drug and expected results
• Instruct patient to change position slowly to
prevent orthostatic hypotension
• Teach patient to turn, cough, deep breathe
after surgery to prevent atelectasis

Evaluation
Positive therapeutic outcome
• Relief of pain

Treatment of overdose: Naloxone
(Narcan) 0.2-0.8 **IV**, O₂, **IV** fluids, vasopressors

---

naloxone (Rx)
(nal-oks'one)
naloxone HCl, Narcan
Func. class.: Opioid antagonist, antidote
Chem. class.: Thebaine derivative

Pregnancy category B

Action: Competes with opioids at opioid
receptor sites

▶ **Therapeutic Outcome:** Absence of
opioid overdose

Uses: Respiratory depression induced by
opioids, pentazocine, propoxyphene; refractory circulatory shock

Dosage and routes
*Opioid-induced respiratory
depression, CNS depression*
Adult: **IV**/SC/IM 0.4-2 mg; repeat q2-3 min
if needed

P *Child:* **IV**/SC/IM 0.5-2 mcg/kg as small,
frequent qmin bolus or as an inf titrated to
response

*Postoperative respiratory
depression*
Adult: **IV** 0.1-0.2 mg q2-3 min prn

P *Child:* **IV**/IM/SC 0.01 mg/kg q2-3 min prn

Asphyxia neonatorum
P *Neonates:* **IV** 0.01 mg/kg given into umbilical vein after delivery; may repeat q2-3
min × 3 doses

Available forms: Inj 0.02, 0.4 mg/ml;
P neonatal inj 0.02 mg/ml

Adverse effects
(*italic* = common; **bold** = life-threatening)
CNS: Drowsiness, nervousness
CV: Rapid pulse, **ventricular tachycardia,
fibrillation,** increased systolic B/P (high
doses)
GI: Nausea, vomiting
RESP: Hyperpnea

Contraindications: Hypersensitivity,
respiratory depression

P **Precautions:** Pregnancy **B**, children, CV disease,
opioid dependency, lactation

◤ **Do Not Confuse:**
Narcan/Norcuron

Pharmacokinetics	
Absorption	Well absorbed (SC, IM); completely absorbed (**IV**)
Distribution	Rapidly distributed; crosses placenta
Metabolism	Liver
Excretion	Kidneys
P **Half-life**	1 hr; up to 3 hr (neonates)

Pharmacodynamics		
	IV	IM/SC
Onset	1 min	2-5 min
Peak	Unknown	Unknown
Duration	45 min	45-60 min

Interactions
Drug classifications
Analgesics (opioids): ↑ withdrawal in those
addicted to opioids
Lab test interferences
Interference: Urine VMA, 5-HIAA, urine
glucose

NURSING CONSIDERATIONS
Assessment
• Assess for signs of opioid withdrawal in
drug-dependent individuals: cramping, hypertension, anxiety, vomiting; may occur up to 2
hr after administration
• Monitor VS q3-5 min; ABGs including Po₂,
Pco₂
• Assess cardiac status: tachycardia,
hypertension; monitor ECG
• Assess for pain: duration, intensity, location
before and after administration; may be used
for respiratory depression

N

- Assess for respiratory dysfunction: respiratory depression, character, rate, rhythm; if respirations are <10/min, probably due to opioid overdose, administer naloxone; monitor LOC

Nursing diagnoses
☑ Breathing pattern, ineffective (uses)
☑ Coping, ineffective (uses)
☑ Pain, acute (adverse reactions)
☑ Knowledge, deficient (teaching)

Implementation
IV IV route
- Give by direct **IV** undiluted; give 0.4 mg or less over 15 sec or titrate inf to response
- Give cont inf **IV** further diluted with 0.9% NaCl and D_5 and give as an inf
- Give only with resuscitative equipment, O_2 nearby
- Use only sol prepared within 24 hr
- Store at room temp in darkness

Syringe compatibilities: Benzquinamide, heparin

Y-site compatibilities: Propofol

Additive compatibilities: Verapamil

Patient/family education
- Explain reason for and expected results of medication when patient alert

Evaluation
Positive therapeutic outcome
- Reversal of respiratory depression
- LOC: alert

---

naproxen (OTC, Rx)
(na-prox′en)
Apo-Naproxen ✦, EC-Naprosyn, Naprelan, Napron X, Naprosyn, Naprosyn-E ✦, Naprosyn-SR ✦, Naxen ✦, Novo-Naprox ✦, Nu-Naprox ✦
naproxen sodium
Aleve, Anaprox, Anaprox DS, Apo-Napro-Na ✦, Apo-Napro-Na DS, Naprelan, Novo-Naprox Sodium ✦, Novo-Naprox Sodium DS ✦, Synflex ✦, Synflex DS ✦
Func. class.: Nonsteroidal antiinflammatory, nonopioid analgesic
Chem. class.: Propionic acid derivative

Pregnancy category B

Action: Inhibits prostaglandin synthesis by decreasing enzyme needed for biosynthesis; analgesic, antiinflammatory

➲ **Therapeutic Outcome:** Decreased pain, inflammation

Uses: Mild to moderate pain, osteoarthritis, rheumatoid arthritis, gouty arthritis, juvenile arthritis, primary dysmenorrhea

Dosage and routes
Adult: PO 250-500 mg bid, not to exceed 1 g/day (base); 550 mg, then 275 mg q6-8h prn, not to exceed 1375 mg (sodium)

P *Child:* PO 10 mg/kg in 2 divided doses

Available forms: Naproxen, tabs 250, 375, 500 mg; del rel tabs 375, 500 mg; oral susp 125 mg/5 ml; naproxen sodium, cont rel tabs 421.5, 550 mg; tabs 275, 550 mg

Adverse effects
(*italic* = common; **bold** = life-threatening)
CNS: Dizziness, drowsiness, fatigue, tremors, confusion, insomnia, anxiety, depression
CV: Tachycardia, peripheral edema, palpitations, **dysrhythmias**
EENT: Tinnitus, hearing loss, blurred vision
GI: Nausea, anorexia, vomiting, diarrhea, jaundice, **cholestatic hepatitis,** constipation, flatulence, cramps, dry mouth, peptic ulcer, **GI ulceration, bleeding, perforation**
GU: Nephrotoxicity: **dysuria, hematuria, oliguria, azotemia**
HEMA: **Blood dyscrasias**
INTEG: Purpura, rash, pruritus, sweating
SYST: **Anaphylaxis**

Contraindications: Hypersensitivity, asthma, severe renal disease, severe hepatic disease, ulcer disease, avoid in 2nd/3rd trimester of pregnancy

Precautions: Pregnancy **B** (1st trimester), **P** lactation, children <2 yr, bleeding disorders, GI disorders, cardiac disorders, hypersensitiv-**G** ity to other antiinflammatory agents, elderly, CCr <25 ml/min

Pharmacokinetics	
Absorption	Completely absorbed
Distribution	Crosses placenta, 99% protein binding
Metabolism	Liver, extensively
Excretion	Breast milk
Half-life	10-20 hr

Pharmacodynamics	
Onset	1 hr
Peak	2-4 hr
Duration	<7 hr

 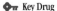

Interactions
Individual drugs
Alcohol, aspirin: ↑ adverse reactions
Aspirin: ↓ effectiveness
Cefamandole, cefoperazone, cefotetan, clopidogrel, eptifibatide, plicamycin, ticlopidine, valproic acid: ↑ bleeding risk
Lithium: ↑ toxicity
Methotrexate: ↑ toxicity
Radiation: ↑ risk of hematologic toxicity
Drug classifications
Anticoagulants, thrombolytics: ↑ risk of bleeding
Antihypertensives: ↓ effect of antihypertensives
Antineoplastics: ↑ risk of hematologic toxicity
Diuretics: ↓ effectiveness of diuretics
NSAIDs: ↑ adverse reactions
Herb/drug
Arginine, gossypol: ↑ gastric irritation
Bearberry, bilberry: ↑ NSAIDs effect
Anise, arnica, bogbean, chamomile, chondroitin, clove, dong quai, fenugreek, feverfew, garlic, ginger, ginkgo, ginseng (Panax), licorice: ↑ bleeding risk
Lab test interferences
↑ BUN, ↑ alkaline phosphatase
False: ↑ 5-HIAA, ↑ 17KS

NURSING CONSIDERATIONS
Assessment
• Monitor liver function, renal function, other blood studies: AST, ALT, bilirubin, creatinine, BUN, CBC, Hct, Hgb, Pro-time, LDH, blood glucose, WBC, platelets; if patient is on long-term therapy
• Check I&O ratio; decreasing output may indicate renal failure (long-term therapy)
• Assess hepatotoxicity: dark urine, clay-colored stools, yellowing of the skin and sclera, itching, abdominal pain, fever, diarrhea if patient is on long-term therapy
• Assess for allergic reactions: rash, urticaria; if these occur, drug may have to be discontinued
• Assess for ototoxicity: tinnitus, ringing, roaring in ears; audiometric testing needed before, after long-term therapy
• Assess for visual changes: blurring, halos; may indicate corneal, retinal damage
• Check for edema in feet, ankles, legs
• Identify prior drug history; there are many drug interactions
• Monitor pain: location, frequency, duration, characteristics, type, intensity before dose and 1 hour after; assess ROM before dose and after
• Assess for asthma, aspirin hypersensitivity, or nasal polyps, increased risk of hypersensitivity

Nursing diagnoses
☑ Pain, acute (uses)
☑ Pain, chronic
☑ Mobility, impaired (uses)
☑ Injury, risk for (adverse reactions)
☑ Knowledge, deficient (teaching)

Implementation
• Administer to patient crushed or whole
• Give with food or milk to decrease gastric symptoms; give ½ hr ac or 2 hr pc for better absorption

Patient/family education
• Teach patient to report any symptoms of hepatotoxicity, renal toxicity, visual changes, ototoxicity, allergic reactions, bleeding (long-term therapy)
• Advise patient to take with 8 oz of water and sit upright for 30 min after dose to prevent ulceration
• Caution patient not to exceed recommended dosage; acute poisoning may result; to take as prescribed, do not double dose
• Advise patient to use sunscreen to prevent photosensitivity reactions
• Teach patient to read label on other OTC drugs; many contain other antiinflammatories; caution patient to avoid alcohol ingestion; GI bleeding may occur
• Inform patient that the therapeutic response takes 2 wk (arthritis)
• Teach patient to report tinnitus, confusion, diarrhea, sweating, hyperventilation, blurred vision, fever, joint aches, black stools, flulike symptoms

Evaluation
Positive therapeutic outcome
• Decreased pain
• Decreased inflammation
• Increased mobility

---

naratriptan (Rx)
(nair'ah-trip-tan)
Amerge
Func. class.: Migraine agent
Chem. class.: 5-HT₁-like receptor agonist
Pregnancy category C

Action: Binds selectively to the vascular 5-HT₁ receptor subtype, exerts antimigraine effect; causes vasoconstriction in cranial arteries
Therapeutic Outcome: Decreased intensity and incidence of migraines
Uses: Acute treatment of migraine with or without aura

Dosage and routes
Adult: PO 1 or 2.5 mg with fluids, if headache returns, repeat once after 4 hr, max 5 mg/24 hr

Hepatic/renal dose
Max 2.5 mg/24 hr

Available forms: Tab 1, 2.5 mg

Adverse effects
(*italic* = common; **bold** = life-threatening)
CV: Increased B/P, palpitations, **tachydys-rhythmias, PR, QT$_C$ prolongation, ST/T wave changes, PVCs, atrial flutter, fibrillation, coronary vasospasm**
EENT: EENT infections, photophobia
GI: Nausea, vomiting
MISC: Temp change sensations, tightness, pressure sensations
MS: Weakness, neck stiffness, myalgia
CNS: Dizziness, sedation, fatigue

Contraindications: Angina pectoris, history of MI, documented silent ischemia, ischemic heart disease, concurrent ergotamine-containing preparations, uncontrolled hypertension, hypersensitivity, severe renal disease (CCr <15 ml/min); severe hepatic disease (Child-Pugh grade C), CV syndromes, hemiplegic or basilar migraines

Precautions: Postmenopausal women, men >40 yr, risk factors for CAD, hypercholesterolemia, obesity, diabetes, impaired hepatic or **P** renal function, pregnancy **C**, lactation, **G** children, elderly, peripheral vascular disease

Pharmacokinetics	
Absorption	Unknown
Distribution	28%-31% protein binding
Metabolism	Liver (metabolite)
Excretion	Urine/feces
Half-life	6 hr

Pharmacodynamics	
Onset	Unknown
Peak	2-3 hr
Duration	Unknown

Interactions
Drug classifications
5-HT agonists, ergot derivatives: ↑ vasospastic effect
MAOIs: ↑ risk of adverse reactions, do not use together
Selective serotonin release inhibitors: ↑ weakness, hyperreflexia, incoordination
Herb/drug
Butterbur: ↑ effect
SAM-e, St. John's wort: ↑ serotonin syndrome

NURSING CONSIDERATIONS
Assessment
• Assess for stress level, activity, recreation, coping mechanisms
• Assess neurologic status: LOC, blurred vision, nausea, tics preceding headache

Nursing diagnoses
☑ Pain, acute (uses)
☑ Knowledge, deficient (teaching)
☑ Noncompliance (teaching)

Implementation
• Give with fluids as soon as symptoms appear, may take another dose after 4 hr; do not take >5 mg in any 24 hr period
• Provide a quiet, calm environment with decreased stimulation for noise, bright light, excessive talking

Patient/family education
• Teach patient to report pain, tightness in chest, neck, throat, or jaw; notify prescriber immediately if sudden, severe abdominal pain occurs
• Teach patient to use contraception while taking drug, to notify prescriber if pregnancy is planned or suspected
• Advise patient not to use if another 5-HT agonist or an ergot preparation has been used in the past 24 hr

Evaluation
Positive therapeutic outcome
• Absence of migraine headaches

---

nedocromil (Rx)
(ned-o-kroe'mil)
Tilade
Func. class.: Antiasthmatic
Chem. class.: Mast cell stabilizer
Pregnancy category B

Action: Stabilizes the membrane of the sensitized mast cell, preventing release of chemical mediators after an antigen-IgE interaction

➔ **Therapeutic Outcome:** Reduced symptoms of asthma

Uses: Allergic rhinitis, severe perennial bronchial asthma, exercise-induced bronchospasm (prevention), prevention of acute bronchospasm induced by environmental pollutants, mastocytosis, not for treatment of acute asthma attacks

Dosage and routes
P *Adult and child >12 yr:* 2 inh 2-4 ×/day at regular intervals to provide 14 g/day

Available forms: 1.75 mg of nedocromil per activation in 16.2-g canisters providing at least 112 metered inhalations

Adverse effects
(*italic* = common; **bold** = life-threatening)
CNS: Headache, dizziness, neuritis, dysphonia
EENT: Throat irritation, cough, nasal congestion, burning eyes, rhinitis
GI: Nausea, vomiting, anorexia, dry mouth, bitter taste
MISC: Anaphylaxis

Contraindications: Hypersensitivity to this drug or lactose, status asthmaticus

Precautions: Pregnancy **B**, lactation, P children

Pharmacokinetics

Absorption	Poorly, 3%
Distribution	Unknown
Metabolism	Not usually metabolized
Excretion	Small amounts in bile, urine unchanged
Half-life	80 min

Pharmacodynamics

Onset	Unknown
Peak	15 min
Duration	4-6 hr

Interactions: None

NURSING CONSIDERATIONS
Assessment
• Assess pulmonary function testing baseline (asthma)
• Assess respiratory status: respiratory rate, rhythm, characteristics, cough, wheezing, dyspnea

Nursing diagnoses
☑ Airway clearance, ineffective (uses)
☑ Knowledge, deficient (teaching)

Implementation
• Give by inh only with spacer device if needed
• Encourage patient to gargle, sip water to decrease irritation in throat

Patient/family education
• Instruct patient to clear mucus before using
• Teach patient proper inhalation technique: exhale; using inhaler, inhale deeply with head tipped back to open airway; remove, hold breath, exhale; use Halermatic or Spinhaler with Intal caps

• Inform patient that therapeutic effect may take up to 4 wk
• Teach patient that drug is preventive only, not restorative

Evaluation
Positive therapeutic outcome
• Decrease in asthmatic symptoms

---

nefazodone (Rx)
(nef-az′oe-done)
Serzone
Func. class.: Antidepressant—misc.
Chem. class.: Phenylpiperazine

Pregnancy category C

Action: Selectively inhibits serotonin uptake by brain, potentiates behavioral changes, occupies central HT₂ receptors

➡ **Therapeutic Outcome:** Decreased symptoms of depression after 2-3 wk

Uses: Major depression

Dosage and routes
Adult: PO 200 mg/day (100 mg bid); dosage may be increased to 300 mg/day (150 bid); max 600 mg/day

G *Elderly:* PO 100 mg/day (50 mg bid); increase to 100 mg bid after 2 wk to desired dose

Available forms: Tabs 50, 100, 150, 200, 250 mg

Adverse effects
(*italic* = common; **bold** = life-threatening)
CNS: Somnolence, dizziness, headache, insomnia
CV: Postural hypotension
EENT: Blurred vision, abnormal vision
GI: Nausea, constipation, dry mouth
GU: Urinary frequency, retention, UTI
RESP: Pharyngitis, cough

Contraindications: Hypersensitivity to this drug or phenylpiperazines

P **Precautions:** Pregnancy C, lactation,
G children, elderly, CV disease, seizure disorder, history of taking digoxin, recent MI, mania, renal disease

Do Not Confuse:
serozone/Seroquel

Pharmacokinetics

Absorption	Well absorbed
Distribution	Widely distributed; crosses placenta
Metabolism	Liver, extensively, to metabolites
Excretion	Kidneys, breast milk
Half-life	2-4 hr

Pharmacodynamics

Onset	Unknown
Peak	1-3 hr
Duration	Unknown

Interactions
Individual drugs
Alcohol: ↑ CNS depression

Alprazolam, carbamazepine, digoxin, midazolam, phenytoin, triazolam: ↑ toxicity

Drug classifications
Benzodiazepines: ↑ plasma concentrations

Barbiturates, CNS depressants: ↑ effects

MAOIs: ↑ toxicity

 Herb/drug

Chamomile, hops, kava, skullcap, valerian: ↑ CNS depression

Corkwood, jimsonweed: ↑ anticholinergic effect

SAM-e, St. John's wort: ↑ serotonin syndrome

NURSING CONSIDERATIONS
Assessment
• Monitor B/P (with patient lying, standing), pulse q4h; if systolic B/P drops 20 mm Hg hold drug, notify prescriber; take B/P q4h in patients with CV disease

• Monitor blood studies: CBC, leukocytes, differential, cardiac enzymes if patient is receiving long-term therapy

• Monitor hepatic studies: AST, ALT, bilirubin; if levels at >3 × upper limit of normal, discontinue drug

• Assess mental status: mood, sensorium, affect, suicidal tendencies; increase in psychiatric symptoms: depression, panic

• Monitor urinary retention, constipation; constipation is more likely to occur in the **G** elderly

• Identify alcohol consumption, if alcohol is consumed, hold dose until am

Nursing diagnoses
✓ Coping, ineffective individual (uses)

✓ Knowledge, deficient (teaching)

✓ Noncompliance (teaching)

Implementation
• Give with food or milk to decrease GI symptoms

• Give crushed if patient is unable to swallow medication whole

• Store at room temp; do not freeze

Patient/family education
• Teach patient that therapeutic effects may take 3-4 wk

• Teach patient to use caution in driving and other activities requiring alertness because of drowsiness, dizziness; to avoid rising quickly **G** from sitting to standing, especially elderly

• Teach patient to avoid alcohol ingestion, other CNS depressants, benzodiazepines

• Teach patient to increase bulk in diet if **G** constipation occurs, especially elderly

• Teach patient to take gum, hard sugarless candy, or frequent sips of water for dry mouth

• To report immediately urinary retention

Evaluation
Positive therapeutic outcome
• Decrease in depression

• Absence of suicidal thoughts

Treatment of overdose: ECG monitoring, induce emesis, lavage, activated charcoal, administer anticonvulsant

---

nelfinavir (Rx)
(nell-fin'a-ver)

Viracept

Func. class.: Antiretroviral

Chem. class.: HIV protease inhibitor

Pregnancy category B

Action: Inhibits HIV protease

➡ **Therapeutic Outcome:** Prevents maturation of the infectious virus

Uses: HIV in combination with other antiretrovirals

Dosage and routes
Adult/child >13 yr: PO 750 mg tid or 1250 mg bid

P *Child 2-13 yr:* PO 20-30 mg/kg tid, max 750 mg tid

Available forms: Tabs 250, 625 mg; oral powder 50 mg/g

Adverse effects
(*italic* = common; **bold** = life-threatening)

CNS: Headache, asthenia, poor concentration, **seizures**

CV: Bleeding

ENDO: Hypoglycemia, hyperlipidemia

GI: Diarrhea, nausea, anorexia, dyspepsia, *flatulence*

HEMA: **Anemia, leukopenia, thrombocytopenia, Hgb abnormalities**
INTEG: Rash, dermatitis
MISC: Asthenia
MS: Pain, arthralgia, myalgia, myopathy

Contraindications: Hypersensitivity to protease inhibitors

Precautions: Liver disease, pregnancy **B**, lactation, hemophilia, PKU, renal disease

Pharmacokinetics

Absorption	Unknown
Distribution	98% protein binding
Metabolism	Liver, (minimal)
Excretion	Feces
Half-life	3½-5 hr

Pharmacodynamics

Onset	Unknown
Peak	2-4 hr
Duration	Unknown

Interactions
Individual drugs
Amiodarone, midazolam, quinidine, triazolam: ↑ serious dysrhythmias
Carbamazepine, nevirapine, phenobarbital, phenytoin, rifamycin: ↓ nelfinavir levels
Indinavir, ketoconazole, ritonavir: ↑ nelfinavir levels
Rifabutin: ↑ effect of rifabutin
Drug classifications
Contraceptives (oral): ↓ effect of contraceptive
Ergots: ↑ serious dysrhythmias
Food/drug
↑ Absorption with food
Herb/drug
St. John's wort: ↓ antiretroviral effect

NURSING CONSIDERATIONS
Assessment
• Assess signs of infection, anemia
• Monitor liver studies: ALT, AST
• Monitor C&S before drug therapy; drug may be taken as soon as culture is performed; repeat C&S after treatment; determine the presence of other sexually transmitted diseases
• Assess bowel pattern before, during treatment; if severe abdominal pain with bleeding occurs, drug should be discontinued; monitor hydration
• Assess skin eruptions, rash, urticaria, itching
• Assess allergies before treatment, reaction of each medication; place allergies on chart
• Monitor viral load, CD$_4$ cell counts baseline and throughout treatment

Nursing diagnoses
✓ Infection, risk for (uses)
✓ Knowledge, deficient (teaching)

Implementation
• Administer with food
• Oral powder can be mixed with fluids, do not mix with juice or acidic fluids, stable mixed for 6 hr

Patient/family education
• Advise patient to take with meal or snack; if dose is missed, take as soon as remembered up to 1 hr before next dose; do not double dose
• Advise patient to avoid taking with other medications, unless directed by prescriber
• Teach patient that drug does not cure, but manages symptoms, does not prevent transmission of HIV to others
• Teach patient to use nonhormonal form of contraception while taking this drug

neomycin (Rx)
(nee-oh-mye'sin)
Mycifradin, Myciguent
Func. class.: Antiinfective
Chem. class.: Aminoglycoside

Pregnancy category C

Action: Interferes with protein synthesis in bacterial cell by binding to 30S ribosomal subunit causing inaccurate peptide sequence to form in protein chain, resulting in bacterial death

⇒ **Therapeutic Outcome:** Bactericidal effects for *Pseudomonas aeruginosa, Escherichia coli, Enterobacter,* enteropathogenic *Escherichia coli, Klebsiella pneumoniae, Proteus vulgaris*

Uses: Severe systemic infections of CNS, respiratory tract, GI tract, urinary tract, eye, bone, skin, soft tissues, also used for hepatic coma, preoperatively to sterilize bowel, infectious diarrhea; minor skin infections (top)

Dosage and routes
Hepatic encephalopathy
Adult: PO 4-12 g/day in divided doses times 5-6 days

P *Child:* PO 50-100 mg/kg/day in divided doses

Preoperative intestinal antisepsis
Adult: PO on 3rd day of a 3-day regimen; give 1 g early PM; repeat in 1 hr; repeat at hs (given with erythromycin); give saline cathartic before giving this drug

P *Child:* PO 14.7 mg/kg or 4.7 mg/m² q4h × 3 days

Available forms: Tabs 500 mg; oral sol 125 mg/5 ml

Adverse effects

(*italic* = common; **bold** = life-threatening)

CNS: Confusion, depression, numbness, tremors, **seizures,** muscle twitching, **neurotoxicity,** dizziness, vertigo

CV: Hypotension, hypertension, palpitations

EENT: Ototoxicity, deafness, visual disturbances, tinnitus

GI: Nausea, vomiting, anorexia, increased ALT, AST, bilirubin, hepatomegaly, **hepatic necrosis,** splenomegaly

GU: **Oliguria, hematuria, renal damage, azotemia, renal failure, nephrotoxicity**

HEMA: **Agranulocytosis, thrombocytopenia,** leukopenia, eosinophilia, anemia

INTEG: Rash, burning, urticaria, photosensitivity, dermatitis, alopecia

Contraindications: Bowel obstruction (PO use), severe renal disease, hypersensitivity, infants, children

Precautions: Mild renal disease, pregnancy **C,** hearing deficits, lactation, myasthenia gravis, Parkinson's disease

Pharmacokinetics

Absorption	Well absorbed (IM); minimally absorbed (top)
Distribution	Unknown
Metabolism	Liver, minimal
Excretion	Feces, unchanged
Half-life	2-3 hr

Pharmacodynamics

	IM
Onset	Rapid
Peak	1-2 hr
Duration	6-8 hr

Interactions

Individual drugs

Amphotericin B, bacitracin, cisplatin, ethacrynic acid, furosemide, mannitol, methoxyflurane, polymyxin, vancomycin: ↑ ototoxicity, neurotoxicity, nephrotoxicity

Digoxin: ↓ effects of digoxin when given with oral neomycin

Penicillin V: ↓ effects of penicillin when given with oral neomycin

Succinylcholine: ↑ effects

Drug classifications

Aminoglycosides, cephalosporins: ↑ ototoxicity, neurotoxicity, nephrotoxicity

Anticoagulants (oral): ↑ effects when given with oral neomycin

Nondepolarizing neuromuscular blockers: ↑ effects

☑ *Herb/drug*

Acidophilus: Do not use with antiinfectives

Lysine (large amounts): ↑ toxicity

NURSING CONSIDERATIONS

Assessment

• Assess patient for previous sensitivity reaction

• Assess patient for signs and symptoms of infection: characteristics of skin; obtain baseline information and during treatment

• Obtain C&S before beginning drug therapy to identify if correct treatment has been initiated

• Assess for allergic reactions: rash, urticaria, pruritus, chills, fever, joint pain

Nursing diagnoses

☑ Infection, risk for (uses)

☑ Knowledge, deficient (teaching)

☑ Noncompliance (teaching)

Implementation

PO route

• Give as a preoperative medication before bowel surgery

Patient/family education

• Instruct patient to take all medication prescribed for the length of time ordered

• Advise patient to report headache, dizziness, symptoms of overgrowth of infection and loss of hearing, ringing or roaring in ears

Evaluation

Positive therapeutic outcome

• Reported improvement in symptoms of infection (top)

Treatment of overdose: Withdraw drug; hemodialysis; monitor serum levels of drug

---

neostigmine (Rx)

(nee-oh-stig′meen)

neostigmine, Prostigmin

Func. class.: Cholinergic stimulant; anticholinesterase

Chem. class.: Quaternary compound

Pregnancy category C

Action: Inhibits destruction of acetylcholine, which increases concentration at sites where acetylcholine is released; this facilitates transmission of impulses across the myoneural junction

Therapeutic Outcome: Increased strength in myasthenia gravis, reversal of nondepolarizing muscular blockers

Uses: Myasthenia gravis, nondepolarizing neuromuscular blocker, antagonist, bladder distention, postoperative ileus

Dosage and routes
Myasthenia gravis
Adult: PO 15 mg q3-4h, may increase to 375 mg/day; IM/**IV** 0.5-2 mg q1-3h

Child: PO 2 mg/kg/day q3-4h

Nondepolarizing neuromuscular blocker antagonist
Adult: **IV** 0.5-2 mg slowly; may repeat if needed (give 0.6-1.2 mg atropine before this drug)

Infant/child: **IV** 0.025-0.1 mg/kg/dose

Abdominal distention/postoperative ileus
Adult: IM/SC 0.25-1 mg (1 : 4000) q4-6h depending on condition × 2-3 days

Renal dose
Adult: PO/IM/**IV** CCr 10-50 ml/min 50% of dose; CCr <10 ml/min 25% of dose

Available forms: Tabs 15 mg; inj 1 : 1000, 1 : 2000, 1 : 4000

Adverse effects
(*italic* = common; **bold** = life-threatening)
CNS: Dizziness, headache, sweating, weakness, **seizures,** incoordination, **paralysis,** drowsiness, LOC
CV: Tachycardia, **dysrhythmias,** bradycardia, hypotension, AV block, ECG changes, **cardiac arrest,** syncope
EENT: Miosis, blurred vision, lacrimation, visual changes
GI: Nausea, diarrhea, vomiting, cramps, increased peristalsis, salivary and gastric secretions
GU: Frequency, incontinence, urgency
INTEG: Rash, urticaria, flushing
RESP: **Respiratory depression, bronchospasm, constriction, laryngospasm, respiratory arrest, dyspnea**

Contraindications: Obstruction of intestine, renal system, bromide sensitivity, peritonitis

Precautions: Bradycardia, hypotension, seizure disorders, bronchial asthma, coronary occlusion, hyperthyroidism, dysrhythmias, peptic ulcer, pregnancy **C,** megacolon, poor GI motility, lactation, children

Pharmacokinetics

Absorption	Poorly absorbed (PO), completely absorbed (**IV**)
Distribution	Unknown
Metabolism	Liver
Excretion	Kidneys
Half-life	40-90 min

Pharmacodynamics

	PO	IM	IV
Onset	45-75 min	10-30 min	4-8 min
Peak	Unknown	30 min	30 min
Duration	2½-4 hr	2½-4 hr	2-4 hr

Interactions
Individual drugs
Atropine: ↓ action of atropine
Disopyramide, haloperidol, quinidine: ↓ neostigmine
Drug classifications
Antidepressants, antihistamines, phenothiazines: ↑ antagonism
Cholinesterase inhibitors: ↑ toxicity
Muscle relaxants, depolarizing: ↑ action of muscle relaxants
Herb/drug
Pill bearing spurge: ↑ effect

NURSING CONSIDERATIONS
Assessment
• Monitor VS, respiration during rest
• Monitor for bradycardia, hypotension, bronchospasm, headache, dizziness, seizures, respiratory depression; drug should be discontinued if toxicity occurs

Nursing diagnoses
☑ Breathing pattern, ineffective (uses)
☑ Knowledge, deficient (teaching)

Implementation
PO route
• Give only after all other cholinergics have been discontinued
• Increased dosage as ordered may be needed if tolerance develops
• Give larger doses as ordered after exercise or fatigue
• Administer on empty stomach for better absorption
• Store at room temp
IV route
• Give direct **IV** undiluted, through Y-tube or 3-way stopcock; give 0.5 mg or less over 1 min
• Give only with atropine sulfate available for cholinergic crisis

Syringe compatibilities: Glycopyrrolate, heparin, pentobarbital, thiopental

N

Y-site compatibilities: Heparin, hydrocortisone sodium succinate, potassium chloride, vit B/C

Additive compatibilities: Netilmicin

Patient/family education
• Teach patient to carry/wear emergency ID specifying myasthenia gravis, drugs taken, prescriber's phone number

Evaluation
Positive therapeutic outcome
• Increased muscle strength, hand grasp
• Improved gait
• Absence of labored breathing (if severe)

Treatment of overdose: Respiratory support, **IV** atropine 1-4 mg

---

nesiritide (Rx)
(nes-eer′ih-tide)
Natrecor
Func. class.: Vasodilator
Chem. class.: Human B-type natriuretic peptide

Pregnancy category C

Action: Uses DNA technology; human B-type natriuretic peptide binds to the receptor in vascular smooth muscle and endothelial cells, leading to smooth muscle relaxation

→ **Therapeutic Outcome:** Improvement in symptoms of congestive heart failure (CHF)

Uses: Acutely decompensated CHF

Dosage and routes
Adult: Bol **IV** 2 mcg/kg, then **IV** inf 0.01 mcg/kg/min

Available forms: Powder for inj, 1.5 mg single-use vial

Adverse effects
(*italic* = common; **bold** = life-threatening)
CNS: Headache, insomnia, dizziness, anxiety, confusion, paresthesia, tremor
CV: Hypotension, **tachycardia,** dysrhythmias, bradycardia, ventricular tachycardia, ventricular extrasystoles, **atrial fibrillation**
GI: Abdominal pain, vomiting, nausea
INTEG: Rash, sweating, pruritus, inj site reaction
MISC: Back pain
RESP: Increased cough, **apnea**

Contraindications: Hypersensitivity, cardiogenic shock or B/P <90 mm Hg as primary therapy

Precautions: Pregnancy **C;** mitral stenosis; significant valvular stenosis, restriction, or obstructive cardiomyopathy, or any condition that depends on venous return; renal disease; P lactation; children

Pharmacokinetics
Absorption	Vascular smooth muscle and endothelial cells
Distribution	Unknown
Metabolism	Unknown
Excretion	Bound to cell surfaces, internalized, and proteolyzed; cleaved by endopeptidases on vascular lumenal surface; renal filtration
Half-life	18 min

Pharmacodynamics
Onset	15 min
Peak	1 hr
Duration	Unknown

Interactions
Drug classifications
ACE inhibitors: ↑ symptomatic hypotension

NURSING CONSIDERATIONS
Assessment
• Assess PCWP, RAP, cardiac index, MPAP
• Assess B/P, pulse during treatment until stable

Nursing diagnoses
☑ Tissue perfusion, ineffective (uses)
☑ Knowledge, deficient (teaching)

Implementation
IV IV route
• Do not administer nesiritide through a central heparin-coated catheter; heparin should be administered through a separate catheter
• Prime **IV** fluid with inf of 25 ml before connecting to patient's vascular access port and before bolus dose or **IV** inf
• Reconstitute one 1.5 mg vial/5 ml of diluent from prefilled 250 ml plastic **IV** bag with diluent of choice (D$_5$, 0.9% NaCl, D$_5$/0.9% NaCl, D$_5$/0.2% NaCl); do not shake vial, roll gently; use only clear sol
• Withdraw all contents of reconstituted vial and add to the 250 ml plastic **IV** bag (6 mcg/ml), invert bag several times
• Use within 24 hr of reconstituting

Patient/family education
• Explain purpose of medication and expected results

Evaluation

Positive therapeutic outcome
• Improvement in CHF with improved PCWP, RAP, MPAP

nevirapine (Rx)
(ne-veer'a-peen)
Viramune
Func. class.: Antiretroviral
Chem. class.: Non-nucleoside reverse transcriptase inhibitor (NNRTI)

Pregnancy category C

Action: Binds directly to reverse transcriptase and blocks RNA, DNA causing a disruption of the enzyme's site

➔ **Therapeutic Outcome:** Improvement of HIV-1 infection

Uses: HIV-1 in combination with other highly active antiretroviral treatments (HAART)

Dosage and routes
Adult: PO 200 mg qd × 2 wk, then 200 mg bid in combination

🅿 *Child ≥8 yr:* PO 4 mg/kg qd × 2 wk, then 4 mg/kg bid

🅿 *Child 2 mo-8 yr:* PO 4 mg/kg qd × 2 wk, then 7 mg/kg bid

Available forms: Tabs 200 mg; oral susp 50 mg/5 ml

Adverse effects
(*italic* = common; **bold** = life-threatening)
CNS: Paresthesia, headache, fever, peripheral neuropathy
GI: Diarrhea, abdominal pain, *nausea, stomatitis,* hepatitis, **hepatotoxicity**
HEMA: **Neutropenia, anemia, thrombocytopenia**
INTEG: Rash, **toxic epidermal necrolysis**
MISC: **Stevens-Johnson syndrome**
MS: Pain, myalgia

Contraindications: Hypersensitivity

Precautions: Liver disease, pregnancy **C**,
🅿 lactation, children, renal disease

🅽 **Do Not Confuse:**
nevirapine/nelfinavir
viramune/viracept

Pharmacokinetics
Absorption	Rapid
Distribution	60% bound to plasma proteins
Metabolism	Liver, by hepatic P450 enzyme system
Excretion	Unknown
Half-life	Unknown

Pharmacodynamics
Unknown

Interactions
Individual drugs
Cimetidine: ↑ nevirapine levels
Methadone: ↓ effect of methadone
Drug classifications
Antiinfectives; macrolides: ↑ nevirapine levels
Oral contraceptives, protease inhibitors: ↓ action
Rifamycins: ↓ nevirapine levels
⚠ *Herb/drug*
St. John's wort: ↓ nevirapine levels, do not use together

NURSING CONSIDERATIONS
Assessment
• Assess signs of infection, anemia
• Assess liver, renal, blood studies: ALT, AST; viral load, CD$_4$, if liver function tests are elevated significantly, drug should be withheld
• Assess C&S before drug therapy; drug may be taken as soon as culture is performed; repeat C&S after treatment; determine the presence of other sexually transmitted disease
• Assess bowel pattern before, during treatment; if severe abdominal pain with bleeding occurs, drug should be discontinued; monitor hydration
◆• Assess skin eruptions; rash, urticaria, itching; if rash is severe or systemic symptoms occur, discontinue immediately
• Assess allergies before treatment, reaction to each medication

Nursing diagnoses
☑ Infection, risk for (uses)
☑ Diarrhea (side effects)
☑ Knowledge, deficient (teaching)

Implementation
• Give without regard to meals

Patient/family education
• Instruct patient to report any right quadrant pain, jaundice, rash immediately
• Inform patient that drug may be taken with food, antacids, didanosine
• Advise patient to take as prescribed; if dose

is missed, take as soon as remembered up to 1 hr before next dose; do not double dose
• Advise patient that drug must be taken in equal intervals around the clock to maintain blood levels for duration of therapy
• Advise patient that drug is not a cure, controls symptoms of HIV
• Instruct patient to avoid OTC agents unless approved by prescriber
• Advise patient to use a nonhormonal form of contraception during treatment

niacin
(nye′a-sin)
Edur-Acin, Nia-Bid, Niac, Niacels, Niacor, Niaspan, Nico-400, Nicobid, Nicolar, Nicotinex
nicotinic acid
(nick-oh-tin′ick)
Novo-Niacin ✤, Slo-Niacin, vitamin B
niacinamide
(nye-a-sin′a-mide)
nicotinamide
(nick-oh-tin′ah-mide)
Func. class.: Vitamin B$_3$
Chem. class.: Water-soluble vitamin, lipid-lowering drug

Pregnancy category C

Action: Needed for conversion of fats, protein, carbohydrates by oxidation-reduction; acts directly on vascular smooth muscle, causing vasodilatation; reduces LDL, HDL, triglycerides, and lipoprotein A

➔ **Therapeutic Outcome:** Decreasing cholesterol and LDL levels, B$_3$ supplementation

Uses: Pellagra, hyperlipidemias (types IV, V), peripheral vascular disease, patients who present a risk for pancreatitis

Dosage and routes
Niacin deficiency
Adult: PO 100-500 mg/day in divided doses; IM/SC 5-100 mg 5 or more times a day; **IV** 25-100 mg bid or tid

P *Child:* PO up to 300 mg/day in divided doses

Adjunct in hyperlipidemia
Adult: 250 mg after evening meal, may increase dose at 1-4 wk intervals to 1-2 g tid, max 6 g/day; ext rel 500 mg hs, ×4 wk, then 1000 mg hs for wk 5-8, do not increase by more than 500 mg q4wk, max 2000 mg/day

Pellagra
Adult: PO 300-500 mg qd in divided doses
P *Child:* PO 100-300 mg qd in divided doses

Peripheral vascular disease
Adult: PO 250-800 mg qd in divided doses

Available forms: Niacin, tabs 25, 50, 100, 500, 1000 mg; time rel caps 250, 500 mg; time rel tabs 250, 375, 500 mg; elixir 50 mg/5 ml; ext rel caps 250, 400 mg; sus rel tabs 500 mg; cont rel tabs 250, 500, 750 mg; sus rel cap 125, 500 mg nicotinamide, tabs 100, 250, 500 mg

Adverse effects
(*italic* = common; **bold** = life-threatening)
CNS: Paresthesias, headache, dizziness, anxiety
CV: Postural hypotension, vasovagal attacks, dysrhythmias, vasodilatation
EENT: Blurred vision, ptosis
GI: Nausea, vomiting, anorexia, flatulence, xerostomia, *jaundice,* diarrhea, peptic ulcer, **hepatotoxicity,** dyspepsia
GU: Hyperuricemia, **glycosuria, hypoalbuminemia**
INTEG: Flushing, dry skin, rash, pruritus, itching, tingling

Contraindications: Hypersensitivity, peptic ulcer, hepatic disease, lactation, hemorrhage, severe hypotension

Precautions: Glaucoma, CV disease, CAD, diabetes mellitus, gout, schizophrenia, pregnancy **C**, lactation

⊠ **Do Not Confuse:**
Nicobid/Nitro-Bid

Pharmacokinetics	
Absorption	Well absorbed (PO)
Distribution	Widely distributed
Metabolism	Converted to niacinamide
Excretion	Urine, unchanged (30%); breast milk
Half-life	45 min

Pharmacodynamics		
	PO	IV
Onset	Unknown	Unknown
Peak	30-70 min	Unknown
Duration	Unknown	Unknown

Interactions
Individual drugs
Alcohol: ↑ flushing, pruritus, avoid use
Guanadrel, guanethidine: ↑ hypotension
Lovastatin: ↑ myopathy
Probenecid, sulfinpyrazone: ↑ uricosuric effects
Drug classifications
HMG-CoA reductase inhibitors: ↑ myopathy, rhabdomyolysis
Ganglionic blockers: ↑ postural hypotension

☑ Herb/drug   Ⓢ Do Not Crush   ✦ Alert   ✤⚕ Key Drug   Ⓖ Geriatric   P Pediatric

Lab test interferences
↑ Bilirubin, ↑ alkaline phosphatase, ↑ liver enzymes, ↑ LDH, ↑ uric acid
↓ Cholesterol
False: ↑ Urinary catecholamines
False positive: Urine glucose

NURSING CONSIDERATIONS
Assessment
• Assess for niacin deficiency (pellagra): nausea, vomiting, stomatitis, confusion, hallucinations before and throughout treatment
• Assess for symptoms of niacin deficiency: nausea, vomiting, anemia, poor memory, confusion, dermatitis
• Assess for lipid, triglyceride, cholesterol level, if using for hyperlipidemia
• Assess nutrition: fat, protein, carbohydrates, nutritional analysis should be completed by dietitian
• Monitor liver function studies: AST, ALT, bilirubin, uric acid, alkaline phosphatase; blood glucose before and during treatment; liver dysfunction: clay-colored stools, itching, dark urine, jaundice
• Monitor niacin levels during administration of this drug
• Monitor cardiac status: rate, rhythm, quality; postural hypotension, dysrhythmias
• Monitor nutritional status: liver, yeast, legumes, organ meat, lean poultry; high-level niacin products should be included in the diet
• Assess for CNS symptoms: headache, paresthesias, blurred vision

Nursing diagnoses
✓ Nutrition: less than body requirements, imbalanced (uses)
✓ Knowledge, deficient (teaching)
✓ Noncompliance (teaching)

Implementation
PO route
• Give with meals or milk for GI symptoms, and 325 mg of aspirin or NSAIDs ½ hr before dose to decrease flushing
🚫• Do not crush, break, or chew ext rel products
IV route
• Give by direct **IV** after diluting to 2 mg/ml at a rate of ≤2 mg/min
• Give by inf by adding 500 ml of 0.9% NaCl at a rate of ≤2 mg/min

Additive incompatibilities: Acids (strong), alkalis, erythromycin, kanamycin, streptomycin

Additive compatibilities: TPN sol

Patient/family education
• Advise patient that flushing and increase in feelings of warmth will occur several hr after taking drug (PO); after 2 wk of therapy these side effects diminish
• Instruct patient to remain recumbent if postural hypotension occurs; to rise slowly from sitting or recumbent
• Caution patient to abstain from alcohol if drug is prescribed for hyperlipidemia
• Caution patient to avoid sunlight if skin lesions are present
• Advise patient to report clay-colored stools, anorexia, jaundiced sclera, skin, dark urine; hepatotoxicity may occur

Evaluation
Positive therapeutic outcome
• Decreased lipid levels
• Warm extremities
• Absence of numbness in extremities

---

*niCARdipine (Rx)
(nye-card′i-peen)
Cardene, Cardene IV, Cardene SR
Func. class.: Calcium channel blocker, antianginal, antihypertensive
Chem. class.: Dihydropyridine
Pregnancy category C

N

Action: Inhibits calcium ion influx across cell membrane during cardiac depolarization, produces relaxation of coronary vascular smooth muscle and peripheral vascular smooth muscle, dilates coronary arteries, increases myocardial oxygen delivery in patients with vasospastic angina

➡ **Therapeutic Outcome:** Decreased angina pectoris, decreased B/P in hypertension

Uses: Chronic stable angina pectoris, hypertension

Dosage and routes
Hypertension
Adult: PO 20 mg tid initially; may increase after 3 days (range 20-40 mg tid) or 30 mg bid sus rel, may increase to 60 mg bid **IV** 5 mg/hr, may increase by 2.5 mg/hr q15min, max 15 mg/hr

Angina
Adult: PO 20 mg tid, may be adjusted q3d, may use 20-40 mg tid

Renal dose
Adult: PO 20 mg tid; or 30 mg bid (sus rel)

Hepatic dose
Adult: PO 20 mg bid

Available forms: Caps 20, 30 mg; sus rel caps 30, 45, 60 mg; inj 2.5 mg/ml

Adverse effects
(*italic* = common; **bold** = life-threatening)
CNS: Headache, dizziness, anxiety, depression, confusion, paresthesia, somnolence
CV: Edema, bradycardia, hypotension, palpitations, **pulmonary edema,** chest pain, tachycardia, increased angina
GI: Nausea, vomiting, gastric upset, constipation, **hepatitis,** abdominal cramps
GU: Nocturia, polyuria
INTEG: Rash
MISC: Blurred vision, flushing, sweating, shortness of breath

Contraindications: Sick sinus syndrome, 2nd- or 3rd-degree heart block, hypersensitivity

Precautions: CHF, hypotension, hepatic **P** injury, pregnancy **C,** lactation, children, renal **G** disease, elderly

N **Do Not Confuse:**
Cardene/Cardizem, Cardene SR/Cardizem SR
niCARdipine/NIFEdipine

Pharmacokinetics

Absorption	Well absorbed (PO); bioavailability poor
Distribution	Unknown
Metabolism	Liver, extensively
Excretion	Kidneys 60%, feces 35%
Half-life	2-5 hr

Pharmacodynamics

	PO	PO-SUS REL
Onset	½ hr	Unknown
Peak	1-2 hr	2-6 hr
Duration	8 hr	10-12 hr

Interactions
Individual drugs
Alcohol: ↑ hypotension
Carbamazepine, cimetidine, cycloSPORINE, prazosin, quinidine: ↑ risk of toxicity
Digoxin: ↑ digoxin levels, bradycardia, CHF
Phenobarbital, phenytoin: ↓ effectiveness
Propranolol: ↑ toxicity
Rifampin: ↓ niCARdipine effect
Drug classifications
Antihypertensives, nitrates: ↑ hypotension
β-Adrenergic blockers: ↑ bradycardia, CHF
NSAIDs: ↓ antihypertensive effect
Food/drug
Grapefruit juice: ↑ hypotensive effect
☑ *Herb/drug*
Barberry, betel palm, burdock, goldenseal,

khat, khella, lily of the valley, plantain: ↑ effect
Yohimbe: ↓ effect

NURSING CONSIDERATIONS
Assessment
• Assess fluid volume status (I&O ratio) and record weight, color, quality and sp gr of urine, skin turgor, adequacy of pulses, moist mucous membranes, bilateral lung sounds, peripheral pitting edema; dehydration symptoms of decreasing output, thirst, hypotension, dry mouth, and mucous membranes should be reported
• Monitor for CHF: weight gain, rales, jugular venous distention, dyspnea
• Monitor B/P and pulse
• Assess anginal pain: intensity, location, duration, alleviating factors
• Monitor potassium, liver function tests, renal studies periodically

Nursing diagnoses
☑ Cardiac output, decreased (uses)
☑ Knowledge, deficient (teaching)

Implementation
PO route
S • Do not open, break, crush, chew sus rel cap
• Give with or without regard to meals
• Store in airtight container at room temp
IV **IV route**
• Dilute each 25 mg/240 ml of compatible sol (0.1 mg/ml), give slowly, stable for 24 hr at room temp

Y-site compatibilities: Diltiazem, DOBUTamine, DOPamine, epINEPHrine, fentanyl, hydromorphone, labetalol, lorazepam, midazolam, milrinone, morphine, nitroglycerin, norepinephrine, ranitidine, vecuronium

Patient/family education
• Advise patient to avoid hazardous activities until stabilized on drug and dizziness is no longer a problem
• Instruct patient to limit caffeine consumption; to avoid alcohol and OTC drugs unless directed by a prescriber
• Instruct patient to comply in all areas of medical regimen: diet, exercise, stress reduction, drug therapy; to notify prescriber of irregular heart beat, shortness of breath, swelling of feet and hands, pronounced dizziness, constipation, nausea, hypotension
• Teach patient to use medication as directed even if feeling better; may be taken with other cardiovascular drugs (nitrates, β-blockers)
• Teach patient to take medication exactly as prescribed

☑ Herb/drug   **S** Do Not Crush   **◆** Alert   **◆—** Key Drug   **G** Geriatric   **P** Pediatric

- Advise patient to contact prescriber if anginal attacks continue or become worse

Evaluation
Positive therapeutic outcome
- Decreased angina attacks
- Decreased B/P

Treatment of overdose: Defibrillation, atropine for AV block, vasopressor for hypotension

---

nicotinamide
See niacin

---

nicotine (OTC)
(nik'o-teen)
nicotine chewing gum (OTC)
Nicorette
nicotine inhaler (Rx)
Nicotrol Inhaler
nicotine nasal spray (Rx)
Nicotrol NS
nicotine transdermal (OTC)
Clear Nicoderm CQ, Habitrol, NicoDerm CQ, Nicotrol
Func. class.: Smoking deterrent
Chem. class.: Ganglionic cholinergic agonist

Pregnancy category D

Action: Agonist at nicotinic receptors in the peripheral and central nervous systems; acts at sympathetic ganglia, on chemoreceptors of the aorta and carotid bodies; also affects adrenalin-releasing catecholamines

Therapeutic Outcome: Decreased withdrawal effects when smoking cessation is attempted

Uses: Deter cigarette smoking

Investigational uses: Gilles de la Tourette's syndrome

Dosage and routes
Habitrol, NicoDerm
Adult: 21 mg/day × 4-8 wk; 14 mg/day × 2-4 wk; 7 mg/day × 2-4 wk

Nicotine chewing gum
Adult: Gum 1 piece chewed × 30 min as needed to abstain from smoking; not to exceed 30/day

Nicotine inhaler
Adult: Inhale 6 cartridges/day for first 3-6 wk, max 16/day × 12 wk

Nicotine nasal spray
Adult: 1 spray in each nostril 1-2 ×/hr, max 5 ×/hr or 40 ×/day, max 3 mo

Nicotrol
Adult: 15 mg/day × 12 wk; 10 mg/day × 2 wk; 5 mg/day × 2 wk

Nicotrol Inhaler
Adult: Delivers 30% of what a smoker receives from an actual cigarette

Gilles de la Tourette's Syndrome (off-label)
Adult/child: Chewing gum 2 mg chewed × ½ hr bid × 1-6 mo; TD 7 or 10 mg patch qd × 2 days

Available forms: Gum 2 mg/piece; nicotine transdermal system 7, 14, 21 mg/day delivered (Habitrol, NicoDerm, Nicotine Transdermal System); NicoDerm 5, 10, 15 mg/day; nicotine inhaler 4 mg delivered; nasal spray 0.5 mg of nicotine/actuation

Adverse effects
(*italic* = common; **bold** = life-threatening)
CNS: Dizziness, vertigo, insomnia, headache, confusion, convulsions, depression, euphoria, numbness, tinnitus, strange dreams
CV: **Dysrhythmias,** tachycardia, palpitations, edema, flushing, hypertension
EENT: Jaw ache, irritation in buccal cavity
GI: *Nausea, vomiting, anorexia, indigestion,* diarrhea, abdominal pain, constipation, eructation
RESP: Breathing difficulty, cough, hoarseness, sneezing, wheezing

Contraindications: Hypersensitivity, immediate post-MI recovery period, severe angina pectoris, pregnancy (X) gum; transdermal **D**

Precautions: Vasospastic disease, dysrhythmias, diabetes mellitus, hyperthyroidism, pheochromocytoma, coronary disease, esophagitis, peptic ulcer, lactation, hepatic/renal disease

Pharmacokinetics	
Absorption	Slowly absorbed, buccal cavity
Distribution	Unknown
Metabolism	Liver; some by lungs, kidneys
Excretion	Kidneys, unchanged (20%); breast milk
Half-life	1-2 hr

Pharmacodynamics	
Onset	Rapid
Peak	½ hr
Duration	Unknown

Interactions
Individual drugs

Acetaminophen, caffeine, furosemide, imipramine, oxazepam, pentazocine, propranolol: ↑ effects of each specific drug

Glutethimide: ↓ absorption

Insulin (SC): ↑ absorption

Propoxyphene: ↓ propoxyphene metabolism

Theophylline: ↑ blood levels with cessation of smoking

Herb/drug

Blue cohosh, lobelia: ↑ effect

Oats: ↓ effect

NURSING CONSIDERATIONS
Assessment

• Assess for adverse reaction to gum: irritation of buccal cavity, dislike of taste, jaw ache

• Assess for withdrawal symptoms: headache, fatigue, drowsiness, restlessness, irritability, severe cravings for nicotine products before, during, and after treatment

• Obtain a nicotine assessment: brand of cigarettes, chewing tobacco, cigars, number of each used per day; what increases need or activities performed when each is used

• Gum should not be used if temporomandibular condition exists

• Assess for nicotine toxicity: GI symptoms (nausea, vomiting, diarrhea), cardiopulmonary symptoms (decreased B/P, dyspnea, change in pulse), weakness, abdominal cramping, headache, blurred vision, tinnitus; drug should be discontinued

Nursing diagnoses

☑ Coping, ineffective individual (uses)

☑ Knowledge, deficient (teaching)

☑ Noncompliance (teaching)

Implementation

• Give only prescribed amount, or toxicity may occur

• Protect gum from light and heat

Patient/family education
Gum

• Advise patient to chew gum slowly for 30 min to promote buccal absorption of the drug; do not chew over 45 min

Transdermal patch

• Caution patient that patch is as toxic as cigarettes; to be used only to deter smoking

• Caution patient not to use during pregnancy; birth defects may occur

• Instruct patient to keep used and unused system out of reach of children and pets

• Instruct patient to apply once a day to a nonhairy, clean, dry area of skin on upper body or upper outer arm; to rotate sites to prevent skin irritation

• Instruct patient to stop smoking immediately when beginning patch treatment

• Teach patient to apply promptly after removing from protective pouch; system may lose strength

Inhaler

• Advise patient that puffing on mouthpiece delivers nicotine through the mouth lining

• Instruct patient to chew gum slowly for 30 min to promote buccal absorption of the drug; do not chew over 45 min

• Advise patient to begin drug withdrawal after 3 mo use; do not exceed 6 mo

• Teach patient all aspects of drug; give package insert to patient and explain; caution patient not to exceed prescribed dose

• Inform patient that gum will not stick to dentures, dental appliances

• Caution patient that gum is as toxic as cigarettes; it is to be used only to deter smoking

• Caution patient not to use during pregnancy; birth defects may occur

Evaluation
Positive therapeutic outcome

• Decrease in urge to smoke

• Decreased need for gum after 3-6 mo

---

*NIFEdipine (Rx)
(nye-fed′i-peen)

Adalat, Adalat CC, Apo-Nifed ♣, Novo-Nifedin ♣, Nu-Nifed ♣, Nu-Nifedin ♣, NIFEdipine, Procardia, Procardia XL

Func. class.: Calcium channel blocker, antianginal, antihypertensive

Chem. class.: Dihydropyridine

Pregnancy category C

Action: Inhibits calcium ion influx across cell membrane during cardiac depolarization, produces relaxation of coronary vascular smooth muscle and peripheral vascular smooth muscle, dilates coronary vascular arteries, increases myocardial oxygen delivery in patients with vasospastic angina

⮕ **Therapeutic Outcome:** Decreased angina pectoris, decreased B/P in hypertension

Uses: Chronic stable angina pectoris, vasospastic angina, hypertension

---

☑ Herb/drug   Ⓢ Do Not Crush   ◆ Alert   ◆⫪ Key Drug   Ⓖ Geriatric   Ⓟ Pediatric

Investigational uses: Migraines, CHF, Raynaud's disease, anal fissures

Dosage and routes
Adult: PO immediate release, 10 mg tid; increase in 10 mg increments q7-14 days, max 180 mg/24 hr or single dose of 30 mg; sus rel, 30-60 mg/day; may increase q7-14 days; doses >120 mg not recommended

P *Child:* PO 0.25-0.5 mg/kg/dose q4-6h, max 1-2 mg/kg/day

Anal fissures (off-label)
Adult: TOP 0.2% gel q12h × 21 days

Available forms: Caps 5, 10, 20 mg; ext rel tabs 10, 20, 30, 60, 90 mg; tabs 10 mg, gel 0.2%

Adverse effects
(*italic* = common; **bold** = life-threatening)
CNS: Headache, fatigue, drowsiness, *dizziness,* anxiety, depression, weakness, insomnia, *lightheadedness,* paresthesia, tinnitus, blurred vision, nervousness, tremor
CV: **Dysrhythmias,** edema, hypotension, palpitations, tachycardia
GI: Nausea, vomiting, diarrhea, gastric upset, constipation, increased liver function studies, dry mouth, flatulence
GU: Nocturia, polyuria
INTEG: Rash, pruritus, *flushing,* hair loss
MISC: Sexual difficulties, cough, fever, chills
SYST: **Stevens-Johnson syndrome**

Contraindications: Hypersensitivity

Precautions: CHF, hypotension, sick sinus syndrome, 2nd- or 3rd-degree heart block, hypotension less than 90 mm Hg systolic, hepatic injury, pregnancy **C**, lactation, **P** children, renal disease

N **Do Not Confuse:**
NIFEdipine/niCARdipine

Pharmacokinetics	
Absorption	Well absorbed (PO)
Distribution	Unknown
Metabolism	Liver, extensively
Excretion	Unknown
Half-life	2-5 hr

Pharmacodynamics		
	PO	PO–EXT REL
Onset	½ hr	Unknown
Peak	Unknown	Unknown
Duration	6-8 hr	24 hr

Interactions
Individual drugs
Alcohol: ↑ hypotension
Cimetidine, cycloSPORINE, prazosin: ↑ risk of toxicity
Digoxin: ↑ digoxin levels, bradycardia, CHF
Propranolol: ↑ toxicity
Theophylline: ↑ theophylline effect
Drug classifications
β-Adrenergic blockers: ↑ bradycardia, CHF
NSAIDs: ↓ antihypertensive effect
Food/drug
Grapefruit juice: ↑ NIFEdipine level
Herb/drug
Barberry, betel palm, burdock, goldenseal, khat, khella, lily of the valley, plaintain: ↑ effect
Yohimbe: ↓ effect
Lab test interferences
Positive: ANA titer, direct Coombs' test

NURSING CONSIDERATIONS
Assessment
• Assess anginal pain: location, intensity, duration, character, alleviating, aggravating factors
• Monitor potassium, liver function tests, renal studies periodically during treatment
• Assess fluid volume status (I&O ratio) and record weight, distended red veins, crackles in lung, color, quality and sp gr of urine, skin turgor, adequacy of pulses, moist mucous membranes, bilateral lung sounds, peripheral pitting edema; dehydration symptoms of decreasing output, thirst, hypotension, dry mouth, and mucous membranes should be reported
• Monitor ALT, AST, bilirubin daily; if these are elevated, hepatotoxicity is suspected
• Monitor cardiac status: B/P, pulse, respirations, ECG

Nursing diagnoses
✓ Cardiac output, decreased (uses)
✓ Pain (uses)
✓ Knowledge, deficient (teaching)

Implementation
PO route
• Give without regard to meals
• Store in airtight container at room temp
Sublingual route
• Using a sterile needle puncture the cap and squeeze medication in buccal area (not an FDA-approved use)

Patient/family education
• Advise patient to avoid hazardous activities until stabilized on drug and dizziness is no longer a problem
• Instruct patient to limit caffeine consump-

tion; to avoid alcohol and OTC drugs unless directed by prescriber
- Tell patient that ext rel tab has nonabsorbable shell, may appear in stools
- Instruct patient to comply in all areas of medical regimen: diet, exercise, stress reduction, drug therapy; to notify prescriber of irregular heart beat, shortness of breath, swelling of feet and hands, pronounced dizziness, constipation, nausea, hypotension, severe rash
- Teach patient to use as directed even if feeling better; may be taken with other cardiovascular drugs (nitrates, β-blockers)

Evaluation
Positive therapeutic outcome
- Decreased angina attacks
- Decreased B/P

Treatment of overdose: Defibrillation, atropine for AV block, vasopressor for hypotension

---

nilutamide (Rx)
(nil-u'ta-mide)
Anandron ✤, Nilandron
Func. class.: Antineoplastic, hormone
Chem. class.: Antiandrogen

Pregnancy category C

Action: Interferes with testosterone uptake in the nucleus or testosterone activity in target tissues; arrests tumor growth in androgen-sensitive tissue, i.e., prostate gland, prostatic carcinoma is androgen-sensitive, so tumor growth is arrested

➔ **Therapeutic Outcome:** Decreased tumor size

Uses: Metastatic prostatic carcinoma, stage D2 in combination with surgical castration

Dosage and routes
Adult: PO 300 mg qd × 30 days, then 150 mg qd

Available forms: Tabs 100 ✤, 150 mg

Adverse effects
(*italic* = common; **bold** = life-threatening)
CNS: Hot flashes, drowsiness, insomnia, dizziness, hyperthesia, depression
EENT: Delay in adaptation to dark
GI: Diarrhea, nausea, vomiting, elevated liver function studies, constipation, dyspepsia, **hepatotoxicity**
GU: Decreased libido, impotence, testicular atrophy, UTI, hematuria, nocturia, gynecomastia

HEMA: Anemia
INTEG: Rash, sweating, alopecia, dry skin
MISC: Edema
RESP: Dyspnea, URI, pneumonia, **interstitial pneumonitis**

Contraindications: Hypersensitivity, severe hepatic impairment, severe respiratory disease, women

Precautions: Pregnancy C

Pharmacokinetics	
Absorption	Rapidly, completely
Distribution	Unknown
Metabolism	Unknown
Excretion	Urine, feces
Half-life	Unknown

Pharmacodynamics
Unknown

Interactions
Individual drugs
Phenytoin, theophylline, vitamin K: ↑ toxicity

NURSING CONSIDERATIONS
Assessment
◆● - Monitor liver function studies: AST, ALT, alkaline phosphatase, which may be elevated; if elevated 3 × normal, discontinue drug
- Monitor for CNS symptoms: drowsiness, insomnia, dizziness
- Monitor chest x-rays routinely, baseline pulmonary function studies, dyspnea, cough, may indicate interstitial pneumonitis, discontinue treatment if this condition is suspected
- Monitor for hyperglycemia, increased BUN, creatinine, alkaline phosphatase leukopenia

Nursing diagnoses
✓ Infection, risk of (side effects)
✓ Knowledge, deficient (teaching)

Implementation
- Administer without regard to meals
- Store at room temp

Patient/family education
◆● - Advise patient to report side effects: decreased libido, impotence, breast enlargement, hot flashes, diarrhea, dyspnea, cough; symptoms of hepatotoxicity (dark urine, abdominal pain, clay-colored stools, jaundiced eyes, skin); notify prescriber immediately if shortness of breath occurs
- Advise patient to wear tinted lens to alleviate delay in adapting to the dark
- Advise patient that drug is started on day of or day after surgical castration
- Advise patient to avoid alcohol consumption

Evaluation
Positive therapeutic outcome
• Decrease in prostatic tumor size, decrease in spread of cancer

Treatment of overdose: Induce vomiting, provide supportive care

---

nimodipine (Rx)
(ni-moe'dip-een)
Nimotop
Func. class.: Calcium channel blocker
Chem. class.: Dihydropyridine

Pregnancy category C

Action: Unknown, may have greater effect on cerebral arteries

→ **Therapeutic Outcome:** Prevention of vascular spasm (subarachnoid hemorrhage)

Uses: Prevention of cerebral vascular spasm in subarachnoid hemorrhage

Dosage and routes
Adult: PO Begin therapy within 96 hr, 60 mg q4h × 21 days

Available forms: Caps 30 mg

Adverse effects
(*italic* = common; **bold** = life-threatening)
CNS: Headache, fatigue, drowsiness, dizziness, anxiety, depression, weakness, insomnia, confusion, paresthesia, somnolence
CV: Dysrhythmia, edema, CHF, bradycardia, hypotension, palpitations, **MI, pulmonary edema**
GI: Nausea, vomiting, diarrhea, gastric upset, constipation, ***hepatitis***, abdominal cramps
GU: Nocturia, polyuria, **acute renal failure**
INTEG: Rash, pruritus, urticaria, photosensitivity, hair loss
MISC: Blurred vision, flushing, nasal congestion, sweating, shortness of breath, gynecomastia, hyperglycemia, sexual difficulties

Contraindications: Sick sinus syndrome, 2nd- or 3rd-degree heart block, hypotension less than 90 mm Hg systolic, hypersensitivity

Precautions: CHF, hypotension, hepatic
P injury, pregnancy **C**, lactation, children, renal
G disease, elderly

Pharmacokinetics
Absorption	Well absorbed, bioavailability poor
Distribution	Crosses blood-brain barrier
Metabolism	Liver, extensively
Excretion	Kidneys
Half-life	1-2 hr

Pharmacodynamics
Onset	Unknown
Peak	1 hr
Duration	Unknown

Interactions
Individual drugs
Alcohol: ↑ hypotension
Digoxin: ↑ digoxin levels, bradycardia
Phenobarbital, phenytoin: ↓ effectiveness
Propranolol: ↑ toxicity
Drug classifications
Antihypertensives: ↑ hypotension
β-Adrenergic blockers: ↑ bradycardia
Nitrates: ↑ nitrates
Herb/drug
Barberry, betel palm, burdock, goldenseal, khat, khella, lily of the valley, plaintain: ↑ effect
Yohimbe: ↓ effect

NURSING CONSIDERATIONS
Assessment
• Assess fluid volume status (I&O ratio) and record weight, distended red veins, crackles in lung, color, quality and sp gr of urine, skin turgor, adequacy of pulses, moist mucous membranes, bilateral lung sounds, peripheral pitting edema; dehydration symptoms of decreasing output, thirst, hypotension, dry mouth and mucous membranes should be reported
• Monitor B/P and pulse; if B/P drops 30 mm Hg, call prescriber
• Monitor ALT, AST, bilirubin daily; if these are elevated, hepatotoxicity is suspected

Nursing diagnoses
✓ Injury, risk for (uses)
✓ Knowledge, deficient (teaching)

Implementation
• May puncture cap and dilute in water and give through nasogastric tube; flush tube with 0.9% NaCl
• Store in airtight container at room temp

Evaluation
Positive therapeutic outcome
• Prevention of neurologic damage from subarachnoid hemorrhage

N

---

nisoldipine (Rx)
(nye'sol-dye-peen)
Sular
Func. class.: Antihypertensive, calcium channel blocker
Chem. class.: Dihydropyridine

Pregnancy category C

Action: Inhibits calcium ion influx across cell membrane, resulting in dilation of peripheral arteries

➔ **Therapeutic Outcome:**
Decreased B/P in hypertension

Uses: Essential hypertension, alone or with other antihypertensives

Dosage and routes
Adult: PO 20 mg qd initially, may increase by 10 mg/wk, usual dose 20-40 mg qd, max 60 mg/day

G *Elderly/hepatic dose:* PO 10 mg/day, increase by 10 mg/wk

Available forms: Tabs, ext rel 10, 20, 30, 40 mg

Adverse effects
(*italic* = common; **bold** = life-threatening)
CNS: Headache, fatigue, drowsiness, dizziness, anxiety, depression, nervousness, insomnia, light-headedness, paresthesia, tinnitus, psychosis, somnolence, ataxia, confusion, malaise, migraine
CV: **Dysrhythmias,** edema, **CHF,** hypotension, palpitations, **MI, pulmonary edema,** tachycardia, syncope, AV block, angina, chest pain, ECG abnormalities
GI: Nausea, vomiting, diarrhea, gastric upset, constipation, elevated liver function studies, dry mouth, dyspepsia, dysphagia, flatulence
GU: Nocturia, hematuria, dysuria
HEMA: Anemia, leukopenia, petechiae
INTEG: Rash, pruritus
MISC: Sexual difficulties, gingival hyperplasia, chills, fever, gout, sweating, cough, nasal congestion, shortness of breath, wheezing, epistaxis

Contraindications: Hypersensitivity, sick sinus syndrome, 2nd- or 3rd-degree heart block

Precautions: CHF, hypotension <90 mm Hg
P systolic, hepatic injury, pregnancy **C,** lactation,
G children, renal disease, elderly, acute MI, unstable angina

Pharmacokinetics
Absorption	Well absorbed
Distribution	Highly protein bound
Metabolism	Liver
Excretion	Kidneys
Half-life	Unknown

Pharmacodynamics
Peak	6-12 hr

Interactions
Individual drugs
Alcohol: ↑ hypotension
Carbamazepine, propranolol: ↑ toxicity
Digoxin: ↑ digoxin levels, ↑ bradycardia, CHF
Phenobarbital, phenytoin: ↓ effectiveness
Drug classifications
Antifungals (azole): ↑ nisoldipine level
Antihypertensives: ↑ hypotension
β-Adrenergic blockers: ↑ bradycardia, CHF
Hydantoins: ↓ nisoldipine effect
Nitrates: ↑ nitrates
Herb/drug
Angelica, cat's claw, chicory: ↑ antidysrhythmic effect
Barberry, betel palm, burdock, goldenseal, khat, khella, lily of the valley, plaintain: ↑ effect
Yohimbe: ↓ effect
Food/drug
Grapefruit juice: ↑ hypotension
High-fat: ↑ nisoldipine level

NURSING CONSIDERATIONS
Assessment
• Assess fluid volume status: I&O ratio and record; weight; skin turgor; adequacy of pulses; moist mucous membranes; bilateral lung sounds; peripheral pitting edema; dehydration symptoms of decreasing output, thirst, hypotension, dry mouth, and mucous membranes should be reported
• Monitor ALT, AST, bilirubin daily, if these are elevated and hepatotoxicity is suspected
• Monitor cardiac status: B/P, pulse, respiration, ECG

Nursing diagnoses
✓ Cardiac output, decreased (uses)
✓ Knowledge, deficient (teaching)

Implementation
• Give once a day, with food to decrease GI symptoms, avoid high-fat foods, grapefruit

Patient/family education
• Caution patient to avoid hazardous activities until stabilized on drug, and dizziness is no longer a problem
• Instruct patient to limit caffeine

 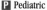

consumption; to avoid alcohol and OTC drugs unless directed by prescriber
• Urge patient to comply in all areas of medical regimen: diet, exercise, stress reduction, drug therapy; to notify prescriber of irregular heart beat, shortness of breath, swelling of feet and hands, pronounced dizziness, constipation, nausea, hypotension
• Teach patient to use as directed even if feeling better; may be taken with other cardiovascular drugs (nitrates, β-blockers)
• Advise patient to rise slowly to prevent orthostatic hypotension
• Teach patient to report nausea, dizziness, edema, shortness of breath, palpitations

Evaluation
Positive therapeutic outcome
• Decreased B/P

---

nitazoxanide (Rx)
(nye-taz-ox′a-nide)
Alinia
Func. class.: Antiprotozoal
Pregnancy category B

Action: Interferes with DNA/RNA synthesis in protozoa

⇒ **Therapeutic Outcome:** C&S negative for organism

Uses: Diarrhea caused by *Cryptosporidium parvum* or *Giardia lamblia*

Dosage and routes
P *Child 4-11 yr:* **PO** 10 ml q12h × 3 days
P *Child 12-47 mo:* **PO** 5 ml q12h × 3 days

Available forms: Powder for oral susp 100 mg/5 ml

Adverse effects
(*italic* = common; **bold** = life-threatening)
CNS: Dizziness, fever, headache
CV: Hypotension
GI: Nausea, anorexia, flatulence, increased appetite, enlarged salivary glands, abdominal pain, diarrhea, vomiting
HEMA: Anemia, **leukopenia,** neutropenia
INTEG: Pruritus, sweating
MISC: Increased creatinine, pale yellow eye discoloration, rhinitis, discolored urine, infection, malaise

Contraindications: Hypersensitivity

Precautions: Renal, hepatic disease,
P pregnancy (B), lactation, children <1 yr or >11 yr

Pharmacokinetics
Absorption	Unknown
Distribution	Metabolite protein binding >99%
Metabolism	Hydrolyzed to active metabolite, undergoes conjugation
Excretion	Urine, bile, feces
Half-life	Unknown

Pharmacodynamics
Unknown

NURSING CONSIDERATIONS
Assessment
• Assess for signs of infection
• Assess bowel pattern before, during treatment

Nursing diagnoses
☑ Risk for infection (uses)
☑ Knowledge, deficient (teaching)

Implementation
PO route
• Give with food

Patient/family education
• Advise to take with food; shake susp well before each dose

Evaluation
Positive therapeutic outcome
• C&S negative for organism

N

nitroglycerin ◆π (Rx)
(nye-troe-gli'ser-in)
transmucosal tablets (Rx)
Nitrogard, Nitrogard SR ✦
sustained-release (Rx)
Nitrocot, Nitroglyn E-R, Nitro-par, Nitro-Time
intravenous (Rx)
Nitro-Bid IV, Tridil
spray (Rx)
Nitrolingual
sublingual (Rx)
Nitrostat, NitroQuick
topical ointment (Rx)
Nitro-Bid, Nitrol
transdermal (Rx)
Deponit, Minitran, Nitrek, Nitrocine, Nitrodisc, Nitro-Dur, Transderm-Nitro,
translingual (Rx)
Nitrolingual
Func. class.: Coronary vasodilator, antianginal
Chem. class.: Nitrate

Pregnancy category C

Action: Decreases preload and afterload, which thus decreases left ventricular end-diastolic pressure and systemic vascular resistance; dilates coronary arteries and improves blood flow through coronary vasculature, dilates arterial, venous beds systemically

➡**Therapeutic Outcome:** Prevention of anginal attack

Uses: Chronic stable angina pectoris, prophylaxis of angina pain, CHF associated with acute MI, controlled hypotension in surgical procedures

Dosage and routes
Adult: SL dissolve tab under tongue when pain begins; may repeat q5 min until relief occurs; take no more than 3 tab/15 min; use 1 tab prophylactically 5-10 min before activities; sus rel cap q6-12h on empty stomach; top 1-2 in q8h; increase to 4 in q4h as needed; **IV** 5 mcg/min, then increase by 5 mcg/min q3-5 min; if no response after 20 mcg/min, increase by 10-20

mcg/min until desired response; TD apply a pad qd to a site free from hair; remove patch hs to provide 10-12 hr nitrate-free interval to avoid tolerance; translingual spray 1-2 metered doses onto or under the tongue, max 3 sprays; transmucosal insert between lip and gums above incisors or between gum and cheek 1 mg q3-5 hr during waking hr

P *Child:* **IV** initial 0.25-0.5 mg/kg/min, titrate to patient response, usual dose 1-3 mg/kg/min

Available forms: Transmucosal tabs cont rel 2, 3 mg; translingual aerosol 0.4 mg/m spray; sus rel caps 2.5, 6.5, 9, 13 mg; sus rel tabs 2.6, 6.5, 9 mg; SL tabs 0.3, 0.4, 0.6 mg; oint 2%; trans syst 0.1, 0.2, 0.3, 0.4, 0.6, 0.8 mg/hr; inj 25, 50, 100 mg/250 ml, 100, 200 mg/500 ml

Adverse effects
(*italic* = common; **bold** = life-threatening)
CNS: *Headache, flushing, dizziness*
CV: *Postural hypotension,* tachycardia, **collapse,** syncope
GI: Nausea, vomiting
INTEG: Pallor, sweating, rash

Pharmacokinetics

Absorption	Well absorbed (PO, buccal, SL)
Distribution	Unknown
Metabolism	Liver, extensively
Excretion	Kidney
Half-life	1-4 min

Contraindications: Hypersensitivity to this drug or nitrites, severe anemia, increased ICP, cerebral hemorrhage, closed-angle glaucoma

Precautions: Postural hypotension, pregnancy **C,** lactation, children, severe renal/hepatic disease

◣ **Do Not Confuse:**
Nitro-Bid/Nicobid

Interactions
Individual drugs
Alcohol: ↑ hypotension, CV collapse
Haloperidol, sildenafil: ↑ hypotension

Pharmacodynamics

	SUS REL	SL	TD	IV	TRANSMU-COSAL	AEROSOL	TOP OINT
Onset	20-45 min	1-3 min	½-1 hr	1-2 min	1-2 min	2 min	½-1 hr
Peak	Unknown	Unknown	Unknown	Unknown	Unknown	Unknown	Unknown
Duration	3-8 hr	½ hr	12-24 hr	3-5 min	3-5 hr	½-1 hr	2-12 hr

⬚ Herb/drug   ◎ Do Not Crush   ◆ Alert   ◆π Key Drug   ᴳ Geriatric   ᴾ Pediatric

Drug classifications

Antidepressants (tricyclic), antihistamines, phenothiazines: ↓ absorption of SL, transmucosal

Antihypertensives, β-adrenergic blockers, calcium channel blockers: ↑ hypotension

NURSING CONSIDERATIONS
Assessment
• Monitor orthostatic B/P, pulse
• Assess pain: duration, time started, activity being performed, character; check for tolerance if taken over long period
• Monitor for headache, lightheadedness, decreased B/P; may indicate a need for decreased dosage

Nursing diagnoses
☑ Cardiac output, decreased (uses)
☑ Poisoning (uses)
☑ Tissue perfusion, ineffective (uses)
☑ Knowledge, deficient (teaching)
☑ Noncompliance (teaching)

Implementation
IV **IV route**
• Give **IV** diluted in amount specified D₅W, or 0.9% NaCl for inf; use glass inf bottles, non–polyvinyl chloride inf tubing; titrate to patient response; do not use filters

Y-site compatibilities: Amiodarone, amphotericin B cholesteryl, amrinone, atracurium, cefmetazole, cisatracurium, diltiazem, DOBUTamine, DOPamine, epINEPHrine, esmolol, famotidine, fentanyl, fluconazole, furosemide, haloperidol, heparin, hydromorphone, regular insulin, labetalol, lidocaine, lorazepam, midazolam, milrinone, morphine, niCARdipine, nitroprusside, norepinephrine, pancuronium, ranitidine, remifentanil, streptokinase, tacrolimus, theophylline, vecuronium

Y-site incompatibilities: Alteplase

Additive compatibilities: Alteplase, aminophylline, DOBUTamine, DOPamine, enalaprilat, furosemide, lidocaine, verapamil

Additive incompatibilities: Manufacturer recommends that nitroglycerin not be admixed with other medications

SL route
• Keep tab in original container
• If 3 SL tab in 15 min do not relieve pain, consider diagnosis of MI
• SL tab should be held under tongue until dissolved (a few min); do not take anything by mouth when SL tab is in place

PO route
• Give 1 hr ac or 2 hr pc with 8 oz of water
⊘ • Sus rel tab should not be chewed, broken or crushed

Transmucosal route
• Tab should be placed between cheek and gum line
• Do not take anything PO when tab is in place

Topical route
• Apply ointment using dose-measuring papers supplied; apply to an area without hair; ointment should cover 2-3 in area; may apply an occlusive dressing as directed

Transdermal route
• Apply TD patches to area without hair; press hard to adhere; if patch becomes dislodged, apply a new one

Patient/family education
• Teach patient to place buccal tab between lip and gum above incisors or between cheek and gum; sus rel tab must be swallowed whole, do not chew; SL should be dissolved under tongue
• Instruct patient to avoid alcohol
• Advise patient that drug may cause headache; tolerance usually develops; use nonopioid analgesic
• Teach patient that drug may be taken before stressful activity, exercise, sexual activity
• Inform patient that SL tab may sting when drug comes in contact with mucous membranes
• Caution patient to avoid hazardous activities if dizziness occurs
• Instruct patient to comply with complete medical regimen
• Advise patient to make position changes slowly to prevent fainting

Evaluation
Positive therapeutic outcome
• Decreased, prevention of anginal pain

N

⚠ HIGH ALERT

nitroprusside (Rx)
(nye-troe-pruss′ide)
Nitropress, Sodium nitroprusside
Func. class.: Antihypertensive, vasodilator

Pregnancy category C

Action: Directly relaxes arteriolar, venous smooth muscle, resulting in reduction in cardiac preload, afterload

➡ **Therapeutic Outcome:** Decreased B/P

in hypertensive crisis, decreased preload, afterload

Uses: Hypertensive crisis, to decrease bleeding by creating hypotension during surgery, acute CHF

Dosage and routes

Adult: **IV** inf dissolve 50 mg in 2-3 ml of D$_5$W, then dilute in 250-1000 ml of D$_5$W; run at 0.5-8 mcg/kg/min

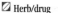 *Child:* **IV** 0.3-0.5 mg/kg/min, titrate to response

Available forms: Inj 50 mg

Adverse effects

(*italic* = common; **bold** = life-threatening)
CNS: *Dizziness, headache,* agitation, twitching, decreased reflexes, restlessness
CV: Bradycardia, ECG changes, tachycardia
GI: Nausea, vomiting, abdominal pain
INTEG: Pain, irritation at inj site, sweating
MISC: **Cyanide, thiocyanate toxicity,** flushing, hypothyroidism

Contraindications: Hypersensitivity, hypertension (compensatory) due to aortic coarctation or AV shunting, acute CHF associated with reduced peripheral vascular resistance

Precautions: Pregnancy **C**, lactation, children, fluid, electrolyte imbalances, hepatic disease, renal disease, hypothyroidism, elderly

Pharmacokinetics

Absorption	Complete bioavailability
Distribution	Not known
Metabolism	RBCs, tissues
Excretion	Kidneys
Half-life	3 days; circulating half-life 2 min

Pharmacodynamics

Onset	1-2 min
Peak	Rapid
Duration	1-10 min

Interactions

Drug classifications
Anesthetics, enflurane, halothane, volatile liquid: Severe hypotension
Ganglionic blockers: ↑ hypotension

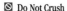 *Herb/drug*
Aconite: ↑ toxicity, death
Angelica: ↑ nitroprusside effect
Astragalus, cola tree: ↑ or ↓ antihypertensive effect
Barberry, betony, black catechu, black cohosh, bloodroot, broom, burdock, cat's claw, dande-

lion, goldenseal, Irish moss, Jamaica dogwood, kelp, khella, mistletoe, parsley: ↑ antihypertensive effect
Coltsfoot, guarana, khat, licorice: ↓ antihypertensive effect

NURSING CONSIDERATIONS
Assessment

• Monitor B/P q5 min × 2 hr, then q1h × 2 hr; monitor pulse q4h; monitor jugular venous distention q4h; ECG should be monitored continuously; monitor PCWP; rebound hypertension may occur after nitroprusside is discontinued

• Monitor electrolytes, blood studies: potassium, sodium, chloride, CO_2, CBC, serum glucose, serum methemoglobin if pulmonary oxygen levels are decreased

• Check weight, I&O, edema in feet and legs daily; assess skin turgor, dryness of mucous membranes for hydration status

• Assess for signs of CHF: dyspnea, edema, wet rales

 • Monitor for increased lactate, cyanide, thiocyanate levels if on long-term treatment, thiocyanate level should be ≤1 millimole/L

• Monitor for decrease in bicarbonate, P_{CO_2} and blood pH; acidosis may occur with this drug

Nursing diagnoses

☑ Tissue perfusion, ineffective (uses)
☑ Injury, risk for (adverse reactions)
☑ Knowledge, deficient (teaching)

Implementation

• Give by cont inf after diluting 50 mg/2-3 ml of D$_5$W; further dilute in 250 ml of D$_5$W; use an infusion pump only; wrap bottle with aluminum foil to protect from light; observe for color change in inf; discard if highly discolored (blue, green, red); titrate to patient response; avoid extravasation

Syringe compatibilities: Heparin

Y-site compatibilities: Amrinone, atracurium, diltiazem, DOBUTamine, DOPamine, enalaprilat, famotidine, lidocaine, nitroglycerin, pancuronium, tacrolimus, theophylline, vecuronium

Additive incompatibilities: Do not give with any other drugs

Patient/family education

• Teach patient to report headache, dizziness, loss of hearing, blurred vision, dyspnea, faintness; may indicate adverse reactions

---

 Herb/drug   Do Not Crush   ◆ Alert   ◆☎ Key Drug   **G** Geriatric   **P** Pediatric

Evaluation
Positive therapeutic outcome
• Decreased B/P in hypertension
• Absence of bleeding in surgery

Treatment of overdose: Administer amyl nitrate inh until 3% sodium nitrate sol can be prepared for **IV** administration, then inject sodium thiosulfate **IV**; correct drop in B/P with vasopressor

---

nizatidine (Rx, OTC)
(ni-za′ti-deen)
Axid, Axid AR
Func. class.: H₂-Receptor antagonist
Chem. class.: Substituted thiazole

Pregnancy category B

Action: Blocks H_2 receptors thereby reducing gastric acid output

⇒ **Therapeutic Outcome:** Healing of duodenal ulcers or gastric ulcers; prevention of duodenal ulcers; decreases symptoms of gastroesophageal reflex disease (GERD)

Uses: Benign gastric and duodenal ulceration, prevention of duodenal ulcer recurrence, symptomatic relief of gastroesophageal reflux, heartburn prevention

Dosage and routes
Prophylaxis of duodenal ulcer
Adult: PO 150 mg qd hs

Gastric and duodenal ulcer disease
Adult: PO 300 mg at night or 150 mg bid for 4-8 wk; maintenance 150 mg at night

Gastroesophageal reflux
Adult: PO 150 mg bid

Heartburn prevention
Adult: PO 75 mg ac

Renal dose
Adult: PO CCr 20-50 ml/min give 150 mg/day; CCr <20 ml/min give 150 mg qod

Available forms: Caps 150, 300 mg; tabs 75 mg

Adverse effects
(*italic* = common; **bold** = life-threatening)
CNS: Headache, somnolence, confusion, abnormal dreams, dizziness
CV: **Dysrhythmias, cardiac arrest**
ENDO: Gynecomastia
GI: Elevated liver enzymes, hepatitis, jaundice, nausea
HEMA: **Thrombocytopenia, agranulocytosis, aplastic anemia**

INTEG: Pruritus, sweating, urticaria, exfoliative dermatitis
METAB: Hyperuricemia
MS: Myalgia
RESP: **Bronchospasm, laryngeal edema**

Contraindications: Hypersensitivity

Precautions: Renal or hepatic impairment (reduce dose in renal impairment), pregnancy **B**, lactation

Pharmacokinetics
Absorption	PO 70%
Distribution	Breast milk, crosses placenta
Metabolism	Liver, partially
Excretion	Kidney
Half-life	1½ hr

Pharmacodynamics
Onset	Variable
Peak	½-3 hr
Duration	Unknown

NURSING CONSIDERATIONS
Assessment
• Assess patient with ulcers or suspected ulcers: epigastric or abdominal pain, hematemesis, occult blood in stools, blood or gastric aspirate before and throughout treatment, monitor gastric pH (5 should be maintained)
◆● Monitor I&O ratio, BUN, creatinine, CBC with differential monthly; agranulocytosis may occur

Nursing diagnoses
☑ Pain, chronic (uses)
☑ Knowledge, deficient (teaching)

Implementation
• May be given with or without meals
• Give antacids 1 hr before or 1 hr after this drug

Patient/family education
• Caution patient that gynecomastia, impotence may occur and are reversible after treatment is discontinued
• Advise patient to avoid driving, other hazardous activities until stabilized on this medication; drowsiness or dizziness may occur
• Caution patient to avoid black pepper, caffeine, alcohol, harsh spices, extremes in temp of food; tell patient to avoid OTC preparations: aspirin, cough, cold preparations because condition may worsen
• Caution patient not to take OTC and ℞ forms concurrently
• Inform patient that smoking decreases the

N

effectiveness of the drug; that smoking cessation should be considered

• Instruct patient that drug must be continued for prescribed time to be effective and taken exactly as prescribed; doses should not be doubled; a missed dose should be taken as soon as remembered up to 1 hr before next dose

• Advise patient to report bruising, fatigue, malaise; blood dyscrasias may occur

• Advise patient to report diarrhea, black tarry stools, sore throat, rash, dizziness, confusion, or delirium to prescriber immediately

Evaluation

Positive therapeutic outcome

• Decreased pain in abdomen
• Healing of ulcers
• Absence of gastroesophageal reflux

---

norfloxacin (Rx)

(nor-flox'a-sin)

Noroxin

Func. class.: Antiinfective—urinary
Chem. class.: Fluoroquinolone antibacterial

Pregnancy category C

Action: Interferes with conversion intermediate DNA fragments into high-molecular weight DNA in bacteria

➡ **Therapeutic Outcome:** Bactericidal action against gram-positive *Staphylococcus epidermidis,* methicillin-resistant strains of *Staphylococcus aureus,* group D streptococci; gram-negative *Escherichia coli, Klebsiella pneumoniae, Enterobacter cloacae, Proteus mirabilis, Proteus vulgaris, Providencia rettgeri, Morganella morganii, Pseudomonas aeruginosa, Citrobacter freundii*

Uses: Adult UTIs (including complicated), uncomplicated gonorrhea

Dosage and routes
Uncomplicated infections
Adult: PO 400 mg bid × 3-10 days 1 hr ac or 2 hr pc

Complicated infections
Adult: PO 400 mg bid × 10-21 days; 400 mg qd × 7-10 days in impaired renal function

Uncomplicated gonorrhea
Adult: PO 800 mg as a single dose

Prostatitis
Adult: PO 400 mg bid × 4 wk

Occular infection
P *Adult and child:* Ophth ĩ gtt qid; may increase to ĩ gtt q2h for severe infections
Renal dose
Adult: PO CCr ≤30 ml/min 400 mg PO qd

Available forms: Tabs 400 mg

Adverse effects

(*italic* = common; **bold** = life-threatening)

CNS: *Headache, dizziness,* fatigue, somnolence, depression, insomnia
EENT: Visual disturbances
GI: *Nausea,* constipation, increased ALT, AST, flatulence, heartburn, vomiting, diarrhea, dry mouth
INTEG: Rash

Contraindications: Hypersensitivity to quinolones

Precautions: Pregnancy C, lactation,
P children, renal disease, seizure disorders

Pharmacokinetics	
Absorption	30% (PO)
Distribution	Concentration in urinary system
Metabolism	Liver (minimal)
Excretion	Kidneys, unchanged (30%)
Half-life	3-4 hr; increased in renal disease

Pharmacodynamics	
	PO
Onset	Unknown
Peak	1 hr

Interactions
Individual drugs

Cyclosporine, probenecid: ↑ serum concentrations
Nitrofurantoin: ↓ effectiveness; monitor closely
Sucralfate: ↓ absorption of norfloxacin, give 2 hr apart
Theophylline: Possible ↑ toxicity; do not use together
Drug classifications

Antacids, iron salts: ↓ absorption of norfloxacin; give 2 hr apart
Anticoagulants (oral): ↑ effect of anticoagulants
Lab test interferences
↑ AST, ↑ ALT, ↑ BUN, ↑ creatinine, ↑ alkaline phosphatase

NURSING CONSIDERATIONS
Assessment

• Assess patient for previous sensitivity reaction
• Assess patient for signs and symptoms of

    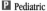

infection including characteristics of urine, WBC >10,000/mm³, temp; obtain baseline information before and during treatment
• Obtain C&S before beginning drug therapy to identify if correct treatment has been initiated
• Assess for allergic reactions: rash, urticaria, pruritus
• Monitor blood studies: AST, ALT, BUN, creatinine, alkaline phosphatase monthly if patient is on long-term therapy
• Assess bowel pattern qd; if severe diarrhea occurs, drug should be discontinued
• Assess for overgrowth of infection: perineal itching, fever, malaise, redness, pain, swelling, drainage, rash, diarrhea, change in cough, sputum

Nursing diagnoses
✓ Infection, risk for (uses)
✓ Diarrhea (adverse reactions)
✓ Injury, risk for (adverse reactions)
✓ Knowledge, deficient (teaching)
✓ Noncompliance (teaching)

Implementation
PO route
• Give in equal intervals q12h around the clock to maintain proper blood levels; give with food to increase absorption of drug; do not give within 3 hr of other agents; drug interactions may occur; give with 8 oz of water
• Do not give with iron, zinc products, or antacids, which decrease absorption

Patient/family education
• Instruct patient to take all medication prescribed for the length of time ordered; drug must be taken at same time of day to maintain blood levels; do not give medication to others; do not double doses; take any missed dose when remembered
• Advise patient to increase fluids to 2 L/day to prevent crystalluria
• Caution patient to avoid driving and other hazardous activities until response is known; dizziness may occur
• Instruct patient to use sunglasses to prevent photophobia
• Have patient use hard candy, frequent sips of water for dry mouth
• Teach patient correct instillation procedure (ophth)

Evaluation
Positive therapeutic outcome
• Reported improvement in symptoms of infection
• Absence of red or itching eyes (ophth)

nortriptyline (Rx)
(nor-trip′ti-leen)
Aventyl, Pamelor
Func. class.: Antidepressant, tricyclic
Chem. class.: Dibenzocycloheptene, secondary amine
Pregnancy category C

Action: Blocks reuptake of norepINEPHrine, serotonin into nerve endings, increasing action of norepINEPHrine, serotonin in nerve cells; has anticholinergic effects

Therapeutic Outcome: Decreased symptoms of depression after 2-3 wk

Uses: Major depression

Investigational uses: Chronic pain management

Dosage and routes
Adult: PO 25 mg tid or qid; may increase to 150 mg/day; may give daily dose hs
Adolescents and elderly: PO 10-25 mg qhs, increase by 10-25 mg at weekly intervals to desired dose; usual maintenance 75 mg qd

Available forms: Caps 10, 25, 50, 75 mg; sol 10 mg/5 ml

Adverse effects
(*italic* = common; **bold** = life-threatening)
CNS: Dizziness, drowsiness, confusion, headache, anxiety, tremors, stimulation, weakness, insomnia, nightmares, EPS (elderly), increased psychiatric symptoms
CV: Orthostatic hypotension, ECG changes, tachycardia, **hypertension,** palpitations
EENT: Blurred vision, tinnitus, mydriasis
GI: Constipation, dry mouth, nausea, vomiting, **paralytic ileus,** increased appetite, cramps, epigastric distress, jaundice, **hepatitis,** stomatitis
GU: Retention, **acute renal failure**
HEMA: **Agranulocytosis, thrombocytopenia, eosinophilia, leukopenia**
INTEG: Rash, urticaria, sweating, pruritus, photosensitivity

Contraindications: Hypersensitivity to tricyclic antidepressants, recovery phase of MI, seizure disorders, prostatic hypertrophy

Precautions: Suicidal patients, severe depression, increased intraocular pressure, narrow-angle glaucoma, urinary retention, cardiac disease, hepatic disease, hyperthyroidism, electroshock therapy, elective surgery, pregnancy **C,** lactation, children

N Do Not Confuse:

nortriptyline/amitriptyline

Pharmacokinetics	
Absorption	Well absorbed
Distribution	Widely distributed; crosses placenta
Metabolism	Liver, extensively
Excretion	Kidneys, breast milk
Half-life	18-28 hr; steady state 4-19 days

Pharmacodynamics	
Unknown	

Interactions

Individual drugs

Alcohol: ↑ CNS depression
Clonidine: Severe hypotension; avoid use
Guanethidine: ↓ effects

Drug classifications

Barbiturates, benzodiazepines, CNS
depressants: ↑ effects
MAOIs: Hypertensive crisis, convulsions
Sympathomimetics (direct-acting): ↑ effects
Sympathomimetics, indirect-acting: ↓ effects

⊘ Herb/drug

Belladonna, corkwood, henbane, jimsonweed,
scopolia: ↑ antidepressant effect
Hops, lavender: ↑ CNS effect
SAM-e, St. John's wort: Serotonin syndrome

Lab test interferences

↑ Serum bilirubin, ↑ blood glucose, ↑ alka-
line phosphatase
↓ VMA, ↓ 5-HIAA
False: ↑ Urinary catecholamines

NURSING CONSIDERATIONS
Assessment

• Monitor B/P (with patient lying, standing),
pulse q4h; if systolic B/P drops 20 mm Hg,
hold drug, notify prescriber; take VS q4h of
patients with CV disease
• Monitor blood studies: CBC, leukocytes,
differential, cardiac enzymes if patient is
receiving long-term therapy
• Monitor hepatic studies: AST, ALT, bilirubin
• Check weight weekly; appetite may increase
with drug
• Assess ECG for flattening of ↑ wave, bundle
branch block, AV block, dysrhythmias in
cardiac patients
• Assess for extrapyramidal symptoms
G primarily in elderly: rigidity, dystonia, akathisia
• Assess mental status: mood, sensorium,
affect, suicidal tendencies; increase in psychiatric symptoms: depression, panic
• Monitor urinary retention, constipation;

P constipation is more likely to occur in children
G or elderly
◆ • Assess for withdrawal symptoms: headache,
nausea, vomiting, muscle pain, weakness; do
not usually occur unless drug was discontinued abruptly
• Identify alcohol consumption; if alcohol is
consumed, hold dose until AM

Nursing diagnoses

☑ Coping, ineffective (uses)
☑ Injury, risk for (adverse reactions)
☑ Knowledge, deficient (teaching)
☑ Noncompliance (teaching)

Implementation

• Give with food or milk to decrease GI
symptoms; mix conc with water, milk, fruit
juice to disguise taste
• Give dose hs if oversedation occurs during
G day; may take entire dose hs; elderly may not
tolerate once/day dosing
• Store at room temp; do not freeze

Patient/family education

• Teach patient that therapeutic effects may
take 2-3 wk
• Teach patient to use caution in driving and
other activities requiring alertness because of
drowsiness, dizziness, blurred vision; to avoid
rising quickly from sitting to standing, espe-
G cially elderly
• Teach patient to avoid alcohol ingestion,
other CNS depressants; teach patient not to
discontinue medication quickly after long-term
use; may cause nausea, headache, malaise
• Teach patient to wear sunscreen or large hat
to avoid burns, because photosensitivity occurs
• Teach patient to increase fluids, bulk in diet
if constipation, urinary retention occur, espe-
G cially elderly
• Teach patient to take gum, hard sugarless
candy, or frequent sips of water for dry mouth

Evaluation

Positive therapeutic outcome
• Decrease in depression
• Absence of suicidal thoughts

Treatment of overdose: ECG monitoring, induce emesis, lavage, activated charcoal,
administer anticonvulsant

⊘ Herb/drug   Ⓢ Do Not Crush   ◆ Alert   ◆ₜₜ Key Drug   **G** Geriatric   **P** Pediatric

nystatin (Rx, OTC)
(nis′ta-tin)

Mycostatin, Mycostatin Pastilles, Nadostine ♣, Nyaderm ♣, PMS-Nystatin ♣, nystatin, Nystex; topical: Mycostatin, Nilstat, Nodostine ♣, Nyoderm ♣, Nystatin, Nystex; vaginal: Mycostatin, Nilstat, Nadostine ♣, Nyoderm ♣, O-V Statin

Func. class.: Antiinfective
Chem. class.: Antifungal

Pregnancy category B; A (vaginal)

Action: Interferes with fungal DNA replication; binds sterols in fungal cell membrane, which increases permeability, resulting in leaking of cell nutrients

➔ **Therapeutic Outcome:** Fungistatic/fungicidal against *Candida* organisms

Uses: *Candida* species causing oral, vaginal, intestinal infections; vag: cutaneous vulvovaginal candidiasis; top: mucocutaneous fungal [P] infections, infant eczema, pruritus ani and vulvae

Dosage and routes
Oral infection
Adult: Susp 400,000-600,000 units qid, use ½ dose in each side of mouth, swish and swallow

[P] **Infants:** 200,000 units qid (100,000 units in each side of mouth)

[P] **Newborn and premature infants:** Susp 100,000 units qid

[P] **Adult and child:** Troches 200,000-400,000 units qid × up to 2 wk

GI infection
Adult: PO 500,000-1,000,000 units tid

Topical
[P] **Adult and child:** Apply to affected area bid-tid × 14 days, not to exceed 4 wk

Vaginal: 1-2 tabs (100,000 units each) inserted into vagina

Available forms: Tabs 500,000 units; powder 50, 150, 500 million, 1, 2, 5 billion units; troches 200,000 units; susp 100,000 units/ml; cream, oint, powder, spray, vag tab 100,000 units; vag cream, lotion 2%

Adverse effects
(*italic* = common; **bold** = life-threatening)
GI: Nausea, vomiting, anorexia, diarrhea, cramps
INTEG: Rash, urticaria (rare)

Contraindication: Hypersensitivity
Precautions: Pregnancy **B**

Pharmacokinetics
Absorption	Poorly absorbed
Distribution	Unknown
Metabolism	Not metabolized
Excretion	Feces, unchanged
Half-life	Unknown

Pharmacodynamics
Onset	Rapid
Peak	Unknown
Duration	6-12 hr

Interactions: None

NURSING CONSIDERATIONS
Assessment
• Assess for allergic reaction: rash, urticaria; drug may have to be discontinued
• Assess for predisposing factors for candidal infection: antibiotic therapy, pregnancy, diabetes mellitus, sexual partner infection (vag infections), AIDS

Nursing diagnoses
☑ Skin integrity, impaired (uses)
☑ Infection, risk for (uses)
☑ Knowledge, deficient (teaching)

Implementation
PO route
• Give oral susp dose by placing ½ in each cheek, swish for several min, then swallow; shake susp before use
• Store oral susp in refrigerator, tab in airtight, light-resistant containers at room temp
Topical route
• Administer by moistening lesions with a swab coated with cream or ointment; use enough medication to cover lesions completely; give after cleansing with soap, water before each application; dry well
Vaginal route
• Insert vag tab high into vagina with applicator provided; administer in gravid client 3-6 wk before term to decrease candidiasis in the [P] newborn
• Store at room temp in dry place; protect from light, air, heat

Patient/family education
• Instruct patient that long-term therapy may be needed to clear infection; to complete entire course of medication
• Teach patient proper hygiene: use no commercial mouthwashes for mouth infection

N

- Advise patient to avoid getting preparation on hands
- Instruct patient to wear light-day pad for vag preparations to avoid soiling clothing; to avoid sexual contact during treatment to minimize reinfection
- Instruct patient to notify prescriber if irritation occurs; drug may have to be discontinued
- Inform patient that relief from itching may occur after 24-72 hr

Topical
- Advise patient to discontinue use and notify prescriber if irritation occurs
- Teach patient to apply with glove to prevent further infection; drug may stain
- Caution patient not to use occlusive dressings; to avoid use of OTC creams, ointments, lotions unless directed by prescriber

Evaluation
Positive therapeutic outcome
- Culture negative for *Candida*
- Decrease in size, number of lesions
- Decreased itching, white patches on vulva (vag)

---

octreotide (Rx)
(ok-tree´-o-tide)
Sandostatin, Sandostatin LAR Depot
Func. class.: Hormone, antidiarrheal
Chem. class.: Octapeptide

Pregnancy category B

Action: Action similar to somatostatin

➡ Therapeutic Outcome: Decreased diarrhea; decreased symptoms of acromegaly, carcinoid tumors, vasoactive intestinal peptide tumors (VIPomas)

Uses: Sandostatin: acromegaly, carcinoid tumors, VIPomas; LAR Depot: long-term maintenance of acromegaly, carcinoid tumors, VIPomas

Investigational uses: GI fistula, variceal bleeding, diarrheal conditions, pancreatic fistula, irritable bowel syndrome, dumping syndrome, acromegaly

Dosage and routes
Acromegaly
Adult: SC 50 mcg tid, adjust q2 wk based on growth hormone levels (Sandostatin) or IM 20 mg q4 wk × 3 mo, adjust by growth hormone levels (Sandostatin LAR)

VIPomas
Adult: SC/**IV** 0.2-0.3 mg qd in 2-4 doses for 2 wk, not to exceed 0.45 mg qd (Sandostatin) or IM 20 mg q2 wk × 2 mo, adjust dose (Sandostatin LAR)

Carcinoid tumors
Adult: SC/**IV** 0.1-0.6 mg qd in 2-4 doses for 2 wk, titrated to patient response (Sandostatin) or IM 20 mg q4 wk × 2 mo, adjust dose (Sandostatin LAR)

GI fistula
Adult: SC 50-200 mcg q8h

Irritable bowel syndrome
Adult: SC 100 mcg single dose to 125 mcg bid

Antidiarrheal in AIDs patients
Adult: SC/**IV** 100-1800 mcg/day

Dumping syndrome
Adult: SC 50-150 mcg/day

Variceal bleeding
Adult: **IV** 25-50 mcg/hr cont **IV** inf for 18 hr-5 days

Available forms: Sandostatin: inj 0.05, 0.1, 0.2, 0.5, 1 mg/ml; LAR Depot: inj 10 mg, 20, 30 mg/5 ml

Adverse effects
(*italic* = common; **bold** = life-threatening)
CNS: Headache, dizziness, fatigue, weakness, depression, anxiety, tremors, **seizures,** paranoia
CV: Sinus bradycardia, conduction abnormalities, **dysrhythmias,** chest pain, shortness of breath, thrombophlebitis, ischemia, **CHF,** hypertension, palpitations
ENDO: Hyperglycemia, ketosis, hypothyroidism, hypoglycemia, galactorrhea, diabetes insipidus
GI: Diarrhea, nausea, abdominal pain, vomiting, flatulence, distension, constipation, **hepatitis,** elevated liver function tests, **GI bleeding, pancreatitis**
GU: UTI, pollakiuria
HEMA: Hematoma of inj site, bruise
INTEG: Rash, urticaria, pain, inflammation at inj site
MS: Joint and muscle pain

Contraindications: Hypersensitivity

Precautions: Diabetes mellitus, hypothyroidism, pregnancy **B**, elderly, lactation, children, renal disease

---

 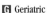

Pharmacokinetics

Absorption	Rapidly, completely
Distribution	Unknown
Metabolism	Little
Excretion	Urine, unchanged
Half-life	1.7 hr

Pharmacodynamics

Onset	Unknown
Peak	½ hr
Duration	12 hr

Interactions
Individual drugs
Cyclosporine: Possible ↑ rejection
Food/drug
↓ Absorption of dietary fat, ↓ vit B_{12} levels

NURSING CONSIDERATIONS
Assessment
• Identify growth hormone antibodies, IGF-1, 1-4 hr intervals for 8-12 hr after dose in acromegaly; 5-HIAA, plasma serotonin, plasma substance P in carcinoid; VIP in VIPomas
• Fecal fat, serum carotene
• Monitor thyroid function tests: T_3, T_4, T_7, TSH to identify hypothyroidism
• Assess for allergic reaction: rash, itching, fever, nausea, wheezing
• Assess for cardiac status: bradycardia, conduction abnormalities, dysrhythmias; monitor ECG for QT prolongation, low voltage, axis shifts, early repolarization, R/S transition, early wave progression

Nursing diagnoses
✓ Body image, disturbed (uses)
✓ Knowledge, deficient (teaching)

Implementation
• Store unopened amps, vials in refrigerator; or room temp for 2 wk, protect from light; do not use discolored or cloudy sol
SC route
• Rotate inj sites, use hip, thigh, abdomen
• Avoid using medication that is cold; allow to reach room temperature
IM route
• Reconstitute with diluent provided; give into gluteal muscle
IV route
• May use **IV** bolus if required; give over 3 min
• To use by intermittent infusion, dilute in 50-200 ml D_5W, 0.9% NaCl, give over 15-30 min

Patient/family education
• Explain reason for medication and expected results
• Advise patient that routine follow-up is needed
• Instruct parents on procedure for medication preparation and inj use; request demonstration, return demonstration; provide written instructions
• Advise patient to change position slowly to prevent orthostatic hypotension

Evaluation
Positive therapeutic outcome
• Decreased symptoms of acromegaly, carcinoid, VIPoma
• Decreased diarrhea in AIDS

ofloxacin (Rx)
(o-flox'a-sin)
Floxin, Ocuflox
Func. class.: Antiinfective
Chem. class.: Fluoroquinolone
Pregnancy category C

Action: Interferes with conversion of intermediate DNA fragments into high molecular weight DNA in bacteria

▶ **Therapeutic Outcome:** Bactericidal action against gram-positive pathogens *Staphylococcus epidermidis,* methicillin-resistant strains of *Staphylococcus aureus, Streptococcus pyogenes, Streptococcus pneumoniae;* gram-negative pathogens *Escherichia coli, Klebsiella* species, *Enterobacter, Salmonella, Shigella, Proteus vulgaris, Proteus rettgeri, Providencia stuartii, Morganella morganii, Pseudomonas aeruginosa, Serratia, Haemophilus* species, *Acinetobacter, Neisseria gonorrhoeae, Neisseria meningitidis, Yersinia, Vibrio, Brucella, Campylobacter,* and *Aeromonas* species; anaerobic pathogens *Bacteroides fragilis intermedius, Clostridium perfringens, Gardnerella vaginalis, Peptococcus niger, Peptostreptococcus* species; *Chlamydia pneumoniae, Chlamydia trachomatis, Legionella pneumoniae, Mycobacterium tuberculosis, Mycoplasma pneumoniae*

Uses: Treatment of lower respiratory tract infections (pneumonia, bronchitis), genitourinary infections (prostatitis, UTIs), skin and skin structure infections, conjunctivitis (ophth)

Dosage and routes
Lower respiratory tract infection/ skin and skin structure infections
Adult: PO/**IV** 400 mg q12h × 10 days

Cervicitis, urethritis
Adult: PO/**IV** 300 mg q12h × 7 days

Prostatitis
Adult: PO 300 mg q12h × 6 wk

Acute, uncomplicated gonorrhea
Adult: PO/**IV** 400 mg as a single dose

Urinary tract infection
Adult: PO/**IV** 200-400 mg q12h × 3-10 days

Conjunctivitis
P *Adult and child:* Ophth 1-2 gtt q2-4h × 2 days, then qid × 5 days

Renal dose
Adult: PO CCr 10-50 ml/min give q24h; CCr <10 ml/min give ½ of dose q24h

Available forms: Tabs 200, 300, 400 mg; inj 20, 40 mg/ml; ophth sol 0.3%

Adverse effects
(*italic* = common; **bold** = life-threatening)
CNS: Dizziness, headache, fatigue, somnolence, depression, insomnia, lethargy, malaise, **seizures**
EENT: Visual disturbances
GI: Diarrhea, nausea, vomiting, anorexia, flatulence, heartburn, dry mouth, increased AST, ALT, abdominal pain, constipation, **pseudomembranous colitis**
INTEG: Rash, pruritus
SYST: **Anaphylaxis, Stevens-Johnson syndrome**

Contraindication: Hypersensitivity to quinolones

Precautions: Pregnancy **C**, lactation,
P children, elderly, renal disease, seizure
G disorders, excessive sunlight

N Do Not Confuse:
Ocuflox/Ocufen

Pharmacokinetics	
Absorption	Well absorbed (PO)
Distribution	Widely distributed
Excretion	Kidneys, unchanged; breast milk
Half-life	5-9 hr; increased in renal disease

Pharmacodynamics			
	PO	IV	OPHTH
Onset	Rapid	Rapid	Unknown
Peak	1-2 hr	Inf end	Unknown

Interactions
Individual drugs
Calcium: ↓ ofloxacin effect
Cimetidine: ↑ ofloxacin effect
Nitrofurantoin: ↓ effectiveness
Probenecid: ↑ blood levels
Procainamide: ↑ procainamide level
Sucralfate, zinc sulfate: ↓ absorption of ofloxacin
Theophylline: ↑ toxicity
Drug classifications
Antacids with aluminum, iron salts: ↓ absorption of ofloxacin
Anticoagulants, oral: ↑ effect of anticoagulants
Antidiabetics: Altered blood glucose levels
NSAIDs: ↑ CNS stimulation, seizures
Food/drug
↓ absorption
☑ *Herb/drug*
Cola nut: ↑ effect

NURSING CONSIDERATIONS
Assessment
• Assess patient for previous sensitivity reaction
• Assess patient for signs and symptoms of infection including characteristics of wounds, sputum, urine, stool, WBC >10,000/mm^3, fever; obtain baselines and monitor during treatment
• Obtain C&S before beginning drug therapy to identify if correct treatment has been initiated
• Assess for allergic reactions: rash, urticaria, pruritus
• Monitor blood studies: AST, ALT, CBC, serum glucose monthly if patient is on long-term therapy
• Assess bowel pattern qd; if severe diarrhea occurs, drug should be discontinued
• Assess for overgrowth of infection: perineal itching, fever, malaise, redness, pain, swelling, drainage, rash, diarrhea, change in cough, sputum
• Assess for CNS symptoms: seizures, vertigo, drowsiness, agitation, confusion, tremors

Nursing diagnoses
✓ Infection, risk for (uses)
✓ Diarrhea (adverse reactions)
✓ Injury, risk for (adverse reactions)
✓ Knowledge, deficient (teaching)
✓ Noncompliance (teaching)

Implementation
PO route
• Give in equal intervals q12h around the clock to maintain proper blood levels; do not give within 2 hr of other agents, since drug

interactions are possible: give with 8 oz of water

• Do not give with iron, aluminum, zinc products or antacids, which decrease absorption and form insoluble chelate

IV IV route

• For intermittent inf, dilute to 4 mg/ml with D$_5$W, D$_5$/0.9% NaCl, 0.9% NaCl, D$_5$/LR, sodium bicarbonate, sodium lactate, D$_5$/Plasmalyte 56; give over 1 hr or more

Syringe compatibilities: Cefotaxime

Y-site compatibilities: Ampicillin, cisatracurium, docetaxel, etoposide, gemcitabine, granisetron, linezolid, propofol, remifentanil, thiotepa

Additive compatibilities: Amoxicillin, ceftazidime, clindamycin, gentamicin, piperacillin, tobramycin, vancomycin

Patient/family education

• Store for 2 wk refrigerated or 6 mo frozen, after reconstitution

• Instruct patient to take all medication prescribed for the length of time ordered; drug must be taken around the clock to maintain blood levels; do not give medication to others

• Teach patient to use sunscreen when outdoors to decrease phototoxicity

• Advise patient to increase fluids to 2 L/day to prevent crystalluria

• Caution patient to avoid driving and other hazardous activities until response is known; dizziness, confusion, drowsiness may occur

Evaluation

Positive therapeutic outcome

• Absence of signs/symptoms of infection

• Reported improvement in symptoms of infection

• Absence of red or itching eyes (ophth)

---

olanzapine (Rx)
(oh-lanz′a-peen)
Zyprexa, Zyprexa Zydis
Func. class.: Antipsychotic/neuroleptic
Chem. class.: Thienbenzodiazepine

Pregnancy category C

Action: Unknown; may mediate antipsychotic activity by both dopamine and serotonin type 2 (5-HT$_2$) antagonism; also, may antagonize muscarinic receptors, histaminic (H$_1$)- and α-adrenergic receptors

➡ **Therapeutic Outcome:** Decreased psychotic symptoms

Uses: Schizophrenia, acute manic episodes in bipolar disorder

Investigational uses: Dementia related to Alzheimer's disease

Dosage and routes

Schizophrenia

Adult: PO 5-10 mg initially qd, may increase dosage by 5 mg at 1 wk or more intervals; orally disintegrating tabs: open blister pack, place tab on tongue, let disintegrate, swallow

G *Elderly:* PO 5 mg, may increase cautiously at 1 wk intervals

Bipolar mania

Adult: PO 10-15 mg qd, may increase dose after 24 hr, by 5 mg

Available forms: Tabs 2.5, 5, 7.5, 10, 15 mg; orally disintegrating tabs 5, 10, 15, 20 mg

Adverse effects

(*italic* = common; **bold** = life-threatening)

CNS: Extrapyramidal symptoms (EPS) (pseudoparkinsonism, akathisia, dystonia, tardive dyskinesia), **seizures,** headache, **neuroleptic malignant syndrome (rare),** somnolence, agitation, nervousness, hostility, dizziness, hypertonia, tremor, euphoria

GI: Dry mouth, nausea, vomiting, anorexia, constipation, abdominal pain, weight gain

GU: Urinary retention, urinary frequency, enuresis, impotence, amenorrhea, gynecomastia, breast engorgement, premenstrual syndrome

INTEG: Rash

MS: Joint pain, twitching

Contraindications: Hypersensitivity

Precautions: Pregnancy **C,** lactation, hypertension, hepatic disease, cardiac **G** disease, elderly

O

Pharmacokinetics	
Absorption	Well
Distribution	93% plasma protein binding
Metabolism	Liver
Excretion	Kidneys
Half-life	Unknown

Pharmacodynamics	
Onset	Unknown
Peak	6 hr
Duration	Unknown

Interactions

Individual drugs

Alcohol: ↑ sedation

Bromocriptine, levodopa: ↓ antiparkinson activity

Carbamazepine, omeprazole, rifampin: ↓ levels of olanzapine

Diazepam: ↑ hypotension

Drug classifications

Anesthetics (barbiturates), antidepressants, antihistamines, CNS depressants: ↑ sedation

Anticholinergics: ↑ anticholinergic effects

Antihypertensives: ↑ hypotension

Herb/drug

Betel palm, kava: ↑ EPS

Cola tree, hops, nettle, nutmeg: ↑ action

Lab test interferences

↑ Liver function tests, ↑ prolactin, ↑ CPK

NURSING CONSIDERATIONS
Assessment
- Assess mental status, orientation, mood, behavior, presence of hallucinations and type before initial administration and monthly
- Monitor swallowing of PO medication: check for hoarding or giving of medication to other patients
- Monitor I&O ratio; palpate bladder if low urinary output occurs, especially in elderly
- Monitor bilirubin, CBC
- Monitor urinalysis; recommended before, during prolonged therapy
- Assess affect, orientation, LOC, reflexes, gait, coordination, sleep pattern disturbances
- Monitor B/P sitting, standing, lying; take pulse and respirations q4h during initial treatment; establish baseline before starting treatment; report drops of 30 mm Hg; obtain baseline ECG
- Assess dizziness, faintness, palpitations, tachycardia on rising
- Assess for neuroleptic malignant syndrome: hyperpyrexia, muscle rigidity, increased CPK, altered mental status, for acute dystonia (check chewing, swallowing, eyes, pin rolling)
- EPS including akathisia (inability to sit still, no pattern to movements), tardive dyskinesia (bizarre movements of the jaw, mouth, tongue, extremities), pseudoparkinsonism (rigidity, tremors, pill rolling, shuffling gait)
- Monitor skin turgor daily
- Monitor constipation, urinary retention daily; increase bulk, H_2O in diet

Nursing diagnoses
☑ Thought processes, disturbed (uses)
☑ Knowledge, deficient (teaching)
☑ Noncompliance (teaching)

Implementation
- Give antiparkinsonian agent for EPS
- **G** • Give decreased dose in elderly
- Give PO with full glass of water, milk; or with food to decrease GI upset
- Provide decreased stimuli by dimming light, avoiding loud noises
- Provide supervised ambulation until stabilized on medication; do not involve in strenuous exercise program because fainting is possible; patients should not stand still for long periods
- Give increased fluids to prevent constipation
- Give sips of water, candy, gum for dry mouth
- Store in airtight, light-resistant container
- Give orally disintegrating tabs: open blister pack, place tab on tongue until dissolved, swallow; no water needed

Patient/family education
- Teach patient to use good oral hygiene; frequent rinsing of mouth, candy, ice chips, sugarless gum for dry mouth
- Advise patient to avoid hazardous activities until drug response is determined
- Advise patient that orthostatic hypotension occurs often and to rise from sitting or lying position gradually
- Advise patient to avoid hot tubs, hot showers, tub baths, since hypotension may occur
- Advise patient to avoid abrupt withdrawal of this drug, or EPS may result; drug should be withdrawn slowly
- Advise patient to avoid OTC preparations (cough, hay fever, cold) unless approved by prescriber, since serious drug interactions may occur; avoid use with alcohol, CNS depressants, increased drowsiness may occur
- Advise patient that in hot weather, heat stroke may occur; take extra precautions to stay cool

Evaluation
Positive therapeutic outcome
- Decrease in emotional excitement, hallucinations, delusions, paranoia, reorganization of patterns of thought, speech

Treatment of overdose: Lavage if orally ingested; provide airway; do not induce vomiting or use epINEPHrine

---

olmesartan medoxomil (Rx)
(ol-meh-sar'tan)
Benicar
Func. class.: Antihypertensive

Pregnancy category D

Action: Blocks the vasoconstrictor and aldosterone-secreting effects of angiotensin II; selectively blocks the binding of angiotensin II to the AT₁ receptor found in tissues

→**Therapeutic Outcome:** Decreased B/P

Uses: Hypertension, alone or in combination with other antihypertensives

Dosage and routes
Adult: **PO** single agent 20 mg qd initially in patients who are not volume depleted, may be increased to 40 mg qd if needed after 2 wk

Available forms: Tabs 5, 20, 40 mg

Adverse effects
(*italic* = common; **bold** = life-threatening)
CNS: *Dizziness,* fatigue, headache, insomnia
GI: *Diarrhea,* abdominal pain
MS: Arthralgia, pain
RESP: *Upper respiratory infection,* bronchitis
SYST: **Angioedema**
CV: Chest pain, peripheral edema, tachycardia
EENT: Sinusitis, rhinitis, pharyngitis

Contraindications: Hypersensitivity, pregnancy **D** 2nd/3rd trimesters

Precautions: Hypersensitivity to ACE inhibitors; pregnancy **C** 1st trimester, lactation; children; elderly; hepatic disease

Pharmacokinetics
Absorption	Unknown
Distribution	Unknown
Metabolism	Unknown
Excretion	Urine, feces
Half-life	Unknown

Pharmacodynamics
Unknown

Interactions
☑*Herb/drug*
Aconite: ↑ toxicity, death
Astragalus, cola tree: ↑ or ↓ antihypertensive effect
Barberry, betony, black catechu, black cohosh, bloodroot, broom, burdock, cat's claw, dandelion, goldenseal, Irish moss, Jamaican dogwood, kelp, khella, mistletoe, parsley: ↑ antihypertensive effect

Coltsfoot, guarana, khat, licorice: ↓ antihypertensive effect

NURSING CONSIDERATIONS
Assessment
• Assess for pregnancy; this drug can cause fetal death when given in pregnancy
• Assess response and adverse reactions, especially in renal disease
• Monitor B/P, pulse q4h; note rate, rhythm, quality; electrolytes: K, Na, Cl; baselines in renal tests, liver function tests before therapy begins
• Assess skin turgor, dryness of mucous membranes for hydration status; for angioedema: facial swelling, dyspnea

Nursing diagnoses
☑ Tissue perfusion, ineffective (uses)
☑ Cardiac output, decreased (uses)
☑ Knowledge, deficient (teaching)
☑ Noncompliance (teaching)

Implementation
• Give without regard to meals

Patient/family education
• Advise to comply with dosage schedule, even if feeling better
• Advise patient to notify prescriber of mouth sores, fever, swelling of hands or feet, irregular heartbeat, chest pain
• Teach that excessive perspiration, dehydration, vomiting, diarrhea may lead to fall in B/P; to consult prescriber if these occur
• Teach that drug may cause dizziness, fainting; light-headedness may occur
• Advise to rise slowly to sitting or standing position to minimize orthostatic hypotension
• Teach to notify prescriber immediately if pregnant; not to use during lactation
• Advise to avoid all OTC medications, unless approved by prescriber
• Advise to inform all health care providers of medication use
• Advise to use proper technique for obtaining B/P and acceptable parameters

Evaluation
Positive therapeutic outcome
• Decreased B/P

omalizumab
Xolair
See Appendix A, Selected New Drugs

omeprazole (Rx)

(oh-mep'ra-zole)

Losec ✦, Prilosec

Func. class.: Antiulcer, proton pump inhibitor

Chem. class.: Benzimidazole

Pregnancy category C

Action: Suppresses gastric secretion by inhibiting hydrogen/potassium ATPase enzyme system in the gastric parietal cell; characterized as a gastric acid pump inhibitor, since it blocks the final step of acid production

➡ **Therapeutic Outcome:** Absence of duodenal ulcers; decreased gastroesophageal reflux

Uses: Gastroesophageal reflux disease (GERD), severe erosive esophagitis, poorly responsive systemic GERD, pathologic hypersecretory conditions (Zollinger-Ellison syndrome, systemic mastocytosis, multiple endocrine adenomas); possibly effective for treatment of duodenal ulcers with or without antiinfectives for *Helicobacter pylori*

Investigational uses: Posterior laryngitis, enhancing pancreatin

Dosage and routes
Active duodenal ulcers

Adult: PO 20 mg qd × 4-8 wk; associated with *H. pylori* 40 mg qAM and clarithromycin 500 mg tid on days 1-14, then 20 mg qd days 15-28

Severe erosive esophagitis/poorly responsive GERD

Adult: PO 20 mg qd × 4-8 wk

Pathologic hypersecretory conditions

Adult: PO 60 mg/day; may increase to 120 mg tid; daily doses >80 mg should be divided

Gastric ulcer

Adult: PO 40 mg qd × 4-8 wk

G *Elderly:* Max 20 mg/day

Laryngitis (unlabeled)

Adult: PO 20-40 mg qhs × 6-24 wk or 20 mg bid × 4-12 wk

Available forms: Sus rel caps 10, 20, 40 mg

Adverse effects

(*italic* = common; **bold** = life-threatening)

CNS: Headache, dizziness, asthenia

CV: Chest pain, angina, tachycardia, bradycardia, palpitations, peripheral edema

EENT: Tinnitus, taste perversion

GI: Diarrhea, abdominal pain, vomiting, nausea, constipation, flatulence, acid regurgitation, abdominal swelling, anorexia, irritable colon, esophageal candidiasis, dry mouth

GU: UTI, frequency, increased creatinine, **proteinuria, hematuria,** testicular pain, glycosuria

HEMA: **Pancytopenia, thrombocytopenia, neutropenia, leukocytosis,** anemia

INTEG: Rash, dry skin, urticaria, pruritus, alopecia

META: Hypoglycemia, increased hepatic enzymes, weight gain

MISC: Back pain, fever, fatigue, malaise

RESP: Upper respiratory tract infections, cough, epistaxis

Contraindications: Hypersensitivity

Precautions: Pregnancy **C**, lactation, **P** children

🔲 **Do Not Confuse:**

Prilosec/Prinivil, Prilosec/predniSONE, Prilosec/Prozac

Pharmacokinetics

Absorption	Rapidly absorbed
Distribution	Protein binding (95%); gastric parietal cells
Metabolism	Liver, extensively; by CYP450 enzyme system
Excretion	Kidneys, feces
Half-life **G**	½-1 hr; increased in the elderly, hepatic disease

Pharmacodynamics

Onset	1 hr
Peak	½-3½ hr
Duration	3-4 days

Interactions
Individual drugs

Ampicillin: ↓ ampicillin absorption

Cyanocobalamin: ↓ absorption of cyanocobalamin

CycloSPORINE: ↑ cycloSPORINE levels

Diazepam: ↑ serum levels of diazepam

Digoxin: ↓ absorption of digoxin

Disulfiram: ↑ disulfiram levels

Flurazepam: ↑ omeprazole level

Iron salts: ↓ absorption

Ketoconazole: ↓ absorption of ketoconazole

Phenytoin: ↑ serum levels of phenytoin

Triazolam: ↑ triazolam level

Warfarin: ↑ bleeding tendencies

Drug classifications

Iron products: ↓ absorption of iron

☑ Herb/drug   Ⓢ Do Not Crush   ◆ Alert   ☀ₙ Key Drug   **G** Geriatric   **P** Pediatric

NURSING CONSIDERATIONS
Assessment
- Assess GI system: bowel sounds q8h, abdomen for pain and swelling, anorexia
- Monitor hepatic enzymes: AST, ALT, increased alkaline phosphatase during treatment

Nursing diagnoses
✓ Pain, chronic (uses)
✓ Knowledge, deficient (teaching)

Implementation
- Give before patient eats; patient should swallow cap whole
🚫 • Do not open, chew, or crush; may give with antacids

Patient/family education
- Advise patient to report severe diarrhea; drug may have to be discontinued
- Caution patient to avoid driving and other hazardous activities until response to drug is known
- Caution patient to avoid alcohol, salicylates, ibuprofen; may cause GI irritation

Evaluation
Positive therapeutic outcome
- Absence of epigastric pain, swelling, fullness

---

ondansetron (Rx)
(on-dan′sa-tron)
Zofran
Func. class.: Antiemetic
Chem. class.: 5-HT receptor antagonist
Pregnancy category B

Action: Prevents nausea, vomiting by blocking serotonin (5-HT) peripherally, centrally, and in the small intestine

Therapeutic Outcome: Control of nausea, vomiting

Uses: Prevention of nausea, vomiting associated with cancer chemotherapy and prevention of postopertive nausea, vomiting

Investigational uses: Bulimia, pruritus, rectal use

Dosage and routes
Prevention of nausea/vomiting associated with cancer chemotherapy
P *Adult/child 4-18 yr:* **IV** 0.15 mg/kg infused over 15 min, 30 min before start of cancer chemotherapy; 0.15 mg/kg is given 4 and 8 hr after first dose or 32 mg as a single dose; dilute in 50 ml of D$_5$ or 0.9% NaCl

before giving; **rectal** (off-label) 16 mg qd 2 hr before chemotherapy
Adult: PO 8 mg ½ hr prior to chemotherapy repeat 8 hr later
P *Child 4-18 yr:* **IV** 0.15 mg/kg ½ hr prior to chemotherapy, repeat 4, 8 hr later

Prevention of nausea/vomiting of radiotherapy
Adult: PO 8 mg tid

Prevention of postoperative nausea/vomiting
Adult: **IV** 4 mg undiluted over >30 sec prior to induction of anesthesia
P *Child 2-12 yr:* **IV** 0.1 mg/kg (≤40 kg); 4 mg (≥40 kg) give ≥30 sec

Hepatic dose
Adult: PO/IM/**IV** max dose 8 mg qd

Bulimia (unlabeled)
Adult: PO 4 mg tid (base dose) prn during bingeing/purging

Pruritus (unlabeled)
Adult: PO 4 mg bid

Available forms: Inj 2 mg/ml, 32 mg/50 ml (premixed); tabs 4, 8 mg; oral sol 4 mg/5 ml; oral disintegrating tabs 4, 8 mg

Adverse effects
(*italic* = common; **bold** = life-threatening)
CNS: *Headache*, dizziness, drowsiness, fatigue, extrapyramidal symptoms (EPS)
GI: *Diarrhea, constipation, abdominal pain*
MISC: Rash, **bronchospasm** (rare), *musculoskeletal pain, wound problems, shivering, fever, hypoxia, urinary retention*

Contraindications: Hypersensitivity

P **Precautions:** Pregnancy B, lactation, children, elderly

Do Not Confuse:
Zofran/Zantac

Pharmacokinetics	
Absorption	Completely absorbed (**IV**)
Distribution	Unknown
Metabolism	Liver, extensively
Excretion	Kidneys
Half-life	3.5-4.7 hr

Pharmacodynamics
Unknown

Interactions: Unknown

NURSING CONSIDERATIONS
Assessment
- Assess for absence of nausea, vomiting during chemotherapy
- Assess for hypersensitivity reaction: rash, bronchospasm
- Assess for EPS shuffling gait, tremors, grimacing, rigidity

Nursing diagnoses
☑ Knowledge, deficient (teaching)
☑ Noncompliance (teaching)

Implementation
IV **IV route**
- Give **IV** after diluting a single dose in 50 ml of 0.9% NaCl or D$_5$W, 0.45% NaCl; give over 15 min
- Store at room temp for 48 hr after dilution

Y-site compatibilities: Aldesleukin, amifostine, amikacin, aztreonam, bleomycin, carboplatin, carmustine, cefazolin, ceforanide, cefotaxime, cefoxitin, ceftazidime, ceftizoxime, cefuroxime, chlorproMAZINE, cimetidine, cisatracurium, cisplatin, cladribine, clindamycin, cyclophosphamide, cytarabine, dacarbazine, dactinomycin, DAUNOrubicin, dexamethasone, diphenhydrAMINE, DOXOrubicin, DOXOrubicin liposome, doxycycline, droperidol, etoposide, famotidine, filgrastim, floxuridine, fluconazole, fludarabine, gentamicin, haloperidol, heparin, hydrocortisone, hydromorphone, hydrOXYzine, ifosfamide, imipenem/cilastatin, magnesium sulfate, mannitol, mechlorethamine, melphalan, meperidine, mesna, methotrexate, metoclopramide, miconazole, mitomycin, mitoxantrone, morphine, paclitaxel, pentostatin, potassium chloride, prochlorperazine, ranitidine, remifentanil, streptozocin, teniposide, thiotepa, ticarcillin, ticarcillin/clavulanate, vancomycin, vinBLAStine, vinCRIStine, vinorelbine, zidovudine

Y-site incompatibilities: Acyclovir, aminophylline, amphotericin B, ampicillin, ampicillin/sulbactam, cefoperazone, furosemide, ganciclovir, lorazepam, methylPREDNISolone, mezlocillin, piperacillin, sargramostim, sodium bicarbonate

Additive compatibilities: Cisplatin, cyclophosphamide, cytarabine, dacarbazine, dexamethasone, DOXOrubicin, etoposide, meperidine, methotrexate

Solution compatibilities: May also be diluted with D$_5$W, LR, D$_5$/0.9% NaCl, D$_5$/0.45% NaCl

Patient/family education
- Instruct patient to report diarrhea, constipation, rash, changes in respirations, or discomfort at insertion site
- Teach patient reason for medication and expected results

Evaluation
Positive therapeutic outcome
- Absence of nausea, vomiting during cancer chemotherapy

---

oral contraceptives (Rx)
Func. class.: Hormone
Chem. class.: Estrogen/progestin combinations

Pregnancy category X

Action: Prevents ovulation by suppressing FSH, LH; **monophasic:** estrogen/progestin (fixed dose) used during a 21-day cycle; ovulation is inhibited by suppression of FSH and LH; thickness of cervical mucus and endometrial lining prevents pregnancy; **biphasic:** ovulation is inhibited by suppression of FSH and LH; alteration of cervical mucus, endometrial lining prevents pregnancy; **triphasic:** ovulation is inhibited by suppression of FSH and LH; change of cervical mucus, endometrial lining prevents pregnancy; variable doses of estrogen/progestin combinations may be similar to natural hormonal fluctuations; **progestin-only pill and implant:** change of cervical mucus and endometrial lining prevents pregnancy; ovulation may be suppressed

⇒ Therapeutic Outcome: Prevention of pregnancy, decreased severity of endometriosis, hypermenorrhea

Uses: To prevent pregnancy, endometriosis, hypermenorrhea

Dosage and routes
Adult: PO 1 qd starting on day 5 of menstrual cycle; day 1 is 1st day of period

21-tablet packs
Adult: PO 1 qd starting on day 7 of menstrual cycle; day 1 is 1st day of period; then on 20 or 21 days, off 7 days

28-tablet packs
Adult: PO 1 qd continuously

Biphasic
Adult: 1 qd × 10 days, then next color 1 qd × 11 days

Triphasic
Adult: 1 qd; check package insert for each brand

Implant
Adult: Subdermal 6 cap implanted during the first wk of menses

Endometriosis
Adult: PO 1 qd × 20 days from day 5 to day 24 of cycle

Available forms: Check specific brand

Adverse effects
(*italic* = common; **bold** = life-threatening)

CNS: Depression, fatigue, dizziness, nervousness, anxiety, headache
CV: Increased B/P, **cerebral hemorrhage, thrombosis, pulmonary embolism,** fluid retention, edema
EENT: Optic neuritis, retinal thrombosis, cataracts
ENDO: Decreased glucose tolerance, increased TBG, PBI, T_4, T_3
GI: *Nausea,* vomiting, cramps, diarrhea, bloating, constipation, change in appetite, **cholestatic jaundice**
GU: Breakthrough bleeding, amenorrhea, spotting, dysmenorrhea, galactorrhea, endocervical hyperplasia, vaginitis, cystitis-like syndrome, breast change
HEMA: Increased fibrinogen, clotting factor
INTEG: *Chloasma, melasma,* acne, rash, urticaria, erythema, pruritus, hirsutism, alopecia, photosensitivity

Contraindications: Pregnancy **X**, lactation, reproductive cancer, thrombophlebitis, MI, hepatic tumors, hepatic disease, CAD, women 40 yr and over, CVA

Precautions: Depression, hypertension, renal disease, seizure disorders, lupus erythematosus, rheumatic disease, migraine headache, amenorrhea, irregular menses, breast cancer (fibrocystic), gallbladder disease, diabetes mellitus, heavy smoking, acute mononucleosis, sickle cell disease

Pharmacokinetics	
Absorption	Well absorbed
Distribution	Unknown
Metabolism	Liver, extensively
Excretion	Kidneys
Half-life	Unknown

Pharmacodynamics			
	PO	IM	IMPLANT
Onset	1 mo	1 mo	1 mo
Peak	1 mo	1 mo	1 mo
Duration	1 mo	3 mo	5 yr

Interactions
Individual drugs
Carbamazepine, griseofulvin, phenylbutazone, phenytoin, rifampin: ↓ effectiveness of oral contraceptive
Drug classifications
Analgesics, antibiotics, anticoagulants (oral), anticonvulsants, antihistamines, glucocorticoids: ↓ action of oral contraceptives
Food/drug
Grapefruit juice: ↑ peak level
Lab test interferences
↑ Pro-time; ↑ clotting factors VII, VIII, IX, X; ↑ TBG, ↑ PBI, ↑ T_4, ↑ platelet aggregation, ↑ BSP, ↑ triglycerides, ↑ bilirubin, ↑ AST, ↑ ALT
↓ T_3, ↓ antithrombin III, ↓ folate, ↓ metyrapone test, ↓ GTT, ↓ 17-OHCS
Herb/drug
Alfalfa, black cohosh, chaste tree: altered action
Saw palmetto, St. John's wort: ↓ oral contraceptive effect

NURSING CONSIDERATIONS
Assessment
• Assess for reproductive changes: change in breasts, tumors, positive Pap smear; drug should be discontinued if changes occur
• Monitor glucose, thyroid function, liver function tests, B/P

Nursing diagnoses
☑ Injury, risk for (adverse reactions)
☑ Body image, disturbed (adverse reactions)
☑ Knowledge, deficient (teaching)
☑ Noncompliance (teaching)

Implementation
PO route
• If GI symptoms occur, medication may be taken with food; take at same time each day
Implant route
• Inject 6 cap subdermally
• Implant is effective for 5 yr, should be removed after that
IM route
• Administer inj deep in large muscle mass after shaking susp well; ensure pregnancy has not occurred if inj are 2 wk or more apart

Patient/family education
• Teach patient about detection of clots using

Homans' sign; teach monitoring technique for heat, redness, pain, swelling
• Teach patient to use sunscreen or to avoid sunlight; photosensitivity can occur
• Teach patient to take at same time each day to ensure equal drug level; to take another tab as soon as possible if one is missed
• Teach patient that after drug is discontinued, pregnancy may not occur for several mo
• Instruct patient to report GI symptoms that occur after 4 mo
• Advise patient to use another birth control method during first 3 wk of oral contraceptive use
• Teach patient to report abdominal pain, change in vision, shortness of breath, change in menstrual flow, spotting, breakthrough bleeding, breast lumps, swelling, headache, severe leg pain, mental changes; that continuing medical care is needed: Pap smear and gynecologic exam q6 mo
• Teach patient to notify physicians and dentist of oral contraceptive use

Evaluation
Positive therapeutic outcome
• Absence of pregnancy
• Decreased severity of endometriosis
• Decreased severity of hypermenorrhea

---

orlistat (Rx)
(or-li'-stat)
Xenical
Chem. class.: Weight control agent, lipase inhibitor

Pregnancy category B

Action: Inhibits the absorption of dietary fat

Therapeutic Outcome: Decrease in weight

Uses: Obesity management

Dosage and routes
Adult: PO 120 mg tid with each main meal containing fat

Available forms: Caps 120 mg

Adverse effects
(*italic* = common; **bold** = life-threatening)
CNS: Insomnia, dizziness, headache, depression, anxiety, fatigue
GI: Oily spotting, flatus with discharge, fecal urgency, fatty/oily stool, oily evacuation, fecal incontinence, nausea, vomiting, abdominal pain, infectious diarrhea, rectal pain, tooth disorder
GU: UTI, vaginitis, menstrual irregularity

INTEG: Dry skin, rash
MS: Back pain, arthritis, myalgia, tendinitis
RESP: Influenza, upper, lower respiratory tract infection, EENT symptoms

Contraindications: Hypersensitivity, malabsorption syndrome, cholestasis, lactation

Precautions: Hypothyroidism, other organic causes of obesity, lactation, children, pregnancy **B**

Pharmacokinetics	
Absorption	Minimal
Distribution	99% protein binding
Metabolism	Unknown
Excretion	Feces
Half-life	1-2 hr

Pharmacodynamics	
Onset	Unknown
Peak	8 hr
Duration	Unknown

Interactions
Individual drugs
Cyclosporine: ↓ absorption
Pravastatin: ↑ lipid-lowering effect
Drug classifications
Fat-soluble vitamins: ↓ absorption

NURSING CONSIDERATIONS
Assessment
• Monitor weight weekly, diabetic patients may need reduction in oral hypoglycemics
• Assess for misuse in certain populations (anorexia nervosa, bulimia)

Nursing diagnoses
☑ Knowledge, deficient (teaching)
☑ Noncompliance (teaching)

Implementation
• Patient should be on a diet with 30% of calories from fat, omit dose of orlistat if a meal contains no fat

Patient/family education
• Warn patient that safety and effectiveness beyond 2 yr have not been determined
• Instruct patient to read patient's information sheet, discuss unpleasant GI side effects
• Advise patient to avoid hazardous activities until stabilized on medication
• Instruct patient to take a multivitamin containing fat-soluble vitamins, take 2 hr before or after orlistat; psyllium taken with each dose or at bedtime may decrease GI symptoms
• Instruct patient/family to notify prescriber if significant side effects occur

- Advise prescriber if pregnancy is planned or suspected

Evaluation
Positive therapeutic outcome
- Decreased weight

---

oseltamivir (Rx)
(oh-sell-tam'ih-ver)
Tamiflu
Func. class.: Antiviral
Chem. class.: Neuramidase inhibitor

Pregnancy category C

Action: Inhibits influenza virus neuraminidase with possible alteration of virus particle aggregation and release

⊃ **Therapeutic Outcome:** Decreased symptoms of influenza type A

Uses: Prevention/treatment of influenza type A

Dosage and routes
Treatment
🄿 *Adult/child >40 kg:* PO 75 bid mg × 5 days, begin treatment within 2 days of onset of symptoms

🄿 *Child 23-40 kg and ≥1 yr:* PO 60 mg bid

🄿 *Child 15-23 kg and ≥1 yr:* PO 45 mg bid

🄿 *Child ≤15 kg or ≥1 yr:* PO 30 mg bid

Renal dose
Adult: PO CCr <30 ml/min 75 mg qd × 5 days

Prevention
🄿 *Adult/child ≥13 yr:* PO 75 mg qd × ≥7 days

Renal dose
🄿 *Adult/child ≥13 yr:* PO CCr 10-30 ml/min 75 mg qod

Available forms: Caps 75 mg; powder for oral susp 12 mg/ml after reconstitution

Adverse effects
(*italic* = common; **bold** = life-threatening)
CNS: Headache, fatigue, insomnia, vertigo
GI: *Nausea, vomiting,* diarrhea, abdominal pain
RESP: Cough

Contraindications: Hypersensitivity

Precautions: Hepatic disease, renal disease, elderly, pregnancy **C**

Pharmacokinetics
Absorption	Rapidly absorbed
Distribution	Protein binding is low
Metabolism	Converted to oseltamivir carboxylate
Excretion	Eliminated by conversion
Half-life	1-3 hr

Pharmacodynamics
Unknown

NURSING CONSIDERATIONS
Assessment
- Assess for symptoms of influenza A: increased temperature, malaise, aches and pains

Nursing diagnoses
☑ Infection, risk for (uses)
☑ Knowledge, deficient (teaching)

Implementation
- Give within 2 days of symptoms of influenza; continue for 5 days
- Give at least 4 hr before hs to prevent insomnia
- Administer after meals for better absorption, to decrease GI symptoms: caps may be opened and mixed with food for easy swallowing
- Store in airtight, dry container

Patient/family education
- Teach patient about aspects of drug therapy: the need to report dyspnea, weight gain, dizziness, poor concentration, dysuria, behavioral changes
- Teach patient to avoid hazardous activities if dizziness occurs
- Advise patient to take missed dose as soon as remembered if within 2 hr of next dose

Evaluation
Positive therapeutic outcome
- Absence of fever, malaise, cough, dyspnea in influenza A

---

oxacillin (Rx)
(ox-a-sill'in)
Bactocill, oxacillin sodium
Func. class.: Broad-spectrum antiinfective
Chem. class.: Penicillinase-resistant penicillin

Pregnancy category B

Action: Interferes with cell wall replication of susceptible organisms; osmotically unstable cell wall swells, bursts from osmotic pressure

O

➥**Therapeutic Outcome:** Bactericidal effects for gram-positive cocci *Staphylococcus aureus, Streptococcus pneumoniae,* infections caused by penicillinase-producing staphylococci

Uses: Infections caused by penicillinase-producing staphylococci, streptococci; respiratory tract, skin, skin structure, urinary tract, bone, joint infections, sinusitis, endocarditis, septicemia, meningitis

Dosage and routes
Adult: PO 2-6 g/day in divided doses q4-6h; IM/**IV** 2-12 g/day in divided doses q4-6h

P *Child:* PO 50-100 mg/kg/day in divided doses q6h; IM/**IV** 50-100 mg/kg/day in divided doses q4-6h

Available forms: Caps 250, 500 mg; powder for oral susp 250 mg/5 ml; powder for inj 250, 500 mg, 1, 2, 4, 10 g

Adverse effects
(*italic* = common; **bold** = life-threatening)
CNS: Lethargy, hallucinations, anxiety, depression, twitching, **coma, seizures**
GI: Nausea, vomiting, diarrhea, increased AST, ALT, abdominal pain, glossitis, colitis, **pseudomembranous colitis**
GU: **Oliguria, proteinuria, hematuria,** vaginitis, moniliasis, **glomerulonephritis**
HEMA: Anemia, increased bleeding time, **bone marrow depression, granulocytopenia**
SYST: **Anaphylaxis, serum sickness**

Contraindications: Hypersensitivity to penicillins

Precautions: Pregnancy **B,** hypersensitivity
P to cephalosporins, neonates

⬖ **Do Not Confuse:**
Bactocill/Pathocil

Pharmacokinetics

Absorption	Rapid, incomplete (PO); well absorbed (IM); completely (**IV**)
Distribution	Widely distributed; crosses placenta
Metabolism	Liver
Excretion	Kidneys, unchanged (51%); breast milk
Half-life	20-50 min; increased in severe hepatic disease

Pharmacodynamics

	PO	IM	IV
Onset	Rapid	Rapid	Rapid
Peak	½-1 hr	½ hr	Inf end

Interactions
Individual drugs
Aspirin, probenecid: ↑ oxacillin levels, ↓ renal excretion
Chloramphenicol: ↑ half-life of chloramphenicol
Chloramphenicol, cholestyramine, colestipol: ↓ effectiveness of oxacillin
Disulfiram: ↑ oxacillin effect
Rifampin: ↓ oxacillin effect
Drug classifications
Contraceptives (oral): ↓ contraceptive effectiveness
Erythromycins, tetracyclines: ↓ antimicrobial effectiveness
⬛*Herb/drug*
Acidophilus: Do not use with antiinfectives
Khat: ↓ absorption
Lab test interferences
False positive: Urine glucose, urine protein

NURSING CONSIDERATIONS
Assessment
• Assess patient for previous sensitivity reaction to penicillins or other cephalosporins; cross-sensitivity between penicillins and cephalosporins is common
• Assess patient for signs and symptoms of infection including characteristics of wounds, sputum, urine, stool, WBC >10,000/mm³, fever; obtain baseline information and during treatment
• Obtain C&S before beginning drug therapy to identify if correct treatment has been initiated
• Assess for allergic reactions: rash, urticaria, pruritus, chills, fever, joint pain; angioedema may occur a few days after therapy begins; epINEPHrine, resuscitation equipment should be available for anaphylactic reaction
⬖• Assess urine output; if decreasing, notify prescriber (may indicate nephrotoxicity); also check for increased BUN, creatinine
• Monitor blood studies: AST, ALT, CBC, Hct, bilirubin, LDH, alkaline phosphatase, Coombs' test monthly if patient is on long-term therapy
• Monitor electrolytes: potassium, sodium, chloride monthly if patient is on long-term therapy
• Assess bowel pattern qd; if severe diarrhea occurs, drug should be discontinued; may indicate pseudomembranous colitis
• Monitor for bleeding: ecchymosis, bleeding gums, hematuria, stool guaiac daily if on long-term therapy
• Assess for overgrowth of infection: perineal itching, fever, malaise, redness, pain, swelling,

---

⬛ Herb/drug   ◻ Do Not Crush   ⬖ Alert   ⬤┬ Key Drug   G Geriatric   P Pediatric drainage, rash, diarrhea, change in cough, sputum

Nursing diagnoses
✓ Infection, risk for (uses)
✓ Diarrhea (adverse reactions)
✓ Injury, risk for (adverse reactions)
✓ Knowledge, deficient (teaching)
✓ Noncompliance (teaching)

Implementation
PO route
• Give in even doses around the clock; if GI upset occurs, give with food; drug must be given for 10-14 days to ensure organism death and prevent superinfection; store in airtight container
• Shake susp; store in refrigerator for 2 wk, 1 wk at room temp

IM route
• Reconstitute 250 mg/1.4 ml, 500 mg/2.7-2.8 ml, 1 g/5.7 ml, 2 g/11.4-11.5 ml, 4 g/21.8-23 ml of sterile water for a conc of 250 mg/1.5 ml; store unused portion in refrigerator for 1 wk or 3 days at room temp
• Inject deeply in large muscle mass

IV IV route
• Reconstitute 250 mg/1.4 ml, 500 mg/2.7-2.8 ml, 1 g/5.7 ml, 2 g/11.4-11.5 ml, 4 g/21.8-23 ml of sterile water for a conc of 250 mg/1.5 ml; store unused portion in refrigerator for 1 week or 3 days at room temp
• Give direct **IV** by diluting reconstituted sol with 250-500 mg/5 ml, 1 g/10 ml, 2 g/20 ml, 4 g/40 ml of sterile water or 0.9% NaCl, give over 10 min
• Give intermittent inf by diluting to a conc of 0.5-40 mg/ml with D_5W, 0.9% NaCl, D_5/0.9% NaCl, LR; give over 6 hr or less

Y-site compatibilities: Acyclovir, cyclophosphamide, diltiazem, famotidine, fluconazole, foscarnet, heparin, hydrocortisone, hydromorphone, labetalol, magnesium sulfate, meperidine, methotrexate, morphine, perphenazine, potassium chloride, tacrolimus, vit B with C, zidovudine

Y-site incompatibilities: Verapamil

Additive compatibilities: Cephapirin, chloramphenicol, DOPamine, potassium chloride, sodium bicarbonate

Additive incompatibilities: Cytarabine, tetracycline

Patient/family education
• Teach patient to report sore throat, bruising, bleeding, joint pain; may indicate blood dyscrasias (rare)

• Advise patient to contact prescriber if vaginal itching, loose foul-smelling stools, furry tongue occur; may indicate superinfection
• Instruct patient to take all medication prescribed for the length of time ordered
• Advise patient to notify prescriber of diarrhea with blood or pus, which may indicate pseudomembranous colitis

Evaluation
Positive therapeutic outcome
• Absence of signs/symptoms of infection (WBC <10,000/mm³, temp WNL, absence of red, draining wounds)
• Reported improvement in symptoms of infection

Treatment of anaphylaxis: Withdraw drug, maintain airway, administer epINEPHrine, aminophylline, O_2, **IV** corticosteroids

oxaliplatin (Rx)
(ox-al-i′plat-in)
Eloxatin
Func. class.: Antineoplastic

Pregnancy category D

Action: Forms cross links, inhibiting DNA replication and transcription, cell-cycle nonspecific

Therapeutic Outcome: Decreased size of tumor, spread of malignancy

Uses: Metastatic carcinoma of the colon or rectum in combination with 5-FU/leucovorin

Dosage and routes
Dosage protocols may vary

Adult: IV INF *Day 1:* oxaliplatin 85 mg/m² in 250-500 ml D_5W and leucovorin 200 mg/m² in D_5W, give both over 2 hr at the same time in separate bags using a Y-line, followed by 5-FU 400 mg/m² **IV BOL** over 2-4 min, then 5-FU 600 mg/m² **IV INF** in 500 ml D_5W as a 22-hr **CONT INF;** *Day 2:* leucovorin 200 mg/m² **IV INF** over 2 hr, then 5-FU 400 mg/m² **IV BOL** over 2-4 min, then 5-FU 600 mg/m² **IV INF** in 500 D_5W as a 22-hr **CONT INF;** repeat cycle q2wk

Available forms: Powder for inj 50, 100 mg single-use vials

Adverse effects
(*italic* = common; **bold** = life-threatening)
CNS: Peripheral neuropathy, fatigue, headache, dizziness, insomnia
CV: Cardiac abnormalities

EENT: *Decreased visual acuity, tinnitus, hearing loss*
GI: *Severe nausea, vomiting, diarrhea, weight loss,* stomatitis, anorexia, gastroesoph- ageal reflux, constipation, dyspepsia, mucosi- tis, flatulence
GU: Hematuria, dysuria, creatinine
HEMA: Thrombocytopenia, leukopenia, pancytopenia, neutropenia, anemia, hemolytic uremic syndrome
INTEG: *Alopecia,* rash, flushing, extravasation, redness, swelling, pain at inj site
META: Hypokalemia
RESP: Fibrosis, dyspnea, cough, rhinitis, URI, pharyngitis
SYST: Anaphylaxis, angioedema

Contraindications: Hypersensitivity to this drug or other platinum products, radiation therapy or chemotherapy within 1 mo, throm- bocytopenia, smallpox vaccination, preg- nancy **D**

P G Precautions: Pneumococcus vaccination, lactation, children, elderly

Pharmacokinetics	
Absorption	Unknown
Distribution	15% of platinum in systemic circulation; 85% is either in tissues or being eliminated in urine
Metabolism	Liver
Excretion	Urine
Half-life	40 days

Pharmacodynamics	
Unknown	

Interactions
Individual drugs
Alcohol: ↑ risk of bleeding
Radiation: ↑ myelosuppression
Drug classifications
Aminoglycosides, diuretics (loop): ↑ nephro- toxicity
Live virus vaccines: ↓ antibody response
Myelosuppressives: ↑ myelosuppression
NSAIDs: ↑ risk of bleeding

NURSING CONSIDERATIONS
Assessment
For bone marrow depression
• Monitor CBC, differential, platelet count weekly; withhold drug if WBC is <4000 or platelet count is <100,000; notify prescriber of results
• Monitor renal function studies: BUN, creati- nine, serum uric acid, urine CCr before, electrolytes during therapy; dose should not

be given if BUN <25 mg/dl; creatinine <1.5 mg/dl; I&O ratio; report fall in urine output of <30 ml/hr
◆● Assess for anaphylaxis: wheezing, tachycar- dia, facial swelling, fainting; discontinue drug and report to prescriber; resuscitation equip- ment should be nearby
• Monitor temp q4h (may indicate beginning infection)
• Monitor liver function tests before, during therapy (bilirubin, AST, ALT, LDH) as needed or monthly
• Assess for bleeding: hematuria, guaiac, bruising or petechiae, mucosa or orifices q8h; obtain prescription for viscous lidocaine (Xylocaine)
• Assess effects of alopecia on body image; discuss feelings about body changes
• Assess for jaundice of skin, sclera; dark urine; clay-colored stools; itchy skin; abdomi- nal pain; fever; diarrhea
• Assess for edema in feet, joint pain, stomach pain, shaking

Nursing diagnoses
☑ Risk for infection (adverse reactions)
☑ Nutrition: less than body requirements, imbal- anced (adverse reactions)
☑ Knowledge, deficient (teaching)

Implementation
• Provide comprehensive oral hygiene
• Provide all medications PO, if possible, avoid IM inj when platelets <100,000/mm³
• Increase fluid intake to 2-3 L/day to prevent urate deposits, calculi formation; elimination of drug
IV IV route
• Do not reconstitute or dilute with sodium chloride or any chloride-containing solutions
• Do not use aluminum equipment during any preparation or administration, will degrade platinum; do not refrigerate unopened powder or solution
• Prepare in biologic cabinet using gown, gloves, mask; do not allow drug to come in contact with skin, use soap and water if contact occurs
• Hydrate patient with 0.9% NaCl over 8-12 hr before treatment
• Have epinephrine, antihistamines, cortico- steroids for hypersensitivity reaction
• Give antiemetic 30-60 min before giving drug and prn
• Give allopurinol to maintain uric acid levels, alkalinization of urine
• Give diuretic (furosemide 40 mg **IV**) or mannitol after infusion

Patient/family education
- Advise to report signs of infection: increased temp, sore throat, flulike symptoms
- Advise to report signs of anemia: fatigue, headache, faintness, shortness of breath, irritability
- Advise to report bleeding; avoid use of razors, commercial mouthwash
- Advise to avoid aspirin, ibuprofen, NSAIDs, alcohol; may cause GI bleeding
- Advise to report any complaints or side effects to nurse or prescriber
- Advise to report any changes in breathing, coughing
- Advise that hair may be lost during treatment; a wig or hairpiece may make patient feel better; new hair may be different in color, texture
- Advise to report numbness, tingling in face or extremities, poor hearing or joint pain, swelling
- Advise not to receive vaccines during treatment
- Advise to use contraception during treatment and 4 mo after; this drug may cause infertility

Evaluation
Positive therapeutic outcome
- Decreased tumor size, spread of malignancy

---

oxaprozin (Rx)
(ox-a-proe′zin)
Daypro
Func. class.: Nonsteroidal antiinflammatory, antirheumatic
Chem. class.: Propionic acid derivative
Pregnancy category C

Action: Inhibits prostaglandin synthesis by decreasing an enzyme needed for biosynthesis; analgesic, antiinflammatory

➡ **Therapeutic Outcome:** Decreased pain, inflammation

Uses: Acute and long-term management of osteoarthritis, rheumatoid arthritis

Dosage and routes
Adult: PO 600-1200 mg qd; maximum dose 1800 mg/day or 26 mg/kg, whichever is lower in divided doses

Available forms: Tabs 600 mg

Adverse effects
(*italic* = common; **bold** = life-threatening)
CNS: Dizziness, headache, drowsiness, fatigue, tremors, confusion, insomnia, anxiety, malaise, depression
CV: Tachycardia, peripheral edema, palpitations, dysrhythmias
EENT: Tinnitus, hearing loss, blurred vision
GI: Nausea, *anorexia,* vomiting, *diarrhea,* jaundice, **cholestatic hepatitis,** constipation, flatulence, *cramps,* dry mouth, peptic ulcer, **GI bleeding**
GU: **Nephrotoxicity: dysuria, hematuria, oliguria, azotemia**
HEMA: Increased bleeding time
INTEG: Purpura, rash, pruritus, sweating
SYST: **Anaphylaxis, angioneurotic edema**

Contraindications: Hypersensitivity, asthma, patients in whom aspirin and iodides have induced symptoms of allergic reactions or asthma

Precautions: Pregnancy C, avoid in late pregnancy, lactation, children, bleeding disorders, GI disorders, cardiac disorders, CHF, hypersensitivity to other antiinflammatory agents, severe renal and hepatic disease, elderly

Ⓝ **Do Not Confuse:**
Daypro/Diupres

Pharmacokinetics	
Absorption	Well absorbed
Distribution	Unknown
Metabolism	Liver, extensively
Excretion	Breast milk
Half-life	40-50 hr

Pharmacodynamics	
Onset	Unknown
Peak	2 hr
Duration	Unknown

Interactions
Individual drugs
Alcohol: ↑ adverse reactions
Aspirin: ↓ effectiveness, ↑ adverse reactions
Cefamandole, cefotetan, cefoperazone, clopidine, clopidogrel, eptifibatide, plicamycin, tirofiban: ↑ bleeding risk
Cyclosporine, lithium, methotrexate: ↑ toxicity
Phenytoin: ↑ phenytoin level
Radiation: ↑ risk of hematologic toxicity
Drug classifications
Anticoagulants, thrombolytics: ↑ risk of bleeding
Antihypertensives: ↓ effect of antihypertensives
Antineoplastics: ↑ risk of hematologic toxicity
Diuretics: ↓ effectiveness of diuretics

NSAIDs: ↑ adverse reactions
Potassium supplements: ↑ adverse reactions
Herb/drug

Anise, arnica, bogbean, chamomile, chondroitin, clove, dong quai, fenugreek, feverfew, garlic, ginger, ginkgo, ginseng (Panax), licorice: ↑ bleeding risk
Arginine, gossypol: ↑ gastric irritation
Bearberry, bilberry: ↑ NSAIDs effect
Lab test interferences
↑ BUN, ↑ alkaline phosphatase
False positive: ↑ 5-HIAA, false ↑ 17KS

NURSING CONSIDERATIONS
Assessment

• Assess for pain and ROM: intensity, location, duration
• Monitor blood studies: alkaline phosphatase, LDH, AST, ALT, and bleeding time (may be increased)
• Assess for asthma, aspirin hypersensitivity, nasal polyps; increased hypersensitivity reactions

Nursing diagnoses
☑ Pain, chronic (uses)
☑ Mobility, impaired (uses)
☑ Injury, risk for (adverse reactions)
☑ Knowledge, deficient (teaching)

Implementation

• Give with food, antacids, milk to decrease gastric symptoms

Patient/family education

• Teach patient that drug must be continued for prescribed time to be effective; to avoid aspirin, alcoholic beverages
• Instruct patient to use caution when driving; drowsiness, dizziness may occur
• Teach patient to take with a full glass of water to enhance absorption; patient should sit upright for 30 min to prevent stomach irritation and ulceration
🚫 • Do not crush, break, or chew
• Instruct patient to use sunscreen and protective clothing to prevent burns
• Advise patient to report to prescriber severe abdominal pain, rash, itching, yellowing of skin or eyes, depression

Evaluation
Positive therapeutic outcome
• Decreased pain
• Decreased inflammation
• Increased mobility

---

oxazepam (Rx)
(ox-az′e-pam)
Apo-Oxazepam ✦, Novoxapam ✦, oxazepam, Serax
Func. class.: Sedative/hypnotic; antianxiety
Chem. class.: Benzodiazepine

Pregnancy category D
Controlled substance schedule IV

Action: Depresses subcortical levels of CNS, including limbic system, reticular formation; potentiates GABA

➡ **Therapeutic Outcome:** Decreased anxiety, successful alcohol withdrawal, relaxation

Uses: Anxiety, alcohol withdrawal

Dosage and routes
Anxiety
Adult: PO 10-30 mg tid-qid
Alcohol withdrawal
Adult: PO 15-30 mg tid-qid

Available forms: Caps 10, 15, 30 mg; tabs 10, 15, 30 mg

Adverse effects
(*italic* = common; **bold** = life-threatening)
CNS: Dizziness, drowsiness, confusion, headache, anxiety, tremors, fatigue, depression, insomnia, hallucinations, paradoxic excitement, transient amnesia
CV: Orthostatic hypotension, **ECG changes, tachycardia,** hypotension
EENT: Blurred vision, tinnitus, mydriasis
GI: Nausea, vomiting, anorexia
INTEG: Rash, dermatitis, itching
HEMA: Leukopenia

Contraindications: Hypersensitivity to benzodiazepines, narrow-angle glaucoma, psychosis, pregnancy **D**, child <12 yr, lactation
Precautions: Elderly, debilitated, hepatic disease, renal disease

Pharmacokinetics
Absorption	Well absorbed
Distribution	Widely distributed; crosses placenta, blood-brain barrier
Metabolism	Liver
Excretion	Kidneys, breast milk
Half-life	5-15 hr

Pharmacodynamics
Onset	½-1½ hr
Peak	Unknown
Duration	6-12 hr

 Herb/drug   Do Not Crush   Alert   Key Drug   Geriatric   **P** Pediatric

Interactions
Individual drugs
Alcohol: ↑ CNS depression
Disulfiram: ↑ oxazepam effects
Valproic acid: ↓ oxazepam effects
Drug classifications
Antidepressants, antihistamines, opiates: ↑
CNS depression
Oral contraceptives: ↑ effect
🖉 *Herb/drug*
Black cohosh: ↑ hypotension
Catnip, chamomile, clary, cowslip, hops, kava, lavender, mistletoe, nettle, pokeweed, poppy, Queen Anne's lace, senega, skullcap, valerian: ↑ CNS depression
Lab test interferences
↑ AST, ↑ ALT, ↑ serum bilirubin
False: ↑ 17-OHCS
↓ Radioactive iodine uptake

NURSING CONSIDERATIONS
Assessment
• Assess mental status: mood, sensorium, anxiety, affect, sleeping pattern, drowsiness, 🅖 dizziness, especially elderly; physical dependency, withdrawal symptoms: anxiety, panic attacks, agitation, convulsions, headache, nausea, vomiting, muscle pain, weakness; suicidal tendencies; indications of increasing tolerance and abuse
• Monitor B/P with patient lying, standing, pulse; if systolic B/P drops 20 mm Hg, hold drug, notify prescriber
• Monitor blood studies: CBC during long-term therapy; blood dyscrasias have occurred rarely; decreased hematocrit, neutropenia may occur
• Monitor hepatic studies: AST, ALT, bilirubin, creatinine LDH, alkaline phosphatase if taking long term
• Monitor I&O; indicate renal dysfunction

Nursing diagnoses
✓ Anxiety (uses)
✓ Depression (uses)
✓ Injury, risk for (adverse reactions)
✓ Knowledge, deficient (teaching)

Implementation
• Give with food or milk for GI symptoms; tab may be crushed if patient is unable to swallow medication whole; give sugarless gum, hard candy, frequent sips of water for dry mouth

Patient/family education
• Teach patient that drug may be taken with food or fluids; tab may be crushed or swallowed whole
• Caution patient not to use for everyday stress or longer than 3 mo unless directed by prescriber; not to take more than prescribed amount; not to double doses or skip doses
• Advise patient to avoid OTC preparations unless approved by prescriber; alcohol and CNS depressants will increase CNS depression
• Caution patient to avoid driving and activities that require alertness, since drowsiness may occur; to avoid alcohol and other psychotropic medications; to rise slowly or fainting may oc-🅖 cur, especially elderly; that drowsiness may worsen at beginning of treatment
• Caution patient not to discontinue medication abruptly after long-term use; withdrawal symptoms include vomiting, cramping, tremors, seizures

Evaluation
Positive therapeutic outcome
• Decreased anxiety, restlessness, sleeplessness (short-term treatment only)

Treatment of overdose: Lavage, VS, supportive care

---

oxcarbazepine (Rx)
ox'kar-baz'uh-peen)
Trileptal
Func. class.: Anticonvulsant
Pregnancy category C

Action: May inhibit nerve impulses by limiting influx of sodium ions across cell membrane in motor cortex

➡ **Therapeutic Outcome:** Absence of seizures

Uses: Partial seizures

Investigational uses: Trigeminal neuralgia, atypical panic disorder

Dosage and routes
Seizures adjunctive therapy
Adult: PO 300 mg bid, may be increased to 600 mg/day in divided doses bid; maintenance 1200 mg/day

🅟 *Child 4-16 yr:* PO 8-10 mg/kg/day divided bid, max 600 mg/day; dose is determined by weight

Conversion to monotherapy in partial seizures
Adult: PO 300 mg bid with reduction in other anticonvulsants, increase oxcarbazepine to max 600 mg/day q1wk over 2-4 wk; withdraw other anticonvulsants over 3-6 wk

Initiation of monotherapy in partial seizures
Adult: PO 300 mg bid, increase by 300 mg/day q3 days to 1200 mg divided bid

Renal dose
Adult: PO CCr <30 ml/min 150 mg bid and increase slowly

Available forms: Tabs, film-coated, 150, 300, 600 mg

Adverse effects
(*italic* = common; **bold** = life-threatening)
CNS: *Headache, dizziness, confusion, fatigue,* feeling abnormal, ataxia, abnormal gait, tremors, anxiety, agitation, **worsening of seizures**
CV: *Hypotension,* chest pain, edema
EENT: *Blurred vision, diplopia, nystagmus,* rhinitis, sinusitis
GI: *Nausea, constipation, diarrhea,* anorexia, vomiting, abdominal pain, gastritis, dry mouth, thirst, **rectal hemorrhage**
GU: *Frequency,* UTI, vaginitis
INTEG: Purpura, rash, acne

Contraindications: Hypersensitivity

Precautions: Hypersensitivity to carbamazepine, pregnancy **C**, lactation, child <4 yr, renal disease, fluid restriction

Pharmacokinetics	
Absorption	Unknown
Distribution	Unknown
Metabolism	Liver
Excretion	Unknown
Half-life	Unknown

Pharmacodynamics	
Onset	Unknown
Peak	Unknown
Duration	Unknown

Interactions
Individual drugs
Alcohol: ↑ CNS depression
Carbamazepine: ↓ carbamazepine level
Felodipine: ↓ effects of felodipine
Phenobarbital, valproic acid, verapamil: ↓ oxcarbazepine level
Phenobarbital: ↑ phenobarbital level
Phenytoin: ↓ oxcarbazepine level, ↑ phenytoin level
Drug classifications
Contraceptives (oral): ↓ oral contraceptive level
Herb/drug
Ginkgo: ↑ anticonvulsant effect
Ginseng, santonica: ↓ anticonvulsant effect

NURSING CONSIDERATIONS
Assessment
• Assess seizure activity including frequency, duration, and aura; provide seizure precautions
• Assess mental status including mood, sensorium, affect, behavioral changes; if mental status changes, notify prescriber
• Assess eye problems: ophthalmic examinations (slit lamp, funduscopy, tonometry) are needed before, during, after treatment

Nursing diagnoses
☑ Injury, risk for (side effects)
☑ Knowledge, deficient (teaching)

Implementation
• Store drug at room temp
• Provide assistance with ambulation during early part of treatment; dizziness may occur
PO route
• Give drug with food, milk to decrease GI symptoms

Patient/family education
• Caution patient to avoid driving, other activities that require alertness
• Advise patient not to discontinue medication quickly after long-term use
• Caution patient to inform prescriber if hypersensitive to carbamazepine
• Instruct patient to avoid use of alcohol while taking this medication
• Instruct patient to use alternate contraception if using hormonal method
• Advise patient to use hard candy or gum for dry mouth, rinse mouth frequently
• Advise patient to carry/wear emergency ID stating name, drugs taken, condition, prescriber's name and phone number

Evaluation
Positive therapeutic outcome
• Decreased seizure activity

---

oxtriphylline (Rx)
(ox-trye'fi-lin)
Choledyl SA
Func. class.: Bronchodilator, spasmolytic
Chem. class.: Choline salt of theophylline
Pregnancy category C

Action: Relaxes smooth muscle of respiratory system by blocking phosphodiesterase, which increases cAMP; 64% theophylline

⇒ **Therapeutic Outcome:** Bronchodilation with ease of breathing

Uses: Acute bronchial asthma, reversible

bronchospasm in chronic bronchitis and COPD

Dosage and routes

P *Adult and child >16 yr:* PO 4.7 mg/kg q8h or ext action q12h

P *Child 9-16 yr and smokers (adult):* 4.7 mg/kg q6h

P *Child 1-9 yr:* 6.2 mg/kg q6h

Available forms: Elixir 100 mg/5 ml ♣; syr 50 mg/5 ml; tabs 100, 200 mg; ext rel tabs 400, 600 mg

Adverse effects

(*italic* = common; **bold** = life-threatening)

CNS: Anxiety, restlessness, insomnia, dizziness, seizures, headache, lightheadedness

CV: Palpitations, sinus tachycardia, hypotension

GI: Nausea, vomiting, anorexia, diarrhea, bitter taste, dyspepsia

INTEG: Flushing, urticaria, alopecia

RESP: Increased rate, **respiratory arrest**

Contraindications: Hypersensitivity to xanthines, tachydysrhythmias, active peptic ulcer

G **Precautions:** Elderly, CHF, cor pulmonale, hepatic disease, diabetes mellitus, hyperthy-

P roidism, hypertension, children, pregnancy **C**

Pharmacokinetics	
Absorption	Well absorbed (PO); slow (PO-SUS REL)
Distribution	Widely distributed; crosses placenta
Metabolism	Liver to caffeine
Excretion	Kidneys, breast milk
Half-life	3-13 hr; increased in renal disease, CHF

Pharmacodynamics		
	PO	PO-SUS REL
Onset	15-60 min	Unknown
Peak	1-5 hr	4-8 hr
Duration	6-8 hr	8-12 hr

Interactions

Individual drugs

Allopurinol, cimetidine, disulfiram, mexiletine: ↓ metabolism

Cimetidine, disulfiram, fluvoxamine, mexiletine: ↑ toxicity

Ketoconazole, phenytoin, rifampin: ↑ metabolism, ↓ effect

Lithium: ↓ effect of lithium

Nicotine: ↓ oxtriphylline level

Drug classifications

Barbiturates: ↓ effect of oxtriphylline

β-Adrenergic blockers, fluoroquinolones, glucocorticoids: ↓ metabolism, ↑ toxicity

Calcium channel blockers: ↑ oxtriphylline level

Contraceptives (oral): ↑ toxicity

Food/drug

Caffeinated foods (cola, coffee, tea, chocolate): ↑ CNS, CV adverse reactions

Charbroiled foods: ↓ effect

Smoking

↑ metabolism, ↓ effect

Herb/drug

Cayenne: ↑ oxtriphylline toxicity

Cola tree: ↑ action of both

St. John's wort: ↓ oxtriphylline level

Lab test interferences

↑ Plasma free fatty acids

NURSING CONSIDERATIONS

Assessment

• Monitor blood levels (therapeutic level is 10-20 mcg/ml); toxicity may occur with small

G increase above 20 mcg/ml, especially elderly; check whether theophylline was given recently (24 hr); watch for toxicity: nausea, vomiting, diarrhea, restlessness, tachycardia

G • Monitor I&O; diuresis can occur; dehydra-

P tion may result in elderly or children

• Monitor respiratory rate, rhythm, depth; auscultate lung fields bilaterally; notify prescriber of abnormalities

• Monitor allergic reactions: rash, urticaria; if these occur, drug should be discontinued

• Monitor pulmonary function studies baseline and during treatment

O

Nursing diagnoses

☑ Airway clearance, ineffective (uses)

☑ Activity intolerance (uses)

☑ Injury, risk for (uses, adverse reactions)

☑ Knowledge, deficient (teaching)

Implementation

• Give PO pc to decrease GI symptoms; absorption may be affected with a full glass of water; do not crush or chew enteric coated or sus rel tab

Patient/family education

• Teach patient to take doses as prescribed, not to skip dose; to check OTC medications, current prescription medications for epHEDrine, which will increase CNS stimulation; not to drink alcohol or caffeine products (tea, coffee, chocolate, colas)

• Caution patient to avoid hazardous activities; dizziness may occur

• Instruct patient if GI upset occurs, to take drug with 8 oz of water or food

• Teach patient to notify prescriber of change

in smoking habit; a change in dosage may be required
• Teach patient to increase fluids to 2 L/day to decrease viscosity of secretions

Evaluation
Positive therapeutic outcome
• Decreased dyspnea
• Clear lung fields bilaterally

---

oxybutynin (Rx)
(ox-i-byoo'ti-nin)
Ditropan, Ditropan XL, oxybutynin
Func. class.: Anticholinergic
Chem. class.: Synthetic tertiary amine

Pregnancy category B

Action: Relaxes smooth muscles in urinary tract by inhibiting acetylcholine at postganglionic sites

➡ Therapeutic Outcome: Decreased symptoms of urgency, nocturia, incontinence

Uses: Antispasmodic for neurogenic bladder

Dosage and routes
Adult: PO 5 mg bid-tid, not to exceed 5 mg qid; ext rel tabs 5 mg qd, may increase by 5 mg, max 30 mg/day

G *Elderly:* PO 2.5-5 mg tid, increase by 2.5 mg q several days

P *Child >5 yr:* PO 5 mg bid, not to exceed 5 mg tid

P *Child 1-5 yrs:* PO 0.2 mg/kg/dose 2-4 ×/day

Available forms: Syr 5 mg/5 ml; tabs 5 mg; ext rel tabs 5, 10, 15 mg

Adverse effects
(*italic* = common; **bold** = life-threatening)
CNS: *Anxiety, restlessness, dizziness,* **seizures,** headache, drowsiness, confusion
CV: *Palpitations, sinus tachycardia,* hypotension
EENT: Blurred vision, increased intraocular tension, dry mouth, throat
GI: *Nausea, vomiting, anorexia,* abdominal pain, constipation
GU: Dysuria, retention, hesitancy

Contraindications: Hypersensitivity, GI obstruction, GI hemorrhage, GU obstruction, glaucoma, severe colitis, myasthenia gravis, unstable CV status in acute hemorrhage

P **Precautions:** Pregnancy **B**, lactation,
G suspected glaucoma, children <12 yr, elderly

◣ Do Not Confuse:
Ditropan/diazepam

Pharmacokinetics
Absorption	Rapidly absorbed
Distribution	Unknown
Metabolism	Liver
Excretion	Unknown
Half-life	Unknown

Pharmacodynamics
Onset	½-1 hr
Peak	3-4 hr
Duration	6-10 hr

Interactions
Individual drugs
Acetaminophen: ↓ levels of acetaminophen
Digoxin: ↑ levels of digoxin
Haloperidol: ↑ anticholinergic effects
Levodopa: ↓ levels of levodopa
Nitrofurantoin: ↑ levels of nitrofurantoin
Drug classifications
Phenothiazines: ↑ anticholinergic effects
▨ *Herb/drug*
Black catechu: ↑ constipation
Butterbur, jimsonweed, scopolia: ↑ anticholinergic action
Jamborandi tree, pill-bearing spurge: ↓ anticholinergic effect

NURSING CONSIDERATIONS
Assessment
• Assess for allergic reactions: rash, urticaria; if these occur, drug should be discontinued
• Assess urinary patterns: distention, nocturia, frequency, urgency, incontinence; catheterization may be required to remove residual urine

Nursing diagnoses
☑ Urinary elimination, impaired (uses)
☑ Pain, acute (uses)
☑ Knowledge, deficient (teaching)

Implementation
• May be given with meals or fluids or given on an empty stomach

Patient/family education
• Advise patient to avoid hazardous activities until response to drug is known; dizziness, blurred vision may occur
• Caution patient to avoid OTC medication with alcohol or other CNS depressants
• Advise patient to prevent photophobia by wearing sunglasses
• Caution patient to stay cool, since overheating may occur

- Teach patient to use frequent rinsing of mouth, sips of water for dry mouth
- Teach patient to avoid hot weather, strenuous activity; drug decreases perspiration
- Advise patient to report CNS effects: confusion, anxiety, anticholinergic effect in the
G elderly
⊘ • Do not crush, break, or chew ext rel product

Evaluation
Positive therapeutic outcome
- Absence of dysuria, frequency, nocturia, incontinence

⚠ HIGH ALERT

oxycodone (Rx)
(ox-i-koe'done)
Endocodone, M-oxy, Oxycontin, OxyFast, Oxyl R, Percolone, Roxicodone, Roxicodone Supeudol ✦

oxycodone/acetaminophen
Endocet ✦, Oxycocet ✦, Percocet, Roxicet, Roxilox, Tylox

oxycodone/aspirin
Endodan ✦, Oxycodan ✦, Percodan, Percodan-Demi, Roxiprin
Func. class.: Opiate analgesic
Chem. class.: Semisynthetic derivative

Pregnancy category B
Controlled substance schedule II

Action: Inhibits ascending pain pathways in CNS, increases pain threshold, alters pain perception

➡ Therapeutic Outcome: Decreased pain

Uses: Moderate to severe pain

Investigational uses: Postherpetic neuralgia (cont rel)

Dosage and routes
Adult: PO 10-30 mg q4h (5 mg q6h for Oxyl R, OxyFast) OxyFast conc sol is extremely concentrated, do not use interchangeably

P *Child:* PO 0.05-0.15 mg/kg/dose up to 5 mg/dose q4-6h; not recommended in children

Available forms: *Oxycodone:* Cont rel tabs 10, 20, 40, 80, 160 mg; immediate rel tabs 5, 15, 30 mg; tabs 5 mg; caps, oral sol 5 mg/5 ml, 20 mg/ml; *oxycodone with acetaminophen:* tabs 5 mg/325 mg; caps 5 mg/500 mg; oral sol 5 mg/325 mg/5 ml; *oxycodone with aspirin:* 2.44, 4.88 mg/325 mg

Adverse effects
(*italic* = common; **bold** = life-threatening)
CNS: *Drowsiness, dizziness, confusion, headache, sedation, euphoria*
CV: Palpitations, bradycardia, change in B/P
EENT: Tinnitus, blurred vision, miosis, diplopia
GI: *Nausea, vomiting, anorexia, constipation, cramps*
GU: Increased urinary output, dysuria, urinary retention
INTEG: *Rash,* urticaria, bruising, flushing, diaphoresis, pruritus
RESP: **Respiratory depression**

Contraindications: Hypersensitivity, addiction (opiate)

Precautions: Addictive personality, pregnancy **B**, lactation, increased ICP, MI (acute), severe heart disease, respiratory depression,
P hepatic disease, renal disease, child <18 yr

⚠ Do Not Confuse:
Percodan/Decadron, Roxicet/Roxanol, Tylox/Trimox, Tylox/Wymox, Tylox/Xanax

Pharmacokinetics	
Absorption	Well absorbed
Distribution	Widely distributed; crosses placenta
Metabolism	Liver, extensively
Excretion	Kidneys, breast milk
Half-life	2-3 hr

Pharmacodynamics		
	PO	REC
Onset	15-30 min	Unknown
Peak	½-1 hr	Unknown
Duration	4-6 hr	4-6 hr

Interactions
Individual drugs
Alcohol: ↑ respiratory depression, hypotension, sedation
Nalbuphine, pentazocine: ↓ analgesia
Drug classifications
Antihistamines, CNS depressants, phenothiazines, sedative/hypnotics: ↑ respiratory depression, hypotension
MAOIs: Do not use 2 wk before oxycodone
⊘ *Herb/drug*
Corkwood: ↑ anticholinergic effect
Jamaican dogwood, lavender, mistletoe, nettle, pokeweed, poppy, senega, valerian: ↑ sedative effect
Lab test interferences
↑ Amylase

NURSING CONSIDERATIONS
Assessment
• Monitor VS after parenteral route; note muscle rigidity, drug history, liver, kidney function tests, respiratory dysfunction: respiratory depression, character, rate, rhythm; notify prescriber if respirations are <10/min
• Monitor CNS changes: dizziness, drowsiness, hallucinations, euphoria, LOC, pupil reaction
• Monitor allergic reactions: rash, urticaria

Nursing diagnoses
☑ Pain, acute (uses)
☑ Pain, chronic
☑ Sensory perception, disturbed: visual, auditory (adverse reactions)
☑ Breathing pattern, ineffective (adverse reactions)
☑ Injury, risk for (adverse reactions)
☑ Knowledge, deficient (teaching)

Implementation
• Give with antiemetic if nausea, vomiting occur
• Give when pain is beginning to return; determine dosage interval by patient response; continuous dosing of medication is more effective than when given prn
• Medication should be slowly withdrawn after long-term use to prevent withdrawal symptoms
• Store in light-resistant container at room temp
PO route
• May be given with food or milk to lessen GI upset
• Use 80, 160 mg cont rel tabs only in opioid-tolerant patients
🚫 • Do not break, crush, or chew cont rel tabs
Rectal route
• Store supp in the refrigerator; run under warm water before insertion

Patient/family education
• Advise patients to avoid CNS depressants: alcohol, sedative/hypnotics
• Discuss with patient that dizziness, drowsiness, and confusion are common; to avoid getting up without assistance
• Discuss in detail all aspects of the drug, including purpose and what to expect
• Advise patient to make position changes slowly to lessen orthostatic hypotension

Evaluation
Positive therapeutic outcome
• Decreased pain

Treatment of overdose: Naloxone 0.2-0.8 **IV**, O_2, **IV** fluids, vasopressors

---

❗ HIGH ALERT

oxymorphone (Rx)
(ox-i-mor′fone)
Num orphan
Func. class.: Opiate analgesic
Chem. class.: Semisynthetic phenanthrene derivative

Pregnancy category B
Controlled substance schedule II

Action: Depresses pain impulse transmission at the spinal cord level by interacting with opioid receptors

➡ **Therapeutic Outcome:** Decreased pain

Uses: Moderate to severe pain

Dosage and routes
Adult: IM/SC 1-1.5 mg q4-6h prn; **IV** 0.5 mg q4-6h prn; rec 5 mg q4-6h prn

Labor analgesia
Adult: IM 0.5-1 mg

Available forms: Inj 1, 1.5 mg/ml; supp 5 mg

Adverse effects
(*italic* = common; **bold** = life-threatening)
CNS: *Drowsiness, dizziness, confusion, headache, sedation, euphoria,* **seizures**
CV: Palpitations, **bradycardia,** change in B/P
EENT: Tinnitus, blurred vision, miosis, diplopia
GI: *Nausea, vomiting, anorexia, constipation, cramps*
GU: Increased urinary output, dysuria, urinary retention
INTEG: *Rash,* urticaria, bruising, flushing, diaphoresis, pruritus
RESP: **Respiratory depression**

Contraindications: Hypersensitivity, addiction (opioid)

Precautions: Addictive personality, pregnancy **B** (short- term), lactation, increased ICP, MI (acute), severe heart disease, respiratory depression, hepatic disease, renal
🅿 disease, child <18 yr

Pharmacokinetics

Absorption	Well absorbed (rec, IM, SC); completely absorbed (**IV**)
Distribution	Widely distributed; crosses placenta
Metabolism	Liver, extensively
Excretion	Kidneys
Half-life	2½-4 hr

🖉 Herb/drug   🚫 Do Not Crush   ◆ Alert   ◆═ Key Drug   🅖 Geriatric   🅟 Pediatric

Pharmacodynamics			
	IM/SC	IV	REC
Onset	15 min	10 min	30 min
Peak	1-1½ hr	15-30 min	Unknown
Duration	3-6 hr	3-4 hr	3-6 hr

Interactions
Individual drugs
Alcohol: ↑ respiratory depression, hypotension, sedation
Nalbuphine, pentazocine: ↓ analgesia
Drug classifications
Antihistamines, CNS depressants, sedative/hypnotics: ↑ respiratory depression, hypotension
MAOIs: Do not use 2 wk before oxymorphone
✒ Herb/drug
Corkwood: ↑ anticholinergic effect
Jamaican dogwood, lavender, mistletoe, nettle, pokeweed, poppy, senega, valerian: ↑ sedative effect
Lab test interferences
↑ Amylase, ↑ lipase

NURSING CONSIDERATIONS
Assessment
• Monitor VS after parenteral route; note muscle rigidity, drug history, liver, kidney function tests, respiratory dysfunction: respiratory depression, character, rate, rhythm; notify prescriber if respirations are <10/min
• Monitor CNS changes: dizziness, drowsiness, hallucinations, euphoria, LOC, pupil reaction
• Monitor allergic reactions: rash, urticaria

Nursing diagnoses
✓ Pain, acute (uses)
✓ Sensory perception, disturbed: visual, auditory (adverse reactions)
✓ Breathing pattern, ineffective (adverse reactions)
✓ Injury, risk for (adverse reactions)
✓ Knowledge, deficient (teaching)

Implementation
• Give with antiemetic if nausea, vomiting occur
• Give when pain is beginning to return; determine dosage interval by patient response; continuous dosing of medication is more effective than when given prn
• Medication should be slowly withdrawn after long-term use to prevent withdrawal symptoms
• Store in light-resistant container at room temp
Rectal route
• Store in refrigerator

IV route
• Give by direct **IV** undiluted over 2-3 min

Y-site compatibilities: Glycopyrrolate, hydrOXYzine, ranitidine

Patient/family education
• Advise patients to avoid CNS depressants: alcohol, sedative/hypnotics
• Discuss with patient that dizziness, drowsiness, and confusion are common; to avoid getting up without assistance
• Discuss in detail all aspects of the drug, including purpose and what to expect
• Advise patient to make position changes slowly to lessen orthostatic hypotension

Evaluation
Positive therapeutic outcome
• Decreased pain

Treatment of overdose: Naloxone (Narcan) 0.2-0.8 mg **IV**, O₂, **IV** fluids, vasopressors

⚠ HIGH ALERT

oxytocin ⚗ (Rx)
(ox-i-toe'sin)
Pitocin, Syntocinon
Func. class.: Oxytocic hormone
Pregnancy category N/A

Action: Acts directly on myofibrils, producing uterine contraction; stimulates breast milk letdown

➜ **Therapeutic Outcome:** Stimulation of labor, control of bleeding; stimulation of milk letdown

Uses: Stimulation, induction of labor; missed or incomplete abortion, postpartum bleeding, postpartum breast engorgement

Dosage and routes
Labor induction
Adult: IV 1-2 mU/min, increase by 1-2 mU q15-60 min until regular contractions occur, then decrease dosage

Postpartum hemorrhage
Adult: IV 10 units infused at 20-40 mU/min
Adult: IM 10 units after placenta delivery

Incomplete abortion
Adult: IV inf 10 units/500 ml D₅W or 0.9% NaCl run at 20-40 mU/min

Fetal stress test
Adult: IV 0.5 mU/min; increase q20 min until 3 contractions occur at 10 min

Available forms: Inj 10 units/ml

Adverse effects
(*italic* = common; **bold** = life-threatening)

CNS: **Seizures, tetanic contractions**

CV: Hypotension, hypertension, dysrhythmias, increased pulse, bradycardia, tachycardia, premature ventricular contractions

FETUS: Dysrhythmias, jaundice, hypoxia, **intracranial hemorrhage**

GI: Anorexia, nausea, vomiting, constipation

GU: **Abruptio placentae, decreased uterine blood flow**

HEMA: Increased hyperbilirubinemia

INTEG: Rash

RESP: **Asphyxia**

Contraindications: Hypersensitivity, pregnancy-induced hypertension, cephalopelvic disproportion, fetal distress, hypertonic uterus

Precautions: Cervical/uterine surgery, uterine sepsis, primipara >35 yr, 1st, 2nd stage of labor

Pharmacokinetics

Absorption	Well absorbed (nasal); completely absorbed (**IV**)
Distribution	Widely distributed (extracellular fluid)
Metabolism	Liver, rapidly
Excretion	Kidneys
Half-life	3-12 min

Pharmacodynamics

	NASAL	IV	IM
Onset	5 min	Rapid	3-7 min
Peak	Unknown	Unknown	Unknown
Duration	20 min	1 hr	1 hr

Interactions
Drug classifications
Vasopressors: ↑ hypertension

NURSING CONSIDERATIONS
Assessment
• Assess labor contractions: fetal heart tones, frequency, duration, intensity of contractions; if fetal heart tones increase or decrease significantly or if contractions are longer than 1 min, notify prescriber; turn patient on left side to increase oxygen to fetus

◆• Assess for water intoxication: confusion, anuria, drowsiness, headache; notify prescriber

• Watch for fetal distress, acceleration, deceleration, fetal presentation, pelvic dimensions

• Monitor B/P, pulse, respiratory rate, rhythm, depth

• Monitor I&O ratio

• Provide an environment conducive to letdown reflex

Nursing diagnoses
☑ Breastfeeding (uses)
☑ Injury, risk for (uses)
☑ Knowledge, deficient (teaching)

Implementation
IV **IV route**
• Use an infusion pump; rotate sol for mixing; have magnesium sulfate available

• For labor induction administer after diluting 10 units/L of D_5W, 0.9% NaCl, 0.45% NaCl, LR, Ringer's for a conc of 10 units/ml; start at 1-2 units/min (0.1-0.2 ml); may increase by 1-2 units/min q15-30 min until labor begins

• For threatened abortion administer after diluting 10 units/500 ml of D_5W, $D_{10}W$, 0.9% NaCl, 0.45% NaCl, LR, Ringer's for a conc of 20 units/ml; give at 10-40 units/min

• For postpartum bleeding administer after diluting 10-40 units/L of D_5W, $D_{10}W$, 0.9% NaCl, 0.45% NaCl, LR, Ringer's for a conc of 10-40 units/ml; may titrate to response

Y-site compatibilities: Heparin, regular insulin, hydrocortisone, meperidine, morphine, potassium chloride, vit B/C, warfarin

Additive compatibilities: Chloramphenicol, metaraminol, netilmicin, sodium bicarbonate, thiopental, verapamil

Additive incompatibilities: Fibrinolysin, warfarin

Patient/family education
• Teach patient to report increased blood loss, abdominal cramps, increased temp or foul-smelling lochia

• Advise patient that contractions will be similar to menstrual cramps, gradually increasing in intensity

Evaluation
Positive therapeutic outcome
• Stimulation of milk letdown (nasal)
• Induction of labor
• Decreased postpartum bleeding

paclitaxel (Rx)
(pa-kli-tax'el)
Onxol, Taxol
Func. class.: Antineoplastic—misc.
Chem. class.: Natural diterpene, antimicrotubule

Pregnancy category D

Action: Inhibits the reorganization of the microtubule network needed for interphase and mitotic cellular functions; also causes abnormal bundles of microtubules during cell cycle and multiple esters of microtubules during mitosis

➔ **Therapeutic Outcome:** Prevention of rapidly growing malignant cells

Uses: Taxol: metastatic carcinoma of the ovary unresponsive to other treatment, breast carcinoma; AIDS-related Kaposi's sarcoma (2nd-line), non–small-cell lung cancer, adjuvant treatment for node-positive breast cancer; Onxol: failure of other treatment in breast cancer, advanced ovarian cancer

Investigational uses: Advanced head, neck, small-cell lung cancer; non-Hodgkin's lymphoma, adenocarcinoma of the upper GI tract, hormone-refractory prostate cancer

Dosage and routes
Ovarian carcinoma
Adults: IV inf 135 mg/m^2 given over 24 hr q3 wk, then cisplatin 75 mg/m^2 or 175 mg/m^2 over 3 hr q3 wk or 175 mg/m^2 over 3 hr

Advanced ovarian carcinoma
Adult: IV inf 175 mg/m^2 with cisplatin 75 mg/m^2 over 3 hr q3 wk

Breast carcinoma
Adult: IV inf 175 mg/m^2 over 3 hr q3 wk × 4 courses

AIDS-related Kaposi's sarcoma
Adult: IV inf 135 mg/m^2 over 3 hr q3 wk or 100 mg/m^2 over 3 hr q2 wk

1st line non–small-cell lung cancer
Adult: Inf 135 mg/m^2/24 hr with cisplatin 75 mg/m^2 × 3 wk

Available forms: Inj 30 mg/5 ml vial (6 mg/ml)

Adverse effects
(*italic* = common; **bold** = life-threatening)
CV: Bradycardia, hypotension, abnormal ECG
GI: Nausea, vomiting, diarrhea, mucositis; increased bilirubin, alkaline phosphatase, AST

HEMA: **Neutropenia, leukopenia, thrombocytopenia, anemia,** bleeding, infections
INTEG: Alopecia
MS: Arthralgia, myalgia
NEURO: Peripheral neuropathy
SYST: Hypersensitivity reactions, **anaphylaxis**

Contraindications: Hypersensitivity to paclitaxel or other drugs with polyoxyethylated castor oil, neutropenia (neutrophils <1500/mm^3), pregnancy **D**

P Precautions: Children, lactation, hepatic disease, CV disease, CNS disorder

Do Not Confuse:
paclitaxel/paroxetine, paclitaxel/Paxil, Taxol/Paxil, Taxol/Taxotera

Pharmacokinetics
Absorption	Completely absorbed
Distribution	89%-98% protein binding
Metabolism	Liver, extensively
Excretion	Unknown
Half-life	5-17 hr

Pharmacodynamics
Onset	Unknown
Peak	1-2 wk
Duration	3 wk

Interactions
Individual drugs
Cyclosporine, dexamethasone, diazepam, etoposide, ketoconazole, quinidine, teniposide, testosterone, verapamil, vinCRIStine: ↓ metabolism of paclitaxel
DOXOrubicin: ↑ levels of DOXOrubicin
Radiation: ↑ myelosuppression
Drug classifications
Antineoplastics: ↑ myelosuppression
Live virus vaccines: ↓ immune response

NURSING CONSIDERATIONS
Assessment
• Assess CNS changes: confusion, paresthesias, psychosis, tremors, seizures, neuropathies; drug should be discontinued
• Check buccal cavity q8h for dryness, sores or ulceration, white patches, oral pain, bleeding, dysphagia; obtain prescription for viscous lidocaine (Xylocaine) to use in mouth
• Assess symptoms indicating severe allergic reaction, anaphylaxis: rash, pruritus, urticaria, purpuric skin lesions, itching, flushing
• Monitor CBC, differential, platelet count weekly; withhold drug if WBC is <1500/mm^3 or platelet count is <100,000/mm^3, notify prescriber of results

P

- Monitor renal function studies: BUN, creatinine, serum uric acid, urine CCr before and during therapy; check I&O ratio; report fall in urine output to <30 ml/hr
- Monitor temp q4h (may indicate beginning of infection)
- Monitor liver function tests before and during therapy (bilirubin, AST, ALT, LDH) as needed or monthly; check for jaundice of skin and sclera, dark urine, clay-colored stools, itchy skin, abdominal pain, fever, diarrhea
- Assess for bleeding: hematuria, stool guaiac, bruising or petechiae, mucosa or orifices q8h; check for inflammation of mucosa, breaks in skin
- Assess effects of alopecia on body image; discuss feelings about body changes

Nursing diagnoses
☑ Injury, risk for (adverse reactions)
☑ Body image, disturbed (adverse reactions)
☑ Infection, risk for (adverse reactions)
☑ Knowledge, deficient (teaching)

Implementation
IV IV route

- Give after diluting in 0.9% NaCl, D_5, D_5 and 0.9% NaCl, D_5LR to a concentration of 0.3-1.2 mg/ml
- Use an in-line filter ≤0.22 μm
- Give after premedicating with dexamethasone 20 mg PO 12 and 6 hr before paclitaxel, diphenhydrAMINE 50 mg **IV** ½-1 hr before paclitaxel and cimetidine 300 mg or ranitidine 50 mg **IV** ½-1 hr before paclitaxel
- Use only glass bottles, polypropylene, polyolefin bags and administration sets; do not use PVC infusion bags or sets
- Use gloves and cytotoxic handling precautions
- Give fluids PO before chemotherapy to hydrate patient
- Give antacid before oral agent; give drug after evening meal, before hs; provide antiemetic 30-60 min before giving drug and prn to prevent vomiting; administer antibiotics for prophylaxis of infection
- Give top or systemic analgesics for pain to lessen effects of stomatitis
- Give liq diet: carbonated beverages; gelatin may be added if patient is not nauseated or vomiting
- Encourage patient to rinse mouth tid-qid with water, club soda; brush teeth bid-qid with soft brush or cotton-tipped applicators for stomatitis; use unwaxed dental floss

Y-site compatiblilities: Acyclovir, amikacin, aminophylline, bleomycin, butorphanol, calcium chloride, carboplatin, cefepime, cefotetan, ceftazidime, ceftriaxone, cimetidine, cisplatin, cyclophosphamide, cytarabine, dacarbazine, dexamethasone, diphenhydrAMINE, DOXOrubicin, droperidol, etoposide, famotidine, floxuridine, fluconazole, fluorouracil, furosemide, ganciclovir, gentamicin, haloperidol, heparin, mannitol, meperidine, mesna, methotrexate, metoclopramide, morphine, nalbuphine, ondansetron, pentostatin, potassium chloride, prochlorperazine, propofol, ranitidine, sodium bicarbonate, vancomycin, vinBLAStine, vinCRIStine, zidovudine

Patient/family education
- Inform patient that nonhormonal contraceptive measures are recommended during therapy and >4 mo after; teratogenic effects are possible
- Teach patient to avoid use of products containing aspirin or ibuprofen, razors, commercial mouthwash, since bleeding may occur; to report symptoms of bleeding (hematuria, tarry stools)
- Instruct patient to report signs of anemia (fatigue, headache, irritability, faintness, shortness of breath) and CNS reactions (confusion, psychosis, nightmares, seizures, severe headaches)
- Inform patient that hair may be lost during treatment; a wig or hairpiece may make patient feel better; new hair may be different in color, texture
- Inform patient that receiving vaccinations during therapy may cause serious reactions

Evaluation
Positive therapeutic outcome
- Prevention of rapid division of malignant cells

palivizumab (Rx)
(pal-ih-viz′uh-mab)
Synagis
Func. class.: Monoclonal antibody

Pregnancy category C

Action: A humanized monoclonal antibody that exhibits neutralizing and fusion-inhibitory activity against respiratory syncytial virus (RSV)

▷ Therapeutic Outcome: Absence of RSV

Uses: Prevention of serious lower respiratory tract disease caused by RSV in pediatric patients

---

Dosage and routes

P *Child:* IM 15 mg/kg, those patients who develop RSV should receive monthly doses during RSV season

Available forms: Lyophilized inj 100 mg

Adverse effects

(*italic* = common; **bold** = life-threatening)
EENT: Otitis media, rhinitis, pharyngitis
GI: Nausea, vomiting, diarrhea, increased AST
INTEG: Rash, inj site reaction
RESP: Upper respiratory tract infection, **apnea**
SYST: **Anaphylaxis**

Contraindications: Hypersensitivity, adults, cyanotic congenital heart disease

Precautions: Thrombocytopenia, coagulation disorders, established RSV, congenital heart disease, chronic lung disease, systemic allergic reactions, pregnancy **C**

Pharmacokinetics

Absorption	Unknown
Distribution	Unknown
Metabolism	Unknown
Excretion	Unknown
Half-life	20 days

Pharmacodynamics

Onset	Unknown
Peak	Unknown
Duration	Unknown

Interactions

Unknown

NURSING CONSIDERATIONS
Assessment

• Assess for presence of RSV infection, drug is given to prevent infection
• Assess for side effects and report if allergic reaction is evident
◆● Assess for anaphylaxis: difficulty breathing, drug should be discontinued, have emergency equipment nearby

Nursing diagnoses

☑ Infection, risk for (uses)
☑ Knowledge, deficient (teaching)

Implementation

• Give IM only
• Give after adding 1 ml of sterile water for inj per 100 mg vial, gently swirl, let stand at room temperature for 20 min until sol clarifies; given within 6 hr of reconstitution

Patient/family education

• Teach patient to report upper respiratory infections, earaches, rash, sore throat

Evaluation

Positive therapeutic outcome
• Absence of RSV

---

palonosetron
Aloxi
See Appendix A, Selected New Drugs

---

pamidronate (Rx)
(pam-i-drone'ate)
Aredia
Func. class.: Bone resorption inhibitor, electrolyte modifier
Chem. class.: Bisphosphonate

Pregnancy category D

Action: Inhibits bone resorption, apparently without inhibiting bone formation and mineralization; absorbs calcium phosphate crystals in bone and may directly block dissolution of hydroxyapatite crystals of bone

→**Therapeutic Outcome:** Serum calcium at normal level

Uses: Moderate to severe Paget's disease associated with malignancy with or without bone metastases; osteolytic bone metastases in breast cancer patients, multiple myeloma

Dosage and routes   **P**
Hypercalcemia of malignancy
Adult: **IV** inf 60-90 mg in moderate hypercalcemia, 90 mg in severe hypercalcemia given over 24 hr

Osteolytic lesions from multiple myeloma
Adult: **IV** 90 mg over 4 hr qmo

Paget's disease
Adult: **IV** 90-180 mg/treatment, may use 30 mg qd × 3 days

Available forms: Inj 30, 60, 90 mg/vial pamidronate disodium and 470 mg of mannitol

Adverse effects

(*italic* = common; **bold** = life-threatening)
CNS: *Fatigue*
CV: *Hypertension*
GI: *Abdominal pain, anorexia, constipation, nausea, vomiting,* diarrhea, dyspepsia
GU: *UTI,* fluid overload

INTEG: Redness, swelling, induration, pain on palpation at site of catheter insertion
META: Anemia, hypokalemia, hypomagnesemia, hypophosphatemia, hypocalcemia
RESP: Coughing, dyspnea, URI
MS: Bone pain, myalgia

Contraindications: Hypersensitivity to bisphosphonates, pregnancy **D**

P Precautions: Children, nursing mothers, renal dysfunction

\ Do Not Confuse:
Aredia/Adriamycin

Pharmacokinetics

Absorption	Rapidly cleared from circulation
Distribution	Mainly to bones, primarily in areas of high bone turnover
Metabolism	Unknown
Excretion	Kidneys, unchanged (50%)
Half-life	Biphasic 1½ hr; 27 hr; from bone to 300 days

Pharmacodynamics

Onset	1 day
Peak	1 wk
Duration	Unknown

Interactions:
Individual drugs
Calcium, vitamin D: ↓ pamidronate effect
Digoxin: ↑ hypomagnesemia, hypokalemia

NURSING CONSIDERATIONS
Assessment
• Assess for hypocalcemia: Chvostek's, Trousseau's sign, paresthesia, twitching, laryngospasm
• Monitor manifestations of hypocalcemia: personality changes, anxiety, disturbances, depression, psychosis; nausea, vomiting, constipation, abdominal pain from muscle spasm; decreased contractility, decreased cardiac output, hypotension, lengthened ST segment, prolonged QT interval; scaling eczema, alopecia, hyperpigmentation; tetany, muscle twitching, cramping, grimacing, seizure, altered deep tendon reflexes, spasm
• Monitor manifestations of hypomagnesemia: agitation; muscle twitching, paresthesia, hyperactive reflexes, positive Babinski reflex, dysphagia, nystagmus, seizures, tetany; nausea, vomiting, diarrhea, anorexia, abdominal distention; ectopy, tachycardia, broad, flat, or inverted T waves, depressed ST segment, prolonged QT interval, decreased cardiac output, hypotension

• Monitor manifestations of hypokalemia: acidic urine, reduced urine osmolality, nocturia, polyuria, polydipsia; hypotension, broad T wave, U wave, ectopy, tachycardia, weak pulse; muscle weakness, altered LOC, drowsiness, apathy, lethargy, confusion, depression; anorexia, nausea, cramps, constipation, distention, paralytic ileus; hypoventilation, respiratory muscle weakness
• Assess fluid volume status: check I&O ratio and record, assess for distended red veins, crackles in lung, color, quality, and sp gr of urine, skin turgor, adequacy of pulses, moist mucous membranes, bilateral lung sounds, peripheral pitting edema
• Monitor electrolytes: phosphorus, potassium, sodium, calcium, magnesium; also include BUN, creatinine, CBC, platelets, hemoglobin
• Assess B/P before and during therapy
• Assess for pain: in joints or on exertion, duration and characteristics; analgesics may be ordered
• Assess for phlebitis at **IV** site: swelling, redness, pain, warmth

Nursing diagnoses
✓ Injury, risk for (uses, adverse reactions)
✓ Fluid volume, excess (side effects)
✓ Knowledge, deficient (teaching)

Implementation
• Give by **IV** inf after reconstituting by adding 10 ml of sterile water for inj to each vial, then adding to 1000 ml of sterile 0.45%, 0.9% NaCl, D₅W, run over 24 hr for hypercalcemia or 60 mg ≥4 hr, 90 mg/24 hr; dilute reconstituted sol in 500 ml of 0.9% NaCl, 0.45% NaCl, or D₅W, give over 4 hr (multiple myeloma, Paget's disease)
• Store inf sol for up to 24 hr at room temp
• Reconstituted sol with sterile water may be stored under refrigeration for up to 24 hr

Additive incompatibilities:
Calcium products, sol

Patient/family education
• Advise patient to report hypercalcemic relapse: nausea, vomiting, bone pain, thirst
• Advise patient to continue with dietary recommendations, including calcium and vit D

Evaluation
Positive therapeutic outcome
• Decreased calcium levels to normal

 Herb/drug   Do Not Crush   ♦ Alert   ♦꜀ Key Drug   **G** Geriatric   **P** Pediatric

pancrelipase (Rx)

(pan-kre-li'pase)

Cotazym, Cotazym-65B ♣, Cotazym E.C.S.
8, Cotazym E.C.S. 20, Cotazym Capsules,
Cotazym-S Capsules, Creon, Ilozyme, Ku-
Zyme HP, Lipram-PN16, Lipram-CR20,
Lipram-UL12, Lipram-PN10, Pancrease
Capsules, Pancrease MT 4, Pancrease MT
10, Pancrease MT 16, Protilase, Ultrase MT
12, Ultrase MT 20, Viokase, Zymase

Func. class.: Digestant

Chem. class.: Pancreatic enzyme (bovine/
porcine)

Pregnancy category C

Action: Pancreatic enzyme needed for
breakdown of substances released from the
pancreas

➡ **Therapeutic Outcome:** Increases
protein, fat, carbohydrate digestion

Uses: Exocrine pancreatic secretion insufficiency, cystic fibrosis (digestive aid), steatorrhea, pancreatic enzyme deficiency

Dosage and routes

Ⓟ *Adult and child:* PO 1-3 cap/tab ac or with
meals, or 1 cap/tab with snack or 1-2 powder
packets ac

Available forms: Powder 16,800 units
lipase/70,000 units protease and amylase; caps
8000 units lipase/30,000 units protease and
amylase; delayed rel caps, 4000 units lipase/
12,000 units protease and amylase, 4000 units
lipase/25,000 units protease/20,000 units
amylase, 5000 units lipase/20,000 units
protease and amylase, 10,000 units lipase/
30,000 units protease and amylase, 12,000
units lipase/24,000 units protease and amylase, 12,000 units lipase/39,000 units protease
and amylase, 16,000 units lipase/48,000 units
protease and amylase 20,000 units lipase/
65,000 units protease and amylase, 24,000
units lipase/78,000 units protease and amylase

Adverse effects

(italic = common; **bold** = life-threatening)

GI: Anorexia, nausea, vomiting, diarrhea

GU: Hyperuricuria, hyperuricemia

Contraindications: Allergy to pork

Precautions: Pregnancy **C**

Pharmacokinetics

Absorption	Unknown
Distribution	Unknown
Metabolism	Unknown
Excretion	Unknown
Half-life	Unknown

Pharmacodynamics

Unknown

Interactions

Individual drugs

Cimetidine, iron (oral): ↓ absorption of
pancrelipase

Drug classifications

Antacids: ↓ absorption of pancrelipase

Lab test interferences

↑ Uric acid (serum, urine)

NURSING CONSIDERATIONS

Assessment

• Monitor I&O ratio; watch for increasing
urinary output

• Monitor fecal fat, nitrogen, Pro-time, during
treatment

• Monitor for polyuria, polydipsia, polyphagia
(may indicate diabetes mellitus)

• Assess for allergy to pork; patient may also
be sensitive to this drug

• Assess for appropriate weight, height,
development; there may be a developmental
lag

• Check stools for steatorrhea, which signifies
undigested fat content

Nursing diagnoses

☑ Nutrition: less than body requirements, imbalanced (uses)

☑ Knowledge, deficient (teaching)

Implementation

• Give after antacid or cimetidine; decreased
pH inactivates drug

Ⓟ • Give powder mixed in prepared fruit for
infants, children

• Administer low-fat diet to decrease GI
symptoms

• Store in airtight container at room temp

Patient/family education

• Teach patient to take tab with 8 oz or more
water, not to let tab sit in mouth; have patient
take tab sitting up only

• Advise patient to notify prescriber of allergic
reactions, abdominal pain, cramping, or
hematuria

• Teach patient not to inhale powder, very
irritating to mucous membranes, some powder
may irritate skin

P

Evaluation
Positive therapeutic outcome
- Absence of steatorrhea
- Improved digestion of carbohydrates, proteins, fat

! HIGH ALERT

pancuronium (Rx)
(pan-cure-oh'nee-yum)
pancuronium bromide, Pavulon
Func. class.: Neuromuscular blocker
(nondepolarizing)
Chem. class.: Synthetic curariform

Pregnancy category C

Action: Inhibits transmission of nerve impulses by binding with cholinergic receptor sites, antagonizing action of acetylcholine; no analgesic response

⇒ **Therapeutic Outcome:** Paralysis of all skeletal muscles

Uses: Facilitation of endotracheal intubation, skeletal muscle relaxation during mechanical ventilation, surgery, or general anesthesia

Dosage and routes
Adult: **IV** 0.04-0.1 mg/kg, then 0.01 mg/kg q30-60 min

P *Child >10 yr:* **IV** 0.04-0.1 mg/kg, then 1/5 initial dose q30-60 min

Available forms: Inj 1, 2 mg/ml

Adverse effects
(*italic* = common; **bold** = life-threatening)
CV: Bradycardia, tachycardia, increased, decreased B/P, ventricular extrasystoles
EENT: Increased secretions
INTEG: Rash, flushing, pruritus, urticaria, sweating, salivation
MS: Weakness to prolonged skeletal muscle relaxation
RESP: **Prolonged apnea, bronchospasm, cyanosis, respiratory depression**
SYST: **Anaphylaxis**

Contraindications: Hypersensitivity to bromide ion

Precautions: Pregnancy **C**, renal disease,
P cardiac disease, lactation, children <2 yr, electrolyte imbalances, dehydration, neuromuscular disease, respiratory disease

Pharmacokinetics

Absorption	Complete bioavailability
Distribution	Extracellular space; crosses placenta
Metabolism	Plasma
Excretion	Kidneys, unchanged
Half-life	2 hr

Pharmacodynamics

Onset	3-5 min, dose dependent
Peak	3-5 min
Duration	35-40 min

Interactions
Individual drugs
Clindamycin, enflurane, isoflurane, lincomycin, lithium, polymyxin B, quinidine: ↑ neuromuscular blockade
Theophylline: Dysrhythmias
Drug classifications
Aminoglycosides, anesthetics (local, opioid), thiazides: ↑ neuromuscular blockade

NURSING CONSIDERATIONS
Assessment
- Monitor vital signs (B/P, pulse, respirations, airway) until fully recovered; note rate, depth, pattern of respirations, strength of hand grip; patient should be intubated before use
- Monitor for electrolyte imbalances (potassium, magnesium) before drug is used; electrolyte imbalances may lead to increased action of this drug
- Monitor for recovery: decreased paralysis of face, diaphragm, leg, arm, rest of body; residual weakness and respiratory problems may occur during recovery period
◆• Assess for hypersensitive reactions, anaphylaxis: rash, fever, respiratory distress, pruritus; drug should be discontinued

Nursing diagnoses
☑ Breathing pattern, ineffective (uses)
☑ Communication, impaired verbal (adverse reactions)
☑ Fear (adverse reactions)
☑ Knowledge, deficient (teaching)

Implementation
- Use peripheral nerve stimulator (anesthesiologist) to determine neuromuscular blockade; deep tendon reflexes should be monitored during extended periods
- Give direct **IV** undiluted over 1-2 min, or diluted in D$_5$W or 0.9% NaCl and give as an inf at prescribed rate; titrate to patient response; should be administered only by qualified person, usually an anesthesiologist; do not administer IM

- Store in light-resistant area
- Give anticholinesterase to reverse neuro-muscular blockade

Syringe compatibilities: Heparin

Y-site compatibilities: Aminophylline, cefazolin, cefuroxime, cimetidine, DOBU-Tamine, DOPamine, epINEPHrine, esmolol, fentanyl, fluconazole, gentamicin, heparin, hydrocortisone, isoproterenol, lorazepam, midazolam, morphine, nitroglycerin, nitroprusside, ranitidine, sulfamethoxazole/trimethoprim, vancomycin

Y-site incompatibilities: Diazepam

Additive compatibilities: Verapamil

Additive incompatibilities: Barbiturates

Patient/family education

- Provide reassurance if communication is difficult during recovery from neuromuscular blockade
- Provide explanation to patients regarding all procedures or treatments; patient will remain conscious if anesthesia is not given also

Evaluation

Positive therapeutic outcome

- Paralysis of jaw, eyelid, head, neck, rest of body as evaluated by peripheral nerve stimulator

Treatment of overdose: Edrophonium or neostigmine, atropine; monitor VS; may require mechanical ventilation

---

pantoprazole (Rx)

(pan-toe-pray′zole)
Protonix, Protonix IV
Func. class.: Proton pump inhibitor
Chem. class.: Benzimidazole

Pregnancy category C

Action: Suppresses gastric secretion by inhibiting hydrogen/potassium ATPase enzyme system in gastric parietal cell; characterized as gastric acid pump inhibitor, since it blocks final step of acid production

➡ **Therapeutic Outcome:** Absence of epigastric fullness, pain, swelling

Uses: Gastroesophageal reflux disease (GERD), severe erosive esophagitis, maintenance, long-term pathological hypersecretory conditions including Zollinger-Ellison syndrome

Dosage and routes
GERD
Adult: PO 40 mg qd × 8 wk, may repeat course

Erosive esophagitis
Adult: **IV** 40 mg qd × 7-10 days; PO 40 mg qd × 8 wk; may repeat PO course

Pathological hypersecretory conditions
Adult: IV 80 mg q12h; max 240 mg/day

Available forms: Tabs, delayed rel 20, 40 mg; powder for inj, freeze dried 40 mg/vial

Adverse effects
(*italic* = common; **bold** = life-threatening)
CNS: *Headache,* insomnia
GI: *Diarrhea, abdominal pain,* flatulence
INTEG: *Rash*
META: Hyperglycemia

Contraindications: Hypersensitivity

P **Precautions:** Pregnancy **C,** lactation, children

Pharmacokinetics	
Absorption	Unknown
Distribution	Protein binding 97%
Metabolism	Unknown
G **Excretion**	Urine-metabolites, feces, ↓ rate in elderly
Half-life	1½ hr

Pharmacodynamics	
Onset	Unknown
Peak	2.4 hr
Duration	>24 hr

Interactions
Individual drugs
Clarithromycin, diazepam, flurazepam, phenytoin, triazolam: ↑ levels of pantoprazole
Sucralfate: ↓ absorption of pantoprazole
Warfarin: ↑ risk of bleeding

NURSING CONSIDERATIONS
Assessment

- Assess GI system: bowel sounds q8h, abdomen for pain, swelling, anorexia
- Monitor hepatic enzymes: AST, ALT, alkaline phosphatase during treatment

Nursing diagnoses
✓ Knowledge, deficient (teaching)

Implementation

- May take with or without food
- Do not crush del rel tabs, swallow whole

IV IV route
- Reconstitute with 10 ml of 0.9% NaCl, further dilute with 80 ml of LR, D_5 (0.8 mg/ml), given over 15 min (≤6 mg/ml) using in-line filter provided

Patient/family education
- Advise patient to report severe diarrhea; drug may have to be discontinued
- Advise patient with diabetes that hypoglycemia may occur
- Advise patient to avoid hazardous activities; dizziness may occur
- Advise patient to avoid alcohol, salicylates, ibuprofen; may cause GI irritation

Evaluation
Positive therapeutic outcome
- Absence of epigastric pain, swelling, fullness

---

paricalcitol (Rx)
(par-ih-cal'sih-tol)
Zemplar
Func. class.: Vitamin D analog
Chem. class.: Fat-soluble vitamin
Pregnancy category C

Action: Reduces parathyroid hormone (PTH) levels; suppresses PTH levels in patients with chronic renal failure with absence of hypercalcemia/hyperphosphatemia; serum PO_4, Ca, calcium-phosphate product (Ca × P) may increase

➡ Therapeutic Outcome:
Decreased symptoms of hyperparathyroidism

Uses: Hyperparathyroidism in chronic renal failure

Dosage and routes
Adult: **IV** bol 0.04-0.1 mcg/kg (2.8-7 mcg) no more than qod during dialysis; may increase by 2-4 mcg q2-4 wk until target serum intact PTH (1.5-3 × nonuremic upper limit of normal) is achieved

Available forms: Inj 5 mcg/ml

Adverse effects
(*italic* = common; **bold** = life-threatening)
CNS: Light-headedness
CV: Palpitations
GI: Nausea, vomiting, anorexia, dry mouth
MISC: Pneumonia, edema, chills, fever, flu, sepsis

Contraindications: Hypersensitivity, hypercalcemia

G Precautions: CV disease, renal calculi,
P pregnancy **C**, elderly, lactation, children

Pharmacokinetics

Absorption	Unknown
Distribution	Unknown
Metabolism	Unknown
Excretion	Unknown
Half-life	Unknown

Pharmacodynamics

Onset	Unknown
Peak	Unknown
Duration	Unknown

Interactions
Individual drugs
Digitalis: ↑ toxicity

NURSING CONSIDERATIONS
Assessment
- Monitor Ca, PO_4, 2 ×/wk qwk during initial therapy; after dose is established measure calcium and phosphorus q mo

Nursing diagnoses
✓ Knowledge, deficient (teaching)

Implementation
IV IV route
- Give by **IV** bol only

Patient/family education
- Advise patient to report weakness, lethargy, headache, anorexia, loss of weight
- Teach patient to report nausea, vomiting, palpitations

Evaluation
Positive therapeutic outcome
- Decreased hypoparathyroidism in chronic renal disease

---

paroxetine (Rx)
(par-ox'e-teen)
Paxil, Paxil CR
Func. class.: Antidepressant, selective serotonin reuptake inhibitor (SSRI)
Chem. class.: Phenylpiperidine derivative
Pregnancy category B

Action: Inhibits CNS neuron reuptake of serotonin but not of norepinephrine or DOPamine

➡ Therapeutic Outcome: Relief of depression

Uses: Major depressive disorder, obsessive-compulsive disorder, panic disorder, generalized anxiety disorder

Investigational uses: Diabetic neuropa-

⬛ Herb/drug   ⬟ Do Not Crush   ◆ Alert   ◆ᴛᴛ Key Drug   G Geriatric   P Pediatric

thy, headache, premature ejaculation, premenstrual disorders, bipolar depression with lithium, fibromyalgia, posttraumatic stress disorder

Dosage and routes
Depression
Adult: PO 20 mg qd in AM; after 4 wk if no clinical improvement is noted, dosage may be increased by 10 mg/day weekly to desired response; not to exceed 60 mg/day; or controlled rel 25 mg/day, may increase by 12.5 mg/day weekly up to 62.5 mg/day

G *Elderly:* PO 10 mg qd, increase by 10 mg to desired dose, max 40 mg/day; cont rel 12.5 mg/day

Obsessive-compulsive disorder
Adults: PO 40 mg/day in AM; start with 20 mg/day, increase 10 mg/day increments, max 60 mg/day

Panic disorder
Adults: PO 40 mg/day; start with 10 mg/day and increase in 10 mg/day increments, max 60 mg/day or controlled rel 12.5 mg/day max 75 mg/day

Renal dose
Adult: PO 10 mg qd in AM, may increase by 10 mg/day q wk, max 50 mg qd or controlled rel 12.5 mg/day max 50 mg/day

Premenstrual disorders (off-label)
Adult: PO 10-30 mg qd

Available forms: Tabs 10, 20, 30, 40 mg; susp 10 mg/5 ml; oral susp 10 mg/5 ml; controlled rel 12.5, 25, 37.5 mg

Adverse effects
(*italic* = common; **bold** = life-threatening)
CNS: Headache, nervousness, insomnia, drowsiness, anxiety, tremor, dizziness, fatigue, sedation, abnormal dreams, agitation, apathy, euphoria, hallucinations, delusions, psychosis
CV: Vasodilatation, postural hypotension, palpitations
EENT: Visual changes
GI: Nausea, diarrhea, constipation, dry mouth, anorexia, dyspepsia, vomiting, taste changes, flatulence, decreased appetite, cramps
GU: Dysmenorrhea, decreased libido, urinary frequency, UTI, amenorrhea, cystitis, impotence, *abnormal ejaculation*
INTEG: Sweating, rash
MS: Pain, arthritis, myalgia, myopathy, myasthenia

RESP: Infection, pharyngitis, nasal congestion, sinus headache, sinusitis, cough, dyspnea
SYST: Asthenia, fever

Contraindications: Hypersensitivity, patients taking MAOIs, alcohol use

Precautions: Pregnancy **B**, lactation, P children, elderly, seizure history, patients with G history of mania, renal and hepatic disease

N **Do Not Confuse:**
paroxetine/paclitaxel, Paxil/paclitaxel, Paxil/Taxol

Pharmacokinetics
Absorption	Well absorbed
Distribution	Widely distributed; crosses blood-brain barrier, protein-binding 95%
Metabolism	Liver, mostly by CPY450 enzyme system
Excretion	Kidneys, unchanged (2%); breast milk
Half-life	21 hrs

Pharmacodynamics
Onset	Unknown
Peak	5.2 hr
Duration	Unknown

Interactions
Individual drugs
Alcohol: ↑ CNS depression
Cimetidine: ↑ paroxetine levels
Digoxin: ↓ effect of digoxin
Phenytoin: ↓ effect of paroxetine
Theophylline: ↑ theophylline levels
Thioridazine: Do not use with paroxetine, hypertensive crisis, seizures
Warfarin: ↑ warfarin levels
Drug classifications
Antidepressants: ↓ metabolism
Barbiturates, benzodiazepines, CNS depressants: ↑ effects
MAOIs: Hypertensive crisis, seizures; do not use together
Ⓗ *Herb/drug*
Corkwood, jimsonweed: ↑ anticholinergic effect
Hops, lavender: ↑ sedation
SAM-e, St. John's wort: possible serotonin syndrome
Yohimbe: ↑ CNS stimulation
Lab test interferences
↑ Serum bilirubin, ↑ blood glucose, ↑ alkaline phosphatase
↓ VMA, ↓ 5-HIAA, ↓ blood glucose
False: ↑ Urinary catecholamines

P

NURSING CONSIDERATIONS
Assessment

- Assess mental status: mood, sensorium, affect, suicidal tendencies; increase in psychiatric symptoms: depression, panic
- Assess for withdrawal symptoms: headache, nausea, vomiting, muscle pain, weakness; do not usually occur unless drug was discontinued abruptly
- Monitor B/P (with patient lying, standing), pulse q4h; if systolic B/P drops 20 mm Hg, hold drug, notify prescriber; take VS q4h in patients with CV disease
- Monitor blood studies: CBC, leukocytes, differential, cardiac enzymes if patient is receiving long-term therapy
- Monitor hepatic studies: AST, ALT, bilirubin
- Check weight weekly; appetite may increase with drug
- Assess ECG for flattening of T wave, bundle branch block, AV block, dysrhythmias in cardiac patients
- **G** Assess for EPS primarily in elderly: rigidity, dystonia, akathisia
- Monitor urinary retention, constipation; constipation is more likely to occur in children **P** **G** or elderly
- Identify alcohol consumption; if alcohol is consumed, hold dose until AM

Nursing diagnoses

☑ Coping, ineffective (uses)
☑ Injury, risk for (adverse reactions)
☑ Knowledge, deficient (teaching)
☑ Noncompliance (teaching)

Implementation

- Give with food or milk for GI symptoms; store at room temp; do not freeze
- Give crushed if patient is unable to swallow whole

Patient/family education

- Advise patient that therapeutic effects may take 1-4 wk
- Teach patient to use caution in driving and other activities requiring alertness because of drowsiness, dizziness, blurred vision; to avoid rising quickly from sitting to standing, especially elderly **G**
- Caution patient to avoid alcohol ingestion, other CNS depressants, and OTC medication unless prescribed
- Caution patient not to discontinue medication quickly after long-term use; may cause nausea, anxiety, headache, malaise; do not double doses if one is missed
- Advise patient to use gum, hard sugarless candy, or frequent sips of water for dry mouth; if dry mouth continues an artificial saliva product may be used

Evaluation
Positive therapeutic outcome
- Decrease in depression
- Absence of suicidal thoughts

Treatment of overdose: Maintain airway, for seizures give diazepam, symptomatic treatment

---

⚠ HIGH ALERT

pegaspargase (Rx)
(peg-as'per-gase)
Oncaspar, PEG-L-asparaginase
Func. class.: Antineoplastic
Chem. class.: Escherichia coli enzyme

Pregnancy category C

Action: Indirectly inhibits protein synthesis in tumor cells; without amino acid, DNA, RNA synthesis is halted; asparagine, protein synthesis is halted; G_1 phase of cell cycle specific; a nonvesicant

→**Therapeutic Outcome:** Prevention of rapidly growing malignant cells

Uses: Acute lymphocytic leukemia unresponsive to other agents in combination with other antineoplastics

Dosage and routes
In combination
P *Adult and child with BSA ≥0.6 m²:*
IV/IM 2500 international units/m² q14d, run **IV** over 1-2 hr in 100 ml of NaCl or D_5 through a running **IV**; IM should be no more than 2 ml in one inj site

P *Child with BSA <0.6 m²:* **IV**/IM 82.5 international units/kg q14 days

Sole induction
Adult: **IV** 2500 international units/m² q14d

Available forms: Inj 750 international units/ml in a phosphate-buffered saline sol

Adverse effects
(*italic* = common; **bold** = life-threatening)
CNS: Neuritis, dizziness, headache, **coma,** depression, fatigue, confusion, hallucinations, **seizures**
CV: Chest pain, **hypertension**
ENDO: Hyperglycemia
GI: *Nausea, vomiting, anorexia, cramps, stomatitis,* **hepatotoxicity, pancreatitis,** *diarrhea*
GU: Urinary retention, **renal failure,** glycosuria, polyuria, azotemia, uric acid neuropathy

---

HEMA: **Thrombocytopenia, leukopenia, myelosuppression, anemia, decreased clotting factors, pancytopenia**
INTEG: *Rash,* urticaria, chills, fever
RESP: **Fibrosis, pulmonary infiltrate, severe bronchospasm**
SYST: **Anaphylaxis, hypersensitivity**

Contraindications: Hypersensitivity, ☐infants, lactation, pancreatitis

Precautions: Renal disease, hepatic disease, pregnancy **C**, CNS disease

Pharmacokinetics

Absorption	Complete bioavailability
Distribution	Intravascular spaces
Metabolism	Unknown
Excretion	Reticuloendothelial system
Half-life	5½ days

Pharmacodynamics

Onset	Rapid
Peak	Unknown
Duration	2 wks

Interactions
Individual drugs
Aspirin, heparin, warfarin: Coagulation factor imbalances
Methotrexate: ↓ action of methotrexate
Radiation: do not use together
Drug classifications
NSAIDs: Coagulation factor imbalances

NURSING CONSIDERATIONS
Assessment
◆• Assess for signs and symptoms of pancreatitis (nausea, vomiting, severe abdominal pain), anaphylaxis (bronchospasm, dyspnea), cyanosis; monitor amylase, glucose
◆• Assess symptoms indicating severe allergic reaction: rash, pruritus, urticaria, purpuric skin lesions, itching, flushing; monitor for joint pain, bronchospasm, hypotension; epINEPHrine and crash carts should be nearby
• Monitor for frequency of stools, characteristics: cramping, acidosis; signs of dehydration: rapid respirations, poor skin turgor, decreased urine output, dry skin, restlessness, weakness
• Monitor CBC, differential, platelet count weekly; withhold drug if WBC is <4000/mm³ or platelet count is <100,000/mm³; notify physician of results; also assess Pro-time, PTT, and thrombin time, which may be increased
• Monitor renal function studies: BUN, creatinine, serum uric acid, urine CCr before and during therapy; check I&O ratio; report fall in urine output to <30 ml/hr; patient should be well hydrated with 2-3 L/day to prevent urate deposits
• Monitor temp q4h (may indicate beginning of infection)
• Monitor liver function tests before and during therapy (bilirubin, AST, ALT, LDH) as needed or monthly; check for jaundice of skin and sclera, dark urine, clay-colored stools, itchy skin, abdominal pain, fever, diarrhea; also monitor cholesterol, alkaline phosphatase
• Assess for bleeding: hematuria, stool guaiac, bruising or petechiae, mucosa or orifices q8h; check for inflammation of mucosa, breaks in skin
• Identify edema in feet, joint pain, stomach pain, shaking

Nursing diagnoses
☑Injury, risk for (adverse reactions)
☑Infection, risk for (adverse reactions)
☑Knowledge, deficient (teaching)

Implementation
• Preparation by trained personnel is required in controlled environment
• Give fluids **IV** or PO before chemotherapy to hydrate patient
• Provide antiemetic 30-60 min before giving drug and prn to prevent vomiting; administer antibiotics for prophylaxis of infection
• Provide a liq diet: carbonated beverages; gelatin may be added if patient is not nauseated or vomiting
Intradermal route
• After intradermal skin testing and desensitization, give 0.1 ml (2 international units) intradermally after reconstituting with 5 ml of sterile water or 0.9% NaCl for inj; then add 0.1 ml of reconstituted drug to 9.9 ml of diluent (20 international units/ml); observe for 1 hr, check for wheal; desensitization may be required
• For direct **IV** dilute 10,000 international units/5 ml of sterile water for inj or 0.9% NaCl without preservatives; give through 5-μm filter if fibers are present; do not use if sol cloudy or discolored, give over 30 min through Y-site of full-flowing **IV** of 0.9% NaCl or D₅W; run **IV** sol for at least 2 hr after direct administration
• Give **IV** inf using 21-, 23-, 25-G needle; administer by slow **IV** inf via Y-tube or 3-way stopcock of flowing D₅W or 0.9% NaCl inf over 30 min after diluting 10,000 international units/5 ml of sterile water or 0.9% NaCl (no preservatives) to 2000 international units/ml; filter may be necessary if fibers are present
• Provide allopurinol or sodium bicarbonate to reduce uric acid levels, alkalinization of urine

P

IM route
- Dilute 10,000 international units/2 ml of 0.9% NaCl with preservatives; give 2 ml or less per site

Patient/family education
- Advise patient that contraceptive measures are recommended during therapy; drug is teratogenic
- Teach patient to avoid use of products containing aspirin or NSAIDs, razors, commercial mouthwash, since bleeding may occur; to report symptoms of bleeding (hematuria, tarry stools)
- Teach patient to report signs of anemia (fatigue, headache, irritability, faintness, shortness of breath)
- Tell patient to avoid crowds and persons with respiratory tract infections to prevent patient infection
- Advise patient to avoid vaccinations, since serious reactions can occur
- Teach patient to report nausea, vomiting, bruising, bleeding, stomatitis, severe diarrhea, jaundice, chest pain, abdominal pain, trouble breathing, rash

Evaluation
Positive therapeutic outcome
- Prevention of rapid division of malignant cells

pegfilgrastim (Rx)
(peg-fill-grass'stim)
Neulasta
Func. class.: Hematopoietic agent

Pregnancy category C

Action: Stimulates proliferation and differentiation of neutrophils

➲ **Therapeutic Outcome:** Absence of infection

Uses: To decrease infection in patients receiving antineoplastics that are myelosuppressive; to increase WBC in patients with drug-induced neutropenia

Dosage and routes
Adult: SC 6 mg give once per chemotherapy cycle

Available forms: Sol for inj 10 mg/ml

Adverse effects
(*italic* = common; **bold** = life-threatening)
CNS: Fever, fatigue, headache, dizziness, insomnia, peripheral edema
GI: *Nausea*, vomiting, diarrhea, mucositis, anorexia, constipation, dyspepsia, abdominal pain, stomatitis
***HEMA:* Leukocytosis, granulocytopenia**
INTEG: Alopecia
MS: Skeletal pain
RESP: Respiratory distress syndrome

Contraindications: Hypersensitivity to proteins of *E. coli,* filgrastim; ARDS

Precautions: Pregnancy (C), lactation, children, myeloid malignancies, sickle cell disease

Pharmacokinetics	
Absorption	Unknown
Distribution	Unknown
Metabolism	Unknown
Excretion	Unknown
Half-life	15-80 hr

Pharmacodynamics
Unknown

Interactions
Individual drug
Lithium: ↑ release of neutrophils
Drug classification
Cytotoxic chemotherapy agents: Do not use this drug concomitantly or 2 wk before or 24 hr after administration of cytotoxics

Lab test interferences
↑ Uric acid, LDH, alk phosphatase

NURSING CONSIDERATIONS
Assessment
- Assess for allergic reactions, anaphylaxis: rash, urticaria; discontinue this drug, have emergency equipment nearby
- Monitor blood studies: CBC, platelet count before treatment and twice weekly; neutrophil counts may be increased for 2 days after therapy
- Monitor B/P, respirations, pulse before and during therapy
- Assess for bone pain, give mild analgesics

Nursing diagnoses
☑ Infection, risk for (uses)
☑ Knowledge, deficient (teaching)

Implementation
- Give using single-use vials; after dose is withdrawn, do not reenter vial
- Do not use 6-mg fixed dose in infants, children, or others <45 kg
- Inspect sol for discoloration, particulates; if present, do not use
- Do not administer in the period 14 days before and 24 hr after cytotoxic chemotherapy

- Store in refrigerator; do not freeze; may store at room temperature up to 6 hr, avoid shaking, protect from light

Patient/family education
- Teach the technique for self-administration: dose, side effects, disposal of containers and needles; provide instruction sheet

Evaluation
Positive therapeutic outcome
- Absence of infection

---

peginterferon alfa-2a (Rx)
(peg-in-ter-feer'on)
Pegasys
Func. class.: Immunomodulator

Pregnancy category C

Action: Stimulates genes to modulate many biologic effects, including inhibition of viral replication; inhibits ion cell proliferation, immunomodulation, stimulates effector proteins, decreases leukocyte, platelet counts

➡**Therapeutic Outcome:** Undetectable viral load; decreasing signs, symptoms of chronic hepatitis C

Uses: Chronic hepatitis C infections in adults with compensated liver disease

Dosage and routes
Adult: **SC** 180 mcg qwk × 48 wk; if poorly tolerated, reduce dose to 135 mcg qwk; in some cases reduction to 90 mcg may be needed

Available forms: Inj 180 mcg/ml

Adverse effects
(*italic* = common; **bold** = life-threatening)
CNS: *Headache, insomnia, dizziness,* anxiety, hostility, lability, nervousness, depression, fatigue, poor concentration, pyrexia
GI: *Abdominal pain, nausea, diarrhea, anorexia, vomiting,* dry mouth
INTEG: *Alopecia, pruritus, rash,* dermatitis
HEMA: **Thrombocytopenia,** neutropenia
MS: *Back pain,* myalgia, arthralgia

Contraindications: Hypersensitivity to interferons, neonates, infants, autoimmune hepatitis, decompensated hepatic disease before use of this drug

Precautions: Thyroid disorders, myelosuppression, hepatic, cardiac disease, lactation,
🄿 children <18 yr, depression/suicide, preexisting ophthalmologic disorders, pancreatitis,
🄶 renal disease, pregnancy (C), elderly

Pharmacokinetics	
Absorption	Large variability
Distribution	Large variability
Metabolism	Large variability
Excretion	Large variability
Half-life	15-80 hr

Pharmacodynamics	
Unknown	

Interactions
Drug classifications
Myelosuppressives, xanthines: Use caution if giving together

NURSING CONSIDERATIONS
Assessment
- Monitor ALT, HCV viral load; patients who show no reduction in ALT, HCV are unlikely to show benefit of treatment after 6 mo
- Monitor platelet counts, heme concentration, ANC, serum creatinine concentration, albumin, bilirubin, TSH, T_4, AFP
- Assess for myelosuppression, hold dose if neutrophil count is <500 × 10^6/L or if platelets are <50 × 10^9/L
- Assess for hypersensitivity: discontinue immediately if hypersensitivity occurs

Nursing diagnoses
✓ Infection, risk for (uses)
✓ Knowledge, deficient (teaching)

Patient/family education
- Provide patient or family member with written, detailed information about drug
- Give instructions for home use if appropriate
- Advise to take in evening to reduce discomfort, sleep through some side effects

Evaluation
Positive therapeutic outcome
- Decreased chronic hepatitis C signs/symptoms, undetectable viral load

---

pegvisomant
Somavert
See Appendix A, Selected New Drugs

pemoline (Rx)

(pem'oh-leen)

Cylert, PemADD, pemoline

Func. class.: Cerebral stimulant
Chem. class.: Oxazolidinone derivative

Pregnancy category B

Controlled substance schedule IV

Action: Exact mechanism unknown; may act through DOPaminergic mechanisms; produces CNS stimulation and a paradoxic effect in attention deficit hyperactivity disorder (ADHD)

➔ Therapeutic Outcome: Increased alertness, increased attention span, decreased hyperactivity (ADHD)

P Uses: ADHD for children >6 yr when other treatments have failed

Investigational uses: Narcolepsy, fatigue, excessive daytime sleepiness

Dosage and routes

P *Child >6 yr:* PO 37.5 mg in AM, increasing by 18.75 mg/wk, max 112.5 mg/day

Available forms: Tabs 18.75, 37.5, 75 mg; chewable tabs 37.5 mg

Adverse effects

(*italic* = common; **bold** = life-threatening)

CNS: *Hyperactivity, insomnia, restlessness,* dizziness, depression, headache, stimulation, irritability, aggressiveness, hallucinations, **seizures, masking or worsening of Gilles de la Tourette's syndrome,** drowsiness, dyskinetic movements

CV: Tachycardia

GI: Nausea, *anorexia,* diarrhea, abdominal pain, increased liver enzymes, **hepatitis,** jaundice, weight loss, **life-threatening hepatic failure**

MISC: Rashes, growth suppression in **P** children

Contraindications: Hypersensitivity, hepatic insufficiency

Precautions: Renal disease, pregnancy **B,** **P** lactation, drug abuse, child <6 yr, psychosis, tics, seizure disorders

Pharmacokinetics

Absorption	Well absorbed
Distribution	Widely distributed; crosses placenta
Metabolism	Liver
Excretion	Kidneys, pH dependent; increased pH, increased reabsorption
Half-life	12 hr; increased when urine is alkaline

Pharmacodynamics

Onset	Unknown
Peak	2-4 hr
Duration	8 hr

Interactions

Drug classifications

Adrenergic blockers, CNS stimulants, decongestants: ↑ stimulation

Anticonvulsants: ↓ seizure threshold

Antihypertensives: ↓ effect of pemoline

Food/drug

Caffeine (coffee, teas, chocolate): ↑ stimulation

☑ *Herb/drug*

Horsetail, yohimbe: ↑ CNS stimulation

Melatonin: synergistic effect

NURSING CONSIDERATIONS
Assessment

• Monitor VS, B/P, since this drug may reverse effects of antihypertensives; check patients with cardiac disease more often for increased B/P

• Monitor height and weight q3 mo, since **P** growth rate in children may be decreased; appetite is suppressed; weight loss is common during the first few mo of treatment

• Monitor mental status: mood, sensorium, affect, stimulation, insomnia; aggressiveness may occur; depression with crying spells may occur after drug has worn off

• Assess for tolerance; should not be used for extended time except in ADHD; dosage should be diminished gradually to prevent withdrawal symptoms

P • In children or adults with ADHD, monitor for improved organizational skills, attention span, attending to tasks, impulse control, socialization, and ability to get along better with others

• Assess for withdrawal symptoms: headache, nausea, vomiting, muscle pain, weakness; drug tolerance will develop after long-term use; dosage should not be increased if tolerance develops

• Monitor hepatic and renal function studies: ALT, AST, bilirubin, creatinine, before treatment and periodically thereafter; life-threatening hepatic failure has occurred; discontinue drug if symptoms of hepatic failure occur

Nursing diagnoses

☑ Thought processes, disturbed (uses, adverse reactions)

☑ Coping, ineffective (uses)

☑ Knowledge, deficient (teaching)

☑ Coping, compromised family (uses)

Implementation
- Give in AM; titrate to patient's response; lowest dosage should be used to control symptoms
- Provide gum, hard candy, frequent sips of water for dry mouth at beginning of treatment; these symptoms tend to lessen with time

Patient/family education
- Teach patient to decrease caffeine consumption (coffee, tea, cola, chocolate), which may increase irritability and stimulation; to avoid OTC preparations unless approved by prescriber; to avoid alcohol ingestion; these may cause serious drug interactions
- Instruct patient to taper off drug over several wk, or depression, increased sleeping, lethargy may occur
- Caution patient to avoid hazardous activities until stabilized on medication
- Instruct patient not to double doses if medication is missed; prescriber may suggest drug holidays (ADHD) during the school year to assess progress and determine continued drug necessity
- Teach patient/family to notify prescriber if significant side effects occur: tremors, insomnia, palpitations, restlessness, jaundice, bleeding, dark urine; drug changes may be needed
- Inform patient that if dry mouth occurs to use frequent sips of water, sugarless gum, hard candy during beginning therapy; dry mouth lessens with continued treatment
- Advise patient to get needed rest; patients will feel more tired at end of day; to take last dose at least 6 hr before hs to avoid insomnia
- Teach patient about the possibility of hepatotoxicity

Evaluation
Positive therapeutic outcome
- Decreased activity in ADHD

Treatment of overdose: Administer fluids, hemodialysis, peritoneal dialysis, antihypertensives for increased B/P; ammonium chloride for increased excretion

PENICILLINS

penicillin G benzathine (Rx)
(pen-i-sill'in)
Bicillin L-A, Megacillin ♣, Permapen
penicillin G (Rx)
Penicillin G Potassium, Pfizerpen
penicillin G procaine (Rx)
Ayercillin ♣, Duracillin A.S., Wycillin
penicillin V potassium (Rx)
Apo-Pen-VK ♣, Deltapen-VK, Nadopen-V ♣, Novopen-VK ♣, Pen-Vee K ♣, PVFK ♣, Veetids
Func. class.: Broad-spectrum antiinfective
Chem. class.: Natural penicillin
Pregnancy category B

Action: Interferes with cell wall replication of susceptible organisms; osmotically unstable cell wall swells and bursts from osmotic pressure, resulting in cell death

➡**Therapeutic Outcome:** Bactericidal effects on the gram-positive cocci *Staphylococcus, Streptococcus pyogenes, Streptococcus viridans, Streptococcus faecalis, Streptococcus bovis, Streptococcus pneumoniae;* gram-negative cocci *Neisseria gonorrhoeae;* gram-positive bacilli *Bacillus anthracis, Clostridium perfringens, Clostridium tetani, Corynebacterium diphtheriae, Listeria monocytogenes;* gram-negative bacilli *Escherichia coli, Proteus mirabilis, Salmonella, Shigella, Enterobacter, Streptobacillus moniliformis,* spirochete *Treponema pallidum; Actinomyces*

Uses: Respiratory tract infections, scarlet fever, erysipelas, otitis media, pneumonia, skin and soft tissue infections, gonorrhea; prevention of rheumatic fever, glomerulonephritis

Dosage and routes
Penicillin G benzathine
Early syphilis
Adult: IM 2.4 million units in single dose

Congenital syphilis
P *Child <2 yr:* IM 50,000 units/kg in single dose

Prophylaxis of rheumatic fever, glomerulonephritis
P *Adult and child:* IM 1.2 million units in single dose qmo or 600,000 units q2 wk

Upper respiratory tract infections (group A streptococcal)
Adult: IM 1.2 million units in single dose

P

P *Child >27 kg:* IM 900,000 units in single dose

P *Child <27 kg:* IM 300,000-600,000 units in single dose

Available forms: Inj 300,000 units/ml; 600,000; 1,200,000; 2,400,000 units/dose

Penicillin G
Pneumococcal/streptococcal infections (serious)
Adult: IM/**IV** 5-24 million units in divided doses q4-6h

P *Child <12 yr:* IV 150,000 units/kg/day in 4-6 divided doses

Renal dose
CCr <50 ml/min dosage reduction indicated

Available forms: Inj 1, 2, 3 million units/50 ml; powder for inj 1, 5, 20 million units/vial

Penicillin G procaine
Moderate to severe infections
P *Adult and child:* IM 600,000-1.2 million units in 1 or 2 doses/day for 10 days to 2 wk

P *Newborn:* 50,000 units/kg IM once daily (avoid use in newborns)

Gonorrhea
P *Adult and child >12 yr:* IM 4.8 million units in two injections given 30 min after probenecid 1 g

Pneumococcal pneumonia
Adult/child >12 yr: IM 600,000-1.2 million units/day × 7-10 days

Renal dose
CCr 10-30 ml/min q8-12h; CCr <10 ml/min q12-18h

Available forms: Inj 300,000, 500,000, 600,000, 1,200,000, 2,400,000 units/dose

Penicillin V potassium
Pneumococcal/staphylococcal infections
Adult: PO 250-500 mg q6h

P *Child <12 yr:* PO 25-50 mg/kg/day in divided doses q6-8h

Streptococcal infections
Adult: PO 125 mg q6-8h × 10 days

Prevention of recurrence of rheumatic fever/chorea
Adult: PO 125-250 mg bid continuously

P *Child <5 yr:* PO 125 mg bid

P *Child >5 yr:* PO 250 mg bid

Vincent's gingivitis/pharyngitis
Adult: PO 250 mg q6-8h

Renal dose
CCr <50 ml/min dosage reduction indicated

Available forms: Tabs 125, 250, 500 mg; powder for oral sol 125, 250 mg/5 ml

Adverse effects
(*italic* = common; **bold** = life-threatening)
CNS: Lethargy, hallucinations, anxiety, depression, twitching, **coma, seizures**
GI: *Nausea, vomiting, diarrhea,* increased AST, ALT, abdominal pain, glossitis, colitis
GU: **Oliguria, proteinuria, hematuria,** *vaginitis, moniliasis,* **glomerulonephritis**
HEMA: Anemia, increased bleeding time, **bone marrow depression, granulocytopenia**
META: Hyperkalemia, hypokalemia, alkalosis, hypernatremia
MISC: Local pain, tenderness and fever with IM inj, **anaphylaxis serum sickness**

Contraindications: Hypersensitivity to
P penicillins; neonates

Precautions: Hypersensitivity to cephalosporins, pregnancy **B**, severe renal disease, lactation

Penicillin G benzathine

Pharmacokinetics

Absorption	Delayed; prolonged drug levels
Distribution	Widely distributed; crosses placenta
Metabolism	Liver, minimally
Excretion	Kidneys, unchanged; breast milk
Half-life	½-1 hr

Pharmacodynamics

Onset	Slow
Peak	12-24 hr
Duration	1-4 wk

Penicillin G

Pharmacokinetics

Absorption	Variably absorbed (PO); well absorbed (IM)
Distribution	Widely distributed; crosses placenta
Metabolism	Liver, minimally
Excretion	Kidneys, unchanged; breast milk
Half-life	½-1 hr

Pharmacodynamics

	PO	IM	IV
Onset	Rapid	Rapid	Rapid
Peak	1 hr	¼-½ hr	Immediate

 Herb/drug   Do Not Crush   Alert   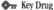 Key Drug   **G** Geriatric   **P** Pediatric

Penicillin G procaine

Pharmacokinetics

Absorption	Delayed; prolonged drug levels
Distribution	Widely distributed; crosses placenta
Metabolism	Liver, minimally
Excretion	Kidneys, unchanged; breast milk
Half-life	½-1 hr

Pharmacodynamics

Onset	Slow
Peak	1-4 hr
Duration	15 hr

Penicillin V potassium

Pharmacokinetics

Absorption	Widely absorbed
Distribution	Widely distributed; crosses placenta
Metabolism	Liver, minimally
Excretion	Kidneys, unchanged; breast milk
Half-life	½-1 hr

Pharmacodynamics

Onset	Rapid
Peak	½ hr

Interactions
Individual drugs
Aspirin, probenecid: ↑ penicillin levels
Aspirin: ↓ renal excretion
Drug classifications
Anticoagulants (oral): ↑ anticoagulant effects
Contraceptives (oral): ↓ contraceptive effectiveness
Erythromycins, tetracyclines: ↓ antimicrobial effectiveness
Herb/drug
Acidophilus: do not use with antiinfectives
Khat: ↓ absorption of penicillin; separate doses by 2 hr or more
Lab test interferences
False positive: Urine glucose, urine protein

NURSING CONSIDERATIONS
Assessment
• Assess patient for previous sensitivity reaction to penicillins or cephalosporins; cross-sensitivity between penicillins and cephalosporins is common
• Assess patient for signs and symptoms of infection including characteristics of wounds, sputum, urine, stool, WBC >10,000/mm³, earache, fever; obtain baseline information and during treatment
• Obtain C&S before beginning drug therapy

to identify if correct treatment has been initiated
• Assess for allergic reactions: rash, urticaria, pruritus, chills, fever, joint pain; angioedema may occur a few days after therapy begins; epINEPHrine, resuscitation equipment should be available for anaphylactic reaction
• Identify urine output; if decreasing, notify prescriber (may indicate nephrotoxicity); also check for increased BUN, creatinine
• Monitor blood studies: AST, ALT, CBC, Hct, bilirubin, LDH, alkaline phosphatase, Coombs' test monthly if patient is on long-term therapy
• Monitor electrolytes: potassium, sodium, chloride monthly if patient is on long-term therapy
• Assess bowel pattern daily; if severe diarrhea occurs, drug should be discontinued; may indicate pseudomembranous colitis
• Monitor for bleeding: ecchymosis, bleeding gums, hematuria, stool guaiac daily if on long-term therapy
• Assess for overgrowth of infection: perineal itching, fever, malaise, redness, pain, swelling, drainage, rash, diarrhea, change in cough, sputum

Nursing diagnoses
☑ Infection, risk for (uses)
☑ Diarrhea (adverse reactions)
☑ Injury, risk for (adverse reactions)
☑ Knowledge, deficient (teaching)
☑ Noncompliance (teaching)

Implementation
Penicillin G benzathine
PO route
• Give in even doses around the clock; if GI upset occurs, give with food, avoid acidic juices; carbonated beverages may decrease PO absorption; drug must be given for 10-14 days to ensure organism death and prevent superinfection
• Shake susp
IM route
• Do not give **IV**
• Give inj deep in large muscle mass
• Reconstitute with 0.9% NaCl, sterile water for inj, D₅W; refrigerate unused portion

Penicillin G
IM route
• Reconstitute with D₅W, 0.9% NaCl, sterile water for inj; shake well
• Give deep in large muscle mass; massage
• Do not give SC; may cause severe pain
• If injected near a nerve, loss of function and severe pain may occur

IV **IV route**
- Change **IV** sites q48h to prevent pain and phlebitis
- Give by intermittent inf by diluting 3 million units or less/50 ml or more; dilute 3 million units or more/100 ml of D_5W, $D_{10}W$, 0.45% NaCl, 0.9% NaCl, LR, Ringer's, or any combination run over 1-2 hr (adult), 15-30 min **P** (child)
- Give by cont inf by diluting and infusing over 24 hr

Syringe compatibilities: Heparin

Syringe incompatibilities: Metoclopramide

Y-site compatibilities: Acyclovir, amiodarone, cyclophosphamide, diltiazem, enalaprilat, esmolol, fluconazole, foscarnet, heparin, hydromorphone, labetalol, magnesium sulfate, meperidine, morphine, perphenazine, potassium chloride, tacrolimus, theophylline, verapamil, vit B/C

Additive compatibilities: Ascorbic acid, calcium chloride, calcium gluconate, cephapirin, chloramphenicol, cimetidine, clindamycin, colistimethate, corticotropin, dimenhyDRINATE, diphenhydrAMINE, epHEDrine, erythromycin, furosemide, hydrocortisone, kanamycin, lidocaine, magnesium sulfate, methicillin, methylPREDNISolone, metronidazole, polymyxin B, prednisoLONE, potassium chloride, procaine, prochlorperazine, verapamil

Additive incompatibilities: Aminoglycosides, aminophylline, amphotericin B, chlorproMAZINE, DOPamine, floxacillin, hydrOXYzine, metaraminol, oxytetracycline, pentobarbital, prochlorperazine mesylate, promazine, tetracycline, thiopental

Penicillin G procaine
- Do not give **IV**
- Give deeply in large muscle mass
- Reconstitute with 0.9% NaCl, sterile water for inj, D_5W; refrigerate unused portion
- Shake medication before administering
- IM route may include procaine reactions: fear of death, depression, seizures, anxiety, confusion, hallucinations

Penicillin V potassium
- Give in even doses around the clock; if GI upset occurs, give with food; drug must be given for 10-14 days to ensure organism death and prevent superinfection; store in tight container

- Shake susp; store in refrigerator for 2 wk or for 1 wk at room temp

Patient/family education
- Teach patient to report sore throat, bruising, bleeding, joint pain; may indicate blood dyscrasias (rare)
- Advise patient to contact prescriber if vaginal itching, loose foul-smelling stools, furry tongue occur; may indicate superinfection
- Instruct patient to take all medication prescribed for the length of time ordered
- Advise patient to notify prescriber of diarrhea with blood or pus, which may indicate pseudomembranous colitis

Evaluation
Positive therapeutic outcome
- Absence of signs/symptoms of infection (WBC <10,000/mm^3, temp WNL, absence of red, draining wounds, earache)
- Reported improvement in symptoms of infection

Treatment of anaphylaxis: Withdraw drug, maintain airway, administer epINEPHrine, aminophylline, O_2, **IV** corticosteroids

---

pentamidine (Rx)
(pen-tam'i-deen)
Nebupent, Pentam 300, Pentacarinat ✤, Pneumopent ✤
Func. class.: Antiprotozoal
Chem. class.: Aromatic diamide derivative
Pregnancy category C

Action: Interferes with DNA/RNA synthesis in protozoa; has direct effect on islet cells in the pancreas

Therapeutic Outcome: Protozoa death

Uses: Treatment/prevention of *Pneumocystis carinii* infections

Investigational uses: Babesiosis, leishmaniasis, African trypanosomiasis

Dosage and routes
P *Adult and child:* **IV**/IM 4 mg/kg/day × 2-3 wk; neb 300 mg via specific nebulizer given q4 wk for prevention

Available forms: Inj; aerosol 300 mg/vial; sol for aerosol 60 mg/vial ✤

Adverse effects
(*italic* = common; **bold** = life-threatening)
CNS: Disorientation, hallucinations, dizziness, confusion

CV: Hypotension, ventricular tachycardia, ECG abnormalities; **dysrhythmias**
GI: Nausea, vomiting, anorexia, increased AST, ALT, **acute pancreatitis,** metallic taste
GU: **Acute renal failure, increased serum creatinine, renal toxicity**
HEMA: Anemia, **leukopenia, thrombocytopenia**
INTEG: Sterile abscess, pain at inj site, pruritus, urticaria, rash
META: Hyperkalemia, hypocalcemia, *hypoglycemia, hyperglycemia*
MISC: Fatigue, chills, night sweats, **anaphylaxis, Stevens-Johnson syndrome**
RESP: Cough, shortness of breath, **bronchospasm** (with aerosol)

Precautions: Blood dyscrasias, hepatic disease, renal disease, diabetes mellitus, cardiac disease, hypocalcemia, pregnancy **C,** hypertension, hypotension, lactation, children

Pharmacokinetics

Absorption	Well absorbed (IM); minimally absorbed (inh); completely absorbed **(IV)**
Distribution	Widely distributed; does not appear in CSF
Metabolism	Not known
Excretion	Kidneys, unchanged (up to 30%)
Half-life	6½-9½ hr; increased in renal disease

Pharmacodynamics

	IM	IV	INH
Onset	Unknown	Unknown	Unknown
Peak	½-1 hr	Inf end	Unknown

Interactions
Individual drugs
Amphotericin B, cisplatin, colistin, foscarnet, methoxyflurane, polymyxin B, radiation, vancomycin: ↑ nephrotoxicity
Erythromycin **IV:** fatal dysrhythmias
Radiation: bone marrow suppression
Drug classifications
Aminoglycosides: ↑ nephrotoxicity
Antineoplastics: ↑ bone marrow depression

NURSING CONSIDERATIONS
Assessment
◆• Assess any patient with compromised renal system: drug is excreted slowly in poor renal system function; toxicity may occur rapidly
• Assess patient for infection including increased temp, thick sputum, WBC >10,000/mm³; monitor these signs of infection throughout treatment; obtain C&S before beginning therapy; treatment may begin after culture is obtained

• Assess respiratory system including rate, rhythm, bilateral lung sounds, shortness of breath, wheezing, dyspnea
• Monitor ECG for cardiac dysrhythmias; ECG and pulse should be checked frequently during treatment, since cardiotoxicity can occur
• Assess for hypoglycemia including nausea, tremors, anxiety, chills, diaphoresis, headache, hunger, cold, pale skin; this side effect can last for several mo after treatment is completed
• Monitor for hyperglycemia including flushed, dry skin, acetone breath, thirst, anorexia, drowsiness, polyuria; this side effect can last for several mo after treatment is completed
• Monitor renal function studies including BUN, urinalysis, creatinine; obtain at baseline and frequently during treatment; nephrotoxicity may occur; check I&O, report hematuria, oliguria
• Monitor blood studies including blood glucose, CBC, platelets; blood glucose fluctuations are common; anemia, leukopenia, thrombocytopenia can occur
• Monitor liver function studies including AST, ALT, alkaline phosphatase, bilirubin before beginning treatment and every 3 days during therapy
• Monitor calcium and magnesium before beginning treatment and every 3 days during therapy; hypocalcemia may occur

Nursing diagnoses
✓ Infection, risk for (uses)
✓ Knowledge, deficient (teaching)

Implementation
IM route
• Reconstitute 300 mg/3 ml of sterile water for inj; give deep in large muscle mass by Z-track; IM is a painful route
• Do not mix in normal saline
IV IV route
• For intermittent inf reconstitute 300 mg/3-5 ml of sterile water for inj, D₅W; withdraw dose and further dilute in 50-250 ml of D₅W; diluted sol is stable for 48 hr; discard unused sol; give over 1 hr or more

Y-site compatibilities: Zidovudine

Y-site incompatibilities: Foscarnet, fluconazole
Inhalation route
• Dilute 300 mg/600 ml sterile water for inj; put reconstituted sol into nebulizer; do not use with other drugs or sol precipitate may occur; sol stable for 48 hr at room temp; protect from light; administer over 30-45 min

Patient/family education
• Teach patient to report sore throat, fever, fatigue; could indicate superinfection
• Advise patient not to drink alcohol or take aspirin, since gastric bleeding may occur
• Teach patient to make position changes slowly to prevent orthostatic hypotension
• Advise patient to maintain adequate fluid intake

Evaluation
Positive therapeutic outcome
• Decreased signs and symptoms of protozoan infections
• Decreased signs and symptoms of *Pneumocystis carinii* pneumonia in HIV infections

---

! HIGH ALERT

pentazocine (Rx)
(pen-taz'oh-seen)
Talwin, Talwin NX
Func. class.: Opiate analgesic
Chem. class.: Synthetic benzomorphan (agonist/antagonist)

Pregnancy category C
Controlled substance schedule IV

Action: Inhibits ascending pain pathways in limbic system, thalamus, midbrain, hypothalamus by binding to opiate receptor sites, altering pain perception and response

Therapeutic Outcome: Relief of pain

Uses: Moderate to severe pain

Dosage and routes
Adult: PO 50-100 mg q3-4h prn, not to exceed 600 mg/day; **IV**/IM/SC 30 mg q3-4h prn, not to exceed 360 mg/day

Labor
Adult: IM 60 mg; **IV** 30 mg q2-3h when contractions are regular

Renal dose
Adult: CCr 10-50 ml/min q24-36h; CCr <10 ml/min q48h

Available forms: SC, IM, **IV** 30 mg/ml; tabs 50 mg

Adverse effects
(*italic* = common; **bold** = life-threatening)
CNS: Drowsiness, dizziness, confusion, headache, sedation, euphoria, hallucinations, dreaming
CV: Palpitations, bradycardia, change in B/P, tachycardia, increased B/P (high doses)
EENT: Tinnitus, blurred vision, miosis, diplopia

GI: Nausea, vomiting, anorexia, constipation, cramps, dry mouth
GU: Urinary retention, increased urinary output, dysuria
INTEG: Rash, urticaria, bruising, flushing, diaphoresis, pruritus, severe irritation at inj sites
***RESP:* Respiratory depression**

Contraindications: Hypersensitivity, addiction (opioid)

Precautions: Addictive personality, pregnancy **C**, lactation, increased ICP, MI (acute), severe heart disease, respiratory depression, hepatic disease, renal disease, seizure disorder, child <18 yr, head trauma

Pharmacokinetics
Absorption	Well absorbed (PO, SC, IM); completely absorbed (**IV**)
Distribution	Widely distributed; crosses placenta
Metabolism	Liver, extensively
Excretion	Kidneys, small amounts (unchanged)
Half-life	2-3 hr

Pharmacodynamics
	PO	SC/IM	IV
Onset	15-30 min	15-30 min	Rapid
Peak	1-3 hr	1-2 hr	15 min
Duration	3 hr	2-4 hr	1 hr

Interactions
Individual drugs
Alcohol: ↑ side effects
Drug classifications
Antipsychotics, CNS depressants, sedative/hypnotics, skeletal muscle relaxants: ↑ side effects
MAOIs: Use cautiously; results are unpredictable
Opiates: ↓ effects
Lab test interferences
↑ Amylase

NURSING CONSIDERATIONS
Assessment
• Assess pain characteristics: location, intensity, type of pain before medication administration and after treatment
• Monitor VS after parenteral route; note muscle rigidity, drug history, liver, kidney function tests, respiratory dysfunction: respiratory depression, character, rate, rhythm; notify prescriber if respirations are <10/min
• Monitor CNS changes: dizziness, drowsiness, hallucinations, euphoria, LOC, pupil reaction
• Monitor allergic reactions: rash, urticaria

 Herb/drug Do Not Crush Alert   Key Drug **G** Geriatric **P** Pediatric

- Assess for withdrawal symptoms in opiate-dependent patients

Nursing diagnoses
☑ Pain, acute (uses)
☑ Sensory-perceptual, disturbed: visual, auditory (adverse reactions)
☑ Breathing pattern, ineffective (adverse reactions)
☑ Knowledge, deficient (teaching)

Implementation
- Give by inj (IM, **IV**), only when resuscitative equipment available; give slowly to prevent rigidity
- Store in light-resistant area at room temp

PO route
- Tabs made in the United States contain naloxone 0.5 mg to prevent abuse if the PO preparation is used **IV**

SC/IM route
- Give IM inj deeply in large muscle mass; rotate inj sites; repeated SC inj may cause necrosis

IV **IV route**
- Give by direct **IV** after diluting 5 mg/ml of sterile water for inj; give 5 mg or less over 1 min

Syringe compatibilities: Atropine, benzquinamide, butorphanol, chlorproMA-ZINE, cimetidine, dimenhyDRINATE, diphenhydrAMINE, droperidol, fentanyl, hydromorphone, hydrOXYzine, meperidine, metoclopramide, morphine, perphenazine, prochlorperazine, promazine, promethazine, propiomazine, ranitidine, scopolamine

Syringe incompatibilities: Glycopyrrolate, heparin, pentobarbital, other barbiturates

Y-site compatibilities: Heparin, hydrocortisone, potassium chloride, vit B/C

Y-site incompatibilities: Nafcillin

Additive incompatibilities: Aminophylline, amobarbital, pentobarbital, phenobarbital, secobarbital, sodium bicarbonate

Patient/family education
- Teach patient to report any symptoms of CNS changes, allergic reactions
- Advise patients to avoid CNS depressants: alcohol, sedative/hypnotics for at least 24 hr after taking this drug
- Discuss with patient that dizziness, drowsiness, and confusion are common; to avoid getting up without assistance
- Discuss in detail all aspects of the drug
- Instruct patient to change position slowly to prevent orthostatic hypotension

- Teach patient to turn, cough, deep breathe after surgery to prevent atelectasis

Evaluation
Positive therapeutic outcome
- Relief of pain

Treatment of overdose: Naloxone (Narcan) 0.2-0.8 mg **IV**, O_2, **IV** fluids, vasopressors

---

⚠ HIGH ALERT

pentobarbital (Rx)
(pen-toe-bar'bi-tal)
Nembutal, Novopentobarb ✦, Nova-Rectal ✦, pentobarbital sodium
Func. class.: Sedative/hypnotic barbiturate; anticonvulsant
Chem. class.: Barbitone, short acting

Pregnancy category D

Controlled substance schedule II (USA), schedule G (Canada)

Action: Depresses activity in brain cells, primarily in reticular activating system in brainstem; also selectively depresses neurons in posterior hypothalamus, limbic structures; may decrease cerebral blood flow, intracranial pressure (**IV**) and cerebral edema; may potentiate GABA, an inhibitory neurotransmitter

➔ **Therapeutic Outcome:** Sedation, sleep

Uses: Insomnia, sedation, preoperative medication, increased intracranial pressure, dental anesthetic

Dosage and routes
Adult: PO 100-200 mg hs; IM 150-200 mg hs; **IV** 100 mg initially, then up to 500 mg; rec 120-200 mg hs

🅿 *Child:* IM 2-6 mg/kg, not to exceed 100 mg; PO 2-6 mg/kg/day in divided doses; PO preoperatively 2-6 mg/kg, max 100 mg/dose; **IV** 100 mg (hypnotic/anticonvulsant)

Available forms: Caps 50, 100 mg; elixir 20 mg/5 ml; rec supp 25, 30, 50, 60, 120, 200 mg; inj 50 mg/ml

Adverse effects
(*italic* = common; **bold** = life-threatening)
CNS: Lethargy, drowsiness, hangover, dizziness, paradoxic stimulation in elderly and children, light-headedness, dependence, **CNS**

depression, mental depression, slurred speech
CV: Hypotension, bradycardia
GI: Nausea, vomiting, diarrhea, constipation
HEMA: **Agranulocytosis, thrombocytopenia, megaloblastic anemia** (long-term treatment)
INTEG: *Rash,* urticaria, pain, abscesses at inj site, angioedema, thrombophlebitis
RESP: **Respiratory depression, apnea, laryngospasm, bronchospasm**
SYST: **Stevens-Johnson syndrome**

Contraindications: Hypersensitivity to barbiturates, respiratory depression, addiction to barbiturates, severe liver, renal impairment, porphyria, uncontrolled pain, pregnancy **D**

Precautions: Anemia, lactation, hepatic
G disease, renal disease, hypertension, elderly, acute/chronic pain

N **Do Not Confuse:**
pentobarbital/phenobarbital

Pharmacokinetics

Absorption	Well absorbed
Distribution	Widely distributed; crosses placenta, enters breast milk
Metabolism	Liver
Excretion	Kidneys, unchanged (minimally)
Half-life	15-48 hr

Pharmacodynamics

	PO	IM	IV	REC
Onset	15-30 min	10-25 min	Immediate	Slow
Peak	3-4 hr	Unknown	1 min	Unknown
Duration	4-6 hr	1-4 hr	15 min	4-6 hr

Interactions:
Individual drugs
Alcohol: ↑ CNS depression
Doxycycline: ↑ half-life
Griseofulvin, quinidine: ↓ effectiveness
Drug classifications
Anticoagulants: ↓ effectiveness
Antihistamines, CNS depressants, MAOIs, opiates, sedative/hypnotics: ↑ CNS depression
Corticosteroids: ↓ effectiveness
⊘ *Herb/drug*
Eucalyptus, Jamaican dogwood, kava, lemon balm, nettle, pill-bearing spurge, poppy, quinidine, senega, valerian: ↑ pentobarbital level

NURSING CONSIDERATIONS
Assessment
• Assess mental status: mood, sensorium, affect, memory (long, short), especially

G elderly; if using as a hypnotic, assess sleep patterns during therapy; drug suppresses REM sleep with dreaming; withdrawal insomnia may occur after short-term use; do not start using drug again; insomnia will improve in 1-3 nights; may experience increased dreaming
• Monitor for respiratory dysfunction: respiratory depression, character, rate, rhythm (when using **IV**); hold drug if respirations are <10/min or if pupils are dilated; also check VS q30 min after parenteral route for 2 hr
• Assess for blood dyscrasias: fever, sore throat, bruising, rash, jaundice, epistaxis (long-term treatment only)
• Assess seizure activity including type, location, duration, and character; provide seizure precaution
• Assess for pain in postoperative patients; pain threshold is lowered when patients are taking this medication

Nursing diagnoses
✓ Injury, risk for (side effects)
✓ Knowledge, deficient (teaching)

Implementation
• Administer only after removal of cigarettes, to prevent fires
• Reserve use until after trying conservative measures for insomnia
PO route
• Give 30 min before bedtime for expected sleeplessness
• May dilute elixir in juice, milk, or water if needed
• Give on empty stomach for best absorption
IM route
• Give deeply in muscle mass (gluteal) to minimize irritation to tissues; split inj >5 ml into 2 inj since irritation to tissues may occur; do not administer SC
IV **IV route**
• Use large vein to prevent extravasation; if extravasation occurs, use moist heat to the area and 5% procaine sol injected into area; give at 50 mg/1 min or more
• Give **IV** only with resuscitative equipment available (and only by qualified personnel)

Syringe compatibilities: Aminophylline, epHEDrine, hydromorphone, neostigmine, scopolamine, sodium bicarbonate, thiopental

Syringe incompatibilities: Benzquinamide, butorphanol, chlorproMAZINE, cimetidine, dimenhyDRINATE, diphenhydrAMINE, droperidol, fentanyl, glycopyrrolate, hydrOXYzine, meperidine, midazolam, nalbuphine, pentazocine, perphenazine, prochlorperazine, promazine, promethazine, ranitidine

---

⊘ Herb/drug　　**S** Do Not Crush　　**◆** Alert　　**◆⊓** Key Drug　　**G** Geriatric　　**P** Pediatric

Y-site compatibilities: Acyclovir, propofol, regular insulin

Additive compatibilities: Amikacin, aminophylline, calcium chloride, cephapirin, chloramphenicol, dimenhyDRINATE, erythromycin, lidocaine, thiopental, verapamil

Additive incompatibilities: Chlorpheniramine, codeine, ePHEDrine, erythromycin gluceptate, hydrocortisone, hydrOXYzine, levorphanol, methadone, norepinephrine, pentazocine, penicillin G potassium, phenytoin, promazine, promethazine, regular insulin, sodium succinate, streptomycin, triflupromazine, vancomycin

Patient/family education
- Teach patient to carry/wear emergency ID stating name, drugs taken, condition, prescriber's name, phone number
- Caution patient to avoid driving and other activities that require alertness
- Caution patient to avoid alcohol ingestion and CNS depressants; increased sedation may occur
- Teach patient not to discontinue medication quickly after long-term use; taper off over several wk

Evaluation
Positive therapeutic outcome
- Improved sleeping patterns
- Decreased seizure activity
- Improved energy

Treatment of overdose: Lavage, activated charcoal, warming blanket, vital signs, hemodialysis

! HIGH ALERT

pentostatin (Rx)
(pen'toe-sta-tin)
Nipent
Func. class.: Antineoplastic, enzyme inhibitor
Chem. class.: *Streptomyces antibioticus* derivative

Pregnancy category D

Action: Inhibits the enzyme adenosine deaminase (ADA), which is able to block DNA synthesis and some RNA synthesis

Therapeutic Outcome: Prevention of rapidly growing malignant cells

Uses: α-Interferon–refractory hairy cell leukemia, chronic lymphocytic leukemia

Dosage and routes
Adult: **IV** 4 mg/m² every other wk; may be given **IV** bol or diluted in a larger volume and given over 20-30 min

Available forms: Inj 10 mg/vial

Adverse effects
(*italic* = common; **bold** = life-threatening)
CNS: Headache, anxiety, confusion, depression, dizziness, insomnia, nervousness, paresthesia
GI: Nausea, vomiting, anorexia, diarrhea, constipation, flatulence, stomatitis, elevated liver function tests
GU: **Hematuria,** dysuria, increased BUN/creatinine
HEMA: **Leukopenia, anemia, thrombocytopenia, ecchymosis, lymphadenopathy,** petechiae
INTEG: Rash, eczema, dry skin, pruritus, sweating, herpes simplex/zoster
RESP: Cough, upper respiratory tract infection, bronchitis, dyspnea, epistaxis, pneumonia, pharyngitis, rhinitis, sinusitis
SYST: Fever, infection, fatigue, pain, allergic reaction, chills, **death, sepsis,** chest pain, flu-like symptoms

Contraindications: Hypersensitivity to this drug or mannitol, pregnancy **D**

Precautions: Renal disease, lactation, children, bone marrow depression

Pharmacokinetics
Absorption	Completely absorbed
Distribution	Unknown; low protein binding
Metabolism	Unknown
Excretion	Kidneys
Half-life	5-7 hr; increased in renal disease

Pharmacodynamics
Onset	4-5 mo
Peak	Unknown
Duration	1½-34 mo

Interactions
Individual drugs
Fludarabine: Fatal pulmonary reaction
Vidarabine: ↑ adverse reactions

NURSING CONSIDERATIONS
Assessment
- Assess CNS changes: confusion, paresthesias, psychosis, tremors, seizures, neuropathies; drug should be discontinued
- Assess for toxicity: facial flushing, epistaxis,

increased Pro-time, thrombocytopenia; drug should be discontinued

• Assess acidosis, signs of dehydration: rapid respirations, poor skin turgor, decreased urine output, dry skin, restlessness, weakness

• Check buccal cavity q8h for dryness, sores or ulceration, white patches, oral pain, bleeding, dysphagia; obtain prescription for viscous lidocaine (Xylocaine) to use in mouth

• Assess symptoms indicating severe allergic reaction: rash, pruritus, urticaria, purpuric skin lesions, itching, flushing

• Assess tachypnea, ECG changes, dyspnea, edema, fatigue; respiratory and cardiovascular reaction can be severe

• Monitor CBC, differential, platelet count weekly; withhold drug if WBC is <2000/mm³ or platelet count is <100,000/mm³, notify prescriber of results

• Monitor renal function studies: BUN, creatinine, serum uric acid, urine CCr before and during therapy; I&O ratio; report fall in urine output to <30 ml/hr

• Monitor temp q4h (may indicate beginning of infection)

• Monitor liver function tests before and during therapy (bilirubin, AST, ALT, LDH) as needed or monthly; check for jaundice of skin and sclera, dark urine, clay-colored stools, itchy skin, abdominal pain, fever, diarrhea

• Assess for bleeding: hematuria, stool guaiac, bruising or petechiae, mucosa or orifices q8h; check for inflammation of mucosa, breaks in skin

• Assess effects of alopecia on body image; discuss feelings about body changes

Nursing diagnoses

✓ Injury, risk for (adverse reactions)
✓ Body image, disturbed (adverse reactions)
✓ Infection, risk for (adverse reactions)
✓ Knowledge, deficient (teaching)

Implementation

• Give fluids **IV** or PO before chemotherapy to hydrate patient

• Give antacid before oral agent, antiemetic 30-60 min before giving drug and prn to prevent vomiting; administer antibiotics for prophylaxis of infection

• Give top or systemic analgesics for pain to lessen effects from stomatitis

• Give liq diet: carbonated beverages; gelatin may be added if patient is not nauseated or vomiting

• Encourage patient to rinse mouth tid-qid with water, club soda; brush teeth bid-qid with soft brush or cotton-tipped applicators for stomatitis; use unwaxed dental floss

• Preparation should be done by personnel knowledgeable in preparing antineoplastics wearing gloves, gown, mask in biologic cabinet

• Give by direct **IV** by reconstituting 10 mg/5 ml of sterile water for inj (2 mg/ml); shake well

• Give over 5 min

• Give by intermittent inf after diluting 10 mg/25-50 ml of 0.9% NaCl, D₅W; give over 30 min

• Diluted sol should be used within 8 hr at room temp

Y-site compatibilities: Fludarabine, melphalan, ondansetron, paclitaxel, sargramostim

Solution compatibilities: D₅W, 0.9% NaCl, LR

Patient/family education

• Teach patient to avoid use of products containing aspirin or NSAIDs, razors, commercial mouthwash, since bleeding may occur; to report symptoms of bleeding (hematuria, tarry stools)

• Advise patient to report signs of anemia (fatigue, headache, irritability, faintness, shortness of breath); CNS reactions including confusion, psychosis, nightmares, seizures, severe headaches

• Inform patient that hair may be lost during treatment; a wig or hairpiece may make patient feel better; new hair may be different in color, texture

• Advise patient to use sunscreen and protective clothing to prevent photosensitive reactions

Evaluation

Positive therapeutic outcome

• Prevention of rapid division of malignant cells

• Decreased bone marrow hairy cells

---

pentoxifylline (Rx)

(pen-tox-if′i-lin)
Trental
Func. class.: Hemorheologic agent
Chem. class.: Dimethylxanthine derivative

Pregnancy category C

Action: Decreases blood viscosity, stimulates prostacyclin formation, increases blood flow by increasing flexibility of RBCs; decreases RBC hyperaggregation; reduces platelet aggregation, decreases fibrinogen concentration

---

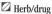 Herb/drug   Ⓢ Do Not Crush   ◆ Alert   Key Drug   Ⓖ Geriatric   Ⓟ Pediatric

Therapeutic Outcome: Decreased claudication and improved blood flow

Uses: Intermittent claudication related to chronic occlusive vascular disease

Investigational uses: Cerebrovascular insufficiency, diabetic neuropathies, TIAs, leg ulcers, CVA, aphthous stomatitis

Dosage and routes
Adult: PO 400 mg tid with meals

Stomatitis (off-label)
Adult: PO 400 mg tid × 1-6 mo

Available forms: Cont rel tabs 400 mg; ext rel tabs 400 mg

Adverse effects
(*italic* = common; **bold** = life-threatening)
CNS: Headache, anxiety, *tremors,* confusion, *dizziness*
CV: Angina, dysrhythmias, palpitations, hypotension, chest pain, dyspnea, edema
EENT: Blurred vision, earache, increased salivation, sore throat, conjunctivitis
GI: Dyspepsia, nausea, vomiting, anorexia, bloating, belching, constipation, cholecystitis, dry mouth, thirst, bad taste
INTEG: Rash, pruritus, urticaria, brittle fingernails
MISC: Epistaxis, flulike symptoms, laryngitis, nasal congestion, **leukopenia,** malaise, weight changes

Contraindications: Hypersensitivity to this drug or xanthines, retinal/cerebral hemorrhage

Precautions: Pregnancy **C,** angina pectoris, cardiac disease, lactation, children, impaired renal function, recent surgery, peptic ulcer

Pharmacokinetics	
Absorption	Well absorbed
Distribution	Unknown
Metabolism	Liver, degradation
Excretion	Kidneys
Half-life	½-1 hr

Pharmacodynamics	
Onset	Unknown
Peak	1 hr
Duration	Unknown

Interactions
Individual drugs
Plicamycin, valproic acid, warfarin: ↑ bleeding risk
Theophylline: ↑ theophylline level
Drug classifications
Antihypertensives, nitrates: ↑ hypotension

NSAIDs, salicylates, thrombolytics: ↑ bleeding risk
Herb/drug
Anise, arnica, chamomile, clove, dong quai, fenugreek, feverfew, garlic, ginger, ginkgo, ginseng (Panax), licorice: ↑ bleeding risk

NURSING CONSIDERATIONS
Assessment
• Monitor B/P, respirations in patient taking antihypertensives
• Assess for intermittent claudication baseline and during treatment

Nursing diagnoses
☑ Pain, chronic (uses)
☑ Activity intolerance (uses)
☑ Knowledge, deficient (teaching)
☑ Noncompliance (teaching)

Implementation
• Give with meals to prevent GI upset
⊘ • Tab should not be crushed or chewed

Patient/family education
• Teach patient that therapeutic response may take 2-4 wk
• Instruct patient to observe feet for arterial insufficiency
• Instruct patient to use cotton socks, well-fitted shoes; not to go barefoot
• Advise patient to watch for bleeding, bruises, petechiae, epistaxis

Evaluation
Positive therapeutic outcome
• Decreased pain, cramping
• Increased ambulation

P

perindopril (Rx) 🔑🚫
(per-in-doe-pril)
Aceon
Func. class.: Antihypertensive
Chem. class.: Angiotensin-converting enzyme (ACE) inhibitor

Pregnancy category
C (1st trimester),
D (2nd/3rd trimesters)

Action: Selectively suppresses renin-angiotensin-aldosterone system; inhibits ACE; prevents conversion of angiotensin I to angiotensin II, resulting in dilatation of arterial and venous vessels

Therapeutic Outcome: Decreased B/P in hypertension

Uses: Hypertension alone or in combination

Dosage and routes
Adult: PO 4 mg/day, may increase or decrease to desired response; range 4-8 mg/day may give in 2 divided doses or as a single dose

Patients taking diuretics
Discontinue diuretic 2-3 days before perindopril, then resume diuretic if needed

Renal dose
Adult: PO CCr <30 ml/min 2 mg/day, max 8 mg/day

Available forms: Tabs 2, 4, 8 mg scored

Adverse effects
(*italic* = common; **bold** = life-threatening)
CNS: Insomnia, dizziness, paresthesias, headache, fatigue, anxiety
CV: Hypotension, chest pain, tachycardia, dysrhythmias, syncope
EENT: Tinnitus, visual changes, sore throat, double vision, dry burning eyes
GI: Nausea, vomiting, colitis, cramps, diarrhea, constipation, flatulence, dry mouth, loss of taste
GU: **Proteinuria, renal failure,** increased frequency of polyuria or oliguria
HEMA: **Agranulocytosis, neutropenia**
INTEG: Rash, purpura, alopecia, hyperhidrosis
META: Hyperkalemia
RESP: Dyspnea, dry cough, rales
SYST: **Angioedema**

Contraindications: Hypersensitivity, history of angioedema, pregnancy **D** (2nd/3rd trimesters)

Precautions: Renal disease, hyperkalemia, pregnancy **C** (1st trimester), lactation, hepatic failure, dehydration, bilateral renal artery stenosis

Pharmacokinetics	
Absorption	Well absorbed
Distribution	Unknown
Metabolism	Liver
Excretion	Kidneys
Half-life	Unknown

Pharmacodynamics
Unknown

Interactions
Individual drugs
Allopurinol: ↑ hypersensitivity
Lithium: ↑ serum levels
Drug classifications
Antihypertensives, diuretics, ganglionic blockers: ↑ hypotension
Diuretics (potassium-sparing), potassium supplements, sympathomimetics: ↑ toxicity
Salt substitutes: ↑ potassium levels
Herb/drug
Aconite: ↑ toxicity, death
Astragalus, cola tree: ↑ or ↓ antihypertensive effect
Barberry, betony, black catechu, black cohosh, bloodroot, broom, burdock, cat's claw, dandelion, goldenseal, Irish moss, Jamaican dogwood, kelp, khella, mistletoe, parsley: ↑ antihypertensive effect
Coltsfoot, guarana, khat, licorice: ↓ antihypertensive effect

Lab test interferences
Interference: Glucose/insulin tolerance tests

NURSING CONSIDERATIONS
Assessment
• Monitor blood studies: neutrophils, decreased platelets
• Monitor B/P, orthostatic hypotension, syncope; if changes occur dosage change may be required
• Monitor renal studies: protein, BUN, creatinine; increased levels may indicate nephrotic syndrome and renal failure
• Monitor renal symptoms: polyuria, oliguria, frequency, dysuria
• Establish baselines in renal, liver function tests before therapy begins
• Check potassium levels throughout treatment, although hyperkalemia rarely occurs
• Check for edema in feet, legs daily
• Assess for allergic reactions: rash, fever, pruritus, urticaria; drug should be discontinued if antihistamines fail to help

Nursing diagnoses
☑ Cardiac output, decreased (uses)
☑ Injury, potential for (adverse reactions)
☑ Knowledge, deficient (teaching)
☑ Noncompliance (teaching)

Implementation
PO route
• Store in airtight container at 86° F (30° C) or less
• Severe hypotension may occur after 1st dose of this medication; decreased hypotension may be prevented by reducing or discontinuing diuretic therapy 3 days before beginning perindopril therapy
• Give by **IV** inf of 0.9% NaCl (as ordered) to expand fluid volume if severe hypotension occurs

Patient/family education
• Advise patient not to discontinue drug

 Herb/drug   Do Not Crush   Alert   Key Drug   Geriatric   **P** Pediatric

abruptly; advise patient to tell all persons associated with health care
- Teach patient not to use OTC products (cough, cold, allergy medications) unless directed by physician; serious side effects can occur; xanthines, such as coffee, tea, chocolate, cola can prevent action of drug
- Instruct patient on the importance of complying with dosage schedule, even if feeling better; to continue with medical regimen to decrease B/P: exercise, cessation of smoking, decreasing stress, diet modifications
- Emphasize the need to rise slowly to sitting or standing position to minimize orthostatic hypotension; not to exercise in hot weather, which can cause increased hypotension
- Advise patient to notify prescriber of mouth sores, sore throat, fever, swelling of hands or feet, irregular heartbeat, chest pain, coughing, shortness of breath
- Caution patient to report excessive perspiration, dehydration, vomiting, diarrhea; may lead to fall in B/P
- Caution patient that drug may cause dizziness, fainting, light-headedness; may occur during 1st few days of therapy; to avoid activities that may be hazardous
- Teach patient how to take B/P, and normal readings for age-group

Evaluation
Positive therapeutic outcome
- Decreased B/P in hypertension

Treatment of overdose: Lavage, **IV** atropine for bradycardia, **IV** theophylline for bronchospasm, digitalis, O₂; diuretic for cardiac failure, hemodialysis

---

perphenazine (Rx)
(per-fen'a-zeen)
Apo-Perphenazine ✤, Trilafon, Trilafon concentrate, perphenazine, Phenazine ✤, PMS Perphenazine ✤
Func. class.: Antipsychotic/neuroleptic
Chem. class.: Phenothiazine piperidine
Pregnancy category C

Action: Depresses cerebral cortex, hypothalamus, limbic system, which control activity, aggression; blocks neurotransmission produced by DOPamine at synapse; exhibits strong α-adrenergic, anticholinergic blocking action; as antiemetic inhibits medullary chemoreceptor trigger zone; mechanism for antipsychotic effects is unclear

→ **Therapeutic Outcome:** Decreased signs and symptoms of psychosis; decreased nausea and vomiting

Uses: Psychotic disorders, schizophrenia, nausea, vomiting

Dosage and routes
🅖 *Elderly:* PO 2-4 mg qd-bid, increase by 2-4 mg/wk to desired dose

Nausea/vomiting/alcoholism
🅟 *Adult and child >12 yr:* IM 5-10 mg prn, max 15 mg in ambulatory patients, 30 mg in hospitalized patients; PO 8-16 mg/day in divided doses, up to 24 mg; **IV** max 5 mg; give diluted or slow **IV** drip

Psychiatric use in hospitalized patients
Adults: PO 8-16 mg bid-qid, gradually increased to desired dose, max 64 mg/day; IM 5 mg q6h, max 30 mg/day

🅟 *Child >12 yr:* PO 6-12 mg in divided doses

Nonhospitalized patients
Adult: PO 4-8 mg tid

Available forms: Tabs 2, 4, 8, 16 mg; oral sol 16 mg/5 ml; inj 5 mg/ml; syr 2 mg/5 ml ✤

Adverse effects
(*italic* = common; **bold** = life-threatening)
CNS: *EPS (pseudoparkinsonism, akathisia, dystonia, tardive dyskinesia),* **neuroleptic malignant syndrome, seizures,** *headache,* dizziness
CV: *Orthostatic hypotension,* **cardiac arrest,** ECG changes, **tachycardia**
EENT: *Blurred vision, glaucoma*
GI: *Dry mouth, nausea, vomiting, anorexia, constipation,* diarrhea, jaundice, weight gain
GU: Urinary retention, urinary frequency, enuresis, impotence, amenorrhea, gynecomastia
HEMA: Anemia, **leukopenia, leukocytosis, agranulocytosis**
INTEG: *Rash,* photosensitivity, dermatitis
RESP: **Laryngospasm,** dyspnea, **respiratory depression**

Contraindications: Hypersensitivity, blood dyscrasias, coma, child <12 yr, brain damage, bone marrow depression

Precautions: Pregnancy **C,** lactation, seizure disorders, hypertension, hepatic disease, cardiac disease, elderly , narrow-angle glaucoma

Pharmacokinetics

Absorption	Variably absorbed (PO); well absorbed (IM)
Distribution	Widely distributed; high concentrations in CNS; crosses placenta
Metabolism	Liver, extensively; GI mucosa
Excretion	Kidneys

Pharmacodynamics

	PO	IM	IV
Onset	Erratic	10 min	Rapid
Peak	2-4 hr	1-2 hr	Unknown
Duration	6-12 hr	6-12 hr	Unknown

Interactions
Individual drugs
Alcohol: ↑ effects of both drugs, oversedation
Aluminum hydroxide, magnesium hydroxide: ↓ absorption
Epinephrine: ↑ toxicity
Levodopa: ↓ antiparkinson activity
Drug classifications
Anesthetics (barbiturates), antidepressants, antihistamines, opiates, sedative/hypnotics: ↑ CNS depression
Antacids, antidiarrheals (adsorbent): ↓ absorption
Anticholinergics: ↑ anticholinergic effects
β-Adrenergic blockers: ↑ effects of both drugs
CNS depressants: ↑ sedation
☑ Herb/drug
Betel palm, kava: ↑ extrapyramidal symptoms (EPS)
Cola tree, hops, nettle, nutmeg: ↑ action
Henbane: ↑ anticholinergic effect
Lab test interferences
↑ Liver function tests, ↑ cardiac enzymes, ↑ cholesterol, ↑ blood glucose, ↑ prolactin, ↑ bilirubin, ↑ PBI, ↑ cholinesterase, ↑ iodine, ↓ Hormones (blood and urine)
False positive: Pregnancy tests, PKU
False negative: Urinary steroids, 17-OHCS

NURSING CONSIDERATIONS
Assessment
• Assess mental status: orientation, mood, behavior, presence and type of hallucinations before initial administration and monthly; this drug should significantly reduce psychotic behavior
• Check for swallowing of PO medication; check for hoarding or giving medication to other patients
• Monitor I&O ratio; palpate bladder if low
G urinary output occurs, especially in elderly; urinalysis recommended before, during prolonged therapy

• Monitor bilirubin, CBC, liver function studies monthly
• Assess affect, orientation, LOC, reflexes, gait, coordination, sleep pattern disturbances
• Monitor B/P with patient sitting, standing, and lying; take pulse and respirations q4h during initial treatment; establish baseline before starting treatment; report drops of 30 mm Hg; obtain baseline ECG, with Q- and T-wave changes
• Check for dizziness, faintness, palpitations, tachycardia on rising; severe orthostatic hypotension is common
◆ • Identify for neuroleptic malignant syndrome: hyperpyrexia, muscle rigidity, increased CPK, altered mental status; drug should be discontinued
• Assess for EPS including akathisia (inability to sit still, no pattern to movements), tardive dyskinesia (bizarre movements of the jaw, mouth, tongue, extremities), pseudoparkinsonism (ragged tremors, pill rolling, shuffling gait); an antiparkinsonian drug should be prescribed
• Assess for constipation, urinary retention daily; if these occur, increase bulk, water in diet

Nursing diagnoses
☑ Thought processes, disturbed (uses)
☑ Coping, ineffective (uses)
☑ Knowledge, deficient (teaching)
☑ Noncompliance (teaching)

Implementation
PO route
• Administer drug in liq form mixed in glass of juice or cola if hoarding is suspected; do not mix in caffeine drinks, tannics, pectins
G • Administer decreased dose in elderly, in whom metabolism is slowed
• Administer PO with full glass of water, milk; or give with food to decrease GI upset
• Store in airtight, light-resistant container; oral sol in amber bottle
IM route
• Inject in deep muscle mass; do not give SC; do not administer sol with a precipitate
IV route
• Give by direct **IV** after diluting with 0.9% NaCl to a conc of 0.5 mg/1 ml; administer at 1 mg/min; may be further diluted and given as an inf

Syringe compatibilities: Atropine, benztropine, butorphanol, chlorproMAZINE, cimetidine, dimenhyDRINATE, diphenhydrAMINE, droperidol, fentanyl, hydrOXYzine, meperidine, methotrimeprazine, metoclopra-

---

☑ Herb/drug   ◎ Do Not Crush   ◆ Alert   ◆⚏ Key Drug   **G** Geriatric   **P** Pediatric mide, morphine, pentazocine, prochlorperazine, promethazine, ranitidine, scopolamine

Syringe incompatibilities: Midazolam, opium alkaloids, pentobarbital, thiethylperazine

Y-site compatibilities: Acyclovir, amikacin, ampicillin, azlocillin, cefamandole, cefazolin, cefotaxime, cefoxitin, cefuroxime, cephalothin, cephapirin, chloramphenicol, clindamycin, cotrimoxazole, doxycycline, erythromycin, famotidine, gentamicin, kanamycin, metronidazole, mezlocillin, minocycline, moxalactam, nafcillin, oxacillin, penicillin G potassium, piperacillin, sulfamethoxazole, tacrolimus, ticarcillin, ticarcillin/clavulanate, tobramycin, trimethoprim, vancomycin

Additive compatibilities: Ascorbic acid, ethacrynate, netilmicin

Additive incompatibilities: Cefoperazone

Patient/family education
• Teach patient to use good oral hygiene; frequent rinsing of mouth, sugarless gum for dry mouth
• Advise patient to avoid hazardous activities until drug response is determined, dizziness, blurred vision may occur
• Inform patient that orthostatic hypotension occurs often and to rise from sitting or lying position gradually; to remain lying down after IM inj for at least 30 min; tell patient to avoid hot tubs, hot showers, tub baths, since hypotension may occur; teach patient that in hot weather heat stroke may occur; take extra precautions to stay cool
• Teach patient to avoid abrupt withdrawal of this drug, or EPS may result; drug should be withdrawn slowly
• Teach patient to avoid OTC preparations (cough, hay fever, cold) unless approved by prescriber, since serious drug interactions may occur; avoid use with alcohol, CNS depressants; increased drowsiness may result
• Caution patient to use a sunscreen and sunglasses to prevent burns
• Teach patient about EPS and necessity of meticulous oral hygiene, since oral candidiasis may occur
• Instruct patient to take antacids 2 hr before or after taking this drug
• Teach patient to report sore throat, malaise, fever, bleeding, mouth sores; if these occur, CBC should be performed and drug discontinued

• Teach patient that urine may turn pink or red

Evaluation
Positive therapeutic outcome
• Decrease in emotional excitement, hallucinations, delusions, paranoia
• Reorganization of patterns of thought, speech

Treatment of overdose: Lavage if orally ingested; provide airway; *do not induce vomiting or use epINEPHrine*

phenazopyridine (Rx, OTC)
(fen-az-o-peer'i-deen)
AZO-Standard, Baridium, Eridium, Geridium, Phenazo ✦, Phenazodine, phenazopyridine, Prodium, Pyridiate, Pyridium, Urodine, Urogesic, Viridium
Func. class.: Nonopioid analgesic, urinary
Chem. class.: Azodye

Pregnancy category B

Action: Exerts analgesic, anesthetic action on the urinary tract mucosa

Uses: Urinary tract irritation, infection (for symptoms only of pain, burning, itching) used with urinary antiinfectives

Dosage and routes
Adult: PO 200 mg tid × 2 days or less when used with antibacterial for UTI
P *Child 6-12 yr:* PO 4 mg/kg tid × 2 days
Renal dose
Adult: PO CCr <50 ml/min do not use

Available forms: Tabs 100, 200 mg

Adverse effects
*(italic = common; **bold** = life-threatening)*
CNS: Headache
GI: Nausea, vomiting, diarrhea, heartburn, anorexia, **hepatic toxicity**
GU: **Renal toxicity,** *orange-red urine*
HEMA: **Thrombocytopenia, agranulocytosis, leukopenia, neutropenia, hemolytic anemia, methemoglobinemia**
INTEG: Rash, pruritus, skin pigmentation

Contraindications: Hypersensitivity, renal insufficiency

Precautions: Pregnancy **B**, lactation, **P** children <12 yr

Pharmacokinetics	
Absorption	Well absorbed
Distribution	Unknown; crosses placenta
Metabolism	Unknown
Excretion	Kidneys, unchanged
Half-life	Unknown

Pharmacodynamics	
Onset	Unknown
Peak	5-6 hr
Duration	8 hr

Interactions: None
Lab test interferences
Interference: Urinalysis

NURSING CONSIDERATIONS
Assessment
• Assess urinary status: burning, pain, itching, urgency, frequency, hematuria before, during, and after completion of drug therapy
• Monitor liver function studies: AST, ALT, bilirubin if patient is on long-term therapy
 • Assess for hepatotoxicity: dark urine, clay-colored stools, yellowing of skin and sclera, itching, abdominal pain, fever, diarrhea if patient is on long-term therapy
• Assess for allergic reactions: rash, urticaria; if these occur, drug may have to be discontinued

Nursing diagnoses
☑ Pain, acute (uses)
☑ Urinary elimination, impaired (uses)
☑ Knowledge, deficient (teaching)

Implementation
• Give to patient crushed or whole; chew tab may be chewed
• Give with food or milk to decrease gastric symptoms

Patient/family education
• Advise patient to report any symptoms of hepatotoxicity
• Caution patient not to exceed recommended dosage and to take with meals; to read label on other OTC drugs
• Teach patient not to discontinue after pain is relieved but continue to take concurrent prescribed antiinfective until finished
• Inform patient urine may turn red-orange, may stain clothing or contact lens

Evaluation
Positive therapeutic outcome
• Decrease in pain, burning, itching when urinating

Treatment of overdose: Methylene blue 1-2 mg/kg **IV** or vit C 100-200 mg PO

---

phenelzine (Rx)
(fen′el-zeen)
Nardil
Func. class.: Antidepressant, MAOI
Chem. class.: Hydrazine
Pregnancy category C

Action: Increases concentrations of endogenous epinephrine, norepinephrine, serotonin, dopamine in storage sites in CNS by inhibition of MAO; increased concentration reduces depression

➲ **Therapeutic Outcome:** Decreased symptoms of depression after 2-3 wk

Uses: Depression, when uncontrolled by other means

Dosage and routes
Adult: PO 45 mg/day in divided doses; may increase to 60 mg/day

G *Elderly:* PO 7.5 mg qd, increase by 7.5-15 mg q3-4 days; usual dose 15-60 mg/day in divided doses

Available forms: Tabs 15 mg

Adverse effects
(*italic* = common; **bold** = life-threatening)
CNS: Dizziness, drowsiness, confusion, headache, anxiety, tremors, stimulation, weakness, hyperreflexia, mania, insomnia, fatigue, weight gain
CV: Orthostatic hypotension, hypertension, **dysrhythmias, hypertensive crisis,** tachycardia, peripheral edema
EENT: Blurred vision
***ENDO:* Syndrome of inappropriate antidiuretic hormone–like syndrome**
GI: Constipation, dry mouth, nausea, vomiting, *anorexia,* diarrhea, weight gain
GU: Change in libido, frequency of urination
HEMA: Anemia
INTEG: Rash, flushing, increased perspiration

Contraindications: Hypersensitivity to MAOIs, hypertension, CHF, severe hepatic disease, pheochromocytoma, severe renal disease, severe cardiac disease, active alcoholism

Precautions: Suicidal patients, seizure disorders, severe depression, schizophrenia, hyperactivity, diabetes mellitus, pregnancy **C**, **P** child <16 yr

---

Pharmacokinetics

Absorption	Well absorbed
Distribution	Crosses placenta
Metabolism	Liver, extensively
Excretion	Kidneys, breast milk
Half-life	Unknown

Pharmacodynamics

Unknown

Interactions

Individual drugs

Alcohol: ↑ CNS depression
Clonidine: Severe hypotension; avoid use
Guanethidine: ↓ effects
Levodopa: ↑ effect of levodopa
L-Tryptophan: ↑ confusion, shivering, hyperreflexia
Meperidine: Hypertensive crisis, seizures, hypertensive episode
Methylphenidate: Seizures, do not use together
Sumatriptan: ↑ toxicity

Drug classifications

Amphetamines, appetite suppressants, asthma inhalants, nasal decongestants, selective serotonin reuptake inhibitors: ↑ hyperpyretic crisis, seizures, hypertensive episode
Anticholinergics: ↑ side effects
Antidepressants (tricyclics), meperidine, methylphenidate, nasal decongestants, sinus medications: Hypertensive crisis
Antidepressants (tricyclics), meperidine, nasal decongestants, sinus medications: Convulsions
Antidepressants (tricyclics), meperidine, nasal decongestants, sinus medications: selective serotonin reuptake inhibitors: Hypertensive episode
Antidiabetics: ↑ hypoglycemia
Barbiturates: ↑ effects of barbiturates
Benzodiazepines: ↑ effects of benzodiazepines
CNS depressants: ↑ effects of CNS depressants
Diuretics (thiazide): ↑ hypotension
Rauwolfia alkaloids: ↓ serotonin, norepinephrine
Sulfonamides: ↑ toxicity
Sympathomimetics (direct-acting): ↑ effects
Sympathomimetics (indirect-acting, mixed): ↑ pressor effect

Food/drug

Caffeine: ↑ hypertension
Tyramine-containing foods: Hypertensive crisis

⬛ Herb/drug

Betel palm, butcher's broom, capsicum peppers, galanthamine, green tea (large amounts), guarana (large amounts), night-blooming cereus: ↑ sympathomimetic effect
Brewer's yeast, cola tree, khat: ↑ hypertension
Ginkgo, nutmeg, yohimbe: ↑ effect
Ginseng: ↑ tension headache, irritability, visual hallucinations, mania
Jimsonweed: ↑ anticholinergic effect
Parsley, St. John's wort: Serotonin syndrome
Valerian: ↓ effect

NURSING CONSIDERATIONS
Assessment

• Monitor B/P (with patient lying, standing), pulse q4h; if systolic B/P drops 20 mm Hg, hold drug, notify prescriber; take VS q4h in patients with CV disease
• Monitor hepatic studies: AST, ALT, bilirubin if patient is on long-term therapy
• Check weight weekly; appetite may increase with drug
• Assess ECG for flattening of T wave, bundle branch block, AV block, dysrhythmias in cardiac patients
• Assess mental status: mood, sensorium, affect, suicidal tendencies; increase in psychiatric symptoms: depression, panic
• Monitor urinary retention, constipation; ⬛ constipation is more likely to occur in elderly
• Assess for withdrawal symptoms: headache, nausea, vomiting, muscle pain, weakness; do not usually occur unless drug was discontinued abruptly
• Identify alcohol consumption; if alcohol is consumed, hold dose until AM

Nursing diagnoses

✓ Coping, ineffective (uses)
✓ Injury, risk for (adverse reactions)
✓ Knowledge, deficient (teaching)
✓ Noncompliance (teaching)

Implementation

• Give with food or milk for GI symptoms; crush if patient is unable to swallow medication whole and mix with food or fluids
• Store at room temp; do not freeze

Patient/family education

• Teach patient that therapeutic effects may take 2-3 wk
• Advise patient to use caution in driving and other activities requiring alertness because of drowsiness, dizziness, blurred vision; to avoid rising quickly from sitting to standing, especially elderly
• Caution patient to avoid alcohol ingestion, other CNS depressants; serious reaction can occur
• Advise patient not to discontinue medication quickly after long-term use: may cause nausea, headache, malaise, sweating, hallucinations
• Instruct patient to increase fluids, bulk in diet if constipation, urinary retention occur,

G especially elderly; a stool softener may be ordered
- Teach patient to take gum, hard sugarless candy, or frequent sips of water for dry mouth
- Teach patient that therapeutic effects may take 1-4 wk
- Teach patient to avoid alcohol ingestion, CNS depressants, OTC medications: cold, weight loss, hay fever, cough syrup
- Teach patient not to discontinue medication quickly after long-term use
- Teach patient to avoid high-tyramine foods: cheese (aged), sour cream, beer, wine, pickled products, liver, raisins, bananas, figs, avocados, meat tenderizers, chocolate, yogurt; increased caffeine
- Teach patient to report headache, palpitations, neck stiffness, dizziness, constriction in chest, throat; rash, insomnia, change in strength, changes in urinary patterns, color of urine

Evaluation
Positive therapeutic outcome
- Decrease in depression
- Absence of suicidal thoughts

Treatment of overdose: Lavage, activated charcoal, monitor electrolytes, VS, diazepam **IV**, sodium bicarbonate

---

! HIGH ALERT

phenobarbital ⊙π (Rx)
(fee-noe-bar′bit-tal)
Ancalixir ✤, Barbita, Luminal, phenobarbital sodium, Solfoton
Func. class.: Anticonvulsant, sedative/hypnotic
Chem. class.: Barbiturate

Pregnancy category D

Controlled substance schedule IV

Action: Depresses activity in brain cells primarily in reticular activating system in brainstem; also selectively depresses neurons in posterior hypothalamus, limbic structures; able to decrease seizure activity by inhibition of impulses in CNS; decreases motor activity

➡ **Therapeutic Outcome:** Sedation, anticonvulsant, improved energy

Uses: All forms of epilepsy, status epilepticus,
P febrile seizures in children, sedation, insomnia

Investigational uses: Hyperbilirubinemia, chronic cholestasis

Dosage and routes
Seizures
Adult: PO 60-200 mg/day in divided doses tid or total dose hs
P *Child:* PO 4-6 mg/kg/day in divided doses q12h; may be given as single dose

Status epilepticus
Adult: **IV** inf 10 mg/kg; run no faster than 50 mg/min; may give up to 20 mg/kg
P *Child:* **IV** inf 5-10 mg/kg; may repeat q10-15 min up to 20 mg/kg; run no faster than 50 mg/min

Insomnia
Adult: PO/IM 100-320 mg
P *Child:* PO/IM 3-5 mg/kg

Sedation
Adult: PO 30-120 mg/day in 2-3 divided doses
P *Child:* PO 3-5 mg/kg/day in 3 divided doses

Preoperative sedation
Adult: IM 100-200 mg 1-1½ hr before surgery
P *Child:* IM 16-100 mg or PO/IM/**IV** 1-3 mg/kg 1-1½ hr before surgery

Available forms: Caps 15 mg; elixir 15 ✤, 20 mg/5 ml; tabs 8, 15, 30, 60, 100 mg; inj 30, 60, 130 mg/ml

Adverse effects
(*italic* = common; **bold** = life-threatening)
G *CNS:* Paradoxic excitement (elderly), drowsiness, lethargy, *hangover headache,* flushing, hallucinations, **coma**
GI: Nausea, vomiting, diarrhea, constipation
INTEG: Rash, urticaria, **Stevens-Johnson syndrome, angioedema,** local pain, swelling, necrosis, **thrombophlebitis**

Contraindications: Hypersensitivity to barbiturates, porphyria, hepatic disease, respiratory disease, nephritis, hyperthyroidism, diabetes mellitus, elderly, lactation, pregnancy **D**

Precautions: Anemia

🗅 **Do Not Confuse:**
phenobarbital/pentobarbital

Pharmacokinetics	
Absorption	Slow (70%-90%) (PO/IM/**IV**)
Distribution	Not known; crosses placenta
Metabolism	Liver (75%)
Excretion	Kidneys (25% unchanged)
Half-life	2-6 days

Pharmacodynamics			
	PO	IM	IV
Onset	30-60 min	10-30 min	5 min
Peak	Unknown	Unknown	30 min
Duration	6-8 hr	4-6 hr	4-6 hr

Interactions
Individual drugs
Alcohol: ↑ CNS depression

Chloramphenicol, disulfiram, theophylline: ↑ effects

Doxycycline: ↓ effects

Furosemide: ↑ orthostatic hypotension

Quinidine: ↓ effectiveness

Valproic acid: ↑ sedation

Drug classifications
Anticoagulants, glucocorticoids: ↓ effectiveness

Antidepressants, antihistamines, MAOIs, opiates, sedative/hypnotics: ↑ CNS depression

Skeletal muscle relaxants (nondepolarizing): ↑ effects

Sulfonamides: ↑ alpha effects

Herb/drug
Chamomile, eucalyptus, hops, Jamaican dogwood, kava, lemon balm, nettle, pill-bearing spurge, poppy, quinidine, senega, skullcap, valerian: ↑ phenobarbital level

St. John's wort: ↓ barbiturate effect

NURSING CONSIDERATIONS
Assessment
• Assess mental status: mood, sensorium, affect, memory (long, short), especially elderly; if using as a hypnotic, assess sleep patterns during therapy; drug suppresses REM sleep with dreaming

• Withdrawal insomnia may occur after short-term use; do not start using drug again; insomnia improves in 1-3 nights; may experience increased dreaming

• Assess respiratory dysfunction: respiratory depression, character, rate, rhythm when using **IV**; hold drug if respirations are <10/min or if pupils are dilated; also check VS q30 min after parenteral route for 2 hr

• Assess for barbiturate toxicity: hypotension, pulmonary constriction, cold, clammy skin, cyanosis of lips, CNS depression, nausea, vomiting, hallucinations, delirium, weakness, coma, pupillary constriction; mild symptoms occur in 8-12 hr without drug

• Assess for pain in postoperative patients; pain threshold is lowered when patients are taking this medication

• Assess for blood dyscrasias: fever, sore throat, bruising, rash, jaundice, epistaxis (long-term treatment only)

• Assess seizure activity including type, location, duration, and character; provide seizure precaution

Nursing diagnoses
☑ Sleep pattern, disturbed (uses)

☑ Injury, risk for (adverse reactions)

☑ Knowledge, deficient (teaching)

Implementation
• Give medication after removal of cigarettes to prevent fires

• Give medication after trying conservative measures for insomnia

PO route

• Tab may be crushed and mixed with food if swallowing is difficult; also may be mixed with other fluids 30-60 min before bedtime for expected sleeplessness; on empty stomach for best absorption

IM route

• Give inj in deep muscle mass (gluteal) to minimize irritation to tissues

• Split inj of >5 ml into two, since irritation to tissues may occur

Direct IV route

• Use large vein to prevent extravasation; if extravasation occurs, use moist heat to the area and 5% procaine sol injected into area; give at 65 mg or less/min; titrate to patient response

Syringe compatibilities: Heparin

Syringe incompatibilities: Benzquinamide, ranitidine

Y-site compatibilities: Enalaprilat, meropenem, propofol, sufentanil

Y-site incompatibilities: Hydromorphone

Additive compatibilities: Amikacin, aminophylline, calcium chloride, calcium gluceptate, cephapirin, colistimethate, dimenhyDRINATE, meropenem, polymyxin B, sodium bicarbonate, thiopental, verapamil

Additive incompatibilities: Cephalothin, chlorproMAZINE, codeine, epHEDrine, hydrALAZINE, hydrocortisone sodium succinate, hydrOXYzine, insulin, levorphanol, meperidine, methadone, morphine, norepinephrine, pentazocine, procaine, prochlorazine mesylate, promazine, promethazine, streptomycin, vancomycin

Solution compatibilities: D$_5$W, D$_{10}$W, 0.45% NaCl, 0.9% NaCl, Ringer's, dextrose/saline combinations, dextrose/Ringer's, dextrose/LR combinations, sodium lactate

P

Patient/family education
- Teach patient that hangover is common
- Instruct patient that drug is indicated only for short-term treatment of insomnia and is probably ineffective after 2 wk
- Inform patient that physical dependency may result when used for extended time (45-90 days depending on dosage)
- Teach patient to avoid driving and other activities requiring alertness
- Caution patient to avoid alcohol ingestion and CNS depressants; serious CNS depression may result
- Instruct patient not to discontinue medication quickly after long-term use; may cause seizures; drug should be tapered over 1 wk; take exactly as prescribed
- Emphasize the need to tell all prescribers that a barbiturate is being taken
- Teach the patient to make position changes slowly; orthostatic hypotension may occur
- Teach patient that response may take 4 days to 2 wk
- Instruct patient to notify prescriber immediately if bruising, bleeding occur, which may indicate blood dyscrasias

Evaluation
Positive therapeutic outcome
- Improved sleeping patterns
- Decreased seizure activity
- Sedative preoperatively

Treatment of overdose: Lavage, activated charcoal, warming blanket, VS, hemodialysis, alkalinize urine, give **IV** volume expanders, **IV** fluids

---

phenolphthalein (OTC)
(fee-nol-thay'leen)
Alophen, Correctol, Espotabs, Evac-U-Gen, Evac-U-Lax, Ex-Lax, Feen-A-Mint, Lax-Pills, Modane, Medilax, Phenolax, Prulet
Func. class.: Laxative, stimulant/irritant
Chem. class.: Diphenylmethane

Pregnancy category C

Action: Directly acts on intestinal smooth muscle by increasing motor activity; thought to irritate colonic intramural plexus; increases fluid in small intestine; alters fluid and electrolytes; action requires presence of bile

⇒**Therapeutic Outcome:** Decreased constipation

Uses: Constipation, preparation for bowel surgery or examination

Dosage and routes
Adult: PO 30-270 mg hs
P *Child >6 yr:* 30-60 mg/day
P *Child 2-5 yr:* 15-20 mg/day

Available forms: Tabs 60, 90, 97.2, 130 mg; chew tabs 65, 90, 97.2 mg; chew gum 97.2 mg; wafers 64.8 mg; chew wafers 80 mg

Adverse effects
(*italic* = common; **bold** = life-threatening)
GI: Nausea, vomiting, anorexia, diarrhea, abdominal cramps, rectal burning
INTEG: Rash, urticaria, **Stevens-Johnson syndrome**
META: Hypokalemia, electrolyte and fluid imbalances

Contraindications: Hypersensitivity, GI obstructions, abdominal pain, nausea/vomiting, fecal impaction, rectal fissures, hemorrhoids (ulcerated)

Precautions: Pregnancy C, lactation

Pharmacokinetics
Absorption	Minimally absorbed (15%)
Distribution	Unknown
Metabolism	Not metabolized
Excretion	Kidneys, feces
Half-life	Unknown

Pharmacodynamics
Onset	6-8 hr
Peak	Unknown
Duration	3-4 days

Interactions
Drug classifications
Oral drugs (any): ↓ absorption
Lab test interferences
Interference: BSP test

NURSING CONSIDERATIONS
Assessment
- Monitor blood, urine electrolytes if drug used often by patient; check I&O ratio to identify fluid loss
- Assess for cramping, rectal bleeding, nausea, vomiting; if these symptoms occur, drug should be discontinued; identify cause of constipation; identify whether fluids, bulk, or exercise is missing from lifestyle
- Assess stool for color, consistency, amount, presence of flatulence

---

Nursing diagnoses
☑ Constipation (uses)
☑ Diarrhea (adverse reaction)
☑ Knowledge, deficient (teaching)
☑ Noncompliance (teaching)

Implementation
• Chew well before swallowing; follow with 4 oz of water to prevent undissolved tab entering small intestine
• Give with 8 oz of water (tab); administer on empty stomach for more rapid results; do not give hs

Patient/family education
• Discuss with patient that adequate fluid consumption is necessary
• Teach patient that normal bowel movements do not always occur daily
• Caution patient not to use in presence of abdominal pain, nausea, vomiting; tell patient to notify prescriber if constipation is unrelieved or if symptoms of electrolyte imbalance occur (muscle cramps, pain, weakness, dizziness, excessive thirst)
• Teach patient not to use laxatives for long-term therapy; bowel tone will be lost
• Shake susp well as needed
• Teach patient not to take hs as a laxative; may interfere with sleep; also can cause problems with lipid pneumonia
• Teach patient not to use with food or vitamin preparations; delays digestion and absorption of fat-soluble vitamins

Evaluation
Positive therapeutic outcome
• Decreased constipation in 8-10 hr

---

phentolamine (Rx)
(fen-tole´a-meen)
Regitine, Rogitine ✦
Func. class.: Antihypertensive
Chem. class.: α-Adrenergic blocker

Pregnancy category C

Action: α-Adrenergic blocker, binds to α-adrenergic receptors, dilating peripheral blood vessels, lowering peripheral resistances, lowering blood pressure

▸**Therapeutic Outcome:** Decreased B/P, reversal of vasoconstriction (dermal necrosis)

Uses: Hypertension, pheochromocytoma, prevention, treatment of dermal necrosis after extravasation of norepinephrine or DOPamine, impotence

Investigational uses: Impotence, hypertensive crisis due to MAOIs

Dosage and routes
Treatment of hypertensive episodes in pheochromocytoma
Adult: **IV**/IM 5 mg; repeat if necessary

P Child: **IV**/IM 1 mg; repeat if necessary

Diagnosis of pheochromocytoma
Adult: **IV** 2.5 mg; if negative, repeat with 5 mg **IV**

P Child: **IV** 0.5 mg; if negative, repeat with 1 mg **IV**

Prevention of dermal necrosis
Adult: **IV** 10 mg/L of norepinephrine-containing sol

P Child: **IV** 0.1-0.2 mg/kg, max 10 mg

Available forms: Inj 5 mg/ml

Adverse effects
(*italic* = common; **bold** = life-threatening)
CNS: *Dizziness,* flushing, weakness, **cerebrovascular spasm**
CV: *Hypotension,* **tachycardia,** *angina,* **dysrhythmias, MI**
EENT: Nasal congestion
GI: *Dry mouth, nausea, vomiting, diarrhea, abdominal pain*

Contraindications: Hypersensitivity, MI, coronary insufficiency, angina

Precautions: Pregnancy **C**, lactation

Pharmacokinetics	
Absorption	Well absorbed (IM); completely absorbed (**IV**)
Distribution	Unknown
Metabolism	Unknown
Excretion	Kidneys, unchanged (10%)
Half-life	Unknown

Pharmacodynamics		
	IM	IV
Onset	Unknown	Rapid
Peak	20 min	2 min
Duration	½-1 hr	½ hr

Interactions
Individual drugs
Epinephrine: ↑ effects of epINEPHrine, hypotension
Drug classifications
Antihypertensives: ↑ effects of antihypertensives
☑ *Herb/drug*
Aconite: ↑ toxicity, death

✦ Canada Only   ◼ Do Not Confuse   * "Tall Man" lettering (See Preface)

Astragalus, cola tree: ↑ or ↓ antihypertensive effect

Barberry, betony, black catechu, black cohosh, bloodroot, broom, burdock, cat's claw, dandelion, goldenseal, Irish moss, Jamaican dogwood, kelp, khella, mistletoe, parsley: ↑ antihypertensive effect

Coltsfoot, guarana, khat, licorice: ↓ antihypertensive effect

NURSING CONSIDERATIONS
Assessment
• Monitor B/P, orthostatic hypotension, syncope, pulse and ECG until stable

Nursing diagnoses
☑ Cardiac output, decreased (uses)
☑ Injury, risk for (adverse reactions)
☑ Knowledge, deficient (teaching)
☑ Noncompliance (teaching)

Implementation
• Give with vasopressor nearby
IV **IV route**
• Give by direct **IV** after diluting 5 mg/1 ml of sterile water for inj or 0.9% NaCl; give 5 mg or less/min
• Give by cont inf by further diluting 5-10 mg/500 ml of D_5W, titrate to patient response

Syringe compatibilities: Papaverine

Y-site compatibilities: Amiodarone

Additive compatibilities: Dobutamine, verapamil

Prevention of dermal necrosis
• Add 10 mg/L to norepINEPHrine in **IV** sol

Patient/family education
• Caution patient not to discontinue drug abruptly
• Teach patient not to use OTC products (cough, cold, allergy) unless directed by prescriber
• Teach patient the importance of complying with dosage schedule, even if feeling better
• Emphasize the need to rise slowly to sitting or standing position to minimize orthostatic hypotension
• Teach patient to notify prescriber of mouth sores, sore throat, fever, swelling of hands or feet, irregular heartbeat, chest pain
• Caution patient to report excessive perspiration, dehydration, vomiting, diarrhea; may lead to fall in B/P
• Caution patient that drug may cause dizziness, fainting, light-headedness; may occur during 1st few days of therapy
• Teach patient how to take B/P, and normal readings for age-group

Evaluation
Positive therapeutic outcome
• Decreased B/P in hypertension
• Resolution of impotence
• Prevention of dermal necrosis

Treatment of overdose: Administer norepinephrine; discontinue drug

phenylephrine (Rx)
(fen-ill-ef′rin)
Neo-Synephrine
Func. class.: Adrenergic, direct acting
Chem. class.: Direct sympathomimetic amine (α-agonist)

Pregnancy category C

Action: Powerful and selective receptor agonist causing contraction of blood vessels, vasoconstriction of eye arterioles; decreases eye engorgement by stimulation of α-adrenergic receptors

⇒ **Therapeutic Outcome:** Increased B/P, decreased nasal congestion, decreased eye irritation

Uses: Hypotension, paroxysmal supraventricular tachycardia, shock, B/P maintenance during spinal anesthesia, topical ocular vasoconstrictor in uveitis, open-angle glaucoma, preoperatively, diagnostic procedures, refraction without cycloplegia, nasal congestion

Dosage and routes
Hypotension
Adult: SC/IM 2-5 mg; may repeat q10-15 min if needed, do not exceed initial dose; **IV** 50-100 mcg; may repeat q10-15 min if needed, do not exceed initial dose

P *Child:* IM/SC 0.1 mg/kg/dose q1-2h prn

Supraventricular tachycardia
Adult: **IV** bol 0.5-1 mg given rapidly, not to exceed prior dose by >0.1 mg; total dose ≤1 mg

Shock
Adult: **IV** inf 10 mg/500 ml of D_5W given 100-180 mcg/min (if 20 gtt/ml device is used), then maintenance of 40-60 mcg/min (if 20 gtt/ml device is used)

P *Child:* **IV** bol 5-20 mcg/kg/dose q10-15 min; **IV** inf 0.1-0.5 mg/kg/min

Available forms: Inj 1% (10 mg/ml)

Adverse effects

(*italic* = common; **bold** = life-threatening)

CNS: Headache, dizziness, weakness, anxiety, tremor, insomnia

CV: Reflex bradycardia, **dysrhythmias,** *hypertension,* **tachycardia,** CV collapse, palpitations, ectopic beats, angina

GI: Nausea, vomiting

INTEG: Necrosis, tissue sloughing with extravasation, **gangrene**

MISC: Anaphylaxis

Contraindications: Hypersensitivity, narrow-angle glaucoma, ventricular fibrillation, tachydysrhythmias, pheochromocytoma, severe hypertension

G **Precautions:** Hyperthyroidism, elderly, severe arteriosclerosis, cardiac disease, P infants, pregnancy **C,** lactation, arterial embolism, peripheral vascular disease, bradycardia, myocardial disease, partial heart block

Pharmacokinetics

Absorption	Well absorbed (IM); completely absorbed (**IV**); minimally absorbed (nasal, ophth)
Distribution	Unknown
Metabolism	Liver
Excretion	Unknown
Half-life	Unknown

Pharmacodynamics

	IV	SC/IM
Onset	Rapid	15 min
Peak	Unknown	Unknown
Duration	20-30 min	45-60 min

Interactions

Individual drugs

Bretylium, digoxin, halothane: ↑ dysrhythmias

Drug classifications

α-blockers: ↓ phenylephrine action

Antidepressants (tricyclic), β-adrenergic blockers, H₁ antihistamines, MAOIs: ↑ pressor effect

General anesthetics: ↑ dysrhythmias

Oxytocics: ↑ B/P

NURSING CONSIDERATIONS
Assessment

• Monitor I&O ratio; notify prescriber if output <30 ml/hr

• Monitor ECG during administration continuously; if B/P increases, drug is decreased

• Monitor B/P and pulse q5 min after parenteral route; CVP or PWP during inf if possible

• Assess for paresthesias and coldness of extremities; peripheral blood flow may decrease

Nursing diagnoses

☑ Tissue perfusion, ineffective (uses)

☑ Cardiac output, decreased (uses)

☑ Knowledge, deficient (teaching)

Implementation

IV **IV route**

• Give plasma expanders for hypovolemia

• Give **IV** after diluting 1 mg/9 ml of sterile water for inj; give dose over 30-60 sec; may be diluted 10 mg/500 ml of D₅W or 0.9% NaCl; titrate to patient response; low normal B/P; check for extravasation; check site for infiltration; use infusion pump

• Store reconstituted sol in refrigerator for no longer than 24 hr

• Do not use discolored sol

Y-site compatibilities: Amrinone, famotidine, haloperidol, zidovudine

Additive compatibilities: Chloramphenicol, DOBUTamine, lidocaine, potassium chloride, sodium bicarbonate

Patient/family education

• Inform patient of reason for drug administration and expected result

• Advise patient to report pain at inf site immediately

• Instruct patient to report change in vision, blurring, loss of sight; breathing trouble, sweating, flushing

Evaluation
Positive therapeutic outcome

• Increased B/P with stabilization

P

---

phenytoin ⚫☍ (Rx)

(fen′i-toyn)

Diphenylhydantoin, Dilantin, Dilantin-125, Dilantin Kapseals, Dilantin Infatab, Diphenylan, DPH, Phenytoin Oral Suspension, Phenytex

Func. class.: Anticonvulsant/antidysrhythmic (class IB)

Chem. class.: Hydantoin

Pregnancy category C

Action: Inhibits spread of seizure activity in motor cortex by altering ion transport; increases AV conduction to decrease dysrhythmias

→ **Therapeutic Outcome:** Decreased seizures, absence of dysrhythmias

Uses: Generalized tonic-clonic seizures, status epilepticus, nonepileptic seizures associated with Reye's syndrome or after head trauma, migraines, trigeminal neuralgia, Bell's palsy, ventricular dysrhythmias uncontrolled by anti-dysrhythmics

Dosage and routes
Seizures

Adult: PO 1 g or 20 mg/kg (ext rel) in 3-4 divided doses given q2h or 400 mg, then 300 mg q2h × 2 doses, maintenance 300-400 mg/day; max 600 mg/day; **IV** 15-20 mg/kg, max 25-50 mg/min then 100 mg q6-8h

 Child: PO 5 mg/kg/day in 2-3 divided doses, maintenance 4-8 mg/kg/day in 2-3 divided doses, max 300 mg/day; **IV** 15-20 mg/kg at 1-3 mg/kg/min

Status epilepticus

Adult: **IV** 15-20 mg/kg, max 25-50 mg/min; may give 100 mg q6-8h thereafter

 Child: **IV** 15-20 mg/kg given 1-3 mg/kg/min

Neuritic pain

Adult: PO 200-600 mg/day in divided doses

Ventricular dysrhythmias

Adult: PO loading dose 1 g divided over 24 hr, then 500 mg/day × 2 days; **IV** 250 mg given over 5 min until dysrhythmias subside or 1 g is given, or 100 mg q15 min until dysrhythmias subside or 1 g is given

 Child: PO 3-8 mg/kg or 250 mg/m²/day as single dose or divided in 2 doses; **IV** 3-8 mg/kg given over several min, or 250 mg/m²/day as single dose or divided in 2 doses

Renal dose

Adult: Do not use loading dose CCr <10 ml/min or hepatic failure

Available forms: Susp 30, 125 mg/5 ml; chew tabs 50 mg; inj 50 mg/ml; ext rel caps 100 mg; prompt rel caps 30, 100 mg

Adverse effects
(*italic* = common; **bold** = life-threatening)

CNS: Drowsiness, dizziness, insomnia, paresthesias, depression, suicidal tendencies, aggression, headache, confusion, slurred speech

CV: Hypotension, **ventricular fibrillation**

EENT: Nystagmus, diplopia, blurred vision

GI: Nausea, vomiting, constipation, anorexia, weight loss, **hepatitis,** jaundice, gingival hyperplasia

GU: **Nephritis,** urine discoloration

HEMA: **Agranulocytosis, leukopenia, aplastic anemia, thrombocytopenia, megaloblastic anemia**

INTEG: Rash, **lupus erythematosus,** **Stevens-Johnson syndrome,** hirsutism

ENDO: Diabetes insipidus

SYST: Hypocalcemia

Contraindications: Hypersensitivity, psychiatric condition, bradycardia, SA and AV block, Stokes-Adams syndrome, hepatic failure, acute intermittent porphyria

Precautions: Allergies, hepatic disease, renal disease, elderly, petit mal seizures, pregnancy **C,** hypotension, myocardial insufficiency

Pharmacokinetics

Absorption	Slowly absorbed from GI tract; erratic (IM)
Distribution	Crosses placenta, highly protein bound
Metabolism	Liver, extensively
Excretion	Kidneys, minimally; enters breast milk
Half-life	22 hr, dose dependent

Pharmacodynamics

	PO	PO–EXT REL	IM	IV
Onset	2-24 hr	2-24 hr	Erratic	1-2 hr
Peak	1.5-3 hr	4-12 hr	Erratic	Unknown
Duration	6-12 hr	12-36 hr	12-24 hr	12-24 hr

Interactions
Individual drugs

Cimetidine, valproic acid: ↑ phenytoin effect

Folic acid, rifampin: ↓ effects of phenytoin

Drug classifications

Antacids, barbiturates: ↓ effect of phenytoin

Anticonvulsants, antidepressants (tricyclics), benzodiazepines, salicylates: ↑ phenytoin level

Barbiturates: ↑ CNS depression

 Herb/drug

Aloe, buckthorn, cascara sagrada, senna: ↑ hypokalemia

Ginkgo: ↑ effect

Ginseng, santonica, valerian: ↓ anticonvulsant effect

Lab test interferences

↑ Glucose, ↑ alkaline phosphatase, ↑ BSP

↓ Dexamethasone, ↓ metyrapone test serum, ↓ PBI, ↓ urinary steroids

NURSING CONSIDERATIONS
Assessment

• Assess drug level: toxic level 30-50 mcg/ml; therapeutic level 7.5-20 mcg/ml, wait ≥1 wk to determine level

• Assess mental status: mood, sensorium, affect, memory (long, short), especially elderly

• Assess for beginning rash that may lead to

Stevens-Johnson syndrome or toxic epidermal necrolysis; phenytoin should not be used again
• Assess for blood dyscrasias: fever, sore throat, bruising, rash, jaundice, epistaxis (long-term treatment only)
• Assess seizure activity including type, location, duration, and character; provide seizure precaution
• Assess renal studies: urinalysis, BUN, urine creatinine
• Monitor blood studies: RBC, Hct, Hgb, reticulocyte counts weekly for 4 wk then monthly; also check thyroid function tests, serum calcium
• Monitor hepatic studies: ALT, AST, bilirubin, creatinine; for renal failure
• Assess for signs of physical withdrawal if medication suddenly discontinued
• Assess eye problems: need for ophth exam before, during, after treatment (slit lamp, funduscopy, tonometry)
• Assess allergic reaction: red raised rash, increased temp, lymphadenopathy; if this occurs, drug should be discontinued, usually occurs 3-12 wk after start of treatment; may also cause hepatotoxicity, rhabdomyolysis
• Monitor for toxicity: bone marrow depression, nausea, vomiting, ataxia, diplopia, CV collapse, slurred speech, confusion

Nursing diagnoses
☑ Injury, risk for (uses, adverse reactions)
☑ Knowledge, deficient (teaching)
☑ Noncompliance (teaching)

Implementation
PO route
• Give with meals to decrease GI upset
• Chew tab can be crushed or chewed; cap can be opened and mixed with foods or fluids; cap and tab are not interchangeable, only ext rel cap can be used for once a day dosing
• Give by gastric/NG tube: dilute susp before administration, flush tube with 20 ml of H_2O after dose
• Shake oral susp well; use measuring device for correct dose

IV IV route
• Administer by direct **IV** after diluting with special diluent provided (1 ml/50 mg, 2.2 ml/100 mg, 5.2 ml/250 mg); shake; give through Y-tube or 3-way stopcock; inject slowly <50 mg/min
• Give intermittent **IV** after diluting to a conc of 1-10 mg/ml
• Clear **IV** tubing first with 0.9% NaCl sol; use in-line filter; discard sol 4 hr after preparation; inject into large veins to prevent purple glove syndrome

Additive compatibilities: Bleomycin, verapamil

Y-site compatibilities: Esmolol, famotidine, fluconazole, foscarnet, tacrolimus

Y-site incompatibilities: Enalaprilat, potassium chloride, vit B/C

Patient/family education
• Teach patient to carry/wear emergency ID stating name, drugs taken, condition, prescriber's name and phone number
• Advise patient to avoid driving and other activities that require alertness until drug response is known; dizziness, drowsiness can occur
• Advise patient to avoid alcohol ingestion and CNS depressants unless approved by prescriber; increased sedation may occur
• Teach patient not to discontinue medication quickly after long-term use; taper off over several wk
• Advise patient that urine may turn pink, red, or brown
• Caution patient to avoid antacids or antidiarrheals within 2-3 hr of taking phenytoin
• Instruct patient in proper oral hygiene to prevent gingival hyperplasia; to visit dentist routinely

Evaluation
Positive therapeutic outcome
• Decreased seizure activity
• Decreased dysrhythmias
• Relief of pain

P

---

phytonadione (Rx)
(fye-toe-na-dye′one)
AquaMEPHYTON, Mephyton
Func. class.: Vitamin K₁, fat-soluble vitamin

Pregnancy category C

Action: Needed for adequate blood clotting (factors II, VII, IX, X)

⇒ Therapeutic Outcome: Prevention of bleeding

Uses: Vitamin K malabsorption, hypoprothrombinemia, prevention of hypoprothrombinemia caused by oral anticoagulants, prevention of hemorrhagic disease of the newborn

---

Dosage and routes
Hypoprothrombinemia caused by vitamin K malabsorption
Adult: PO/IM 2.5-25 mg; may repeat or increase to 50 mg

🅿 *Child:* PO/IM 5-10 mg

🅿 *Infants:* PO/IM 2 mg

Prevention of hemorrhagic disease of the newborn

🅿 *Neonate:* IM 0.5-1 mg within 1 hr after birth; repeat in 2-3 wk if required

Hypoprothrombinemia caused by oral anticoagulants

🅿 *Adult and child:* PO/SC/IM 2.5-10 mg, may repeat 12-48 hr after PO dose or 6-8 hr after SC/IM dose, based on prothrombin time

Available forms: Tabs 5 mg; inj 2 mg/ml; aqueous colloidal (IM, **IV**); inj aqueous dispersion 10 mg/ml (IM)

Adverse effects
(*italic* = common; **bold** = life-threatening)
CNS: Headache, **brain damage** (large doses)
GI: Nausea, decreased liver function tests
HEMA: **Hemolytic anemia, hemoglobin-uria, hyperbilirubinemia**
INTEG: Rash, urticaria

Contraindications: Hypersensitivity, severe hepatic disease, last few wk of pregnancy

🅿 **Precautions:** Pregnancy **C**, neonates

Pharmacokinetics
Absorption	Well absorbed (PO, IM, SC)
Distribution	Crosses placenta
Metabolism	Liver, rapidly
Excretion	Breast milk
Half-life	Unknown

Pharmacodynamics
	PO	SC/IM
Onset	6-12 hr	1-2 hr
Peak	Unknown	6 hr
Duration	Unknown	14 hr

Interactions
Individual drugs
Cholestyramine, mineral oil: ↓ action of phytonadione
Drug classifications
Oral anticoagulants: ↓ anticoagulant effect
Food/drug
Olestra: ↓ Vit K levels

NURSING CONSIDERATIONS
Assessment
• Monitor Pro-time during treatment (2-sec deviation from control time, bleeding time, and clotting time); monitor for bleeding, pulse, and B/P
• Assess nutritional status: liver (beef), spinach, tomatoes, coffee, asparagus, broccoli, cabbage, lettuce, greens
• Assess for bleeding or bruising: hematuria, black tarry stools, hematemesis

Nursing diagnoses
☑ Nutrition: less than body requirements, imbalanced (uses)
☑ Tissue perfusion, ineffective (uses)
☑ Knowledge, deficient (teaching)

Implementation
Ⓘ**IV route**
• Give **IV** after diluting with D₅ NS 10 ml or more; give 1 mg/min or more
• Give **IV** only when other routes not possible (deaths have occurred)
• Store in airtight, light-resistant container

Syringe compatibilities: Doxapram

Y-site compatibilities: Ampicillin, epINEPHrine, famotidine, heparin, hydrocortisone, potassium chloride, tolazoline, vit B/C

Additive compatibilities: Amikacin, calcium glucceptate, cephapirin, chloramphenicol, cimetidine, netilmicin, sodium bicarbonate

Patient/family education
• Teach patient not to take other supplements, unless directed by prescriber; to take this medication as directed
• Teach patient necessary foods high in vit K to be included in diet
• Advise patient to avoid IM inj, hard toothbrush, flossing; use electric razor until treatment is terminated
• Instruct patient to report symptoms of bleeding: bruising, nosebleeds, blood in urine, heavy menstruation, black tarry stools
• Caution patient not to use OTC medications unless approved by prescriber
• Stress the need for periodic lab tests to monitor coagulation levels
• Stress the need for patient to carry/wear emergency ID with condition, treatment, and medications taken

Evaluation
Positive therapeutic outcome
• Decreased bleeding tendencies

 Herb/drug   Do Not Crush   ◆ Alert   ◆ₜ Key Drug   🄶 Geriatric   🅿 Pediatric

- Decreased Pro-time
- Decreased clotting time

pindolol (Rx)
(pin′doe-lole)
Novo-Pindol ♣, Syn-Pindol ♣, Visken
Func. class.: Antihypertensive
Chem. class.: Nonselective β-blocker

Pregnancy category B

Action: Competitively blocks stimulation of β-adrenergic receptor within vascular smooth muscle; produces chronotropic, inotropic activity (decreases rate of SA node discharge, increases recovery time), slows conduction of AV node, decreases heart rate, which decreases O_2 consumption in myocardium; also decreases renin-aldosterone-angiotensin system and at high doses inhibits $β_2$ receptors in bronchial system

➥ **Therapeutic Outcome:** Decreased B/P in hypertension, heart rate

Uses: Mild to moderate hypertension

Dosage and routes
Adult: PO 5 mg bid; usual dose 15 mg/day (5 mg tid); may increase by 10 mg/day q3-4 wk to a max of 60 mg/day

G *Elderly:* PO 5 mg qd increase by 5 mg q3-4 wk

Available forms: Tabs 5, 10 mg

Adverse effects
(*italic* = common; **bold** = life-threatening)
CNS: Insomnia, dizziness, hallucinations, anxiety, fatigue, headache, depression
CV: Hypotension, bradycardia, **CHF,** edema, chest pain, palpitations, claudication, tachycardia, **AV block, pulmonary edema, bradycardia, dysrhythmias**
EENT: Visual changes, sore throat, *double vision,* dry burning eyes, nasal stuffiness
GI: Nausea, vomiting, **ischemic colitis,** diarrhea, *abdominal pain,* **mesenteric arterial thrombosis,** flatulence, constipation
GU: Impotence, frequency
HEMA: **Agranulocytosis, thrombocytopenia, purpura**
INTEG: Rash, alopecia, pruritus, fever
MISC: Joint pain, muscle pain
RESP: **Bronchospasm,** *dyspnea,* cough, rales

Contraindications: Hypersensitivity to β-blockers, cardiogenic shock, 2nd- or 3rd-degree heart block, sinus bradycardia, CHF, cardiac failure, bronchial asthma, severe COPD

Precautions: Major surgery, pregnancy **B,** lactation, diabetes mellitus, renal disease, thyroid disease, COPD, well-compensated heart failure, CAD, nonallergic bronchospasm, peripheral vascular disease, hepatic disease

🔃 **Do Not Confuse:**
pindolol/Parlodel, pindolol/Plendil

Pharmacokinetics
Absorption	Well absorbed
Distribution	Crosses placenta; some penetration in CNS, protein binding 40%
Metabolism	Liver, moderately (60%-65%)
Excretion	Kidneys, unchanged (30%-45%)
Half-life	3-4 hr

Pharmacodynamics
Onset	Unknown
Peak	2-4 hr
Duration	8-24 hr

Interactions
Individual drugs
Hydralazine, methyldopa, prazosin, reserpine: ↑ hypotension, bradycardia
Thyroid: ↓ effect of β-blockers
Verapamil: ↑ cardiac depression
Drug classifications
Anticholinergics, nitrates: ↑ hypotension
Anticholinergics, cardiac glycosides: ↑ bradycardia
Antihypertensives: ↑ hypertension
$β_2$-Adrenergic agonists: ↑ effect of β-blockers
NSAIDs, sympathomimetics: ↓ antihypertensive effect
Sulfonylureas: ↓ hypoglycemic effect
Theophyllines: ↓ bronchodilatation
🌿 *Herb/drug*
Aconite: ↑ toxicity, death
Astragalus, cola tree: ↑ or ↓ antihypertensive effect
Barberry, betony, black catechu, black cohosh, bloodroot, broom, burdock, cat's claw, dandelion, goldenseal, Irish moss, Jamaica dogwood, kelp, khella, mistletoe, parsley: ↑ antihypertensive effect
Coltsfoot, guarana, khat, licorice: ↓ antihypertensive effect
Lab test interferences
↑ liver function tests
↑ renal function tests
False: ↑ Urinary catecholamines
Interference: Glucose, insulin tolerance test

P

NURSING CONSIDERATIONS
Assessment
- Monitor B/P during beginning treatment, periodically thereafter; pulse q4h; note rate, rhythm, quality: apical/radial pulse before administration; notify prescriber of any significant changes (pulse <50 bpm)
- Obtain baselines in renal, liver function tests before therapy begins
- Assess for edema in feet, legs daily; monitor I&O, daily weight; check for jugular vein distention, rales bilaterally, dyspnea (CHF)
- Monitor skin turgor, dryness of mucous membranes for hydration status, especially
G elderly

Nursing diagnoses
☑ Cardiac output, decreased (uses)
☑ Injury, risk for (adverse reactions)
☑ Knowledge, deficient (teaching)
☑ Noncompliance (teaching)

Implementation
- Given ac, hs, tab may be crushed or swallowed whole; give with food to prevent GI upset
- Store protected from light, moisture; place in cool environment

Patient/family education
◆• Teach patient not to discontinue drug abruptly; taper over 2 wk; may cause precipitate angina if stopped abruptly
- Teach patient not to use OTC products containing α-adrenergic stimulants (such as nasal decongestants, cold preparations); to avoid alcohol, smoking, and to limit sodium intake as prescribed
- Teach patient how to take pulse and B/P at home; advise when to notify prescriber
- Instruct patient to comply with weight control, dietary adjustments, modified exercise program
- Tell patient to carry/wear emergency ID to identify drug being taken, allergies; tell patient drug controls symptoms but does not cure
- Caution patient to avoid hazardous activities if dizziness, drowsiness present
- Teach patient to report symptoms of CHF: difficult breathing, especially on exertion or when lying down, night cough, swelling of extremities or bradycardia, dizziness, confusion, depression, fever
- Teach patient to take drug as prescribed, not to double doses, skip doses; take any missed doses as soon as remembered if at least 4 hr until next dose; to take with or immediately after meals if GI symptoms occur

Evaluation
Positive therapeutic outcome
- Decreased B/P in hypertension (after 1-2 wk)

Treatment of overdose: Lavage, **IV** atropine for bradycardia, **IV** theophylline for bronchospasm, digitalis, O_2, diuretic for cardiac failure, hemodialysis, **IV** glucose for hyperglycemia, **IV** diazepam (or phenytoin) for seizures

---

pioglitazone (Rx)
(pie-oh-glye′ta-zone)
Actos
Func. class.: Antidiabetic, oral
Chem. class.: Thiazolidinedione
Pregnancy category C

Action: Improves insulin resistance by hepatic glucose metabolism, insulin receptor kinase activity, insulin receptor phosphorylation

→Therapeutic Outcome: Decreased symptoms of diabetes mellitus

Uses: Stable adult-onset diabetes mellitus, type 2

Dosage and routes
Monotherapy
Adult: PO 15-30 mg qd, may increase to 45 mg/day

Combination therapy
Adult: PO 15-30 mg qd with a sulfonylurea, metformin, or insulin; decrease sulfonylurea dose if hypoglycemia occurs; decrease insulin dose by 10%-25% if hypoglycemia occurs or if plasma glucose is <100 mg/dl, max 45 mg/day

Hepatic dose
Do not use in active liver disease or if ALT >2.5 × ULN

Available forms: Tabs 15, 30, 45 mg
Adverse effects
(*italic* = common; **bold** = life-threatening)
CNS: Headache
ENDO: Aggravated diabetes mellitus
MISC: Myalgia, sinusitis, upper respiratory tract infection, pharyngitis

Contraindications: Hypersensitivity to thiazolidinediones, diabetic ketoacidosis,
P lactation, children

G Precautions: Pregnancy **C**, elderly, thyroid disease, hepatic, renal disease, edema, CHF

Pharmacokinetics

Absorption	Unknown
Distribution	Unknown
Metabolism	Unknown
Excretion	Kidneys
Half-life	3-7 hr, terminal 16-24 hr

Pharmacodynamics

Onset	Unknown
Peak	6-12 wk
Duration	Unknown

Interactions
Individual drugs
Ketoconazole: ↓ pioglitazone effect
Drug classifications
Oral contraceptives: ↓ effect, use an alternate contraceptive method
⚠ *Herb/drug*
Alfalfa, aloe, basil, bay, bilberry, bitter melon, black catechu, buchu, burdock, coriander, dandelion, eyebright (po), fenugreek, garlic, ginseng, glucomannan, glucosamine, goat's rue, gymnema, horehound, horse chestnut, jambul, myrrh, myrtle: ↑ antidiabetic effect
Bee pollen, blue cohosh, broom, chromium, elecampane, eucalyptus, gotu kola: ↓ antidiabetic effect
Chromium, coenzyme Q10, fenugreek: ↑ hypoglycemia
Glucosamine: ↓ blood glucose control

NURSING CONSIDERATIONS
Assessment
• Assess for hypoglycemic reactions (sweating, weakness, dizziness, anxiety, tremors, hunger), hyperglycemic reactions soon after meals
• Assess CBC (baseline, q3 mo) during treatment; check liver function tests periodically; check AST, LDH, FBS, glycosylated Hgb, fasting plasma insulin, plasma lipids, lipoproteins, B/P, body weight during treatment

Nursing diagnoses
✓ Nutrition: more than body requirements, imbalanced (uses)
✓ Knowledge, deficient (teaching)

Implementation
• Convert from other oral hypoglycemic agents; change may be made without gradual dosage change; monitor serum or urine glucose and ketones tid during conversion
• Give once a day; give with meals to decrease GI upset and provide best absorption
• Give tabs crushed and mixed with meal or fluids for patients with difficulty swallowing

• Store in airtight container in cool environment

Patient/family education
• Teach patient to use capillary blood glucose test or Chemstrip tid
• Teach patient symptoms of hypo/hyperglycemia, what to do about each
• Advise patient that drug must be continued on daily basis; explain consequence of discontinuing drug abruptly
• Advise patient to avoid OTC medications or herbal preparations unless approved by prescriber
• Advise patient that diabetes is life-long illness; that this drug is not a cure, only controls symptoms
• Advise patient that all food included in diet plan must be eaten to prevent hypoglycemia
• Advise patient to carry/wear emergency ID and glucagon emergency kit for emergencies
• Instruct patient to notify prescriber if oral contraceptives are used
• Teach patient not to use if breast-feeding

Evaluation
Positive therapeutic outcome
• Decrease in polyuria, polydipsia, polyphagia; clear sensorium; absence of dizziness; stable gait; blood glucose at normal level

---

⚠ **HIGH ALERT**

pipecuronium (Rx)
(pip-e-kyoor'oh'nee-um)
Arduran
Func. class.: Neuromuscular blocker (nondepolarizing)
Chem. class.: Synthetic curariform

Pregnancy category C

Action: Inhibits transmission of nerve impulses by binding with cholinergic receptor sites, antagonizing action of acetylcholine; no analgesic response

→ **Therapeutic Outcome:** Paralysis of all skeletal muscles

Uses: Facilitation of endotracheal intubation, skeletal muscle relaxation during mechanical ventilation, surgery, or general anesthesia

Dosage and routes
Adult: **IV** dosage is individualized; in patients with normal renal function who are not obese, initial dose 70-85 mcg/kg; maintenance dose 10-15 mcg/kg
▣ *Child 1-14 yr:* **IV** 57 mcg/kg

P *Child 3 mo-1 yr:* **IV** 40 mcg/kg

Available forms: Inj 10-mg vials

Adverse effects

(*italic* = common; **bold** = life-threatening)

CNS: Hypesthesia, CNS depression

CV: Bradycardia, tachycardia, increased or decreased B/P, ventricular extrasystole, **myocardial ischemia, CVA, thrombosis, atrial fibrillation**

EENT: Increased secretions

GU: Anuria

INTEG: Rash, urticaria

META: Hypoglycemia, hyperkalemia, increased creatinine

MS: Weakness to prolonged skeletal muscle relaxation

RESP: **Prolonged apnea, bronchospasm, cyanosis, respiratory depression**

Contraindications: Hypersensitivity to bromide ion

Precautions: Pregnancy **C**, renal disease,
P cardiac disease, lactation, children <3 mo, fluid and electrolyte imbalances, neuromuscular diseases, respiratory disease, obesity

Pharmacokinetics	
Absorption	Complete bioavailability
Distribution	Unknown
Metabolism	Unknown
Excretion	Kidneys, unchanged (>75%)
Half-life	1½ hr; increased in renal disease

Pharmacodynamics	
Onset	30-45 sec
Peak	3-5 min
Duration	1-2 hr

Interactions

Individual drugs

Colistin, magnesium, polymyxin B, quinidine: ↑ paralysis length and intensity

Drug classifications

Aminoglycosides, anesthetics (general): ↑ paralysis length and intensity

Tetracyclines: ↑ neuromuscular blockade

NURSING CONSIDERATIONS

Assessment

• Monitor vital signs (B/P, pulse, respirations, airway) until fully recovered; rate, depth, pattern of respirations, strength of hand grip; patient should be intubated before use

• Monitor for electrolyte imbalances (potassium, magnesium) before drug is used; electrolyte imbalances may lead to increased action of this drug

• Monitor for recovery: decreased paralysis of face, diaphragm, leg, arm, rest of body; residual weakness and respiratory problems may occur during recovery period

• Assess for hypersensitive reactions: rash, fever, respiratory distress, pruritus; drug should be discontinued

Nursing diagnoses

☑ Breathing pattern, ineffective (uses)

☑ Communication, impaired verbal (adverse reactions)

☑ Fear (adverse reactions)

☑ Knowledge, deficient (teaching)

Implementation

• Use peripheral nerve stimulator (anesthesiologist) to determine neuromuscular blockade; deep tendon reflexes should be monitored during extended periods

• Give **IV** after reconstituting with 0.9% NaCl, D₅W, D₅/0.9% NaCl, LR, sterile water for inj; sol with benzyl alcohol should not be used for
P newborns; should be administered only by qualified person, usually an anesthesiologist; do not administer IM

• Store in light-resistant area (powder); refrigerate unused portions (sterile water); use within 24 hr

Patient/family education

• Provide reassurance to patient if communication is difficult during recovery from neuromuscular blockade

• Provide patient with explanation of all procedures or treatments; patient will remain conscious if anesthesia is not given also

Evaluation

Positive therapeutic outcome

• Paralysis of jaw, eyelid, head, neck, rest of body as evaluated by peripheral nerve stimulator

Treatment of overdose: Edrophonium or neostigmine, atropine, monitor VS; may require mechanical ventilation

---

piperacillin (Rx)

(pi-per′a-sill-in)

Pipracil

Func. class.: Broad-spectrum antiinfective

Chem. class.: Extended-spectrum penicillin

Pregnancy category B

Action: Interferes with cell wall replication of susceptible organisms; osmotically unstable cell wall swells and bursts from osmotic pressure

---

 Herb/drug   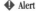 Do Not Crush   ◆ Alert   ◆ᵤ Key Drug   **G** Geriatric   **P** Pediatric

⮞ Therapeutic Outcome: Bactericidal effects for gram-positive cocci *Staphylococcus aureus, Streptococcus pyogenes, Streptococcus viridans, Streptococcus faecalis, Streptococcus bovis, Streptococcus pneumoniae;* gram-negative cocci *Neisseria gonorrhoeae, Neisseria meningitidis;* gram-positive bacilli *Clostridium perfringens, Clostridium tetani;* gram-negative bacilli *Bacteroides, Fusobacterium nucleatum, Escherichia coli, Klebsiella, Proteus mirabilis, Proteus vulgaris, Proteus rettgeri, Morganella morganii, Enterobacter, Citrobacter, Pseudomonas aeruginosa, Serratia, Acinetobacter, Peptococcus, Peptostreptococcus, Eubacterium*

Uses: Respiratory tract, skin, skin structure, urinary tract, bone, and joint infections; gonorrhea, pneumonia, endocarditis, septicemia, meningitis, sinusitis; infections caused by penicillinase-producing staphylococci, streptococci; may be combined with an aminoglycoside for *Pseudomonas* infection

Dosage and routes
Urinary tract infections
Adult: **IV** 8-16 g/day (125-200 mg/kg/day) in divided doses q6-8h

Serious systemic infections
P *Adult and child >12 yr:* IM/**IV** 2-4 g q4-6h (2 g/site IM)

P *Child <12 yr:* IM/**IV** 200-300 mg/kg/day in divided doses q4-6h

P *Neonates <36 wk:* **IV** 75 mg/kg q12h in the 1st wk of life, then q8h in 2nd wk

P *Full term infants:* **IV** 75 mg/kg q8h in 1st wk of life, then q6h thereafter

Prophylaxis of surgical infections
Adult: **IV** 2 g 30-60 min before procedure; may be repeated during or after surgery

Renal dose
Adult: **IV** CCr 20-40 ml/min give q8h, CCr <20 ml/min give q12h; CCr 10-50 ml/min give q6-8h, CCr <10 ml/min give q8h

Available forms: Powder for inj 2, 3, 4, 40 g

Adverse effects
(*italic* = common; **bold** = life-threatening)
CNS: Lethargy, hallucinations, anxiety, depression, twitching, **coma, seizures**
GI: Nausea, vomiting, diarrhea, increased AST, ALT, abdominal pain, glossitis, colitis, **pseudomembranous colitis**
GU: Oliguria, proteinuria, hematuria, **vaginitis, moniliasis, glomerulonephritis**
HEMA: Anemia, increased bleeding time, **bone marrow depression, thrombocytopenia**
META: Hypokalemia, hypernatremia
SYST: **Serum sickness, anaphylaxis**

Contraindications: Hypersensitivity to
P penicillins; neonates

Precautions: Pregnancy **B,** hypersensitivity to cephalosporins, CHF, renal disease, seizures, lactation

Pharmacokinetics
Absorption	Well absorbed (80%)
Distribution	Widely distributed; crosses placenta
Metabolism	Not metabolized
Excretion	Kidneys, unchanged (90%); bile (10%); breast milk
Half-life	0.7-1.3 hr

Pharmacodynamics
	IM	IV
Onset	Rapid	Rapid
Peak	30-50 min	Inf end

Interactions
Individual drugs
Aspirin, probenecid: ↑ piperacillin levels, ↓ renal excretion
Drug classifications
Aminoglycosides: ↓ half-life in renal disease
Contraceptives (oral): ↓ contraceptive effectiveness
Diuretics, glucocorticoids: ↑ hypokalemia
Hepatotoxic agents: ↑ hepatotoxicity
Tetracyclines: ↓ antimicrobial effectiveness
Herb/drug
Acidophilus: Do not give with antiinfective
Khat: ↓ absorption
Lab test interferences
False positive: Urine glucose, urine protein, Coombs' test

P

NURSING CONSIDERATIONS
Assessment
• Assess patient for previous sensitivity reaction to penicillins or other cephalosporins; cross-sensitivity between penicillins and cephalosporins is common
• Assess patient for signs and symptoms of infection including characteristics of wounds, sputum, urine, stool, WBC >10,000/mm^3, fever; obtain baseline information and during treatment
• Obtain C&S before beginning drug therapy to identify if correct treatment has been initiated
• Assess for allergic reactions: rash, urticaria, pruritus, chills, fever, joint pain; angioedema

may occur a few days after therapy begins; epINEPHrine, resuscitation equipment should be available for anaphylactic reaction

 • Identify urine output; if decreasing, notify prescriber (may indicate nephrotoxicity); also check for increased BUN, creatinine
• Monitor blood studies: AST, ALT, CBC, Hct, bilirubin, LDH, alkaline phosphatase, Coombs' test monthly if patient is on long-term therapy
• Monitor electrolytes: potassium, sodium, chloride monthly if patient is on long-term therapy
• Assess bowel pattern daily; if severe diarrhea occurs, drug should be discontinued; may indicate pseudomembranous colitis
• Monitor for bleeding: ecchymosis, bleeding gums, hematuria, stool guaiac daily if on long-term therapy
• Assess for overgrowth of infection: perineal itching, fever, malaise, redness, pain, swelling, drainage, rash, diarrhea, change in cough, sputum

Nursing diagnoses
☑ Infection, risk for (uses)
☑ Diarrhea (adverse reactions)
☑ Injury, risk for (adverse reactions)
☑ Knowledge, deficient (teaching)
☑ Noncompliance (teaching)

Implementation
IM route
• Reconstitute 2 g/4 ml, 3 g/6 ml, 4 g/7.8 ml with sterile water, 0.9% NaCl, bacteriostatic water, 0.5% or 1% lidocaine without epINEPHrine
• Inject deep in large muscle mass, massage; split inj >2 g into 2 inj

IV IV route
• Reconstitute with 5 ml or more 0.9% NaCl, bacteriostatic water; shake sol to dissolve
• Change **IV** sites q48h to prevent phlebitis and pain
• Give direct **IV** over 3-5 min
• Give by intermittent inf by diluting in 50 ml or more D_5W, 0.9% NaCl, D_5/0.9% NaCl, LR, give over 20-30 min by Y-site; discontinue primary inf during intermittent inf

Syringe compatibilities: Heparin

Y-site compatibilities: Acyclovir, aldesleukin, allopurinol, amifostine, aztreonam, ciprofloxacin, cyclophosphamide, diltiazem, enalaprilat, esmolol, famotidine, fludarabine, foscarnet, heparin, hydromorphone, IL-2, labetalol, lorazepam, magnesium sulfate, melphalan, meperidine, midazolam, morphine, perphenazine, propofol, ranitidine,

tacrolimus, teniposide, theophylline, thiotepa, verapamil, zidovudine

Y-site incompatibilities: Ondansetron, fluconazole, sargramostim, vinorelbine

Additive compatibilities: Ciprofloxacin, clindamycin, fluconazole, hydrocortisone sodium succinate, ofloxacin, potassium chloride, verapamil

Additive incompatibilities: Aminoglycosides

Patient/family education
• Teach patient to report sore throat, bruising, bleeding, joint pain; may indicate blood dyscrasias (rare)
• Advise patient to contact prescriber if vaginal itching, loose foul-smelling stools, furry tongue occur; may indicate superinfection
• Advise patient to notify prescriber of diarrhea with blood or pus, which may indicate pseudomembranous colitis

Evaluation
Positive therapeutic outcome
• Absence of signs/symptoms of infection (WBC <10,000/mm^3, temp WNL, absence of red, draining wounds)
• Reported improvement in symptoms of infection

Treatment of anaphylaxis: Withdraw drug, maintain airway, administer epINEPHrine, aminophylline, O_2, **IV** corticosteroids

---

piperacillin/tazobactam (Rx)
Zosyn
Func. class.: Broad-spectrum antiinfective
Chem. class.: Extended-spectrum penicillin
Pregnancy category B

Action: Interferes with cell wall replication of susceptible organisms; osmotically unstable cell wall swells and bursts from osmotic pressure

➡ **Therapeutic Outcome:** Bactericidal effects for piperacillin-resistant β-lactamase, *Escherichia coli, Staphylococcus aureus, Bacteroides fragilis, Haemophilus influenzae*

Uses: Respiratory tract, skin, skin structure, urinary tract, bone, and joint infections; gonorrhea, pneumonia, infections from penicillinase-producing staphylococci, streptococci

---

Dosage and routes
Nosocomial pneumonia
Adult: **IV** 3.375 g q6-8h with an aminoglycoside × 1-2 wk; continue aminoglycoside only if *Pseudomonas aeruginosa* is isolated

Other infections
Adult: **IV** inf 6-12 g/day, given 2.25 g q8h to 3.375 g q6h over 30 min × 7-10 days

Renal dose
Adult: **IV** CCr 20-40 ml/min 2.25 g q6h; CCr <20 ml/min 2.25 g q8h

Available forms: Powder for inj 2 g piperacillin/0.25 g tazobactam; 3 g piperacillin/0.375 g tazobactam, 4 g piperacillin/0.5 g tazobactam, 36 g piperacillin/4.5 g tazobactam

Adverse effects
(*italic* = common; **bold** = life-threatening)
CNS: Headache, insomnia, agitation, dizziness, fever, lethargy, hallucinations, anxiety, depression, twitching
GI: *Nausea, vomiting, diarrhea,* increased AST, ALT, abdominal pain, glossitis, constipation, **pseudomembranous colitis**
INTEG: Rash, pruritus
SYST: **Serum sickness, anaphylaxis**
GU: **Oliguria, proteinuria, hematuria,** *vaginitis, moniliasis,* **glomerulonephritis**
HEMA: Anemia, ↑ bleeding time, **bone marrow depression**
META: Hypokalemia, hypernatremia

Contraindications: Hypersensitivity to penicillins; neonates

Precautions: Pregnancy **B,** CHF, renal disease, lactation, children, seizures, hypersensitivity to cephalosporins, renal insufficiency in children

Pharmacokinetics
Absorption	Well absorbed (80%)
Distribution	Widely distributed; crosses placenta
Metabolism	Not metabolized
Excretion	Kidneys, unchanged (90%); bile (10%); breast milk
Half-life	0.7-1.3 hr

Pharmacodynamics
Onset	Rapid
Peak	Inf end

Interactions
Individual drugs
Aminoglycosides (**IV**): ↓ piperacillin effect
Aspirin, probenecid: ↑ piperacillin levels

Drug classifications
Anticoagulants (oral): ↑ anticoagulant effects
Contraceptives (oral): ↓ contraceptive effectiveness
Tetracyclines: ↓ antimicrobial effectiveness

Herb/drug
Acidophilus: Do not use with antiinfectives
Khat: ↓ absorption

Lab test interferences
False positive: Urine glucose, urine protein, Coombs' test

NURSING CONSIDERATIONS
Assessment
- Assess patient for previous sensitivity reaction to penicillins or other cephalosporins, cross-sensitivity between penicillins and cephalosporins is common
- Assess patient for signs and symptoms of infection including characteristics of wounds, sputum, urine, stool, WBC >10,000/mm^3, fever; obtain baseline information and during treatment
- Obtain C&S before beginning drug therapy to identify if correct treatment has been initiated
- Assess for allergic reactions: rash, urticaria, pruritus, chills, fever, joint pain; angioedema may occur a few days after therapy begins; epINEPHrine, resuscitation equipment should be available for anaphylactic reaction
- Identify urine output; if decreasing, notify prescriber (may indicate nephrotoxicity); also check for increased BUN, creatinine
- Monitor blood studies: AST, ALT, CBC, Hct, bilirubin, LDH, alkaline phosphatase, Coombs' test monthly if patient is on long-term therapy
- Monitor electrolytes: potassium, sodium, chloride monthly if patient is on long-term therapy
- Assess bowel pattern daily; if severe diarrhea occurs, drug should be discontinued; may indicate pseudomembranous colitis
- Monitor for bleeding: ecchymosis, bleeding gums, hematuria, stool guaiac daily if on long-term therapy
- Assess for overgrowth of infection: perineal itching, fever, malaise, redness, pain, swelling, drainage, rash, diarrhea, change in cough, sputum

Nursing diagnoses
☑ Infection, risk for (uses)
☑ Diarrhea (adverse reactions)
☑ Injury, risk for (adverse reactions)
☑ Knowledge, deficient (teaching)
☑ Noncompliance (teaching)

P

Implementation

- Reconstitute with 5 ml or more 0.9% NaCl, bacteriostatic water; shake sol to dissolve
- Give by intermittent inf by diluting in 50 ml or more D_5W, 0.9% NaCl, D_5/0.9% NaCl, LR; give over 20-30 min by Y-site; discontinue primary inf during intermittent inf
- Change **IV** sites q48h to prevent phlebitis and pain
- Give direct **IV** over 3-5 min

Y-site compatibilities: Aminophylline, aztreonam, bleomycin, bumetanide, buprenorphine, butorphanol, calcium gluconate, carboplatin, carmustine, cefepime, cimetidine, clindamycin, cyclophosphamide, cytarabine, dexamethasone, diphenhydrAMINE, DOPamine, enalaprilat, etoposide, floxuridine, fluconazole, fludarabine, fluorouracil, furosemide, gallium, granisetron, heparin, hydrocortisone, hydromorphone, ifosfamide, leucovorin, lorazepam, magnesium sulfate, mannitol, meperidine, mesna, methotrexate, methylPREDNISolone, metoclopramide, metronidazole, morphine, ondansetron, plicomycin, potassium chloride, ranitidine, sargramostim, sodium bicarbonate, thiotepa, trimethoprim/sulfamethoxazole, vinBLAStine, vinCRIStine, zidovudine

Y-site incompatibilities: Fluconazole, ondansetron, sargramostim, vinorelbine

Patient/family education

- Teach patient to report sore throat, bruising, bleeding, joint pain; may indicate blood dyscrasias (rare)
- Advise patient to contact prescriber if vaginal itching, loose foul-smelling stools, furry tongue occur; may indicate superinfection
- Advise patient to notify prescriber of diarrhea with blood or pus, which may indicate pseudomembranous colitis

Evaluation

Positive therapeutic outcome
- Absence of signs/symptoms of infection (WBC <10,000/mm³, temp WNL, absence of red, draining wounds)
- Reported improvement in symptoms of infection

Treatment of anaphylaxis: Withdraw
drug, maintain airway, administer epINEPHrine, aminophylline, O_2, **IV** corticosteroids

pirbuterol (Rx)
(peer-byoo'ter-ole)
Maxair
Func. class.: Bronchodilator
Chem. class.: β-Adrenergic agonist

Pregnancy category C

Action: Relaxes bronchial smooth muscle by direct action on $β_2$-adrenergic receptors, with increased levels of cAMP and increased bronchodilatation, diuresis, and cardiac and CNS stimulation

➡ **Therapeutic Outcome:** Bronchodilatation with ease of breathing

Uses: Reversible bronchospasm (prevention, treatment), including asthma, may be given with theophylline or steroids

Dosage and routes

P *Adult and child >12 yr:* INH 1-2 (0.4 mg) q4-6h; max 12 inh/day

Available forms: Aerosol delivers 0.2 mg pirbuterol/actuation

Adverse effects
(*italic* = common; **bold** = life-threatening)
CNS: Tremors, anxiety, insomnia, headache, dizziness, stimulation, restlessness, hallucinations, drowsiness, irritability
CV: Palpitations, tachycardia, hypertension, angina, hypotension, **dysrhythmias**
EENT: Dry nose and mouth, irritation of nose, throat
GI: Gastritis, nausea, vomiting, anorexia
MS: Muscle cramps
RESP: **Paradoxical bronchospasm,** dyspnea, coughing

Contraindications: Hypersensitivity to sympathomimetics, tachycardia

Precautions: Lactation, pregnancy **C**, cardiac disorders, hyperthyroidism, diabetes mellitus, prostatic hypertrophy

Pharmacokinetics	
Absorption	Minimally absorbed
Distribution	Unknown
Metabolism	Liver
Excretion	Unknown
Half-life	2 hr

Pharmacodynamics	
Onset	5-15 min
Peak	1-1½ hr
Duration	5 hr

Interactions
Drug classifications
Antidepressants (tricyclics), antihistamines, thyroid hormones: ↑ pirbuterol action
β-Adrenergic blockers: Block therapeutic effect
Bronchodilators, aerosol: ↑ action of bronchodilator
MAOIs: ↑ chance of hypertensive crisis
🗹 *Herb/drug*
Cola nut, guarana, yerba maté: ↑ action of both
Green tea (large amounts), guarana: ↑ effect

NURSING CONSIDERATIONS
Assessment
• Monitor respiratory function: vital capacity, FEV, ABGs, lung sounds, heart rate, rhythm (baseline)
• Monitor for evidence of allergic reactions, paradoxic bronchospasm (can occur rapidly); withhold dose and notify prescriber

Nursing diagnoses
✓ Airway clearance, ineffective (uses)
✓ Gas exchange, impaired (uses)
✓ Knowledge, deficient (teaching)

Implementation
• Give after shaking; have patient exhale, place mouthpiece in mouth, inhale slowly, hold breath, remove, exhale slowly; allow at least 1 min between inhalations
• Store in light-resistant container; do not expose to temp over 86° F (30° C)

Patient/family education
• Advise patient not to use OTC medications; extra stimulation may occur; to use this medication before other medications and allow at least 1 min between each to prevent overstimulation
• Teach patient use of inhaler; to avoid getting aerosol in eyes; blurring may result; to wash inhaler in warm water and dry daily; to avoid smoking, smoke-filled rooms, persons with respiratory tract infections; review package insert with patient
• Teach patient that paradoxic bronchospasm may occur and to stop drug immediately and notify prescriber; to limit caffeine products such as chocolate, coffee, tea, and colas
• Instruct patient on administration of dose; not to use more than prescribed; serious side effects may occur

Evaluation
Positive therapeutic outcome
• Absence of dyspnea, wheezing after 1 hr
• Improved airway exchange
• Improved ABGs

Treatment of overdose: Administer a β₂-adrenergic blocker

---

piroxicam (Rx)
(peer-ox′i-kam)
Apo-Piroxicam ✦, Feldene, Novopirocam ✦, Nu-Pirox, PMS-Piroxicam ✦
Func. class.: Nonsteroidal antiinflammatory
Chem. class.: Oxicam derivative

Pregnancy category B

Action: Inhibits prostaglandin synthesis by decreasing an enzyme needed for biosynthesis; analgesic, antiinflammatory

⮊ **Therapeutic Outcome:** Decreased pain, inflammation

Uses: Mild to moderate pain, osteoarthritis, rheumatoid arthritis

Dosage and routes
Adult: PO 20 mg qd or 10 mg bid

Available forms: Caps 10, 20 mg

Adverse effects
(*italic* = common; **bold** = life-threatening)
CNS: Dizziness, *drowsiness,* fatigue, tremors, confusion, insomnia, anxiety, depression, *headache*
CV: Tachycardia, peripheral edema, palpitations, **dysrhythmias**
EENT: Tinnitus, hearing loss, blurred vision
GI: Nausea, anorexia, vomiting, diarrhea, jaundice, **cholestatic hepatitis,** constipation, flatulence, cramps, dry mouth, peptic ulcer, **bleeding, ulceration, perforation**
GU: Nephrotoxicity: dysuria, hematuria, oliguria, azotemia
HEMA: Blood dyscrasias
INTEG: Purpura, rash, pruritus, sweating, photosensitivity
SYST: **Anaphylaxis**

Contraindications: Hypersensitivity, asthma, severe renal disease, severe hepatic disease, ulcer disease, cardiac disease

Precautions: Pregnancy **B,** lactation, children, bleeding disorders, GI disorders, cardiac disorders, hypersensitivity to other antiinflammatory agents, CHF, avoid in late pregnancy

P

Pharmacokinetics

Absorption	Well absorbed
Distribution	Unknown
Metabolism	Liver, extensively
Excretion	Kidneys, minimal; breast milk
Half-life	30-80 hr

Pharmacodynamics

Onset	1 hr
Peak	Unknown
Duration	48-72 hr

Interactions
Individual drugs
Alcohol, cycloSPORINE, lithium, methotrexate: ↑ toxicity
Drug classifications
Antidiabetics (oral): Hypoglycemia
Antihypertensives: ↓ effect of antihypertensives
Corticosteroids: ↑ toxicity
Diuretics: ↓ effectiveness of diuretics
☑ **Herb/drug**

Arginine, gossypol: ↑ gastric irritation
Bearberry, bilberry: ↑ NSAIDs effect
Bogbean, chondroitin: ↑ bleeding risk

NURSING CONSIDERATIONS
Assessment
• Monitor blood counts during therapy; watch for decreasing platelets; if low, therapy may need to be discontinued, restarted after hematologic recovery; check for blood dyscrasia (thrombocytopenia): bruising, fatigue, bleeding, poor healing
• Assess for pain: location, duration, ROM, before and 1-2 hr after administration
• Assess for aspirin sensitivity, asthma, nasal polyps; these may develop into allergic reactions

Nursing diagnoses
☑ Pain, chronic (uses)
☑ Mobility, impaired (uses)
☑ Knowledge, deficient (teaching)
☑ Injury, risk for (adverse reactions)

Implementation
• Administer to patient whole; give with food or milk to decrease gastric symptoms
🚫• Do not crush, chew caps

Patient/family education
• Teach patient that drug must be continued for prescribed time to be effective; to avoid aspirin, alcoholic beverages, and other OTC medications unless approved by prescriber
• Caution patient to report bleeding, bruising, fatigue, malaise, since blood dyscrasias do occur

• Instruct patient to use caution when driving; drowsiness, dizziness may occur
• Teach patient to take with a full glass of water to enhance absorption; do not crush, break, or chew

Evaluation
Positive therapeutic outcome
• Decreased pain
• Decreased inflammation
• Increased mobility

plasma protein fraction (Rx)
Plasmanate, Plasma Plex, Plasmatein, Protenate
Func. class.: Blood derivative
Chem. class.: Human plasma in sodium chloride

Pregnancy category C

Action: Exerts similar oncotic pressure as human plasma, expands blood volume, shifts water from extravascular space to intravascular space

➔**Therapeutic Outcome:** Shift of fluid from extravascular into intravascular space

Uses: Hypovolemic shock, hypoproteinemia, ARDS, preoperative cardiopulmonary bypass, acute liver failure, nephrotic syndrome

Dosage and routes
Hypovolemia
Adult: **IV** inf 250-500 ml (12.5-25 g of protein), max 10 ml/min
P *Child:* **IV** inf 22-33 ml/kg at 5-10 ml/min

Hypoproteinemia
Adult: **IV** inf 1000-1500 ml qd, max 8 ml/min

Available forms: Inj 5%

Adverse effects
(*italic* = common; **bold** = life-threatening)
CNS: Fever, chills, headache, paresthesias, flushing
CV: **Fluid overload,** hypotension, erratic pulse
GI: Nausea, vomiting, increased salivation
INTEG: Rash, urticaria, cyanosis
RESP: Altered respirations, dyspnea, **pulmonary edema**

Contraindications: Hypersensitivity, CHF, severe anemia, renal insufficiency

Precautions: Decreased salt intake, decreased cardiac reserve, lack of albumin deficiency, hepatic disease, renal disease, pregnancy **C**

Pharmacokinetics

Absorption	Completely absorbed
Distribution	Intravascular space
Metabolism	Unknown
Excretion	Unknown
Half-life	Unknown

Pharmacodynamics

Onset	15-30 min
Peak	Unknown
Duration	Unknown

Interactions: None
Lab test interferences
False: ↑ Alkaline phosphatase

NURSING CONSIDERATIONS
Assessment
- Monitor blood studies: Hct, Hgb; electrolytes, serum protein, if serum protein declines, dyspnea, hypoxemia can result
- Monitor B/P (decreased), pulse (erratic), respiration during inf; CVP, jugular vein distention, PWP (increases if overload occurs); shortness of breath, anxiety, insomnia, expiratory rales, frothy blood-tinged cough, cyanosis indicate pulmonary overload
- Monitor I&O ratio; urinary output may decrease
- Assess for allergy: fever, rash, itching, chills, flushing, urticaria, nausea, vomiting, or hypotension requires discontinuation of inf; use new lot if therapy reinstituted, premedicate with diphenhydrAMINE

Nursing diagnoses
- ☑ Fluid volume, deficient (uses)
- ☑ Cardiac output, decreased (uses)
- ☑ Fluid volume, excess (adverse reactions)

Implementation
- Give by **IV**; no dilution required; use infusion pump, large-gauge needle (≥20 G); discard unused portion; infuse slowly within 4 hr of opening
- Provide adequate hydration before administration
- When storing, check type of albumin, date; may have to refrigerate

Additive compatibilities:
Carbohydrate and electrolyte sol, whole blood, packed RBCs, chloramphenicol, tetracycline

Additive incompatibilities:
Protein hydrolysate sol, amino acids sol, alcohol, norepinephrine

Patient/family education
- Explain reason for and expected result of medication

Evaluation
Positive therapeutic outcome
- Increased B/P
- Decreased edema
- Increased serum albumin

❗ HIGH ALERT

plicamycin (Rx)
(plik-a-mi′cin)
Mithramycin, Mithracin
Func. class.: Antineoplastic, antibiotic; hypocalcemic
Chem. class.: Crystalline aglycone

Pregnancy category X

Action: Inhibits DNA, RNA, protein synthesis; derived from *Streptomyces plicatus;* replication is decreased by binding to DNA; demonstrates calcium-lowering effect not related to its tumoricidal activity; also acts on osteoclasts and blocks action of parathyroid hormone; a vesicant

➡ Therapeutic Outcome: Prevention of rapidly growing malignant cells, decreased calcium levels

Uses: Testicular cancer, hypercalcemia, hypercalciuria, symptomatic treatment of advanced neoplasms

Dosage and routes
Testicular tumors
Adult: **IV** 25-30 mcg/kg/day × 8-10 days, max 30 mcg/kg/day

Hypercalcemia/hypercalciuria
Adult: **IV** 25 mcg/kg/day × 3-4 days; repeat at intervals of 1 wk

Available forms: Inj 2500 mcg/vial powder

Adverse effects
(*italic* = common; **bold** = life-threatening)
CNS: Drowsiness, weakness, lethargy, headache, flushing, fever, depression
GI: Nausea, vomiting, anorexia, diarrhea, stomatitis, increased liver enzymes
GU: Increased BUN, creatinine, **proteinuria**
HEMA: **Hemorrhage, thrombocytopenia,** decreased Pro-time, WBC count
INTEG: Rash, cellulitis, **extravasation,** facial flushing
META: Decreased serum calcium, potassium, phosphorus

Contraindications: Hypersensitivity, thrombocytopenia, bone marrow depression, bleeding disorders, pregnancy **X,** child <15 yr

---

Precautions: Renal disease, hepatic disease, electrolyte imbalances, lactation

Pharmacokinetics

Absorption	Completely absorbed
Distribution	Crosses blood-brain barrier; concentration in bone, liver, renal system
Metabolism	Unknown
Excretion	Kidneys
Half-life	Unknown

Pharmacodynamics
Unknown

Interactions
Individual drugs
Radiation: ↑ toxicity, bone marrow suppression
Drug classifications
Antineoplastics: ↑ toxicity, bone marrow suppression
◩ *Herb/drug*
Anise, arnica, chamomile, clove, dong quai, fenugreek, garlic, ginger, ginkgo, ginseng (Panax), licorice: ↑ bleeding risk

NURSING CONSIDERATIONS
Assessment
• Assess buccal cavity q8h for dryness, sores or ulceration, white patches, oral pain, bleeding, dysphagia; obtain prescription for viscous lidocaine (Xylocaine)
• Assess symptoms indicating severe allergic reaction: rash, pruritus, urticaria, purpuric skin lesions, itching, flushing
• Monitor CBC, differential, platelet count weekly; withhold drug if WBC is <4000/mm^3 or platelet count is <100,000/mm^3; notify prescriber of results if WBC <20,000/mm^3, platelets <150,000/mm^3
• Monitor renal function studies: BUN, creatinine, serum uric acid, urine CCr before and during therapy; I&O ratio; report fall in urine output to <30 ml/hr
• Monitor temp q4h (may indicate beginning of infection)
• Monitor liver function tests before and during therapy (bilirubin, AST, ALT, LDH) as needed or monthly; check for jaundice of skin and sclera, dark urine, clay-colored stools, itchy skin, abdominal pain, fever, diarrhea
• Assess for bleeding: hematuria, stool guaiac, bruising or petechiae, mucosa or orifices q8h, may progress to severe bleeding; check for inflammation of mucosa, breaks in skin

Nursing diagnoses
☑ Injury, risk for (adverse reactions)
☑ Body image, disturbed (adverse reactions)
☑ Infection, risk for (adverse reactions)
☑ Knowledge, deficient (teaching)

Implementation
• Avoid contact with skin; very irritating; wash completely to remove
• Give fluids **IV** or PO before chemotherapy to hydrate patient
• Give antacid before oral agent; give drug after evening meal, before bedtime; provide antiemetic 30-60 min before giving drug and prn to prevent vomiting; administer antibiotics for prophylaxis of infection
• Give top or systemic analgesics for pain
• Give in AM so drug can be eliminated before bedtime
• Provide liq diet: carbonated beverages; gelatin may be added if patient is not nauseated or vomiting
• Encourage patient to rinse mouth tid-qid with water, club soda; brush teeth bid-qid with soft brush or cotton-tipped applicators for stomatitis; use unwaxed dental floss
• Make sure drug is prepared by experienced personnel using proper precautions
• Give **IV** intermittent inf by diluting 2.5 mg/4.9 ml of sterile water (1 ml = 500 mcg); dilute single dose in 1000 ml of D$_5$W run over 4-6 hr; give slow **IV** inf using 20- or 21-G needle
• Administer EDTA for extravasation; apply ice compress

Y-site compatibilities: Allopurinol, amifostine, aztreonam, filgrastim, melphalan, piperacillin/tazobactam, teniposide, thiotepa, vinorelbine

Patient/family education
• Teach patient to avoid use of products containing aspirin or NSAIDs, razors, commercial mouthwash, since bleeding may occur; to report symptoms of bleeding (hematuria, tarry stools)
• Caution patient to report signs of anemia (fatigue, headache, irritability, faintness, shortness of breath)
• Advise patient to report any changes in breathing or coughing even several mo after treatment; to avoid crowds or persons with respiratory tract and other infections
• Advise patient that hair may be lost during treatment; a wig or hairpiece may make patient feel better; new hair may be different in color, texture
• Caution patient not to have any vaccinations without the advice of the prescriber; serious reactions can occur
• Advise patient that contraception is needed

◩ Herb/drug   Ⓢ Do Not Crush   ◆ Alert   ●π Key Drug   Ⓖ Geriatric   Ⓟ Pediatric during treatment and for several mo after completion of therapy

Evaluation
Positive therapeutic outcome
• Prevention of rapid division of malignant cells

porfirmer (Rx)
(pour'fur-meer)
Photofrin
Func. class.: Antineoplastic—misc.
Chem. class.: Photosensitizing agent

Pregnancy category C

Action: Used in photodynamic treatment (PDT) of tumors; antitumor and cytotoxic actions are light and O_2 dependent; used with 630 nm laser light

➡ **Therapeutic Outcome:** Prevention of growth of tumor

Uses: Esophageal cancer (completely obstructing), endobronchial non–small-cell lung cancer

Dosage and routes
Refer to guide for complete instructions

Adult: **IV** 2 mg/kg, then illumination with laser light 40-50 hr after inj; a second laser light application may be given 96-120 hr after inj; may repeat q30 days × 3

Endobronchial cancer
Adult: 200 joules/cm of tumor length

Available forms: Cake/powder for inj 75 mg

Adverse effects
(*italic* = common; **bold** = life-threatening)
CNS: Anxiety, confusion, insomnia
CV: Hypotension, hypertension, **atrial fibrillation, cardiac failure,** *tachycardia*
GI: Abdominal pain, constipation, diarrhea, dyspepsia, dysphagia, eructation, esophageal edema/bleeding, hematemesis, melena, nausea, vomiting, anorexia
MISC: Dehydration, weight decrease, anemia, photosensitivity reaction, UTI, moniliasis
RESP: **Pleural effusion,** *pneumonia, dyspnea, respiratory insufficiency,* **tracheoesophageal fistula**

Contraindications: Porphyria, porphyrin allergy (porfirmer); tracheoesophageal, bronchoesophageal fistula; major blood vessels with eroding tumors (PDT)

G **Precautions:** Elderly, pregnancy **C,**
P lactation, children

Pharmacokinetics
Absorption	Unknown
Distribution	Unknown
Metabolism	Unknown
Excretion	Unknown
Half-life	250 hr

Pharmacodynamics
Unknown

Interactions
Drug classifications
Phenothiazines, sulfonamides, sulfonylureas, tetracyclines, thiazides: ↑ photosensitivity

NURSING CONSIDERATIONS
Assessment
• Assess for ocular sensitivity; sensitivity to sun, bright lights, car headlights; patients should wear dark sunglasses with an average white light transmittance of <4%
• Assess for chest pain: may be so severe as to necessitate opiate analgesics
• Assess for extravasation at inj site: take care to protect from light

Nursing diagnoses
☑ Infection, risk for (adverse reactions)
☑ Knowledge, deficient (teaching)

Implementation
• Give as a single slow **IV** inj over 3-5 min at 2 mg/kg; reconstitute each vial with 31.8 ml of D_5 or 0.9% NaCl (2.5 mg/ml), shake well, do not mix with other drugs or sol, protect from light, and use immediately
• Laser light is initiated 630 nm wavelength laser light
• Wipe spills with damp cloth, avoid skin/eye contact, use rubber gloves, eye protection; dispose of material in polyethylene bag according to policy

Patient/family education
• Advise patient to report chest pain, eye sensitivity
• Advise patient to wear sunglasses; avoid exposure to sunlight or bright light for 30 days

P

**potassium acetate/
potassium bicarbonate** (Rx)
K+Care ET, K-Electrolyte, K-Ide, Klor-Con EF, K-Lyte, K-Vescent

**potassium bicarbonate/
potassium chloride** (Rx)
Klorvess, Klorvess Effervescent Granules, K-Lyte/Cl, Neo-K ✦

**potassium bicarbonate/
potassium citrate** (Rx)
Effer-K, K-Lyte DS

potassium chloride (R)
Apo-K ✦, Cena-K, Gen-K, K+care, K+10, Kalium Durules ✦, Kaochlor, Kaochlor S-F, Kaon-Cl, Kay Ciel, KCl, K-Dur, K-Lease, K-Long ✦, K-Lor, Klor-Con, Klorvess, Klotrix, K-Lyte/Cl powder, K-med, K-Norm, K-Sol, K-Tab, Micro-K, Micro-LS, Potasalan, Roychlor, Rum-K, Slow-K, Ten-K

**potassium chloride/
potassium bicarbonate/
potassium citrate**
Kaochlor Eff

potassium gluconate
Kaon, Kaylixir, K-G Elixir, Potassium-Rougier ✦

**potassium gluconate/
potassium chloride**
Kolyum

**potassium gluconate/
potassium citrate**
Twin-K
Func. class.: Electrolyte, mineral replacement
Chem. class.: Potassium

Pregnancy category C

Action: Needed for adequate transmission of nerve impulses and cardiac contraction, renal function, intracellular ion maintenance

⇒**Therapeutic Outcome:** Potassium level 3.0-5.0 mg/dl

Uses: Prevention and treatment of hypokalemia

Dosage and routes
Potassium bicarbonate
Adult: PO dissolve 25-50 mEq in water qd-qid

Hypokalemia (prevention)
P *Adult and child:* PO 20 mEq/day in 2-4 divided doses

Potassium acetate—hypokalemia
P *Adult and child:* PO 40-100 mEq/day in divided doses × 2-4 days

Potassium chloride
Adult: PO 40-100 mEq in divided doses tid-qid; **IV** 20 mEq/hr when diluted as 40 mEq/1000 ml, max 150 mEq/day

P *Child:* PO 2-4 mEq/kg/day

Potassium gluconate
Adult: PO 40-100 mEq in divided doses tid-qid

Potassium phosphate
Adult: **IV** 1 mEq/hr in sol of 60 mEq/L, max 150 mEq/day; PO 40-100 mEq/day in divided doses

P *Child:* **IV** max rate of infusion 1 mEq/kg/min

Available forms: Tabs for sol 6.5, 25 mEq; ext rel caps 8, 10 mEq; powder for sol 3.3, 5, 6.7, 10, 13.3 mEq/5 ml; tabs 4, 13.4 mEq; ext rel tabs 6.7, 8, 10 mEq; elixir 6.7 mEq/5 ml; tabs 2, 5 mEq; oral sol 2.375 mEq/5 ml; inj for prep of **IV** 1.5, 2, 2.4, 3, 3.2, 4.4, 4.7 mEq

Adverse effects
(*italic* = common; **bold** = life-threatening)
CNS: Confusion
CV: Bradycardia, *cardiac depression,* **dysrhythmias, arrest, peaking T waves, lowered R and depressed RST, prolonged PR interval, widened QRS complex**
GI: *Nausea, vomiting, cramps,* pain, *diarrhea,* ulceration of small bowel
GU: Oliguria
INTEG: Cold extremities, rash

Contraindications: Renal disease (severe), severe hemolytic disease, Addison's disease, hyperkalemia, acute dehydration, extensive tissue breakdown

Precautions: Cardiac disease, potassium-sparing diuretic therapy, systemic acidosis, pregnancy C

Pharmacokinetics	
Absorption	Unknown
Distribution	Unknown
Metabolism	Unknown
Excretion	Kidneys, feces
Half-life	Unknown

Pharmacodynamics		
	PO	IV
Onset	30 min	Immediate

Interactions
Drug classifications
Angiotensin converting enzyme inhibitors, calcium, diuretics (potassium-sparing), magnesium, potassium phosphate, **IV**: ↑ hyperkalemia

NURSING CONSIDERATIONS
Assessment
• Assess ECG for peaking T waves, lowered R, depressed RST, prolonged PR interval, widening QRS complex, hyperkalemia; drug should be reduced or discontinued
• Monitor potassium level during treatment (3.5-5.0 mg/dl is normal level)
• Monitor I&O ratio; watch for decreased urinary output; notify prescriber immediately; check urinary pH in patients receiving the drug as a urinary acidifier
• Assess cardiac status: rate, rhythm, CVP, PWP, PAWP if being monitored directly

Nursing diagnoses
✓ Nutrition: less than body requirements, imbalanced (uses)
✓ Knowledge, deficient (teaching)

Implementation
IV IV route
• Give through large-bore needle to decrease vein inflammation; check for extravasation; administer in large vein, avoiding scalp vein in P child
• After diluting in large volume of **IV** sol give as an **IV** inf slowly to prevent toxicity; never give **IV** bol or IM

Potassium acetate
Additive compatibilities: Metoclopramide

Potassium chloride
Y-site compatibilities: Acyclovir, aldesleukin, allopurinol, amifostine, aminophylline, amiodarone, ampicillin, amrinone, atropine, aztreonam, betamethasone, calcium gluconate, cefmetazole, cephalothin, cephapirin, chlordiazepoxide, chlorproMAZINE, ciprofloxacin, cladribine, cyanocobalamin, dexamethasone, digoxin, diltiazem, diphenhydrAMINE, DOBUTamine, DOPamine, droperidol, edrophonium, enalaprilat, epINEPHrine, esmolol, estrogens, ethacrynate, famotidine, fentanyl, filgrastim, fludarabine, fluorouracil, furosemide, gallium, granisetron, heparin, hydrALAZINE, idarubicin, indomethacin, insulin, regular, isoproterenol, kanamycin, labetalol, lidocaine, lorazepam, magnesium sulfate, melphalan, meperidine, methicillin, methoxamine, methylergonovine, midazolam, minocycline, morphine, neostigmine, norepi-

nephrine, ondansetron, oxacillin, oxytocin, paclitaxel, penicillin G potassium, pentazocine, phytonadione, piperacillin/tazobactam, prednisoLONE, procainamide, prochlorperazine, propofol, propranolol, pyridostigmine, sargramostim, scopolamine, sodium bicarbonate, succinylcholine, tacrolimus, teniposide, theophylline, thiotepa, trimethaphan, trimethobenzamide, vinorelbine, zidovudine

Additive compatibilities: Aminophylline, amiodarone, atracurium, bretylium, calcium chloride, cefepime, cephalothin, cephapirin, chloramphenicol, cimetidine, ciprofloxacin, clindamycin, cloxacillin, corticotropin, cytarabine, dimenhyDRINATE, DOPamine, enalaprilat, erythromycin, floxacillin, fluconazole, furosemide, heparin, hydrocortisone, isoproterenol, lidocaine, metaraminol, methicillin, methyldopate, metoclopramide, mitoxantrone, nafcillin, netilmicin, norepinephrine, oxacillin, penicillin G potassium or sodium, phenylephrine, piperacillin, ranitidine, sodium bicarbonate, thiopental, vancomycin, verapamil, vit B/C

Potassium chloride
Y-site compatibilities: Aldesleukin, amifostine, granisetron, lorazepam, midazolam, thiotepa
PO route
• Give with meal or pc; dissolve effervescent tab, powder in 8 oz of cold water or juice; do not give IM, SC
🚫 • Do not crush, break, or chew ext rel tabs/caps or enteric products
• Store at room temp

Patient/family education
• Teach patient to eat foods rich in potassium after medication is discontinued
• Advise patient to avoid OTC products: antacids, salt substitutes, analgesics, vit preparations, unless specifically directed by prescriber
• Advise patient to report hyperkalemia symptoms or continued hypokalemia symptoms
• Tell patient to take cap with full glass of liq; to dissolve powder or tab completely in at least 🚫 120 ml of water or juice; not to chew time rel or ext rel preparations
• Emphasize importance of regular follow-up

Evaluation
Positive therapeutic outcome
• Absence of fatigue, muscle weakness, and decreased thirst and urinary output, cardiac changes
• Potassium level normal

pramipexole (Rx)
(pra-mi-pex'ol)
Mirapex
Func. class.: Antiparkinsonian agent
Chem. class.: Dopamine receptor agonist, nonergot

Pregnancy category C

Action: Selective agonist for D_2 receptors (presynaptic/postsynaptic sites); binding at D_3 receptor contributes to antiparkinson effects

➡ **Therapeutic Outcome:** Decreased symptoms of Parkinson's disease (involuntary movements)

Uses: Parkinsonism

Investigational uses: Restless legs syndrome

Dosage and routes
Initial treatment
Adult: PO from a starting dose of 0.375 mg/day given in 3 divided doses; increase gradually by 0.125 mg/dose at 5–7–day intervals until total daily dose of 4.5 mg is reached

Maintenance treatment
Adult: PO 1.5-4.5 mg qd in 3 divided doses

Renal dose
Adult: PO CCr 35-59 ml/min 0.125 mg bid, may increase q5-7 days to 1.5 mg bid; CCr 15-34 ml/min 0.125 mg qd, may increase q5-7 days to 1.5 mg qd

Restless legs syndrome (off-label)
Adult: PO 0.125-0.375 mg 1-2h before bedtime, increase gradually

Available forms: Tabs 0.125, 0.25, 1, 1.5 mg

Adverse effects
(*italic* = common; **bold** = life-threatening)
CNS: *Agitation, insomnia,* psychosis, hallucinations, depression, dizziness, headache, confusion, **sleep attacks**
CV: *Orthostatic hypotension,* edema, syncope, tachycardia
EENT: Blurred vision
GI: *Nausea, anorexia,* constipation, dysphagia, dry mouth
GU: Impotence, urinary frequency
HEMA: **Hemolytic anemia, leukopenia, agranulocytosis**

Contraindications: Hypersensitivity

Precautions: Renal disease, cardiac disease, MI with dysrhythmias, affective disorders, psychosis, pregnancy **C**, preexisting dyskinesias

Pharmacokinetics

Absorption	Well absorbed
Distribution	Widely distributed
Metabolism	Liver, minimally
Excretion	Kidneys, unchanged
G Half-life	8 hr, 12 hr in elderly

Pharmacodynamics

Onset	Unknown
Peak	2 hr
Duration	Unknown

Interactions
Individual drugs
Cimetidine, diltiazem, levodopa, quinidine, ranitidine, triamterine, verapamil: ↑ pramipexole levels
Metoclopramide: ↓ pramipexole levels

Drug classifications
Butyrophenones, DOPamine agonists, phenothiazines: ↓ pramipexole effect
Herb/drug
Chaste tree fruit, kava: ↓ pramipexole effect

NURSING CONSIDERATIONS
Assessment
• Monitor B/P, ECG, respiration during initial treatment; hypotension or hypertension should be reported
• Assess mental status: affect, mood, behavioral changes, depression; complete suicide assessment
• Monitor renal function studies
• Assess for involuntary movements in parkinsonism: akinesia, tremors, staggering gait, muscle rigidity, drooling; these symptoms should improve with therapy
◆• Assess for sleep attacks: may fall asleep during activities, without warning; may need to discontinue medication

Nursing diagnoses
☑ Mobility, impaired (uses)
☑ Injury, risk for (uses)
☑ Knowledge, deficient (teaching)
☑ Noncompliance (teaching)

Implementation
PO route
• Adjust dosage to patient response
• Give with meals to decrease GI upset

Patient/family education
• Advise patient that therapeutic effects may take several wk to a few mo
• Caution patient to change positions slowly to prevent orthostatic hypotension
• Instruct patient to use drug exactly as prescribed; if drug is discontinued abruptly,

---

 Herb/drug   Do Not Crush   Alert   Key Drug   Geriatric   **P** Pediatric

parkinsonian crisis may occur; if treatment is
to be discontinued, taper over 1 wk; avoid
alcohol, OTC sleeping products
• Advise patient to notify prescriber if pregnancy is planned or suspected

Evaluation
Positive therapeutic outcome
• Decreased akathisia, other involuntary
movements
• Improved mood

---

pravastatin (Rx)
(pra′va-sta-tin)
Pravachol
Func. class.: Antilipidemic
Pregnancy category X

Action: Inhibits biosynthesis of VLDL, LDL,
which are responsible for cholesterol development, by inhibiting the enzyme HMG-CoA
reductase

➡ **Therapeutic Outcome:** Decreasing
cholesterol levels and LDL, increased HDL

Uses: As an adjunct in primary hypercholesterolemia types IIa, IIb, III, IV, arthero-
sclerosis, to reduce the risk of recurrent MI

Dosage and routes
Adult: PO 40-80 mg qd hs (range 20-80
mg qd)
G *Elderly/renal/hepatic dose:* PO 10
mg/day, initially

Available forms: Tabs 10, 20, 40, 80 mg

Adverse effects
(*italic* = common; **bold** = life-threatening)
CNS: Headache, dizziness, fatigue
EENT: Lens opacities
GI: Nausea, constipation, diarrhea, flatus,
abdominal pain, heartburn, **liver dysfunc-
tion, pancreatitis, hepatitis**
INTEG: Rash, pruritus, photosensitivity
MS: Muscle cramps, myalgia, **myositis,
rhabdomyolysis**
MISC: Chest pain, rash, pruritis, photosensitiv-
ity
RESP: Common cold, rhinitis, cough

Contraindications: Hypersensitivity,
pregnancy **X**, lactation, active liver disease

Precautions: Past liver disease, alcoholism,
severe acute infections, trauma, severe metabolic disorders, electrolyte imbalances

Do Not Confuse:
Pravachol/Prevacid

Pharmacokinetics
Absorption	Poorly absorbed, erratic
Distribution	Protein binding 80%
Metabolism	Liver, extensively
Excretion	Feces (70%-75%); kidneys, unchanged (20%), breast milk (minimal)
Half-life	2 hr

Pharmacodynamics
Onset	Unknown
Peak	1-1½ hr
Duration	Unknown

Interactions
Individual drugs
Clarithromycin, clofibrate, cycloSPORINE,
erythromycin, gemfibrozil, itraconazole,
niacin: ↑ risk for myopathy
Cyclosporine, erythromycin, gemfibrozil,
niacin: Rhabdomyolysis
Digoxin: ↑ effects of digoxin
Warfarin: ↑ bleeding
Drug classifications
Bile acid sequestrants: ↓ pravastat in bioavail-
ability
Protease inhibitors: ↑ risk of myopathy
Herb/drug
Glucomannan: ↑ effect
Gotu kola: ↓ effect
Lab test interferences
↑ CPK, ↑ AST, ↑ ALT, ↑ alkaline phosphatase,
↑ bilirubin
Altered: Thyroid function tests

NURSING CONSIDERATIONS
Assessment
• Assess nutrition: fat, protein, carbohydrates;
nutritional analysis should be completed by
dietitian before treatment
• Monitor triglycerides, esterol, cholesterol at
baseline and throughout treatment; LDL and
HDL should be watched closely; if increased,
drug should be discontinued
• Assess for muscle tenderness, pain, obtain
CPK; rhabdomyolysis may occur, therapy
should be discontinued
• Monitor ophthal status qyr

Nursing diagnoses
✓ Knowledge, deficient (teaching)
✓ Noncompliance (teaching)

Implementation
• Give hs only; give 1 hr before or 2 hr after
bile acid sequestrants
• Store in cool environment in airtight,
light-resistant container

Patient/family education
- Inform patient that compliance is needed for positive results to occur; not to double doses or skip doses
- Teach patient that risk factors should be decreased: high-fat diet, smoking, alcohol consumption, absence of exercise
- Advise patient to notify prescriber of weakness, tenderness, or limited mobility
- Explain to patient that contraception is necessary, since drug produces teratogenic effects
- Advise patient to use sunscreen, protective clothing to prevent burns

Evaluation
Positive therapeutic outcome
- Decreased cholesterol, serum triglyceride levels and improved ratio with HDL

---

prazosin ⦿ℼ (Rx)
(pra'zoe-sin)
Minipress, prazosin
Func. class.: Antihypertensive
Chem. class.: α₁-Adrenergic blocker

Pregnancy category C

Action: Blocks α-mediated vasoconstriction of adrenergic receptors, inducing peripheral vasodilatation

⟶ **Therapeutic Outcome:** Decreased B/P in hypertension; decreased cardiac preload, afterload

Uses: Hypertension

Investigational uses: Benign prostatic hypertrophy to decreased urine outflow obstruction

Dosage and routes
Hypertension
Adult: PO 1 mg bid or tid, increasing to 20 mg qd in divided doses if required, usual range 6-15 mg/day, not to exceed 1 mg initially; max 20-40 mg/day

P *Child:* PO 0.5-7 mg bid

Benign prostatic hypertrophy
Adult: PO 1-5 mg bid

Available forms: Caps 1, 2, 5 mg

Adverse effects
(*italic* = common; **bold** = life-threatening)
CNS: Dizziness, headache, drowsiness, anxiety, depression, vertigo, weakness, fatigue
CV: Palpitations, orthostatic hypotension, tachycardia, edema, rebound hypertension

EENT: Blurred vision, epistaxis, tinnitus, dry mouth, red sclera
GI: Nausea, vomiting, diarrhea, constipation, abdominal pain
GU: Urinary frequency, incontinence, impotence, priapism, water and sodium retention

Contraindications: Hypersensitivity

P **Precautions:** Pregnancy **C,** children, lactation

Pharmacokinetics
Absorption	60%
Distribution	Widely distributed
Metabolism	Liver, extensively; protein binding 97%
Excretion	Kidneys, unchanged (10%), bile (90%)
Half-life	2-3 hr

Pharmacodynamics
Onset	2 hr
Peak	1-3 hr
Duration	6-12 hr

Interactions
Individual drugs
Alcohol, nitroglycerin, verapamil: ↑ hypotension
Clonidine: ↓ antihypertensive effect
Drug classifications
Antihypertensives, β-adrenergic blockers: ↑ hypotension
NSAIDs: ↓ antihypertensive effect
⧄ *Herb/drug*
Aconite: ↑ toxicity, death
Astragalus, cola tree: ↑ or ↓ antihypertensive effect
Barberry, betony, black catechu, black cohosh, bloodroot, broom, burdock, cat's claw, dandelion, goldenseal, Irish moss, Jamaican dogwood, kelp, khella, mistletoe, parsley: ↑ antihypertensive effect
Coltsoot, guarana, khat, licorice: ↓ antihypertensive effect
Lab test interferences
↑ Urinary norepinephrine, ↑ VMA

NURSING CONSIDERATIONS
Assessment
- Monitor B/P, orthostatic hypotension, syncope; check for edema in feet, legs daily; monitor I&O, weight daily; notify prescriber of changes
- Assess for allergic reactions: rash, fever, pruritus, urticaria; drug should be discontinued if antihistamines fail to help
- Assess for orthostatic hypotension; tell patient to rise slowly from sitting or lying position

---

Nursing diagnoses
☑ Cardiac output, decreased (uses)
☑ Injury, risk for (adverse reactions)
☑ Knowledge, deficient (teaching)
☑ Noncompliance (teaching)

Implementation
• Severe hypotension may occur after 1st dose of this medication; hypotension may be prevented by reducing or discontinuing diuretic therapy 3 days before beginning prazosin therapy
• Store in airtight container at 86° F (30° C) or less

Patient/family education
• Instruct patient not to discontinue drug abruptly; stress the importance of complying with dosage schedule, even if feeling better; if dose is missed, take as soon as remembered; take at same time each day
• Advise patient not to use OTC products (cough, cold, allergy) unless directed by prescriber; also to avoid large amounts of caffeine
• Emphasize the need to rise slowly to sitting or standing position to minimize orthostatic hypotension
• Teach patient to notify prescriber of mouth sores, sore throat, fever, swelling of hands or feet, irregular heartbeat, chest pain
• Caution patient to report excessive perspiration, dehydration, vomiting, diarrhea; may lead to fall in B/P
• Caution patient that drug may cause dizziness, fainting, light-headedness; may occur during 1st few days of therapy; to avoid hazardous activities
• Teach patient how to take B/P and normal readings for age group; instruct to take B/P q7 days

Evaluation
Positive therapeutic outcome
• Decreased B/P in hypertension

Treatment of overdose: Administer
volume expanders or vasopressors, discontinue drug, place in supine position

*prednisoLONE (Rx)
(pred-niss'oh-lone)
Articulose-50, Delta-Cortef, prednisoLONE, Prelone, Key-Pred 25, Key-Pred 50, Predaject-50, Predalone 50, Predcor-25, Predcor-50, Prednisolone Acetate, Orapred, Hydeltrasol, Key-Pred-SP, Pediapred, Hydeltra-T.B.A., Predalone-T.B.A., Prednisol TBA
Func. class.: Corticosteroid
Chem. class.: Intermediate-acting glucocorticoid

Pregnancy category C

Action: Decreases inflammation by suppressing migration of polymorphonuclear leukocytes, fibroblasts; reversal to increase capillary permeability and lysosomal stabilization, minimal mineralocorticoid

Therapeutic Outcome: Decreased inflammation, decreased adrenal insufficiency

Uses: Severe inflammation, immunosuppression, neoplasms

Dosage and routes
Adult: PO 2.5-15 mg bid-qid; IM 2-30 mg (acetate, phosphate) q12h; **IV** 2-30 mg (phosphate) q12h, 2-30 mg in joint or soft tissue (phosphate), 4-40 mg in joint of lesion (tebutate)

Asthma/antiinflammatory
Child: PO 1-2 mg/kg/day; **IV** 2-4 mg/kg/day

Available forms: *PrednisoLONE:* tabs 5 mg, syr 5 mg/5 ml, 15 mg/5 ml; *prednisoLONE acetate:* inj 25, 50 mg/ml; *prednisoLONE tebutate:* inj 20 mg/ml; *prednisoLONE phosphate:* inj 20 mg/ml, oral liq 5 mg/5 ml; tabs 1, 2.5, 5, 10, 20, 50 mg, oral sol 5 mg/ml, 5 mg/5 ml, syr 5 mg/5 ml

Adverse effects
(*italic* = common; **bold** = life-threatening)
CNS: Depression, flushing, sweating, headache, mood changes
CV: Hypertension, **circulatory collapse, thrombophlebitis, embolism,** tachycardia
EENT: Fungal infections, increased intraocular pressure, blurred vision
GI: Diarrhea, nausea, abdominal distention, **GI hemorrhage,** increased appetite, **pancreatitis**
HEMA: **Thrombocytopenia**
INTEG: Acne, poor wound healing, ecchymosis, petechiae
MS: Fractures, osteoporosis, weakness

Contraindications: Psychosis, hypersensitivity, idiopathic thrombocytopenia, acute glomerulonephritis, amebiasis, fungal infec-tions, nonasthmatic bronchial disease, child <2 yr

Precautions: Pregnancy **C,** diabetes mellitus, glaucoma, osteoporosis, seizure disorders, ulcerative colitis, CHF, myasthenia gravis

⊠ Do Not Confuse:
prednisoLONE/predniSONE

Pharmacokinetics

Absorption	Well absorbed (PO, IM), completely absorbed (**IV**)
Distribution	Widely distributed; crosses placenta
Metabolism	Liver, extensively
Excretion	Kidney, breast milk
Half-life	2-4 hr

Pharmacodynamics

	PO	IM (phosphate)	IV	IA/IL
Onset	1 hr	Rapid	Rapid	Slow
Peak	2 hr	1 hr	Unknown	Unknown
Duration	1½ days	Unknown	Unknown	Up to 1 mo

Interactions
Individual drugs
Alcohol, amphotericin B, cycloSPORINE, digitalis, indomethacin: ↑ side effects
Ambenonium, isoniazid, neostigmine, somatrem: ↓ effects of each specific drug
Cholestyramine, colestipol, epHEDrine, theophylline: ↓ action of prednisoLONE
Indomethacin, ketoconazole: ↑ action of prednisoLONE
Phenytoin, rifampin: ↓ action
Piperacillin: ↑ hypokalemia
Drug classifications
Antibiotics (macrolide), contraceptives (oral), estrogens, salicylates: ↑ action of prednisoLONE
Anticholinesterases: ↓ effects of cholinesterases
Anticoagulants, anticonvulsants, antidiabetics, salicylates, toxoids, vaccines: ↓ effects of each specific drug
Barbiturates: ↓ action of prednisoLONE
Diuretics, salicylates: ↑ side effects
⊘ Herb/drug
Aloe, buckthorn, cascara sagrada, Chinese rhubarb, senna: ↑ hypokalemia
Aloe, licorice, perilla: ↑ effect
Lab test interferences
↑ Cholesterol, ↑ sodium, ↑ blood glucose, ↑ uric acid, ↑ calcium, ↑ urine glucose

↓ Calcium, ↓ potassium, ↓ T₄, ↓ T₃, ↓ thyroid ^{131}I uptake test, ↓ urine 17-OHCS, ↓ 17-KS, ↓ PBI
False negative: Skin allergy tests

NURSING CONSIDERATIONS
Assessment
• Monitor potassium, blood glucose, urine glucose while patient is on long-term therapy; hypokalemia and hyperglycemia may occur
• Monitor weight daily; notify prescriber of weekly gain >5 lb; monitor I&O ratio; be alert for decreasing urinary output and increasing edema
• Monitor B/P q4h, pulse; notify prescriber if chest pain occurs
• Monitor plasma cortisol levels during long-term therapy (normal level; 138-635 nmol/L [SI units] when measured at 8 AM)
• Assess adrenal function periodically for hypothalamic-pituitary-adrenal axis suppression
• Assess infection: increased temp, WBC even after withdrawal of medication; drug masks infection symptoms
• Assess for potassium depletion: paresthesias, fatigue, nausea, vomiting, depression, polyuria, dysrhythmias, weakness, edema, hypertension, cardiac symptoms
• Assess mental status: affect, mood, behavioral changes, aggression
• Monitor temp; if fever develops, drug should be discontinued
• Assess for systemic absorption: increased temp, inflammation, irritation (top)

Nursing diagnoses
☑ Infection, risk for (adverse reactions)
☑ Knowledge, deficient (teaching)
☑ Noncompliance (teaching)

Implementation
Ⅳ IV route
• Give by direct **IV** only sodium phosphate product; give over >1 min; may be given by **IV** inf in D₅W, 0.9% NaCl
• Give after shaking susp (parenteral)
• Give titrated dose; use lowest effective dosage

Y-site compatibilities: Ciprofloxacin, potassium chloride, vit B/C

Additive compatibilities: Ascorbic acid, cephalothin, cytarabine, erythromycin, fluorouracil, heparin, methicillin, penicillin G potassium, penicillin G sodium, vit B/C

Additive incompatibilities: Calcium gluceptate, methotrexate, polymyxin B sulfate

PO route

• Give with food or milk to decrease GI symptoms

IM route

• Give IM inj deep in large muscle mass; rotate sites; avoid deltoid; use 21-G needle

• Give in one dose in ᴀᴍ to prevent adrenal suppression; avoid SC administration; may damage tissue

Patient/family education

• Advise patient to carry/wear emergency ID as steroid user

• Advise patient to notify prescriber if therapeutic response decreases; dosage adjustment may be needed

• Caution patient not to discontinue abruptly; adrenal crisis can result; take exactly as prescribed

• Caution patient to avoid OTC products: salicylates, cough products with alcohol, cold preparations unless directed by prescriber

• Teach patient all aspects of drug usage including cushingoid symptoms

• Teach patient symptoms of adrenal insufficiency: nausea, anorexia, fatigue, dizziness, dyspnea, weakness, joint pain

• Advise patient that long-term therapy may be needed to clear infection (1-2 mo depending on type of infection)

Evaluation

Positive therapeutic outcome

• Decreased inflammation

---

*prednISONE ⊙ₙ (Rx)
(pred'ni-sone)

Apo-Prednisone ✤, Deltasone, Liquid Pred, Meticorten, Orasone, Panasol-S, Prednicen-M, prednISONE, Sterapred, Winpred

Func. class.: Corticosteroid
Chem. class.: Intermediate-acting glucocorticoid

Pregnancy category C

Action: Decreases inflammation by suppressing migration of polymorphonuclear leukocytes, fibroblasts; reversal to increase capillary permeability and lysosomal stabilization

⮕**Therapeutic Outcome:** Decreased inflammation, decreased adrenal insufficiency

Uses: Severe inflammation, immunosuppression, neoplasms, multiple sclerosis, collagen disorders, dermatologic disorders

Dosage and routes

Adult: PO 5-60 mg qd or divided bid-qid

Ⓟ *Child:* PO 0.05-2 mg/kg/day divided 1-4 ✕/day

Nephrosis

Ⓟ *Child 18 mo-4 yr:* 7.5-10 mg qid initially

Ⓟ *Child 4-10 yr:* 15 mg qid initially

Ⓟ *Child >10 yr:* 20 mg qid initially

Multiple sclerosis

Adult: PO 200 mg/day × 1 wk, then 80 mg qod × 1 mo

Available forms: Tabs 1, 2.5, 5, 10, 20, 25, 50 mg; oral sol 5 mg/5 ml; syr 5 mg/5 ml

Adverse effects

(*italic* = common; **bold** = life-threatening)

CNS: Depression, flushing, sweating, headache, mood changes

CV: Hypertension, **circulatory collapse, thrombophlebitis, embolism,** tachycardia

EENT: Fungal infections, increased intraocular pressure, blurred vision

GI: Diarrhea, nausea, abdominal distention, **GI hemorrhage,** increased appetite, **pancreatitis**

HEMA: **Thrombocytopenia**

INTEG: Acne, poor wound healing, ecchymosis, petechiae

MS: Fractures, osteoporosis, weakness

Contraindications: Psychosis, hypersensitivity, idiopathic thrombocytopenia, acute glomerulonephritis, amebiasis, fungal infecⓅtions, nonasthmatic bronchial disease, child <2 yr, AIDS, TB

Precautions: Pregnancy **C**, diabetes mellitus, glaucoma, osteoporosis, seizure disorders, ulcerative colitis, CHF, myasthenia gravis, renal disease, esophagitis, peptic ulcer

◥ **Do Not Confuse:**
prednISONE/methylPREDNISolone, prednISONE/prednisoLONE, prednISONE/Prilosec

Pharmacokinetics	
Absorption	Well absorbed
Distribution	Widely distributed; crosses placenta
Metabolism	Liver, extensively
Excretion	Kidney, breast milk
Half-life	3-4 hr

Pharmacodynamics	
Onset	Unknown
Peak	1-2 hr
Duration	1½ days

Interactions
Individual drugs
Alcohol, amphotericin B, cycloSPORINE, digitalis, indomethacin: ↑ side effects

Ambenonium, isoniazid, neostigmine, sometrem: ↓ effects of each specific drug

EpHEDrine, phenytoin, theophylline: ↓ action of predniSONE

Indomethacin, ketoconazole: ↑ action of predniSONE

Drug classifications
Anticholinesterases, anticoagulants, anticonvulsants, antidiabetics, toxoids, vaccines: ↓ effects of each specific drug

Antiinfectives (macrolide), contraceptives (oral), estrogens: ↑ action of predniSONE

Barbiturates, colestipol, rifampin: ↓ action of predniSONE

Diuretics: ↑ side effects

Hypoglycemic agents: ↑ need for hypoglycemic agents

Salicylates: ↓ effects of salicylates, ↑ side effects, ↑ action of predniSONE

☑ Herb/drug
Aloe, buckthorn, Chinese rhubarb, senna: ↑ hypokalemia

Lab test interferences
↑ Cholesterol, ↑ sodium, ↑ blood glucose, ↑ uric acid, ↑ calcium, ↑ urine glucose

↓ Calcium, ↓ potassium, ↓ T_4, ↓ T_3, ↓ thyroid ^{131}I uptake test, ↓ urine 17-OHCS, ↓ 17-KS, ↓ PBI

False negative: Skin allergy tests

NURSING CONSIDERATIONS
Assessment
• Monitor potassium, blood glucose, urine glucose while on long-term therapy; hypokalemia and hyperglycemia may occur

• Monitor weight daily; notify prescriber of weekly gain >5 lb; monitor I&O ratio; be alert for decreasing urinary output and increasing edema

• Monitor B/P q4h, pulse; notify prescriber if chest pain occurs

• Monitor plasma cortisol levels during long-term therapy (normal level 138-635 nmol/L when measured at 8 AM)

• Assess adrenal function periodically for hypothalamic-pituitary-adrenal axis suppression

• Assess infection: increased temp, WBC even after withdrawal of medication; drug masks infection symptoms

• Assess for potassium depletion: paresthesias, fatigue, nausea, vomiting, depression, polyuria, dysrhythmias, weakness, edema, hypertension, cardiac symptoms

• Assess mental status: affect, mood, behavioral changes, aggression

• Monitor temp; if fever develops, drug should be discontinued

• Assess for systemic absorption: increased temp, inflammation, irritation (top)

Nursing diagnoses
☑ Infection, risk for (adverse reactions)
☑ Knowledge, deficient (teaching)
☑ Noncompliance (teaching)

Implementation
• Give with food or milk to decrease GI symptoms; use measuring device for liq route

• For long-term use, alternative drug therapy is recommended, to decrease adverse reactions

Patient/family education
• Advise patient that emergency ID as steroid user should be carried or worn

• Advise patient to notify prescriber if therapeutic response decreases; dosage adjustment may be needed

• Caution patient not to discontinue abruptly; adrenal crisis can result

• Caution patient to avoid OTC products: salicylates, cough products with alcohol, cold preparations unless directed by prescriber

• Teach patient all aspects of drug usage including cushingoid symptoms

• Teach patient symptoms of adrenal insufficiency: nausea, anorexia, fatigue, dizziness, dyspnea, weakness, joint pain

• Advise patient that long-term therapy may be needed to clear infection (1-2 mo depending on type of infection)

Evaluation
Positive therapeutic outcome
• Decreased inflammation

primidone (Rx)
(pri'mi-done)
Apo-Primidone ♣, Mysoline, PMS-Primidone ♣, primidone, Sertan ♣
Func. class.: Anticonvulsant
Chem. class.: Barbiturate derivative

Pregnancy category D

Action: Raises seizure threshold by conversion of drug to phenobarbital; decreases neuron firing

Therapeutic Outcome: Reduction in seizure activity

Uses: Generalized tonic-clonic (grand mal), complex-partial, psychomotor seizures

Dosage and routes
P *Adult and child >8 yr:* PO 100-125 mg hs on days 1, 2, 3; then 100-125 mg bid on days 4, 5, 6; then 100-125 mg tid on days 7, 8, 9; then maintenance 250 mg tid-qid, max 2 g/day in divided doses

P *Child <8 yr:* PO 50 mg hs on days 1, 2, 3; then 50 mg bid on days 4, 5, 6; then 100 mg bid on days 7, 8, 9; maintenance 125-250 mg tid or 10-25 mg/kg/day in divided doses

Available forms: Tabs 50, 250 mg; susp 250 mg/5 ml; chew tabs 125 mg ♣

Adverse effects
(*italic* = common; **bold** = life-threatening)
CNS: *Stimulation, drowsiness,* irritability, fatigue, emotional disturbances, mood changes, paranoia, psychosis, ataxia, *vertigo*
EENT: Diplopia, nystagmus, edema of eyelids
GI: *Nausea, vomiting, anorexia,* **hepatitis**
GU: Impotence
HEMA: **Thrombocytopenia, leukopenia, neutropenia, eosinophilia, megaloblastic anemia,** decreased serum folate level, lymphadenopathy
INTEG: Rash, edema, alopecia, lupus-like syndrome

Contraindications: Hypersensitivity, porphyria, pregnancy **D**

Precautions: COPD, hepatic disease, renal
P disease, hyperactive children

Pharmacokinetics
Absorption	60%-80%
Distribution	Widely distributed; crosses placenta
Metabolism	Liver, converted to phenobarbital + PEMA
Excretion	Kidneys, breast milk
Half-life	3-24 hr

Pharmacodynamics
Onset	Unknown
Peak	4 hr
Duration	Unknown

Interactions
Individual drugs
Acebutolol, metoprolol, propranolol: ↓ effectiveness
Acetazolamide, carbamazepine: ↓ primidone levels
Alcohol: ↑ CNS depression
Heparin: ↑ blood levels
Isoniazid, nicotinamide: ↑ primidone levels
Phenobarbital: ↑ toxicity
Drug classifications
Antidepressants (tricyclic), antihistamines, opiates, sedative/hypnotics: ↑ CNS depression
Hydantoins: ↑ primidone levels
Oral contraceptives: ↓ effectiveness
Phenothiazines: ↓ CNS depression
Succinimides: ↓ primidone levels
Herb/drug
Ginkgo: ↑ effect
Ginseng, santonica: ↓ effect

NURSING CONSIDERATIONS
Assessment
• Assess mental status: mood, sensorium, affect, memory (long, short), especially
G elderly
• Assess for blood dyscrasias: fever, sore throat, bruising, rash, jaundice, epistaxis (long-term treatment only)
• Assess seizure activity including type, location, duration, and character; provide seizure precaution
• Assess renal studies: urinalysis, BUN, urine creatinine
• Monitor blood studies: RBC, Hct, Hgb, reticulocyte counts weekly for 4 wk then monthly
• Monitor hepatic studies: ALT, AST, bilirubin, creatinine
• Monitor drug levels during initial treatment
• Assess for signs of physical withdrawal if medication is suddenly discontinued
• Assess eye problems: need for ophthal exam before, during, after treatment (slit lamp, funduscopy, tonometry)
• Assess allergic reaction: red raised rash; if this occurs, drug should be discontinued
• Monitor for toxicity: bone marrow depression, nausea, vomiting, ataxia, diplopia, CV collapse

P

Nursing diagnoses
☑ Injury, risk for (side effects)
☑ Knowledge, deficient (teaching)

Implementation
- May give with food to decrease gastric irritation
- May crush tab and mix with food or fluid

Patient/family education
- Teach patient to carry/wear emergency ID stating name, drugs taken, condition, prescriber's name, phone number
- Advise patient to avoid driving and other activities that require alertness
- Caution patient to avoid alcohol and CNS depressants; increased sedation may occur
- Teach patient not to discontinue medication quickly after long-term use; taper off over several wk

Evaluation
Positive therapeutic outcome
- Decreased seizure activity

---

probenecid (Rx)
(proe-ben'e-sid)
Benemid, Benuryl ✦, Probalan, probenecid
Func. class.: Uricosuric; antigout
Chem. class.: Sulfonamide derivative

Pregnancy category B

Action: Inhibits tubular reabsorption of urates, with increased excretion of uric acids

➡ **Therapeutic Outcome:** Decreased uric acid levels

Uses: Hyperuricemia in gout, gouty arthritis; adjunct to cephalosporin or penicillin treatment (gonorrhea)

Dosage and routes
Gonorrhea
Adult: PO 1 g with 3.5 g of ampicillin or 1 g 30 min before 4.8 million units of aqueous penicillin G procaine injected into 2 sites IM

Gout/gouty arthritis
Adult: PO 250 mg bid for 1 wk, then 500 mg bid, not to exceed 2 g/day; maintenance 500 mg/day × 6 mo

Adjunct in penicillin/cephalosporin treatment
P *Adult and child >50 kg:* PO 500 mg qid

P *Child <50 kg:* PO 25 mg/kg, then 40 mg/kg in divided doses qid

Renal dose
Adult: PO CCr <30 ml/min avoid use

Available forms: Tabs 0.5 g

Adverse effects
(*italic* = common; **bold** = life-threatening)
CNS: Drowsiness, headache
CV: Bradycardia
GI: *Gastric irritation, nausea, vomiting, anorexia,* **hepatic necrosis**
GU: *Glycosuria, thirst, frequency,* **nephrotic syndrome**
INTEG: *Rash, dermatitis, pruritus, fever*
META: *Acidosis, hypokalemia, hyperchloremia,* hyperglycemia
RESP: **Apnea,** irregular respirations

Contraindications: Hypersensitivity, severe hepatic disease, severe renal disease, CCr <50 mg/min, history of uric acid calculus

P **Precautions:** Pregnancy **B,** child <2 yr

Pharmacokinetics	
Absorption	Well absorbed
Distribution	Crosses placenta
Metabolism	Liver
Excretion	Kidneys
Half-life	5-8 hr

Pharmacodynamics	
Onset	½ hr
Peak	2-4 hr
Duration	8 hr

Interactions
Individual drugs
Acyclovir, allopurinol, dyphylline, zidovudine: ↑ effect
Clofibrate, dapsone, indomethacin, methotrexate, naproxen, rifampin: ↑ toxicity
Drug classifications
Barbiturates, benzodiazepines: ↑ effect
Salicylates: ↓ action of probenecid
Sulfa drugs: ↑ toxicity
Lab test interferences
↑ BSP/urinary PSP, ↑ theophylline levels
False positive: Urine glucose with copper sulfate test

NURSING CONSIDERATIONS
Assessment
- Monitor I&O ratio; observe for decrease in urinary output; increase fluids to 2-3 L/day; urine may be alkalized with sodium bicarbonate acetaZOLAMIDE
- Assess mobility, joint pain, and swelling in the joints
- Monitor CBC, urine pH, uric acid and BUN, creatinine before and periodically during treatment

---

 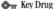

Nursing diagnoses
☑ Pain, chronic (uses)
☑ Mobility, impaired (uses)
☑ Knowledge, deficient (teaching)

Implementation
• Give with food or antacid to decrease GI upset
• Reduce dosage gradually if uric acid levels are normal after 6 mo

Patient/family education
• Advise patient to increase fluids to 2-3 L/day, avoid caffeine, alcohol
• Caution patient to avoid salicylates; probenecid levels will be decreased
• Advise patient to report any pain, redness, or hard area, usually in legs
• Instruct patient in importance of complying with medical regimen including weight loss program, diet restrictions, and alcohol intake

Evaluation
Positive therapeutic outcome
• Decreased pain in joints
• Normal serum uric acid levels
• Increased duration of antiinfectives

---

procainamide ⚛ (Rx)
(proe'kane-ah-mide)
Procan SR, Promine, procainamide, Procanbid, Pronestyl, Pronestyl-SR
Func. class.: Antidysrhythmic (class IA)
Chem. class.: procaine HCl amide analog

Pregnancy category C

Action: Depresses excitability of cardiac muscle to electrical stimulation and slows conduction in atrium, bundle of His, and ventricle increases refractory period

➡ **Therapeutic Outcome:** Prevention of dysrhythmias

Uses: Life-threatening ventricular dysrhythmias

Dosage and routes
Atrial fibrillation/PAT
Adult: PO 1-1.25 g; may give another 750 mg if needed; if no response, 500 mg-1g q2h until desired response; maintenance 50 mg/kg in divided doses q6h

Ventricular tachycardia
Adult: PO 1 g; maintenance 50 mg/kg/day given in 3-hr intervals; sus rel tab 500 mg-1.25 g q6h

Other dysrhythmias
Adult: **IV** bol 100 mg q5 min, given 25-50 mg/min, max 500 mg; or 17 mg/kg total, then **IV** inf 2-6 mg/min

Renal dose
Adult: **IV** CCr 10-50 ml/min give q6-12h; CCr <10 ml/min give q8-24h

Available forms: Caps 250, 375, 500 mg; tabs 250, 375, 500 mg; sus rel tabs 250, 500, 750, 1000 mg; inj **IV** 100, 500 mg/ml

Adverse effects
(*italic* = common; **bold** = life-threatening)
CNS: *Headache, dizziness,* confusion, psychosis, restlessness, irritability, weakness
CV: *Hypotension,* **heart block, cardiovascular collapse, arrest**
GI: Nausea, vomiting, anorexia, diarrhea, hepatomegaly, pain, bitter taste
HEMA: Systemic lupus erythematosus syndrome, **agranulocytosis, thrombocytopenia, neutropenia, hemolytic anemia**
INTEG: Rash, urticaria, edema, swelling (rare), pruritus, flushing

Contraindications: Hypersensitivity, severe heart block, lupus erythromatosis, torsades de pointes

Precautions: Pregnancy **C**, lactation, children, renal disease, liver disease, CHF, respiratory depression, cytopenia, bone marrow failure, dysrhythmia associated with digitalis toxicity, myasthenia gravis

Pharmacokinetics
Absorption	Well absorbed
Distribution	Rapidly distributed
Metabolism	Liver
Excretion	Kidneys, unchanged (50%-70%)
Half-life	2½-4½ hr; increased in renal disease

Pharmacodynamics
	PO	PO-EXT REL	IV
Onset	½ hr	Unknown	Rapid
Peak	1-1½ hr	Unknown	½-1 hr
Duration	3 hr	Up to 8 hr	3-4 hr

Interactions
Individual drugs
Cimetidine: ↑ procainamide effect
Haloperidol: ↑ anticholinergic effect
Quinidine: ↑ levels
Quinidine, thioridazine: ↑ toxicity
Trimethoprim: ↑ procainamide action

Drug classifications
Antidysrhythmics, quinolones: ↑ toxicity
Antihistamines: ↑ antihistamine action
β-Adrenergic blockers: ↑ dysrhythmias, arrest
Neuromuscular blockers: ↑ neuromuscular blocking effect

🗹 *Herb/drug*
Aconite: ↑ toxicity, death
Aloe, broom, buckthorn (chronic use), cascara sagrada (chronic use), Chinese rhubarb, figwort, fumitory, goldenseal, kudzu, licorice: ↑ effect
Coltsfoot: ↓ effect
Horehound: ↑ serotonin effect

Lab test interferences
↑ ALT, ↑ AST, ↑ Alkaline phosphatase, ↑ LDH, ↑ bilirubin

NURSING CONSIDERATIONS
Assessment
• Assess for oxygenation or perfusion deficit: decreased B/P, chest pain, dizziness, loss of consciousness
• Assess respiratory status: auscultate lung fields for bibasilar crackles in patients with advanced CHF
• Monitor I&O ratio; electrolytes: potassium, sodium, chloride; watch for decreasing urinary output, possible retention
• Monitor liver function studies: AST, ALT, bilirubin, alkaline phosphatase
◆• Monitor ECG continuously to determine drug effectiveness; measure PR, QRS, QT intervals; check for PVCs, other dysrhythmias; check B/P continuously for hypotension, hypertension; for rebound hypertension after 1-2 hr; prolonged PR/QT intervals, QRS complex; if QT or QRS increases by 50% or more, withhold next dose, notify prescriber
• Monitor ANA titer; during long-term treatment, watch for lupuslike symptoms
• Monitor for dehydration or hypovolemia
◆• Monitor for CNS symptoms: confusion, seizures, psychosis, numbness, depression, involuntary movements; if these occur, drug should be discontinued
• Monitor blood levels (therapeutic level 3-10 mcg/ml), ANA titer or *N*-acetylprocainamide levels 10-20 mcg/ml; notify prescriber of abnormal results; assess for toxicity: confusion, drowsiness, nausea, vomiting, tachydysrhythmias, oliguria
• Assess cardiac rate, respiration: rate, rhythm, character, chest pain, ventricular tachycardia, supraventricular tachycardia or fibrillation

Nursing diagnoses
✓ Cardiac output, decreased (uses)

✓ Gas exchange, impaired (adverse reactions)
✓ Knowledge, deficient (teaching)

Implementation
PO route
• Give on an empty stomach with a full glass of water
• May be given with meals if GI irritation occurs; absorption will be decreased
🚫 Tab may be crushed and mixed with fluid or foods for patients with swallowing difficulties; do not break, chew, or crush sus rel tab

ⅣV IV route
• Give by direct **IV** after diluting 100 mg/10 ml of D_5W or sterile water for inj; give 50 mg/min or less
• Give by intermittent inf after diluting to a conc of 2-4 mg/ml, 200 mg up to 1 g/50-500 ml of D_5W; give over 30 min (2-6 mg/min maintenance); use infusion pump for correct dosage
• Do not use if sol is dark or if precipitate is present

Y-site compatibilities: Amiodarone, famotidine, heparin, hydrocortisone, potassium chloride, ranitidine, vit B/C

Y-site incompatibilities: Milrinone

Additive compatibilities: Amiodarone, DOBUTamine, flumazenil, lidocaine, netilmicin, verapamil

Additive incompatibilities: Esmolol, ethacrynate, milrinone

Solution compatibilities: D_5W, D_5/0.9% NaCl, 0.45% NaCl, 0.9% NaCl, water for inj

Patient/family education
• Advise patient to report side effects immediately to prescriber; to take exactly as prescribed; if dose is missed take when remembered if within 3-4 hr of next dose, do not double doses
• Caution patient that dark glasses may be needed for photophobia; to use sunscreen or stay out of sun to prevent burns; avoid temp extremes; impairment of heat-regulating mechanism can occur
• Advise patient to complete follow-up appointment with prescriber including pulmonary function studies, chest x-ray
• Instruct patient that dry mouth may be relieved by frequent sips of water, hard candy, sugarless gum
• Caution patient to make position changes from lying to standing slowly to prevent orthostatic hypotension

---

🗹 Herb/drug   🚫 Do Not Crush   ◆ Alert   ◆ₐ Key Drug   Ⓖ Geriatric   Ⓟ Pediatric

• Advise prescriber immediately if lupuslike symptoms appear (joint pain, butterfly rash, fever, chills, dyspnea), or leukopenia (sore mouth, gums, throat) or thrombocytopenia (bleeding, bruising)
• Teach patient how to take pulse and when to report to prescriber

Evaluation
Positive therapeutic outcome
• Decreased PVCs, ventricular tachycardia

Treatment of overdose: O₂, artificial ventilation, ECG, administer DOPamine for circulatory depression, diazepam or thiopental for convulsions, isoproterenol

---

procarbazine (Rx)
(proe-kar′ba-zeen)
Matulane, Natulan ✤
Func. class.: Antineoplastic, alkylating agent
Chem. class.: Hydrazine derivative

Pregnancy category D

Action: Inhibits DNA, RNA, protein synthesis, cell cycle S phase specific; has multiple sites of action; a nonvesicant

⊟ **Therapeutic Outcome:** Prevention of rapidly growing malignant cells

Uses: Lymphoma, Hodgkin's disease, cancers resistant to other therapy

Investigational uses: Brain, lung malignancies, other lymphomas, multiple myeloma, malignant melanoma, polycythemia vera

Dosage and routes
Adult: PO 2-4 mg/kg/day for first wk; maintain dosage of 4-6 mg/kg/day until platelets and WBC fall; after recovery, 1-2 mg/kg/day

🄿 *Child:* PO 50 mg/m²/day for 7 days, then 100 mg/m² until desired response, leukopenia, or thrombocytopenia occurs; 50 mg/day is maintenance after bone marrow recovery

Available forms: Caps 50 mg

Adverse effects
(*italic* = common; **bold** = life-threatening)
CNS: Headache, dizziness, **seizures**, insomnia, hallucinations, confusion, **coma**, pain, chills, fever, sweating, paresthesias
EENT: Retinal hemorrhage, nystagmus, photophobia, diplopia
GI: *Nausea, vomiting,* anorexia, diarrhea, constipation, dry mouth, stomatitis
GU: Azoospermia, cessation of menses
HEMA: **Thrombocytopenia, anemia, leukopenia, myelosuppression, bleeding tendencies,** purpura, petechiae, epistaxis
INTEG: *Rash,* pruritus, dermatitis, alopecia, herpes, hyperpigmentation
MS: Arthralgias, myalgias
RESP: Cough, pneumonitis

Contraindications: Hypersensitivity, thrombocytopenia, bone marrow depression, pregnancy **D**

Precautions: Renal disease, hepatic disease, radiation therapy

Pharmacokinetics	
Absorption	Well absorbed
Distribution	Widely distributed; crosses blood-brain barrier
Metabolism	Liver
Excretion	Kidneys
Half-life	1 hr

Pharmacodynamics
Unknown

Interactions
Individual drugs
Alcohol: ↑ CNS depression, disulfiram reaction
Guanethidine, levodopa, reserpine: ↑ hypertensive crisis
Radiation: ↑ toxicity, bone marrow suppression
Drug classifications
Antidepressants, local anesthetics, sympathomimetic amines: ↑ hypertensive crisis
Antihistamines, CNS depressants, opiates, sedative/hypnotics: ↑ CNS depression
Antineoplastics: ↑ toxicity, bone marrow suppression
MAOIs: ↑ seizures, temperature
Food/drug
Tyramine-foods: ↑ disulfiram-like reaction

NURSING CONSIDERATIONS
Assessment
• Monitor CBC, differential, platelet count weekly; withhold drug if WBC is <4000/mm³ or platelet count is <75,000/mm³; notify prescriber of results if WBC <20,000/mm³, platelets <150,000/mm³
• Monitor pulmonary function tests, chest x-ray films before, during therapy; chest film should be obtained q2 wk during treatment; check for dyspnea, rales, unproductive cough, chest pain, tachypnea
• Monitor renal function studies: BUN, serum uric acid, urine CCr before, during therapy;

P

I&O ratio; report fall in urine output of 30 ml/hr; check for decreased hyperuricemia
- Monitor for cold, fever, sore throat (may indicate beginning of infection); identify edema in feet, joint and stomach pain, shaking; prescriber should be notified
- Assess for bleeding: hematuria, guaiac, bruising or petechiae, mucosa or orifices q8h, no rectal temp
- Assess for tyramine-containing foods in the diet; hypertensive crisis can occur

Nursing diagnoses
☑ Injury, risk for (adverse reactions)
☑ Body image, disturbed (adverse reactions)
☑ Infection, risk for (adverse reactions)
☑ Knowledge, deficient (teaching)

Implementation
- Give with foods, fluids for GI upset; open cap and give with food/fluids for swallowing difficulty; administer as directed

Patient/family education
- Teach patient to avoid use of products containing aspirin or NSAIDs, razors, commercial mouthwash, since bleeding may occur; to report symptoms of bleeding (hematuria, tarry stools)
- Caution patient to report signs of anemia (fatigue, headache, irritability, faintness, shortness of breath)
- Advise patient to report any changes in breathing or coughing even several mo after treatment; to avoid crowds and persons with respiratory tract or other infections
- Inform patient hair loss is common; discuss the use of wigs or hairpieces
- Caution patient not to have any vaccinations without the advice of the prescriber; serious reactions can occur
- Advise patient that contraception is needed during treatment and for several mo after the completion of therapy
- To avoid sunlight, or UV exposure, wear sunscreen or protective clothing

Evaluation
Positive therapeutic outcome
- Absence of swelling at night
- Increased appetite, increased weight

---

prochlorperazine (Rx)
(proe-klor-pair'a-zeen)
Chlorpazine, Compa-Z, Compazine, Contranzine, Provazin ✦, Stemetil ✦, Ultrazine
Func. class.: Antiemetic/antipsychotic
Chem. class.: Phenothiazine, piperazine derivative

Pregnancy category C

Action: Depresses cerebral cortex, hypothalamus, limbic system, which control activity aggression; blocks neurotransmission produced by DOPamine at synapse; exhibits a strong α-adrenergic, anticholinergic blocking action; mechanism for antipsychotic effects is unclear; acts centrally by blocking chemoreceptor trigger zone, which in turn acts on vomiting center

→**Therapeutic Outcome:** Decreased nausea, vomiting, decreased signs and symptoms of psychosis

Uses: Nausea, vomiting, psychosis

Dosage and routes
Postoperative nausea/vomiting
Adult: IM 5-10 mg 1-2 hr before anesthesia; may repeat in 30 min; **IV** 5-10 mg 15-30 min before anesthesia; **IV** inf 20 mg/L D₅W or 0.9% NaCl 15-30 min before anesthesia, max 40 mg/day

Severe nausea/vomiting
Adult: PO 5-10 mg tid-qid; sus rel 15 mg qd in ᴀᴍ or 10 mg q12h; rec 25 mg/bid; IM 5-10 mg; may repeat q4h, max 40 mg/day

P *Child 18-39 kg:* PO 2.5 mg tid or 5 mg bid; max 15 mg/day; IM 0.132 mg/kg

P *Child 14-17 kg:* PO/rec 2.5 mg bid-tid, max 10 mg/day; IM 0.132 mg/kg

P *Child 9-13 kg:* PO/rec 2.5 mg qd-bid, max 7.5 mg/day; IM 0.132 mg/kg

Antipsychotic
P *Adult and child ≥12 yr:* PO 5-10 mg tid-qid; may increase q2-3 day, max 150 mg/day; IM 10-20 mg q2-4h up to 4 doses, then 10-20 mg q4-6h, max 200 mg/day; rec 10 mg tid-qid may increase by 5-10 mg q2-3 days as needed

P *Child 2-12 yr:* PO 2.5 mg bid-tid; IM 0.132 mg/kg, max 10 mg/dose

Antianxiety
P *Adult and child ≥12 yr:* 5 mg tid-qid, max 20 mg/day or >12 wk; IM 5-10 mg q3-4h, max 40 mg/day; **IV** 2.5-10 mg; max 40 mg/day

---

☒ Herb/drug   Ⓢ Do Not Crush   ✦ Alert   ✦ₜᵣ Key Drug   Ⓖ Geriatric   Ⓟ Pediatric

P *Child 2-12 yr:* IM 132 mcg/kg

Available forms: Syr 5 mg/ml; inj 5 mg/ml; tabs 5, 10, 25 mg; sus rel caps 10, 15, 30 mg; supp 2.5, 5, 25 mg

Adverse effects

(*italic* = common; **bold** = life-threatening)

CNS: Tardive dyskinesia, *euphoria*, **depression, extrapyramidal symptoms (EPS),** restlessness, tremor, dizziness, **neuroleptic malignant syndrome,** drowsiness

CV: **Circulatory failure, tachycardia**

EENT: Blurred vision

HEMA: **Agranulocytosis**

GI: Nausea, vomiting, anorexia, dry mouth, diarrhea, constipation, weight loss, metallic taste, cramps

RESP: **Respiratory depression**

Contraindications: Hypersensitivity to phenothiazines, coma, seizure, encephalopathy, bone marrow depression, narrow-angle glaucoma

P **Precautions:** Children <2 yr, pregnancy **C**,
G elderly

N **Do Not Confuse:**

Compazine/Coumadin, prochlorperazine/chlorproMAZINE

Pharmacokinetics

Absorption	Variably absorbed (PO); well absorbed (IM)
Distribution	Widely distributed; high concentration in CNS; crosses placenta
Metabolism	Liver, extensively; GI mucosa
Excretion	Kidneys, breast milk
Half-life	Unknown

Pharmacodynamics

	PO	PO–SUS REL	REC	IM	IV
Onset	½ hr	½ hr	1 hr	10-20 min	4-5 min
Peak	Unkn	Unkn	Unkn	Unkn	Unkn
Duration	3-4 hr	10-12 hr	3-4 hr	3-4 hr	3-4 hr

Interactions

Drug classifications

Antacids: ↓ absorption

Anticholinergics: ↑ anticholinergic effects

Antidepressants, antihistamines, barbiturates: ↑ CNS depression

Antidiarrheals (adsorbent): ↓ absorption

Antihypertensives: ↑ hypotension

Antiparkinson agents: ↑ anticholinergic action, ↑ parkinson symptoms

Antithyroid agents: ↑ agranulocytosis

☑ *Herb/drug*

Betel palm, kava: ↑ EPS

Chamomile, cola nut, hops, kava, nettle, nutmeg, skullcap, valerian: ↑ CNS depression

Henbane, jimsonweed, scopolia: ↑ anticholinergic effect

Lab test interferences

↑ Liver function tests, ↑ cardiac enzymes, ↑ cholesterol, ↑ blood glucose, ↑ prolactin, ↑ bilirubin, ↑ PBI, ↑ cholinesterase, ↑ ^{131}I, ↑ alkaline phosphatase, ↑ leukocytes, ↑ granulocytes, ↑ platelets

↓ Hormones (blood and urine)

False positive: Pregnancy tests, PKU, urine bilirubin

False negative: Urinary steroids, 17-OHCS, pregnancy tests

NURSING CONSIDERATIONS

Assessment

• Assess mental status: orientation, mood, behavior, presence and type of hallucinations before initial administration and monthly; this drug should significantly reduce psychotic behavior

• Check for swallowing of PO medication; check for hoarding or giving of medication to other patients

• Monitor I&O ratio; palpate bladder if low
G urinary output occurs, especially in elderly; urinalysis recommended before, during prolonged therapy

◆● Monitor bilirubin, CBC, liver function studies monthly; blood dyscrasias hepatotoxicity may occur

• Assess affect, orientation, LOC, reflexes, gait, coordination, sleep pattern disturbances

• Monitor B/P with patient sitting, standing, and lying; take pulse and respirations q4h during initial treatment; establish baseline before starting treatment; report drops of 30 mm Hg; obtain baseline ECG, Q-wave and T-wave changes

• Check for dizziness, faintness, palpitations, tachycardia on rising; severe orthostatic hypotension is common

◆● Identify neuroleptic malignant syndrome: hyperpyrexia, muscle rigidity, increased CPK, altered mental status, seizures, fever, tachycardia, dyspnea, fatigue, loss of bladder control; notify prescriber immediately; drug should be discontinued

• Assess for EPS including akathisia (inability to sit still, no pattern to movements), tardive dyskinesia (bizarre movements of the jaw, mouth, tongue, extremities), pseudoparkinsonism (ragged tremors, pill rolling, shuffling

P

gait); an antiparkinsonism drug should be prescribed

• Assess for constipation, urinary retention daily; if these occur, increase bulk, water in diet

Nursing diagnoses
☑ Thought processes, disturbed (uses)
☑ Coping, ineffective (uses)
☑ Knowledge, deficient (teaching)
☑ Noncompliance (teaching)

Implementation
PO route
• Give drug in liq form mixed in glass of juice or cola if hoarding is suspected; do not mix in caffeine drinks, tannics, pectins
G • Give decreased dosage in elderly since metabolism is slowed
• Give PO with full glass of water, milk; or give with food to decrease GI upset
• Store in airtight, light-resistant container; oral sol in amber bottle
🚫 • Do not crush or chew sus rel cap
IM route
• Inject slowly in deep muscle mass; do not give SC; aspirate to avoid **IV** administration; do not administer sol with a precipitate; have patient lie down afterward for at least 30 min
IV **IV route**
• Give by direct **IV** after diluting **IV** using 0.9% NaCl to 1 mg/1 ml; administer at 1 mg/min or less
• Administer by intermittent inf after diluting 20 mg/L or less LR, Ringer's, dextrose, saline, or any combination

Syringe compatibilities: Atropine, butorphanol, chlorproMAZINE, cimetidine, diamorphine, diphenhydrAMINE, droperidol, fentanyl, glycopyrrolate, hydrOXYzine, meperidine, metoclopramide, nalbuphine, pentazocine, perphenazine, promazine, promethazine, ranitidine, scopolamine, sufentanil

Syringe incompatibilities: Dimenhydrinate, midazolam, pentobarbital, thiopental

Y-site compatibilities: Amsacrine, calcium gluconate, cisplatin, cladribine, cyclophosphamide, cytarabine, DOXOrubicin, fluconazole, granisetron, heparin, hydrocortisone, melphalan, methotrexate, ondansetron, paclitaxel, potassium chloride, propofol, sargramostim, sufentanil, teniposide, thiotepa, vinorelbine, vit B/C

Y-site incompatibilities: Foscarnet

Additive compatibilities: Amikacin, ascorbic acid, dexamethasone, dimenhydrinate, erythromycin, ethacrynate, lidocaine, nafcillin, netilmicin, sodium bicarbonate, vit B/C

Additive incompatibilities: Aminophylline, amphotericin B, ampicillin, calcium gluceptate, cefoperazone, cephalothin, chloramphenicol, chlorothiazide, floxacillin, furosemide, hydrocortisone sodium succinate, methohexital sodium, penicillin G sodium, phenobarbital, thiopental

Patient/family education
• Teach patient to use good oral hygiene; frequent rinsing of mouth, sugarless gum for dry mouth
• Caution patient to avoid hazardous activities until drug response is determined; dizziness, blurred vision may occur
• Inform patient that orthostatic hypotension occurs often and to rise from sitting or lying position gradually; to remain lying down after IM inj for at least 30 min; tell patient to avoid hot tubs, hot showers, tub baths, since hypotension may occur; tell patient that in hot weather heat stroke may occur; take extra precautions to stay cool
• Advise patient to avoid abrupt withdrawal of this drug, or EPS may result; drug should be withdrawn slowly
• Teach patient to avoid OTC preparations (cough, hay fever, cold) unless approved by prescriber, since serious drug interactions may occur; avoid use with alcohol, CNS depressants; increased drowsiness may occur; avoid activities requiring mental alertness
• Instruct patient to use a sunscreen and sunglasses to prevent burns
• Teach patient about EPS and necessity of meticulous oral hygiene, since oral candidiasis may occur
• Advise patient to take antacids 2 hr before or after taking this drug
• Advise patient to report sore throat, malaise, fever, bleeding, mouth sores; if these occur, CBC should be done and drug discontinued
• Teach patient not to double or skip doses
• Teach patient urine may turn pink to reddish brown
• Instruct patient to report dark urine, clay-colored stools, bleeding, bruising, rash, blurred vision
• Teach patient to avoid sun or use sunscreen, protective clothing

Evaluation
Positive therapeutic outcome
• Relief of nausea and vomiting

 Herb/drug   Do Not Crush   Alert   Key Drug   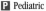 Geriatric   **P** Pediatric

- Decrease in emotional excitement, hallucinations, delusions, paranoia
- Reorganization of patterns of thought, speech

Treatment of overdose: Lavage if orally ingested; provide airway; *do not induce vomiting or use epINEPHrine*

---

progesterone 🔄 (Rx)
(proe-jess′ter-one)
Crinone, progesterone, Prometrium
Func. class.: Progestogen
Chem. class.: Progesterone derivative
Pregnancy category D

Action: Inhibits secretion of pituitary gonadotropins, which prevents follicular maturation, ovulation; stimulates growth of mammary tissue; antineoplastic action against endometrial cancer

➡**Therapeutic Outcome:** Decreased abnormal uterine bleeding, absence of amenorrhea

Uses: Contraception, amenorrhea, premenstrual syndrome, abnormal uterine bleeding, endometrial hyperplasia prevention

Investigational uses: Corpus luteum dysfunction

Dosage and routes
Infertility
Adult: VAG 90 mg qd

Amenorrhea/uterine bleeding
Adult: IM 5-10 mg qd × 6-8 doses

Endometrial hyperplasia prevention
Adult: PO 200 mg/day

Available forms: Caps 100, 200 mg; inj 50 mg/ml; powder micronized, vag gel 8%

Adverse effects
(*italic* = common; **bold** = life-threatening)
CNS: Dizziness, headache, migraines, depression, fatigue
CV: Hypotension, thrombophlebitis, edema, **thromboembolism, stroke, pulmonary embolism, MI**
EENT: Diplopia, retinal thrombosis
GI: *Nausea,* vomiting, anorexia, cramps, increased weight, **cholestatic jaundice**
GU: Amenorrhea, cervical erosion, breakthrough bleeding, dysmenorrhea, vaginal candidiasis, breast changes, *gynecomastia, testicular atrophy, impotence,* endometriosis, **spontaneous abortion**
INTEG: Rash, urticaria, acne, hirsutism,

alopecia, oily skin, seborrhea, purpura, melasma
META: Hyperglycemia
SYST: Angioedema, anaphylaxis

Contraindications: Breast cancer, hypersensitivity, thromboembolic disorders, reproductive cancer, genital bleeding (abnormal, undiagnosed), cerebral hemorrhage, pregnancy **D**

Precautions: Lactation, hypertension, asthma, blood dyscrasias, gallbladder disease, CHF, diabetes mellitus, bone disease, depression, migraine headache, seizure disorders, hepatic disease, renal disease, family history of breast or reproductive tract cancer

Pharmacokinetics

Absorption	Unknown
Distribution	Unknown
Metabolism	Unknown
Excretion	Breast milk
Half-life	Unknown

Pharmacodynamics

	IM	REC	VAG
Onset	Unknown	Unknown	Unknown
Peak	Unknown	Unknown	Unknown
Duration	24 hr	24 hr	24 hr

Interactions
Drug classifications
Barbiturates, phenytoins: ↓ progesterone effect
Herb/drug
Alfalfa: ↑ hormonal effect
Lab test interferences
↑ Alkaline phosphatase, ↑ nitrogen (urine), ↑ pregnanediol, ↑ amino acids, ↑ factors VII, VIII, IX, X
↓ GTT, ↓ HDL

NURSING CONSIDERATIONS
Assessment
- Monitor B/P at beginning of treatment and periodically; check weight daily; notify prescriber of weekly weight gain >5 lb
- Monitor I&O ratio: be alert for decreasing urinary output, increasing edema, hypertension
- Assess liver function studies: ALT, AST, bilirubin periodically during long-term therapy
- Assess edema, hypertension, cardiac symptoms, jaundice
- Assess mental status: affect, mood, behavioral changes, depression
- Assess for hypercalcemia

P

Nursing diagnoses

✓ Sexual dysfunction (uses)
✓ Tissue perfusion, ineffective (adverse reactions)
✓ Injury, risk for (adverse reactions)
✓ Knowledge, deficient (teaching)

Implementation
IM route

- Store in dark area
- Give titrated dose; use lowest effective dosage; give oil sol deep in large muscle mass; rotate sites; use after warming to dissolve crystals

Patient/family education

- Teach patient to report breast lumps, vaginal bleeding, edema, jaundice, dark urine, clay-colored stools, dyspnea, headache, blurred vision, abdominal pain, numbness or stiffness in legs, chest pain
- Teach patient to report suspected pregnancy

Evaluation
Positive therapeutic outcome

- Decreased abnormal uterine bleeding
- Absence of amenorrhea
- Prevented pregnancy

---

promethazine (Rx)
(proe-meth′a-zeen)
Anergan, Antinaus, Histanil ✦, Pentazine, Phenazine, Phenecen-50, Phenergan, Phenergan Fortis, Phenergan Plain, Phenerzine, Phenoject, Pro-50, Promacot, Pro-med, Promet, promethazine HCl, Prorex, Shogan, V-Gan
Func. class.: Antihistamine, H_1-receptor antagonist; antiemetic; sedative/hypnotic
Chem. class.: Phenothiazine derivative

Pregnancy category C

Action: Acts on blood vessels, GI, respiratory system by competing with histamine for H_1-receptor site; decreases allergic response by blocking histamine; also acts on chemoreceptor trigger zone to decrease vomiting; increases CNS stimulation, has anticholinergic response

➔ **Therapeutic Outcome:** Absence of allergy symptoms and rhinitis, absence of nausea/vomiting, sedation

Uses: Motion sickness, rhinitis, allergy symptoms, sedation, nausea, preoperative and postoperative sedation

Dosage and routes
Nausea
Adult: PO/IM/**IV**/REC 10-25 mg; may repeat 12.5-25 mg q4-6h

P *Child >2 yr:* PO/IM/**IV**/REC 0.25-0.5 mg/kg q4-6h

Motion sickness
Adult: PO 25 mg bid; give 30-60 min before departure

P *Child >2 yr:* PO/IM/REC 12.5-25 mg bid; give 30-60 min before departure

Allergy/rhinitis
Adult: PO 12.5 mg qid, or 25 mg hs

P *Child >2 yr:* PO 6.25-12.5 mg tid or 25 mg hs

Sedation
Adult: PO/IM/**IV**/REC 25-50 mg hs

P *Child >2 yr:* PO/IM/REC 12.5-25 mg hs

Sedation (preoperative/postoperative)
Adult: PO/IM/**IV** 25-50 mg

P *Child >2 yr:* PO/IM/**IV** 12.5-25 mg

Available forms: Tabs 10, 12.5, 25, 50 mg; supp 2.5, 5, 25 mg; inj 25, 50 mg/ml; syr 6.25, 10, 25 mg/5 ml

Adverse effects
(*italic* = common; **bold** = life-threatening)
CNS: *Dizziness, drowsiness,* poor coordination, fatigue, anxiety, euphoria, confusion, paresthesia, neuritis, extrapyramidal symptoms (EPS), **neuroleptic malignant syndrome**
CV: Hypotension, palpitations, tachycardia
EENT: Blurred vision, dilated pupils, tinnitus, nasal stuffiness, dry nose, throat, mouth, photosensitivity
GI: *Constipation,* dry mouth, nausea, vomiting, anorexia, diarrhea
GU: *Retention,* dysuria, frequency
HEMA: **Thrombocytopenia, agranulocytosis, hemolytic anemia**
INTEG: Rash, urticaria, photosensitivity
RESP: Increased thick secretions, wheezing,
P chest tightness, **apnea in pediatric patients**

Contraindications: Hypersensitivity to H_1-receptor antagonist, acute asthma attack, lower respiratory tract disease

Precautions: Increased intraocular pressure, renal disease, cardiac disease, hypertension, bronchial asthma, seizure disorder, stenosed peptic ulcers, hyperthyroidism, prostatic hypertrophy, bladder neck obstruction, pregnancy C

⊘ Herb/drug   ⊘ Do Not Crush   ✦ Alert   ✦ₜₜ Key Drug   G Geriatric   P Pediatric

Do Not Confuse:
Phenergan/Theragran

Pharmacokinetics

Absorption	Well absorbed (PO, IM); erratically absorbed (rec)
Distribution	Widely distributed; crosses the blood-brain barrier, placenta
Metabolism	Liver
Excretion	Kidneys, breast milk
Half-life	Unknown

Pharmacodynamics

	PO/IM/REC	IV
Onset	20 min	3-5 min
Peak	Unknown	Unknown
Duration	4-6 hr	4-6 hr

Interactions
Individual drugs
Alcohol: ↑ CNS depression
Drug classifications
Anticoagulants, oral: ↓ anticoagulant effect
Antidepressants (tricyclics), antihistamines, MAOIs: ↑ anticholinergic reactions
Barbiturates, CNS depressants, opiates, sedative/hypnotics: ↑ CNS depression
Herb/drug
Henbane, jimsonweed, scopolia: ↑ anticholinergic effect
Lab test interferences
False negative: Skin allergy tests (discontinue antihistamines 3 days before testing)
False-positive: Urine pregnancy test

NURSING CONSIDERATIONS
Assessment
• Assess respiratory status: rate, rhythm, increase in bronchial secretions, wheezing, chest tightness; provide fluids to 2 L/day to decrease secretion thickness
• Monitor I&O ratio: be alert for urinary retention, frequency, dysuria, especially elderly; drug should be discontinued if these occur
• Monitor CBC during long-term therapy; blood dyscrasias may occur but are rare

Nursing diagnoses
☑ Airway clearance, ineffective (uses)
☑ Injury, risk for (adverse reactions)
☑ Knowledge, deficient (teaching)
☑ Noncompliance (teaching, overuse)

Implementation
PO route
• Give with meals to decrease GI upset
• Store in airtight, light-resistant container

IM route
• Give IM inj in large muscle mass; aspirate to avoid **IV** administration; do not give SC; necrosis may occur
IV route
• Give **IV** directly; give 25 mg or less over 1 min; rapid drop in B/P may occur with rapid administration

Syringe compatibilities: Atropine, butorphanol, chlorproMAZINE, cimetidine, diphenhydramine, droperidol, fentanyl, glycopyrrolate, hydromorphone, hydrOXYzine, meperidine, metoclopramide, midazolam, pentazocine, perphenazine, prochlorperazine, promazine, ranitidine, scopolamine

Syringe incompatibilities: Dimenhydrinate, heparin, pentobarbital, thiopental

Y-site compatibilities: Amifostine, amsacrine, aztreonam, ciprofloxacin, cisplatin, cladribine, cyclophosphamide, cytarabine, DOXOrubicin, filgrastim, fluconazole, fludarabine, granisetron, melphalan, ondansetron, sargramostim, teniposide, thiotepa, vinorelbine

Y-site incompatibilities: Cefoperazone, foscarnet, heparin

Additive compatibilities: Amikacin, ascorbic acid, chloroquine, hydromorphone, netilmicin, vit B/C

Additive incompatibilities: Aminophylline, carbenicillin, chloramphenicol, chlorothiazide, floxacillin, furosemide, heparin, hydrocortisone sodium succinate, methicillin, methohexital, penicillin G, pentobarbital, phenobarbital, thiopental

Patient/family education
• Inform patient that a false negative result may occur with skin testing; these procedures should not be scheduled until 3 days after discontinuing use
• Advise patient to take 30 min before departure to prevent motion sickness
• Caution patient to avoid hazardous activities, activities requiring alertness, since dizziness may occur; instruct patient to request assistance with ambulation
• Advise patient to avoid alcohol, other depressants; serious CNS depression may occur
• Teach patient all aspects of drug use; to notify prescriber if confusion, sedation, hypotension occur; to avoid driving and other hazardous activity if drowsiness occurs

- Advise patient to take 1 hr ac or 2 hr pc to facilitate absorption
- Caution patient not to exceed recommended dosage; dysrhythmias may occur
- Inform patient hard candy, gum, frequent rinsing of mouth may be used for dryness

Evaluation
Positive therapeutic outcome
- Absence of motion sickness
- Absence of nausea, vomiting

Treatment of overdose: Administer ipecac syrup or lavage, diazepam, vasopressors, barbiturates (short-acting)

---

propantheline (Rx)
(proe-pan'the-leen)
Pro-Banthine, Propanthel ✦
Func. class.: GI anticholinergic; antiulcer agent
Chem. class.: Synthetic quaternary ammonium compound

Pregnancy category C

Action: Inhibits muscarinic actions of acetylcholine at postganglionic parasympathetic neuroeffector sites

➡ **Therapeutic Outcome:** Absence of peptic ulcer disease symptoms

Uses: Treatment of peptic ulcer disease, irritable bowel syndrome, duodenography, urinary incontinence

Investigational uses: Antispasmodic uses

Dosage and routes
Adult: PO 15 mg tid ac, 30 mg hs

G *Elderly/small patients:* PO 7.5 mg tid ac

Available forms: Tabs 7.5, 15 mg

Adverse effects
(*italic* = common; **bold** = life-threatening)
G *CNS: Confusion, stimulation in elderly,* headache, insomnia, dizziness, drowsiness, anxiety, weakness, hallucinations
CV: Palpitations, tachycardia, orthostatic
G hypotension (elderly)
EENT: Blurred vision, photophobia, mydriasis, cycloplegia, increased ocular tension
GI: Dry mouth, constipation, **paralytic ileus,** heartburn, nausea, vomiting, dysphagia, absence of taste
GU: Hesitancy, retention, impotence
INTEG: Urticaria, rash, pruritus, anhidrosis, fever, allergic reactions

Contraindications: Hypersensitivity to anticholinergics, narrow-angle glaucoma, GI obstruction, myasthenia gravis, paralytic ileus, GI atony, toxic megacolon

Precautions: Hyperthyroidism, CAD, dysrhythmias, CHF, ulcerative colitis, hypertension, hiatal hernia, hepatic disease, renal disease, pregnancy **C**, urinary retention, prostatic hypertrophy

Pharmacokinetics
Absorption	Moderately absorbed
Distribution	Unknown
Metabolism	Unknown
Excretion	Unknown
Half-life	Unknown

Pharmacodynamics
Onset	½ hr
Peak	2-6 hr
Duration	4-6 hr

Interactions
Individual drugs
Amantadine: ↑ anticholinergic effect
Drug classifications
Antidepressants (tricyclic), antihistamines, MAOIs, phenothiazines: ↑ anticholinergic effect
☑ *Herb/drug*
Henbane, jimsonweed, scopolia: ↑ anticholinergic effect

NURSING CONSIDERATIONS
Assessment
- Assess for the pain of peptic ulcer disease before, during, and after treatment

Nursing diagnoses
☑ Pain, chronic (uses)
☑ Constipation (adverse reactions)
☑ Thought processes, disturbed (adverse reactions)
☑ Knowledge, deficient (teaching)

Implementation
- Give 30 min ac and hs; do not give with antacids; separate by at least 1 hr

Patient/family education
- Teach patient to report blurred vision, chest pain, allergic reactions
- Advise patient not to perform strenuous activity in high temp; heat stroke may result due to decreased perspiration
- Instruct patient to take as prescribed; not to skip doses
- Instruct patient to report change in vision; blurring or loss of sight; drug should be discontinued

---

 Herb/drug   Do Not Crush   Alert   Key Drug **G** Geriatric **P** Pediatric

- Advise patient not to operate machinery or drive if dizziness occurs
- Caution patient not to take OTC products without approval of prescriber

Evaluation
Positive therapeutic outcome
- Decreased pain in peptic ulcer disease

! HIGH ALERT

propoxyphene (Rx)
(proe-pox'i-feen)
Darvon, Darvon-N, Dolene, Novapropoxyn ♣
Func. class.: Opiate analgesics
Chem. class.: Synthetic opiate

Pregnancy category C

Controlled substance schedule IV

Action: Depresses pain impulse transmission at the spinal cord level by interacting with opioid receptors

➔ **Therapeutic Outcome:** Decreased pain

Uses: Mild to moderate pain

Dosage and routes
Adult: PO 65 mg q4h prn (HCl)

Adult: PO 100 mg q4h prn (napsylate)

Available forms: *Propoxyphene HCl:* caps 32, 65 mg; *propoxyphene napsylate:* tabs 100 mg; oral susp 50 mg/5 ml

Adverse effects
(*italic* = common; **bold** = life-threatening)
CNS: Drowsiness, dizziness, confusion, headache, sedation, euphoria, **seizures,**
🅖 **hyperthermia** (elderly)
CV: Palpitations, bradycardia, change in B/P, **dysrhythmias**
EENT: Tinnitus, blurred vision, miosis, diplopia
GI: Nausea, vomiting, anorexia, constipation, cramps
GU: Urinary retention, dysuria
INTEG: Rash, urticaria, bruising, flushing, diaphoresis, pruritus
RESP: **Respiratory depression**

Contraindications: Hypersensitivity to acetylsalicylic acid products (some preparations), addiction (opioid)

Precautions: Addictive personality, pregnancy **C**, lactation, increased ICP, MI (acute), severe heart disease, respiratory depression,
🅟 hepatic disease, renal disease, child <18 yr,
🅖 elderly

Pharmacokinetics
Absorption	Well absorbed
Distribution	Widely distributed; crosses placenta
Metabolism	Liver, extensively
Excretion	Kidneys, breast milk
Half-life	6-12 hr

Pharmacodynamics
Onset	½-1 hr
Peak	2-2½ hr
Duration	4-6 hr

Interactions
Individual drugs
Alcohol: ↑ respiratory depression, hypotension, sedation
Nalbuphine, pentazocine: ↓ analgesia
Drug classifications
Antihistamines, CNS depressants, sedative/hypnotics: ↑ respiratory depression, hypotension
MAOIs: Possible fatal reactions
⬚ *Herb/drug*
Chamomile, hops, kava, skullcap, valerian: ↑ CNS depression
Corkwood: ↑ anticholinergic effects
Lab test interferences
↑ Amylase

NURSING CONSIDERATIONS
Assessment
- Assess pain: location, duration, intensity before and 1 hr after administration
- Monitor CNS changes: dizziness, drowsiness, euphoria, LOC, pupil reaction
- Monitor allergic reactions: rash, urticaria

Nursing diagnoses
☑ Pain (uses)
☑ Sensory perception, disturbed: visual, auditory (adverse reactions)
☑ Breathing pattern, ineffective (adverse reactions)
☑ Injury, risk for (adverse reactions)
☑ Knowledge, deficient (teaching)

Implementation
- Give with antiemetic if nausea, vomiting occur
- Give when pain is beginning to return; determine dosage interval by patient response; continuous dosing of medication is more effective than when given prn
- Withdraw medication slowly after long-term use to prevent withdrawal symptoms
- Store in light-resistant container at room temp

• May be given with food or milk to lessen GI upset

Patient/family education

• Teach patient to avoid CNS depressants: alcohol, sedative/hypnotics for at least 24 hr after taking this drug
• Discuss with patient that dizziness, drowsiness, and confusion are common; to avoid getting up without assistance
• Discuss in detail all aspects of the drug, including purpose and what to expect after anesthesia
• Advise patient to make position changes slowly to lessen orthostatic hypotension

Evaluation

Positive therapeutic outcome

• Decreased pain

Treatment of overdose: Naloxone 0.2-0.8 mg **IV**, O_2, **IV** fluids, vasopressors

---

propranolol ⊶ (Rx)

(proe-pran'oh-lole)

Apo-Propranolol ✤, Betaclinron E-R ✤, Detensol ✤, Inderal, Inderal LA, NovoPranol ✤, PMS-Propranol, propranolol HCl

Func. class.: Antihypertensive, antianginal, antidysrhythmic (class III)
Chem. class.: β-Adrenergic blocker

Pregnancy category C

Action: Competitively blocks stimulation of β-adrenergic receptor within vascular smooth muscle; produces chronotropic, inotropic activity (decreases rate of SA node discharge, increases recovery time), slows conduction of AV node, decreased heart rate, which decreases O_2 consumption in myocardium; also suppresses renin-aldosterone-angiotensin system at high doses, inhibits $β_2$-receptors in bronchial system (high doses)

⮑ **Therapeutic Outcome:** Decreased B/P, heart rate

Uses: Chronic stable angina pectoris, hypertension, supraventricular dysrhythmias, migraine prophylaxis, MI, pheochromocytoma, essential tremor, cyanotic spells related to hypertrophic subaortic stenosis

Investigational uses: Parkinson's tremor, prevention of variceal bleeding caused by portal hypertension, akathisia induced by antipsychotics, anxiety

Dosage and routes

Dysrhythmias
Adult: PO 10-30 mg tid-qid; **IV** bol 0.5-3 mg given 1 mg/min; may repeat in 2 min; may repeat q4h thereafter
P *Child:* PO 0.5-1 mg/kg/day divided in 2 doses, **IV** 0.01-0.1 mg/kg over 5 min

Hypertension
Adult: PO 40 mg bid or 80 mg qd (sus rel) initially; usual dosage 120-240 mg/day bid-tid or 120-160 mg qd (sus rel)
P *Child:* PO 0.5-1 mg/kg/day divided q6-12h

Angina
Adult: PO 80-320 mg in divided doses bid-qid or 80 mg qd (sus rel); usual dosage 160 mg qd (sus rel)

MI prophylaxis
Adult: PO 180-240 mg/day tid-qid starting 5 days to 3 wk after MI

Pheochromocytoma
Adult: PO 60 mg/day × 3 days preoperatively in divided doses or 30 mg/day in divided doses (inoperable tumor)

Migraine
Adult: PO 80 mg/day (sus rel) or in divided doses; may increase to 160-240 mg/day in divided doses
P *Child:* PO 0.6-1.5 mg/kg/day divided q8h

Essential tremor
Adult: PO 40 mg bid; usual dosage 120 mg/day

Available forms: Sus rel caps 60, 80, 120, 160 mg; tabs 10, 20, 40, 60, 80, 90 mg; inj 1 mg/ml; oral sol 4 mg, 8 mg/ml; conc oral sol 80 mg/ml

Adverse effects

(*italic* = common; **bold** = life-threatening)

CNS: Depression, hallucinations, dizziness, fatigue, lethargy, paresthesia, bizarre dreams, disorientation
CV: **Bradycardia,** *hypotension,* **CHF,** palpitations, AV block, peripheral vascular insufficiency, vasodilatation, **pulmonary edema, dysrhythmias,** cold extremities
EENT: Sore throat, **laryngospasm,** blurred vision, dry eyes
GI: Nausea, vomiting, diarrhea, colitis, constipation, cramps, dry mouth, hepatomegaly, gastric pain, acute pancreatitis
GU: Impotence, decreased libido, UTIs
HEMA: **Agranulocytosis, thrombocytopenia**

INTEG: Rash, pruritus, fever
META: Hyperglycemia, hypoglycemia
MISC: Facial swelling, weight change, Raynaud's phenomenon
MS: Joint pain, arthralgia, muscle cramps, pain
RESP: Dyspnea, respiratory dysfunction, **bronchospasm,** cough

Contraindications: Hypersensitivity to this drug, cardiac failure, cardiogenic shock, 2nd- or 3rd-degree heart block, bronchospastic disease, sinus bradycardia, CHF

Precautions: Diabetes mellitus, pregnancy **C,** renal disease, lactation, hyperthyroidism, P COPD, hepatic disease, children, myasthenia gravis, peripheral vascular disease, hypotension, CHF

N Do Not Confuse:
Inderal/Toradol, Inderal LA/IMDUR

Pharmacokinetics

Absorption	Well absorbed (PO); slowly absorbed (ext rel); completely absorbed (**IV**)
Distribution	Widely distributed; crosses blood-brain barrier, protein binding 90%
Metabolism	Liver, extensively
Excretion	Kidneys
Half-life	3-5 hr; EXT REL 8-11 hr

Pharmacodynamics

	PO	PO–EXT REL	IV
Onset	½ hr	Unknown	Rapid
Peak	1-1½ hr	6 hr	1 min
Duration	6-12 hr	24 hr	4-6 hr

Interactions
Individual drugs
Alcohol: ↑ hypotension (large amounts)
Cimetidine: ↑ β-blocking effect
Clonidine: ↑ B/P may be fatal after discontinuing β-blocker
Disopyramide: Difficult to predict
Epinephrine: α-Adrenergic stimulation
Haloperidol, prazosin, quinidine, reserpine: ↑ hypotension
Prazosin, reserpine: ↑ bradycardia
Thyroid hormones: ↓ effect of propranolol
Verapamil: ↑ myocardial depression
Drug classifications
Anticoagulants: ↑ bleeding risk
Barbiturates: ↓ β-blocking effect
Calcium channel blockers: ↑ or ↓ effect
Neuromuscular blockers: ↑ effects
SSRIs: ↓ metabolism, ↑ propranolol effect
Theophyllines: ↓ or ↑ effect

☑ Herb/drug
Aconite: ↑ toxicity, death
Astragalus, cola tree: ↑ or ↓ antihypertensive effect
Barberry, betony, black catechu, black cohosh, bloodroot, broom, burdock, cat's claw, dandelion, goldenseal, Irish moss, Jamaican dogwood, kelp, khella, mistletoe, parsley: ↑ antihypertensive effect
Coltsfoot, guarana, khat, licorice: ↓ antihypertensive effect
Lab test interferences
False: ↑ Urinary catecholamines
Interference: Glaucoma testing

NURSING CONSIDERATIONS
Assessment
• Monitor B/P during beginning treatment, periodically thereafter; pulse q4h; note rate, rhythm, quality; check apical/radial pulse before administration; notify prescriber of any significant changes (pulse <50 bpm)
• Check for baselines in renal, liver function tests before therapy begins and periodically thereafter
• Assess for edema in feet, legs daily; monitor I&O, weight daily; check for jugular vein distention, rales bilaterally; dyspnea (CHF)
• Monitor skin turgor, dryness of mucous membranes for hydration status, especially **G** elderly

Nursing diagnoses
☑ Cardiac output, decreased (uses)
☑ Injury, risk for (adverse reactions)
☑ Knowledge, deficient (teaching)
☑ Noncompliance (teaching)

Implementation
PO route
• Given ac, hs, tab may be crushed or swallowed whole; do not crush or chew ext rel cap; give with food to prevent GI upset; reduce dosage in renal dysfunction
• May mix oral sol with liquid or semisolid food, rinse container to get entire dose
• Store protected from light, moisture; placed in cool environment
IV route
• Give by direct **IV** undiluted or diluted 1 mg/10 ml of D₅W for inj; administer over 1 min or more
• Give by intermittent inf after diluting in 50 ml of D₅W, 0.9% NaCl, D₅/0.45% NaCl, D₅/0.9% NaCl, LR; administer over 15 min

Y-site compatibilities:
Amrinone, heparin, hydrocortisone, meperi-

P

dine, milrinone, morphine, potassium chloride, tacrolimus, vit B/C

Y-site incompatibilities: Diazoxide

Additive compatibilities: Dobutamine, verapamil

Solution compatibilities: 0.9% NaCl, 0.45% NaCl, Ringer's, D_5W, $D_5/0.9\%$ NaCl, $D_5/0.45\%$ NaCl

Patient/family education
• Teach patient not to discontinue drug abruptly, taper over 2 wk; may cause precipitate angina if stopped abruptly
• Teach patient not to use OTC products containing α-adrenergic stimulants (such as nasal decongestants, cold preparations); to avoid alcohol, smoking and to limit sodium intake as prescribed
• Teach patient how to take pulse and B/P at home; advise when to notify prescriber
• Instruct patient to comply with weight control, dietary adjustments, modified exercise program
• Instruct patient to carry/wear emergency ID to identify drug being taken, allergies; tell patient drug controls symptoms but does not cure
• Caution patient to avoid hazardous activities if dizziness, drowsiness is present
• Teach patient to report symptoms of CHF: difficult breathing, especially on exertion or when lying down, night cough, swelling of extremities or bradycardia, dizziness, confusion, depression, fever
• Teach patient to take drug as prescribed, not to double doses, skip doses; take any missed doses as soon as remembered if at least 8 hr until next dose
• Advise patient that sensitivity to cold may occur

Evaluation
Positive therapeutic outcome
• Decreased B/P in hypertension (after 1-2 wk)
• Decreased tremors
• Absence of dysrhythmias
• Decreased migraine headaches

Treatment of overdose: Lavage, **IV** atropine for bradycardia, **IV** theophylline for bronchospasm, digitalis, O_2, diuretic for cardiac failure, hemodialysis, **IV** glucose for hyperglycemia, **IV** diazepam (or phenytoin) for seizures

propylthiouracil (Rx)
(proe-pill-thye-oh-yoor'a-sill)
propylthiouracil, Propyl-Thyracil ✦, PTU
Func. class.: Thyroid hormone antagonist (antithyroid)
Chem. class.: Thioamide
Pregnancy category D

Action: Blocks synthesis peripherally of T_3, T_4, inhibits organification of iodine

⇒**Therapeutic Outcome:** Decreased T_3, T_4 levels, hyperthyroid symptoms

Uses: Preparation for thyroidectomy, thyrotoxic crisis, hyperthyroidism, thyroid storm

Dosage and routes
Thyrotoxic crisis
P *Adult and child:* PO same as hyperthyroidism with iodine and propranolol

Preparation for thyroidectomy
Adult: PO 600-1200 mg/day

P *Child:* PO 10 mg/kg/day in divided doses

Hyperthyroidism
Adult: PO 100 mg tid increasing to 300 mg q8h if condition is severe; continue to euthyroid state, then 100 mg qd-tid

P *Child >10 yr:* PO 100 mg tid; continue to euthyroid state, then 25 mg tid to 100 mg bid

P *Child 6-10 yr:* PO 50-150 mg in divided doses q8h

P *Neonates:* PO 10 mg/kg/day in divided doses

Available forms: Tabs 50, 100 mg

Adverse effects
(*italic* = common; **bold** = life-threatening)
CNS: Drowsiness, headache, vertigo, fever, paresthesias, neuritis
GI: Nausea, diarrhea, vomiting, jaundice, hepatitis, loss of taste
GU: **Nephritis**
HEMA: **Agranulocytosis, leukopenia, thrombocytopenia, hypothrombinemia, lymphadenopathy,** bleeding, vasculitis, periarteritis
INTEG: Rash, urticaria, pruritus, alopecia, hyperpigmentation, lupus-like syndrome
MS: Myalgia, arthralgia, nocturnal muscle cramps, osteoporosis

Contraindications: Hypersensitivity, pregnancy **D**, lactation

Precautions: Infection, bone marrow depression, hepatic disease

---

⊘ Herb/drug   ⓢ Do Not Crush   ✦ Alert   ✦ᴛᴛ Key Drug   Ⓖ Geriatric   Ⓟ Pediatric

Pharmacokinetics

Absorption	Rapidly absorbed
Distribution	Crosses placenta; concentration in thyroid gland
Metabolism	Liver
Excretion	Urine, bile, breast milk
Half-life	1-2 hr

Pharmacodynamics

Onset	30-40 min
Peak	Unknown
Duration	2-4 hr

Interactions
Individual drugs
Heparin: ↑ anticoagulant effect
Lithium: ↑ antithyroid effect
Potassium/sodium iodide: ↑ effects
Radiation: ↑ bone marrow depression
Drug classifications
Anticoagulants (oral): ↑ anticoagulant effect
Antineoplastics: ↑ bone marrow depression
Phenothiazines: ↑ agranulocytosis
Lab test interferences
↑ Pro-time, ↑ AST, ↑ ALT, ↑ alkaline phosphatase

NURSING CONSIDERATIONS
Assessment
- Monitor pulse, B/P, temp; I&O ratio; check for edema (puffy hands, feet, periorbits); indicates hypothyroidism
- Check weight daily with same clothing, scale, time of day
- Monitor T_3, T_4, which are increased; check serum TSH, which is decreased; assess free thyroxine index, which is increased if dosage is too low; discontinue drug 3-4 wk before radioactive iodine uptake test
- Monitor blood work: CBC for blood dyscrasias (leukopenia, thrombocytopenia, agranulocytosis); liver function tests
- Assess overdose (peripheral edema, heat intolerance, diaphoresis, palpitations, dysrhythmias, severe tachycardia, increased temp, delirium, CNS irritability); drug should be discontinued
- Assess for hypersensitivity (rash, enlarged cervical lymph nodes); drug may have to be discontinued
- Assess for hypoprothrombinemia (bleeding, petechiae, ecchymosis)
- Monitor clinical response: after 3 wk should include increased weight, decreased pulse, decreased T_4
- Assess for bone marrow depression: sore throat, fever, fatigue

Nursing diagnoses
☑ Knowledge, deficient (teaching)
☑ Noncompliance (teaching)
Implementation
- Give with meals to decrease GI upset
- Give at same time each day to maintain drug level
- Give lowest dosage that relieves symptoms
- Store in light-resistant container
- Increase fluids to 3-4 L/day, unless contraindicated

Patient/family education
- Advise patient to abstain from breastfeeding after delivery; drug appears in breast milk
- Teach patient to take pulse daily and to keep graph of weight, pulse, mood
- Advise patient to report redness, swelling, sore throat, mouth lesions, which indicate blood dyscrasias
- Caution patient to avoid OTC products that contain iodine; that seafood, other iodine-containing foods may be restricted by prescriber
- Caution patient not to discontinue this medication abruptly; thyroid crisis may occur; stress patient compliance
- Teach patient that response may take several mo if thyroid is large
- Teach patient symptoms/signs of overdose: periorbital edema, cold intolerance, mental depression; notify prescriber at once
- Teach patient symptoms of inadequate dose: tachycardia, diarrhea, fever, irritability; prescriber should be notified to adjust dosage
- Teach patient to take medication exactly as prescribed, not to skip or double doses; missed doses should be taken when remembered up to 1 hr before next dose
- Instruct patient to carry/wear emergency identification indicating medication taken and condition being treated

Evaluation
Positive therapeutic outcome
- Weight gain
- Decreased pulse
- Decreased T_4
- Decreased B/P

P

protamine (Rx)

(proe′ta-meen)

Func. class.: Heparin antagonist
Chem. class.: Low molecular weight protein

Pregnancy category C

Action: Binds heparin, making it ineffective

⮕ **Therapeutic Outcome:** Prevention of heparin overdose

Uses: Heparin overdose; neutralizes heparin in procedures

Dosage and routes

P *Adult and child:* **IV** 1 mg of protamine/90-115 units of heparin given; administer slowly over 1-3 min; not to exceed 50 mg/10 min

Available forms: Inj 10 mg/ml

Adverse effects

(*italic* = common; **bold** = life-threatening)

CNS: Lassitude

CV: Hypotension, bradycardia, **circulatory collapse**

GI: Nausea, vomiting, anorexia

INTEG: *Rash*, dermatitis, urticaria

HEMA: Bleeding

RESP: Dyspnea, **pulmonary edema, severe respiratory distress**

SYST: **Anaphylaxis, angioedema**

Contraindication: Hypersensitivity

Precautions: Pregnancy **C**, lactation, **P** children, allergy to salmon

Pharmacokinetics

Absorption	Completely absorbed
Distribution	Unknown
Metabolism	Unknown
Excretion	Unknown
Half-life	Unknown

Pharmacodynamics

Onset	5 min
Peak	Unknown
Duration	2 hr

Interactions: None

NURSING CONSIDERATIONS

Assessment

- Monitor blood studies (Hct, platelets, occult blood stools) q3 mo
- Monitor coagulation tests (APTT, ACT) 15 min after dose, then in several hr
- Monitor VS, B/P, pulse q30 min, plus 3 hr after dose
- Assess for hypersensitivity: skin rash, urticaria, dermatitis, cough, wheezing, have emergency equipment nearby; men that have had a vasectomy may be more prone to hypersensitivity
- Assess for allergy to salmon; use with caution in these patients

Nursing diagnoses

☑ Injury, risk for (uses)
☑ Tissue perfusion, ineffective (uses)
☑ Knowledge, deficient (teaching)

Implementation

- Give by direct **IV** after diluting 50 mg/5 ml of sterile bacteriostatic water for inj; shake; give 20 mg or less over 1-3 min
- Give by intermittent inf after further diluting with equal volume of NaCl or D$_5$W and run over 2-3 hr; titrate to APTT, ACT; use infusion pump
- Store at 36-46° F (2-8° C)

Additive compatibilities:
Cimetidine, ranitidine, verapamil

Additive incompatibilities:
Penicillins, cephalosporins

Patient/family education

- Explain reason for medication and expected results
- Caution patient to avoid contact activities that may result in bleeding

Evaluation

Positive therapeutic outcome

- Reversal of heparin overdose

pseudoephedrine (OTC)

(soo-doe-e-fed′rin)

Afrin, Allermed, Canafed, Cenafed, Children's Congestion Relief, Children's Silfedrine, Congestion Relief, Decofed Syrup, DeFed-60, Dorcol Children's Decongestant, Drixoral Non-Drowsy Formula, Dynafed, Efidac/24, Eltor ♣, Genaphed, Halofed, Mini Thin Pseudo, Pedia Care Infant's Decongestant, pseudoepHEDrine HCl, Pseudogest, Seudotabs, Sinustop Pro, Sudafed, Sudafed 12 hour, Sudex, Triaminic AM Decongestant Formula

Func. class.: Adrenergic
Chem. class.: Substituted phenylethylamine

Pregnancy category B

Action: Primary activity through α-adrenergic effects on respiratory mucosal membranes reducing congestion, hyperemia, edema; minimal bronchodilatation secondary to β-adrenergic effects

→ **Therapeutic Outcome:** Decreased nasal congestion, swelling

Uses: Nasal decongestant, otitis media adjustment, adjunct with antihistamines

Dosage and routes
P *Adult and child >12 yr:* PO 60 mg q6h; ext rel 120 mg q12h or 240 mg q24h

G *Elderly:* PO 30-60 mg q6h prn

P *Child 6-12 yr:* PO 30 mg q6h, max 120 mg/day

P *Child 2-6 yr:* PO 15 mg q6h, max 60 mg/day

Available forms: Ext rel caps 120, 240 mg; oral sol 15 mg, 30 mg/5 ml; drops 7.5 mg/0.8 ml; tabs 30, 60 mg; caps 60 mg; ext rel tabs 120, 240 mg

Adverse effects
(*italic* = common; **bold** = life-threatening)
CNS: *Tremors, anxiety,* insomnia, headache,
G dizziness, hallucinations, **seizures** (elderly)
CV: Palpitations, tachycardia, hypertension, chest pain, **dysrhythmias, CV collapse**
EENT: Dry nose, irritation of nose and throat
GI: *Anorexia, nausea, vomiting,* dry mouth
GU: Dysuria

Contraindications: Hypersensitivity to sympathomimetics, narrow-angle glaucoma

Precautions: Pregnancy **B**, cardiac disorders, hyperthyroidism, diabetes mellitus, prostatic hypertrophy, lactation, hypertension

Pharmacokinetics
Absorption	Well absorbed
Distribution	Enters CSF, crosses placenta
Metabolism	Liver, partially
Excretion	Kidneys, unchanged (75%); breast milk
Half-life	7 hr

Pharmacodynamics
	PO	PO–EXT REL
Onset	15-30 min	1 hr
Peak	Unknown	Unknown
Duration	4-6 hr	12 hr

Interactions
Individual drugs
Methyldopa: ↓ effect of pseudoephedrine
Drug classifications
Antidepressants (tricyclics), MAOIs: Hypertensive crisis, do not use together
Urinary acidifiers: ↓ effect of pseudoephedrine
Urinary alkalizers: ↑ effect of pseudoephedrine

NURSING CONSIDERATIONS
Assessment
G • Assess for CNS side effects in the elderly: excitation, seizures, hallucinations
• Monitor for nasal congestion; auscultate lung sounds; check for tenacious bronchial
P secretions; children with otitis media should be assessed for eustachian tube congestion
• Monitor B/P and pulse throughout treatment

Nursing diagnoses
✓ Airway clearance, ineffective (uses)
✓ Knowledge, deficient (teaching)

Implementation
• Give ext rel cap and tab whole
⊘ • Do not crush, break or chew
• Give several hr before bedtime if insomnia occurs
• Store at room temp

Patient/family education
• Teach patient reason for drug administration and expected results
• Instruct patient not to use continuously, or more than recommended dose; rebound congestion may occur
• Advise patient to check with prescriber before using other drugs, as drug interactions may occur
• Advise patient to avoid taking near bedtime; stimulation can occur
• Caution patient not to use if stimulation, restlessness, tremors occur
P • Notify parents of possible excessive agitation in children
◆ • Advise patient to notify prescriber of anxiety, slow or fast heart rate, dyspnea, seizures

Evaluation
Positive therapeutic outcome
• Decreased nasal congestion

P

psyllium (OTC)

(sill'i-um)

Alramucil, Fiberall, Fiberall Natural Flavor and Orange Flavor, Genifiber, Hydrocil Instant, Karacil ✤, Konsyl, Konsyl Orange, Maalox Daily Fiber Therapy, Metamucil, Metamucil Lemon Lime, Metamucil Orange Flavor, Metamucil Sugar Free, Metamucil Sugar Free Orange Flavor, Modane Bulk, Mylanta Natural Fiber Supplement, Natural Fiber Laxative, Natural Fiber Laxative Sugar Free, Natural Vegetable Reguloid, Perdiem, Prodiem Plain ✤, Reguloid Natural, Reguloid Orange, Reguloid Sugar Free Orange, Reguloid Sugar Free Regular, Restore, Restore Sugar Free, Serutan, Syllact, V-Lax

Func. class.: Laxative, bulk-forming
Chem. class.: Psyllium colloid

Pregnancy category C

Action: Promotes peristalsis by combining with water in the intestine to form a gel-like substance that is easily evacuated

⟹ **Therapeutic Outcome:** Decreased constipation, decreased diarrhea in colitis

Uses: Chronic constipation, ulcerative colitis, irritable bowel syndrome

Dosage and routes

Adult: PO 1-2 tsp in 8 oz of water bid or tid, then 8 oz of water or 1 premeasured packet in 8 oz of water bid or tid, then 8 oz of water

P *Child >6 yr:* 1 tsp in 4 oz of water hs

Available forms: Chew pieces 1.7, 3.4 g/piece; powder effervescent 3.4, 3.7 g/packet; granules 2.5, 4.03 g/tsp; powder 3.3, 3.4, 3.5, 4.94 g/tsp; wafers 3.4 g/wafer

Adverse effects

(*italic* = common; **bold** = life-threatening)
GI: Nausea, vomiting, anorexia, diarrhea, cramps, intestinal/esophageal blockage

Contraindications: Hypersensitivity, intestinal obstruction, abdominal pain, nausea/vomiting, fecal impaction

Precautions: Pregnancy **C**

Pharmacokinetics

Absorption	None
Distribution	None
Excretion	Feces
Half-life	Unknown

Pharmacodynamics

Onset	12-24 hr
Peak	2-4 days
Duration	Unknown

Interactions

Drug classifications
Cardiac glycosides, oral anticoagulants, salicylates: ↓ absorption of each specific drug
⬜ *Herb/drug*
Flax, senna: ↑ laxative
Lab test interferences
↑ Blood glucose

NURSING CONSIDERATIONS
Assessment

• Monitor blood, urine electrolytes if used often by patient; check I&O ratio to identify fluid loss

• Assess for cramping, rectal bleeding, nausea, vomiting; if these symptoms occur, drug should be discontinued; identify cause of constipation; identify whether fluids, bulk, or exercise is missing from lifestyle

• Assess stool for color, consistency, amount, presence of flatulence

Nursing diagnoses

☑ Constipation (uses)
☑ Knowledge, deficient (teaching)
☑ Noncompliance (teaching)

Implementation

• Give alone for better absorption; give after mixing with water immediately before use; administer with 8 oz of water or juice followed by another 8 oz of fluid

• Administer in AM or PM (oral dose)

Patient/family education

• Discuss with patient that adequate fluid consumption is necessary

• Teach patient that normal bowel movements do not always occur daily

• Caution patient not to use in presence of abdominal pain, nausea, vomiting; tell patient to notify prescriber if constipation is unrelieved or if symptoms of electrolyte imbalance occur (muscle cramps, pain, weakness, dizziness, excessive thirst)

• Teach patient not to use laxatives for long-term therapy; bowel tone will be lost and will decrease

• Teach patient to shake susp well as needed

• Teach patient not to take hs as a laxative;

may interfere with sleep; also problems with lipid pneumonia
• Teach patient not to use with food or vitamin preparations; delays digestion and absorption of fat-soluble vitamins

Evaluation
Positive therapeutic outcome
• Decreased constipation in 12-24 hr

---

pyrazinamide (Rx)
(peer-a-zin′a-mide)
PMS Pyrazinamide ♣, pyrazinamide, Tebrazid ♣
Func. class.: Antitubercular agent
Chem. class.: Pyrazinoic acid amine/nicoturimide analog

Pregnancy category C

Action: Bactericidal interference with lipid; nucleic acid biosynthesis is possible

⮊ **Therapeutic Outcome:** Bactericidal for *Mycobacterium* species

Uses: Tuberculosis, as an adjunct when other drugs are not feasible

Dosage and routes
🅟 *Adult and child:* PO 15-30 mg/kg qd, max 2 g/day

Available forms: Tabs 500 mg

Adverse effects
(*italic* = common; **bold** = life-threatening)
CNS: Headache
GI: **Hepatotoxicity,** abnormal liver function tests, peptic ulcer, nausea, vomiting, anorexia, cramps, diarrhea
GU: Urinary difficulty, increased uric acid
HEMA: **Hemolytic anemia**
INTEG: Photosensitivity, urticaria

Contraindications: Hypersensitivity, severe hepatic damage, acute gout

🅟 **Precautions:** Pregnancy **C,** child <13 yr, renal failure, diabetes, porphyria, chronic gout

Pharmacokinetics
Absorption	Well absorbed
Distribution	Widely distributed
Metabolism	Liver, extensively
Excretion	Kidneys, breast milk
Half-life	9-10 hr

Pharmacodynamics
Onset	Unknown
Peak	2 hr
Duration	9½ hr; metabolites 12 hr

Interactions: None
Lab test interferences
↑ PBI
↓ 17 KS

NURSING CONSIDERATIONS
Assessment
• C&S studies should be done before treatment begins, and periodically during treatment
• Monitor serum uric acid, which may be elevated and cause gout symptoms
• Monitor liver studies weekly: ALT, AST, bilirubin; hepatic status: decreased appetite, jaundice, dark urine, fatigue
• Monitor renal status before treatment and monthly thereafter: BUN, creatinine, output, sp gr, urinalysis, uric acid
• Monitor mental status often: affect, mood, behavioral changes; psychosis may occur

Nursing diagnoses
☑ Infection, risk for (uses)
☑ Diarrhea (adverse reactions)
☑ Injury, risk for (adverse reactions)
☑ Knowledge, deficient (teaching)
☑ Noncompliance (teaching)

Implementation
• Give with meals to decrease GI symptoms
• Give antiemetic if vomiting occurs
• May be given with other antitubercular drugs

Patient/family education
• Instruct patient that compliance with dosage schedule, duration is necessary; that scheduled appointments must be kept or relapse may occur
• Advise diabetic patient to use blood glucose monitor to obtain correct result
• Advise patient to report weakness, fatigue, loss of appetite, nausea, vomiting, yellowing of skin or eyes, tingling/numbness of hands/feet

Evaluation
Positive therapeutic outcome
• Decreased symptoms of TB
• Sputum culture negative × 3

P

---

pyridostigmine (Rx)

(peer-id-oh-stig'meen)

Mestinon, Mestinon SR, Mestinon Timespan, Regonol

Func. class.: Cholinergic, anticholinesterase
Chem. class.: Tertiary amine carbamate

Pregnancy category C

Action: Inhibits destruction of acetylcholine, which increases concentration at sites where acetylcholine is released; this facilitates transmission of impulses across myoneural junction

→ **Therapeutic Outcome:** Decreased action of nondepolarizing muscle relaxant; increased muscle strength in myasthenia gravis

Uses: Nondepolarizing muscle relaxant antagonist, myasthenia gravis

Dosage and routes

Myasthenia gravis
Adult: PO 60-180 mg bid-qid, not to exceed 1.5 g/day; IM/**IV** 2 mg or 1/30 of PO dose; sus rel 180-540 mg qd or bid at intervals of at least 6 hr

P *Child:* 7 mg/kg/day in 5-6 divided doses

Nondepolarizing neuromuscular blocker antagonist
Adult: 0.6-1.2 mg **IV** atropine, then 10-30 mg

P *Child:* 0.1-0.25 mg/kg/dose

Available forms: Tabs 60 mg; ext rel tabs 180 mg; syr 60 mg/5 ml; inj 5 mg/ml

Adverse effects

(*italic* = common; **bold** = life-threatening)
CNS: Dizziness, headache, sweating, weakness, **seizures,** uncoordination, paralysis, drowsiness, LOC
CV: Tachycardia, dysrhythmias, bradycardia, AV block, hypotension, ECG changes, **cardiac arrest,** syncope
EENT: Miosis, blurred vision, lacrimation, visual changes
GI: Nausea, diarrhea, vomiting, cramps, increased salivary and gastric secretions, peristalsis
GU: Frequency, incontinence, urgency
INTEG: Rash, urticaria, flushing
RESP: **Respiratory depression, bronchospasm, constriction, laryngospasm, respiratory arrest**

Contraindications: Bradycardia, hypotension, obstruction of intestine, renal system, bromide sensitivity

Precautions: Seizure disorders, bronchial asthma, coronary occlusion, hyperthyroidism, dysrhythmias, peptic ulcer, megacolon, poor GI motility, pregnancy **C**

Pharmacokinetics

Absorption	Poorly absorbed (PO)
Distribution	Widely distributed; crosses placenta
Metabolism	Liver, plasma cholinesterase
Excretion	Kidneys
Half-life	2 hr (**IV**); 4 hr (PO)

Pharmacodynamics

	PO	IM/IV	PO-EXT REL
Onset	20-30 min	2-15 min	½-1 hr
Peak	Unknown	Unknown	Unknown
Duration	3-6 hr	2-4 hr	3-6 hr

Interactions

Individual drugs
Atropine, gallamine, metocurine, tubocurarine: ↓ action
Magnesium, mecamylamine, polymyxin, procainamide, quinidine: ↓ action of pyridostigmine
Decamethonium, succinylcholine: ↑ action of succinylcholine

Drug classifications
Aminoglycosides, anesthetics, antidysrhythmics, corticosteroids: ↓ action of pyridostigmine

Herb/drug
Jaborandi tree, pill-bearing spurge: ↑ effect

NURSING CONSIDERATIONS

Assessment

- Monitor VS, respiration; increased B/P during test and at baseline
- Monitor diabetic patient carefully, since this drug lowers blood glucose

Nursing diagnoses

☑ Breathing pattern, ineffective (uses)
☑ Knowledge, deficient (teaching)

Implementation

IV IV route
- Give **IV** undiluted, give through Y-tube or 3-way stopcock; give 0.5 mg or less/min
- Give only when atropine sulfate available for cholinergic crisis

Syringe compatibilities: Glycopyrrolate

Y-site compatibilities: Heparin, hydrocortisone, potassium chloride, vit B/C

PO route
- Give only after all other cholinergics have been discontinued
- Give increased doses as ordered if tolerance occurs

- Give larger doses as ordered after exercise or fatigue
- Give on empty stomach for better absorption
- Store at room temp

Patient/family education
- Advise patient to carry/wear emergency ID specifying myasthenia gravis, drugs taken

Evaluation
Positive therapeutic outcome
- Increased muscle strength, hand grasp
- Improved gait
- Absence of labored breathing (if severe)

Treatment of overdose: Discontinue drug, atropine 1-4 mg **IV**

---

pyridoxine (vitamin B$_6$) (OTC, Rx)
(peer-i-dox'een)
Beesix, Doxine, Nestrex, pyridoxine HCl, Pyri, Rodex, Vitabee 6, Vitamin B$_6$
Func. class.: Vitamin B$_6$, water soluble

Pregnancy category A

Action: Needed for fat, protein, carbohydrate metabolism; enhances glycogen release from liver and muscle tissue; needed as coenzyme for metabolic transformations of a variety of amino acids

Therapeutic Outcome: Absence of vit B$_6$ deficiency

Uses: Vitamin B$_6$ deficiency associated with the following: inborn errors of metabolism, seizures, cycloSERINE, hydrALAZINE penicillamine, isoniazid therapy, oral contraceptives, alcoholism, polyneuritis

Investigational uses: Palmar-plantar erythrodysesthesia syndrome

Dosage and routes
RDA
Adult: PO male 1.7-2 mg; female 1.4-1.6 mg
Vitamin B$_6$ deficiency
Adult: PO/IM/**IV** 5-25 mg qd × 3 wk
P *Child:* PO/IM/**IV** 100 mg until desired response
Deficiency caused by isoniazid, cycloSERINE, hydrALAZINE, penicillamine
Adult: PO 6-100 mg qd
P *Child:* PO 5-25 mg/day

Prevention of deficiency caused by isoniazid, cycloSERINE, hydrALAZINE, penicillamine
Adult: PO 6-50 mg qd
P *Child:* PO 0.5-1.5 mg qd
P *Infant:* PO 0.1-0.5 mg qd
Palmar-plantar erythrodysesthesia syndrome (off-label)
Adult: PO 50-150 mg qd

Available forms: Tabs 10, 25, 50, 100 mg; ext rel tabs 100 mg; inj 100 mg/ml; ext rel caps 150 mg

Adverse effects
(*italic* = common; **bold** = life-threatening)
CNS: Paresthesia
INTEG: Pain at inj site

Contraindication: Hypersensitivity

Precautions: Pregnancy **A**, lactation,
P children, Parkinson's disease, patients taking levodopa should avoid supplemental vitamins with >5 mg pyridoxine

Pharmacokinetics

Absorption	Well absorbed (PO)
Distribution	Stored in liver, muscle, brain; crosses placenta
Metabolism	Unknown
Excretion	Kidneys, unchanged (not used)
Half-life	Unknown

Pharmacodynamics
Unknown

Interactions
Individual drugs
Chloramphenicol, cycloSERINE, hydrALAZINE, isoniazid, penicillamine: ↓ effects of pyridoxine
Levodopa: ↓ effects of levodopa
Drug classifications
Contraceptives (oral), immunosuppressants: ↓ effects of pyridoxine

NURSING CONSIDERATIONS
Assessment
- Monitor pyridoxine levels throughout treatment
- Assess nutritional status: yeast, liver, legumes, bananas, green vegetables, whole grains
- Assess for pyridoxine (B$_6$) deficiency: nausea, vomiting, dermatitis, cheilosis, seizures, irritability, dermatitis before and during treatment

Nursing diagnoses
☑ Nutrition: less than body requirements, imbalanced (uses)
☑ Knowledge, deficient (teaching)
☑ Noncompliance (teaching, overuse)

Implementation
PO route
🚫 • Do not crush, break, chew ext rel tabs, caps
IM route
• Rotate sites; burning or stinging at site may occur; give by Z-track to minimize pain
• Store in airtight, light-resistant container
IV IV route
• Give IV undiluted or added to most IV sol; give 50 mg or less/1 min if undiluted

Syringe compatibilities:
Doxapram

Additive incompatibilities:
Erythromycin, iron salts, kanamycin, riboflavin, streptomycin

PO route
🚫 • Ext rel cap and tab should be swallowed whole; do not break, crush, or chew
IM/SC route
• Administer in different site each time to avoid pain

Patient/family education
• Teach patient to avoid other vitamin supplements unless directed by prescriber
• Advise patient to increase meat, bananas, potatoes, lima beans, whole grain cereals in diet which are high in vit B_6
• Caution patient not to increase dosage, since serious reactions may occur

Evaluation
Positive therapeutic outcome
• Absence of nausea, vomiting, anorexia, skin lesions, glossitis, stomatitis, edema, seizures, restlessness, paresthesia

---

pyrimethamine (Rx)
(peer-i-meth'a-meen)
Daraprim, Fansidar (with sulfadoxine)
Func. class.: Antimalarial, antiprotozoal
Chem. class.: Folic acid antagonist

Pregnancy category C

Action: Inhibits folic acid metabolism in parasite; prevents transmission by stopping growth of fertilized gametes

➔ **Therapeutic Outcome:** Prevention of malaria

Uses: Malaria prophylaxis, antiprotozoal action against *Plasmodium vivax*

Investigational uses: *Pneumocystis carinii* pneumonia as an adjunct

Dosage and routes
Prophylaxis of malaria
P *Adult and child >10 yr:* PO 25 mg qwk
P *Child 4-10 yr:* PO 12.5 mg qwk
P *Child <4 yr:* PO 6.25 mg qwk

Toxoplasmosis
Adult: PO 100 mg, then 25 mg qd × 4-5 wk, with 1 g sulfADIAZINE q6h
P *Child:* PO 1 mg/kg/day in 2 divided doses or 2 mg/kg/day × 3 days, then 1 mg/kg/day or divided twice qd × 4 wk, max 25 mg/day

Toxoplasmosis in AIDS patients
Adult: PO 100-200 mg/day × 1-2 days, then 50-100 mg/day × 3-6 wk, then 25-50 mg/day for life (given with clindamycin or sulfADIAZINE)

Available forms: Tabs 25 mg; combo tabs 500 mg sulfadoxine/25 mg pyrimethamine

Adverse effects
(*italic* = common; **bold** = life-threatening)
CNS: Stimulation, irritability, **seizures,** tremors, ataxia, fatigue
CV: **Dysrhythmias**
GI: Nausea, vomiting, cramps, anorexia, diarrhea, atrophic glossitis, gastritis
HEMA: **Thrombocytopenia, leukopenia, pancytopenia, megaloblastic anemia,** decreased folic acid, **agranulocytosis**
INTEG: Skin eruptions, photosensitivity
RESP: **Respiratory failure**

Contraindications: Hypersensitivity, chloroquine-resistant malaria, megaloblastic anemia caused by folate deficiency

Precautions: Blood dyscrasias, seizure disorder, pregnancy **C**, lactation, glucose-6-phosphate dehydrogenase disease, renal/hepatic disease

Pharmacokinetics
Absorption	Well absorbed
Distribution	Widely; crosses placenta
Metabolism	Liver, extensively
Excretion	Kidneys, unchanged (30%); breast milk
Half-life	4 days

Pharmacodynamics
Onset	Unknown
Peak	2 hr
Duration	Unknown

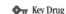

☑ Herb/drug   🚫 Do Not Crush   ◆ Alert   ◆━ Key Drug   G Geriatric   P Pediatric

Interactions
Individual drugs
Folic acid: ↑ synergistic action
Radiation: ↑ bone marrow suppression
Drug classifications
Bone marrow depressants: ↑ bone marrow suppression

NURSING CONSIDERATIONS
Assessment
- C&S studies should be done before treatment begins and periodically during treatment
- Monitor serum uric acid, which may be elevated and cause gout symptoms
- Monitor liver studies weekly: ALT, AST, bilirubin; hepatic status: decreased appetite, jaundice, dark urine, fatigue
- Monitor renal status before therapy and monthly thereafter: BUN, creatinine, output, sp gr, urinalysis
- Monitor mental status often: affect, mood, behavioral changes; psychosis may occur

Nursing diagnoses
☑ Infection, risk for (uses)
☑ Diarrhea (adverse reactions)
☑ Injury, risk for (adverse reactions)
☑ Knowledge, deficient (teaching)
☑ Noncompliance (teaching)

Implementation
- Give with meals to decrease GI symptoms
- Give antiemetic if vomiting occurs

Patient/family education
- Instruct patient that compliance with dosage schedule, duration is necessary; that scheduled appointments must be kept or relapse may occur
- Advise diabetic patient to use blood glucose monitor to obtain correct result
- Advise patient to report weakness, fatigue, loss of appetite, nausea, vomiting, yellowing of skin or eyes, sore throat, glossitis

Evaluation
Positive therapeutic outcome
- Decreased symptoms of toxoplasmosis
- Decreased symptoms of *Pneumocystis carinii* pneumonia

---

quetiapine (Rx)
(kwe-tie'a-peen)
Seroquel
Func. class.: Antipsychotic

Pregnancy category C

Action: Functions as an antagonist at multiple neurotransmitter receptors in the brain including 5-HT$_{1A}$, 5-HT$_2$, dopamine D$_1$, D$_2$, H$_1$, adrenergic α$_1$, α$_2$ receptors

⤷ **Therapeutic Outcome:** Decreased hallucination and disorganized thought

Uses: Psychotic disorders

Dosage and routes
Adult: PO 25 mg bid, with incremental increases of 25-50 mg bid-tid on days 2 and 3 to a dose of 300-400 mg qd given bid-tid; max 800 mg/day

Available forms: Tabs 25, 100, 200, 300 mg

Adverse effects
(*italic* = common; **bold** = life-threatening)
CNS: Extrapyramidal symptoms (EPS), pseudoparkinsonism, akathisia, dystonia, tardive dyskinesia, drowsiness, insomnia, agitation, anxiety, *headache*, **neuroleptic malignant syndrome**, dizziness
CV: Orthostatic hypotension, **tachycardia**
GI: Nausea, anorexia, constipation, abdominal pain, dry mouth
INTEG: Rash
MISC: Asthenia, back pain, fever, ear pain
RESP: Rhinitis

Contraindications: Hypersensitivity

P **Precautions:** Children, lactation, long-term use, seizures, dementia, pregnancy **C,** hepatic
G disease, elderly, breast cancer

Pharmacokinetics	
Absorption	Rapidly
Distribution	Widely
Metabolism	Liver, extensively; inhibits P450 CYP3A4 enzyme system
Excretion	Urine, feces
Half-life	≥6 hr

Pharmacodynamics	
Onset	Unknown
Peak	1.5 hr
Duration	Up to 12 hr

Interactions
Individual drugs
Alcohol: ↑ CNS depression
Carbamazepine, phenytoin, rifampin, thioridazine: ↑ quetiapine clearance
Cimetidine: ↓ quetiapine clearance
Erythromycin: Erythromycin level may be ↑
Fluconazole, itraconazole, ketoconazole: ↑ quetiapine action
Levodopa: ↓ effect of levodopa
Lorazepam: ↓ clearance of lorazepam

Drug classifications

Analgesics (opioid), antihistamines, sedative/hypnotics: ↑ CNS depression

Barbiturates, glucocorticoids: ↑ clearance of quetiapine

DOPamine agonists: ↓ effects of DOPamine agonists

🖉 *Herb/drug*

Cola tree, hops, nettle, nutmeg: ↑ action
Betel palm, kava: ↑ EPS

NURSING CONSIDERATIONS
Assessment

• Assess mental status: orientation, mood, behavior, presence and type of hallucinations before initial administration and monthly; this drug should significantly reduce psychotic behavior

• Check that patient swallows all PO medication; check for hoarding or giving of medication to other patients

• Monitor I&O ratio, palpate bladder if low 🅖 urinary output occurs, especially in elderly; urinalysis recommended before, during prolonged therapy

• Monitor bilirubin, CBC, liver function studies monthly

• Assess affect, orientation, LOC, reflexes, gait, coordination, sleep pattern disturbances

• Monitor B/P with patient in sitting, standing, and lying positions; take pulse and respirations q4h during initial treatment; establish baseline before starting treatment; report drops of 30 mm Hg; obtain baseline ECG and monitor Q- and T-wave changes

• Check for dizziness, faintness, palpitations, tachycardia on rising; severe orthostatic hypotension is common

◈• Identify for neuroleptic malignant syndrome: hyperpyrexia, muscle rigidity, increased CPK, altered mental status, seizures, tachycardia, diaphoresis, hyper/hypotension, fatigue; drug should be discontinued and prescriber notified immediately

• Assess for EPS including akathisia (inability to sit still, no pattern to movements), tardive dyskinesia (bizarre movements of the jaw, mouth, tongue, extremities), pseudoparkinsonism (rigidity, tremors, pill rolling, shuffling gait); an antiparkinson drug should be prescribed

• Assess for constipation, urinary retention daily; if these occur, increase bulk, water in diet

Nursing diagnoses

☑ Thought processes, disturbed (uses)
☑ Coping, individual (uses)
☑ Knowledge, deficient (teaching)
☑ Noncompliance (teaching)

Implementation

• PO with full glass of water, milk; or give with food to decrease GI upset

• Store in airtight, light-resistant container

Patient/family education

• Teach patient to use good oral hygiene; frequent rinsing of mouth, sugarless gum for dry mouth

• Caution patient to avoid hazardous activities until drug response is determined; dizziness, blurred vision may occur

• Inform patient that orthostatic hypotension occurs often; patient should rise from sitting or lying position gradually

• Instruct patient to avoid hot tubs, hot showers, tub baths; hypotension may occur

• Inform patient that heat stroke may occur in hot weather, and to take extra precautions to stay cool

• Advise patient to avoid abrupt withdrawal of this drug or EPS may result; drug should be withdrawn slowly

• Teach patient to avoid OTC preparations (cough, hayfever, cold) unless approved by prescriber; serious drug interactions may occur; avoid use with alcohol, CNS depressants because increased drowsiness may occur

Evaluation
Positive therapeutic outcome

• Decrease in emotional excitement, hallucinations, delusions, paranoia

• Reorganization of patterns of thought, speech

Treatment of overdose: Lavage, provide airway

---

quinapril (Rx)
(kwin′a-pril)

Accupril
Func. class.: Antihypertensive
Chem. class.: Angiotensin-converting enzyme (ACE) inhibitor

Pregnancy category
D (2nd/3rd trimesters);
C (1st trimester)

Action: Selectively suppresses renin-angiotensin-aldosterone system; inhibits ACE, prevents conversion of angiotensin I to angiotensin II; results in dilation of arterial, venous vessels

---

🖉 Herb/drug   🚫 Do Not Crush   ◈ Alert   ◆ℼ Key Drug   🅖 Geriatric   🅟 Pediatric

➔ **Therapeutic Outcome:** Decreased B/P in hypertension

Uses: Hypertension, alone or in combination with thiazide diuretics, systolic CHF

Dosage and routes
Hypertension (monotherapy)
Adult: PO 10-20 mg qd initially, then 20-80 mg/day divided bid or qd

G *Elderly:* PO 10 mg qd, titrate to desired response

Congestive heart failure
Adult: PO 5 mg bid, may increase qwk unitl 20-40 mg/day in 2 divided doses

Renal dose
Adult: PO CCr 30-60 ml/min 5 mg/day initially; CCr <30 ml/min 2.5 mg/day initially

Available forms: Tabs 5, 10, 20, 40 mg

Adverse effects
(*italic* = common; **bold** = life-threatening)
CNS: Headache, dizziness, fatigue, somnolence, depression, malaise, nervousness, vertigo
CV: Hypotension, postural hypotension, syncope, palpitations, angina pectoris, **MI, tachycardia,** vasodilation
GI: Nausea, diarrhea, constipation, vomiting, gastritis, GI hemorrhage, dry mouth
GU: Increased BUN, creatinine, decreased libido, impotence
HEMA: **Thrombocytopenia, agranulocytosis**
INTEG: **Angioedema,** rash, sweating, photosensitivity, pruritus
META: Hyperkalemia
MISC: Back pain, amblyopia, pharyngitis
MS: Arthralgia, arthritis, myalgia
RESP: Cough, pharyngitis, dyspnea

Contraindications: Hypersensitivity to ACE inhibitors, pregnancy **D** (2nd/3rd **P** trimesters), children

Precautions: Impaired renal and liver function, dialysis patients, hypovolemia, blood **G** dyscrasias, COPD, asthma, elderly, lactation, pregnancy **C** (1st trimester), bilateral renal stenosis

Pharmacokinetics
Absorption	Well absorbed
Distribution	Unknown, crosses placenta
Metabolism	Unknown
Excretion	Urine (60%), feces (37%)
Half-life	2 hr

Pharmacodynamics
Onset	½-1 hr
Peak	2-6 hr
Duration	12-24 hr

Interactions
Individual drugs
Alcohol: ↑ hypotension (large amounts)
Allopurinol: ↑ hypersensitivity
Digoxin, hydralazine, lithium, prazosin: ↑ toxicity
Indomethacin: ↓ antihypertensive effect
Drug classifications
Adrenergic blockers, antihypertensives, diuretics, diuretics (potassium sparing), ganglionic blockers, nitrates, phenothiazines: ↑ hypotension
Antacids: ↓ absorption
Diuretics (potassium sparing), potassium supplements, sympathomimetics: ↑ toxicity
Vasodilators: Use caution
☑ *Herb/drug*
Aconite: ↑ toxicity, death
Astragalus, cola tree: ↑ or ↓ antihypertensive effect
Barberry, betony, black catechu, black cohosh, bloodroot, broom, burdock, cat's claw, dandelion, goldenseal, Irish moss, Jamaican dogwood, kelp, khella, mistletoe, parsley: ↑ antihypertensive effect
Coltsfoot, guarana, khat, licorice: ↓ antihypertensive effect
Lab test interferences
False positive: Urine acetone, ANA titer

NURSING CONSIDERATIONS
Assessment
• Monitor blood studies: neutrophils, decreased platelets; WBC with differential baseline and periodically q3 mo; if neutrophils <1000/mm^3 discontinue treatment
• Monitor B/P, check for orthostatic hypotension, syncope; if changes occur dosage change may be required
• Monitor renal studies (protein, BUN, creatinine); and periodically liver function tests, uric acid, also glucose may be elevated; watch for increased levels that may indicate nephrotic syndrome and renal failure; monitor renal symptoms: polyuria, oliguria, frequency, dysuria
• Check potassium levels throughout treatment, although hyperkalemia rarely occurs
• Check for edema in feet, legs daily, weight daily in CHF

Q

• Assess for allergic reactions: rash, fever, pruritus, urticaria; drug should be discontinued if antihistamines fail to help

Nursing diagnoses
☑ Cardiac output, decreased (uses)
☑ Injury, risk for (adverse reactions)
☑ Knowledge, deficient (teaching)
☑ Noncompliance (teaching)

Implementation
PO route
• Tabs may be crushed if necessary
• Store in airtight container at 86° F (30° C) or less
• Severe hypotension may occur after 1st dose of this medication; may be prevented by reducing or discontinuing diuretic therapy 3 days before beginning quinapril therapy

Patient/family education
• Advise patient not to discontinue drug abruptly; advise patient to tell all persons associated with care
• Teach patient not to use OTC products (cough, cold, allergy) unless directed by physician; serious side effects can occur
• Inform patient that xanthines such as coffee, tea, chocolate, cola can prevent action of drug
• Caution patient on the importance of complying with dosage schedule, even if feeling better; to continue with medical regimen to decrease B/P: exercise, cessation of smoking, decreasing stress, diet modifications
• Emphasize the need to rise slowly to sitting or standing position to minimize orthostatic hypotension; not to exercise in hot weather or increased hypotension can occur
• Teach patient to notify prescriber of mouth sores, sore throat, fever, swelling of hands or feet, irregular heartbeat, chest pain, coughing, shortness of breath
• Caution patient to report excessive perspiration, dehydration, vomiting, diarrhea; may lead to fall in B/P
• Caution patient that drug may cause dizziness, fainting, light-headedness; may occur during 1st few days of therapy; to avoid activities that may be hazardous
• Teach patient how to take B/P, and normal readings for age-group

Evaluation
Positive therapeutic outcome
• Decreased B/P in hypertension

Treatment of overdose: 0.9% NaCl **IV** inf, hemodialysis

quinidine (Rx)
(kwin'i-deen)
quinidine gluconate
Quinaglute Dura-Tabs, Quinalan, Quinate ✦
quinidine polygalacturonate
cardioquin
quinidine sulfate
Apo-Quinidine ✦, Cin-Quin, Novoquinidine ✦, Quinidex Extentabs, Quinora
Func. class.: Antidysrhythmic (class IA)
Chem. class.: Quinine dextro isomer

Pregnancy category C

Action: Prolongs action potential duration and effective refractory period, thus decreasing myocardial excitability; anticholinergic properties

⇒ **Therapeutic Outcome:** Treatment of dysrhythmias

Uses: Premature ventricular contractions (PVCs), atrial fibrillation, flutter; paroxysmal atrial tachycardia, ventricular tachycardia, malaria/**IV** quinidine gluconate

Dosage and routes
Quinidine sulfate
Atrial fibrillation/flutter
Adult: PO 200 mg q2-3h × 5-8 doses; may increase qd until sinus rhythm is restored; max 4 g/day given only after digitalization, maintenance 200-300 mg tid-qid or 300-600 mg q8-12 hr (sus rel)

Paroxysmal supraventricular tachycardia
Adult: PO 400-600 mg q2-3h, then 200-300 mg q6-8h or 300-600 mg q8-12h (sus rel)

Premature atrial/ventricular contraction
Adult: PO 200-300 mg q6-8h or 300-600 mg (sus rel) q8-12h, not to exceed 4 g/day
P *Child:* PO 30 mg/kg/day or 900 mg/m^2/day in 5 divided doses

Quinidine gluconate
Adult: PO 324-660 mg q6-12h (sus rel); IM 600 mg, then 400 mg q2h; **IV** give 16 mg/min

---

 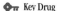

Available forms: *Gluconate:* sus rel tabs 324, 330 mg; inj gluconate 80 mg/ml; *sulfate:* tabs 200, 300 mg; sus rel tabs 300 mg; *polygalacturonase:* tabs 275 mg

Adverse effects
(*italic* = common; **bold** = life-threatening)
CNS: Headache, dizziness, involuntary movement, confusion, psychosis, restlessness, irritability, syncope, excitement, depression, ataxia
CV: **Hypotension,** *bradycardia, PVCs,* **heart block, cardiovascular collapse, arrest, torsade de pointes,** widening QRS complex, **ventricular tachycardia**
EENT: Cinchonism: tinnitus, blurred vision, hearing loss, mydriasis, disturbed color vision
GI: Nausea, vomiting, anorexia, *diarrhea,* **hepatotoxicity,** abdominal pain
HEMA: **Thrombocytopenia,** hemolytic anemia, agranulocytosis, hypoprothrombinemia
INTEG: Rash, urticaria, **angioedema,** swelling, photosensitivity, flushing with severe pruritus
RESP: Dyspnea, **respiratory depression**

Contraindications: Hypersensitivity or idiosyncratic response, digitalis toxicity, history of long QT syndrome, drug induced torsades de pointes, blood dyscrasias, severe heart block, myasthenia gravis

Precautions: Pregnancy **C**, lactation, children, renal disease, potassium imbalance, liver disease, CHF, respiratory depression (elderly)

Pharmacokinetics

Absorption	Well absorbed (PO, IM), slowly absorbed (sus rel)
Distribution	Widely distributed, crosses placenta, protein binding (80%-90%)
Metabolism	Liver
Excretion	Kidney unchanged, 10%-50% breast milk
Half-life	6-8 hr

Interactions
Individual drugs
Amiodarone, cimetidine, nifedipine, propranolol: ↑ quinidine level
Digoxin: ↑ digoxin level

Nifedipine, phenytoin, rifampin, sucralfate: ↓ effects of quinidine
Reserpine: ↑ cardiac depression
Sodium bicarbonate, verapamil: ↑ quinidine effect
Warfarin: ↑ levels of warfarin

Drug classifications
Antacids, carbonic anhydrase inhibitors, diuretics (thiazide), hydroxide suspensions: ↑ effects of quinidine
Anticholinergics: ↑ vagolytic effects
Anticoagulants (oral): ↑ levels of anticoagulant
Antidepressants (tricyclics): ↑ effect of antidepressant
Antidysrhythmics: ↑ cardiac depression
Barbiturates, cholinergics: ↓ effects of quinidine
Neuromuscular blockers: ↑ neuromuscular blocking
Phenothiazines: ↑ cardiac depression
Herb/drug
Aconite: ↑ toxicity, death
Aloe, broom, buckthorn (chronic use), cascara sagrada (chronic use), Chinese rhubarb, figwort, fumitory, goldenseal, kudzu, licorice: ↑ effect
Aloe, buckthorn, cascara sagrada, senna: ↑ hypokalemia, ↑ antidysrhythmic action
Coltsfoot: ↓ effect
Horehound: ↑ serotonin effect
Food/drug
Grapefruit juice: ↓ absorption, ↓ metabolism
Lab test interferences
↑ CPK
Interference: Triamterene therapy interferes with quinidine test levels

NURSING CONSIDERATIONS
Assessment
• Monitor ECG continuously to determine drug effectiveness, measure PR, QRS, QT intervals, check for PVCs, other dysrhythmias; monitor B/P continuously for hypotension, hypertension; for rebound hypertension after 1-2 hr; check for dehydration or hypovolemia
• Monitor blood levels (therapeutic level 2-7 mcg/ml)
• Monitor I&O ratio, electrolytes (potassium, sodium, chloride); check weight daily; check for signs of CHF or pulmonary toxicity: dys-

Pharmacodynamics

	PO (SULFATE)	PO-SUS REL	PO (GLUCONATE)	IM	IV
Onset	½ hr	Unknown	Unknown	½ hr	5 min
Peak	1-1½ hr	4 hr	4 hr	½-1½ hr	Unknown
Duration	6-8 hr	8-12 hr	6-8 hr	6-8 hr	6-8 hr

Q

pnea, fatigue, cough, fever, chest pain; if these occur, drug should be discontinued
• Monitor liver function studies: AST, ALT, bilirubin, alkaline phosphatase
• Assess for CNS symptoms: confusion, psychosis, numbness, depression, involuntary movements; if these occur, drug should be discontinued
• Monitor cardiac rate, respiration: rate, rhythm, character, chest pain; watch for ventricular tachycardia, supraventricular tachycardia, or fibrillation that indicates toxicity

Nursing diagnoses
☑ Cardiac output, decreased (uses)
☑ Gas exchange, impaired (adverse reactions)
☑ Knowledge, deficient (teaching)

Implementation
PO route
• Give on an empty stomach with a full glass of water
• May be given with meals if GI irritation occurs, absorption will be decreased
• Sus rel forms not interchangeable
• Tab may be crushed and mixed with fluid or foods for patients with swallowing
🚫 difficulties; do not break, chew or crush sus rel tab
Ⅳ IV route
• Give by intermittent inf after diluting 800 mg/50 ml of D_5W; gluconate: (16 mg/ml) give at 1 ml/min or less using an infusion pump for correct dose
• Do not use colored sol or sol with precipitate
• Diluted quinidine is stable for 24 hr at room temp

Y-site compatibilities: Diazepam, milrinone

Y-site incompatibilities: Furosemide

Additive compatibilities: Bretylium, cimetidine, milrinone, ranitidine, verapamil

Additive incompatibilities: Amiodarone

Patient/family education
• Instruct patient to report adverse effects immediately to prescriber
• Caution patient that sunglasses may be needed for photophobia; to use sunscreen, protective clothing, or stay out of sun to prevent burns
• Instruct patient to complete follow-up

appointments with health care provider including pulmonary function studies, chest x-ray, ophth and otoscopic exams

---

rabeprazole (Rx)
(rab-ee-pray′zole)
Aciphex
Func. class.: Proton pump inhibitor
Chem. class.: Benzimidazole
Pregnancy category C

Action: Suppresses gastric secretion by inhibiting hydrogen/potassium ATPase enzyme system in the gastric parietal cell; characterized as a gastric acid pump inhibitor, since it blocks the final step of acid production

➡ **Therapeutic Outcome:** Absence of duodenal ulcers; decreased gastroesophageal reflux

Uses: Gastroesophageal reflux disease (GERD), severe erosive esophagitis, poorly responsive systemic GERD, pathologic hypersecretory conditions (Zollinger-Ellison syndrome, systemic mastocytosis, multiple endocrine adenomas); possibly effective for treatment of duodenal ulcers with or without antiinfectives for *Helicobacter pylori;* daytime, nighttime heartburn

Dosage and routes
Healing of duodenal ulcers
Adult: PO 20 mg qd × ≤4 wk, to be taken after breakfast

Erosive esophagitis/GERD
Adult: PO 20 mg qd × 4-8 wk

Pathologic hypersecretory conditions
Adult: PO 60 mg/day; may increase to 120 mg in 2 divided doses

Available forms: Tabs, delayed rel 20 mg

Adverse effects
(*italic* = common; **bold** = life-threatening)
CNS: Headache, dizziness, asthenia
CV: Chest pain, angina, tachycardia, bradycardia, palpitations, peripheral edema
EENT: Tinnitus, taste perversion
GI: Diarrhea, abdominal pain, vomiting, nausea, constipation, flatulence, acid regurgitation, abdominal swelling, anorexia,

---

irritable colon, esophageal candidiasis, dry mouth
GU: UTI, frequency, increased creatinine, **proteinuria, hematuria,** testicular pain, glycosuria
HEMA: **Pancytopenia, thrombocytopenia, neutropenia, leukocytosis,** anemia
INTEG: Rash, dry skin, urticaria, pruritus, alopecia
META: Hypoglycemia, increased hepatic enzymes, weight gain
MISC: Back pain, fever, fatigue, malaise
RESP: Upper respiratory tract infections, cough, epistaxis

Contraindications: Hypersensitivity

Precautions: Pregnancy **C,** lactation, [P] children

Pharmacokinetics

Absorption	Unknown
Distribution	Unknown
Metabolism	Liver, extensively
Excretion	Kidneys, feces
Half-life	Unknown

Pharmacodynamics
Unknown

Interactions
Individual drugs
Clarithromycin, phenytoin: ↑ levels of rapeprazole
Sucralfate: ↓ rapeprazole levels
Drug classifications
Benzodiazepines: ↑ levels of rapeprazole

NURSING CONSIDERATIONS
Assessment
• Assess GI system: bowel sounds q8h, abdomen for pain and swelling, anorexia
• Monitor hepatic enzymes: AST, ALT, increased alkaline phosphatase during treatment

Nursing diagnoses
☑ Pain, chronic (uses)
☑ Knowledge, deficient (teaching)

Implementation
⊘• Give after breakfast qd; do not crush, break, chew delayed rel tab

Patient/family education
• Advise patient to report severe diarrhea; drug may have to be discontinued
• Caution patient to avoid driving and other hazardous activities until response to drug is known
• Caution patient to avoid alcohol, salicylates, NSAIDs; may cause GI irritation

• Advise patient to wear sunscreen, protective clothing to prevent burns

Evaluation
Positive therapeutic outcome
• Absence of epigastric pain, swelling, fullness

---

raloxifene (Rx)
(ral-ox'ih-feen)
Evista
Func. class.: Bone resorption inhibitor, selective estrogen receptor modulator (SERM)
Chem. class.: Benzothiophene
Pregnancy category X

Action: Reduces resorption of bone and decreases bone turnover; mediated through estrogen receptor binding

➔**Therapeutic Outcome:** Absence, or decrease of osteoporosis in postmenopausal women

Uses: Prevention, treatment of osteoporosis in postmenopausal women

Dosage and routes
Hormone replacement
Adult: PO 60 mg qd

Available forms: Tabs 60 mg

Adverse effects
(*italic* = common; **bold** = life-threatening)
CNS: Insomnia, migraines, depression
CV: Hot flashes
GI: Nausea, vomiting, diarrhea, anorexia, cramps
GU: Vaginitis, UTI, leukorrhea, *hot flashes,* cystitis
INTEG: Rash, sweating
META: Weight gain, peripheral edema
MS: Arthralgia, myalgia, *leg cramps,* arthritis
RESP: Sinusitis, pharyngitis, increased cough, pneumonia, laryngitis, rhinitis, bronchitis

Contraindications: Hypersensitivity, pregnancy **X,** lactation, women with active or history of venous thromboembolic events

Precautions: Venous thromboembolic events, hepatic disease

Pharmacokinetics

Absorption	Unknown
Distribution	Highly protein bound
Metabolism	Unknown
Excretion	Feces, breast milk
Half-life	28-32 hr (elimination)

[R]

Pharmacodynamics	
Onset	Unknown
Peak	Unknown
Duration	Unknown

Interactions
Individual drugs
Ampicillin, cholestyramine: ↓ action of raloxifene
Drug classifications
Anticoagulants: ↓ action of anticoagulants
Highly protein-bound drugs: Administer cautiously
Lab test interferences
↑ Apolipoproteins A_1 and B
↓ lipoprotein, ↓ fibrinogen, ↓ LDL cholesterol, ↓ total cholesterol
↑ corticosteroid-binding globulin,
↑ thyroxine-binding globulin (TBG)
↓ Calcium, ↓ total protein, ↓ albumin,
↓ platelets

NURSING CONSIDERATIONS
Assessment
• Obtain bone density test baseline and periodically throughout treatment; bone-specific alkaline phosphatase; osteocalcin, collagen breakdown
• Monitor weight daily, notify prescriber of weekly weight gain >5 lb
• Monitor B/P q4h, watch for increase caused by H_2O and sodium retention
• Monitor liver function studies: AST, ALT, bilirubin, alkaline phosphatase
• Monitor I&O ratio; decreasing urinary output, increasing edema

Nursing diagnoses
☑ Immobility, risk for (uses)
☑ Knowledge, deficient (teaching)

Implementation
PO route
• Administer without regard to meals
• Add calcium supplement, vit D if lacking

Patient/family education
• Teach patient to weigh weekly, report gain >5 lb
• Teach patients to discontinue drug 72 hr before prolonged bedrest
• Advise patient to avoid maintaining one position for long periods
• Advise patient to take calcium supplements, vit D if intake is inadequate
• Advise patient to increase exercise using weights
• Advise patient to stop smoking and to decrease alcohol consumption
• Inform patient that this drug does not help control hot flashes
• Teach patient to report fever, acute migraine, insomnia, emotional distress; UTI or vaginal burning/itching; swelling, warmth, or pain in calves

Evaluation
Positive therapeutic outcome
• Prevention, treatment of osteoporosis

---

ramipril (Rx)
(ra-mi'pril)
Altace
Func. class.: Antihypertensive
Chem. class.: Angiotensin-converting enzyme (ACE) inhibitor

Pregnancy category
D (2nd/3rd trimesters),
C (1st trimester)

Action: Selectively suppresses renin-angiotensin-aldosterone system; inhibits ACE; prevents conversion of angiotensin I to angiotensin II; results in dilation of arterial, venous vessels

➡ Therapeutic Outcome: Decreased B/P in hypertension

Uses: Hypertension, alone or in combination with thiazide diuretics; CHF (after MI), reduction in risk of MI, stroke, death from CV disorders

Dosage and routes
Hypertension
Adult: PO 2.5 mg qd initially, then 2.5-20 mg/day divided bid or qd; renal impairment: 1.25 mg qd with CCr <40 ml/min/1.73 m^2, increase as needed to max 5 mg/day

CHF/Post MI
Adult: PO 1.25-2.5 mg bid, may increase to 5 mg bid

Reduction in risk of MI, stroke, death
Adult: PO 2.5 mg qd × 7 days, then 5 mg qd × 21 days, then may increase to 10 mg/day

Renal dose
Adult: PO CCr <40 ml/min 1.73 m^2

Available forms: Caps 1.25, 2.5, 5, 10 mg

Adverse effects
(*italic* = common; **bold** = life-threatening)
CNS: Headache, dizziness, anxiety, insomnia, paresthesia, fatigue, depression, malaise, vertigo, **seizures**

EENT: Hearing loss
CV: *Hypotension,* chest pain, palpitations, angina, syncope, **dysrhythmia**
GI: Nausea, constipation, vomiting, dyspepsia, dysphagia, anorexia, diarrhea, abdominal pain
GU: **Proteinuria,** increased BUN, creatinine, impotence
HEMA: Decreased Hct, Hgb, **eosinophilia, leukopenia**
INTEG: Rash, sweating, photosensitivity, pruritus
META: Hyperkalemia
MS: Arthralgia, arthritis, myalgia
RESP: Cough, dyspnea
MISC: **Angioedema**

Contraindications: Hypersensitivity to ACE inhibitors, pregnancy **D** (2nd/3rd trimesters), lactation, children

Precautions: Impaired renal and liver function, dialysis patients, hypovolemia, blood dyscrasias, COPD, CHF, asthma, elderly, renal artery stenosis, pregnancy **C** (1st trimester)

Do Not Confuse:
Altace/alteplase, Altace/Artane, ramipril/enalapril

Pharmacokinetics	
Absorption	Well absorbed
Distribution	Not known, crosses placenta
Metabolism	Liver, extensively, protein binding 73%
Excretion	Urine
Half-life	Ramipril (5 hr), ramiprilat (24 hr)

Pharmacodynamics	
Onset	½-1 hr
Peak	6-8 hr
Duration	24-72 hr

Interactions
Individual drugs
Alcohol: ↑ hypotension (large amounts)
Digoxin, lithium: ↑ serum levels
Hydralazine, prazocin: ↑ toxicity
Indomethacin: ↓ antihypertensive effect
Drug classifications
Adrenergic blockers, antihypertensives, diuretics, ganglionic blockers, nitrates: ↑ hypotension
Antacids: ↓ absorption
Diuretics (potassium sparing), potassium supplements, sympathomimetics: ↑ toxicity
Herb/drug
Aconite: ↑ toxicity, death
Astragalus, cola tree: ↑ or ↓ antihypertensive effect

Barberry, betony, black catechu, black cohosh, bloodroot, broom, burdock, cat's claw, dandelion, goldenseal, Irish moss, Jamaican dogwood, kelp, khella, mistletoe, parsley: ↑ antihypertensive effect
Coltsfoot, guarana, khat, licorice: ↓ antihypertensive effect
Lab test interferences
False positive: Urine acetone, ANA titer

NURSING CONSIDERATIONS
Assessment
● Monitor blood studies: neutrophils, decreased platelets; WBC with differential baseline and periodically q3mo, if neutrophils <1000/mm³, discontinue treatment
● Monitor B/P, check for orthostatic hypotension, syncope; if changes occur, dosage may need to be changed
● Monitor renal studies: protein, BUN, creatinine; watch for increased levels that may indicate nephrotic syndrome and renal failure; monitor renal symptoms: polyuria, oliguria, frequency, dysuria
● Establish baselines in renal, liver function tests before therapy begins and monitor periodically; liver function tests, uric acid, and glucose may be increased
● Check potassium levels throughout treatment, although hyperkalemia rarely occurs
● Check for edema in feet, legs daily, weight daily in CHF
● Assess for allergic reactions: rash, fever, pruritus, urticaria; drug should be discontinued if antihistamines fail to help

Nursing diagnoses
✓ Cardiac output, decreased (uses)
✓ Injury, risk for (side effects)
✓ Knowledge, deficient (teaching)
✓ Noncompliance (teaching)

Implementation
● Caps can be opened and added to food
● Store in airtight container at 86° F (30° C) or less
● Severe hypotension may occur after 1st dose of this medication; decreased hypotension may be prevented by reducing or discontinuing diuretic therapy 3 days before beginning benazepril therapy
● Give **IV** inf of 0.9% NaCl (as ordered) to expand fluid volume if severe hypotension occurs

Patient/family education
● Caution patient not to discontinue drug abruptly; advise patient to tell all persons associated with care
● Teach patient not to use OTC products

R

(cough, cold, allergy) unless directed by physician; serious side effects can occur; xanthines such as coffee, tea, chocolate, cola can prevent action of drug

• Instruct patient on the importance of complying with dosage schedule, even if feeling better; to continue with medical regimen to decrease B/P: exercise, cessation of smoking, decreasing stress, diet modifications

• Emphasize the need to rise slowly to sitting or standing position to minimize orthostatic hypotension; not to exercise in hot weather because increased hypotension can occur

• Teach patient to notify prescriber of mouth sores, sore throat, fever, swelling of hands or feet, irregular heartbeat, chest pain, coughing, shortness of breath

• Caution patient to report excessive perspiration, dehydration, vomiting, diarrhea; may lead to fall in B/P

• Caution patient that drug may cause dizziness, fainting, lightheadedness; may occur during 1st few days of therapy; to avoid activities that may be hazardous

• Teach patient how to take B/P, and normal readings for age group

Evaluation
Positive therapeutic outcome
• Decreased B/P in hypertension

Treatment of overdose: 0.9% NaCl **IV** inf, hemodialysis

---

ranitidine (Rx)
(ra-nit'i-deen)
Apo-Ranitidine ✦, Zantac, Zantac-C ✦, Zantac EFFER-dose, Zantac GELdose
ranitidine bismuth citrate
Tritec
Func. class.: H$_2$ histamine receptor antagonist

Pregnancy category B

Action: Inhibits histamine at H$_2$ receptor site in the gastric parietal cells, which inhibits gastric acid secretion

➡ **Therapeutic Outcome:** Healing of duodenal ulcers or gastric ulcers; prevention of duodenal ulcers; decreases symptoms of gastroesophageal reflux disease (GERD) or Zollinger-Ellison syndrome

Uses: Short-term treatment of duodenal and gastric ulcers and maintenance; management of GERD, Zollinger-Ellison syndrome, active

duodenal ulcers with *Helicobacter pylori* in combination with clarithromycin

Investigational uses: Prevention of aspiration pneumonitis, stress ulcers, upper GI bleeding

Dosage and routes
Renal dose
Adult: CCr <50 ml/min PO q24h, IM/**IV** q8-24h

Erosive esophagitis
Adult: PO 150 mg bid, 300 mg hs; IM 50 mg q6-8h; **IV** bol 50 mg diluted to 20 ml over 5 min q6-8h; **IV** intermittent inf 50 mg/100 ml of D$_5$ over 15-20 min q6-8h

P *Child:* PO 4-5 mg/kg/day divided q8-12h, max 6 mg/kg/day or 300 mg; **IV** 2-4 mg/kg/day divided q6-8h

Duodenal ulcer
Adult: PO 150 mg bid, maintenance 150 mg hs

Zollinger-Ellison syndrome
Adult: PO 150 mg bid, may increase if needed

Gastric ulcer
Adult: PO 150 mg bid × 6 wk, then 150 mg hs

GERD
Adult: PO 150 mg bid

Erosive esophagitis
Adult: PO 150 mg qid

Ranitidine bismuth citrate
Adult: PO 400 mg bid × 4 wk with clarithromycin 500 mg tid × 1st 2 wk

Available forms: *Ranitidine:* tabs 75, 150, 300 mg; inj 25 mg/ml; caps 150, 300 mg; syr 15 mg/ml; sol for inj 25 mg/ml; effervescent tabs 75, 100 mg; effervescent granules 150 mg/packet; *ranitidine bismuth citrate:* tabs 400 mg

Adverse effects
(*italic* = common; **bold** = life-threatening)
CNS: Headache, sleeplessness, dizziness, confusion, agitation, depression; hallucination
G (elderly)
CV: Tachycardia, bradycardia, premature ventricular contractions
EENT: Blurred vision, increased ocular pressure
GI: Constipation, abdominal pain, diarrhea, nausea, vomiting, **hepatotoxicity**
GU: Impotence, gynecomastia
INTEG: Urticaria, rash, fever

Contraindications: Hypersensitivity

P **Precautions:** Pregnancy **B**, lactation, child <12 yr, hepatic disease, renal disease

N **Do Not Confuse:**
ranitidine/amantadine, Zantac/Xanax, Zantac/Zofran

Pharmacokinetics	
Absorption	Well absorbed (PO, IM), completely absorbed (**IV**)
Distribution	Widely distributed, crosses placenta
Metabolism	Liver (30%)
Excretion	Kidneys unchanged (70%)
Half-life	2-3 hr, ↑ renal disease

Pharmacodynamics		
	PO	IV/IM
Onset	Unknown	Unknown
Peak	2-3 hr	15 min
Duration	8-12 hr	8-12 hr

Interactions
Individual drugs
Diazepam, ketoconazole, metoclopramide: ↓ absorption of ranitidine
Procainamide: ↑ absorption, toxicity
Drug classifications
Anticoagulants, sulfonylureas: ↑ absorption, toxicity
Anticholinergics, antacids: ↓ rantidine absorption
Smoking
↓ Effectiveness
Lab test interferences
↑ Alkaline phosphatase, ↑ AST, ↑ creatinine
False positive: Gastric bleeding test

NURSING CONSIDERATIONS
Assessment
• Assess patient with ulcers or suspected ulcers: epigastric or abdominal pain, hematemesis, occult blood in stools, blood in gastric aspirate before and throughout treatment, monitor gastric pH (5 should be maintained)
• Monitor I&O ratio, BUN, creatinine, CBC with differential monthly

Nursing diagnoses
☑ Pain, chronic (uses)
☑ Knowledge, deficient (teaching)

Implementation
PO route
• May be given with or without meals
• Give antacids 1 hr before or 1 hr after this drug

IV **IV route**
Direct **IV**
• Give by direct **IV** after diluting 50 mg/20 ml of 0.9% D$_5$W, NaCl over 5 min or more
Intermittent infusion
• Give by intermittent inf over 15 min after diluting 50 mg/100 ml of D$_5$W, 0.9% NaCl
Continuous infusion
• Give by continuous inf for a concentration 150 mg/250 ml, give 6.25 mg/hr
• Give Zollinger-Ellison patients up to a conc of 2.5 mg/ml at 1 mg/kg/hr initially

Syringe compatibilities: Atropine, cyclizine, dexamethasone, dimenhyDRINATE, diphenhydrAMINE, DOBUTamine, DOPamine, fentanyl, glycopyrrolate, hydromorphone, meperidine, metoclopramide, morphine, nalbuphine, oxymorphone, pentazocine, perphenazine, prochlorperazine, promethazine, scopolamine

Syringe incompatibilities: Hydroxyzine, methotrimeprazine, midazolam, pentobarbital, phenobarbital

Y-site compatibilities: Acyclovir, aldesleukin, allopurinol, amifostine, aminophylline, atracurium, aztreonam, bretylium, DOBUTamine, DOPamine, DOXOrubicin, enalaprilat, epINEPHrine, esmolol, fentanyl, filgrastim, fluconazole, fludarabine, foscarnet, furosemide, gallium, granisetron, heparin, hydromorphone, idarubicin, labetalol, lorazepam, melphalan, meperidine, methotrexate, midazolam, milrinone, morphine, niCARdipine, nitroglycerin, norepinephrine, ondansetron, paclitaxel, pancuronium, piperacillin, piperacillin/tazobactam, procainamide, propofol, sargramostim, vecuronium, zidovudine

Additive compatibilities: Acetazolamide, amikacin, aminophylline, chloramphenicol, chlorothiazide, ciprofloxacin, colistimethate, dexamethasone, digoxin, DOBUTamine, DOPamine, doxycycline, furosemide, gentamicin, heparin, lidocaine, penicillin G sodium, potassium chloride, ticarcillin, tobramycin, vancomycin

Additive incompatibilities: Amphotericin B, clindamycin

Patient/family education
• Caution patient that gynecomastia, impotence may occur and are reversible after treatment is discontinued
• Advise patient to avoid driving, other hazardous activities until stabilized on this medication; drowsiness or dizziness may occur
• Caution patient to avoid black pepper,

R

---

caffeine, alcohol, harsh spices, extremes in temp of food; tell patient to avoid OTC preparations (aspirin, cough, cold preparations) because condition may worsen
• Inform patient that smoking decreases the effectiveness of the drug; that smoking cessation should be considered
• Instruct patient that drug must be continued for prescribed time to be effective and taken exactly as prescribed; doses should not be doubled; a missed dose should be taken when remembered up to 1 hr before next dose
• Advise patient to report bruising, fatigue, malaise; blood dyscrasias may occur
• Inform patient to report diarrhea, black tarry stools, sore throat, rash, dizziness, confusion, rash, or delirium to prescriber immediately

Evaluation
Positive therapeutic outcome
• Decreased pain in abdomen
• Healing of ulcers
• Absence of gastroesophageal reflux

---

rasburicase (Rx)
(rass-burr'i-case)
Elitek
Func. class.: Antineoplastic, antimetabolite

Pregnancy category C

Action: Catalyzes enzymatic oxidation of uric acid into an inactive and a soluble metabolite

Therapeutic Outcome: Uric acid levels are decreased

Uses: To reduce uric acid levels in children with leukemia, lymphoma, solid tumor malignancies who are receiving chemotherapy

Dosage and routes
Adult: **IV INF** 0.15 or 0.2 mg/kg as a single daily dose given as **IV INF** over ½ hr

Available forms: Powder for inj 1.5 mg/vial

Adverse effects
(*italic* = common; **bold** = life-threatening)
CNS: Headache
GI: Nausea, vomiting, anorexia, diarrhea, abdominal pain, constipation, dyspepsia, mucositis
HEMA: **Neutropenia with fever**
SYST: Anaphylaxis, hemolysis, **methemoglobinemia, sepsis**

Contraindications: Hypersensitivity, G6PD deficiency, hemolytic reactions, or methemoglobinemia reactions to this drug

P **Precautions:** Lactation, children <2 yr, pregnancy (C)

Pharmacokinetics	
Absorption	Unknown
Distribution	Unknown
Metabolism	Unknown
Excretion	Unknown
Half-life	Elimination 18 hr

Pharmacodynamics
Unknown

NURSING CONSIDERATIONS
Assessment
• Monitor renal function studies: BUN, serum uric acid, urine CCr, electrolytes before and during therapy
• Monitor temp q4h; fever may indicate beginning infection; no rectal temps
• Assess for anaphylaxis, have emergency equipment nearby
• Assess for G6PD deficiency, hemolytic reactions, methemoglobinemia; these patients should not be given this agent
• Assess for toxicity: severe diarrhea, nausea, vomiting
• Assess GI symptoms: frequency of stools, cramping; if severe diarrhea occurs, fluid and electrolytes may need to be given

Nursing diagnoses
☑ Injury, risk for (adverse reactions, uses)
☑ Knowledge, deficient (teaching)

Implementation
• Give antiemetic 30-60 min before giving drug and prn

Patient/family education
• Advise of reason for therapy, expected results

Evaluation
Positive therapeutic outcome
• Decreased uric acid levels

☑ Herb/drug   Ⓢ Do Not Crush   ◆ Alert   ◆ᴛᴛ Key Drug   Ⓖ Geriatric   Ⓟ Pediatric

! HIGH ALERT

remifentanil (Rx)
(re-me-fin'ta-nill)
Ultiva
Func. class.: Opiate agonist analgesic
Chem. class.: μ-Opioid agonist

Pregnancy category C
Controlled substance schedule II

Action: Inhibits ascending pain pathways in limbic system, thalamus, midbrain, hypothalamus

➡ **Therapeutic Outcome:** Maintenance of anesthesia

Uses: In combination with other drugs in general anesthesia to provide analgesia

Dosage and routes
Adult: Induction **IV** 0.5-1 mcg/kg/min with a hypnotic or volatile agent; maintenance with isoflurane (0.4-1.5 MAC) or propofol (100-200 mcg/kg/min); cont inf 0.25-0.4 mcg/kg/min

Available forms: Powder for inj, lyophilized 1 mg/ml after reconstitution

Adverse effects
(*italic* = common; **bold** = life-threatening)
CNS: Drowsiness, *dizziness,* confusion, *headache,* sedation, euphoria, delirium, agitation, anxiety
CV: Palpitations, **bradycardia,** change in B/P; facial flushing, syncope, **asystole**
EENT: Tinnitus, blurred vision, miosis, diplopia
GI: *Nausea, vomiting,* anorexia, constipation, cramps, dry mouth
GU: Urinary retention, dysuria
INTEG: Rash, urticaria, bruising, flushing, diaphoresis, pruritus
MS: Rigidity
RESP: **Respiratory depression, apnea**

P **Contraindications:** Child <12 yr, hypersensitivity

Precautions: Pregnancy **C,** lactation, increased ICP, acute MI, severe heart disease; renal disease, hepatic disease, asthma, respiratory conditions, seizure disorders, elderly
G

Pharmacokinetics
Absorption	Complete
Distribution	Unknown
Metabolism	Unknown
Excretion	Unknown
Half-life	Unknown

Pharmacodynamics
Onset	Immediate
Peak	Unknown
Duration	Unknown

Interactions
Individual drugs
Alcohol: ↑ respiratory depression, hypotension, profound sedation
Drug classifications
Antihistamines, CNS depressants, phenothiazines, sedative/hypnotics: ↑ respiratory depression, hypotension, profound sedation
☑ *Herb/drug*
Kava: ↑ CNS depression

NURSING CONSIDERATIONS
Assessment
- Monitor I&O ratio, check for decreasing output; may indicate urinary retention, especially in elderly
G
- Assess CNS changes: dizziness, drowsiness, hallucinations, euphoria, LOC pupil reaction
- Assess allergic reactions: rash, urticaria
- Assess respiratory dysfunction: respiratory depression, character, rate, rhythm; notify prescriber if respirations are <12/min; CV status, bradycardia, syncope
- Use pain scoring to determine pain perception

Nursing diagnoses
☑ Knowledge, deficient (teaching)

Implementation
- Give by direct **IV** over 1½-3 min; use tuberculin syringe
- Interruption of infusion results in rapid reversal (no residual opioid effect within 5-10 min)
- Store in light-resistant area at room temperature

R

Y-site compatibilities: Acyclovir, alfentanil, amikacin, aminophylline, ampicillin, ampicillin/sulbactam, amrinone, aztreonam, bretylium, bumetanide, buprenorphine, butorphanol, calcium gluconate, cefazolin, cefotaxime, cefotetan, cefoxitin, ceftazidime, ceftizoxime, ceftriaxone, cefuroxime, cimetidine, ciprofloxacin, cisatracurium, clindamycin, dexamethasone, digoxin, diphenhydrAMINE, DOBUTamine, DOPamine, doxycycline, droperidol, enalaprilat, epINEPHrine, esmolol, famotidine, fentanyl, fluconazole, furosemide, ganciclovir, gentamicin, haloperidol, heparin, hydrocortisone sodium succinate, hydromorphone, hydrOXYzine, imipenem/cilastatin, isoproterenol, ketorolac, lidocaine, lorazepam, magnesium sulfate, mannitol, meperidine, methylprednisoLONE sodium succinate, metoclopramide, metronidazole, mezlocillin, midazolam, minocycline, morphine, nalbuphine, netilmicin, nitroglycerin, norepinephrine, ofloxacin, ondansetron

Patient/family education

• Advise patient to call for assistance when ambulating or smoking; drowsiness, dizziness may occur

• Advise patient to make position changes slowly to prevent orthostatic hypotension

Evaluation

Positive therapeutic outcome

• Maintenance of anesthesia

---

repaglinide (Rx)

(re-pag'lih-nide)

Prandin

Func. class.: Antidiabetic

Chem. class.: Meglitinides

Pregnancy category C

Action: Causes functioning β-cells in pancreas to release insulin, leading to drop in blood glucose levels; closes ATP-dependent potassium channels in the β-cell membrane; this leads to opening of calcium channels; increased calcium influx induces insulin secretion

➔ **Therapeutic Outcome:**
Blood glucose controlled

Uses: Stable adult-onset diabetes mellitus, type 2

Dosage and routes

Adult: PO 1-2 mg with each meal, max 16 mg/day, adjust at weekly intervals

Available forms: Tabs 0.5, 1, 2 mg

Adverse effects

(*italic* = common; **bold** = life-threatening)

CNS: *Headache, weakness,* paresthesia

ENDO: *Hypoglycemia*

GI: Nausea, vomiting, diarrhea, constipation, dyspepsia

INTEG: Rash, allergic reactions

MS: Back pains, arthralgia

RESP: URI, sinusitis, rhinitis, bronchitis

Contraindications: Hypersensitivity to meglitinides, diabetic ketoacidosis, type 1 diabetes

G Precautions: Pregnancy C, elderly, cardiac disease, severe renal disease, severe hepatic disease, thyroid disease, severe hypoglycemic **P** reactions, lactation, children

Pharmacokinetics

Absorption	Complete
Distribution	98% protein binding, crosses placenta
Metabolism	Liver
Excretion	Urine/feces
Half-life	1 hr

Pharmacodynamics

Onset	30 min
Peak	1-1½ hr
Duration	<4 hr

Interactions

Individual drugs

Alcohol: Disulfiram reaction

Carbamazepine, erythromycin: ↑ repaglinide metabolism

Chloramphenicol, probenecid: ↑ effect of repaglinide

Isoniazid, phenobarbital, phenytoin, rifampin: ↓ action of repaglinide

Drug classifications

Antifungals: ↓ repaglinide metabolism

Barbiturates: ↑ repaglinide metabolism

β-Adrenergic blockers, coumarins, MAOIs, NSAIDs, salicylates, sulfonamides: ↑ repaglinide effect

Calcium channel blockers, contraceptives (oral), corticosteroids, diuretics (thiazide), estrogens, phenothiazines, sympathomimetics, thyroid preparations: ↓ repaglinide effect

Herb/drug

Alfalfa, aloe, basil, bay, bilberry, bitter melon, black catechu, buchu, burdock, coriander, dandelion, eyebright (po), fenugreek, garlic, ginseng, glucomannan, glucosamine, goat's rue, gymnema, horehound, horse chestnut, jambul, myrrh, myrtle: ↑ antidiabetic effect

Bee pollen, blue cohosh, broom, chromium, elecampane, eucalyptus, gotu kola: ↓ antidiabetic effect

Broom, buchu, dandelion, juniper: ↓ hypoglycemia

Chromium, fenugreek, ginseng: ↑ or ↓ hypoglycemia

Karela: ↑ glucose tolerance

NURSING CONSIDERATIONS

Assessment

◆• Assess for hypoglycemic or hyperglycemic reaction, which can occur soon after meals; dizziness, weakness, headache, tremor, anxiety, tachycardia, hunger, sweating, abdominal pain

---

- Monitor glycosylated Hgb, fasting glucose during treatment

Nursing diagnoses
✓ Nutrition: more than body requirements, imbalanced (uses)
✓ Knowledge, deficient (teaching)
✓ Noncompliance (teaching)

Implementation
PO route
- 15 min before meals: 2, 3, or 4 ×/day preprandially
- Skip dose if meal is skipped; add dose if meal is added
- Store in airtight container in cool environment

Patient/family education
- Advise patient to avoid alcohol; explain disulfiram reaction
- Teach patient to use a capillary blood glucose test while taking this drug
- Teach patient the symptoms of hypoglycemia and hyperglycemia; what to do about each
- Teach patient that drug must be continued on daily basis; explain consequence of discontinuing drug abruptly
- Advise patient to avoid OTC medications unless ordered by prescriber
- Advise patient that diabetes is a lifelong illness; drug will not cure disease
- Advise patient to eat all food included in diet plan to prevent hypoglycemia; to have glucagon emergency kit available
- Instruct patient to carry/wear emergency ID for emergency purposes

Evaluation
Positive therapeutic outcome
- Decrease in polyuria, polydipsia, polyphagia, clear sensorium, absence of dizziness, stable gait

Treatment of overdose: Glucose 25 g **IV** via D$_{50}$ sol, 50 ml or 1 mg glucagon

---

retinoic acid
See tretinoin

Rh$_o$ (D) immune globulin, standard dose IM (Rx)
Gamulin Rh, HypoRho-D, RhoGAM
Rh$_o$ (D) globulin microdose IM
HypoRho-D Mini-Dose, MICRh$_o$GAM, Mini-Gamulin R
Rh$_o$ (D) immune globulin IV (Rx)
WinRho SD, WinRho SDF
Func. class.: Immune globulins

Pregnancy category C

Action: Suppresses immune response of nonsensitized Rh$_o$ (D or D^u)-negative patients who are exposed to Rh$_o$ (D or D^u)-positive blood

➡ **Therapeutic Outcome:** Absence of Rh factor and transfusion error

Uses: Prevention of isoimmunization in Rh-negative women exposed to Rh-positive blood given after abortions, miscarriages, amniocentesis

Dosage and routes
After delivery
Adult: IM 1 vial (standard dose) if fetal packed RBCs <15 ml, or 2 vials if fetal packed RBCs >15 ml; given within 72 hr of delivery or miscarriage

Before delivery
Adult: IM 1 vial (standard dose) at 26-28 wk, 1 vial (standard dose) 72 hr after delivery

Pregnancy termination <13 wk
Adult: IM 1 vial (micro dose) within 72 hr

Pregnancy termination >13 wk
Adult: IM 1 vial (standard dose) within 72 hr

Fetal-maternal hemorrhage
Adult: IM packed RBCs volume of hemorrhage/15 = needed vials (standard dose)

Transfusion error
Adult: IM (standard dose—1 vial) give within 72 hr

After 34 wk gestation
Adult: IM/**IV** 120 mcg, give within 72 hr (**IV** dose)

Available forms: Inj single-dose vial (50 mcg/vial—microdose, 300 mcg/vial—standard); inj 120, 300 mcg Rh$_o$(D) immune globulin IV, human

Adverse effects
(*italic* = common; **bold** = life-threatening)
CNS: Lethargy

INTEG: Irritation at inj site, fever
MS: Myalgia

Contraindications: Previous immunization with this drug, Rh$_o$ (O)-positive/D^u-positive patient

Precautions: Pregnancy **C**

Do Not Confuse:
Gamulin Rh/MICRh$_o$GAM

Pharmacokinetics	
Absorption	Well absorbed
Distribution	Unknown
Metabolism	Unknown
Excretion	Unknown
Half-life	Unknown

Pharmacodynamics	
Onset	Rapid
Peak	Unknown
Duration	Unknown

Interactions
Drug classifications
Live virus vaccines: ↓ antibody response to vaccine

NURSING CONSIDERATIONS
Assessment
● • Assess for allergies, reactions to immunizations; previous immunization with this drug
● Obtain type and cross-match of mother's blood and of neonate's cord blood; neonate must be Rh$_o$(D)-positive, mother must be Rh$_o$(D)-negative and (D^u)-negative, medication should be given if there is a doubt
● • Assess for intravascular hemolysis: back pain, chills, hemoglobinuria, renal insufficiency, idiopathic thrombocytopenic purpura

Nursing diagnoses
✓ Knowledge, deficient (teaching)

Implementation
IM route
● Reconstitute Rh$_o$ (D) immune globulin IV using 1.25 ml of 0.9% NaCl swirl
● Do not use Rh$_o$ (D) immune globulin or Rh$_o$ (D) immune globulin microdose by **IV**
● Give IM inj in deltoid muscle within 3 hr if possible; aspirate to prevent **IV** administration
● Give only equal lot numbers of drug, cross-match
● Give only MICRh$_o$GAM for abortions or miscarriages <13 wk unless fetus or father is Rh-negative
● Store in refrigerator

IV **IV direct route**
● Reconstitute Rh$_o$ (D) immune globulin IV using 2.5 ml of 0.9% NaCl, swirl, give over 3-5 min
● Do not use Rh$_o$ (D) immune globulin or Rh$_o$ (D) immune globulin microdose by **IV**

Patient/family education
● Teach patient how drug works; that drug must be given after subsequent deliveries if subsequent babies are Rh-positive

Evaluation
Positive therapeutic outcome
● Prevention of Rh$_o$(D) sensitization in transfusion error
● Prevention of erythroblastosis fetalis in subsequent Rh$_o$(D)-positive neonates

---

ribavarin (Rx)
(rye-ba-vye'rin)
Virazole
Func. class.: Synthetic antiviral
Chem. class.: Tricyclic amine

Pregnancy category X

Action: Prevents replication of DNA and RNA synthesis

➔ **Therapeutic Outcome:** Resolution of severe lower respiratory tract infections

Uses: Severe lower respiratory tract infections in infants and children

Investigational uses: Influenza A or B (early)

Dosage and routes
P *Infants and young children:* INH 20 mg/ml × 12-18 hr/day × 3-7 days

Available forms: Powder for reconstitution for aerosol 6 g/vial

Adverse effects
(*italic* = common; **bold** = life-threatening)
CNS: Dizziness, faintness
CV: Hypotension, cardiac arrest
EENT: Eye irritation, conjunctivitis, blurred vision, photosensitivity
INTEG: Rash

Contraindications: Hypersensitivity, lactation, child <1 yr, pregnancy **X**

Precautions: Epilepsy, hepatic disease, renal disease

 Herb/drug   Do Not Crush   Alert   Key Drug   Geriatric   **P** Pediatric

Pharmacokinetics

Absorption	Inh (systemic)
Distribution	To respiratory tract
Metabolism	Liver
Excretion	Respiratory tract
Half-life	9½ hr

Pharmacodynamics

Onset	Unknown
Peak	Inh end
Duration	Unknown

Interactions
Individual drugs
Zidovudine: ↓ antiviral action, ↑ toxicity
Drug classification
Cardiac glycosides: ↑ toxicity

NURSING CONSIDERATIONS
Assessment
• Assess allergies before initiation of treatment, reaction of each medication; list allergies on chart in bright red letters
• Monitor respiratory status: rate, character, wheezing, tightness in chest
• Obtain C&S test results before starting treatment

Nursing diagnoses
☑ Infection, risk for (uses)
☑ Gas exchange, impaired (uses)
☑ Knowledge, deficient (teaching)

Implementation
• Give by the Viratek small particle aerosol generator (SPAG-2), do not use other inhalation equipment
P • May be given by an oxygen hood for infants, or a face mask may be attached to the SPAG-2
• Reconstitute 6 g of sterile water for inj or inh, place sol in the Erlenmeyer flask and dilute further to 20 mg/ml

Patient/family education
• Teach patient and parents aspects of drug therapy

Evaluation
Positive therapeutic outcome
• Absence of respiratory syncytial virus (RSV)

riboflavin
(vitamin B$_2$) (OTC)
(rye′boo-flay-vin)
Func. class.: Vitamin B$_2$, water soluble

Pregnancy category A

Action: Needed for respiratory reactions (catalyzes proteins) and for normal vision

➔ **Therapeutic Outcome:** Prevention or treatment of riboflavin deficiency

Uses: Vitamin B$_2$ deficiency or polyneuritis; cheilosis adjunct with thiamine

Dosage and routes
Deficiency
P *Adult and child >12 yr:* PO 5-25 mg qd
P *Child <12 yr:* PO 2-10 mg qd, then 0.6 mg/1000 cal ingested

RDA
Adult: Males 1.4-1.8 mg; females 1.2-1.3 mg

Available forms: Tabs 5, 10, 25, 50, 100, 250 mg

Adverse effects
(*italic* = common; **bold** = life-threatening)
GU: Yellow discoloration of urine (large doses)

Precautions: Pregnancy **A**

Pharmacokinetics

Absorption	Well absorbed (by active transport)
Distribution	60% protein bound, widely distributed, crosses placenta
Metabolism	Unknown
Excretion	Kidneys (unchanged), excess amounts
Half-life	1-1½ hr

Pharmacodynamics
Unknown

R

Interactions
Individual drugs
Alcohol, probenecid: ↑ riboflavin need
Tetracycline: ↓ action of tetracycline
Drug classifications
Antidepressants (tricyclic), phenothiazines: ↑ riboflavin need
Lab test interferences
False: ↑ Urinary catecholamines, ↑ urobilinogen

NURSING CONSIDERATIONS
Assessment
- Assess patient's nutritional status: liver, eggs, dairy products, yeast, whole grain, green vegetables
- Assess for vit B_2 deficiency: photophobia, cheilosis, stomatitis, ocular swelling

Nursing diagnoses
✓ Nutrition: less than body requirements, imbalanced (uses)
✓ Knowledge, deficient (teaching)

Implementation
- Give with food for better absorption
- Store in airtight, light-resistant container

Patient/family education
- Inform patient that urine may turn bright yellow
- Instruct patient about addition of needed foods that are rich in riboflavin

Evaluation
Positive therapeutic outcome
- Absence of headache, GI problems, cheilosis, skin lesions, depression, burning, itchy eyes, anemia

---

rifabutin (Rx)
(riff′a-byoo-tin)
Mycobutin
Func. class.: Antimycobacterial
Chem. class.: Rifamycin S derivative

Pregnancy category B

Action: Inhibits DNA-dependent RNA polymerase in susceptible strains

→ **Therapeutic Outcome:** Antimycobacterial death of *Escherichia coli, Bacillus subtilis,* and *Mycobacterium avium*

Uses: Prevention of *M. avium* complex (MAC) in patients with advanced HIV infection

Investigational uses: *Helicobacter pylori* that has not responded to other treatment

Dosage and routes
Adult: PO 300 mg qd (may take as 150 mg bid)

Available forms: Caps 150 mg

Adverse effects
(*italic* = common; **bold** = life-threatening)
CNS: Headache, fatigue, anxiety, confusion, insomnia
GI: Nausea, vomiting, anorexia, diarrhea, heartburn, **hepatitis,** discolored saliva
GU: Hematuria, discolored urine
***HEMA:* Hemolytic anemia, eosinophilia, thrombocytopenia, leukopenia**
INTEG: Rash
MISC: Flulike syndrome, shortness of breath, chest pressure
MS: Asthenia, arthralgia, myalgia

Contraindications: Hypersensitivity, active TB, WBC <1000/mm³, platelets <50,000/mm³

Precautions: Pregnancy **B**, lactation,
P hepatic disease, blood dyscrasias, children

▧ **Do Not Confuse:**
rifabutin/rifampin

Pharmacokinetics
Absorption	Well absorbed
Distribution	Widely distributed
Metabolism	Liver
Excretion	Kidney
Half-life	45 hr

Pharmacodynamics
Onset	Unknown
Peak	2-3 hr

Interactions
Individual drugs
Amprenavir, clofibrate, cycloSPORINE, dapsone, delavirdine, digoxin, disopyramide, efavirenz, fluconazole, indinavir, ketoconazole, nelfinavir, nevirapine, phenytoin, quinidine, saquinavir, theophylline, tocainide, verapamil, zidovudine: ↓ action of each specific drug
Ritonavir: ↑ rifabutin level
Drug classifications
Analgesics (opioid), anticoagulants, barbiturates, β-blockers, contraceptives (oral), corticosteroids, estrogens, sulfonylureas: ↓ action of each specific drug
Food/drug
High-fat foods: ↓ absorption

Lab test interferences
Interference: Folate level, vit B_{12}, BSP, gallbladder studies

NURSING CONSIDERATIONS
Assessment
- Assess for active TB: chest x-ray, sputum culture, blood culture, biopsy of lymph nodes, obtain PPD test; drug should be given only for MAC and never for TB

- Monitor CBC for neutropenia, thrombocytopenia, eosinophilia

Nursing diagnoses
✓ Infection, risk for (uses)
✓ Diarrhea (adverse reaction)
✓ Injury, risk for (adverse reaction)
✓ Knowledge, deficient (teaching)
✓ Noncompliance (teaching)

Implementation
- Give with meals to decrease GI symptoms; better to take on empty stomach 1 hr ac or 2 hr pc; high-fat food slows absorption
- Give antiemetic if vomiting occurs

Patient/family education
- Caution patient that compliance with dosage schedule and duration is necessary
- Instruct patient that scheduled appointments must be kept or relapse may occur
- Instruct patient to notify prescriber if hepatitis, neutropenia, or thrombocytopenia occurs: sore throat, fever, bleeding, bruising, yellow sclera, anorexia, nausea, vomiting, fatigue, weakness; myositis: muscle or bone pain
- Advise patient that urine, feces, saliva, sputum, sweat, tears may be colored red-orange; soft contact lens may become permanently stained
- Caution patients using oral contraceptives to use a nonhormonal method of birth control because rifabutin may decrease efficiency of oral contraceptives

Evaluation
Positive therapeutic outcome
- Decreased symptoms of *M. avium* in patients with HIV

---

rifampin (Rx)
(rif'am-pin)
Rifadin, Rimactane, Rofact ♦
Func. class.: Antitubercular
Chem. class.: Rifamycin B derivative

Pregnancy category C

Action: Inhibits DNA-dependent polymerase, decreases replication

➔ **Therapeutic Outcome:** Bactericidal against the following organisms: mycobacteria, *Staphylococcus aureus, Haemophilus influenzae, Neisseria meningitidis, Legionella pneumophila*

Uses: Pulmonary TB, meningococcal carriers (prevention)

Dosage and routes
Tuberculosis
Adult: PO/**IV** max 600 mg/day as single dose 1 hr ac or 2 hr pc or 10 mg/kg/day 2-3 ×/wk

P *Child >5 yr:* PO/**IV** 10-20 mg/kg/day as single dose 1 hr ac or 2 hr pc, max 600 mg/day, with other antitubercular drugs

6-mo regimen: 2-mo treatment of isoniazid, rifampin, pyrazinamide, and possibly streptomycin or ethambutol; then rifampin and isoniazid × 4 mo

9-mo regimen: Rifampin and isoniazid supplemented with pyrazinamide, or streptomycin or ethambutol

Meningococcal carriers
Adult: PO/**IV** 600 mg bid × 2 days

P *Child >5 yr:* PO/**IV** 10-20 mg/kg bid × 2 days, max 600 mg/dose

P *Infant 3 mo-1 yr:* PO 5 mg/kg bid for 2 days

Prevention of H. influenzae *type B infection*
Adult: PO 600 mg/day × 4 days

P *Child:* PO 20 mg/kg/day × 4 days

Available forms: Caps 150, 300 mg; powder for inj 600 mg/vial

Adverse effects
(*italic* = common; **bold** = life-threatening)
CNS: Headache, fatigue, anxiety, drowsiness, confusion
EENT: Visual disturbances
GI: Nausea, vomiting, anorexia, diarrhea, **pseudomembranous colitis,** *heartburn,* sore mouth and tongue, pancreatitis, elevated liver function tests
GU: **Hematuria, acute renal failure, hemoglobinuria**
HEMA: **Hemolytic anemia, eosinophilia, thrombocytopenia, leukopenia**
INTEG: Rash, pruritus, urticaria
MISC: Flulike syndrome, menstrual disturbances, edema, shortness of breath
MS: Ataxia, weakness

Contraindications: Hypersensitivity

Precautions: Pregnancy C, lactation, hepatic disease, blood dyscrasias

◣ **Do Not Confuse:**
rifampin/rifabutin

R

Pharmacokinetics

Absorption	Well absorbed (PO), completely absorbed (IV)
Distribution	Widely distributed, crosses placenta
Metabolism	Liver—extensively
Excretion	Feces
Half-life	3 hr

Pharmacodynamics

	PO	IV
Onset	Rapid	Rapid
Peak	2-3 hr	Inf end

Interactions
Individual drugs
Acetaminophen: ↓ action of acetaminophen
Alcohol: ↓ action of alcohol
Chloramphenicol: ↓ effect of chloramphenicol
Clofibrate: ↓ action of clofibrate
CycloSPORINE: ↓ action of cycloSPORINE
Dapsone: ↓ action of dapsone
Digoxin: ↓ action of digoxin
Diltiazem: ↓ action of diltiazem
Doxycycline: ↓ action of doxycycline
Haloperidol: ↓ action of haloperidol
Imidazole: ↓ antifungal action
Isoniazid: ↑ hepatotoxicity
Lithium: ↑ lithium toxicity
Nifedipine: ↓ action of nifedipine
Phenytoin: ↓ effect of phenytoin
Sodium lactate: drugs are incompatible
Theophylline: ↓ effect of theophylline
Verapamil: ↓ effect of verapamil
Zidovudine: ↓ action of zidovudine
Drug classifications
Antidiabetics: ↓ action of antidiabetics
Barbiturates: ↓ action of barbiturates
Benzodiazepines: ↓ action of benzodiazepines
β-blockers: ↓ action of β-blockers
Contraceptives (oral), glucocorticoids: ↓ effect
Fluroquinolones: ↓ action of fluoroquinolones
Hormones: ↓ action of hormones
Imidazole antifungals: ↓ antifungal action
Sulfonamides: ↓ action of sulfonamides
Protease inhibitors: ↓ action of protease inhibitors

Lab test interferences
Interference: Folate level, vit B$_{12}$ gallbladder studies, dexamethasone suppression test
False positive: Direct Coombs' test

NURSING CONSIDERATIONS
Assessment
• Monitor liver studies qmo: ALT, AST, bilirubin
• Monitor renal status: before, qmo: BUN, creatinine, output, sp gr, urinalysis
• Monitor mental status often: affect, mood, behavioral changes; psychosis may occur
• Monitor hepatic status: decreased appetite, jaundice, dark urine, fatigue
• Assess for infection: sputum culture, lung sounds
• C&S should be performed before beginning treatment, during, and after therapy is completed
Nursing diagnoses
✓ Infection, risk for (uses)
✓ Diarrhea (adverse reactions)
✓ Injury, risk for (adverse reactions)
✓ Knowledge, deficient (teaching)
✓ Noncompliance (teaching)
Implementation
PO route
• Administer with meals to decrease GI symptoms; better to take on empty stomach 1 hr ac or 2 hr pc, with full glass of water
IV IV route
Intermittent IV
• Give by intermittent inf after reconstituting 600 mg/10 ml of sterile water for inj, agitate gently; dilute further in 100 or 500 ml of 0.9% NaCl or D$_5$W; give 100 ml/30 min or 500 ml/3 hr
• Do not mix with other drugs or sols
Patient/family education
• Instruct patient that compliance with dosage schedule, duration is necessary
• Instruct patient that scheduled appointments must be kept or relapse may occur
• Instruct patient to notify prescriber if hepatitis, neutropenia, or thrombocytopenia occurs: sore throat, fever, bleeding, bruising, yellow sclera, anorexia, nausea, vomiting, fatigue, weakness
• Advise patient that urine, feces, saliva, sputum, sweat, tears may be colored red-orange; soft contact lens may be permanently stained
• Caution patients using oral contraceptives to use a nonhormonal method of birth control because rifabutin may decrease the efficiency of oral contraceptives
• Advise patient to avoid alcohol, hepatotoxicity may occur
Evaluation
Positive therapeutic outcome
• Decreased symptoms of TB

rifapentine (Rx)
(riff'ah-pen-teen)
Priftin
Func. class.: Antitubercular
Chem. class.: Rifamycin derivative

Pregnancy category C

Action: Inhibits DNA-dependent polymerase, decreases tubercule bacilli replication

⟳ Therapeutic Outcome: Resolution of pulmonary TB

Uses: Pulmonary TB; must be used with at least one other antitubercular drug

Dosage and routes
Intensive phase
Adult: PO 600 mg (4 150 mg tabs 2 ×/wk), with an interval of 72 hr between doses × 2 mo; must be given with at least one other antitubercular drug

Continuation phase
Adult: 600 mg qwk × 4 mo in combination with isoniazid or other appropriate antitubercular drug

Available forms: Tabs 150 mg

Adverse effects
(*italic* = common; **bold** = life-threatening)
CNS: Headache, fatigue, anxiety, dizziness
EENT: Visual disturbances
GI: *Nausea, vomiting, anorexia, diarrhea,* bilirubinemia, hepatitis, increased ALT, AST, *heartburn,* **pancreatitis**
GU: **Hematuria,** pyuria, proteinuria, urinary casts, urine discoloration
HEMA: **Thrombocytopenia, leukopenia, neutropenia, lymphopenia,** anemia, **leukocytosis,** purpura, hematoma
INTEG: Rash, pruritus, urticaria, acne
MISC: Edema, aggressive reaction, increased B/P
MS: Gout, arthrosis

Contraindications: Hypersensitivity to rifamycins, porphyria

Precautions: Pregnancy **C,** lactation, **P** hepatic disease, blood dyscrasias, children **G** <12 yr, HIV, elderly

Pharmacokinetics	
Absorption	Unknown
Distribution	Unknown
Metabolism	Unknown
Excretion	Unknown
Half-life	Unknown

Pharmacodynamics	
Onset	Unknown
Peak	Unknown
Duration	Unknown

Interactions
Individual drugs
Amitriptyline: ↓ amitriptyline action
Chloramphenicol: ↓ chloramphenicol action
Clarithromycin: ↓ clarithromycin action
Clofibrate: ↓ clofibrate action
CycloSPORINE: ↓ cycloSPORINE action
Dapsone: ↓ dapsone action
Delaviridine: ↓ delaviridine action
Diazepam: ↓ diazepam action
Digoxin: ↓ digoxin action
Diltiazem: ↓ diltiazem action
Disopyramide: ↓ disopyramide action
Doxycycline: ↓ doxycycline action
Fentanyl: ↓ fentanyl action
Fluconazole: ↓ fluconazole action
Haloperidol: ↓ haloperidol action
Indinavir: ↓ indinavir action
Itraconazole: ↓ itraconazole action
Ketoconazole: ↓ ketoconazole action
Methadone: ↓ methadone action
Mexiletine: ↓ mexiletine action
Nelfinavir: ↓ nelfinavir action
NIFEdipine: ↓ NIFEdipine action
Nortriptyline: ↓ nortriptyline action
Phenytoin: ↓ phenytoin action
Quinidine: ↓ quinidine action
Quinine: ↓ quinine action
Ritonavir: ↓ ritonavir action
Saquinavir: ↓ saquinavir action
Sildenafil: ↓ sildenafil action
Tacrolimus: ↓ tacrolimus action
Theophylline: ↓ theophylline action
Tocainide: ↓ tocainide action
Verapamil: ↓ verapamil action
Warfarin: ↓ warfarin action
Zidovudine: ↓ zidovudine action
Drug classifications
Anticoagulants: ↓ anticoagulants action
Antidiabetics: ↓ antidiabetics action
Barbiturates: ↓ barbiturates action
β-Adrenergic blockers: ↓ β-blocker action
Corticosteroids: ↓ corticosteroids action
Fluoroquinolones: ↓ fluoroquinolones action
Oral contraceptives: ↓ oral contraceptives action
Phenothiazines: ↓ phenothiazines action
Progestins: ↓ progestin action
Protease inhibitors: Use extreme caution
Thyroid preparations: ↓ thyroid preparations action

R

Food/drug
Food: ↑ drug concentration by 44% with food
Lab test interferences:
Interference: Folate level, vit B$_{12}$

NURSING CONSIDERATIONS
Assessment
• Obtain baselines in CBC, AST, ALT, bilirubin, platelets
• Assess for infection: sputum culture, lung sounds
• Assess signs of anemia: Hct, Hgb, fatigue
• Monitor liver studies qmo: ALT, AST, bilirubin
• Monitor renal status qmo: BUN, creatinine, output, sp gr, urinalysis
• Assess hepatic status: decreased appetite, jaundice, dark urine, fatigue

Nursing diagnoses
☑ Infection, risk for (uses)
☑ Diarrhea (side effects)
☑ Knowledge, deficient (teaching)
☑ Noncompliance (teaching)

Implementation
PO route
• Give PO, may be given with food for GI upset
• Give antiemetic if vomiting occurs
• Administer after C&S is completed; qmo to detect resistance

Patient/family education
• Advise patient that compliance with dosage schedule, duration is necessary
• Instruct patient that scheduled appointments must be kept; relapse may occur
• Teach patient that urine, feces, saliva, sputum, sweat, tears may be colored red-orange; soft contact lenses, dentures may be permanently stained
• Teach patient to use alternate method of contraception, oral contraceptive action may be decreased
• Teach patient to report flulike symptoms: excessive fatigue, anorexia, vomiting, sore throat; unusual bleeding, jaundice of skin, eyes

Evaluation
Positive therapeutic outcome
• Decreased symptoms of TB
• Negative culture

riluzole (Rx)
(ri-loo'zole)
Rilutek
Func. class.: Amyotropic lateral sclerosis (ALS) agent
Chem. class.: Benzathiazole

Pregnancy category C

Action: Unknown; may act by inhibiting glutamate, interfering with binding of amino acid receptors, inactivation of voltage-dependent sodium channels

⇒ **Therapeutic Outcome:** Decreased symptoms of ALS

Uses: ALS

Dosage and routes
Adult: PO 50 mg q12h, take 1 hr ac or 2 hr pc

Available forms: Tabs 50 mg

Adverse effects
(*italic* = common; **bold** = life-threatening)
CNS: Hypertonia, depression, dizziness, insomnia, somnolence, vertigo
CV: Hypertension, tachycardia, phlebitis, palpitation, postural hypertension
GI: Nausea, vomiting, dyspepsia, anorexia, diarrhea, flatulence, stomatitis, dry mouth
GU: UTI, dysuria
HEMA: Neutropenia
INTEG: Pruritus, eczema, alopecia, **exfoliative dermatitis**
RESP: Decreased lung function; rhinitis, increased cough

Contraindications: Hypersensitivity

Precautions: Neutropenia, renal disease, hepatic disease, elderly, pregnancy **C**, lactation, children

Pharmacokinetics
Absorption	Well
Distribution	Unknown
Metabolism	Extensively—live
Excretion	Urine, feces
Half-life	Unknown

Pharmacodynamics
Unknown

Interactions
Individual drugs
Amitriptyline, caffeine, theophylline: ↓ elimination of riluzole
Cigarette smoke, omeprazole, rifampin: ↑ elimination of riluzole

Drug classifications
Quinolones: ↓ elimination of riluzole
Food/drug
Charcoal-broiled foods: ↑ elimination of riluzole
High-fat meal: ↓ absorption

NURSING CONSIDERATIONS
Assessment
• Monitor liver function tests: AST, ALT, bilirubin, GGT, baseline and qmo × 3 mo, then q3 mo
• Assess for neutropenia (neutrophils <500/mm³)

Nursing diagnoses
☑ Mobility, impaired physical (uses)
☑ Knowledge, deficient (teaching)

Implementation
• Give 1 hr ac or 2 hr pc; a high-fat meal decreases absorption

Patient/family education
• Advise to report febrile illness, may indicate neutropenia
• Teach reason for drug and expected results

---

rimantadine (Rx)
(ri-man'ti-deen)
Flumadine
Func. class.: Synthetic antiviral
Chem. class.: Tricyclic amine

Pregnancy category C

Action: Prevents uncoating of nucleic acid in viral cell, preventing penetration of virus to host; causes release of DOPamine from neurons

➡ **Therapeutic Outcome:** Prevention of influenza type A

Uses: Prophylaxis or treatment of influenza type A

Dosage and routes
Renal/hepatic dose
Reduce as needed

Influenza type A prophylaxis
P **Adult and child >10 yr:** PO 100 mg bid; in renal or hepatic disease, lower dose to 100 mg/day

P **Child <10 yr:** PO 5 mg/kg/day, max 150 mg

Treatment
Adult: PO 100 mg bid; in renal or hepatic disease, lower dose to 100 mg/day; start treatment at onset of symptoms, continue for at least 1 wk

G **Elderly:** PO 100 mg/day

Available forms: Tabs 100 mg; syr 50 mg/5 ml

Adverse effects
(*italic* = common; **bold** = life-threatening)
CNS: *Headache, dizziness,* fatigue, depression, hallucinations, tremors, **seizures,** insomnia, *poor concentration,* asthenia, gait abnormalities, anxiety, confusion
CV: Pallor, palpitations, *hypotension, edema*
EENT: Tinnitus, taste abnormality, eye pain
GI: Nausea, vomiting, constipation, dry mouth, anorexia, abdominal pain, diarrhea, dyspepsia
INTEG: Rash

Contraindications: Hypersensitivity to drugs of adamantance class (this drug, amantadine)

Precautions: Epilepsy, hepatic disease, renal disease, pregnancy **C,** lactation, child
P <1 yr

N **Do Not Confuse:**
rimantadine/amantadine

Pharmacokinetics
Absorption	Minimally absorbed (PO)
Distribution	Widely distributed, crosses placenta, CSF concentration 50% plasma
Metabolism	Liver
Excretion	95% unchanged—kidneys
Half-life	2-3.5 hr, increased in renal disease

Pharmacodynamics
	PO
Onset	Unknown
Peak	1½-2½

Interactions
Individual drugs
Acetaminophen, aspirin: ↓ peak concentration of rimantadine
Cimetidine: ↑ rimantidine concentration

NURSING CONSIDERATIONS
Assessment
• Assess for seizures; if seizures occur, drug should be discontinued
• Assess allergies before initiation of treatment, patient's reaction to each medication; list allergies on chart
• Monitor respiratory status: rate, character, wheezing, tightness in chest

Nursing diagnoses
☑ Infection, risk for (uses)
☑ Knowledge, deficient (teaching)

Implementation
- Give before exposure to influenza; continue for 10 days after contact
- Give at least 4 hr before bedtime to prevent insomnia
- Administer pc for better absorption, to decrease GI symptoms; cap may be opened and mixed with food for easy swallowing
- Give in divided doses to prevent CNS disturbances: headache, dizziness, fatigue, drowsiness
- Store in airtight, dry container

Patient/family education
- Instruct patient about aspects of drug therapy: need to report dyspnea, dizziness, poor concentration, behavioral changes
- Advise patient to avoid hazardous activities if dizziness occurs
- Caution patient to consult prescriber before taking OTC medications, alcohol; serious drug interactions may result

Evaluation
Positive therapeutic outcome
- Absence of fever, malaise, cough, dyspnea

Treatment of overdose: Withdraw drug, maintain airway, administer epINEPHrine, aminophylline, O_2, **IV** corticosteroids, physostigmine

---

risedronate (Rx)
(rih-sed'roh-nate)
Actonel
Func. class: Bone resorption inhibitor
Chem. class.: Bisphosphonate
Pregnancy category C

Action: Inhibits bone resorption; absorbs calcium phosphate crystal in bone and may directly block dissolution of hydroxyapatite crystals of bone

➡ **Therapeutic Outcome:** Increased bone mass, activity without fractures

Uses: Paget's disease, prevention, treatment of osteoporosis in postmenopausal women, glucocorticoid-induced osteoporosis

Dosage and routes
Paget's disease
Adult: PO 30 mg qd × 2 mo; give calcium and vit D if dietary intake is lacking; if relapse occurs, retreatment is advised

Postmenopausal osteoporosis/ glucocorticoid-induced osteoporosis
Adult: PO 35 mg qwk (postmenopausal osteoporosis) or 5 mg qd

Available forms: Tabs 5, 30, 35 mg
Adverse effects
(*italic* = common; **bold** = life-threatening)
CNS: Dizziness, headache, depression
CV: Chest pain, hypertension
GI: *Abdominal pain, anorexia, diarrhea, nausea,* constipation
MS: *Bone pain,* arthralgia
MISC: Rash, UTI, pharyngitis

Contraindications: Hypersensitivity to bisphosphonates, inability to stand or sit upright for ≥30 min

P Precautions: Children, lactation, pregnancy C, renal disease, active upper GI disorders

Pharmacokinetics	
Absorption	Unknown
Distribution	To bones
Metabolism	Unknown
Excretion	Kidneys
Half-life	Unknown

Pharmacodynamics	
Onset	Unknown
Peak	Unknown
Duration	Unknown

Interactions
Drug classifications
Antacids, calcium supplements: ↓ absorption of risedronate
NSAIDs, salicylates: ↑ GI irritation
Food/drug
Food: ↓ bioavailability: take ½ hr before food or drinks other than water

NURSING CONSIDERATIONS
Assessment
- Assess for symptoms of Paget's disease: headache, bone pain, increased head circumference
- Monitor electrolytes; renal function studies (calcium, phosphorus, magnesium, potassium)
- Assess for hypercalcemia: paresthesia, twitching, laryngospasm, Chvostek's/ Trousseau's signs

Nursing diagnoses
✓ Mobility, impaired (uses)
✓ Nutrition: less than body requirements, imbalanced (uses)
✓ Knowledge, deficient (teaching)

Implementation
- Give PO for 2 months to be effective in Paget's disease

- Give with a full glass of water; patient should be in upright position
- Administer supplemental calcium and vit D in Paget's disease
- Give qd ≥30 min ac
- Store in cool environment, out of direct sunlight

Patient/family education

- Advise patient to sit upright for ½ hr after dose to prevent irritation
- Instruct patient to comply with dietary restrictions
- Advise patient to notify prescriber if pregnancy is planned or suspected

Evaluation

Positive therapeutic outcome

- Increased bone mass, absence of fractures

---

risperidone (Rx)

(res-pare'a-done)

Risperdal

Func. class: Antipsychotic

Chem. class.: Benzisoxazole derivative

Pregnancy category C

Action: Unknown; may be mediated through both dopamine type 2 (D_2) and serotinin type 2 (5-HT_2) antagonism

Therapeutic Outcome: Decreased hallucinations and disorganized thought

Uses: Psychotic disorders

Dosage and routes

Adult: PO 1 mg bid, with incremental increases of 1 mg bid on days 2 and 3 to a dose of 3 mg bid by day 3; then do not increase dose for at least 1 wk

G *Elderly:* PO 0.5 mg qd-bid increase by 1 mg qwk

Hepatic dose/renal dose

Adult: PO 0.5 mg, increase by 0.5 mg bid, then increase to 1.5 mg bid

Available forms: Tabs 1, 2, 3, 4 mg; oral sol 1 mg/ml

Adverse effects

(*italic* = common; **bold** = life-threatening)

CNS: *EPS (pseudoparkinsonism, akathisia, dystonia, tardive dyskinesia), drowsiness, insomnia, agitation, anxiety, headache,* **neuroleptic malignant syndrome,** dizziness, **seizures**

CV: Orthostatic hypotension, **tachycardia**

EENT: Blurred vision

GI: *Nausea,* vomiting, *anorexia, constipation,* jaundice, weight gain

RESP: Rhinitis

Contraindications: Hypersensitivity, lactation, seizure disorders

P **Precautions:** Children, renal disease,

G pregnancy **C**, hepatic disease, elderly, breast cancer

N **Do Not Confuse:**

Risperdal/reserpine

Pharmacokinetics

Absorption	Unknown
Distribution	Unknown
Metabolism	Liver, extensively
Excretion	Unknown
Half-life	Unknown

Pharmacodynamics

Onset	Unknown
Peak	Unknown
Duration	Up to 12 hr

Interactions

Individual drugs

Alcohol: ↑ effects of both drugs, oversedation

Carbamazepine: ↓ risperidone effect

Levodopa: ↓ levodopa effect

Drug classifications

Anesthetics (barbiturate, general), antidepressants, antihistamines, MAOIs, opiates, sedative/hypnotics: ↑ CNS depression

☑ *Herb/drug*

Betel palm, kava: ↑ extrapyramidal symptoms (EPS)

Cola tree, hops, nettle, nutmeg: ↑ action

Kava: ↑ CNS depression

Lab test interferences

↑ prolactin levels

R

NURSING CONSIDERATIONS

Assessment

- Assess mental status: orientation, mood, behavior, presence and type of hallucinations before initial administration and monthly; this drug should significantly reduce psychotic behavior
- Check that patient swallows all PO medication; check for hoarding or giving of medication to other patients
- Monitor I&O ratio, palpate bladder if low

G urinary output occurs, especially in elderly; urinalysis recommended before, during prolonged therapy

- Monitor bilirubin, CBC, liver function studies monthly

- Assess affect, orientation, LOC, reflexes, gait, coordination, sleep pattern disturbances
- Monitor B/P with patient in sitting, standing, and lying positions; take pulse and respirations q4h during initial treatment; establish baseline before starting treatment; report drops of 30 mm Hg; obtain baseline ECG and monitor Q- and T-wave changes
- Check for dizziness, faintness, palpitations, tachycardia on rising; severe orthostatic hypotension is common

⬥• Identify for neuroleptic malignant syndrome: hyperpyrexia, muscle rigidity, increased CPK, altered mental status; drug should be discontinued

- Assess for EPS including akathisia (inability to sit still, no desire to movements), tardive dyskinesia (bizarre movements of the jaw, mouth, tongue, extremities), pseudoparkinsonism (rigidity, tremors, pill rolling, shuffling gait); an antiparkinsonian drug should be prescribed
- Assess for constipation, urinary retention daily; if these occur, increase bulk, water in diet

Nursing diagnoses
☑ Thought processes, disturbed (uses)
☑ Coping, ineffective (uses)
☑ Knowledge, deficient (teaching)
☑ Noncompliance (teaching)

Implementation
- PO with full glass of water, milk; or give with food to decrease GI upset
- Store in airtight, light-resistant container

Patient/family education
- Teach patient to use good oral hygiene; frequent rinsing of mouth, sugarless gum for dry mouth
- Caution patient to avoid hazardous activities until drug response is determined; dizziness, blurred vision may occur
- Inform patient that orthostatic hypotension occurs often; patient should rise from sitting or lying position gradually and remain lying down for at least 30 min after IM inj
- Instruct patient to avoid hot tubs, hot showers, tub baths; hypotension may occur
- Inform patient that heat stroke may occur in hot weather, and to take extra precautions to stay cool
- Advise patient to avoid abrupt withdrawal of this drug, or EPS may result; drug should be withdrawn slowly
- Teach patient to avoid OTC preparations (cough, hay fever, cold) unless approved by

prescriber; serious drug interactions may occur; avoid use with alcohol, CNS depressants because increased drowsiness may occur
- Advise patient to use contraception, to inform prescriber if pregnancy is planned or suspected

Evaluation
Positive therapeutic outcome
- Decrease in emotional excitement, hallucinations, delusions, paranoia
- Reorganization of patterns of thought, speech

Treatment of overdose: Lavage, provide airway

---

ritonavir (Rx)
(ri-toe'na-veer)
Norvir
Func. class.: Antiretroviral
Chem. class.: Protease inhibitor

Pregnancy category B

Action: Inhibits HIV protease and prevents maturation of the infectious virus

➡**Therapeutic Outcome:** Improvement of HIV infection

Uses: HIV in combination with other antiretrovirals

Dosage and routes
Adult: PO 600 mg bid; if nausea occurs, begin dose at ½ and gradually increase

Ⓟ *Child:* PO 250 mg/m² bid, titrate upward to 400 mg/m² bid

Available forms: Caps 100 mg; oral sol 80 mg/ml

Adverse effects
(*italic* = common; **bold** = life-threatening)
CNS: Paresthesia, headache, **seizures**, dizziness, insomnia, headache
GI: Diarrhea, buccal mucosa ulceration, abdominal pain, *nausea*, taste perversion, dry mouth, vomiting
INTEG: Rash
MISC: Asthenia, **angioedema, anaphylaxis, Stevens-Johnson syndrome**, increase lipids
MS: Pain

Contraindications: Hypersensitivity

Precautions: Liver disease,
Ⓟ pregnancy **B**, lactation, children

◰ **Do Not Confuse:**
ritonavir/retrovir

☑ Herb/drug   ◎ Do Not Crush   ⬥ Alert   ◆ₜₜ Key Drug   Ⓖ Geriatric   Ⓟ Pediatric

Pharmacokinetics

Absorption	Unknown
Distribution	Unknown
Metabolism	Unknown
Excretion	Unknown
Half-life	Unknown

Pharmacodynamics

Unknown

Interactions
Individual drugs
Amiodarone, bepridil, bupropion, clozapine, desipramine, dihydroergotamine, encainide, ergotamine, flecainide, meperedine, midazolam, pimozide, piroxicam, propafenone, propoxyphene, quinidine, saquinavir, terfenadine, trazolam, zolpidem: toxicity, do not use together
Atovaquone: ↓ levels of atovaquone
Clarithromycin: ↑ level of both drugs
Despiramine, disulfiram, fluconazole, metronidazole: ↑ ritonavir level
Divalproex: ↓ levels of divalproex
Ethinyl estradiol: ↓ levels of ethinyl estradiol
Lamotrigine: ↓ levels of lamotrigine
Phenytoin: ↓ levels of phenytoin
Sulfamethoxazole: ↓ levels of sulfamethoxazole
Theophylline: ↓ levels of theophylline
Zalcitabine: ↑ ritonavir level of both drugs
Zidovudine: ↓ levels of zidovudine
Drug classifications
Anticoagulants: ↓ levels of anticoagulants
Azole antifungals, benzodiazepines, interleukins: toxicity, do not use together
Barbiturates: ↓ ritonavir level
Herb/drug
St. John's wort: ↓ ritonavir levels, avoid concurrent use
Lab test interferences
↑ ALT, ↑ GGT, ↑ AST, ↑ CPK, ↑ cholesterol, ↑ triglycerides, ↑ uric acid
↓ Hct, ↓ RBC, ↓ Hgb, ↓ neutrophils, ↓ WBC

NURSING CONSIDERATIONS
Assessment
- Assess signs of infection, anemia
- Monitor viral load and CD4 baseline and throughout therapy
- Assess liver function studies: ALT, AST
- Monitor C&S before drug therapy; drug may be taken as soon as culture is done; repeat C&S after treatment; determine the presence of other sexually transmitted diseases
- Assess bowel pattern before, during treatment; if severe abdominal pain with

bleeding occurs, drug should be discontinued; monitor hydration
- Assess skin eruptions, rash
- Assess allergies before treatment, reaction to each medication; place allergies on chart
Nursing diagnoses
☑ Infection, risk for (uses)
☑ Knowledge, deficient (teaching)
Implementation
- Administer with food
- Mix oral powder with high-calorie drink
- Store caps in refrigerator
Patient/family education
- Teach patient to take as prescribed; if dose is missed, take as soon as remembered up to 1 hr before next dose; do not double dose
- Teach patient that drug must be taken in equal intervals around the clock to maintain blood levels for duration of therapy
- Teach patient that drug is not a cure for HIV; opportunistic infections may continue to be acquired, and others may continue to contract HIV from the patient
- Advise patient not to use St. John's wort, that it decreases this drug's effect
- Inform that redistribution of body fat or accumulation of body fat may occur

---

rituximab (Rx)
(rih-tuks′ih-mab)
Rituxan
Func. class.: Antineoplastic—misc.
Chem. class.: Murine/human monoclonal antibody

Pregnancy category C

Action: Directed against the CD20 antigen that is found on malignant B lymphocytes; CD20 regulates a portion of cell cycle initiation/differentiation

▶ **Therapeutic Outcome:** Decreased tumor size, prevention of spread of cancer

Uses: Non-Hodgkin's lymphoma (CD20 positive, B-cell), bulky disease (tumors >10 cm)

Dosage and routes
Adult: **IV** inf 375 mg/m² qwk × 4 doses; give at 50 mg/hr for 1st inf; if hypersensitivity does not occur, increase rate by 50 mg/hr q½h, max 400 mg/hr; slow/interrupt inf if hypersensitivity occurs; other inf can be given at 100 mg/hr and increased by 100 mg/hr, max 400 mg/hr

Available forms: Inj 10 mg/ml

R

Adverse effects
(*italic* = common; **bold** = life-threatening)
CV: **Cardiac dysrhythmias**
GI: *Nausea, vomiting, anorexia*
GU: **Renal failure**
HEMA: **Leukopenia, neutropenia, thrombocytopenia**
INTEG: *Irritation at inj site, rash,* **fatal mucocutaneous infections (rare)**
MISC: Fever, chills, asthenia, headache, **angioedema,** hypotension, myalgia, bronchospasm
SYST: **Stevens-Johnson syndrome**

Contraindications: Hypersensitivity, murine proteins

P **Precautions:** Lactation, children, elderly,
G pregnancy **C,** cardiac conditions

Pharmacokinetics
Absorption	Unknown
Distribution	Unknown
Metabolism	Unknown
Excretion	Unknown
Half-life	42-79 min

Pharmacodynamics
Onset	Unknown
Peak	Unknown
Duration	Unknown

Interactions
Unknown

NURSING CONSIDERATIONS
Assessment
◆ • Assess for signs of fatal infusion reaction: hypoxia, pulmonary infiltrates, acute respiratory distress syndrome, MI, ventricular fibrillation, cardiogenic shock; most fatal infusion reactions occur with 1st inf, discontinue drug
◆ • Assess for signs of severe mucocutaneous reactions: Stevens-Johnson syndrome, lichenoid dermatitis, toxic epidermal lysis; signs occur 1-13 wk after drug was given
◆ • Assess for tumor lysis syndrome: acute renal failure requiring hemodialysis, hyperkalemia, hypocalcemia, hyperuricemia, hyperphosphatasemia
• Monitor CBC, differential, platelet count weekly; withhold drug if WBC is <3500/mm³, or platelet count <100,000/mm³; notify prescriber of these results; drug should be discontinued
• Assess food preferences: list likes, dislikes
• Assess GI symptoms: frequency of stools
• Assess signs of dehydration: rapid respirations, poor skin turgor, decreased urine output, dry skin, restlessness, weakness

Nursing diagnoses
☑ Injury, risk for (side effects)
☑ Knowledge, deficient (teaching)

Implementation
IV **IV route**
• Administer after diluting to a final conc of 1-4 mg/ml; use 0.9% NaCl, D₅W, gently invert bag to mix; do not mix with other drugs
• Increase fluid intake to 2-3 L/day to prevent dehydration, unless contraindicated
• Change **IV** site q48h
• Provide nutritious diet with iron, vitamin supplement, low fiber, few dairy products
• Store vials at 36°-40° F, protect vials from direct sunlight, inf sol is stable at 36°-46° F × 24 hr and room temp for another 12 hr

Patient/family education
• Teach patient to report adverse reactions

Evaluation
Positive therapeutic outcome
• Decrease in tumor size, decrease in spread of cancer

---

rivastigmine (Rx)
(riv-as-tig′mine)
Exelon
Func. class.: Anti-Alzheimer agent
Chem. class.: Cholinesterase inhibitor
Pregnancy category B

Action: May enhance cholinergic functioning by increasing acetylcholine

➦ **Therapeutic Outcome:** Decreased signs and symptoms of Alzheimer's dementia

Uses: Alzheimer's dementia

Dosage and routes
Adult: PO 1.5 mg bid for 2 wk or more, may increase to 3 mg bid after 2 wk or more; may increase to 4.5 mg bid and thereafter 6 mg bid

Available forms: Caps 1.5, 3, 4.5, 6 mg; sol 2 mg/ml

Adverse effects
(*italic* = common; **bold** = life-threatening)
CNS: *Tremors, confusion, insomnia,* psychosis, hallucination, depression, dizziness, headache, anxiety, somnolence, fatigue, syncope
GI: *Nausea, vomiting, anorexia, abdominal distress, flatulence,* diarrhea, constipation
MISC: UTI, asthenia, increased sweating,

---

hypertension, influenza-like syncope, weight change

Contraindications: Hypersensitivity to this drug, other carbamates; narrow-angle glaucoma, undiagnosed skin lesions

Precautions: Renal disease, hepatic disease, respiratory disease, seizure disorder, **P** pregnancy **B**, asthma, lactation, children, cardiac disease, urinary obstruction, asthma

Pharmacokinetics

Absorption	Rapidly, completely
Distribution	Not known
Metabolism	To decarbamylated metabolite
G Excretion	Kidney—metabolites, clearance lowered in elderly, hepatic disease, ↑ nicotine use
Half-life	1½ hr

Pharmacodynamics

Unknown

Interactions
Drug classifications
Cholinesterase inhibitors: ↑ synergistic effect
☑ Herb/drug
Pill-bearing spurge: ↑ effect
Food/drug
↓ Rivastigmine absorption

NURSING CONSIDERATIONS
Assessment
• Monitor liver function studies: AST, ALT, alkaline phosphatase, LDH, bilirubin, CBC
• Assess for severe GI effects: nausea, vomiting, anorexia, weight loss
• Monitor B/P, respiration during initial treatment; hypo/hypertension should be reported
• Assess mental status: affect, mood, behavioral changes, depression; complete suicide assessment

Nursing diagnoses
✓ Knowledge, deficient (teaching)

Implementation
• Give with meals; take with AM and PM meal even though absorption may be decreased
• Provide assistance with ambulation during beginning therapy

Patient/family education
• Teach patient procedure for giving oral sol; use instruction sheet provided
• Teach patient to notify prescriber of severe GI effects

Evaluation
Positive therapeutic outcome
• Increased coherence, decreased symptoms of Alzheimer's disease

---

rizatriptan (Rx)
(rye-zah-trip′tan)
Maxalt, Maxalt-MLT
Func. class.: Migraine agent
Chem. class.: 5-HT₁-like receptor agonist

Pregnancy category C

Action: Binds selectively to the vascular serotonin type 1 (5-HT₁) receptor, exerts antimigraine effect; causes vasoconstriction in cranial arteries

➔ Therapeutic Outcome: After treatment, relief of migraine

Uses: Acute treatment of migraine

Dosage and routes
Adult: **PO** 5-10 mg single dose, redosing separate by 2 hr or more; max 30 mg/24 hr

Available forms: *Maxalt:* tabs 5, 10 mg; *Maxalt-MLT:* tabs, orally disintegrating 5, 10 mg

Adverse effects
(*italic* = common; **bold** = life-threatening)
CNS: Dizziness, headache, fatigue, warm/cold sensation, flushing, hot flashes
CV: MI, ventricular fibrillation, ventricular tachycardia, coronary artery vasospasm
GI: Nausea, dry mouth, diarrhea
RESP: Chest tightness, pressure, dyspnea

Contraindications: Angina pectoris, history of MI, documented silent ischemia, Prinzmetal's angina, ischemic heart disease, concurrent ergotamine-containing preparations, uncontrolled hypertension, hypersensitivity, basilar or hemiplegic migraine

Precautions: Postmenopausal women, men >40 yr, risk factors for CAD, hypercholesterolemia, obesity, diabetes, impaired hepatic or **P** renal function, pregnancy **C**, lactation, **G** children, elderly

R

Pharmacokinetics

Absorption	Unknown
Distribution	Unknown
Metabolism	Liver (metabolite)
Excretion	Urine/feces
Half-life	2-3 hr

Pharmacodynamics	
Onset	10 min-2 hr
Peak	Unknown
Duration	Unknown

Interactions
Individual drugs
Cimetidine, isocarboxazide, pargyline, phenelzine, propranolol, trancyclomine: ↑ rizatriptan action

Ergot: ↑ vasospastic effects

Drug classifications
Contraceptives (oral), MAOIs, MAOIs (nonselective types A and B): ↑ rizatriptan action

Ergot derivatives, 5-HT₁ receptor agonists: ↑ vasospastic effects

Selective serotonin reuptake inhibitors: ↑ weakness, hyperreflexia, incoordination

Herb/drug
SAM-e, St. John's wort: Serotonin syndrome

NURSING CONSIDERATIONS
Assessment
- Assess for stress level, activity, recreation, coping mechanisms
- Assess neurologic status: LOC, blurring vision, nausea, vomiting, tingling in extremities preceding headache
- Monitor for ingestion of tyramine-containing foods (pickled products, beer, wine, aged cheese), food additives, preservatives, colorings, artificial sweeteners, chocolate, caffeine, which may precipitate these types of headaches

Nursing diagnoses
☑ Pain, acute (uses)
☑ Knowledge, deficient (teaching)

Implementation
- Provide quiet, calm environment with decreased stimulation for noise, bright light, excessive talking

Patient/family education
- Teach patient use of orally disintegrating tab: instruct patient not to open blister until use, to peel blister open with dry hands, to place tab on tongue, where it will dissolve, and to swallow with saliva (contains phenylalanine)
- Advise patient to report any side effects to prescriber
- Advise patient to use alternate contraception while taking drug if oral contraceptives are being used

Evaluation
Positive therapeutic outcome
- Decrease in frequency, severity of headache

rofecoxib (Rx)
(roh-feh-cock'sib)

Vioxx

Func. class.: Nonsteroidal antiinflammatory
Chem. class.: COX-2 inhibitor

Pregnancy category C

Action: May inhibit prostaglandin synthesis by decreasing enzyme needed for biosynthesis; analgesic, antiinflammatory, antipyretic properties

➡ **Therapeutic Outcome:** Decreased pain, inflammation

Uses: Acute, chronic osteoarthritis, pain, primary dysmenorrhea, relief of rheumatoid arthritis

Dosage and routes
Osteoarthritis
Adult: PO 12.5 mg/day as a single dose, may increase to 25 mg if needed

Primary dysmenorrhea
Adult: PO 50 mg qd, use for <5 days

Rheumatoid arthritis
Adult: PO 25 mg qd, max 25 mg qd

Available forms: Tabs 12.5, 25, 50 mg; susp 12.5, 25 mg/5 ml

Adverse effects
(italic = common, **bold** = life-threatening)
CNS: *Fatigue, anxiety, depression, nervousness, paresthesia*
CV: *Tachycardia, angina,* **MI,** *palpitations,* **dysrhythmias,** *hypertension, fluid retention*
EENT: *Tinnitus, hearing loss, blurred vision, glaucoma, cataract, conjunctivitis, eye pain*
GI: *Nausea, anorexia, vomiting, constipation, dry mouth, diverticulitis, gastritis, gastroenteritis, hemorrhoids, hiatal hernia, stomatitis,* **GI bleeding**
GU: **Nephrotoxicity: dysuria, hematuria,** *oliguria, azotemia, cystitis, UTI*
HEMA: **Blood dyscrasias, epistaxis,** *bruising, anemia*
INTEG: *Purpura, rash, pruritus, sweating, erythema, petechiae, photosensitivity, alopecia*
RESP: *Pharyngitis, shortness of breath, pneumonia, coughing*

Contraindications: Hypersensitivity to aspirin, iodides, other NSAIDs, asthma

Precautions: Pregnancy **C,** avoid in late pregnancy, lactation, children, bleeding disorders, GI disorders, cardiac disorders, hypersensitivity to other antiinflammatory agents

Pharmacokinetics

Absorption	Well absorbed (PO)
Distribution	Crosses placenta, bound to plasma proteins
Metabolism	Liver
Excretion	Kidneys
Half-life	Unknown

Pharmacodynamics
Unknown

Interactions
Individual drugs
Aspirin: ↓ effectiveness, ↑ adverse reactions
Lithium: ↑ toxicity
Warfarin: ↑ anticoagulant effects
Drug classifications
Angiotensin-converting enzyme inhibitors: may ↓ effects of ACE inhibitors
Anticoagulants: ↑ risk of bleeding
Antineoplastics: ↑ risk of hematologic toxicity
Diuretics: ↓ effectiveness of diuretics
Glucocorticoids, NSAIDs: ↑ adverse reactions
Herb/drug
Arginine, gossypol: ↑ gastric irritation
Bearberry, bilberry: ↑ NSAIDs effect
Bogbean, chondroitin: ↑ bleeding risk

NURSING CONSIDERATIONS
Assessment
• Assess patients with asthma, aspirin allergy, or nasal polyps for hypersensitivity
• Assess for pain of osteoarthritis, check ROM, inflammation of joints, characteristics of pain
• Assess for pain, discomfort of dysmenorrhea
• Monitor blood counts during therapy; watch for decreasing platelets; if low, therapy may need to be discontinued, restarted after hematologic recovery; and for blood dyscrasias (thrombocytopenia): bruising, fatigue, bleeding, poor healing
Nursing diagnoses
✓ Pain, acute (uses)
✓ Pain, chronic (uses)
✓ Mobility, impaired physical (uses)
✓ Injury, risk for (side effects)
✓ Knowledge, deficient (teaching)
Implementation
PO route
• Administer with food or milk to decrease gastric symptoms
🚫 • Do not crush, dissolve, or chew
Patient/family education
• Teach patient that drug must be continued

for prescribed time to be effective; to avoid other NSAIDs, aspirin, alcohol
• Caution patient to report bleeding, bruising, fatigue, malaise, since blood dyscrasias do occur
• Teach patient to take with full glass of water to enhance absorption
Evaluation
Positive therapeutic outcome
• Decreased pain and inflammation in arthritic conditions
• Decrease pain in dysmenorrhea

---

ropinirole (Rx)
(roe-pin´e-role)
Requip
Func. class.: Antiparkinsonian agent
Chem. class.: Dopamine-receptor agonist, nonergot

Pregnancy category C

Action: Selective agonist for dopamine D_2 receptors (presynaptic/postsynaptic sites); binding at D_3 receptor contributes to antiparkinson effects

⮞ **Therapeutic Outcome:** Decreased symptoms of Parkinson's disease (involuntary movements)

Uses: Parkinsonism

Dosage and routes
Adult: PO 0.25 mg tid, titrate weekly to max of 24 mg/day

Available forms: Tabs 0.25, 0.5, 1, 2, 4, 5 mg

Adverse effects
(*italic* = common; **bold** = life-threatening)
CNS: Dystonia, *agitation, insomnia,* dizziness, psychosis, hallucinations, depression, somnolence, **sleep attacks**
CV: Orthostatic hypotension, hypotension, syncope, palpitations, **tachycardia,** hypertension
EENT: Blurred vision
GI: Nausea, vomiting, anorexia, dry mouth, constipation, dyspepsia, flatulence
HEMA: **Hemolytic anemia, leukopenia, agranulocytosis**
GU: Impotence, urinary frequency
INTEG: Rash, sweating
RESP: Pharyngitis, rhinitis, sinusitis, bronchitis, dyspnea

Contraindications: Hypersensitivity

R

Precautions: Renal disease, cardiac disease, dysrhythmias, affective disorders, psychosis, pregnancy **C**, hepatic disease

Pharmacokinetics

Absorption	Well absorbed
Distribution	Widely distributed
Metabolism	Liver, extensively by the liver by CYP450 CYP1A2 enzyme system
Excretion	Kidneys
Half-life	6 hr

Pharmacodynamics

Unknown

Interactions
Individual drugs
Cimetidine, ciprofloxacin, digoxin, diltiazem, enoxacin, erythromycin, fluvoxamine, levodopa, mexiletine, norfloxacin, tacrine, theophylline: ↑ effect of ropinirole
Metoclopramide: ↓ ropinirole effect
Drug classifications
Butyrophenones, phenothiazines, thioxanthenes: ↓ ropinirole effect
☑ *Herb/drug*
Chaste tree fruit, kava: ↓ ropinirole action

NURSING CONSIDERATIONS
Assessment
• Monitor B/P, respiration during initial treatment; hypotension or hypertension should be reported
• Assess mental status: affect, mood, behavioral changes, depression; complete suicide assessment
• Assess for involuntary movements in parkinsonism: akinesia, tremors, staggering gait, muscle rigidity, drooling; these symptoms should improve with therapy
◆• Assess for sleep attacks, drowsiness, falling asleep without warning even during hazardous activities

Nursing diagnoses
☑ Mobility, impaired (uses)
☑ Injury, risk for (uses)
☑ Knowledge, deficient (teaching)
☑ Noncompliance (teaching)

Implementation
• Give drug until NPO before surgery
• Adjust dosage to patient response
• Give with meals to decrease GI upset

Patient/family education
• Advise patient that therapeutic effects may take several wk to a few mo

• Caution patient to change positions slowly to prevent orthostatic hypotension
• Instruct patient to use drug exactly as prescribed; if drug is discontinued abruptly, parkinsonian crisis may occur

Evaluation
Positive therapeutic outcome
• Decreased akathisia, other involuntary movements
• Increased mood

---

ropivacaine (Rx)
(roe-pi′va-kane)
Naropin
Func. class.: Local anesthetic
Chem. class.: Amide

Pregnancy category B

Action: Competes with calcium for sites in nerve membrane that control sodium transport across cell membrane; decreases rise of depolarization phase of action potential

▶**Therapeutic Outcome:** Maintenance of local anesthesia

Uses: Peripheral nerve block, caudal anesthesia, central neural block, vaginal, epidural, spinal block

Dosage and routes
Varies with route of anesthesia

Available forms: Inj 2, 5, 7.5 mg/ml

Adverse effects
(*italic* = common; **bold** = life-threatening)
CNS: Anxiety, restlessness, **seizures, loss of consciousness,** drowsiness, disorientation, tremors, shivering
CV: **Myocardial depression, cardiac arrest, dysrhythmias,** bradycardia, hypotension, hypertension, **fetal bradycardia**
EENT: Blurred vision, tinnitus, pupil constriction
GI: Nausea, vomiting
INTEG: Rash, urticaria, allergic reactions, edema, burning, skin discoloration at injection site, tissue necrosis
RESP: **Status asthmaticus, respiratory arrest, anaphylaxis**

🅿 **Contraindications:** Hypersensitivity, child
🅖 <12 yr, elderly, severe liver disease

Precautions: Severe drug allergies, pregnancy **B**, hyperthyroidism, cardiovascular disease

---

☑ Herb/drug   🅢 Do Not Crush   ◆ Alert   ◆ₙ Key Drug   🅖 Geriatric   🅿 Pediatric

Pharmacokinetics	
Absorption	Complete
Distribution	Unknown
Metabolism	Liver
Excretion	Kidneys
Half-life	Unknown

Pharmacodynamics	
Onset	2-8 min
Peak	Unknown
Duration	3 hr, varies with inj site

Interactions
Individual drugs
Chloroprocaine: ↓ action of ropivacaine
Enflurane, epINEPHrine, halothane: ↑ dysrhythmias
Drug classifications
Antidepressants (tricyclic), MAOIs, phenothiazines: ↑ hypertension

NURSING CONSIDERATIONS
Assessment
• Assess B/P, pulse, respiration during treatment
• Assess fetal heart tones during labor
• Assess allergic reactions: rash, urticaria, itching
• Assess cardiac status: ECG for dysrhythmias, pulse, B/P during anesthesia

Nursing diagnoses
✓ Knowledge, deficient (teaching)

Implementation
• Give only with resuscitative equipment nearby
• Give only drugs without preservatives for epidural or caudal anesthesia
• Use new sol; discard unused portions

Evaluation
Positive therapeutic outcome
• Anesthesia necessary for procedure

Treatment of overdose: Airway, O₂, vasopressor, **IV** fluids, anticonvulsants for seizures

---

rosavastatin
Crestor
See Appendix A, Selected New Drugs

---

rosiglitazone (Rx)
(roes-i-glye'ta-zone)
Avandia
Func. class.: Antidiabetic, oral
Chem. class.: Thiazolidinedione
Pregnancy category C

Action: Improves insulin resistance by hepatic glucose metabolism, insulin receptor kinase activity, insulin receptor phosphorylation

⮕ **Therapeutic Outcome:** Decreased symptoms of diabetes mellitus

Uses: Stable adult-onset diabetes mellitus, type 2 alone or in combination with sulfonylureas, metformin, or insulin

Dosage and routes
Monotherapy
Adult: PO 4 mg qd or in 2 divided doses, may increase to 8 mg qd or in 2 divided doses after 12 wk

Combination therapy
Adult: PO this drug should be added to metformin, sulfonylureas at the adult dose

Available forms: Tabs 2, 4, 8 mg

Adverse effects
(*italic* = common; **bold** = life-threatening)
CNS: Fatigue, headache
ENDO: Hyper/hypoglycemia
MISC: Accidental injury, upper respiratory tract infection, sinusitis, anemia, back pain, diarrhea, edema

Contraindications: Hypersensitivity to thiazolidinediones, children, lactation, diabetic ketoacidosis

Precautions: Pregnancy C, elderly, thyroid disease, hepatic, renal disease

Pharmacokinetics	
Absorption	Unknown
Distribution	Protein binding 99.8%
Metabolism	Unknown
Excretion	Urine, feces, breast milk
Half-life	Elimination 3-4 hr

Pharmacodynamics	
Onset	Unknown
Peak	6-12 wk
Duration	Unknown

Interactions
Drug classification
Contraceptives (oral): May decrease effect of oral contraceptive, alternate method advised

⚠ Herb/drug

Alfalfa, aloe, basil, bay, bilberry, bitter melon, black catechu, buchu, burdock, coriander, dandelion, eyebright (po), fenugreek, garlic, ginseng, glucomannan, glucosamine, goat's rue, gymnema, horehound, horse chestnut, jambul, myrrh, myrtle: ↑ antidiabetic effect
Bee pollen, blue cohosh, broom, chromium, elecampane, eucalyptus, gotu kola: ↓ antidiabetic effect
Chromium, coenzyme Q10, fenugreek, glucosamine: ↓ glucose control

NURSING CONSIDERATIONS
Assessment

• Assess for hypoglycemic reactions (sweating, weakness, dizziness, anxiety, tremors, hunger), hyperglycemic reactions soon after meals
• Assess CBC (baseline, q3 mo) during treatment; check liver function tests periodically; AST, LDH, FBS, ALT (if ALT >2.5 × ULN, do not use), HbA$_{2c}$, fasting plasma insulin, plasma lipids, lipoproteins, B/P, body weight during treatment

Nursing diagnoses

✓ Nutrition: more than body requirements, imbalanced (uses)
✓ Knowledge, deficient (teaching)

Implementation

• Convert from other oral hypoglycemic agents if needed; change may be made without gradual dosage change; monitor serum or urine glucose and ketones tid during conversion
• Give tabs crushed and mixed with meal or fluids for patients with difficulty swallowing
• Store in airtight container in cool environment

Patient/family education

• Teach patient to use capillary blood glucose test or Chemstrip tid
• Teach patient symptoms of hypo/hyperglycemia, what to do about each
• Advise patient that drug must be continued on daily basis; explain consequence of discontinuing drug abruptly
• Advise patient to avoid OTC medications or herbal preparations unless approved by prescriber
• Advise patient that diabetes is life-long illness; that this drug is not a cure, only controls symptoms
• Advise patient that all food included in diet plan must be eaten to prevent hypoglycemia

• Advise patient to carry/wear emergency ID and glucagon emergency kit for emergencies
• Instruct patient to notify prescriber if oral contraceptives are used
• Teach patient not to use if breast-feeding, may be secreted in breast milk

Evaluation
Positive therapeutic outcome
• Decrease in polyuria, polydipsia, polyphagia; clear sensorium; absence of dizziness; stable gait; blood glucose at normal level

---

salmeterol (Rx)
(sal-met'er-ole)
Serevent
Func. class.: Adrenergic β$_2$ agonist, bronchodilator

Pregnancy category C

Action: Causes bronchodilatation by action on β$_2$ (pulmonary) receptors by increasing levels of cAMP, which relaxes smooth muscle; with very little effect on heart rate, maintains improvement in FEV from 3 to 12 hr; prevents nocturnal asthma symptoms

➡ **Therapeutic Outcome:** Ease of breathing

Uses: Prevention of exercise-induced asthma, bronchospasm, COPD

Dosage and routes
Adult: INH 2 puffs bid (AM and PM); exercise-induced bronchospasm: 50 mcg (2 inh) ½-1 hr prior to exercise

P *Child 4-12 yr:* INH 50 mcg as dry powder bid; exercise-induced bronchospasm 50 mcg as dry powder ½-1 hr prior to exercise

Available forms: Aerosol 25 mcg/actuation; inhalation powder 50 mcg/blister

Adverse effects
(*italic* = common; **bold** = life-threatening)
CNS: Tremors, anxiety, insomnia, headache, dizziness, stimulation, restlessness, hallucinations, flushing, irritability
CV: Palpitations, **tachycardia**, hypertension, angina, hypotension, **dysrhythmias**
EENT: Dry nose, irritation of nose and throat
GI: Heartburn, nausea, vomiting
MS: Muscle cramps
RESP: **Bronchospasm**

Contraindications: Hypersensitivity to sympathomimetics, tachydysrhythmias, severe cardiac disease

---

⚠ Herb/drug   Ⓢ Do Not Crush   ◆ Alert   ✦π Key Drug   Ⓖ Geriatric   Ⓟ Pediatric

Precautions: Lactation, pregnancy **C**, cardiac disorders, hyperthyroidism, diabetes mellitus, hypertension, prostatic hypertrophy, narrow-angle glaucoma, seizures, acute asthma, as a substitute for corticosteroids

Pharmacokinetics

Absorption	Unknown
Distribution	Unknown
Metabolism	Unknown
Excretion	Unknown
Half-life	Unknown

Pharmacodynamics

Onset	5-15 min
Peak	4 hr
Duration	12 hr

Interactions
Drug classifications
Antidepressants (tricyclics): ↑ salmeterol action
β-Adrenergic blockers: Block therapeutic effect
Bronchodilators, aerosol: ↑ action of bronchodilator
MAOIs: ↑ chance of hypertensive crisis
Sympathomimetics: ↑ adrenergic side effects
☑ *Herb/drug*
Betel palm, butterbur, coffee, cola nut, figwort, fumitory, guarana, hawthorn, lily of the valley, motherwort, plantain, tea (black, green), yerba maté: ↑ stimulation

NURSING CONSIDERATIONS
Assessment
• Monitor respiratory function: vital capacity, FEV, ABGs, lung sounds, heart rate, rhythm (baseline)

Nursing diagnoses
☑ Airway clearance, ineffective (uses)
☑ Gas exchange, impaired (uses)
☑ Knowledge, deficient (teaching)

Implementation
• Shake aerosol container, ask patient to exhale, then place mouthpiece in mouth, inhale slowly, hold breath, remove, exhale slowly; allow at least 1 min between inhalations
P • Use spacing device for pediatric/elderly
G patients
• Store in light-resistant container, do not expose to temp over 86° F (30° C)

Patient/family education
• Caution patient not to use OTC medications because extra stimulation may occur
• Instruct patient to use this medication

before other medications and to allow at least 1 min between each, to prevent overstimulation
• Teach patient how to use inhaler; to avoid getting aerosol in eyes; blurring may result; to wash inhaler in warm water qd and dry; to avoid smoking, smoke-filled rooms, and persons with respiratory infections; review package insert with patient
• Instruct patient on administration of dose, not to use more than prescribed; serious side effects may occur

Evaluation
Positive therapeutic outcome
• Absence of dyspnea, wheezing
• Improved airway exchange
• Improved ABGs

Treatment of overdose: Administer a β₂-adrenergic blocker

---

salsalate (Rx)
(sal-sa'late)
Amigesic, Anaflex, Disalcid, Marthritic, Mono-Gesic, Salflex, Salgesic, Salsalate, Salsitab
Func. class.: Nonopioid analgesic; nonsteroidal antiinflammatory agent
Chem. class.: Salicylate

Pregnancy category   C

Action: Blocks formation of peripheral prostaglandins, which cause pain and inflammation; antipyretic action results from inhibition of hypothalamic heat-regulating center; does not inhibit platelet aggregation

⇒ **Therapeutic Outcome:** Decreased pain, inflammation

Uses: Mild to moderate pain or fever, includ-
P ing arthritis, juvenile rheumatoid arthritis

Dosage and routes
Adult: PO 3 g/day in divided doses

Available forms: Caps 500 mg; tabs 500, 750 mg

Adverse effects
(*italic* = common; **bold** = life-threatening)
CNS: Stimulation, drowsiness, dizziness, confusion, **seizures**, headache, flushing, hallucinations, coma
CV: Rapid pulse, **pulmonary edema**
EENT: Tinnitus, hearing loss
ENDO: Hypoglycemia, hyponatremia, hypokalemia, alteration in acid-base balance
GI: Nausea, vomiting, GI bleeding, diarrhea, heartburn, anorexia, **hepatotoxicity**

S

HEMA: **Thrombocytopenia, agranulocyto-sis, leukopenia, neutropenia, hemolytic anemia,** increased Pro-time
INTEG: Rash, urticaria, bruising
RESP: Wheezing, hyperpnea

Contraindications: Hypersensitivity to salicylates, NSAIDs, GI bleeding, bleeding
P disorders, children <3 yr, vit K deficiency

Precautions: Anemia, hepatic disease, renal disease, Hodgkin's disease, pregnancy **C**
G 1st trimester, lactation, elderly

Pharmacokinetics

Absorption	Absorbed in small intestine
Distribution	Rapidly and widely distributed, crosses placenta
Metabolism	Not metabolized
Excretion	Unchanged—kidneys
Half-life	2-3 hr (low doses), 15-30 hr (high doses)

Pharmacodynamics

Onset	30 min
Peak	1-3 hr
Duration	3-6 hr

Interactions
Individual drugs

Alcohol, heparin, ibuprofen, warfarin: ↑ bleeding
Insulin, methotrexate, phenytoin, probenecid: ↑ effects
p-Aminobenzoic acid: ↑ toxic effects
Spironolactone, sulfinpyrazone: ↓ effects
Drug classifications
Antacids, urinary alkalizers: ↓ effects of salsalate
Anticoagulants, penicillins: ↑ effects
Salicylates: ↓ blood glucose levels
Diuretics (loop), sulfonylamides: ↓ effects
Food/drug
Foods causing acidic urine may ↑ level
Lab test interferences
↑ Coagulation studies, ↑ liver function studies, ↑ serum uric acid, ↑ amylase, ↑ CO_2, ↑ urinary protein
↓ Serum potassium, ↓ PBI, ↓ cholesterol, ↓ blood glucose
Interference: Urine catecholamines, pregnancy test

NURSING CONSIDERATIONS
Assessment

• Monitor liver function studies: AST, ALT, bilirubin, creatinine if patient is on long-term therapy

• Monitor renal function studies: BUN, urine creatinine if patient is on long-term therapy
• Monitor blood studies: CBC, Hct, Hgb, Pro-time if patient is on long-term therapy
• Check I&O ratio; decreasing output may indicate renal failure if patient is on long-term therapy
• Assess hepatotoxicity: dark urine, clay-colored stools, yellowing of the skin and sclera, itching, abdominal pain, fever, diarrhea if patient is on long-term therapy
• Assess for allergic reactions: rash, urticaria; if these occur, drug may have to be discontinued; assess for asthma, aspirin sensitivity, nasal polyps, may develop hypersensitivity
• Assess for ototoxicity: tinnitus, ringing, roaring in ears; audiometric testing needed before, after long-term therapy
• Assess for visual changes: blurring, halos; corneal, retinal damage
• Check edema in feet, ankles, legs
• Identify prior drug history; many drug interactions are possible
• Monitor pain: location, duration, type, intensity, prior to dose and 1 hr after
• Monitor musculoskeletal status: ROM before dose
• Identify fever, length of time, and related symptoms

Nursing diagnoses
☑ Pain, chronic (uses)
☑ Mobility, impaired physical (uses)
☑ Knowledge, deficient (teaching)
☑ Injury, risk for (side effects)

Implementation
• Administer to patient crushed or whole; chewable tab may be chewed
• Give with food or milk to decrease gastric symptoms; give 30 min ac or 2 hr pc; absorption may be slowed
• Give antacids 1-2 hr after enteric products

Patient/family education
• Advise patient to report any symptoms of hepatotoxicity, renal toxicity, visual changes, ototoxicity, allergic reactions, bleeding (long-term therapy)
• Instruct patient to take with 8 oz of water and sit upright for ½ hr after dose
• Caution patient not to exceed recommended dosage; acute poisoning may result
• Advise patient to read label on other OTC drugs; many contain aspirin
• Inform patient that the therapeutic response takes 2 wk (arthritis)
• Teach patient to report tinnitus, confusion, diarrhea, sweating, hyperventilation

---

☑ Herb/drug   ⓢ Do Not Crush   ◆ Alert   ◆⊓ Key Drug   **G** Geriatric   **P** Pediatric

- Caution patient to avoid alcohol ingestion; GI bleeding may occur
- Inform patient that patients who have allergies may develop allergic reactions

Evaluation
Positive therapeutic outcome
- Decreased pain
- Decreased inflammation

Treatment of overdose: Lavage, activated charcoal, monitor electrolytes, VS

---

saquinavir (Rx)
(sa-quen′a-ver)
Fortovase, Invirase
Func. class.: Antiretroviral
Chem. class.: Protease inhibitor

Pregnancy category B

Action: Inhibits HIV protease

Therapeutic Outcome: Prevents maturation of the infectious virus

Uses: HIV in combination with other antiretrovirals

Dosage and routes
Adult: PO 600 mg (hard cap, Invirase) or 1200 mg (soft cap, Fortovase) tid within 2 hr after a full meal

Available forms: Caps 200 mg (soft); 200 mg (hard)

Adverse effects
(*italic* = common; **bold** = life-threatening)
CNS: Paresthesia, headache
GI: Diarrhea, buccal mucosa ulceration, *abdominal pain, nausea*
INTEG: Rash
MISC: Asthenia, *hyperglycemia*
MS: Pain

Contraindications: Hypersensitivity

Precautions: Liver disease, pregnancy **B**, lactation, children

Pharmacokinetics
Absorption	↑ with food
Distribution	Protein-binding 98%
Metabolism	Extensively
Excretion	Unknown
Half-life	Unknown

Pharmacodynamics
Unknown

Interactions
Individual drugs
Clarithromycin, delavirdine, indinavir, ketoconazole, nelfinavir, ritonavir: ↑ saquinavir level
Carbamazepine, dexamethasone, nevirapine, phenobarbital, phenytoin, rifamycins: ↓ saquinavir levels
Clindamycin, dapsone, quinidine: ↑ toxicity
Midazolam, triazolam: ↑ toxicity, ↑ CNS depression; do not use concurrently
Drug classifications
Calcium channel blockers, ergot derivatives: ↑ toxicity
Ergot derivatives: ↑ vasoconstriction, do not use together
HMG-CoA reductase inhibitors: avoid use with saquinavir
Food/drug
↑ bioavailability after high-fat meal
Grapefruit juice: ↑ saquinivir level
Herb/drug
St. John's wort: ↓ saquinavir level, avoid concurrent use
Lab test interferences
Interference: CPK, glucose (low)

NURSING CONSIDERATIONS
Assessment
- Assess signs of infection, anemia
- Monitor liver function studies: ALT, AST
- Monitor C&S before drug therapy; drug may be taken as soon as culture is done; repeat C&S after treatment; determine the presence of other sexually transmitted diseases
- Assess bowel pattern before, during treatment; if severe abdominal pain with bleeding occurs, drug should be discontinued; monitor hydration
- Assess skin eruptions, rash, urticaria, itching
- Assess allergies before treatment, reaction of each medication; place allergies on chart

Nursing diagnoses
☑ Infection, risk for (uses)
☑ Knowledge, deficient (teaching)

Patient/family education
- Advise patient to take as prescribed within 2 hr of a full meal; if dose is missed, take as soon as remembered up to 1 hr before next dose; do not double dose
- Advise patient that drug must be taken in equal intervals around the clock to maintain blood levels for duration of therapy, that Invirase and Fortovase are not interchangeable

S

---

sargramostim (Rx)

(sar-gram'oh-stim)
Leukine, rhu GM-CSF
Func. class.: Biologic modifier: cytokine
Chem. class.: Granulocyte/macrophage colony stimulating factor (GM-CSF)

Pregnancy category C

Action: Stimulates proliferation and differentiation of hematopoietic progenitor cells (granulocyte, macrophage)

Uses: Acceleration of myeloid recovery in patients with non-Hodgkin's lymphoma, acute lymphoblastic leukemia, autologous bone marrow transplantation in Hodgkin's disease; bone marrow transplantation failure or engraftment delay; mobilization and transplant of peripheral blood progenitor cells (PBPCs)

Dosage and routes
Myeloid reconstitution after autologous bone marrow transplantation
Adult: IV 250 mcg/m²/day × 3 wk; give over 2 hr, 2-4 hr after autologous bone marrow inf, and not less than 24 hr after last dose of antineoplastics and 12 hr after last dose of radiotherapy, bone marrow transplantation failure, or engraftment delay

Acceleration of myeloid recovery
Adult: IV 250 mcg/m²/day × 14 days; give over 2 hr; may repeat in 7 days, may repeat 500 mcg/m²/day × 14 days after another 7 days if no improvement

Mobilization of PBPCs
Adult: IV/SC 250 mcg/m²/day during collection of PBPCs

After PBPC transplantation
Adult: IV/SC 250 mcg/m²/day until ANC >1500/mm³ × 3 days

Available forms: Powder for inj lyophilized 250, 500 mcg; liq 500 mcg/ml

Adverse effects
(*italic* = common; **bold** = life-threatening)
CNS: Fever, malaise, CNS disorder, weakness, chills

CV: **Transient supraventricular tachycardia,** peripheral edema, **pericardial effusion**
GI: Nausea, vomiting, diarrhea, anorexia, **GI hemorrhage,** stomatitis, **liver damage**
GU: Urinary tract disorder, abnormal kidney function

HEMA: Blood dyscrasias, **hemorrhage**
INTEG: Alopecia, rash, peripheral edema
RESP: Dyspnea

Contraindications: Hypersensitivity to GM-CSF, yeast products; excessive leukemic myeloid blast in the bone marrow or peripheral blood

Precautions: Pregnancy **C,** lactation, children; renal, hepatic, lung disease; cardiac disease; pleural, pericardial effusions

Do Not Confuse:
Leukine/leucovorin, Leukine/Leukeran

Pharmacokinetics
Absorption	Completely absorbed
Distribution	Unknown
Metabolism	Unknown
Excretion	Unknown
Half-life	2 hr

Pharmacodynamics
Onset	Rapid
Peak	2 hr
Duration	Unknown

Interactions
Individual drugs
Lithium: ↑ myeloproliferation
Drug classifications
Antineoplastics: Do not use together
Corticosteroids: ↑ myeloproliferation

NURSING CONSIDERATIONS
Assessment
• Monitor blood studies: CBC, differential count before treatment and twice weekly; leukocytosis may occur (WBC >50,000 cells/mm³, ANC >20,000 cells/mm³), platelets; if ANC >20,000/mm³ or 10,000/mm³ after nadir has occurred, or platelets >500,000/mm³ reduce dose by ½ or discontinue; if blast cells occur, discontinue
• Monitor renal and hepatic studies before treatment: BUN, creatinine, urinalysis; AST, ALT, alkaline phosphatase; monitoring is needed twice a week in renal, hepatic disease
• Assess for hypersensitivity reactions/rashes, and local inj site reactions; usually transient
• Assess for increased fluid retention in cardiac disease
• Assess for myalgia, arthralgia in legs, feet; use analgesics

Nursing diagnoses
☑ Infection, risk for (uses)
☑ Knowledge, deficient (teaching)

Implementation
• Reconstitute with 1 ml of sterile water for inj without preservative; do not reenter vial;

discard unused portion; direct reconstitution sol at side of vial; rotate contents; do not shake

SC route
• Use reconstituted sol

IV IV route
• Give by intermittent inf after diluting in 0.9% NaCl inj to prepare **IV** inf; if final conc is <10 mcg/ml, add human albumin to make a final conc of 0.1% to the NaCl before adding sargramostim to prevent absorption; for a final conc of 0.1% albumin, add 1 mg of human albumin/1 ml of 0.9% NaCl inj; run over 2 hr (bone marrow transplant or failure of graft); over 4 hr (chemotherapy for acute myeloid leukemia); over 24 hr as cont inf (PBPCs); give within 6 hr after reconstitution
• Store in refrigerator; do not freeze

Y-site compatibilities: Amikacin, aminophylline, aztreonam, bleomycin, butorphanol, calcium gluconate, carboplatin, carmustine, cefazolin, cefepime, cefotaxime, cefotetan, ceftizoxime, ceftriaxone, cefuroxime, cimetidine, cisplatin, clindamycin, cyclophosphamide, cycloSPORINE, cytarabine, dacarbazine, dactinomycin, dexamethasone, diphenhydrAMINE, DOPamine, DOXOrubicin, doxycycline, droperidol, etoposide, famotidine, fentanyl, floxuridine, fluconazole, fluorouracil, furosemide, gentamicin, granisetron, heparin, idarubicin, ifosfamide, immune globulin, magnesium sulfate, mannitol, mechlorethamine, meperidine, mesna, methotrexate, metoclopramide, metronidazole, mezlocillin, miconazole, minocycline, mitoxantrone, netilmicin, pentostatin, piperacillin/tazobactam, potassium chloride, prochlorperazine, promethazine, ranitidine, teniposide, ticarcillin, ticarcillin/clavulanate, trimethoprim/sulfamethoxazole, vinBLAStine, vinCRIStine, zidovudine

Y-site incompatibilities: Acyclovir, ampicillin, ampicillin/sulbactam, cefonicid, cefoperazine, ceftazidime, chlorproMAZINE, ganciclovir, haloperidol, hydrocortisone, hydromorphone, hydrOXYzine, idarubicin, imipenem/cilastatin, lorazepam, methylPREDNISolone sodium succinate, mitomycin, morphine, nalbuphine, ondansetron, piperacillin, sodium bicarbonate, tobramycin

Patient/family education
• Teach patient reason for medication and expected results
• Advise patient to notify nurse or prescriber of side effects

Evaluation
Positive therapeutic outcome
• WBC and differential recovery
• Absence of infection

---

scopolamine (Rx)
(skoe-pol'a-meen)
Scopolamine Hydrobromide Injection, Transderm-Scop, Transderm-V
Func. class.: Antiemetic, anticholinergic, mydriatic
Chem. class.: Belladonna alkaloid

Pregnancy category C

Action: Inhibits acetylcholine at receptor sites in autonomic nervous system, which controls secretions, free acids in stomach; blocks central muscarinic receptors, which decreases involuntary movements; blocks response of iris sphincter muscle, muscle of accommodation of ciliary body to cholinergic stimulation, resulting in dilatation, paralysis of accommodation

➤ **Therapeutic Outcome:** Absence of vomiting, secretions (preoperatively), involuntary movements

Uses: Reduction of secretions before surgery, calm delirium, uveitis, iritis, cycloplegia, mydriasis; prevention of motion sickness, parkinson symptoms

Investigational uses: Drooling (TD)

Dosage and routes
Ophthalmic route
Adult: Instill 1-2 gtt before refraction or 1-2 gtt qd-tid for iritis or uveitis
P *Child:* Instill 1 gtt bid × 2 days before refraction

Prevention of motion sickness
Adult: TD 1 patch placed behind ear 4-5 hr before travel, reapply q3d, alternate ears
P Not recommended for children

Parkinson symptoms
Adult: IM/SC/**IV** 0.3-0.6 mg tid-qid diluted using dilution provided

Preoperatively
Adult: SC 0.4-0.6 mg

Nausea and vomiting
P *Child:* SC 0.006 mg/kg or 0.2 mg/m^2

Drooling (off-label)
Adult: TD 1.5 mg patch q3 days

Available forms: Patch 0.5, 1 mg delivered in 72 hr; inj 0.3, 0.4, 0.86, 1 mg/ml

S

Adverse effects

(*italic* = common; **bold** = life-threatening)

CNS: Confusion, anxiety, restlessness, irritability, delusions, hallucinations, headache, sedation, depression, incoherence, dizziness, excitement, delirium, flushing, weakness, **TD,** memory disturbances

CV: Palpitations, **tachycardia,** postural hypotension, paradoxical bradycardia

EENT TD: Blurred vision, photophobia, dilated pupils, difficulty swallowing, mydriasis, cycloplegia, altered depth perception, *dry mouth,* dry, itchy red eyes, narrow-angle glaucoma

GI: Dryness of mouth, constipation, nausea, vomiting, abdominal distress, **paralytic ileus**

GU: Hesitancy, retention

INTEG: Urticaria, rash, erythema (patch)

MISC: Suppression of lactation, nasal congestion, decreased sweating

Contraindications: Hypersensitivity, narrow-angle glaucoma, myasthenia gravis, GI/GU obstruction, hypersensitivity to belladonna, barbiturates

G Precautions: Pregnancy **C,** elderly, lactation, prostatic hypertrophy, CHF, hypertension, **P** dysrhythmias, children, gastric ulcer; TD: pyloric urinary, bladder neck, intestinal obstruction; liver, kidney disease

Pharmacokinetics

Absorption	Well absorbed (IM, SC, TD)
Distribution	Crosses placenta, blood-brain barrier
Metabolism	Liver
Excretion	Unknown
Half-life	8 hr

Pharmacodynamics

	SC/IM	IV	TD	OPHTH
Onset	30-45 min	10-15 min	4-5 hr	Unknown
Peak	1 hr	1 hr	Unknown	20-30 min
Duration	6 hr	4 hr	72 hr	3-7 days

Interactions

Individual drugs

Alcohol: ↑ anticholinergic effect

Drug classifications

Antidepressants, antidepressants (tricyclic), antihistamines, opiates, phenothiazines: ↑ anticholinergic effect

Herb/drug

Henbane, jimsonweed, scopolia: ↑ anticholinergic effect

NURSING CONSIDERATIONS

Assessment

• Assess for eye pain; discontinue use (opticue)

• Monitor I&O ratio; retention commonly causes decreased urinary output

• Assess for parkinsonism, extrapyramidal symptoms (EPS): shuffling gait, muscle rigidity, involuntary movements

• Assess for urinary hesitancy, retention; palpate bladder if retention occurs

• Assess for constipation; increase fluids, bulk, exercise if this occurs

• Assess for tolerance over long-term therapy; dose may have to be increased or changed

• Assess mental status: affect, mood, CNS depression, worsening of mental symptoms during early therapy

Nursing diagnoses

☑ Fluid volume, deficient (uses)

☑ Knowledge, deficient (teaching)

Implementation

IV SC/IM/IV route

• Administer parenteral dose with patient recumbent to prevent postural hypotension

IV IV route

• Give by direct **IV** after diluting with sterile water; give slowly

Syringe compatibilities: Atropine, benzquinamide, butorphanol, chlorproMAZINE, cimetidine, dimenhyDRINATE, diphenhydrAMINE, droperidol, fentanyl, glycopyrrolate, hydromorphone, hydrOXYzine, meperidine, metoclopramide, midazolam, morphine, nalbuphine, pentazocine, pentobarbital, perphenazine, prochlorperazine, promazine, promethazine, ranitidine, sufentanil, thiopental

Y-site compatibilities: Heparin, hydrocortisone, potassium chloride, propofol, sufentanil, vit B/C

Additive compatibilities: Floxacillin, furosemide, meperidine, succinylcholine

Patient/family education

• Tell patient to avoid hazardous activities, activities requiring alertness; dizziness may occur

TD route

• Instruct patient to wash, dry hands before and after applying to surface behind ear; to change patch q72h; to apply at least 4 hr before traveling

• Advise patient to discontinue use if blurred vision, severe dizziness, drowsiness occurs;

another type of antiemetic may be used or the patch rotated to the other ear
- Instruct patient to read labels of all OTC medications; if any scopolamine is found in product, avoid use
- Advise patient to keep medication out of children's reach
- Caution patient to report change in vision, blurring or loss of sight, trouble breathing, inhibition of sweating, flushing

Ophthalmic route
- Teach patient method of instillation: pressure on lacrimal sac for 1 min; do not touch dropper to eye
- Inform patient that blurred vision will decrease with repeated use of drug
- Advise patient to wait 5 min to use other drops; blink more than usual
- Caution patient not to discontinue this drug abruptly; to taper off over 1 wk

Evaluation
Positive therapeutic outcome
- Decrease in inflammation, cycloplegic refraction
- Decreased secretions
- Absence of motion sickness

---

selegiline (Rx)
(se-le′ji-leen)
Apo-Selegiline, Carbex, Eldepryl, Gen-Selegiline, Novo-Selegiline ✦, Nu-Selegiline, SD-Deprenyl
Func. class.: Antiparkinson agent
Chem. class.: MAOI, type B

Pregnancy category C

Action: Increased DOPaminergic activity by inhibition of MAO type B activity; not fully understood

➡ **Therapeutic Outcome:** Decreased symptoms of Parkinson's disease

Uses: Adjunct management of Parkinson's disease in patients being treated with levodopa/carbidopa who have responded poorly to therapy

Investigational use: Alzheimer's disease

Dosage and routes
Adult: PO 10 mg/day in divided doses, 5 mg at breakfast and lunch with levodopa/carbidopa; after 2-3 days begin to reduce the dose of levodopa/carbidopa 10%-30%

Available forms: Tabs 5 mg, caps 5 mg

Adverse effects
(*italic* = common; **bold** = life-threatening)
CNS: Increased tremors, chorea, restlessness, blepharospasm, increased bradykinesia, grimacing, tardive dyskinesia, dystonic symptoms, involuntary movements, increased apraxia, hallucinations, dizziness, mood changes, nightmares, delusions, lethargy, apathy, overstimulation, sleep disturbances, headache, migraine, numbness, muscle cramps, confusion, anxiety, tiredness, vertigo, personality change, back/leg pain
CV: Orthostatic hypotension, hypertension, **dysrhythmia**, palpitations; angina pectoris, hypotension, tachycardia, edema, sinus bradycardia, syncope
EENT: Diplopia, dry mouth, blurred vision, tinnitus
GI: *Nausea,* vomiting, constipation, weight loss, anorexia, diarrhea, heartburn, rectal bleeding, poor appetite, dysphagia, xerostomia
GU: Slow urination, nocturia, prostatic hypertrophy, hesitation, retention, frequency, sexual dysfunction
INTEG: Increased sweating, alopecia, hematoma, rash, photosensitivity, facial hair
RESP: Asthma, shortness of breath

Contraindications: Hypersensitivity

Precautions: Pregnancy C, lactation,
P children

N **Do Not Confuse:**
Eldepryl/enalapril

Pharmacokinetics	
Absorption	Well absorbed
Distribution	Widely distributed
Metabolism	Rapidly, liver
Excretion	Metabolites-N-desmethyldeprenyl, amphetamine, methamphetamine
Half-life	9 min

Pharmacodynamics	
Onset	Unknown
Peak	½-2 hr
Duration	Unknown

S

Interactions
Individual drugs
Fluoxetine, fluvoxamine, paroxetine, sertraline: ↑ serotonin syndrome (confusion, seizures, fever, hypertension, agitation) discontinue 5 wk before selegiline
Levodopa/carbidopa: ↑ side effects
Meperidine: Do not use—fatal reaction

Drug classifications
Antidepressants (tricyclics), opioids: Do not use—fatal reaction
⚠ *Herb/drug*
Chaste tree fruit, kava: ↓ selegiline action
Lab test interferences
↓ VMA
False positive: Urine ketones, urine glucose
False negative: Urine glucose (glucose oxidase)
False: ↑ Uric acid, ↑ urine protein

NURSING CONSIDERATIONS
Assessment
• Monitor B/P, respiration throughout treatment
• Assess mental status: affect, mood, behavioral changes, depression; perform suicide assessment
• Assess for decreased Parkinson's symptoms: rigidity, unsteady gait, weakness, tremors; these should decrease in severity

Nursing diagnoses
✓ Mobility, impaired physical (uses)
✓ Knowledge, deficient (teaching)

Implementation
• Adjust dosage to patient response
• Give with meals; limit protein taken with drug
• Give at doses <10 mg/day because of risks associated with nonselective inhibition of MAO

Patient/family education
• Caution patient to change positions slowly to prevent orthostatic hypotension
• Advise patient to report side effects: twitching, eye spasms; may indicate overdose
• Caution patient to use drug exactly as prescribed; if drug is discontinued abruptly, parkinsonian crisis may occur
• Instruct patient to avoid foods high in tyramine: cheese, pickled products, wine, beer, large amounts of caffeine
• Instruct patient not to exceed recommended dose of 10 mg; might precipitate a hypertensive crisis; report severe headache or other unusual symptoms

Evaluation
Positive therapeutic outcome
• Decreased symptoms of Parkinson's disease

Treatment of overdose: IV fluids for hypertension, **IV** dilute pressure agent for B/P titration

senna, sennosides (OTC)
(sin'na)
Black Draught, Dr. Caldwell Dosalax, Ex-Lax Gentle, Fletcher's Castoria, Gentlax, Senexon, Senna-Gen, Senokot, Senokotxtra, Senolax
Func. class.: Laxative-stimulant
Chem. class.: Anthraquinone
Pregnancy category C

Action: Stimulates peristalsis by action on Auerbach's plexus; softens feces by increasing water and electrolytes in large intestine

➔ **Therapeutic Outcome:** Decreased constipation

Uses: Acute constipation; bowel preparation for surgery or exam

Dosage and routes
Adult: PO 1-8 tabs (Senokot)/day or 1/2 to 4 tsp of granules added to water or juice; rec supp 1-2 hs; syr 1-4 tsp hs (1 tsp = 4 ml), 7.5-15 ml; Black Draught: 3/4 oz dissolved in 2.5 oz of liq given between 2-4 PM the day before procedure (X-Prep)

P *Child >27 kg:* PO ½ adult dose; do not use Black Draught for children

P *Child 1 mo-1 yr:* Syr 1.25-2.5 ml (Senokot) hs

Available forms: Supp 625 mg, 30 mg sennosides; powder 662 mg/g, 6, 15 mg sennosides/3 g; tabs 8.6 sennosides, 180 mg; oral sol 3 mg sennosides/ml

Adverse effects
(*italic* = common; **bold** = life-threatening)
GI: Nausea, vomiting, anorexia, abdominal cramps, diarrhea, flatulence
GU: Pink-red or brown-black discoloration of urine
META: Hypocalcemia, enteropathy, alkalosis, hypokalemia, **tetany**

Contraindications: Hypersensitivity, GI bleeding, intestinal obstruction, CHF, lactation, abdominal pain, nausea/vomiting, appendicitis, acute surgical abdomen

Precautions: Pregnancy **C**

Pharmacokinetics

Absorption	Minimally absorbed (PO)
Distribution	Unknown
Metabolism	Not metabolized
Excretion	Kidneys, feces
Half-life	Unknown

Pharmacodynamics		
	PO	REC
Onset	6-24 hr	Unknown
Peak	Unknown	Unknown
Duration	3-4 days	Unknown

Interactions
Individual drugs
Disulfiram: Do not use together
Drug classifications
Oral drugs: ↓ absorption
⊘ *Herb/drug*
Flax, senna: ↑ laxative effect

NURSING CONSIDERATIONS
Assessment
• Monitor blood, urine electrolytes if used often by patient; check I&O ratio to identify fluid loss
• Assess cramping, rectal bleeding, nausea, vomiting; if these symptoms occur, drug should be discontinued; identify cause of constipation; identify whether fluids, bulk, or exercise is missing from lifestyle
• Assess for magnesium toxicity: thirst, confusion, decrease in reflexes
• Monitor blood ammonia level (30-70 mg/100 ml); monitor for clearing of confusion, lethargy, restlessness, irritability (hepatic encephalopathy)

Nursing diagnoses
✓ Constipation (uses)
✓ Diarrhea (side effects)
✓ Knowledge, deficient (teaching)
✓ Noncompliance (teaching)

Implementation
PO route
• Administer on empty stomach for more rapid results
• Give with a full glass of water in AM or PM (oral dose); evacuation occurs 6-12 hr later
• Dissolve granules in water or juice before administration
• Shake oral sol before giving

Patient/family education
• Discuss with patient that adequate fluid consumption is necessary
• Inform patient that normal bowel movements do not always occur daily
• Teach patient not to use in presence of abdominal pain, nausea, vomiting; tell patient to notify prescriber if constipation is unrelieved or if symptoms of electrolyte imbalance occur: muscle cramps, pain, weakness, dizziness, excessive thirst

Evaluation
Positive therapeutic outcome
• Decreased constipation in 8-10 hr

---

sertraline (Rx)
(ser'tra-leen)
Zoloft
Func. class.: Antidepressant
Chem. class.: Selective serotonin reuptake inhibitor (SSRI)
Pregnancy category B

Action: Inhibits serotonin reuptake in CNS, thus increasing action of serotonin; does not affect dopamine, norepinephrine

⊅ **Therapeutic Outcome:** Relief of depression, obsessive-compulsive disorder (OCD), posttraumatic stress disorder (PTSD), panic disorder

Uses: Major depression, OCD, PTSD, panic disorder

Investigational uses: Extended interval dosing, premenstrual dysphoric disorder (PMDD)

Dosage and routes
Adult: PO 50 mg qd; may increase to a maximum of 200 mg/day, do not change dose at intervals of <1 wk; administer qd in AM or PM; or 100 mg 3 ×/wk (off-label)

🄶 *Elderly:* PO 25 mg qd, increase by 25 mg q3 days to desired dose

🄿 *Child 6-12 yr:* PO 25 mg qd

🄿 *Child 13-17 yr:* PO 50 mg qd

Premenstrual disorders (off-label)
Adult: PO 50-150 mg qhs

Available forms: Tabs 25, 50, 100 mg; liq 20 mg/ml

Adverse effects
(*italic* = common; **bold** = life-threatening)
CNS: Insomnia, agitation, somnolence, dizziness, headache, tremor, fatigue, paresthesia, twitching, confusion, ataxia, fever, gait
🄶 abnormality (elderly)
CV: Palpitations, chest pain
EENT: Vision abnormalities
ENDO: Syndrome of inappropriate antidiuretic
🄶 hormone (elderly)
GI: Diarrhea, nausea, constipation, anorexia, dry mouth, dyspepsia, *vomiting, flatulence*

S

GU: Male sexual dysfunction, micturition disorder
INTEG: Increased sweating, rash, hot flashes

Contraindications: Hypersensitivity to this drug or SSRIs

Precautions: Pregnancy **B**, lactation, elderly, hepatic, renal disease, epilepsy, recent MI

 Do Not Confuse:
Zoloft/Zocor

Pharmacokinetics

Absorption	Well absorbed
Distribution	Unknown, steady state 1 wk
Metabolism	Liver, extensively
Excretion	Feces (14%)
Half-life	1-4 days

Pharmacodynamics

Onset	Unknown
Peak	4.5-8.4 hr
Duration	Unknown

Interactions
Individual drugs
Cimetidine, warfarin: ↑ sertraline effect
Diazepam: ↑ diazepam effect
Pimozide: Sertraline is contraindicated with pimozide
Sumatriptan: ↑ sumatriptan effects
Drug classifications
Antidepressants (tricyclic), benzodiazepines: ↑ effect
MAOIs: Hypertensive crisis, seizures, do not use together
 Herb/drug
Corkwood, jimsonweed: ↑ anticholinergic effect
Hops, lavender: ↑ CNS effect
SAM-e, St. John's wort: ↑ effect of SSRIs, serotonin syndrome; do not use together
Lab test interferences
↑ AST, ↑ ALT

NURSING CONSIDERATIONS
Assessment
• Assess mental status: mood, sensorium, affect, suicidal tendencies; increase in psychiatric symptoms: depression, panic
• Identify alcohol consumption; if alcohol is consumed, hold dose until ᴀᴍ

Nursing diagnoses
✓ Coping, ineffective (uses)
✓ Injury, risk for (adverse reactions)
✓ Knowledge, deficient (teaching)
✓ Noncompliance (teaching)

Implementation
• Administer dosage hs if oversedation occurs during day; may take entire dose hs; may crush
• Store at room temp; do not freeze

Patient/family education
• Teach patient that therapeutic effects may take 1 wk or longer
• Instruct patient to use caution in driving or other activities requiring alertness because of drowsiness, dizziness, blurred vision; to avoid rising quickly from sitting to standing, especially elderly
• Advise patient to avoid alcohol ingestion, other CNS depressants
• Teach patient not to discontinue medication quickly after long-term use: may cause nausea, headache, malaise
• Caution patient to wear sunscreen or large hat because photosensitivity can occur
• Teach patient to increase fluids, bulk in diet if constipation, urinary retention occur, especially elderly
• Instruct patient to take gum, hard sugarless candy, or frequent sips of water for dry mouth

Evaluation
Positive therapeutic outcome
• Decrease in depression, OCD
• Absence of suicidal thoughts

Treatment of overdose: ECG monitoring, induce emesis, lavage, activated charcoal, administer anticonvulsant

sildenafil (Rx)
(sil-den′a-fill)
Viagra
Func. class.: Erectile agent
Chem. class.: Selective inhibitor of cGMP-PDE5

Pregnancy category B

Action: Enhances the effect of nitric oxide (NO) by inhibiting phosphodiesterase type 5 (PDE5), which is necessary for degrading cGMP in the carpus cavernosum

➔ **Therapeutic Outcome:** Ability to achieve and maintain erection

Uses: Treatment of erectile dysfunction

Dosage and routes
Adult: PO 50 mg 1 hr before sexual activity or may be taken ½-4 hr before sexual activity; may be increased to 100 mg or decreased to 25 mg; max once/day

---

Renal/hepatic dose
Adult: PO 25 mg, take 1 hr before sexual activity, do not use more than 1 ×/day

Available forms: Tabs 25, 50, 100 mg

Adverse effects
(*italic* = common; **bold** = life-threatening)
CNS: Headache, flushing, dizziness
CV: **MI, sudden death, CV collapse**
MISC: Dyspepsia, nasal congestion, UTI, abnormal vision, diarrhea, rash

Contraindications: Hypersensitivity

Precautions: Anatomical penile deformities, sickle cell anemia, leukemia, multiple myeloma, pregnancy **B**

Pharmacokinetics

Absorption	Rapidly, bioavailability (40%)
Distribution	Unknown
Metabolism	Liver (active metabolites)
Excretion	Feces, urine
Half-life	4 hr

Pharmacodynamics

Onset	Unknown
Peak	½-1½ hr
Duration	Unknown

Interactions
Individual drugs
Amlodipine: ↓ B/P
Cimetidine, erythromycin, itraconazole, ketoconazole: ↑ sildenafil levels
Nitrates: Fatal reaction, do not use together
Rifampin: ↓ sildenafil levels

NURSING CONSIDERATIONS
Assessment
• Identify organic nitrates that should not be used with this drug

Nursing diagnoses
✓ Noncompliance (teaching)
✓ Knowledge, deficient (teaching)

Implementation
• Give approximately 1 hr before sexual activity, do not use more than once a day

Patient/family education
• Teach patient that drug does not protect against sexually transmitted diseases, including HIV
• Teach patient that drug absorption is reduced with a high-fat meal
• Teach patient that drug should not be used with nitrates in any form
• Teach patient that tab may be split

Evaluation
Positive therapeutic outcome
• Ability to achieve and maintain an erection

---

simethicone (OTC)
(si-meth'i-kone)
Extra Strength Gas-X, Extra Strength Maalox Anti-Gas, Extra Strength Maalox GRF Gas Relief Formula ♣, Flatulex, Gas Relief, Gas-X, Genasyme, Maalox Anti-Gas, Maalox GRF Gas Relief Formula, Maximum Strength Gas Relief, Maximum Strength Mylanta Gas Relief, Maximum Strength Phazyme, Mylanta Gas, Mylicon ♣, Phazyme, Phazyme-95, Phazyme-125
Func. class.: Antiflatulent

Pregnancy category C

Action: Disperses, prevents gas pockets in GI system; does not decrease gas production

➜ **Therapeutic Outcome:** Belching or flatus

Uses: Flatulence

Dosage and routes
P *Adult and child >12 yr:* PO 40-100 mg pc, hs

P *Child <2 yr:* PO 20 mg qid

Available forms: Chew tabs 40, 80, 125 mg; tabs 60, 80, 95 mg; drops 40 mg/0.6 ml, 40 mg/ml, 95 mg/1.425 ml; caps 95, 125 mg; caps, soft gel 125 mg

Adverse effects
(*italic* = common; **bold** = life-threatening)
GI: Belching, rectal flatus

Contraindications: Hypersensitivity

Precautions: Pregnancy C

◨ **Do Not Confuse:**
Mylicon/Mylanta Gas

S

Pharmacokinetics

Absorption	None
Distribution	None
Metabolism	None
Excretion	None
Half-life	Unknown

Pharmacodynamics

Onset	Rapid
Peak	Unknown
Duration	3 hr

Interactions: None

NURSING CONSIDERATIONS
Assessment
• Identify the reason for excess gas production: decreased bowel sounds, recent surgery, other GI conditions

Nursing diagnoses
☑ Pain, acute (uses)
☑ Knowledge, deficient (teaching)

Implementation
• Give pc and hs
• Shake susp well before administration
• Chew tab should be chewed and not swallowed whole

Patient/family education
• Caution patient that tab must be chewed; to shake susp well before pouring

Evaluation
Positive therapeutic outcome
• Absence of flatulence

---

simvastatin (Rx)
(sim-va-stat'in)
Zocor
Func. class.: Antilipidemic
Chem. class.: HMG-CoA reductase inhibitor

Pregnancy category X

Action: Inhibits HMG-COA reductase enzyme, which reduces cholesterol synthesis; this enzyme is needed for cholesterol production

➡ **Therapeutic Outcome:** Decreasing cholesterol levels and LDLs, increased HDLs

Uses: As an adjunct in primary hypercholesterolemia (types IIa, IIb), mixed hyperlipidemia, CAD, isolated hypertriglyceridemia (Frederickson type IV) and type III hyperlipoproteinemia

Dosage and routes
Adult: PO 5-20 mg qd in PM initially, usual range 5-40 mg/day qd in PM, not to exceed 80 mg/day; dosage adjustments may be made at 4-wk intervals or more; those taking verapamil, max 20 mg/day

G *Elderly/renal dose /those taking cycloSPORINE*
PO 5 mg/day, initially

Available forms: Tabs 5, 10, 20, 40, 80 mg

Adverse effects
(*italic* = common; **bold** = life-threatening)
CNS: Headache
EENT: Lens opacities
GI: Nausea, constipation, diarrhea, dyspepsia, flatus, abdominal pain, **liver dysfunction, pancreatitis**
INTEG: Rash, pruritus, photosensitivity
RESP: Upper respiratory tract infection
MS: Muscle cramps, myalgia, **myositis, rhabdomyolysis**

Contraindications: Hypersensitivity, pregnancy **X,** lactation, active liver disease

Precautions: Past liver disease, alcoholism, severe acute infections, trauma, severe metabolic disorders, electrolyte imbalances,
G elderly, renal disease

⚠ **Do Not Confuse:**
Zocor/Cozaar, Zocor/Zoloft

Pharmacokinetics
Absorption	85%
Distribution	Unknown
Metabolism	Liver—extensively
Excretion	70% feces, 20% kidneys
Half-life	3 hr

Pharmacodynamics
Onset	Unknown
Peak	Unknown
Duration	Unknown

Interactions
Individual drugs
Clarithromycin, clofibrate, itraconazole: ↑ myalgia, myositis
CycloSPORINE, erythromycin, gemfibrozil, niacin: ↑ risk of myopathy
CycloSPORINE, digoxin: ↑ digoxin levels
Gemfibrozil: ↑ risk of rhabdomyolysis
Warfarin: ↑ risk of bleeding

Drug classifications
Protekase inhibitors: ↑ myalgia, myositis
⚠ *Herb/drug*
Glucomannan: ↑ effect
Gotu kola: ↓ effect
Lab test interferences
↑ CPK, ↑ liver function tests

NURSING CONSIDERATIONS
Assessment
• Assess nutrition: fat, protein, carbohydrates; nutritional analysis should be completed by dietitian before treatment is initiated
◆• Assess for rhabdomyolysis: muscle tenderness, increased CPK levels; therapy should be discontinued
• Monitor bowel pattern daily; diarrhea may be a problem
• Monitor triglycerides, cholesterol baseline and throughout treatment; LDL, HDL, triglycer-

---

ides and cholesterol at 6-8 wk and q6 mo should be watched closely; if increased, drug should be discontinued

Nursing diagnoses
☑ Diarrhea (adverse reactions)
☑ Knowledge, deficient (teaching)
☑ Noncompliance (teaching)

Implementation
• Give 30 min before AM and PM meals

Patient/family education
• Inform patient that compliance is needed for positive results to occur; not to double doses
• Advise patient to lower risk factors: high-fat diet, smoking, alcohol consumption, absence of exercise
• Advise patient to notify health care prescriber if the GI symptoms of diarrhea, abdominal or epigastric pain, nausea, vomiting occur; or if chills, fever, sore throat occur

Evaluation
Positive therapeutic outcome
• Decreased cholesterol levels, serum triglycerides and improved ratio with HDLs

---

sirolimus (Rx)
(seer-roe'-li-mus)
Rapamune
Func. class.: Immunosuppressant
Chem. class.: Macrolide
Pregnancy category C

Action: Produces immunosuppression by inhibiting T-lymphocyte activation and proliferation

⇒ **Therapeutic Outcome:** Prevention of rejection in organ transplant

Uses: Organ transplants: to prevent rejection, recommended use is with cyclosporine and corticosteroids

Investigational uses: Psoriasis

Dosage and routes
Adult: PO 2 mg qd with 6 mg loading dose, may use 5 mg qd with a 15 mg loading dose

🄿 *Child >13 yr <40 kg (88 lb):* PO 1 mg/m²/day, 3 mg/m²/loading dose

Hepatic dose
🄿 *Adult/child≥13 yr<40 kg:* PO reduce by 33% in maintenance dose

Available forms: Oral sol 1 mg/ml

Adverse effects
(*italic* = common; **bold** = life-threatening)
CNS: *Tremors, headache, insomnia,* paresthesia, chills, fever
CV: Hypertension, **atrial fibrillation, CHF,** hypotension, palpitations, **tachycardia**
EENT: Blurred vision, photophobia
GI: Nausea, vomiting, diarrhea, constipation
GU: UTI, **albuminuria, hematuria, proteinuria, renal failure**
HEMA: Anemia, **thrombocytopenia purpura, leukopenia**
INTEG: *Rash, acne,* photosensitivity
META: Increased creatinine, edema, hypercholesterolemia, *hyperlipemia,* hypophosphatemia, weight gain, hyperglycemia, hyperkalemia, hyperuricemia, hypokalemia, hypomagnesemia
RESP: **Pleural effusion, atelectasis,** *dyspnea*
SYST: **Lymphoma**

Contraindications: Hypersensitivity to this drug or to components of the drug

Precautions: Severe renal disease, severe hepatic disease, pregnancy **C,** diabetes mellitus, hyperkalemia, hyperuricemia, lymphomas, 🄿 lactation, child <13 yr, hypertension, infection, other malignancies

Pharmacokinetics
Absorption	Rapidly absorbed
Distribution	92% protein binding
Metabolism	Liver; extensively by CYP3A4 enzyme system
Excretion	Unknown
Half-life	Unknown

Pharmacodynamics
	PO
Onset	Unknown
Peak	1 hr single dose, 2 hr multiple dosing
Duration	Unknown

Interactions
Individual drugs
Bromocriptine, cimetidine, cycloSPORINE, danazol, erythromycin, metoclopramide: ↑ blood level
Carbamazepine, phenobarbital, phenytoin, rifamycin, rifapentine: ↓ blood levels
Drug classifications
Antifungal agents, calcium channel blockers: ↑ sirolimus levels
HIV protease inhibitors: ↑ blood levels
Live virus vaccines: ↓ effect of vaccines

S

Food/drug
Food: Alters bioavailability, use consistently with or without food
Grapefruit juice: Do not use with grapefruit juice

⚡ *Herb/drug*
Astragalus, echinacea, melatonin: ↓ immuno-suppression
Ginseng, maitake, mistletoe: ↑ effect
St. John's wort: ↓ sirolimus effect

NURSING CONSIDERATIONS
Assessment
• Monitor blood studies: Hgb, WBC, platelets monthly during treatment; if leukocytes are <3000/mm³, or platelets <100,000/mm³, drug should be discontinued or reduced; decreased Hgb level may indicate bone marrow suppression
• Monitor blood levels in those who may have altered metabolism, trough levels ≥15 ng/ml are associated with increased adverse reactions
• Monitor lipid profile: cholesterol, triglycerides; a lipid-lowering agent may be needed
• Assess for infection and development of lymphoma
• Monitor liver function studies: alkaline phosphatase, AST, ALT, amylase, bilirubin, and for hepatotoxicity: dark urine, jaundice, itching, light-colored stools; drug should be discontinued

Nursing diagnoses
☑ Infection, risk for (uses)
☑ Knowledge, deficient (teaching)

Implementation
• Administer prophylaxis for *Pneumocystis carinii* pneumonia for 1 yr after transplantation; prophylaxis for cytomegalovirus (CMV) is recommended for 90 days after transplantation in those at increased risk for CMV
• Use amber oral dose syringe and withdraw amount of oral sol needed from the bottle, empty correct dose into plastic/glass container holding 60 ml of water/orange juice, stir vigorously and have patient drink at once, refill container with additional 120 ml of water/orange juice, stir vigorously, and have patient drink at once; if using a pouch squeeze entire contents into container and follow above directions
• Give all medications PO if possible; avoid IM inj because bleeding may occur
• Give for 3 days before transplant surgery; patients should be placed in protective isolation

• Store protected from light, refrigerate, stable for 24 months

Patient/family education
• Instruct patient to report fever, rash, severe diarrhea, chills, sore throat, fatigue because serious infections may occur; clay-colored stools, cramping may indicate hepatotoxicity
• Caution patient to avoid crowds or persons with known infections to reduce risk of infection
• Teach patient to use contraception before, during, and 12 wk after drug has been discontinued, avoid breastfeeding
• Teach patient to use sunscreen, protective clothing to prevent burns

Evaluation
Positive therapeutic outcome
• Absence of graft rejection

---

sodium bicarbonate (OTC)
Arm and Hammer Pure Baking Soda, Bell/ans, Citrocarbonate, Neut, Soda Mint
Func. class.: Alkalinizer; antacid
Pregnancy category C

Action: Orally neutralizes gastric acid, which forms water, NaCl, CO_2; increases plasma bicarbonate, which buffers H^+ ion concentration; reverses acidosis **IV**

➤ **Therapeutic Outcome:** Correction of acidosis, gastric acid neutralization

Uses: Acidosis (metabolic), cardiac arrest, alkalinization (systemic/urinary); antacid (PO)

Dosage and routes
Acidosis, metabolic
🅿 *Adult and child:* **IV** inf 2-5 mEq/kg over 4-8 hr depending on CO_2, pH
Cardiac arrest
🅿 *Adult and child:* **IV** bol 1 mEq/kg of 7.5% or 8.4% sol, then 0.5 mEq/kg q10 min, then doses based on ABGs
🅿 *Infant:* **IV** inf not to exceed 8 mEq/kg/day based on ABGs (4.2% sol)
Alkalinization of urine
Adult: PO 325 mg-2 g qid or 48 mEq/kg (4 g), then 12-24 mEq q4h
🅿 *Child:* PO 12-120 mg/kg/day (1-10 mEq/kg)
Antacid
Adult: PO 300 mg-2 g chewed, taken with water qd-qid

⚡ Herb/drug　　🚫 Do Not Crush　　◆ Alert　　◆� Key Drug　　🄶 Geriatric　　🅿 Pediatric

Available forms: Tabs 300, 325, 600, 650 mg; inj 4.2%, 5%, 7.5%, 8.4%

Adverse effects

*(italic = common; **bold** = life-threatening)*

CNS: Irritability, headache, confusion, stimulation, tremors, *twitching, hyperreflexia,* **tetany,** weakness, **seizures** caused by alkalosis

CV: Irregular pulse, **cardiac arrest,** water retention, edema, weight gain

GI: Flatulence, *belching, distention,* **paralytic ileus,** acid rebound

GU: Calculi

META: *Alkalosis*

RESP: Shallow, slow respirations, cyanosis, **apnea**

Contraindications: Hypertension, peptic ulcer, renal disease, hypocalcemia

Precautions: CHF, cirrhosis, toxemia, renal disease, pregnancy **C**

Pharmacokinetics

Absorption	Unknown
Distribution	Widely distributed—extracellular fluids
Metabolism	Unknown
Excretion	Kidneys
Half-life	Unknown

Pharmacodynamics

	PO	IV
Onset	2 min	Rapid
Peak	½ hr	Rapid
Duration	1-3 hr	Unknown

Interactions

Individual drugs

Chlorpropamide, lithium: ↓ effect of each specific drug

Flecainide, pseudoephedrine, quinidine, quinine: ↑ effects of each specific drug

Ketoconazole: ↓ absorption of ketocanazole

Drug classifications

Amphetamines, anorexiants: ↑ effects

Barbiturates: ↓ effects of barbiturates

Benzodiazepines: ↓ effects

Corticosteroids: ↑ sodium, potassium

Fluoroquinolones: ↑ crystalluria

Salicylates: ↓ effect of salicylates

Herb/drug

Oak bark: ↓ action of sodium bicarbonate

Lab test interferences

↑ Urinary urobilinogen

False positive: Urinary protein, blood lactate

NURSING CONSIDERATIONS

Assessment

- Assess respiratory and pulse rate, rhythm, depth, lung sounds; notify prescriber of abnormalities

- Assess for CO_2 in GI tract; may lead to perforation if ulcer is severe

- Monitor fluid balance (I&O ratio, weight qd, edema); notify prescriber of fluid overload

- Monitor electrolytes, blood pH, PO_2, HCO_3, during beginning treatment; ABGs frequently during emergencies

- Monitor urine pH, urinary output, during beginning treatment

- Monitor extravasation with **IV** administration (tissue sloughing, ulceration, and necrosis)

- Assess for alkalosis: irritability, confusion, twitching, hyperreflexia, stimulation, slow respirations, cyanosis, irregular pulse

- Monitor manifestations of hypokalemia: *RENAL:* acidic urine, reduced urine osmolality, nocturia, polyuria, polydipsia; *CV:* hypotension, broad ↑ wave, ∪ wave, ectopy, tachycardia, weak pulse; *NEURO:* muscle weakness, altered LOC, drowsiness, apathy, lethargy, confusion, depression; *GI:* anorexia, nausea, cramps, constipation, distention, paralytic ileus; *RESP:* hypoventilation, respiratory muscle weakness

- Monitor for manifestations of hyponatremia: *CV:* ↑ B/P, cold, clammy skin, hypo- or hypervolemia; *GI:* anorexia, nausea, vomiting, diarrhea, abdominal cramps; *NEURO:* lethargy, increased ICP, confusion, headache, seizures, coma, fatigue, tremors, hyperreflexia

- Assess for milk-alkali syndrome: confusion, headache, nausea, vomiting, anorexia, urinary stones, hypercalcemia

Nursing diagnoses

☑ Gas exchange, impaired (uses)

☑ Fluid volume, excess (adverse reactions)

☑ Knowledge, deficient (teaching)

Implementation

PO route

- Tab must be chewed and taken with 8 oz of water

- Dissolve effervescent tab in water

- May be used to neutralize gastric acid in peptic ulcer disease, given 1 and 3 hr pc and hs

IV route

- Give **IV** bol in cardiac arrest, may be repeated q10 min

- Give by intermittent or continuous inf in prepared sol or diluted in an equal amount of any dextrose/saline combination; administer

S

2-5 mEq/kg over 4-8 hr, not to exceed 50 **P** mEq/hr; slower rate in children

Syringe compatibilities: Milrinone, pentobarbital

Syringe incompatibilities: Glycopyrrolate, metoclopramide, thiopental

Y-site compatibilities: Acyclovir, amifostine, asparaginase, aztreonam, cefepime, cefmetazole, ceftriaxone, cladribine, cyclophosphamide, cytarabine, DAUNOrubicin, dexamethasone, dexchlorpheniramine, DOXOrubicin, etoposide, famotidine, filgrastim, fludarabine, gallium, granisetron, heparin, ifosfamide, indomethacin, insulin, melphalan, mesna, methylPREDNISolone, morphine, paclitaxel, piperacillin/tazobactam, potassium chloride, propofol, tacrolimus, teniposide, thiotepa, tolazoline, vancomycin, vit B/C

Y-site incompatibilities: Amrinone, calcium chloride, idarubicin, sargramostim, verapamil, vinorelbine

Additive compatibilities: Amikacin, aminophylline, amobarbital, amphotericin B, atropine, bretylium, calcium glucceptate, cefoxitin, ceftazidime, cephalothin, cephapirin, chloramphenicol, chlorothiazide, cimetidine, clindamycin, cytarabine, droperidol/fentanyl, ergonovine, erythromycin, esmolol, floxacillin, furosemide, heparin, hyaluronidase, hydrocortisone, kanamycin, lidocaine, mannitol, metaraminol, methotrexate, methyldopate, multivitamins, nafcillin, nalmefene, netilmicin, nizatidine, ofloxacin, oxacillin, oxytocin, phenobarbital, phenylephrine, phenytoin, phytonadione, potassium chloride, prochlorperazine, thiopental, verapamil

Additive incompatibilities: Amoxicillin, ascorbic acid, carboplatin, carmustine, cefotaxime, cisplatin, codeine, DOBUTamine, epINEPHrine, hydromorphone, imipenem/cilastatin, insulin, isoproterenol, labetalol, levorphanol, magnesium sulfate, methadone, morphine, norepinephrine, pentazocine, pentobarbital, procaine, secobarbital, streptomycin, succinylcholine, tetracycline, vit B/C

Patient/family education
• Instruct patient to chew antacid tab and drink 8 oz of water; not to take antacid with milk because milk-alkali syndrome may result; not to use antacid for more than 2 wk
• Advise patient to notify prescriber if indigestion is accompanied by chest pain; dyspnea; diarrhea; dark, tarry stools

• Teach patient about sodium-restricted diet; to avoid use of baking soda for indigestion

Evaluation
Positive therapeutic outcome
• ABGs, electrolytes, blood pH, HCO_3 normal levels
• Decreased gastric pain

**sodium biphosphate/
sodium phosphate** (OTC)
Fleet Enema, Phospho-soda
Func. class.: Laxative, saline
Pregnancy category C

Action: Increases water absorption in the small intestine by osmotic action; laxative effect occurs by increased peristalsis and water retention

⮕ **Therapeutic Outcome:** Absence of constipation

Uses: Constipation, bowel or rectal preparation for surgery, examination

Dosage and routes
Adult: PO 20-30 ml (Phospho-soda)
P *Child:* PO 5-15 ml (Phospho-soda)
P *Adult and child >12 yr:* REC enema (118 ml)
P *Child 2-12 yr:* REC ½ enema (59 ml)

Available forms: Enema 7 g/phosphate and 19 g/biphosphate/118 ml; oral sol 18 g phosphate/48 g biphosphate/100 ml

Adverse effects
(*italic* = common; **bold** = life-threatening)
GI: Nausea, cramps, diarrhea
META: Electrolyte, fluid imbalances
CV: **Dysrhythmias, cardiac arrest,** hypotension, widening QRS complex

Contraindications: Hypersensitivity, rectal fissures, abdominal pain, nausea/vomiting, appendicitis, acute surgical abdomen, ulcerated hemorrhoids, Na-restricted diets, renal failure, hyperphosphatemia, hypocalcemia, hypokalemia, hypernatremia, Addison's disease, CHF, ascites, bowel perforation

Precautions: Pregnancy **C**

Pharmacokinetics

Absorption	Up to 20% (rec)
Distribution	Unknown
Metabolism	Unknown
Excretion	Kidneys
Half-life	Unknown

Pharmacodynamics

	PO	REC
Onset	½-3 hr	5 min
Peak	Unknown	Unknown
Duration	Unknown	Unknown

Interactions: None

NURSING CONSIDERATIONS
Assessment
- Assess stools: color, amount, consistency
- Assess for bowel pattern, bowel sounds (frequency, intensity), flatulence, distention, increased temp, dietary patterns (fluid, bulk), exercise
- Assess for cramping, rectal bleeding, nausea, vomiting; if these symptoms occur, drug should be discontinued

Nursing diagnoses
✓ Constipation (uses)
✓ Knowledge, deficient (teaching)

Implementation
PO route
- Give on empty stomach
- Mix oral sol in cold water
- Take alone for better absorption; do not take within 1 hr of other drugs

Patient/family education
- Advise patient not to use laxatives or enema for long-term therapy; bowel tone will be lost
- Teach patient that normal bowel movements do not always occur daily
- Caution patient not to use in presence of abdominal pain, nausea, vomiting
- Caution patient to notify prescriber if constipation is unrelieved or if symptoms of electrolyte imbalance occur: muscle cramps, pain, weakness, dizziness, excessive thirst
- Instruct patient to maintain adequate fluid consumption to help prevent constipation

Evaluation
Positive therapeutic outcome
- Decrease in constipation

---

sodium polystyrene sulfonate (Rx)
(po-lee-stye′reen)
Kayexalate, K-Exit ♣, Kionex, PMS
Sodium Polystyrene Sulfonate ♣, SPS
Func. class.: Potassium-removing resin
Chem. class.: Cation exchange resin

Pregnancy category C

Action: Removes potassium by exchanging sodium for potassium in body; occurs primarily in large intestine

➔ **Therapeutic Outcome:** Potassium levels within accepted range

Uses: Hyperkalemia in conjunction with other measures

Dosage and routes
Adult: PO 15 g qd-qid; rec enema 30-50 g/100 ml of sorbitol warmed to body temp q6h

☐ *Child:* PO/rec 1 mEq of K exchanged/g of resin, approximate dose 1 g/kg q6h

Available forms: Susp, 15 g polystyrene sulfonate, 21.5 ml sorbitol, 15 g (65 mEq) sodium/60 ml; powder 15 g/4 level tsp

Adverse effects
(*italic* = common; **bold** = life-threatening)
GI: Constipation, anorexia, nausea, vomiting, diarrhea (sorbitol), *fecal impaction,* gastric irritation
META: Hypocalcemia, hypokalemia, hypomagnesemia, sodium retention

Precautions: Pregnancy **C**, renal failure, CHF, severe edema, severe hypertension

---

Pharmacokinetics

Absorption	None
Distribution	None
Metabolism	None
Excretion	Feces
Half-life	Unknown

Pharmacodynamics

	PO	REC
Onset	2-12 hr	2-12 hr
Peak	Unknown	Unknown
Duration	6-24 hr	4-6 hr

S

Interactions
Drug classifications
Antacids (calcium or magnesium), laxatives: ↓ effect of sodium polystyrene

---

NURSING CONSIDERATIONS
Assessment
• Assess bowel function daily: amount of stool, color, characteristics
• Assess for hypotension: confusion, irritability, muscular pain, weakness
• Monitor for manifestations of hypokalemia: *RENAL:* acidic urine, reduced urine osmolality, nocturia, polyuria, polydipsia; *CV:* hypotension, broad T wave, U wave, ectopy, tachycardia, weak pulse; *NEURO:* muscle weakness, altered LOC, drowsiness, apathy, lethargy, confusion, depression; *GI:* anorexia, nausea, cramps, constipation, distention, paralytic ileus; *RESP:* hypoventilation, respiratory muscle weakness
• Monitor for manifestations of hyperkalemia: confusion, dyspnea, weakness, dysrhythmias
• Monitor for manifestations of hypocalcemia: *CNS:* personality changes, anxiety, disturbances, depression, psychosis, nausea, vomiting, *GI:* constipation, abdominal pain from muscle spasm; *CV:* decreased contractility, decreased cardiac output, hypotension, lengthened ST segment, prolonged QT interval; *INTEG:* scaling eczema, alopecia, hyperpigmentation; *NEURO:* tetany, muscle twitching, cramping grimacing, seizure, altered deep tendon reflexes, spasm
• Monitor for manifestations of hypomagnesemia; *CNS:* agitation; *NEURO:* muscle twitching, paresthesias, hyperactive reflexes, positive Babinski reflex, dysphagia, nystagmus, seizures, tetany; *GI:* nausea, vomiting, diarrhea, anorexia, abdominal distention; *CV:* ectopy; tachycardia, broad, flat, or inverted T waves; depressed ST segment; prolonged QT interval; decreased cardiac output; hypotension
• Monitor electrolytes: potassium, sodium, calcium, magnesium; I&O ratio, weight qd
• Monitor ECG for spiked T waves, depressed ST segments, prolonged QT interval and widening QRS complex

Nursing diagnoses
☑ Constipation (adverse reactions)
☑ Diarrhea (adverse reactions)
☑ Knowledge, deficient (teaching)

Implementation
PO route
• Give oral dose as susp mixed with H$_2$O or syr (20-100 ml)
• Give mild laxative as ordered to prevent constipation and fecal impaction; sorbitol as ordered to prevent constipation
Rectal route
• Give by retention enema after mixing with warm water; introduce by gravity, continue stirring, flush with 100 ml of fluid, clamp, and leave in place for at least ½-1 hr
• Complete irrigation of colon after enema with 1-2 qt of nonsodium sol, drain
• Store freshly prepared sol for 24 hr at room temp

Patient/family education
• Explain reason for medication and expected results

Evaluation
Positive therapeutic outcome
• Potassium level 3.5-5 mg/dl

---

somatropin (Rx)
(soe-ma-troe′pin)
Genotropin, Humatrope, Norditropin, Nutropin, Nutropin AQ, Nutropin Depot, Saizen, Serostim
Func. class.: Pituitary hormone
Chem. class.: Growth hormone

Pregnancy category C

Action: Stimulates growth; similar to natural growth hormone—both preparations are developed by recombinant DNA technique

➡ **Therapeutic Outcome:** Increase in height as a result of skeletal growth in pituitary growth hormone deficiency

Uses: Pituitary growth hormone deficiency (hypopituitary dwarfism), children with human growth hormone deficiency, AIDS wasting syndrome, cachexia, adults with somatropin deficiency syndrome (SDS)

Dosage and routes
Genotropin: SC 0.16-0.24 mg/kg/wk, divided into 6 or 7 inj, give in abdomen, thigh, buttocks

Humatrope: SC/IM 0.18 mg/kg divided into equal doses either on 3 alternate days or 6 ×/wk, max wk dose is 0.3 mg/kg

Growth hormone deficiency
Nutropin/Nutropin AQ: SC 0.3 mg/kg/wk

Serostim: SC hs >55 kg 6 mg, 45-55 kg 5 mg, 35-45 kg 4 mg

Norditropin: SC 0.024-0.034 mg/kg 6-7 ×/wk

Available forms: Powder for inj (lyophilized) 1.5 mg (4 international units/ml), 4 mg (12 international units/vial), 5 mg (13 international units/vial), 5 mg (15 international units/vial), 5 mg (15 international units/vial) rDNA origin, 5.8 mg (15 international units/ml), 6 mg (18 international units/ml), 8 mg

---

☑ Herb/drug   Ⓢ Do Not Crush   ✦ Alert   ✦ᴛ Key Drug   🄖 Geriatric   🄿 Pediatric

(24 international units/vial), 10 mg (26 international units/vial), inj 10 mg (30 international units/vial); 5, 10, 15 mg/1.5 ml

Adverse effects
(*italic* = common; **bold** = life-threatening)
CNS: Headache, **growth of intracranial tumor**
ENDO: *Hyperglycemia, ketosis, hypothyroidism*
GU: *Hypercalciuria*
INTEG: Rash, urticaria, pain, inflammation at inj site
MS: Tissue swelling, joint and muscle pain
SYST: *Antibodies to growth hormone*

Contraindications: Hypersensitivity to benzyl alcohol, closed epiphyses, intracranial lesions

Precautions: Diabetes mellitus, hypothyroidism, pregnancy **C**

Pharmacokinetics
Absorption	Well absorbed (SC/IM)
Distribution	Unknown
Metabolism	Unknown
Half-life	15-60 min

Pharmacodynamics
	IM/SC (GROWTH)
Onset	Unknown
Peak	Unknown
Duration	7 days

Interactions
Drug classifications
Androgens, thyroid hormones: ↑ epiphyseal closure
Glucocorticosteroids: ↓ growth

NURSING CONSIDERATIONS
Assessment
• Identify growth hormone antibodies if patient fails to respond to therapy
• Monitor thyroid function tests: T_3, T_4, T_7, TSH to identify hypothyroidism
• Assess for allergic reaction: rash, itching, fever, nausea, wheezing
• Assess for hypercalciuria: urinary stones; groin, flank pain; nausea, vomiting, frequency, hematuria, chills
P • Monitor growth rate of child at intervals during treatment

Nursing diagnoses
✓ Body image, disturbed (uses)
✓ Knowledge, deficient (teaching)

Implementation
• Store in refrigerator for <1 mo; if recon-

stituted, <1 wk; do not use discolored or cloudy sol
IM route
• Norditropin: After reconstituting 4-8 mg/2 ml diluent
• Humetrope: 5 mg/1.5-5 ml dilute, do not shake
• Nutropin/Nutropin AQ: Reconstitute 5 mg/1-5 ml or 10 mg/1-10 ml of bacteriostatic water for inj (benzyl alcohol preserved)

Patient/family education
• Explain reason for medication and expected results; that treatment may continue for yr
• Advise patient that routine follow-up is needed to monitor growth rate
• Instruct parents on procedure for medication preparation and inj use; request demonstration, return demonstration; provide written instructions

Evaluation
Positive therapeutic outcome
• Growth in children until epiphyseal plates close

---

sotalol (Rx)
(soe-ta′lole)
Betapace, Betapace AF, Sotacar ✦
Func. class.: Antidysrhythmic, group III
Chem. class.: Nonselective β-blocker

Pregnancy category B

Action: Competitively blocks stimulation of β-adrenergic receptor within vascular smooth muscle; produces chronotropic, inotropic activity (decreases rate of SA node discharge, increases recovery time), slows conduction of AV node, decreases heart rate, which decreases O_2 consumption in myocardium; also decreases renin-aldosterone-angiotensin system at high doses, inhibits $β_2$ receptors in bronchial system (high doses)

➡**Therapeutic Outcome:** Decreased B/P, heart rate, AV conduction

Uses: Life-threatening ventricular dysrhythmias; Betapace AF: to maintain sinus rhythm in symptomatic atrial fibrillation/flutter

Dosage and routes
Adult: PO initial 80 mg bid, may increase to total of 240-320 mg/day

Renal dose
Adult: PO CCr 30-60 ml/min q24h; CCr 10-29 ml/min q36-48h; CCr <10 ml/min individualize dose

S

Betapace AF
Adult: PO initial 80 mg bid, titrate upward to 120 mg bid during initial hospitalization

Renal dose (Betapace AF)
CCr >60 ml/min q12h; CCr 40-60 ml/min q24h; CCr <40 ml/min do not use

Available forms: Tabs 80, 120, 160, 240 mg; Betapace AF 80, 120, 160 mg

Adverse effects
(*italic* = common; **bold** = life-threatening)
CNS: Dizziness, mental changes, drowsiness, fatigue, headache, catatonia, depression, anxiety, nightmares, paresthesia, lethargy, insomnia, decreased concentration
CV: Orthostatic hypotension, bradycardia, **CHF,** chest pain, **ventricular dysrhythmias,** AV block, peripheral vascular insufficiency, palpitations, **prodysrhythmia, torsades de pointes; Betapace AF: life-threatening ventricular dysrhythmias**
EENT: Tinnitus, visual changes, sore throat, double vision, dry, burning eyes
GI: Nausea, vomiting, diarrhea, dry mouth, flatulence, constipation, anorexia
GU: Impotence, dysuria, ejaculatory failure, urinary retention
HEMA: **Agranulocytosis, thrombocytopenic purpura (rare), thrombocytopenia, leukopenia**
INTEG: Rash, alopecia, urticaria, pruritus, fever
MISC: Facial swelling, decreased exercise tolerance, weight change, Raynaud's disease
MS: Joint pain, arthralgia, muscle cramps, pain
RESP: **Bronchospasm,** dyspnea, wheezing, nasal stuffiness, pharyngitis

Contraindications: Hypersensitivity to β-blockers, cardiogenic shock, heart block (2nd or 3rd degree), sinus bradycardia, CHF, bronchial asthma, congenital or acquired long QT syndrome

Precautions: Major surgery, pregnancy **B,** lactation, diabetes mellitus, renal disease, thyroid disease, COPD, well-compensated heart failure, CAD, nonallergic bronchospasm, electrolyte disturbances, bradycardia, cardiac dysrhythmias, peripheral vascular disease

Absorption	Variable (30%)
Distribution	Crosses placenta, minimal penetration in CNS
Metabolism	Liver, protein binding 0%
Excretion	70% unchanged—kidneys
Half-life	10-24 hr, ↑ in renal disease

Onset	Several hr
Peak	Unknown
Duration	Unknown

Interactions
Individual drugs
Insulin: ↑ hypoglycemia
Lidocaine: ↑ effects of lidocaine
Nitroglycerin: ↑ hypotension
Theophylline: ↓ bronchodilating effects of theophylline
Drug classifications
Antihypertensives, diuretics: ↑ hypotension
β₂-Agonists: ↓ bronchodilating effects
Sulfonylureas: ↓ hypoglycemic effects
Sympathomimetics: ↓ β-blocker effects
Herb/drug
Aconite: ↑ toxicity, death
Aloe, broom, buckthorn (chronic use), cascara sagrada (chronic use), Chinese rhubarb, figwort, fumitory, goldenseal, kudzu, licorice: ↑ effect
Coltsfoot: ↓ effect
Horehound: ↑ serotonin effect
Lab test interferences
False: ↑ Urinary catecholamines
Interference: Glucose, insulin tolerance tests

NURSING CONSIDERATIONS
Assessment
• Monitor B/P during beginning treatment, periodically thereafter; pulse q4h; note rate, rhythm, quality: apical/radial pulse before administration; notify prescriber of any significant changes (pulse <50 bpm); monitor ECG continuously (Betapace AF); use QT interval to determine patient eligibility; baseline QT must be ≤450 msec
• Check for baselines in renal, before therapy begins
• Assess for edema in feet, legs daily, monitor I&O ratio, daily weight; check for jugular vein distention, rales, bilaterally, dyspnea (CHF)
• Monitor skin turgor, dryness of mucous membranes for hydration status, especially in elderly

Nursing diagnoses
☑ Cardiac output, decreased (uses)
☑ Injury, risk for (adverse reactions)
☑ Knowledge, deficient (teaching)
☑ Noncompliance (teaching)

Implementation
• Given ac, hs, tab may be crushed or swallowed whole; give with food to prevent GI upset; reduce dosage in renal dysfunction

- Betapace and Betapace AF are not interchangeable
- Store protected from light, moisture; place in cool environment

Patient/family education
- Teach patient not to discontinue drug abruptly, taper over 2 wk; may cause precipitate angina if stopped abruptly
- Teach patient not to use OTC products containing α-adrenergic stimulants (such as nasal decongestants, cold preparations); to avoid alcohol and smoking and to limit sodium intake as prescribed
- Teach patient how to take pulse and B/P at home, advise when to notify prescriber
- Instruct patient to comply with weight control, dietary adjustments, modified exercise program
- Caution patient to carry/wear emergency ID to identify drug being taken, allergies
- Inform patient that drug controls symptoms but does not cure
- Caution patient to avoid hazardous activities if dizziness, drowsiness is present
- Teach patient to report symptoms of CHF: difficulty breathing, especially on exertion or when lying down; night cough; swelling of extremities; bradycardia; dizziness; confusion; depression; fever
- Teach patient to take drug as prescribed, not to double or skip doses; take any missed doses as soon as remembered if at least 4 hr until next dose

Evaluation
Positive therapeutic outcome
- Absence of dysrhythmias

Treatment of overdose: Lavage; **IV** atropine for bradycardia; **IV** theophylline for bronchospasm; digitalis, O$_2$, diuretic for cardiac failure; hemodialysis; **IV** glucose for hyperglycemia; **IV** diazepam (or phenytoin) for seizures

---

sparfloxacin (Rx)
(spar-floks′a-sin)
Zagam
Func. class.: Antiinfective
Chem. class.: Fluoroquinolone antibacterial

Pregnancy category C

Action: Interferes with conversion of intermediate DNA fragments into high molecular weight DNA in bacteria; DNA gyrase inhibitor

➡ **Therapeutic Outcome:** Bactericidal action against the following organisms: *Chlamydia pneumoniae, Haemophilus influenzae, Haemophilus parainfluenzae, Moraxella catarrhalis*

Uses: Adult infections (including complicated): lower respiratory, community-acquired pneumonia, chronic bronchitis

Dosage and routes
Adult: PO 400 mg loading dose, then 200 mg q24h × 10 days
Renal dose
Adult: PO 400 mg on day 1 if CCr <50 ml/min; then 200 mg qod on days 2-10

Available forms: Tabs 200 mg

Adverse effects
(*italic* = common; **bold** = life-threatening)
CNS: *Headache, dizziness, insomnia*
CV: QT interval prolongation, vasodilation
GI: *Nausea*, flatulence, abdominal pain, **pseudomembranous colitis,** *vomiting*, diarrhea
HEMA: **Leukopenia,** eosinophilia, anemia
INTEG: Rash, pruritus, photosensitivity
SYST: **Anaphylaxis, Stevens-Johnson syndrome**

Contraindications: Hypersensitivity to quinolones, photosensitivity

Precautions: Pregnancy **C,** lactation, children, renal disease, seizure disorder

Pharmacokinetics	
Absorption	Slow-erratic
Distribution	Widely distributed
Metabolism	Liver
Excretion	Kidneys, feces
Half-life	20 hr

Pharmacodynamics	
Unknown	

Interactions
Individual drugs
Amiodarone, bepridil, disopyramide, erythromycin, pentamine: ↑ torsades de pointes
Cyclosporine: ↑ nephrotoxicity
Sucralfate, zinc sulfate: ↓ absorption of sparfloxacin
Theophylline: ↑ theophylline level, toxicity
Warfarin: ↑ warfarin level
Drug classifications
Antacids, iron products: ↓ absorption of sparfloxacin
Antidepressants (tricyclic), antidysrhythmics (class IA/III), phenothiazines: ↑ torsades de pointes

S

Herb/drug
Cola tree: ↑ effect
Lab test interferences
↑ AST, ↑ ALT

NURSING CONSIDERATIONS
Assessment
• Assess patient for previous sensitivity reaction
• Assess patient for signs and symptoms of infection including characteristics of wounds, sputum, urine, stool, WBC >10,000/mm³, fever; obtain baseline information before and monitor during treatment
• Obtain C&S before beginning drug therapy to identify if correct treatment has been initiated
• Assess for allergic reactions, anaphylaxis: rash, urticaria, pruritus, chills, fever, joint pain; may occur a few days after therapy begins; epINEPHrine and resuscitation equipment should be available for anaphylactic reaction
• Identify urine output; if decreasing, notify prescriber (may indicate nephrotoxicity); also check for increased BUN, creatinine
• Monitor blood studies: AST, ALT, CBC, Hct, bilirubin, LDH, alkaline phosphatase, Coombs' test monthly if patient is on long-term therapy
• Assess bowel pattern qd; if severe diarrhea occurs, drug should be discontinued
• Monitor for bleeding: ecchymosis, bleeding gums, hematuria, stool guaiac daily if on long-term therapy
• Assess for overgrowth of infection: perineal itching, fever, malaise, redness, pain, swelling, drainage, rash, diarrhea, change in cough, sputum

Nursing diagnoses
☑ Infection, risk for (uses)
☑ Diarrhea (side effects)
☑ Injury, risk for (side effects)
☑ Knowledge, deficient (teaching)
☑ Noncompliance (teaching)

Implementation
PO route
• Give around the clock to maintain proper blood levels
• Give 4 hr before or after antacids/calcium

IV IV route
• Check for irritation, extravasation, phlebitis daily
• For intermittent inf, dilute to 1-2 mg/ml of D₅W, 0.9% NaCl; give over 60 min; sol will remain stable under refrigeration for 2 wk

Patient/family education
• Advise patient to contact prescriber if vaginal itching, loose foul-smelling stools, furry tongue occur; may indicate superinfection; report itching, rash, pruritus, urticaria
• Instruct patient to take all medication prescribed for the length of time ordered; drug must be taken around the clock to maintain blood levels; do not give medication to others
• Teach patient to avoid direct sunlight or use sunscreen to prevent phototoxicity
• Advise patient to drink plenty of fluids, take 4 hr before or after antacids/calcium
• Advise patient to notify prescriber of diarrhea with blood or pus
• Advise patient to increase fluid intake to 2 L/day to prevent crystalluria
• Advise patient to avoid hazardous activities until response is known
• Advise patient not to use theophylline with this product unless approved by prescriber
• Instruct patient to rinse mouth frequently, use sugarless candy or gum for dry mouth

Evaluation
Positive therapeutic outcome
• Absence of signs/symptoms of infection (WBC <10,000/mm³, temp WNL)
• Reported improvement in symptoms of infection
• C&S negative for organism

spironolactone (Rx)
(speer'on-oh-lak'tone)
Aldactone, Novospiroton ✤
Func. class: Potassium-sparing diuretic
Chem. class.: Aldosterone antagonist
Pregnancy category D

Action: Competes with aldosterone at receptor sites in the distal tubule in the renal system, resulting in excretion of sodium, chloride, water, bicarbonate, and calcium; potassium, phosphate, and hydrogen are retained

→**Therapeutic Outcome:** Diuretic and antihypertensive effect while retaining potassium; lowered aldosterone levels

Uses: Edema of CHF, hypertension, diuretic-induced hypokalemia, primary hyperaldosteronism (diagnosis, short-term treatment, long-term treatment), edema of nephrotic syndrome, cirrhosis of the liver with ascites

Investigational uses: CHF

Dosage and routes
Edema/hypertension
Adult: PO 25-400 mg/qd in single or divided doses

CHF
Adult: PO 12.5-25 mg/day

Edema
P *Child:* PO 3.3 mg/kg/day in single or divided doses

Hypertension
P *Child:* PO 1-2 mg/kg bid

Hypokalemia
Adult: PO 25-100 mg/day; if PO, potassium supplements must not be used

Primary hyperaldosteronism diagnosis
Adult: PO 400 mg/day × 4 days or 4 wk depending on the test, then 100-400 mg/day maintenance

Available forms: Tabs 25, 50, 100 mg

Adverse effects
(*italic* = common; **bold** = life-threatening)
CNS: Headache, confusion, drowsiness, lethargy, ataxia
ELECT: Hyperchloremic metabolic acidosis, **hyperkalemia,** hyponatremia
ENDO: Impotence, gynecomastia, irregular menses, amenorrhea, postmenopausal bleeding, hirsutism, deepening voice
GI: Diarrhea, cramps, bleeding, gastritis, vomiting, anorexia, nausea
HEMA: **Agranulocytosis**
INTEG: *Rash, pruritus,* urticaria

Contraindications: Hypersensitivity, anuria, severe renal disease, hyperkalemia, pregnancy **D**

Precautions: Dehydration, hepatic disease,
G lactation, elderly, renal disease

Pharmacokinetics
Absorption	GI tract; well absorbed
Distribution	Crosses placenta
Metabolism	Liver to canrenone (active metabolite)
Excretion	Renal; breast milk
Half-life	12-24 hr (canrenone)

Pharmacodynamics
Onset	24-48 hr
Peak	48-72 hr
Duration	Unknown

Interactions
Individual drugs
Aspirin: ↓ action of spironolactone
Digoxin: ↑ digoxin action
Lithium: ↑ action, toxicity

Drug classifications
ACE inhibitors, diuretics (potassium-sparing), potassium products, salt substitute: ↑ hyperkalemia
Anticoagulants: ↓ effects of anticoagulants
Antihypertensives: ↑ action

Herb/drug
Bearberry, gossypol: Hypokalemia
Cucumber, dandelion, horsetail, licorice nettle, pumpkin, Queen Anne's lace: ↑ effect
Khella: ↑ hypotension
St. John's wort: severe photosensitivity
Arginine: Fatal hypokalemia

Lab test interferences
False: ↑ Urinary catecholamines
Interference: Glucose, insulin tolerance tests

NURSING CONSIDERATIONS
Assessment
• Monitor for manifestations of hyperkalemia: *MS:* fatigue, muscle weakness; *CV:* arrhythmias, hypotension, *NEURO:* paresthesias, confusion, *RESP:* dyspnea
• Monitor for manifestations of hyponatremia: *CV:* ↑ B/P, cold, clammy skin, hypo- or hypervolemia; *GI:* anorexia, nausea, vomiting, diarrhea, abdominal cramps; *NEURO:* lethargy, increased ICP, confusion, headache, seizures, coma, fatigue, tremors, hyperreflexia
• Monitor for manifestations of hyperchloremia: *NEURO:* weakness, lethargy, coma; *RESP:* deep rapid breathing
• Assess fluid volume status: I&O ratios and record, count or weigh diapers as appropriate, weight, distended red veins, crackles in lung, color, quality, and sp gr of urine, skin turgor, adequacy of pulses, moist mucous membranes, bilateral lung sounds, peripheral pitting edema; dehydration symptoms of decreasing output, thirst, hypotension, dry mouth and mucous membranes should be reported
• Monitor electrolytes: potassium, sodium, calcium, magnesium; also include BUN, ABGs, uric acid, CBC, blood glucose

Nursing diagnoses
✓ Urinary elimination, impaired (adverse reactions)
✓ Fluid volume, deficient (adverse reactions)
✓ Fluid volume, excess (uses)
✓ Knowledge, deficient (teaching)

Implementation
• Give in AM to avoid interference with sleep
• With food, if nausea occurs, absorption may be increased; take at same time each day

S

Patient/family education

- Teach patient to take medication early in day to prevent nocturia
- Instruct patient to take with food or milk if GI symptoms of nausea and anorexia occur
- Teach patient to maintain a record of weight on a weekly basis and notify prescriber of weight loss of >5 lb
- Caution patient that this drug causes an increase in potassium levels, that foods high in potassium should be avoided; refer to dietitian for assistance planning
- Teach patient not to use alcohol, or any OTC medications without prescriber's approval; serious drug reactions may occur
- Emphasize the need to contact prescriber immediately if muscle cramps, weakness, nausea, dizziness, or numbness occurs
- Teach patient to take own B/P and pulse and record
- Advise patient that dizziness and confusion may occur; avoid driving or other hazardous activities if alertness is decreased
- Teach patient to continue taking medication even if feeling better; this drug controls symptoms but does not cure the condition
- Advise patient with hypertension to continue other treatment (exercise, weight loss, relaxation techniques, cessation of smoking)

Evaluation

Positive therapeutic outcome
- Prevention of hypokalemia (diuretic use)
- Decreased edema
- Decreased B/P
- Decreased aldosterone levels
- Increased diuresis

Treatment of overdose:

- Lavage if taken orally, monitor electrolytes
- Administer sodium bicarbonate
- Monitor hydration, CV, renal status

---

stavudine (Rx)

(sta'vu-deen)
d4T, Zerit
Func. class.: Antiretroviral
Chem. class.: nucleoside reverse transcriptase inhibitor

Pregnancy category C

Action: Prevents replication of HIV by the inhibition of the enzyme reverse transcriptase

➔ **Therapeutic Outcome:** Decreasing diarrhea, fatigue, night sweats; increased body weight

Uses: Treatment of HIV-1; used in combination with other antiretrovirals

Dosage and routes

Adult >60 kg: PO 1 40 mg q12h up to 2 mg/kg/day

Adult <60 kg: 30 mg q12h

P *Child <30 kg:* PO 1 mg/kg q12h

P *Child ≥30 kg ≤60 kg:* PO 30 mg q12h

P *Child >60 kg:* PO 40 mg q12h

Renal dose
Adult >60 kg: CCr 26-50 ml/min 20 mg q12h; CCr 10-25 ml/min 20 mg q24h

Adult <60 kg: CCr 26-50 ml/min 15 mg q12h; CCr 10-25 ml/min 15 mg q24h

Available forms: Caps 15, 20, 30, 40 mg; oral powder for sol 1 mg/ml

Adverse effects

(*italic* = common; **bold** = life-threatening)
CNS: *Peripheral neuropathy,* headache, chills/fever, malaise
GI: **Hepatotoxicity,** diarrhea, nausea, vomiting, anorexia, dyspepsia, constipation, stomatitis, **pancreatitis**
HEMA: **Bone marrow suppression,** anemia
INTEG: Rash, sweating, pruritus, benign neoplasms
RESP: Dyspnea, pneumonia, asthma
EENT: Conjunctivitis, abnormal vision
CV: Chest pain, vasodilatation, hypertension
MISC: **Lactic acidosis**
MS: Myalgia, arthralgia

Contraindications: Hypersensitivity to this drug or zidovudine, didanosine, zalcitabine; severe peripheral neuropathy

Precautions: Advanced HIV infections, pregnancy **C**, lactation, bone marrow suppression, renal disease, liver disease, peripheral neuropathy

Pharmacokinetics

Absorption	Rapidly absorbed, 82% bioavailability
Distribution	Cerebrospinal fluid
Metabolism	Unknown
Excretion	Kidneys, breast milk
Half-life	Elimination: 1-1.6 hr, intracellular: 3-3.5 hr

Pharmacodynamics

Onset	Unknown
Peak	1 hr
Duration	Unknown

 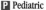

Interactions
Individual drugs
Chloramphenicol, dapsone, didanosine, ethambutol, hydrALAZINE, lithium, phenytoin, vinCRIStine, zalcitabine: ↑ peripheral neuropathy
Drug classifications
Myelosuppressants: ↑ myelosuppressor

NURSING CONSIDERATIONS
Assessment
⚠• Assess for lactic acidosis and severe hepatomegaly with steatosis; death may result
• Monitor viral load and CD4 counts baseline and throughout treatment
• Monitor for peripheral neuropathy: tingling, pain in extremities; if these occur discontinue drug
• Monitor for pancreatitis: severe upper abdominal pain, nausea, vomiting throughout treatment; if these occur discontinue drug
• Monitor blood studies: WBC, differential, RBC, Hct, Hgb, platelets
• Monitor renal studies: urinalysis, protein, blood
• Obtain C&S before drug therapy; drug may be taken as soon as culture is performed; repeat C&S after therapy
• Monitor bowel pattern before, during treatment
• Monitor fluid overload; drug requires large volume to stay in sol
• Assess for weakness, tremors, confusion, dizziness, psychosis; if these occur, drug may have to be decreased or discontinued

Nursing diagnoses
✓ Infection, risk for (uses)
✓ Knowledge, deficient (teaching)

Implementation
• Give with or without meals; absorption does not appear to be lowered when taken with food

Patient/family education
• Teach patient signs of peripheral neuropathy: burning, weakness, pain, pricking feeling in the extremities
• Caution patient that this drug should not be given with antineoplastics
• Inform patient that GI complaints and insomnia resolve after 3-4 wk of treatment
• Inform patient that drug is not a cure for AIDS, but will control symptoms
• Advise patient to call prescriber if sore throat, swollen lymph nodes, malaise, fever occur; may indicate presence of other infections
• Caution patient that even with drug adminis-tration, virus is still infective and may be passed on to others
• Caution patient that follow-up visits must be continued because serious toxicity may occur; blood counts must be done q2 wk
• Teach patient that drug must be taken q4h around the clock even during night
• Caution patient that serious drug interactions with other medications may occur, check with prescriber first if taking chloramphenicol, dapsone, cisplatin, didanosine, ethambutol, lithium, antifungals, antineoplastics
• Inform patient that other drugs may be necessary to prevent other infections
• Inform patient that drug may cause fainting or dizziness

Evaluation
Positive therapeutic outcome
• Decreased symptoms of HIV infection

! HIGH ALERT

streptokinase ⚠ (Rx)
(strep-toe-kye'nase)
Kabikinase, Streptase
Func. class.: Thrombolytic enzyme
Chem. class.: β-Hemolytic *Streptococcus* filtrate (purified)
Pregnancy category C

Action: Activates conversion of plasminogen to plasmin (fibrinolysin): plasmin breaks down clots (fibrin), fibrinogen, factors V, VII; occlusion of venous access lines

➡ **Therapeutic Outcome:** Lysis of emboli, or thrombosis in various parts of the body

Uses: Deep vein thrombosis (DVT), pulmonary embolism, arterial thrombosis, arterial embolism, arteriovenous cannula occlusion, lysis of coronary artery thrombi after MI, acute evolving transmural MI

Dosage and routes
Lysis of coronary artery thrombi
Adult: **IV** inf 20,000 international units, then 2000 international units/min over 1 hr

Arteriovenous cannula occlusion
Adult: **IV** inf 250,000 international units/2 ml sol into occluded limb of cannula run over ½ hr; clamp for 2 hr; aspirate contents; flush with NaCl sol and reconnect

Thrombosis/embolism/DVT/ pulmonary embolism
Adult: **IV** inf 250,000 international units over ½ hr, then 100,000 international units/hr for 72 hr for deep thrombosis; 100,000 interna-

S

---

tional units/hr over 24-72 hr for pulmonary embolism; 100,000 international units/hr × 24-72 hr for arterial thrombosis or embolism

Acute evolving transmural MI
Adult: IV inf 1,500,000 international units diluted to a volume of 45 ml; give within 1 hr; intracoronary inf 20,000 international units by bol, then 2000 international units/min × 1 hr, total dose 140,000 international units

Available forms: Powder for inj, lyophilized 250,000, 600,000, 750,000, 1,500,000 international units vial

Adverse effects
(*italic* = common; **bold** = life-threatening)
CNS: Headache, fever
CV: **Dysrhythmias,** hypotension, noncardiogenic pulmonary edema, **pulmonary embolism**
EENT: Periorbital edema
GI: Nausea
HEMA: Decreased Hct, **bleeding**
INTEG: Rash, urticaria, phlebitis at infusion site, itching, flushing
MS: Low back pain
RESP: Altered respirations, shortness of breath, **bronchospasm**
SYST: **GI, GU, intracranial retroperitoneal bleeding, surface bleeding, anaphylaxis**

Contraindications: Hypersensitivity, active internal bleeding, intraspinal surgery, CNS, neoplasms, uncontrolled severe hypertension, recent CVA, intracranial, intrapleural surgery

Precautions: Arterial emboli from left side of heart, pregnancy **C,** ulcerative colitis, enteritis, severe renal disease, hepatic disease, hypocoagulation, COPD, subacute bacterial endocarditis, rheumatic valvular disease, cerebral embolism/thrombosis/hemorrhage, intraarterial diagnostic procedure or surgery (10 days), recent major surgery

Pharmacokinetics
Absorption	Completely absorbed
Distribution	Unknown
Metabolism	>80%—liver, rapidly cleared by reticuloendothelial system
Excretion	Kidneys
Half-life	35 min

Pharmacodynamics
Onset	Immediate
Peak	Rapid
Duration	<12 hr

Interaction
Individual drugs
Abciximab, aspirin, clopidogrel, dipyridamole, eptifibatide, indomethacin, phenylbutazone, plicamycin, tirofiban, ticlopidine, valproic acid: ↑ bleeding risk
Drug classifications
Anticoagulants (oral), cephalosporins, glycoprotein IIb/IIIa inhibitors, NSAIDs: ↑ bleeding risk
Lab test interferences
↑ Pro-time, ↑ APTT, ↑ TT
↓ Plasminogen, ↓ fibrinogen

NURSING CONSIDERATIONS
Assessment
• Monitor VS, B/P, pulse, respirations (including peripheral), neurologic signs, temp at least q4h; temp >104° F (40° C) indicates internal bleeding; monitor rhythm closely; ventricular dysrhythmias may occur with hyperfusion; monitor heart, breath sounds, neurologic status, peripheral pulses

◆• Assess for bleeding during first hr of treatment: hematuria, hematemesis, bleeding from mucous membranes, epistaxis, ecchymosis; guaiac; all body fluids, stools; may require transfusion (rare); blood studies (Hct, platelets, PTT, Pro-time, TT, APTT) before starting therapy; Pro-time or APTT must be less than 2 × control before starting therapy; TT or Pro-time q3-4h during treatment

• Assess allergy: fever, rash, itching, chills; mild reaction may be treated with antihistamines; report to prescriber

• Monitor ECG on monitor, watch for segment changes, changes in rhythm; sinus bradycardia, ventricular tachycardia, accelerated idioventricular rhythm may occur as a result of reperfusion (coronary thrombosis); cardiac enzymes, radionuclide myocardial scanning/coronary angiography

• Monitor ABGs, respiratory rate (depth, characteristics), pulse, B/P, hemodynamics (pulmonary embolism)

• Monitor peripheral pulses, assess Homan's sign, check for redness, swelling qh; notify prescriber of changes; B/P should not be taken in extremities (deep vein thrombosis)

• Check catheter for ability to aspirate blood from port; patient must exhale and hold breath when inserting and removing syringe to prevent air embolism (catheter/cannula occlusion)

• Assess for Guillain-Barré syndrome that may occur after treatment with this drug

• Assess for respiratory depression

Nursing diagnoses
✓ Tissue perfusion, ineffective (uses)
✓ Injury, risk for (adverse reactions)
✓ Gas exchange, impaired (uses)
✓ Knowledge, deficient (teaching)

Implementation
• Give after reconstituting with provided diluent; add appropriate amount of sterile water for inj (no preservatives) 20-mg vial/20 ml or 50 mg-vial/50 ml to make 1 mg/ml, mix by slow inversion or dilute with NaCl, D_5W to a concentration of 0.5 mg/ml; further dilution, 1.5-<0.5 mg/ml may result in precipitation of drug; use 18-G needle; flush line with NaCl after administration; reconstituted **IV** sol within 8 hr; within 6 hr of coronary occlusion for best results
• Give **IV** loading dose over 30 min to avoid hypotension
• Give **IV** over 1 hr after dilution with 4-5 g/250 ml of 0.9% NaCl, D_5W, LR; may give by continuous inf after loading dose(s) of 1 g/hr diluted in 50-100 ml of compatible sol; use infusion pump; do not give by direct **IV**
• Give heparin therapy after thrombolytic therapy is discontinued, TT, ACT, or APTT less than 2 × control (about 3-4 hr); **IV** heparin with loading dose is recommended after discontinuing streptokinase to prevent redevelopment of thrombis
• Avoid invasive procedures, injection, taking temp via rectal route
• Apply pressure for 30 sec to minor bleeding sites; 30 min to sites of atrial puncture, followed by pressure dressing; inform prescriber if this does not attain hemostasis; apply pressure dressing
• Store powder at room temp or refrigerate; protect from excessive light

Y-site compatibilities: Dobutamine, DOPamine, heparin, lidocaine, nitroglycerin

Additive incompatibilities: Do not mix with other medications

Patient/family education
• Teach patient reason for medication, signs and symptoms of bleeding, allergic reactions, when to notify prescriber
• Explain that patient is to continue bed rest to avoid injury

Evaluation
Positive therapeutic outcome
• Lysis of thrombi or emboli

---

streptomycin (Rx)
(strep-toe-mye′sin)
Func. class.: Antiinfective, antitubercular
Chem. class.: Aminoglycoside
Pregnancy category D

Action: Interferes with protein synthesis in bacterial cell by binding to ribosomal subunit, causing inaccurate peptide sequence to form in protein chain, resulting in bacterial death

▶ **Therapeutic Outcome:** Bactericidal effects for the following organisms: sensitive strains of *Mycobacterium tuberculosis,* nontuberculous infections caused by sensitive strains of *Yersinia pestis, Brucella, Haemophilus influenzae, Klebsiella pneumoniae, Escherichia coli, Enterobacter aerogenes, Streptococcus viridans, Francisella tularensis, Proteus*

Uses: Active TB; used in combination for streptococcal and enterococcal infections; endocarditis, tularemia, plague

Dosage and routes
Tuberculosis
Adult: IM 15 mg/kg (max 1 g) qd × 2-3 mo, then 1 g 2-3 ×/wk given with other antitubercular drugs

P *Child:* IM 20-40 mg/kg/day in divided doses given with other antitubercular drugs; max 15 mg/kg/day

Streptococcal endocarditis
Adult: IM 1 g q12h × 1 wk with penicillin, then 500 mg bid × 1 wk

Enterococcal endocarditis
Adult: IM 1 g q12h × 2 wk, then 500 mg q12h × 4 wk with penicillin, max 15 mg/kg/day

Available forms: Inj 500 mg, 1 g/ml

Adverse effects
(*italic* = common; **bold** = life-threatening)
CNS: Confusion, dizziness, depression, numbness, tremors, **seizures,** muscle twitching, **neurotoxicity**
CV: Hypotension, myocarditis, palpitations
EENT: *Ototoxicity,* tinnitus, deafness, visual disturbances
GI: Nausea, vomiting, anorexia, increased ALT, AST, bilirubin, hepatomegaly, **hepatic necrosis,** splenomegaly
GU: **Oliguria, hematuria, renal damage, azotemia, renal failure, nephrotoxicity**
HEMA: **Agranulocytosis, thrombocytopenia, leukopenia, eosinophilia, anemia**

S

INTEG: *Rash,* burning, urticaria, dermatitis, alopecia

Contraindications: Severe renal disease, hypersensitivity, pregnancy **D**

P **Precautions:** Neonates, mild renal disease, myasthenia gravis, lactation, hearing deficits, **G** elderly, Parkinson's disease

Pharmacokinetics

Absorption	Well absorbed
Distribution	Widely distributed in extracellular fluids, poorly distributed in CSF; crosses placenta
Metabolism	Minimal—liver
Excretion	Mostly unchanged (>90%) kidneys
Half-life	2-2½ hr, increase in renal disease

Pharmacodynamics

Onset	Rapid
Peak	1-2 hr

Interactions
Individual drugs
Amphotericin B, bacitracin, cisplatin, ethacrynic acid, furosemide, mannitol, methoxyflurane, polymyxin, vancomycin: ↑ ototoxicity, neurotoxicity, nephrotoxicity
Succinylcholine, warfarin: ↑ effects of each specific drug
Drug classifications
Aminoglycosides, cephalosporins: ↑ ototoxicity, neurotoxicity, nephrotoxicity
Nondepolarizing neuromuscular blockers: ↑ effects of nondepolarizing muscle relaxants

NURSING CONSIDERATIONS
Assessment
• Assess patient for previous sensitivity reaction
• Assess patient for signs and symptoms of infection including characteristics of sputum, urine, stool WBC >10,000/mm³, temp
• Obtain baseline information before and during treatment
• Complete C&S testing before and after drug therapy to identify if correct treatment has been initiated
• Assess for allergic reactions: rash, urticaria, pruritus, chills, fever, joint pain; angioedema may occur a few days after therapy begins; epINEPHrine, resuscitation equipment should be available for anaphylactic reaction
• Identify urine output; if decreasing, notify prescriber (may indicate nephrotoxicity); also

increased BUN, creatinine, urine CCr <80 ml/min
• Monitor blood studies: AST, ALT, CBC, Hct, bilirubin, LDH, alkaline phosphatase, Coombs' test monthly if patient is on long-term therapy
• Monitor electrolytes: potassium, sodium, chloride, magnesium monthly if patient is on long-term therapy
• Monitor for bleeding: ecchymosis, bleeding gums, hematuria, stool guaiac daily if on long-term therapy
• Assess for overgrowth of infection: perineal itching, fever, malaise, redness, pain, swelling, drainage, rash, diarrhea, change in cough, sputum
• Obtain weight before treatment; calculation of dosage is usually based on ideal body weight, but may be calculated on actual body weight
• Monitor I&O ratio; urinalysis daily for proteinuria, cells, casts; report sudden change in urine output
• Obtain serum peak 60 min after IM inj, trough level obtained just before next dose; blood level should be 2-4 × bacteriostatic level
• Monitor for deafness by audiometric testing, ringing, roaring in ears, vertigo; assess hearing before, during, after treatment
• Monitor for dehydration: high sp gr, decrease in skin turgor, dry mucous membranes, dark urine

Nursing diagnoses
☑ Infection, risk for (uses)
☑ Diarrhea (adverse reactions)
☑ Injury, risk for (adverse reactions)
☑ Knowledge, deficient (teaching)
☑ Noncompliance (teaching)

Implementation
• Give deeply in large muscle mass
• Reconstitute with 4.2-4.5 ml of sterile water for inj or 0.9% NaCl/1 g (200 mg/ml), 3.2-3.5 ml/1 g (250 mg/ml), 17 ml/5 g (250 mg/ml); give at 500 mg/ml or less

Syringe compatibilities: Penicillin G sodium

Syringe incompatibilities: Heparin

Y-site compatibilities: Esmolol

Additive compatibilities: Bleomycin

Patient/family education
• Teach patient to report sore throat, bruising, bleeding, joint pain, may indicate blood dyscrasias (rare); ringing, roaring in the ears

---

- Advise patient to contact prescriber if vaginal itching, loose foul-smelling stools, furry tongue occur; may indicate superinfection

Evaluation
Positive therapeutic outcome
- Absence of signs/symptoms of infection
- Reported improvement in symptoms of infection

Treatment of overdose: Withdraw drug, hemodialysis, monitor serum levels of drug, may give ticarcillin or carbenicillin

---

succimer (Rx)
(sux′i-mer)
Chemet
Func. class: Heavy metal antagonist
Chem. class.: Chelating agent

Pregnancy category C

Action: Binds with ions of lead to form a water-soluble complex that is excreted by kidneys

➡ **Therapeutic Outcome:** Removal of lead from the body

▣ **Uses:** Lead poisoning in children with lead levels above 45 mcg/dl; may be beneficial in mercury, arsenic poisoning

Dosage and routes
▣ *Child:* PO 10 mg/kg or 350 mg/m^2 q8h × 5 days, then 10 mg/kg or 350 mg/m^2 q12h × 2 wk; another course may be required depending on lead levels; allow 2 wk between courses

Available forms: Caps 100 mg

Adverse effects
(*italic* = common; **bold** = life-threatening)
CNS: Drowsiness, dizziness, paresthesia, sensorimotor neuropathy
EENT: Otitis media, watery eyes, film in eyes, plugged ears
GI: Nausea, vomiting, diarrhea, metallic taste, anorexia
GU: **Proteinuria,** decreased urination, voiding difficulties
HEMA: **Increased platelets, intermittent eosinophilia**
INTEG: Rash, urticaria, pruritus
META: Increased AST, ALT, alkaline phosphatase, cholesterol
RESP: Sore throat, rhinorrhea, nasal congestion, cough
SYST: Back, stomach, head, rib, flank pain; abdominal cramps; chills; fever; flulike symptoms, head cold; headache

Contraindications: Hypersensitivity

Precautions: Pregnancy **C**, lactation,
▣ children <1 yr

Pharmacokinetics
Absorption	Rapidly absorbed
Distribution	Unknown
Metabolism	Liver—extensively
Excretion	Kidneys—unchanged
Half-life	2 days

Pharmacodynamics
Onset	Up to 2 hr
Peak	2-4 hr
Duration	8-12 hr

Interactions
Drug classifications
Heavy metal antagonist, others: Do not use together

NURSING CONSIDERATIONS
Assessment
- Assess VS, B/P, pulse, respirations, weigh daily
- Monitor I&O ratio, kidney function studies, BUN, creatinine, CCr; watch for decreasing urine output
- Assess neurologic status: watch for paresthesias, beginning of seizures
- Monitor urine: pH, albumin, casts, blood, coproporphyrins, calcium
- Assess for febrile reactions that may occur 4-8 hr after drug therapy
- Monitor for cardiac abnormalities: dysrhythmias, hypotension, tachycardia
- Assess for allergic reactions (rash, urticaria); if these occur, drug should be discontinued

Nursing diagnoses
☑ Poisoning, risk for (uses)
☑ Injury, risk for (uses, adverse reactions)
☑ Knowledge, deficient (teaching)

Implementation
- Give PO whole or cap contents mixed with food or fluid

Patient/family education
- Explain reason for medication and expected results
- Provide a referral to health department to assess lead levels in home or workplace
- Teach patient to increase fluid intake

S

Evaluation
Positive therapeutic outcome
- Decreased symptoms of lead intoxication
- Decreased lead level <50 mcg/dl

! HIGH ALERT

succinylcholine (Rx)
(suk-sin-ill-koe'leen)
Anectine, Anectine Flo-Pack, Quelicin,
succinylcholine chloride, Sucostrin,
Suxamethonium
Func. class.: Neuromuscular blocker
(depolarizing—ultra short)

Pregnancy category C

Action: Inhibits transmission of nerve
impulses by binding with cholinergic receptor
sites, antagonizing action of acetylcholine;
causes release of histamine

➡ **Therapeutic Outcome:** Paralysis of
skeletal muscles

Uses: Facilitation of endotracheal intubation,
skeletal muscle relaxation during orthopedic
manipulations

Dosage and routes
Adult: IV 0.6 mg/kg, then 2.5 mg/min as
needed; IM 2.5 mg/kg, max 150 mg

P *Child:* IV/IM 1-2 mg/kg, max 150 mg IM

Available forms: Inj 20, 50, 100 mg/ml;
powder for inj 100/vial; powder for inf 500
mg/vial, 1 g/vial

Adverse effects
(*italic* = common; **bold** = life-threatening)
CV: Bradycardia, tachycardia; increased,
decreased B/P, **sinus arrest, dysrhythmias**
EENT: Increased secretions, increased intra-
ocular pressure
HEMA: Myoglobulinemia
INTEG: Rash, flushing, pruritus, urticaria
MS: Weakness, muscle pain, fasciculation,
prolonged relaxation
RESP: **Prolonged apnea, bronchospasm,
cyanosis, respiratory depression**

Contraindications: Hypersensitivity,
malignant hyperthermia, decreased plasma
pseudocholinesterase, penetrating eye injuries,
acute narrow-angle glaucoma

Precautions: Pregnancy **C**, cardiac disease,
severe burns, fractures (fasciculation may
P increase damage), lactation, children <2 yr,
electrolyte imbalances, dehydration, neuromuscular disease, respiratory disease, collagen
diseases, glaucoma, eye surgery, penetrating
G eye wounds, elderly or debilitated patients

Pharmacokinetics
Absorption	Well absorbed (IM)
Distribution	Widely distributed, crosses placenta
Metabolism	Plasma (90%)
Excretion	Hydrolyzed in urine (active/inactive metabolites)
Half-life	Unknown

Pharmacodynamics
	IV	IM
Onset	1 min	2-3 min
Peak	2-3 min	Unknown
Duration	6-10 min	10-30 min

Interactions
Individual drugs
Clindamycin, enflurane, isoflurane, lincomycin, lithium, oxytocin, quinidine: ↑ neuromuscular blockade
Theophylline: Dysrhythmias
Drug classifications
Aminoglycosides, anesthetics (local), antibiotics (polymyxin), β-adrenergic blockers,
diuretics (potassium-losing), magnesium salts,
opioids, thiazides: ↑ neuromuscular blockade
Herb/drug
Melatonin: blocks succinylcholine

NURSING CONSIDERATIONS
Assessment
- Assess for electrolyte imbalances (potassium, magnesium); may lead to increased
action of this drug
- Monitor VS (B/P, pulse, respirations, airway) until fully recovered; rate, depth, pattern
of respirations, strength of hand grip
- Monitor I&O ratio; check for urinary
retention, frequency, hesitancy
- Assess for recovery: decreased paralysis of
face, diaphragm, leg, arm, rest of body
- Assess for allergic reactions: rash, fever,
respiratory distress, pruritus; drug should be
discontinued if these occur

Nursing diagnoses
☑ Communication, impaired verbal (adverse
reactions)
☑ Breathing pattern, ineffective (uses)

Implementation
IV **IV route**
- Use nerve stimulator by anesthesiologist to
determine neuromuscular blockade
- Give anticholinesterase to reverse neuro-
muscular blockade

- Give by **IV** inf; dilute 1-2 mg/ml in D₅, isotonic saline sol, give 0.5-10 mg/min, titrate to patient response; may be given directly over 1 min

Syringe compatibilities: Heparin

Y-site compatibilities: Etomidate, heparin, potassium chloride, propofol, vit B/C

Additive compatibilities: Amikacin, cephapirin, isoproterenol, meperidine, methyldopate, morphine, norepinephrine, scopolamine

Additive incompatibilities: Barbiturates, nafcillin, sodium bicarbonate

IM route
- Give inj deep IM, preferably high in deltoid muscle
- Store in refrigerator; store powder at room temp; close container tightly

Patient/family education
- Explain reason for medication and expected results
- Provide reassurance if communication is difficult during recovery from neuromuscular blockade; postoperative stiffness is normal, soon subsides

Evaluation
Positive therapeutic outcome
- Paralysis of jaw, eyelid, head, neck, rest of body

Treatment of overdose: Edrophonium or neostigmine, atropine, monitor VS; may require mechanical ventilation

---

sucralfate (Rx)
(soo-kral'fate)
Carafate, Sulcrate ♣
Func. class.: Protectant; antiulcer
Chem. class.: Aluminum hydroxide/sulfated sucrose

Pregnancy category B

Action: Forms a complex that adheres to ulcer site, adsorbs pepsin

➔ **Therapeutic Outcome:** Healing of ulcers

Uses: Duodenal ulcer, oral mucositis, stomatitis after radiation of head and neck

Investigational uses: Gastric ulcers, gastroesophageal reflux

Dosage and routes
Ulcers
Adult: PO 1 g qid 1 hr ac, hs

P *Child:* PO 40-80 mg/kg/day

Prevention of ulcers
Adult: PO 1 g bid, 1 hr ac

Gastroesophageal reflux disease (GERD)
Adult: PO 1 g qid 1 hr ac and hs

P *Child:* PO 500 mg-1g qid, 1 hr ac and hs

Available forms: Tabs 1 g; oral susp 500 mg/5 ml

Adverse effects
(*italic* = common; **bold** = life-threatening)
CNS: Drowsiness, dizziness
GI: Dry mouth, constipation, nausea, gastric pain, vomiting
INTEG: Urticaria, rash, pruritus

Contraindications: Hypersensitivity

Precautions: Pregnancy **B**, lactation,
P children, renal failure

⚠ Do Not Confuse:
Carafate/Cafergot

Pharmacokinetics
Absorption	Minimally absorbed
Distribution	Unknown
Metabolism	Not metabolized
Excretion	Feces (90%)
Half-life	6-20 hr

Pharmacodynamics
Onset	½ hr
Peak	Unknown
Duration	6 hr

Interactions
Individual drugs
Cimetidine, digoxin, ketoconazole, phenytoin, ranitidine, tetracycline, theophylline: ↓ action of each specific drug

Drug classifications
Antacids: ↓ absorption of sucralfate
Fat-soluble vitamins: ↓ action of fat-soluble vitamins
Fluoroquinolones: ↓ absorption

NURSING CONSIDERATIONS
Assessment
- Monitor gastric pH (>5 should be maintained); blood in stools

S

Nursing diagnoses
☑ Pain, chronic (uses)
☑ Pain, acute (uses)
☑ Constipation (adverse reactions)
☑ Knowledge, deficient (teaching)

Implementation
- Give on empty stomach 1 hr ac and hs
🚫 • Do not crush, chew tabs
- Store at room temp

Patient/family education
- Instruct patient to take medication on empty stomach
- Caution patient to take full course of therapy, not to use over 8 wk, to avoid smoking
- Caution patient to avoid antacids within ½ hr of drug or 1 hr after this drug

Evaluation
Positive therapeutic outcome
- Absence of pain or GI complaints

---

sulfamethoxazole
See also trimethoprim/sulfamethoxazole

---

sulfamethoxazole (Rx)
(sul-fa-meth-ox'a-zole)
Apo-Sulfamethoxazole ✤, Gantanol, Urobak
Func. class.: Antiinfective
Chem. class.: Sulfonamide, intermediate-acting

Pregnancy category C

Action: Interferes with bacterial biosynthesis of proteins by competitive antagonism of *p*-aminobenzoic acid (PABA)

➡ **Therapeutic Outcome:** Bactericidal action against susceptible organisms: streptococci and staphylococci, *Clostridium perfringens, Clostridium tetani, Nocardia asteroides;* gram-negative pathogens, including *Enterobacter, Escherichia coli, Klebsiella, Proteus mirabilis, Proteus vulgaris, Salmonella, Shigella*

Uses: UTIs, chancroid, inclusion conjunctivitis, malaria, meningococcal meningitis, nocardiosis, acute otitis media, toxoplasmosis, trachoma

Dosage and routes
Adult: PO 2 g, then 1 g bid or tid for 7-10 days

🅿 *Child >2 mo:* PO 50-60 mg/kg then 25-30 mg/kg × 1 dose bid, max 75 mg/kg/day

Renal dose
Adult: PO CCr <50 ml/min 50% of dose

Available forms: Tabs 500 mg; oral susp 500 mg/5 ml

Adverse effects
(*italic* = common; **bold** = life-threatening)
CNS: Headache, insomnia, hallucinations, depression, vertigo, fatigue, anxiety, seizures, drug fever, chills, drowsiness
CV: **Allergic myocarditis**
GI: Nausea, vomiting, abdominal pain, stomatitis, **hepatitis**, glossitis, **pancreatitis,** diarrhea, **enterocolitis**, anorexia
GU: **Renal failure, toxic nephrosis,** increased BUN, creatinine, crystalluria, hematuria, proteinuria
HEMA: **Leukopenia, thrombocytopenia, agranulocytosis, hemolytic anemia, aplastic anemia**
INTEG: Rash, dermatitis, urticaria, erythema, photosensitivity, alopecia
SYST: **Anaphylaxis, Stevens-Johnson syndrome**

Contraindications: Hypersensitivity to sulfonamides, sulfonylureas, thiazide and loop diuretics, salicylates, sunscreen with PABA, 🅿 lactation, infants <2 mo (except congenital toxoplasmosis), pregnancy at term, porphyria, G6PD deficiency

Precautions: Pregnancy **C**, lactation, impaired hepatic/renal function, severe allergy, bronchial asthma

Pharmacokinetics	
Absorption	Well absorbed
Distribution	Widely distributed, crosses placenta
Metabolism	Liver, large amounts
Excretion	Unchanged kidneys (20%), enters breast milk
Half-life	7-12 hr

Pharmacodynamics	
Onset	1 hr
Peak	3-4 hr

Interactions
Individual drugs
Cyclosporine: ↑ nephrotoxicity
Indomethacin, probenecid: ↑ drug-free concentrations
Methotrexate: ↓ renal excretion of methotrexate
Phenytoin: ↓ hepatic clearance of phenytoin
Warfarin: ↑ anticoagulant effect

Drug classifications
Barbiturates, uricosuric agents: ↑ effects
Diuretics (thiazide): ↑ thrombocytopenia
Salicylates: ↑ drug-free concentrations
Sulfonylurea agents: ↑ hypoglycemic response

Lab test interferences
False positive: Urinary glucose test Benedict's method

NURSING CONSIDERATIONS
Assessment
• Assess patient for previous sensitivity reaction
• Assess patient for signs and symptoms of infection including characteristics of wounds, sputum, urine, stool, WBC >10,000/mm³, elevated temp; obtain baseline information before and during treatment
• Complete C&S studies before beginning drug therapy to identify if correct treatment has been initiated
• Assess for allergic reactions: rash, urticaria, pruritus, chills, fever, joint pain; angioedema may occur a few days after therapy begins; epINEPHrine, resuscitation equipment should be on unit for anaphylactic reaction; AIDS patients are more susceptible
• Monitor blood studies: CBC, Hct, bilirubin, alkaline phosphatase monthly if patient is on long-term therapy
• Monitor for bleeding: ecchymosis, bleeding gums, hematuria, stool guaiac daily if patient is on long-term therapy
• Assess for overgrowth of infection: perineal itching, fever, malaise, redness, pain, swelling, drainage, rash, diarrhea, change in cough, sputum

Nursing diagnoses
✓ Infection, risk for (uses)
✓ Diarrhea (adverse reactions)
✓ Injury, risk for (adverse reactions)
✓ Knowledge, deficient (teaching)
✓ Noncompliance (teaching)

Implementation
• Give around the clock to maintain proper blood levels; give on empty stomach to increase absorption of drug; do not give within 3 hr of other agents, drug actions may occur
• Give with 8 oz of water to prevent crystalluria

Patient/family education
• Teach patient to report sore throat, bruising, bleeding, joint pain; may indicate blood dyscrasias (rare)
• Advise patient to contact prescriber if vaginal itching, loose foul-smelling stools, furry tongue occur; may indicate super-

infection; report itching, rash, pruritus, urticaria
• Instruct patient to take all medication prescribed for the length of time ordered; drug must be taken around the clock to maintain blood levels; do not give medication to others

Evaluation
Positive therapeutic outcome
• Absence of signs/symptoms of infection (WBC <10,000/mm³, temp WNL, absence of urinary pain, hematuria)
• Reported improvement in symptoms of infection
• Negative C&S

---

sulfasalazine (Rx)
(sul-fa-sal′a-zeen)
Azulfidine, Azulfidine EN-tabs, PMS-Sulfasalazine ✦, S.A.S. ✦, Salazopyrin ✦, sulfasalazine
Func. class.: GI Antiinflammatory, antirheumatic (DMARD)
Chem. class.: GI Sulfonamide

Pregnancy category C

Action: Prodrug to deliver sulfapyridine and 5-aminosalicylic acid to colon; antinflammatory in connective tissue

→ **Therapeutic Outcome:** Treatment of ulcerative colitis, rheumatoid arthritis

Uses: Ulcerative colitis, rheumatoid arthritis (delayed rel tab) in patients who inadequately respond to or are intolerant of analgesics/NSAIDs, juvenile rheumatoid arthritis (Azulfidine EN-tabs)

Investigational uses: Ankylosing spondylitis, Crohn's disease, psoriasis

Dosage and routes
Bowel disease
Adult: PO 3-4 g/day in divided doses; maintenance 2 g/day in divided doses q6h

Child >2 yr: PO 40-60 mg/kg/day in 4-6 divided doses, then 30 mg/kg/day in 4 doses, max 2 g/day

Rheumatoid arthritis
Adult: PO 2 g/day in evenly divided doses, initiate treatment with a lower dose of enteric-coated tab

Child ≥2 yr: PO 30 mg/kg/24 hr, divided into 4 doses

Renal dose
Adult: PO CCr 10-30 ml/min bid; CCr <10 ml/min qd

S

Available forms: Tabs 500 mg; oral susp 250 mg/5 ml; delayed rel tabs 500 mg

Adverse effects

(*italic* = common; **bold** = life-threatening)

CNS: Headache, confusion, insomnia, hallucinations, depression, vertigo, fatigue, anxiety, **seizures,** drug fever, chills

CV: **Allergic myocarditis**

GI: *Nausea, vomiting, abdominal pain,* stomatitis, **hepatitis,** glossitis, **pancreatitis,** diarrhea, anorexia

GU: **Renal failure, toxic nephrosis,** increased BUN, creatinine, crystalluria

INTEG: Rash, dermatitis, **Stevens-Johnson syndrome,** erythema, photosensitivity

SYST: **Anaphylaxis**

HEMA: **Leukopenia, neutropenia, thrombocytopenia, agranulocytosis, hemolytic anemia**

Contraindications: Hypersensitivity to sulfonamides or salicylates, pregnancy at term, ℗ child <2 yr, intestinal, urinary obstruction

Precautions: Pregnancy **C**, lactation, impaired hepatic function, severe allergy, bronchial asthma, impaired renal function

⊠ Do Not Confuse:
sulfasalazine/sulfiSOXAZOLE

Pharmacokinetics	
Absorption	Partially absorbed
Distribution	Crosses placenta
Metabolism	Liver
Excretion	Kidneys, breast milk
Half-life	6 hr

Pharmacodynamics	
Onset	1 hr
Peak	1½-6 hr
Duration	6-12 hr

Interactions

Individual drugs

Digoxin: ↓ digoxin effect

Methotrexate: ↓ renal excretion

Phenytoin: ↓ hepatic clearance

Drug classifications

Anticoagulants (oral): ↑ anticoagulant effect

Hypoglycemics (oral): ↑ hypoglycemic response

Food/drug

Iron, folic acid will be poorly absorbed

Lab test interferences

False positive: Urinary glucose test

NURSING CONSIDERATIONS

Assessment

• Monitor I&O ratio; note color, amount, character, pH of urine if drug administered for UTIs; output should be 800 ml less than intake; if urine is highly acidic, alkalization may be needed

• Monitor kidney function studies: BUN, creatinine, urinalysis if on long-term therapy

• Monitor blood dyscrasias: skin rash, fever, sore throat, bruising, bleeding, fatigue, joint pain; monitor CBC before, during therapy (q3 mo)

• Assess for allergic reaction: rash, dermatitis, urticaria, pruritus, dyspnea, bronchospasm

Nursing diagnoses

☑ Injury, risk for (uses)

☑ Knowledge, deficient (teaching)

Implementation

• Give with full glass of water to maintain adequate hydration; increase fluids to 2 L/day to decrease crystallization in kidneys; contact lens, urine, skin may be yellow-orange

• Give total daily dose in evenly spaced doses and after meals to help minimize GI intolerance

• Store in airtight, light-resistant container at room temp

Patient/family education

• Advise patient to take each oral dose with full glass of water to prevent crystalluria

• Teach patient to avoid sunlight or to use sunscreen to prevent burns

• Teach patient to avoid OTC medication (aspirin, vit C) unless directed by prescriber

• Advise patient to notify prescriber if skin rash, sore throat, fever, mouth sores, unusual bruising, bleeding occur

• Advise patient to use rectal susp hs and retain all night

Evaluation

Positive therapeutic outcome

• Absence of fever, mucus in stools or pain in joints

---

sulfinpyrazone (Rx)

(sul-fin-peer'a-zone)

Anturan ✦, Anturane, sulfinpyrazone

Func. class.: Uricosuric

Chem. class.: Pyrazolone

Pregnancy category C

Action: Inhibits tubular reabsorption of urates, with increased excretion of uric acid;

---

inhibits prostaglandin synthesis, which decreases platelet aggregation

⮞ **Therapeutic Outcome:** Decreased uric acid levels, absence of platelet aggregation

Uses: Inhibition of platelet aggregation, gout

Dosage and routes
Inhibition of platelet aggregation
Adult: PO 200 mg qid

Gout/gouty arthritis
Adult: PO 100-200 mg bid × 1 wk, then 200-400 mg bid, not to exceed 800 mg/day

Available forms: Tabs 100 mg; caps 200 mg

Adverse effects
(*italic* = common; **bold** = life-threatening)
CNS: Dizziness, **seizures, coma**
EENT: Tinnitus
GI: *Gastric irritation, nausea, vomiting, anorexia,* **hepatic necrosis, GI bleeding**
GU: Renal calculi, hypoglycemia
HEMA: **Agranulocytosis** (rare)
INTEG: Rash, dermatitis, pruritus, fever, photosensitivity
RESP: **Apnea,** irregular respirations

Contraindications: Hypersensitivity to pyrazolone derivatives, blood dyscrasias, CCr <50 ml/min, active peptic ulcer, GI inflammation

Precautions: Pregnancy **C**

Pharmacokinetics	
Absorption	Well absorbed
Distribution	Unknown
Metabolism	Liver
Excretion	Feces (metabolites/active drug)
Half-life	4 hr

Pharmacodynamics	
Onset	Unknown
Peak	1-2 hr
Duration	4-6 hr

Interactions
Individual drugs:
Acetaminophen: ↑ toxicity
Niacin, theophylline, verapamil: ↓ effect of each specific drug
TOLBUTamide, warfarin: ↑ effect of each specific drug
Drug classifications
Salicylates: ↓ effect of sulfinpyrazone
Lab test interferences
↑ PSP, ↑ aminohippuric acid
False positive: Clinitest

NURSING CONSIDERATIONS
Assessment
• Monitor I&O ratio; observe for decrease in urinary output; increase fluids to 2-3 L/day
• Monitor CBC, platelets, reticulocytes before, during therapy (q3 mo)
• Assess mobility, joint pain, and swelling in the joints

Nursing diagnoses
☑ Pain, chronic (uses)
☑ Mobility, impaired physical (uses)
☑ Knowledge, deficient (teaching)

Implementation
• Give with food or antacid to decrease GI upset
• Reduce dose gradually if uric acid levels are normal after 6 mo

Patient/family education
• Advise patient to increase fluids to 3-4 L/day
• Caution patient to avoid alcohol, OTC preparations that contain alcohol; skin rashes may occur
• Advise patient to report any pain, redness, or hard area, usually in legs
• Instruct patient on importance of complying with medical regimen; bone marrow depression may occur

Evaluation
Positive therapeutic outcome
• Decreased pain in joints
• Normal serum uric acid levels
• Increased duration of antiinfectives

---

*sulfiSOXAZOLE (Rx)
(sul-fi-sox′a-zole)
Gantrisin, Gantrisin Pediatric, Novo-Soxazole ✦, sulfiSOXAZOLE
Func. class.: Antiinfective
Chem. class.: Sulfonamide, short-acting

Pregnancy category B

S

Action: Interferes with bacterial biosynthesis of proteins by competitive antagonism of *p*-aminobenzoic acid (PABA)

⮞ **Therapeutic Outcome:** Bactericidal action against susceptible organisms: gram-positive pathogens, including streptococci and staphylococci, *Clostridium perfringens, Clostridium tetani, Nocardia asteroides;* gram-negative pathogens, including *Enterobacter, Escherichia coli, Klebsiella, Proteus mirabilis, Proteus vulgaris, Salmonella, Shigella*

Uses: UTIs; chancroid, trachoma, toxoplasmosis, acute otitis media, malaria, *Haemophilus influenzae* meningitis, meningococcal meningitis, nocardiosis

Dosage and routes
UTIs, other systemic infections
Adult: PO 2-4 g loading dose, then 1-2 g qid × 7-10 days

P *Child >2 mo:* PO 75 mg/kg or 2 g/m^2 loading dose, then 120-150 mg/kg/day or 4 g/m^2/day in divided doses q6h, max 6 g/day

Chlamydia trachomatis
Adult: PO 500 mg-1 g qid × 3 wk

Renal dose
Adult: PO CCr 10-50 ml/min q8-12h; CCr <10 ml/min q12-24h

Available forms: Tabs 500 mg; liq 500 mg/5 ml

Adverse effects
(*italic* = common; **bold** = life-threatening)
CNS: Headache, insomnia, hallucinations, depression, vertigo, fatigue, anxiety, **seizures**, drug fever, chills, drowsiness
CV: **Allergic myocarditis**
GI: *Nausea, vomiting, abdominal pain,* stomatitis, **hepatitis**, glossitis, pancreatitis, diarrhea, **enterocolitis**, anorexia
GU: **Renal failure, toxic nephrosis,** increased BUN, creatinine, crystalluria, hematuria, proteinuria
HEMA: **Leukopenia, thrombocytopenia, agranulocytosis, hemolytic anemia, aplastic anemia**
INTEG: Rash, dermatitis, urticaria, erythema, photosensitivity, alopecia
SYST: **Anaphylaxis, Stevens-Johnson syndrome**

Contraindications: Hypersensitivity to sulfonamides and sulfonylureas, thiazide and loop diuretics, salicylates; sunscreen with
P PABA, lactation, infants <2 mo (except congenital toxoplasmosis); pregnancy at term, porphyria

Precautions: Pregnancy **B**, lactation, impaired hepatic/renal function, severe allergy, bronchial asthma

⚠ Do Not Confuse:
sulfiSOXAZOLE/sulfasalazine
sulfiSOXAZOLE/sulfADIAZINE

Pharmacokinetics	
Absorption	Well absorbed
Distribution	Widely distributed, crosses placenta
Metabolism	Liver, mostly
Excretion	Breast milk
Half-life	4-7 hr

Pharmacodynamics	
Onset	Unknown
Peak	2-4 hr

Interactions
Individual drugs
Cyclosporine: ↑ nephrotoxicity
Indomethacin, probenecid: ↑ drug-free concentrations
Methotrexate: ↓ renal excretion of methotrexate
Phenytoin: ↓ hepatic clearance of phenytoin
Tolbutamide: ↑ effects of tolbutamide
Warfarin: ↑ anticoagulant effect
Drug classifications
Barbiturates, uricosuric agents: ↑ effects of each specific drug
Diuretics (thiazide): ↑ thrombocytopenia
Salicylates: ↑ drug-free concentrations
Sulfonylurea agents: ↑ hypoglycemic response
Lab test interferences
False positive: Urinary glucose test

NURSING CONSIDERATIONS
Assessment
• Assess patient for previous sensitivity reaction
• Assess patient for signs and symptoms of infection including characteristics of wounds, sputum, urine, stool, WBC >10,000/mm^3, temp; obtain baseline information before and during treatment
• Complete C&S testing before beginning drug therapy to identify if correct treatment has been initiated
• Assess for allergic reactions: rash, urticaria, pruritus, chills, fever, joint pain; angioedema may occur a few days after therapy begins; epINEPHrine, resuscitation equipment should be available for anaphylactic reaction
• Monitor blood studies: CBC, Hct, bilirubin, alkaline phosphatase monthly if patient is on long-term therapy
• Monitor for bleeding: ecchymosis, bleeding gums, hematuria, stool guaiac daily if on long-term therapy
• Assess for overgrowth of infection: perineal itching, fever, malaise, redness, pain, swelling, drainage, rash, diarrhea, change in cough, sputum

---

◪ Herb/drug   🚫 Do Not Crush   ◆ Alert   ↻ Key Drug   G Geriatric   P Pediatric

Nursing diagnoses
☑ Infection, risk for (uses)
☑ Diarrhea (adverse reactions)
☑ Injury, risk for (adverse reactions)
☑ Knowledge, deficient (teaching)
☑ Noncompliance (teaching)

Implementation
- Give around the clock to maintain proper blood levels; give on an empty stomach to increase absorption of drug; do not give within 3 hr of other agents; drug interactions may occur
- Give with 8 oz of water

Patient/family education
- Teach patient to report sore throat, bruising, bleeding, joint pain; may indicate blood dyscrasias (rare)
- Advise patient to contact prescriber if vaginal itching; loose foul-smelling stools; or furry tongue occur; may indicate super-infection; report itching, rash, pruritus, urticaria
- Instruct patient to take all medication prescribed for the length of time ordered; drug must be taken around the clock to maintain blood levels; medication should not be shared with others

Evaluation
Positive therapeutic outcome
- Absence of signs/symptoms of infection (WBC <10,000/mm^3, temp WNL, absence of urinary pain, hematuria)
- Reported improvement in symptoms of infection
- Negative C&S

---

sulindac (Rx)
(sul-in'dak)
Apo-Sulin ✦, Clinoril, Novosundac ✦, sulindac
Func. class.: Nonsteroidal antiinflammatory, antirheumatic
Chem. class.: Indeneacetic acid derivative
Pregnancy category C

Action: Inhibits prostaglandin synthesis by decreasing an enzyme needed for biosynthesis; analgesic, antiinflammatory, antipyretic

➜ **Therapeutic Outcome:** Decreased pain, inflammation

Uses: Mild to moderate pain, osteoarthritis, rheumatoid, gouty arthritis, ankylosing spondylitis

Dosage and routes
Arthritis
Adult: PO 150 mg bid, may increase to 200 mg bid
Bursitis/acute arthritis
Adult: PO 200 mg bid × 1-2 wk, then reduce dose

Available forms: Tabs 150, 200 mg

Adverse effects
(*italic* = common; **bold** = life-threatening)
CNS: Dizziness, drowsiness, fatigue, tremors, confusion, insomnia, anxiety, depression, *headache*
CV: Tachycardia, peripheral edema, palpitations, dysrhythmias
EENT: Tinnitus, hearing loss, blurred vision
GI: Nausea, anorexia, vomiting, diarrhea, jaundice, **cholestatic hepatitis,** constipation, flatulence, cramps, dry mouth, peptic ulcer, **bleeding, ulceration, perforation**
GU: **Nephrotoxicity: dysuria, hematuria, oliguria, azotemia**
HEMA: **Blood dyscrasias with prolonged use**
INTEG: Purpura, *rash, pruritus,* sweating, photosensitivity

Contraindications: Hypersensitivity, asthma, severe renal disease, severe hepatic disease, active ulcers

Precautions: Pregnancy **C**, 1st trimester, Ⓟ lactation, children, bleeding disorders, GI disorders, cardiac, renal disorders, hypersensitivity to other antiinflammatory agents

▧ **Do Not Confuse:**
Clinoril/Clozaril, Clinoril/Oruvail

Pharmacokinetics
Absorption	Well absorbed
Distribution	Not known
Metabolism	Converted to active drug—liver
Excretion	Minimal unchanged kidneys, breast milk
Half-life	7.8 hr; 16.4 hr active metabolite

Pharmacodynamics
Onset	Unknown
Peak	2 hr
Duration	Unknown

Interactions
Individual drugs
Aspirin: ↑ GI reactions
Clopidogrel, eptifibatide, plicamycin, tirofiban, ticlopidine, valproic acid: ↑ bleeding risk
CycloSPORINE: ↑ nephrotoxicity

Diflunisal: ↓ sulindac effect; do not use together

Methotrexate, probenecid: ↑ toxicity

Drug classifications

Anticoagulants, cephalosporins, thrombolytics: ↑ bleeding risk

Glucocorticoids, NSAIDs: ↑ GI reactions

Sulfonamides, sulfonylurea: ↑ toxicity

Herb/drug

Arginine, gossypol: ↑ gastric irritation

Bearberry, bilberry: ↑ NSAIDs effect

Bogbean, chondroitin: ↑ bleeding risk

NURSING CONSIDERATIONS

Assessment

• Monitor blood counts during therapy; watch for decreasing platelets; if low, therapy may need to be discontinued, restarted after hematologic recovery; and for blood dyscrasia (thrombocytopenia): bruising, fatigue, bleeding, poor healing

• Assess pain: frequency, intensity, characteristics, relief 1-2 hr after medication

• Assess for asthma, aspirin hypersensitivity, nasal polyps; hypersensitivity may develop

Nursing diagnoses

☑ Pain, chronic (uses)

☑ Mobility, impaired physical (uses)

☑ Knowledge, deficient (teaching)

☑ Injury, risk for (adverse reactions)

Implementation

• Administer with food or milk to decrease gastric symptoms; food slows absorption slightly, does not decrease absorption

Patient/family education

• Advise patient that drug must be continued for prescribed time to be effective; to avoid aspirin, alcoholic beverages

• Caution patient to report bleeding, bruising, fatigue, malaise because blood dyscrasias do occur

• Instruct patient to use caution when driving; drowsiness, dizziness may occur

• Teach patient to take with a full glass of water to enhance absorption; do not crush, break, or chew

Evaluation

Positive therapeutic outcome

• Decreased pain

• Decreased inflammation

• Increased mobility

---

sumatriptan (Rx)

(soo-ma-trip'tan)

Imitrex

Func. class.: Antimigraine agent

Chem. class.: 5-HT₁ receptor agonist

Pregnancy category C

Action: Binds selectively to the vascular 5-HT₁ receptor subtype and exerts antimigraine effect; causes vasoconstriction in cranial arteries

Therapeutic Outcome: Absence of migraines

Uses: Acute treatment of migraine with or without aura and cluster headache

Dosage and routes

Adult: SC 6 mg or less; may repeat in 1 hr; not to exceed 12 mg/24 hr; PO 25 mg with fluids, max 100 mg; nasal: 1 dose of 5, 10, or 20 mg in one nostril, may repeat in 2 hr, max 40 mg/24 hr

Hepatic dose

Adult: PO 25 mg, if no response after 2 hr, give up to 50 mg

Available forms: Inj 6 mg (12 mg/ml); tabs 25, 50, 100 mg; nasal spray 5 mg/100 mcl-units dose spray device 20 mg/100 mcl-units

Adverse effects

(*italic* = common; **bold** = life-threatening)

CNS: Tingling, hot sensation, burning, feeling of pressure, tightness, numbness, dizziness, sedation, headache, anxiety, fatigue, cold sensation

CV: Flushing, **MI**

EENT: Throat, mouth, nasal discomfort, vision changes

GI: Abdominal discomfort

INTEG: Inj site reaction, sweating

MS: Weakness, neck stiffness, myalgia

RESP: Chest tightness, pressure

Contraindications: Angina pectoris, history of MI, documented silent ischemia, Prinzmetal's angina, ischemic heart disease, **IV** use, concurrent ergotamine-containing preparations, uncontrolled hypertension, hypersensitivity, basilar or hemiplegic migraine

Precautions: Postmenopausal women, men >40 yr, risk factors for CAD, hypercholesterolemia, obesity, diabetes, impaired hepatic or renal function, pregnancy **C,** lactation, children, elderly

---

 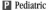

Pharmacokinetics	
Absorption	Well absorbed (SC)
Distribution	10%-20% plasma protein binding
Metabolism	Liver (metabolite)
Excretion	Urine, feces
Half-life	2 hr

Pharmacodynamics	
	SC
Onset	10-20 min
Peak	10 min-2 hr
Duration	Up to 24 hr (pain relief)

Interactions
Individual drugs
Ergotamine: ↑ risk of vasospastic reaction
Drug classifications
MAOIs, SSRIs: ↑ sumatriptan levels
Herb/drug
Butterbur: ↑ effect
SAM-e, St. John's wort: serotonin syndrome

NURSING CONSIDERATIONS
Assessment
• Assess for tingling, hot sensation, burning, feeling of pressure, numbness, flushing, inj site reaction
• Assess B/P; signs/symptoms of coronary vasospasm
• Monitor stress level, activity, reaction, coping mechanisms of patient
• Assess neurologic status: LOC, blurring vision, nausea, vomiting, tingling in extremities preceding headache
• Assess for ingestion of tyramine-containing foods (pickled products, beer, wine, aged cheese), food additives, preservatives, colorings, artificial sweeteners, chocolate, caffeine, which may precipitate these types of headaches

Nursing diagnoses
✓ Pain, chronic (uses)
✓ Knowledge, deficient (teaching)

Implementation
PO route
• Swallow whole; take with fluids as soon as symptoms appear; may take a second dose >4 hr, max 200 mg/24 hr
SC route
• Give by SC route only, avoid IM or **IV** administration, use only for actual migraine attack

Patient/family education
• Caution patient not to take more than 2 doses/day or 12 mg/day; allow at least 1 hr between doses

• Caution patient to avoid driving or hazardous activities if dizziness or drowsiness occurs
• Teach patient to report chest tightness, heat, flushing, drowsiness, dizziness, fatigue, sudden severe abdominal pain or any allergic reactions that occur to prescriber immediately
• Inform patient to report any side effects to prescriber
• Caution patient to use contraception when taking drug, to notify prescriber if pregnancy is suspected or planned
Nasal spray
• Teach patient to spray once in 1 nostril, may repeat if headache returns, do not repeat if pain continues after 1st dose

Evaluation
Positive therapeutic outcome
• Decrease in frequency, severity of headache

---

tacrine (Rx)
(tack'rin)
Cognex
Func. class.: Anti-Alzheimer agent
Chem. class.: Reversible cholinesterase inhibitor

Pregnancy category C

Action: Elevates acetylcholine concentrations (cerebral cortex) by slowing degrading of acetylcholine released in cholinergic neurons; does not alter underlying dementia

⇒**Therapeutic Outcome:** Improvement in symptoms of dementia in Alzheimer's disease

Uses: Treatment of mild to moderate dementia in Alzheimer's disease

Dosage and routes
Adult: PO 10 mg qid × 6 wk, then 20 mg qid × 6 wk, increase at 6-wk intervals if patient tolerates drug well and if transaminase is within normal limits

Available forms: Caps 10, 20, 30, 40 mg

Adverse effects
(*italic* = common; **bold** = life-threatening)
CNS: *Dizziness, confusion, insomnia,* tremor, *ataxia, somnolence, anxiety, agitation, depression, hallucinations, hostility, abnormal thinking,* chills, fever
CV: Hypotension or hypertension
GI: *Nausea, vomiting, anorexia, abdominal pain, constipation,* dyspepsia, flatulence, **hepatotoxicity, GI bleeding**
GU: *Frequency, UTI, incontinence*
INTEG: *Rash,* flushing

RESP: *Rhinitis, upper respiratory tract infection, cough,* pharyngitis

Contraindications: Hypersensitivity to this drug or acridine derivatives, patients treated with this drug who developed jaundice with a total bilirubin of >3 mg/dl

Precautions: Sick sinus syndrome, history of ulcers, GI bleeding, hepatic disease, bladder obstruction, asthma, pregnancy **C**, lactation, **P** children, seizure disorder

Do Not Confuse:
Cognex/Corgard

Pharmacokinetics	
Absorption	Rapidly absorbed, low
Distribution	55% plasma protein bound
Metabolism	Liver, extensively by CYP450 enzyme system
Excretion	Unknown
Half-life	2-4 hr

Pharmacodynamics	
Unknown	

Interactions
Individual drugs
Cimetidine: ↑ tacrine level
Succinylcholine: Synergistic effect
Theophylline: ↑ elimination half-life of theophylline
Drug classifications
Anticholinergics: ↓ activity of anticholinergics
Cholinergic agonists, cholinesterase inhibitors: Synergistic effect

NURSING CONSIDERATIONS
Assessment
• Monitor ALT qo wk × 4-16 wk, then q3 mo; weekly ALT × 6 wk if dose is increased
• Monitor B/P for hypotension or hypertension
• Assess mental status: affect, mood, behavioral changes, depression, hallucinations, confusion; conduct suicide assessment
• Assess GI status: nausea, vomiting, anorexia, constipation, abdominal pain; add bulk and increase fluids for constipation
• Assess GU status: urinary frequency, incontinence

Nursing diagnoses
☑ Injury, risk for (uses)
☑ Thought processes, disturbed (uses)
☑ Knowledge, deficient (teaching)

Implementation
• Give dosage adjusted to patient's response no more than q6 wk

• Provide assistance with ambulation if needed during beginning therapy; dizziness, ataxia may occur
• Give between meals; if GI symptoms occur, may be given with meals

Patient/family education
• Advise patient to report side effects: twitching, eye spasms; may indicate overdose
• Instruct patient to use drug exactly as prescribed at regular intervals, preferably between meals; may be taken with meals for GI upset; drug is not a cure
• Advise patient to notify prescriber of nausea, vomiting, diarrhea (dose increased or beginning treatment) or rash, very dark or very light stools, jaundice (delayed onset)
• Caution patient not to increase or abruptly decrease dose; serious consequences may result

Evaluation
Positive therapeutic outcome
• Decrease in confusion, improved mood

Treatment of overdose: Withdraw drug, administer tertiary anticholinergics, provide supportive care

tacrolimus (Rx)
(tak-roe′li-mus)
Prograf
tacrolimus topical
Protopic
Func. class.: Immunosuppressant
Chem. clas.: Macrolide

Pregnancy category C

Action: Produces immunosuppression by inhibiting lymphocytes (T)

➡ **Therapeutic Outcome:** Prevention of rejection in organ transplant

Uses: Organ transplants, to prevent rejection; topical: atopic dermatitis

Investigational uses:
Autoimmune diseases, severe recalcitrant psoriasis

Dosage and routes
P *Adult and child:* **IV** 0.03-0.05 mg/kg/day × 3 days then PO 0.15 mg/kg bid; adjust dose in renal impairment

P *Adult/child ≥2 yr:* Apply ointment bid × 7 days

Available forms: Inj **IV** 5 mg/ml; caps 0.5, 1, 5 mg; ointment 0.03%, 0.1%

☑ Herb/drug   ⓢ Do Not Crush   ◆ Alert   ◆⊓ Key Drug   Ⓖ Geriatric   Ⓟ Pediatric

Adverse effects

(*italic* = common; **bold** = life-threatening)

CNS: Tremors, headache, insomnia, paresthesia, chills, fever, **seizures**

CV: Hypertension

EENT: Blurred vision, photophobia

GI: Nausea, vomiting, diarrhea, *oral Candida, gum hyperplasia,* **hepatotoxicity,** constipation, GI bleeding

GU: Urinary tract infections, **albuminuria, hematuria, proteinuria, renal failure**

HEMA: Anemia, **leukocytosis, thrombocytopenia purpura**

INTEG: Rash, flushing, itching, alopecia

META: Hirsutism, hyperglycemia, hyperkalemia, hyperuricemia, hypokalemia, hypomagnesemia

RESP: **Pleural effusion, atelectasis,** dyspnea

SYST: **Anaphylaxis**

Contraindications: Hypersensitivity to this drug or to some kinds of castor oil

Precautions: Severe renal disease, severe hepatic disease, pregnancy **C,** diabetes mellitus, hyperkalemia, hyperuricemia, lymphomas, P lactation, children <12 yr; hypertension

Pharmacokinetics

Absorption	Erractically absorbed (PO), completely absorbed (**IV**)
Distribution	Crosses placenta, 75% protein binding
Metabolism	Liver to metabolite
Excretion	Kidney—minimal, breast milk, bile
Half-life	10 hr

Pharmacodynamics

	PO	IV
Onset	Unknown	Unknown
Peak	1-4 hr	Unknown
Duration	12 hr	12 hr

Interactions

Individual drugs

Carbamazepine, phenobarbital, phenytoin, rifampin: ↓ blood levels

Cisplatin, cyclosporine, danazol, erythromycin: ↑ toxicity

Ibuprofen: ↑ oliguria

Mycophenolate, mofetil: ↑ blood levels

Drug classifications

Aminoglycosides: ↑ toxicity

Antifungals, calcium channel blockers: ↑ blood levels

Vaccines: ↓ effect

Herb/drug

Astragalus, echinacea, melatonin: ↓ immunosuppression

Ginseng, maitake, mistletoe: ↓ effect

NURSING CONSIDERATIONS

Assessment

• Monitor blood studies: Hgb, WBC, platelets during treatment monthly; if WBC is <3000/mm^3, or platelet count <100,000/mm^3, drug should be discontinued or reduced; decreased Hgb level may indicate bone marrow suppression

• Monitor liver function studies: alkaline phosphatase, AST, ALT, amylase, bilirubin, and for hepatotoxicity: dark urine, jaundice, itching, light-colored stools; drug should be discontinued

• Assess for anaphylaxis: rash, pruritus, wheezing, laryngeal edema; stop infusion, initiate emergency procedures

Nursing diagnoses

☑ Infection, risk for (uses)

☑ Knowledge, deficient (teaching)

Implementation

PO route

• Give all medications PO if possible; avoid IM inj because bleeding may occur

• Give with meals to reduce GI upset; nausea is common

• Give for several days before transplant surgery; patients should be placed in protective isolation

IV route

• Give after diluting in 0.9% NaCl or D$_5$W to a concentration of 0.004-0.02 mg/ml as a cont inf

Y-site compatibilities: Acyclovir, aminophylline, amphotericin B, ampicillin, ampicillin/sulbactam, benztropine, calcium gluconate, cefazolin, cefotetan, ceftazidime, ceftriaxone, cefuroxime, chloramphenicol, cimetidine, ciprofloxacin, clindamycin, dexamethasone, digoxin, diphenhydrAMINE, dobutamine, DOPamine, doxycycline, erythromycin, esmolol, fluconazole, furosemide, ganciclovir, gentamicin, haloperidol, heparin, hydrocortisone, imipenem/cilastatin, insulin (regular), isoproterenol, leucovorin, lorazepam, methylPREDNISolone, metoclopramide, metronidazole, mezlocillin, multivitamins, nitroglycerin, nitroprusside, oxacillin, penicillin G potassium, perphenazine, phenytoin, piperacillin, potassium chloride, propranolol, ranitidine, sodium bicarbonate, trimethoprim/sulfamethoxazole, vancomycin

T

Patient/family education

• Instruct patient to report fever, rash, severe diarrhea, chills, sore throat, fatigue because serious infections may occur; clay-colored stools, cramping may indicate hepatotoxicity
• Caution patient to avoid crowds or persons with known infections to reduce risk of infection

Evaluation
Positive therapeutic outcome

• Absence of graft rejection
• Immunosuppression in autoimmune disorders

---

tadalafil
Cialis
See Appendix A, Selected New Drugs

---

tamoxifen (Rx)
(ta-mox'i-fen)
Alpha-Tamoxifen ✦, Med Tamoxifen ✦, Nolvadex, Nolvadex-D ✦, Novo-Tamoxifen ✦, Tamofen ✦, Tamone ✦, Tamoplex ✦
Func. class.: Antineoplastic
Chem. class.: Antiestrogen hormone

Pregnancy category D

Action: Inhibits cell division by binding to cytoplasmic estrogen receptors; resembles normal cell complex but inhibits DNA synthesis and estrogen response of target tissue

⊳ **Therapeutic Outcome:** Prevention of rapidly growing malignant cells

Uses: Advanced breast carcinoma that has not responded to other therapy in estrogen receptor-positive patients (usually postmenopausal), prevention of breast cancer, after breast surgery/radiation in ductal carcinoma in situ

Investigational uses: Mastalgia, pain/size of gynecomastia, ovulation stimulation, malignant carcinoid tumor, carcinoid syndrome

Dosage and routes
Breast cancer
Adult: PO 20-40 mg qd, doses >20 mg/day divide AM/PM

High risk for breast cancer
Adult: PO 20 mg qd × 5 yr

Ductal carcinoma in situ
Adult: PO 20 mg qd × 5 yr

Available forms: Tabs 10, 20 mg

Adverse effects
(*italic* = common; **bold** = life-threatening)
CNS: *Hot flashes, headache, lightheadedness,* depression
CV: Chest pain
EENT: Ocular lesions, retinopathy, corneal opacity, blurred vision (high doses)
GI: *Nausea, vomiting,* altered taste (anorexia)
GU: Vaginal bleeding, pruritus vulvae
HEMA: **Thrombocytopenia, leukopenia,** deep vein thrombosis, pulmonary embolism
INTEG: *Rash,* alopecia
META: Hypercalcemia

Contraindications: Hypersensitivity, pregnancy **D**

Precautions: Leukopenia, thrombocytopenia, lactation, cataracts

Pharmacokinetics
Absorption	Adequately absorbed
Distribution	Unknown
Metabolism	Liver—extensively
Excretion	Feces—slowly, small amounts (kidneys)
Half-life	1 wk

Pharmacodynamics
Onset	Unknown
Peak	4-7 hr
Duration	Unknown

Interactions
Individual drugs
Aminoglutethimide, medroxyprogesterone: ↓ tamoxifen levels
Bromocriptine: ↑ tamoxifen level
Letrozole, rifamycin: ↓ levels of each specific drug
Radiation: ↑ myelosuppression
Drug classifications
Anticoagulants: ↑ risk of bleeding
Antineoplastics: ↑ thromboembolic action
Lab test interferences
↑ Serum calcium

NURSING CONSIDERATIONS
Assessment
• Monitor CBC, differential, platelet count weekly; withhold drug if WBC is <4000/mm³ or platelet count is <75,000/mm³; notify prescriber of results; monitor calcium levels (hypercalcemia is common)
◆• Assess for tumor flare: increase in bone, tumor pain during beginning treatment; give analgesics as ordered to decrease pain

---

⊘ Herb/drug 🚫 Do Not Crush ◆ Alert ◆╥ Key Drug 🄶 Geriatric 🄿 Pediatric

- Assess for bleeding: hematuria, guaiac, bruising or petechiae, mucosa or orifices q8h, no rectal temp
◆◆• Assess for uterine malignancies: Symptoms of stroke, pulmonary embolism that may occur in women with ductal carcinoma in situ (DCIS) and women at high risk for breast cancer

Nursing diagnoses
☑ Injury, risk for (adverse reactions)
☑ Knowledge, deficient (teaching)

Implementation
🚫• Give with food or fluids for GI upset; do not break, crush, or chew enteric products; repeat dose may be needed if vomiting occurs
- Store in light-resistant container at room temp

Patient/family education
- Instruct patient to report any complaints, side effects to prescriber; if dose is missed, do not double next dose
- Advise patient that vaginal bleeding, pruritus, hot flashes can occur and are reversible after discontinuing treatment
- Instruct patient to report immediately decreased visual acuity, which may be irreversible; stress need for routine eye exams
- Inform patient about who should be told about tamoxifen therapy
- Advise patient to report vaginal bleeding immediately; that tumor flare (increase in size or tumor, increased bone pain) may occur and will subside rapidly; may take analgesics for pain; that premenopausal women must use mechanical birth control method because ovulation may be induced (teratogenic drug)
- Caution patient to use sunscreen and protective clothing to prevent burns because photosensitivity is common
- Teach patient that hair loss may occur during treatment; a wig or hairpiece may make patient feel better; new hair may be different in color, texture
- Inform patient rash or lesions are temporary and may become large during beginning therapy
- Advise patient to increase fluids to 2 L/day unless contraindicated

Evaluation
Positive therapeutic outcome
- Decreased spread of malignant cells in breast cancer

---

tamsulosin (Rx)
(tam-sue-lo'sen)
Flomax
Func. class.: Selective α-adrenergic blocker
Chem. class.: Sulfamoyl phenethylamine derivative

Pregnancy category B

➡**Therapeutic Outcome:** Decreased symptoms of benign prostatic hyperplasia (BPH)

Uses: Symptoms of BPH

Dosage and routes
Adult: PO 0.4 mg qd, increasing to 0.8 mg qd if required

Available forms: Caps 0.4 mg

Adverse effects
(*italic* = common; **bold** = life-threatening)
CNS: Dizziness, headache, asthenia
CV: Chest pain
EENT: Amblyopia
GI: Nausea, diarrhea
GU: Decreased libido, abnormal ejaculation
MS: Back pain
RESP: Rhinitis, pharyngitis, cough

Contraindications: Hypersensitivity

🅿**Precautions:** Pregnancy **B,** children, lactation, hepatic disease, coronary artery disease, severe renal disease

---

Pharmacokinetics	
Absorption	Well absorbed
Distribution	Not known; 98% plasma protein bound
Metabolism	Liver, extensively
Excretion	Kidneys
Half-life	9-15 hr

Pharmacodynamics
Unknown

Interactions
Drug classifications
α₁-Adrenergic blockers: Do not use together

NURSING CONSIDERATIONS
Assessment
- Monitor CBC with differential and liver function studies; B/P and heart rate
- Monitor urodynamic studies/urinary flow rates, residual volume
- Assess for BPH: change in urinary patterns, baseline and throughout treatment
- Monitor I&O ratios, weight qd, edema, report weight gain or edema

Nursing diagnoses

✓ Cardiac output, decreased (uses)
✓ Injury, risk for (side effects)
✓ Knowledge, deficient (teaching)
✓ Noncompliance (teaching)

Implementation

🚫 • Give whole; do not chew or crush tabs
• Store in airtight container at 86° F (30° C) or less
• May be given with food to prevent GI symptoms; ½ hr after same meal each day

Patient/family education

• Teach patient not to discontinue drug abruptly; emphasize the importance of complying with dosage schedule, even if feeling better; if dose is missed take as soon as remembered; take at same time each day
• Teach patient not to use OTC products (cough, cold, allergy) unless directed by prescriber; also to avoid large amounts of caffeine
• Caution patient that drug may cause dizziness, may occur during 1st few days of therapy; to avoid hazardous activities

Evaluation

Positive therapeutic outcome

• Decreased symptoms of BPH

---

tazobactam
See piperacillin/tazobactam

---

tegaserod (Rx)
(teg-as'er-odd)
Zelnorm
Func. class.: 5-HT₄ receptor partial agonist, GI agent—misc.

Pregnancy category B

Action: A 5-HT₄ receptor partial agonist that binds 5-HT₄ receptors, stimulating peristalsis and intestinal secretion

➡ **Therapeutic Outcome:** Decreased constipation in irritable bowel syndrome (IBS)

Uses: IBS where primary bowel symptom is constipation

Dosage and routes
Adult: **PO** 6 mg bid before meals × 4-6 wk, another 4-6 wk course may be used

Available forms: Tabs 2, 6 mg

Adverse effects
(*italic* = common; **bold** = life-threatening)
CNS: Headache, dizziness, depression,

vertigo, fatigue, suicide attempt, poor concentration
CV: Hypotension, angina, **dysrhythmias, bundle branch block, supraventricular tachycardia**
GI: Nausea, abdominal pain, increased appetite, eructation, increased AST, increased ALT, diarrhea, irritable colon, tenesmus, flatulence
GU: Polyuria, renal pain, ovarian cyst, miscarriage, albuminuria
MISC: Pain, facial edema, increased CPK, asthma, breast carcinoma
MS: Back pain, arthralgia
SYST: **Anaphylaxis**

Contraindications: Hypersensitivity, severe renal disease, moderate to severe hepatic disease, history of bowel obstruction, gallbladder disease, abdominal adhesions, sphincter of Oddi dysfunction

Precautions: Pregnancy (B), lactation,
🅿 children, diarrhea

Pharmacokinetics	
Absorption	Unknown
Distribution	98% protein binding
Metabolism	Unknown
Excretion	⅔ unchanged in feces, remainder in urine as metabolites
Half-life	11 hr

Pharmacodynamics	
Onset	Unknown
Peak	1 hr
Duration	Unknown

Interactions
Individual drug
Digoxin: ↓ effect of digoxin when used with tegaserod
Drug classification
Oral contraceptives: ↓ effect of oral contraceptives when used with tegaserod
Food/drug
Food: ↓ absorption, but is minimized when taken ½ hr before a meal

NURSING CONSIDERATIONS
Assessment

• Assess GI symptoms: nausea, abdominal pain
• Assess CV status: B/P, pulse, chest pain

Nursing diagnoses

✓ Constipation, chronic (uses)
✓ Knowledge, deficient (teaching)

 Herb/drug   Do Not Crush   Alert   Key Drug   Geriatric   🅿 Pediatric

Implementation
- Give before meals, bid
- Store at room temp

Patient/family education
- Advise to notify prescriber of GI symptoms, hypersensitivity reactions

Evaluation
Positive therapeutic outcome
- Decreased constipation in IBS

---

telmisartan (Rx)
(tel-mih-sar'tan)
Micardis
Func. class.: Antihypertensive
Chem. class.: Angiotensin II receptor (type AT₁)

Pregnancy category
C (1st trimester)
D (2nd/3rd trimesters)

Action: Blocks the vasoconstrictor and aldosterone-secreting effects of angiotensin II; selectively blocks the binding of angiotensin II to the AT₁ receptor found in tissues

➔**Therapeutic Outcome:** ↓ B/P

Uses: Hypertension, alone or in combination

Investigational uses: Heart failure

Dosage and routes
Adult: PO 40 mg qd; range 20-80 mg

Available forms: Tabs 20, 40, 80 mg

Adverse effects
(*italic* = common; **bold** = life-threatening)
CNS: Dizziness, insomnia, *anxiety,* headache, fatigue
GI: Diarrhea, dyspepsia, *anorexia, vomiting*
MS: Myalgia, pain
RESP: Cough, *upper respiratory tract infection,* sinusitis, pharyngitis

Contraindications: Hypersensitivity, pregnancy **D** (2nd/3rd trimesters)

Precautions: Hypersensitivity to angiotensin-converting enzyme (ACE)
P inhibitors; pregnancy **C** (1st trimes-
G ter); lactation, children, elderly

Pharmacokinetics

Absorption	Unknown
Distribution	Highly protein bound
Metabolism	Liver (extensively)
Excretion	Urine/feces
Half-life	Terminal 24 hr

Pharmacodynamics

Onset	Unknown
Peak	Unknown
Duration	Unknown

Interactions
Digoxin: ↑ digoxin peak, trough concentrations
Drug classifications
Antihypertensives, diuretics: ↑ antihypertensive action
⊘*Herb/drug*
Aconite: ↑ toxicity, death
Astragalus, cola tree: ↑ or ↓ antihypertensive effect
Barberry, betony, black catechu, black cohosh, bloodroot, broom, burdock, cat's claw, dandelion, goldenseal, Irish moss, Jamaican dogwood, kelp, khella, mistletoe, parsley: ↑ antihypertensive effect
Coltsfoot, guarana, khat, licorice: ↓ antihypertensive effect

NURSING CONSIDERATIONS
Assessment
- Monitor B/P, pulse q4h; note rate, rhythm, quality
- Monitor electrolytes: potassium, sodium, chloride
- Monitor baselines in renal, liver function tests before therapy begins
- Assess edema in feet, legs qd
- Assess skin turgor, dryness of mucous membranes for hydration status

Nursing diagnoses
☑ Tissue perfusion, ineffective (uses)
☑ Knowledge, deficient (teaching)
☑ Noncompliance (teaching)

Implementation
- Give without regard to meals
- Give increased dose to black patients, B/P response may be reduced

Patient/family education
- Instruct patient to comply with dosage schedule, even if feeling better
- Advise patient to notify prescriber of mouth sores, fever, swelling of hands or feet, irregular heartbeat, chest pain
- Teach patient that excessive perspiration, dehydration, vomiting, diarrhea may lead to fall in blood pressure; consult prescriber if these occur
- Teach patient that drug may cause dizziness, fainting; light-headedness may occur
- Advise patient to use contraception while taking this drug

T

• Teach patient to notify prescriber of all prescriptions, OTC preparations, and supplements taken

Evaluation
Positive therapeutic outcome
• Decreased B/P

---

temazepam (Rx)
(tem-az'a-pam)
Razepam, Restoril, Temazepam
Func. class.: Sedative/hypnotic
Chem. class.: Benzodiazepine

Pregnancy category X

Controlled substance schedule IV (USA) schedule F (Canada)

Action: Produces CNS depression at limbic, thalamic, hypothalamic levels of the CNS; may be mediated by neurotransmitter γ-aminobutyric acid (GABA); results are sedation, hypnosis, skeletal muscle relaxation, anticonvulsant activity, anxiolytic action

➡**Therapeutic Outcome:** Decreased insomnia

Uses: Insomnia (short-term)

Dosage and routes
Adult: PO 15-30 mg hs
G *Elderly:* PO 7.5 mg hs

Available forms: Caps 7.5, 15, 30 mg

Adverse effects
(*italic* = common; **bold** = life-threatening)
CNS: Lethargy, drowsiness, daytime sedation, dizziness, confusion, lightheadedness, headache, anxiety, irritability
CV: Chest pain, pulse changes
GI: Nausea, vomiting, diarrhea, heartburn, abdominal pain, constipation, anorexia
***HEMA:* Leukopenia, granulocytopenia** (rare)

Contraindications: Hypersensitivity to benzodiazepines, pregnancy **X**, lactation, intermittent porphyria

Precautions: Anemia, hepatic disease, renal disease, suicidal individuals, drug
P abuse, elderly, psychosis, child <15 yr, acute
G narrow-angle glaucoma, seizure disorders

Pharmacokinetics
Absorption	Well absorbed
Distribution	Widely distributed, crosses placenta, crosses blood-brain barrier
Metabolism	Liver
Excretion	Kidneys, breast milk
Half-life	10-20 hr

Pharmacodynamics
Onset	½ hr
Peak	2-3 hr
Duration	6-8 hr

Interactions
Individual drugs
Alcohol: ↑ CNS depression
Cimetidine, disulfiram: ↑ effect of each specific drug
Propoxyphene, propranolol, valproic acid: ↑ action
Rifampin: ↓ action of temazepam
Theophylline: ↓ sedative effects
Drug classifications
Antidepressants, antihistamines, opiates: ↑ CNS depression
Barbiturates: ↓ effect of temazepam
Contraceptives (oral): ↑ effect
🗹 *Herb/drug*
Black cohosh: ↑ hypotension
Catnip, chamomile, clary, cowslip, hops, kava, lavender, mistletoe, nettle, pokeweed, poppy, Queen Anne's lace, senega, skullcap, valerian: ↑ CNS depression
Lab test interferences
↑ AST/ALT, ↑ serum bilirubin
↓ Radioactive iodine uptake
False: ↑ 17-OHCS

NURSING CONSIDERATIONS
Assessment
• Assess mental status: mood, sensorium, anxiety, affect, sleeping pattern, drowsiness,
G dizziness, especially elderly; physical dependency, withdrawal symptoms: anxiety, panic attacks, agitation, seizures, headache, nausea, vomiting, muscle pain, weakness; suicidal tendencies; for indications of increasing tolerance and abuse
• Monitor B/P (lying, standing), pulse; if systolic B/P drops 20 mm Hg, hold drug, notify prescriber
• Monitor blood studies: CBC during long-term therapy; blood dyscrasias have occurred rarely; decreased hematocrit, neutropenia may occur
• Monitor hepatic studies: AST, ALT, bilirubin, creatinine LDH, alkaline phosphatase

---

🗹 Herb/drug   🚫 Do Not Crush   ◆ Alert   ☗ Key Drug   **G** Geriatric   **P** Pediatric

• Monitor I&O ratio; indicate renal dysfunction

Nursing diagnoses
✓ Anxiety (uses)
✓ Depression (uses)
✓ Injury, risk for (adverse reactions)
✓ Knowledge, deficient (teaching)

Implementation
• Give with food or milk to decrease GI symptoms; if patient is unable to swallow medication whole, tab may be crushed and mixed with foods or fluids
• Give sugarless gum, hard candy, frequent sips of water for dry mouth

Patient/family education
• Inform patient that drug may be taken with food, and that fluids and tab may be crushed or swallowed whole
• Advise patient not to use for everyday stress or longer than 3 mo unless directed by prescriber; not to take more than prescribed amount; may be habit forming; not to double or skip doses
• Caution patient to avoid OTC preparations unless approved by prescriber; alcohol and CNS depressants will increase CNS depression
• Advise patient to avoid driving, activities that require alertness, because drowsiness may occur; to avoid alcohol ingestion or other psychotropic medications; to rise slowly or fainting may occur, especially in elderly; that drowsiness may worsen at beginning of treatment
• Caution patient not to discontinue medication abruptly after long-term use; withdrawal symptoms include vomiting, cramping, tremors, seizures
• Advise patient to use contraception while taking this drug

Evaluation
Positive therapeutic outcome
• Decreased anxiety, restlessness, sleeplessness (short-term treatment only)

Treatment of overdose: Lavage, VS, supportive care

---

temozolomide (Rx)
(tem-oo-zole′oo-mide)
Temodar
Func. class.: Antineoplastic alkylating agents
Chem. class.: Imidazotetrazine derivative

Pregnancy category D

Action: A pro-drug that undergoes conversion to 5-(3-methyl-1-triazeno) imidazole-4-carboxamide (MTIC); MTIC action prevents DNA transcription

➲ **Therapeutic Outcome:** Prevention of rapidly growing malignant cells

Uses: Anaplastic astrocytoma with relapse

Dosage and routes
Adult: PO adjust dose based on nadir neutrophil and platelet counts 150 mg/m^2/day × 5 days during 28-day cycle

Available forms: Caps 5, 20, 100, 250 mg

Adverse effects
(*italic* = common; **bold** = life-threatening)
CNS: **Seizures,** *hemiparesis, dizziness, poor coordination, amnesia, insomnia, paresthesia, somnolence, paresis, ataxia, anxiety, dysphagia, depression, confusion*
GI: *Nausea, anorexia, vomiting*
GU: *Urinary incontinence, UTI, frequency*
HEMA: **Thrombocytopenia, leukopenia,** anemia
INTEG: *Rash, pruritus*
MISC: *Headache, fatigue, asthenia, fever, edema, back pain, weight increase, diplopia*
RESP: *Upper respiratory tract infection, pharyngitis, sinusitis, coughing*

Contraindications: Hypersensitivity to this drug or dacarbazine, pregnancy **D**, lactation

Precautions: Radiation therapy, renal, hepatic disease

Pharmacokinetics

Absorption	Rapid, complete
Distribution	Crosses blood-brain barrier
Metabolism	To MTIC and metabolite
Excretion	Urine, feces
Half-life	1.8 hr

Pharmacodynamics

Onset	Unknown
Peak	1 hr
Duration	Unknown

Interactions
Individual drugs
Radiation: ↑ toxicity, bone marrow suppression
Drug classifications
Antineoplastics: ↑ toxicity
Antineoplastics, bone marrow-suppressing drugs: ↑ bone marrow suppression

Live virus vaccines: ↑ adverse reactions, ↓ antibody reaction

NURSING CONSIDERATIONS
Assessment
• Assess symptoms indicating severe allergic reaction: rash, pruritus, urticaria, purpuric skin lesions, itching, flushing; drug should be discontinued
• Obtain CBC on day 22 (21 days after 1st dose), CBC weekly until recovery if ANC is $<1.5 \times 10^9$/L and platelets $<100 \times 10^9$/L, do not administer to patients that do not tolerate 100 mg/m^2; myelosuppression usually occurs late in the treatment cycle
• Assess for seizures throughout treatment
• Monitor renal function studies: BUN, creatinine, urine CCr before and during therapy; I&O ratio; report fall in urine output to <30 ml/hr
• Monitor temp q4h (may indicate beginning of infection)
• Monitor liver function tests before and during therapy (bilirubin, AST, ALT, LDH) as needed or monthly; note jaundice of skin or sclera, dark urine, clay-colored stools, itchy skin, abdominal pain, fever, diarrhea; hepatotoxicity can be serious and fatal
• Assess for bleeding: hematuria, stool guaiac, bruising or petechiae, mucosa or orifices q8h; check for inflammation of mucosa, breaks in skin

Nursing diagnoses
☑ Injury, risk for (adverse reactions)
☑ Body image, disturbed (adverse reactions)
☑ Infection, risk for (adverse reactions)
☑ Knowledge, deficient (teaching)

Implementation
• Give fluids **IV** or PO before chemotherapy to hydrate patient
• Give antiemetic 30-60 min before giving drug to prevent vomiting, and prn; antibiotics for prophylaxis of infection
• Provide liq diet: carbonated beverages; gelatin may be added if patient is not nauseated or vomiting
• Capsules should not be opened, if accidentally damaged, do not allow contact with skin, or inhale; take caps one at a time with 8 oz of water at the same time of day
• Give on empty stomach to prevent nausea/vomiting

Patient/family education
• Teach patient to avoid use of products containing aspirin or NSAIDs, razors, commercial mouthwash, since bleeding may occur; to

report symptoms of bleeding (hematuria, tarry stools)
• Instruct patient to report signs of anemia (fatigue, headache, irritability, faintness, shortness of breath)
• Caution patient not to have any vaccinations without the advice of prescriber; serious reactions can occur
• Advise patient contraception is needed during treatment and for several months after completion of therapy; drug has teratogenic properties

Evaluation
Positive therapeutic outcome
• Prevention of rapid division of malignant cells

! HIGH ALERT

tenecteplase (Rx)
(ten-ek'ta-place)
TNKase
Func. class.: Thrombolytic enzyme
Chem. class.: Tissue plasminogen activator

Pregnancy category C

Action: Activates conversion of plasminogen to plasmin (fibrinolysin): plasmin breaks down clots (fibrin), fibrinogen, factors V, VII; occlusion of venous access lines

➔ **Therapeutic Outcome:** Resolution of MI

Uses: Acute MI

Dosage and routes
Adult <60 kg: **IV** bol 30 mg, give over 5 sec

Adult ≥60-<70 kg: **IV** bol 35 mg, give over 5 sec

Adult ≥70-<80 kg: **IV** bol 40 mg, give over 5 sec

Adult ≥80-<90 kg: **IV** bol 45 mg, give over 5 sec

Adult ≥90 kg: **IV** bol 50 mg, give over 5 sec

Available forms: Powder for inj, lyophilized 50 mg

Adverse effects
(*italic* = common; **bold** = life-threatening)
CV: Dysrhythmias, hypotension, pulmonary edema, **pulmonary embolism, cardiogenic shock, cardiac arrest, heart failure, myocardial reinfarction, myocardial**

☑ Herb/drug   Ⓢ Do Not Crush   ◆ Alert   ◑ₜₜ Key Drug   Ⓖ Geriatric   Ⓟ Pediatric

rupture, tamponade, pericarditis, pericardial effusion, thrombosis
HEMA: Decreased Hct, **bleeding**
INTEG: Rash, urticaria, phlebitis at **IV** inf site,
itching, flushing
SYST: **GI, GU, intracranial, retroperitoneal bleeding, surface bleeding, anaphylaxis**

Contraindications: Hypersensitivity,
arteriovenous malformation, aneurysm, active
bleeding, intracranial, intraspinal surgery, CNS
neoplasms, severe hypertension, severe renal
disease, hepatic disease

Precautions: Arterial emboli from left side
of heart, pregnancy **C**, lactation, children,
ulcerative colitis, enteritis, hypocoagulation,
COPD, subacute bacterial endocarditis, rheumatic valvular disease, cerebral embolism/
thrombosis/hemorrhage, intraarterial diagnostic procedure or surgery (10 days), recent
major surgery

Pharmacokinetics

Absorption	Unknown
Distribution	Unknown
Metabolism	Liver
Excretion	Unknown
Half-life	20-24 min

Pharmacodynamics

Onset	Immediate
Peak	Unknown
Duration	Unknown

Interactions
Individual drugs
Aspirin, dipyridamole, glycoprotein IIb,
indomethacin, IIIa inhibitors, phenylbutazone:
↑ bleeding potential
Drug classifications
Anticoagulants, antithrombolytics: ↑ bleeding
potential
Herb/drug
Agrimony, alfalfa, angelica, anise, basil, bay,
bilberry, black haw, bogbean, bromelain,
buchu, chondroitin, cinchona bark, dong quai,
fenugreek, feverfew, garlic, ginger, ginkgo,
ginseng, horse chestnut, Irish moss, kelp,
kelpware, khella, lovage, lungwort, meadowsweet, motherwort, mugwort, nettle, papaya,
parsley (large amounts), pau d'arco, pineapple, poplar, prickly ash, safflower, saw palmetto, tonka bean, turmeric, wintergreen,
yarrow: ↑ risk of bleeding
Chamomile, coenzyme Q10, flax, glucoman-

nan, goldenseal, guar gum: ↓ anticoagulant
effect
Lab test interferences
↑ Pro-time, ↑ APTT, ↑ TT
↓ Plasminogen, ↓ fibrinogen

NURSING CONSIDERATIONS
Assessment
• Assess for allergy: fever, rash, itching, chills;
mild reaction may be treated with antihistamines
◆ Assess for bleeding during 1st hr of treatment;
hematuria, hematemesis, bleeding from
mucous membranes, epistaxis, ecchymosis;
may require transfusion (rare), continue to
assess for bleeding for 24 hr
• Monitor blood studies (Hct, platelets, PTT,
Pro-time, TT, APTT) before starting therapy;
Pro-time or APTT must be less than 2 ×
control before starting therapy; PTT or Pro-
time q3-4h during treatment
• Assess for hypersensitivity reactions: fever,
rash, dyspnea; drug should be discontinued
• Monitor VS, B/P, pulse, respirations, neurologic signs, temp at least q4h; temp >104° F
(40° C) indicates internal bleeding; systolic
pressure increase >25 mm Hg should be
reported to prescriber
◆• Assess for neurologic changes that may
indicate intracranial bleeding
◆• Assess for retroperitoneal bleeding: back
pain, leg weakness, diminished pulses
Nursing diagnoses
☑ Knowledge, deficient (teaching)
☑ Cardiac output, decreased (uses)
Implementation
IV route
• Give as soon as thrombi identified; not
useful for thrombi >1 wk old
• Administer cryoprecipitate or fresh frozen
plasma if bleeding occurs
• Give heparin after fibrinogen level >100
mg/dl; heparin infusion to increase PTT to
1.5-2 × baseline for 3-7 days; **IV** heparin with
loading dose is recommended
• Aseptically withdraw 10 ml of sterile H_2O for
inj from diluent vial, use red cannula syringe-
filling device, inject all contents of syringe into
drug vial, direct into powder, swirl, withdraw
correct dose, discard any unused solution;
stand the shield with dose vertically on flat
surface and passively recap the red cannula,
remove entire shield assembly by twisting
counterclockwise, give by **IV** bol
• **IV** therapy: use upper extremity vessel that
is accessible to manual compression

T

- Provide bed rest during entire course of treatment
- Avoid venous or arterial puncture, inj, rectal temp; any invasive treatment
- Treat fever with acetaminophen or aspirin
- Apply pressure for 30 sec to minor bleeding sites; inform prescriber if this does not attain hemostasis; apply pressure dressing

Evaluation
Positive therapeutic outcome
- Resolution of myocardial infarction

---

tenofovir (Rx)
(ten-oh-foh'veer)
Viread
Func. class.: Antiretroviral
Chem. class.: Nucleoside analog reverse transcriptase inhibitor

Pregnancy category B

Action: Inhibits replication of HIV virus by competing with the natural substrate and then incorporating into cellular DNA by viral reverse transcriptase, thereby terminating cellular DNA chain

⇒**Therapeutic Outcome:** Improved symptoms of HIV infection

Uses: HIV-1 infection with other antiretrovirals

Dosage and routes
Adult: PO 300 mg with meal; if used with didanosine, give tenofovir 2 hr before or 1 hr after didanosine

Available forms: Tabs 300 mg (300 mg of fumarate salt equivalent to 245 mg tenofovir disoproxil)

Adverse effects
(*italic* = common; **bold** = life-threatening)
CNS: Headache
GI: Nausea, vomiting, diarrhea, anorexia, *flatulence, abdominal pain*
SYST: Change in body fat distribution

Contraindications: Hypersensitivity, CCr <60 ml/min

🅿**Precautions:** Pregnancy **B**, lactation,
🅖 children, elderly, renal disease, hepatic insufficiency

Pharmacokinetics

Absorption	Rapidly absorbed
Distribution	Extravascular space; bound to serum plasma <0.7%; to serum proteins <7.2%
Metabolism	Unknown
Excretion	Urine, unchanged (70%-80%)
Half-life	Unknown

Pharmacodynamics

Onset	Unknown
Peak	0.6-1.4 hr
Duration	Unknown

Interactions
Individual drugs
Acyclovir, cidofovir, ganciclovir, valacyclovir, valganciclovir: ↑ level of tenofovir
Didanosine: ↑ level of didanosine when coadministered with tenofovir
Drug classifications
↑ levels of tenofovir with any drug that ↓ renal function

NURSING CONSIDERATIONS
Assessment
- Assess liver studies: AST, ALT, bilirubin; amylase, lipase, triglycerides periodically during treatment
- Assess for bone, renal toxicity: if bone abnormalities are suspected, obtain tests: serum phosphorus, creatinine
- Assess for lactic acidosis, severe hepatomegaly with steatosis

Nursing diagnoses
☑ Infection, risk for (uses)
☑ Injury, risk for (adverse reactions)
☑ Knowledge, deficient (teaching)

Implementation
- Administer PO qd with meal
- Store at 25° C (77° F)

Patient/family education
- Instruct patient to take this drug 2 hr before or 1 hr after taking didanosine (if used)
- Instruct patient to take drug with meal
- Advise patients that GI complaints resolve after 3-4 wk of treatment
- Caution patient not to breastfeed while taking this drug
- Inform patient that drug must be taken qd even if patient feels better
- Advise patient to continue follow-up visits since serious toxicity may occur; blood counts must be done q2 wk
- Inform patient that drug will control symp-

toms but is not a cure for HIV; patient is still infectious, may pass HIV virus on to others
- Advise patient that other drugs may be necessary to prevent other infections
- Advise patient that changes in body fat distribution may occur

Evaluation
Positive therapeutic outcome
- Decrease in signs/symptoms of HIV

---

terazosin (Rx)
(ter-ay'zoe-sin)
Hytrin
Func. class.: Antihypertensive
Chem. class.: α-Adrenergic blocker
(peripherally acting)

Pregnancy category C

Action: Peripheral blood vessels are dilated, peripheral resistance lowered; reduction in blood pressure results from α-adrenergic receptors being blocked

⇒ **Therapeutic Outcome:** Decreased B/P in hypertension, decreased symptoms of benign prostatic hyperplasia (BPH)

Uses: Hypertension, as a single agent or in combination with diuretics or β-blockers, BPH

Dosage and routes
Hypertension
Adult: PO 1 mg hs, may increase doses slowly to desired response; max 20 mg/day

Benign prostatic hyperplasia
Adult: PO 1 mg hs, gradually increase up to 5-10 mg

Available forms: Tabs 1, 2, 5, 10 mg

Adverse effects
(*italic* = common; **bold** = life-threatening)
CNS: *Dizziness, headache, drowsiness,* anxiety, depression, vertigo, weakness, fatigue
CV: Palpitations, orthostatic hypotension, tachycardia, edema, rebound hypertension
EENT: Blurred vision, epistaxis, tinnitus, dry mouth, red sclera, nasal congestion, sinusitis
GI: *Nausea,* vomiting, diarrhea, constipation, abdominal pain
GU: Urinary frequency, incontinence, impotence, priapism
RESP: Dyspnea, cough, pharyngitis

Contraindications: Hypersensitivity

P **Precautions:** Pregnancy **C**, children, lactation

Pharmacokinetics
Absorption	Well absorbed
Distribution	Not known
Metabolism	Liver—50%
Excretion	Kidneys unchanged—10%, feces unchanged—20%
Half-life	9-12 hr

Pharmacodynamics
Onset	15 min
Peak	1 hr
Duration	24 hr

Interactions
Individual drugs
Alcohol: ↑ CNS depression
Nitroglycerin: ↑ hypotensive effects
Drug classifications
Antihypertensives (other): ↑ hypotension
β-blockers, nitrates: ↑ hypotensive effects
Estrogens, NSAIDs, sympathomimetics: ↓ antihypertensive effect

NURSING CONSIDERATIONS
Assessment
- Monitor B/P, orthostatic hypotension, syncope; check for edema in feet, legs daily; I&O ratio; weight daily; notify prescriber of changes
- Assess for allergic reactions: rash, fever, pruritus, urticaria; drug should be discontinued if antihistamines fail to help

Nursing diagnoses
✓ Cardiac output, decreased (uses)
✓ Injury, risk for (adverse reactions)
✓ Knowledge, deficient (teaching)
✓ Noncompliance (teaching)

Implementation
- Store in airtight container at 86° F (30° C) or less
- May be used in combination with other antihypertensives
- May be given with food to prevent GI symptoms

Patient/family education
- Caution patient not to discontinue drug abruptly; the importance of complying with dosage schedule, even if feeling better; if dose is missed take as soon as remembered; take medication at same time each day
- Teach patient not to use OTC products (cough, cold, allergy) unless directed by prescriber; also to avoid large amounts of caffeine
- Emphasize the need to rise slowly to sitting or standing position to minimize orthostatic hypotension

T

- Teach patient to notify prescriber of mouth sores, sore throat, fever, swelling of hands or feet, irregular heartbeat, chest pain
- Caution patient to report excessive perspiration, dehydration, vomiting, diarrhea; may lead to fall in B/P
- Caution patient that drug may cause dizziness, fainting, light-headedness; may occur during 1st few days of therapy; to avoid hazardous activities
- Teach patient how to take B/P, and normal readings for age group; to take B/P q7 days

Evaluation

Positive therapeutic outcome
- Decreased B/P in hypertension
- Decreased symptoms of BPH

Treatment of overdose: Administer volume expanders or vasopressors; discontinue drug; place patient in supine position

---

terbutaline (Rx)
(ter-byoo′te-leen)
Brethine, Bricanyl
Func. class.: Selective β_2-agonist; bronchodilator
Chem. class.: Catecholamine

Pregnancy category B

Action: Relaxes bronchial smooth muscle by direct action on β_2-adrenergic receptors through accumulation of cAMP at β-adrenergic receptor sites; results in bronchodilation, diuresis, and CNS and cardiac stimulation; relaxes uterine smooth muscle

➡ **Therapeutic Outcome:** Bronchodilation with ease of breathing

Uses: Bronchospasm

Investigational uses: Premature labor, hyperkalemia

Dosage and routes
Bronchospasm
P *Adult and child >12 yr:* INH 2 puffs q1 min, then q4-6h; PO 2.5-5 mg q8h; SC 0.25 mg q15-30 min, max 0.5 mg in 4 hr

Bronchodilation
P *Adult/child >15 yr:* PO 2.5-5 mg q6h during day, max 15 mg/24 hr

P *Child 12-15 yr:* PO 2.5 mg tid

Renal dose
Adult: PO GFR 10-50 ml/min 50% of dose

Severe renal failure
Adult: PO avoid if GFR <10 ml/min

Available forms: Tabs 2.5, 5 mg; aerosol 0.2 mg/actuation; inj 1 mg/ml

Adverse effects
(*italic* = common; **bold** = life-threatening)
CNS: Tremors, anxiety, insomnia, headache, dizziness, stimulation
CV: Palpitations, tachycardia, hypertension, dysrhythmias, **cardiac arrest**
GI: Nausea, vomiting

Contraindications: Hypersensitivity to sympathomimetics, narrow-angle glaucoma, tachydysrhythmias

Precautions: Pregnancy **B**, cardiac disorders, hyperthyroidism, diabetes mellitus,
G prostatic hypertension, lactation, elderly, hypertension, glaucoma

Pharmacokinetics	
Absorption	Well absorbed (SC), partially absorbed (PO)
Distribution	Unknown
Metabolism	Liver—partially
Excretion	Unknown
Half-life	Unknown

Pharmacodynamics				
	PO	INH	SC	IV
Onset	½ hr	5-15 min	10-15 min	Rapid
Peak	1-2 hr	1-2 hr	½-1 hr	Unknown
Duration	4-8 hr	4-6 hr	1½-4 hr	Unknown

Interactions
Individual drugs
Bleomycin: drugs are incompatible
Drug classifications
β-Adrenergic blockers: Block therapeutic effect
Bronchodilators, aerosol: ↑ action of bronchodilator
MAOIs: ↑ chance of hypertensive crisis
Sympathomimetics: ↑ adrenergic side effects
🗹 *Herb/drug*
Green tea (large amounts), guarana: ↑ effect

NURSING CONSIDERATIONS
Assessment
- Monitor respiratory function: vital capacity, FEV, ABGs, lung sounds, heart rate, rhythm (baseline)
- Determine that patient has not received theophylline therapy before giving dose; assess client's ability to self-medicate
- Monitor for evidence of allergic reactions; withhold dose and notify prescriber
- Assess for paradoxical bronchospasm: dyspnea, wheezing, keep emergency resuscitative equipment nearby

---

🗹 Herb/drug   Ⓢ Do Not Crush   ◆ Alert   ◆⚡ Key Drug   G Geriatric   P Pediatric

- Assess for labor: maternal heart rate, B/P, contractions, fetal heart rate

Nursing diagnoses
☑ Airway clearance, ineffective (uses)
☑ Gas exchange, impaired (uses)
☑ Knowledge, deficient (teaching)
☑ Noncompliance (teaching)

Implementation
Aerosol route
- Give after shaking; ask patient to exhale, place mouthpiece in mouth, then inhale slowly; hold breath, remove, exhale slowly; allow at least 1 min between inhalations
- Store in light-resistant container, do not expose to temp over 86° F (30° C)

PO route
- Give PO with meals to decrease gastric irritation; tab may be crushed and mixed with foods and fluids

IM route
- Do not give by IM route

SC route
- May give by SC route

IV route
- Give at 5 mcg q10 min until contractions are stopped, use infusion pump for correct dose; after ½-1 hr with no contraction decrease dose by 5 mcg; switch to PO dose when possible

Syringe compatibilities: Doxapram

Y-site compatibilities: Regular insulin

Additive compatibilities: Aminophylline

Additive incompatibilities: Bleomycin

Patient/family education
- Advise patient not to use OTC medications; extra stimulation may occur; to use this medication before other medications and allow at least 5 min between each to prevent overstimulation
- Teach patient how to use inhaler; to avoid getting aerosol in eyes because blurring may result; to wash inhaler in warm water qd and dry; to avoid smoking, smoke-filled rooms, persons with respiratory infections; review package insert with patient
- Teach patient that paradoxical bronchospasm may occur; to stop drug immediately and notify prescriber; to limit caffeine products such as chocolate, coffee, tea, and colas
- Instruct patient on administration of dose, not to use more than prescribed; serious side effects may occur; if taking PO regularly and dose is missed, take when remembered; space other doses on new time schedule

Evaluation
Positive therapeutic outcome
- Absence of dyspnea, wheezing after 1 hr
- Improved airway exchange
- Improved ABGs

Treatment of overdose: Administer a β_2-adrenergic blocker

---

teriparatide (Rx)
(tah-ree-par'ah-tide)
Forteo
Func. class.: Parathyroid hormone (rDNA)

Pregnancy category C

Action: Contains human recombinant parathyroid hormone, which stimulates new bone growth

Therapeutic Outcome: Calcium levels at 9-10 mg/dl,
↓ symptoms of hypocalcemia, hypoparathyroidism

Uses: Postmenopausal women with osteoporosis, men with primary or hypogonadal osteoporosis who are at high risk for fracture

Dosage and routes
Adult: **SC** 20 mcg qd, use >2 yr

Available forms: Inj 250 mcg/ml

Adverse effects
(*italic* = common; **bold** = life-threatening)

CNS: Dizziness, headache, insomnia, depression, vertigo
CV: Hypertension, angina, syncope
GI: Nausea, diarrhea, dyspepsia, vomiting, constipation
INTEG: Rash, sweating
MS: Arthralgia, leg cramps
MISC: Pain, asthenia
RESP: Rhinitis, cough, pharyngitis, pneumonia, dyspnea

Contraindications: Hypersensitivity, increased baseline risk of osteosarcoma (Paget's disease, open epiphyses, previous bone radiation), bone metastases, history of skeletal malignancies, other metabolic bone diseases, preexisting hypercalcemia

Precautions: Pregnancy **C**, lactation, urolithiasis, hypotension

T

Pharmacokinetics

Absorption	Extensively, rapidly
Distribution	Unknown
Metabolism	Liver
Excretion	Kidneys
Half-life	Unknown

Pharmacodynamics
Unknown

Interactions
Individual drug
Digoxin: ↑ digoxin toxicity when used with teriparatide
Lab test interferences
Calcium: ↑ levels

NURSING CONSIDERATIONS
Assessment
• Uric acid, chloride, magnesium, electrolytes, urine pH, vit D, phosphate for normal serum levels. Serum calcium may be transiently increased after dosing (max at 4-6 hrs post-dose)
• For bone pain, headache, fatigue, changes in LOC, leg cramps
• For signs of persistent hypercalcemia: nausea, vomiting, constipation, lethargy, muscle weakness
• Nutritional status: diet for sources of vit D (milk, some seafood), calcium (dairy products, dark green vegetables), phosphates (dairy products)

Nursing diagnoses
✓ Injury, risk for (uses)
✓ Mobility, impaired physical (uses)
✓ Knowledge, deficient (teaching)

Implementation
• Store refrigerated, do not freeze
SC route
• Give by SC only, rotate inj sites

Patient/family education
• Advise patient of the symptoms of hypercalcemia
• Teach about foods rich in calcium
• Teach how to use delivery device, dispose of needles, not to share pen with others
• To sit or lie down if dizziness or fast heartbeat occurs after the first few doses

Evaluation
Positive therapeutic outcome
• Increased bone mineral density

testosterone ⬥℞ (Rx)
(tess-toss'te-rone)
testosterone, long acting
testosterone enanthate
Andro LA, Andropository, Andryl, Delatest, Delatestryl, Everone, Malogx ✦, Testone LA, Testrin-PA
testosterone cypionate
Andro-Cyp, Andronate, depAndro, Depotest, Dura-test, T-Cypionate, Testa-C, Testred, Testoject-LA, Virilon IM
testosterone pellets
Testopel
testosterone transdermal
Androderm, Testoderm, Testoderm TTS, Testoderm with Adhesive
testosterone gel
AndroGel 1%
Func. class.: Androgenic anabolic steroid
Chem. class.: Halogenated testosterone derivative

Pregnancy category X
Controlled substance III

Action: Increases weight by building body tissue; increases potassium, phosphorus, chloride, nitrogen levels; increases bone development; responsible for maintenance of secondary sex characteristics (male)

➡ **Therapeutic Outcome:** Increased hormone levels in eunuchoidism, decreased tumor growth in female breast cancer, onset of male puberty

Uses: Female breast cancer, eunuchoidism, male climacteric, oligospermia, impotence, osteoporosis, weight loss in AIDS patients, vulvar dystrophies, low testosterone levels

Dosage and routes
Replacement
Adult: IM 25-50 mg 2-3 ×/wk (base or propionate) or 50-400 mg q2-4 wk (enanthate or cypionate); TD Testoderm 4-6 mg applied q24h; Androderm 5 mg applied q24h; once qd (gel)

Breast cancer
Adult: IM 50-100 mg 3 ×/wk (propionate) or 200-400 mg q2-4 wk (cypionate or enanthate)

Delayed male puberty
P *Child >12 yr:* IM up to 100 mg/mo for up to 6 mo

Available forms: *Enanthate:* inj 200 mg/ml; *cypionate:* inj 100, 200 mg/ml; pellets 75 mg; TD 2.5, 4, 5, 6 mg/24 hr; gel 1%

Adverse effects

(*italic* = common; **bold** = life-threatening)

CNS: Dizziness, headache, fatigue, tremors, paresthesias, flushing, sweating, anxiety, lability, insomnia, carpal tunnel syndrome
CV: Increased B/P
EENT: Conjunctival edema, nasal congestion
ENDO: Abnormal GTT
GI: Nausea, vomiting, constipation, weight gain, **cholestatic jaundice**
GU: Hematuria, amenorrhea, vaginitis, decreased libido, decreased breast size, clitoral hypertrophy, testicular atrophy
INTEG: Rash, acneiform lesions, oily hair and skin, flushing, sweating, acne vulgaris, alopecia, hirsutism
MS: Cramps, spasms

Contraindications: Severe renal disease, severe cardiac disease, severe hepatic disease, hypersensitivity, pregnancy **X,** lactation, genital bleeding (abnormal)

Precautions: Diabetes mellitus, CV disease, MI

Pharmacokinetics

Absorption	Well but slowly absorbed
Distribution	Crosses placenta
Metabolism	Liver
Excretion	Kidneys, breast milk
Half-life	8 days (cypionate)
	10-100 min (base)

Pharmacodynamics

	IM (base)	IM (cypionate)	IM (enanthate)	IM (propionate)
Onset	Unknown	Unknown	Unknown	Unknown
Peak	Unknown	Unknown	Unknown	Unknown
Duration	1-3 days	2-4 wk	2-4 wk	1-3 days

Interactions

Individual drugs

ACTH: ↑ edema
Oxyphenbutazone: ↑ effects of oxyphenbutazone

Drug classifications

Adrenal steroids: ↑ edema
Anticoagulants: ↑ Pro-time
Antidiabetics, oral: ↓ need for oral antidiabetics

Lab test interferences

↑ Serum cholesterol, ↑ blood glucose, ↑ urine glucose

↓ Serum Ca, ↓ serum K, ↓ T$_4$, ↓ T$_3$, ↓ thyroid ^{131}I uptake test, ↓ urine 17-OHCS, ↓ 17-KS, ↓ PBI

NURSING CONSIDERATIONS

Assessment

• Monitor patient's weight daily; notify prescriber if weekly weight gain is >5 lb; assess I&O ratio; be alert for decreasing urinary output, increasing edema
• Monitor B/P q4h
P • Assess growth rate in adolescent because growth rate may be uneven (linear/bone growth) if used for extended periods
• Monitor electrolytes: potassium, sodium, chloride, calcium; cholesterol
• Monitor liver function studies: ALT, AST, bilirubin
• Assess edema, hypertension, cardiac symptoms, jaundice
• Assess mental status: affect, mood, behavioral changes, aggression
• Assess signs of masculinization in female: increased libido, deepening of voice, decreased breast tissue, enlarged clitoris, menstrual irregularities; male: gynecomastia, impotence, testicular atrophy
• Assess hypercalcemia: lethargy, polyuria, polydipsia, nausea, vomiting, constipation; drug may have to be decreased
• Assess hypoglycemia in diabetics because oral antidiabetic action is increased

Nursing diagnoses

✓ Infection, risk for (adverse reactions)
✓ Injury, risk for (adverse reactions)
✓ Knowledge, deficient (teaching)

Implementation

• Administer diet with increased calories, protein; decreased sodium if edema occurs
• Administer supportive drug if anemia occurs
• Give titrated dose; use lowest effective dose
• Give IM inj deep into upper outer quadrant of gluteal muscle; route can be painful
Gel route
• Apply qd to clean, dry area on shoulders, upper arms, or abdomen

Patient/family education

• Inform patient that drug needs to be combined with complete health plan: diet, rest, exercise
• Caution patient to notify prescriber if therapeutic response decreases; not to discontinue this medication abruptly
• Inform women patients to report menstrual irregularities; about changes in sex characteristics

- Discuss that 1-3 mo course is necessary for response in breast cancer
- TD patches: Testoderm to skin of scrotum, Androderm to skin of back, upper arms, thighs, abdomen; area must be dry and free of hair; may be reapplied after bathing, swimming

Evaluation
Positive therapeutic outcome
- Decrease size of tumor in breast cancer
- Increased androgen levels

---

tetracycline (Rx)
(tet-ra-sye′kleen)
Achromycin V, Actisite (dental product), Alatel, Apo-Tetra ✦, Novotetra ✦, Nu-Tetra ✦, Panmycin, Robitet, Sumycin, Teline, Tetracap, tetracycline HCl, Tetracyn, Tetralan, Tetram
Func. class.: Antiinfective—broad-spectrum
Chem. class.: Tetracycline

Pregnancy category D

Action: Inhibits protein synthesis and phosphorylation in microorganisms; bacteriostatic

➲ **Therapeutic Outcome:** Bactericidal action against susceptible organisms: gram-positive pathogens *Bacillus anthracis, Clostridium perfringens, Clostridium tetani, Listeria monocytogenes, Nocardia, Propionibacterium acnes, Actinomyces israelii;* gram-negative pathogens *Haemophilus influenzae, Legionella pneumophila, Yersinia enterocolitica, Yersinia pestis, Neisseria gonorrhoeae, Neisseria meningitidis*

Uses: Syphilis, *Chlamydia trachomatis,* gonorrhea, lymphogranuloma venereum, uncommon gram-positive, gram-negative organisms, rickettsial infections

Dosage and routes
Adult: PO 250-500 mg q6h

P *Child >8 yr:* PO 25-50 mg/kg/day in divided doses q6h

Gonorrhea
Adult: PO 1.5 g, then 500 mg qid for a total of 9 g over 7 days

Chlamydia trachomatis
Adult: PO 500 mg qid × 7 days

Syphilis
Adult: PO 2-3 g in divided doses × 10-15 days; if syphilis duration >1 yr, must treat 30 days

Brucellosis
Adult: PO 500 mg qid × 3 wk with 1 g of streptomycin IM 2 ×/day × 1 wk, and 1 ×/day the 2nd wk

Urethral syndrome in women
Adult: PO 500 mg qid × 7 days

Acne
Adult: 1 g/day in divided doses; maintenance 125-500 mg/day

Available forms: Oral susp 125 mg/5 ml, caps 100, 200, 500 mg; tabs 250, 500 mg

Adverse effects
(*italic* = common; **bold** = life-threatening)
CNS: Fever, headache, paresthesia
CV: **Pericarditis**
EENT: Dysphagia, glossitis, decreased calcification (permanent discoloration) of deciduous teeth, oral candidiasis, oral ulcers
GI: *Nausea,* abdominal pain, *vomiting, diarrhea,* anorexia, enterocolitis, **hepatotoxicity,** flatulence, abdominal cramps, epigastric burning, stomatitis
GU: *Increased BUN*
HEMA: **Eosinophilia, neutropenia, thrombocytopenia, leukocytosis, hemolytic anemia**
INTEG: *Rash, urticaria, photosensitivity, increased pigmentation,* **exfoliative dermatitis,** pruritus, **angioedema**

Contraindications: Hypersensitivity to
P tetracyclines, children <8 yr, pregnancy **D,** lactation

Precautions: Renal disease, hepatic disease

Pharmacokinetics	
Absorption	60%-80% (PO), lower (IM)
Distribution	Widely distributed, some in CSF; crosses placenta
Metabolism	Not metabolized
Excretion	Unchanged—kidneys
Half-life	6-10 hr

Pharmacodynamics	
Onset	1-2 hr
Peak	2-3 hr

Interactions
Individual drugs
Cimetidine, kaolin/pectin, NaHCO$_3$: ↓ tetracycline effect
Digoxin: ↑ digoxin effect
Iron: Forms chelates, ↓ absorption
Methoxyflurane: nephrotoxicity
Warfarin: ↑ warfarin effect

Drug classifications
Alkali products, antacids: ↓ tetracycline effect
Contraceptives (oral): ↓ oral contraceptive effect
Penicillins: ↓ penicillin effect
Food/drug
↓ Absorption with dairy products; forms insoluble chelate
Herb/drug
Dong quai: ↑ photosensitivity
Lab test interferences
False: ↑ Urinary catecholamines
False negative: Urine glucose with Clinistix, Tes-Tape

NURSING CONSIDERATIONS
Assessment
- Assess patient for previous sensitivity reaction
- Assess patient for signs and symptoms of infection including characteristics of wounds, sputum, urine, stool, WBC >10,000/mm³, temp; obtain baseline information before and during treatment
- Complete C&S testing before beginning drug therapy to identify if correct treatment has been initiated
- Assess for allergic reactions: rash, urticaria, pruritus, chills, fever, joint pain; angioedema may occur a few days after therapy begins; epINEPHrine, resuscitation equipment should be available for anaphylactic reaction
- Identify urine output; if decreasing, notify prescriber (may indicate nephrotoxicity); also, increased BUN, creatinine
- Monitor blood studies: AST, ALT, CBC, Hct, bilirubin, LDH, alkaline phosphatase, monthly if patient is on long-term therapy
- Assess bowel pattern qd; if severe diarrhea occurs, drug should be discontinued
- Monitor for bleeding: ecchymosis, bleeding gums, hematuria, stool guaiac daily if on long-term therapy; blood dyscrasias may occur
- Assess for overgrowth of infection: perineal itching, fever, malaise, redness, pain, swelling, drainage, rash, diarrhea, change in cough, sputum

Nursing diagnoses
☑ Infection, risk for (uses)
☑ Diarrhea (adverse reactions)
☑ Injury, risk for (adverse reactions)
☑ Knowledge, deficient (teaching)
☑ Noncompliance (teaching)

Implementation
PO route
- Give around the clock to maintain proper blood levels; give with food to increase absorp-

tion of drug; do not give within 3 hr of other agents; drug actions may occur; take on an empty stomach
- Give with 8 oz of water
- Shake liq preparation well before giving; use calibrated device for proper dosing

Patient/family education
- Teach patient to report sore throat, bruising, bleeding, joint pain; may indicate blood dyscrasias (rare)
- Advise patient to use sunscreen when outdoors to decrease photosensitivity reaction
- Advise patient to contact prescriber if vaginal itching; loose foul-smelling stools; furry tongue occur; may indicate super-infection; report itching, rash, pruritus, urticaria
- Instruct patient to take all medication prescribed for the length of time ordered; drug must be taken around the clock to maintain blood levels; do not give medication to others

Evaluation
Positive therapeutic outcome
- Absence of signs/symptoms of infection (WBC <10,000/mm³, temp WNL, absence of red, draining wounds)
- Reported improvement in symptoms of infection

---

theophylline ⚙π (Rx)
(thee-off'i-lin)
Accurbron, Aquaphyllin, Asmalix, Bronkodyl, Elixomin, Elixophyllin, Lanophyllin, Quibron-T Dividose, Quibron-T/SR, Respbid, Slo-bid Gyrocaps, Slo-Phyllin, Sustaire, Theo-24, Theobid Duracaps, Theochron, Theoclear-80, Theoclear L.A., Theo-Dur, Theolair-SR, Theo-Sav, Theospan-SR, Theostat 80, Theovent, Theo-X, T-Phy, Uni-Dur, Uniphyl
Func. class.: Spasmolytic, bronchodilator
Chem. class.: Xanthine, ethylenediamine

Pregnancy category C

Action: Relaxes smooth muscle of respiratory system by blocking phosphodiesterase, which increases cAMP, which increases bronchodilatation, diuresis, circulation, CNS stimulation

➲ **Therapeutic Outcome:** Ability to breathe without difficulty

Uses: Bronchial asthma, bronchospasm of COPD, chronic bronchitis

T

Dosage and routes
Hepatic dose
Adult: PO 6 mg/kg loading dose, then 2 mg/kg q8h ×2 doses, then 1-2 mg/kg q12h

Adult: **IV** 4.7 mg/kg then 0.39 mg/kg/hr for 12 hr, then 0.08-0.16 mg/kg/hr maintenance

Bronchospasm, bronchial asthma
Adult: PO 100-200 mg q6h; dosage must be individualized; rec 250-500 mg q8-12h

Child: PO 50-100 mg q6h, max 12 mg/kg/24 hr

COPD, chronic bronchitis
Adult: PO 330-660 q6-8h pc

Child 1-9 yr: PO 5 mg/kg loading dose, then 4 mg/kg q6h

Child 9-16 yr: PO 5 mg/kg loading dose, then 3 mg/kg q6h

Apnea of prematurity
Neonate: 2-10 mg/kg/day divided q8-12h (usual loading dose is 4 mg/kg)

Available forms: Caps 50, 100, 200, 250 mg; tabs 100, 125, 200, 225, 250, 300 mg; time rel tabs 100, 200, 250, 300, 400, 500 mg; time rel caps 50, 65, 100, 125, 130, 200, 250, 260, 300, 400, 500 mg; elixir 80, 11.25 mg/15 mg; sol 80 mg/15 ml; liq 80, 150, 160 mg/15 ml; susp 300 mg/15 ml

Adverse effects
(*italic* = common; **bold** = life-threatening)

CNS: *Anxiety, restlessness, insomnia, dizziness, seizures,* headache, light-headedness, muscle twitching, tremors

CV: *Palpitations, sinus tachycardia,* hypotension, **dysrhythmias,** fluid retention with tachycardia

ENDO: Hyperglycemia

GI: *Nausea, vomiting, anorexia,* diarrhea, bitter taste, dyspepsia, gastric distress

INTEG: Flushing, urticaria

RESP: Increased rate

Contraindications: Hypersensitivity to xanthines, tachydysrhythmias

Precautions: Elderly, CHF, cor pulmonale, hepatic disease, active peptic ulcer disease, diabetes mellitus, hyperthyroidism, hypertension, children, pregnancy **C**

Pharmacokinetics

Absorption	Well absorbed (PO), slowly absorbed (ext rel)
Distribution	Crosses placenta, widely distributed
Metabolism	Liver
Excretion	Kidneys, breast milk
Half-life	3-13, increased in liver disease, CHF, elderly

Pharmacodynamics

	PO	POTIME REL	IV
Onset	Rapid	Slow	Immediate
Peak	1 hr	4-8 hr	Inf end
Duration	6 hr	12-24 hr	6-8 hr

Interactions
Individual drugs
Carbamazepine: ↓ theophylline level

Cimetidine, ciprofloxacin, disulfiram, erythromycin, fluvoxamine, influenza vaccine, mexiletine, propranolol: ↑ theophylline action

Lithium: ↓ effect of lithium

Phenobarbital, phenytoin, rifampin: ↓ theophylline

Drug classifications
Anticoagulants: ↑ anticoagulant level

β-Adrenergic blockers: cardiotoxicity

Contraceptives (oral), corticosteroids, fluoroquinolones, interferons: ↑ theophylline action

Smoking: ↓ theophylline level

Herb/drug
Coffee, cola nut, guarana, tea (black, green), yerba maté: ↑ toxicity

St. John's wort: ↓ theophylline level

Ma Huang: ↑ toxicity

NURSING CONSIDERATIONS
Assessment
• Monitor theophylline blood levels (therapeutic level is 5-15 mcg/ml); toxicity may occur with small increase above 15 mcg/ml

• Monitor I&O; diuresis occurs; dehydration may result in elderly or children

• Assess for signs of toxicity: irritability, insomnia, restlessness, tremors, nausea, vomiting

• Monitor respiratory rate, rhythm, depth; auscultate lung fields bilaterally; notify prescriber of abnormalities

• Assess for allergic reactions: rash, urticaria; if these occur, drug should be discontinued

Nursing diagnoses
☑ Airway clearance, ineffective (uses)

☑ Knowledge, deficient (teaching)

 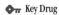

Implementation

PO route

- Give PO pc to decrease GI symptoms; absorption may be affected

IV IV route

- Give loading dose over 20-30 min, max 20-25 mg/min, do not give by rapid **IV**, use only by cont inf

Y-site compatibilities: Acyclovir, ampicillin, aztreonam, cefazolin, cefotetan, ceftazidime, ceftriaxone, cimetidine, clindamycin, dexamethasone, diltiazem, DOBUTamine, DOPamine, doxycycline, erythromycin, famotidine, fluconazole, gentamicin, haloperidol, heparin, hydrocortisone, lidocaine, methyldopate, methylPREDNISolone, metronidazole, midazolam, nafcillin, nitroglycerin, nitroprusside, penicillin G potassium, piperacillin, potassium chloride, ranitidine, ticarcillin, ticarcillin/clavulanate, tobramycin, vancomycin

Additive compatibilities: Cefepime, chlorproMAZINE, fluconazole, methylPREDNISolone, verapamil

Patient/family education

- Advise patient to check OTC medications, current prescription medications for epHEDrine, which will increase stimulation, and to avoid alcohol, caffeine
- Caution patient to avoid hazardous activities; dizziness may occur
- Inform patient that if GI upset occurs, to take drug with 8 oz of water; avoid food; absorption may be decreased
- Teach patient not to crush, dissolve, or chew slow-release products
- Teach patient that contents of bead-filled cap may be sprinkled over food for children's use
- Advise patient to notify prescriber of toxicity: nausea, vomiting, anxiety, insomnia, seizures
- Advise patient to notify prescriber of change in smoking habit; dosage may have to be changed

Evaluation

Positive therapeutic outcome

- Ability to breathe more easily

---

thiamine (vitamin B₁) (PO, OTC; IV Rx)

Betaxin ✦, Betalin S, Biamine, Revitonus, Thiamilate, thiamine HCl, vitamin B₁
Func. class.: Vitamin B₁
Chem. class.: Water soluble

Pregnancy category A

Action: Needed for pyruvate metabolism, carbohydrate metabolism

⮕ **Therapeutic Outcome:** Prevention and treatment of thiamine deficiency

Uses: Vit B₁ deficiency or polyneuritis, cheilosis adjunct with thiamine beriberi, Wernicke-Korsakoff syndrome, pellagra, metabolic disorders

Dosage and routes

RDA
Adult: Male 1.2-1.5 mg; females 1.1 mg; pregnancy 1.5 mg; lactation 1.6 mg

P *Child 7-10 yr:* 1.3 mg

P *Child 4-6 yr:* 0.9 mg

P *Child 1-3 yr:* 0.7 mg

P *Infants 6 mo-1 yr:* 0.4 mg

P *Neonates and infants to 6 mo:* 0.3 mg

Beriberi
Adult: IM 10-20 mg tid × 2 wk, then 5-10 mg qd × 1 mo

Beriberi with cardiac failure
P *Adult and child:* **IV** 10-30 mg tid

Available forms: Tabs 50, 100, 250, 500 mg; inj 100 mg/ml; enteric-coated tabs 20 mg

Adverse effects

(*italic* = common; **bold** = life-threatening)
CNS: Weakness, restlessness
CV: **Collapse, pulmonary edema,** hypotension
EENT: Tightness of throat
GI: Hemorrhage, *nausea, diarrhea*
INTEG: **Angioneurotic edema,** cyanosis, sweating, warmth
SYST: **Anaphylaxis**

Contraindications: Hypersensitivity

Precautions: Pregnancy **A**

◣ Do Not Confuse:
thiamine/Tenormin

T

Pharmacokinetics

Absorption	Well absorbed (PO, IM), completely absorbed (**IV**)
Distribution	Widely distributed
Metabolism	Liver
Excretion	Kidneys (unchanged—excess amounts)
Half-life	Unknown

Pharmacodynamics

Unknown

Interactions

None known

NURSING CONSIDERATIONS
Assessment

• Monitor thiamine levels throughout treatment
• Assess nutritional status: yeast, beef, liver, whole or enriched grains, legumes

Nursing diagnoses

☑ Nutrition: less than body requirements, imbalanced (uses)
☑ Knowledge, deficient (teaching)

Implementation
IM route

• Give by IM inj; rotate sites if pain and inflammation occur; do not mix with alkaline sol; Z-track to minimize pain
• Application of cold may decrease pain
• Store in airtight, light-resistant container

IV IV route

• **IV** undiluted given over 5 min or diluted with **IV** sol and given as an inf at a rate of 100 mg or less/5 min or more

Syringe compatibilities: Doxapram

Y-site compatibilities: Famotidine

Additive incompatibilities: Barbiturates; sol with neutral or alkaline pH, such as carbonates, bicarbonates, citrates and acetates; erythromycin, kanamycin, or streptomycin

Patient/family education

• Teach patient necessary foods to be included in diet: yeast, beef, liver, legumes, whole grains

Evaluation
Positive therapeutic outcome

• Absence of nausea, vomiting, anorexia, insomnia, tachycardia, paresthesias, depression, muscle weakness

---

thiethylperazine (Rx)
(thye-eth-il-per′a-zeen)
Norzine, Torecan
Func. class.: Antiemetic
Chem. class.: Phenothiazine, piperazine derivative

Pregnancy category X

Action: Acts centrally by blocking chemoreceptor trigger zone, which in turn acts on vomiting center

➡ **Therapeutic Outcome:** Control of nausea, vomiting

Uses: Nausea, vomiting

Dosage and routes
Adult: PO/IM 10 mg/qd-tid

Available forms: Tabs 10 mg; inj 5 mg/ml

Adverse effects
(*italic* = common; **bold** = life-threatening)
CNS: Euphoria, depression, restlessness, tremor, extrapyramidal symptoms (EPS), **seizures,** drowsiness, confusion, **neuroleptic malignant syndrome**
CV: **Circulatory failure, tachycardia,** postural hypotension, ECG changes
GI: Nausea, vomiting, anorexia, dry mouth, diarrhea, constipation, weight loss, metallic taste, cramps
GU: Urinary retention, dark urine
HEMA: **Agranulocytosis, leukopenia**
RESP: **Respiratory depression**

Contraindications: Hypersensitivity to phenothiazines, coma, seizure, encephalopathy, bone marrow depression, pregnancy **X**

P Precautions: Children <2 yr, elderly, **G** lactation

Do Not Confuse:
Torecan/Toradol

Pharmacokinetics

Absorption	Readily absorbed
Distribution	Crosses placenta
Metabolism	Liver
Excretion	Kidneys, breast milk
Half-life	Unknown

Pharmacodynamics

	PO	IM
Onset	45-60 min	Unknown
Peak	Unknown	Unknown
Duration	4 hr	Unknown

Interactions
Drug classifications
Anesthetics (barbiturate, general), antidepressants, antihistamines, MAOIs, opiates, sedative/hypnotics: ↑ CNS depression
Antacids: ↓ absorption
Anticholinergics: ↑ anticholinergic effects
Antidiarrheals, adsorbent: ↓ absorption
Antihypertensives: ↑ hypotension
Antithyroid agents: ↑ agranulocytosis
β-Adrenergic blockers: ↑ effects of both drugs

NURSING CONSIDERATIONS
Assessment
• Monitor I&O ratio, palpate bladder if low
 G urinary output occurs, especially in elderly; urinalysis recommended before, during prolonged therapy
• Monitor bilirubin, CBC, liver function studies monthly
• Assess affect, orientation, LOC, reflexes, gait, coordination, sleep pattern disturbances
• Monitor B/P with patient in sitting, standing, and lying positions; take pulse and respirations q4h during initial treatment; establish baseline before starting treatment; report drops of 30 mm Hg
• Check for dizziness, faintness, palpitations, tachycardia on rising; severe orthostatic hypotension is common
◆• Identify for neuroleptic malignant syndrome: hyperpyrexia, muscle rigidity, increased CPK, altered mental status, seizures, fatigue, loss of urinary control, tachycardia; drug should be discontinued; have emergency equipment nearby
• Assess for EPS including akathisia (inability to sit still, no pattern to movements), tardive dyskinesia (bizarre movements of the jaw, mouth, tongue, extremities), pseudoparkinsonism (tremors, pill rolling, shuffling gait); antiparkinsonian drug should be prescribed
• Assess for constipation, urinary retention daily; if these occur, increase bulk, water in diet

Nursing diagnoses
☑ Thought processes, disturbed (uses)
☑ Coping, ineffective (uses)
☑ Knowledge, deficient (teaching)
☑ Noncompliance (teaching)

Implementation
IM route
• Give IM inj in large muscle mass; aspirate to avoid **IV** administration; give slowly; have patient remain supine for 1 hr after administration

Syringe compatibilities: Butorphanol, hydromorphone, midazolam, ranitidine

Y-site compatibilities: Aldesleukin

Patient/family education
• Teach patient to use good oral hygiene; frequent rinsing of mouth, sugarless gum for dry mouth
• Caution patient to avoid hazardous activities until drug response is determined; dizziness, blurred vision may occur
• Inform patient that orthostatic hypotension occurs often and to rise from sitting or lying position gradually
• Instruct patient to remain lying down after IM inj for at least 30 min
• Advise patient to avoid hot tubs, hot showers, tub baths, since hypotension may occur
• Inform patient that heat stroke may occur in hot weather, and to take extra precautions to stay cool
• Teach patient to avoid OTC preparations (cough, hay fever, cold) unless approved by prescriber because serious drug interactions may occur; avoid use with alcohol, CNS depressants because increased drowsiness may occur
• Inform patient to use sunglasses and sunscreen to prevent burns
• Teach patient about EPS
• Instruct patient to report sore throat, malaise, fever, bleeding, mouth sores; if these occur, CBC should be performed and drug discontinued

Evaluation
Positive therapeutic outcome
• Absence of nausea, vomiting

---

thioridazine (Rx)
(thye-or-rid′a-zeen)
Apo-Thioridazine ✦, Mellaril, Mellaril Concentrate, Mellaril-S, Novo-Ridazine ✦, PMS-Thioridazine ✦, thioridazine HCl
Func. class.: Antipsychotic/neuroleptic
Chem. class.: Phenothiazine, piperidine
Pregnancy category C

Action: Depresses cerebral cortex, hypothalamus, limbic system, which control activity, aggression; blocks neurotransmission produced by dopamine at synapse; exhibits strong α-adrenergic, anticholinergic blocking action; mechanism for antipsychotic effects is unclear

T

⊋ Therapeutic Outcome: Decreased signs and symptoms of psychosis

Uses: Psychotic disorders, schizophrenia, behavioral problems in children, alcohol withdrawal as adjunct, anxiety, major depressive disorders, organic brain syndrome, **G** dementia in elderly

Dosage and routes
Psychosis
Adult: PO 25-100 mg tid, max dose 800 mg/day; dose is gradually increased to desired response, then reduced to minimum maintenance

Depression/behavioral problems/ organic brain syndrome
Adult: PO 25 tid, range from 10 mg bid-qid to 50 mg tid-qid

G *Geriatric:* PO 10-25 mg qd-bid, increase 4-7 days by 10-25 mg to desired dose

P *Child 2-12 yr:* PO 0.5-3 mg/kg/day in divided doses

Available forms: Tabs 10, 15, 25, 50, 100, 150, 200 mg; conc 30, 100 mg/ml; susp 25, 100 mg/5 ml; syr 10 mg/15 ml

Adverse effects
(*italic* = common; **bold** = life-threatening)
CNS: Extrapyramidal symptoms (EPS) (rare) (pseudoparkinsonism, akathisia, dystonia, tardive dyskinesia), **seizures,** *headache,* confusion, **neuroleptic malignant syndrome, dizziness**
CV: Orthostatic hypotension, **cardiac arrest,** ECG changes, **tachycardia**
EENT: Blurred vision, glaucoma, dry eyes
GI: Dry mouth, nausea, vomiting, anorexia, constipation, diarrhea, jaundice, weight gain
GU: Urinary retention, urinary frequency, enuresis, impotence, amenorrhea, gynecomastia
HEMA: Anemia, **leukopenia, leukocytosis, agranulocytosis**
INTEG: Rash, photosensitivity, dermatitis
RESP: **Laryngospasm,** dyspnea, **respiratory depression**

Contraindications: Hypersensitivity,
P blood dyscrasias, coma, child <2 yr, brain damage, bone marrow depression

Precautions: Pregnancy C, lactation, seizure disorders, hypertension, hepatic disease, cardiac disease

◪ Do Not Confuse:
Mellaril/Elavil

Pharmacokinetics

Absorption	Variably absorbed (tab)
Distribution	Widely distributed, high concentrations in CNS, crosses placenta
Metabolism	Liver, extensively, GI mucosa
Excretion	Kidneys, breast milk
Half-life	26-36 hr

Pharmacodynamics

Onset	Erratic
Peak	2-4 hr
Duration	8-12 hr

Interactions
Individual drugs
Alcohol: ↑ oversedation
Aluminum hydroxide, magnesium hydroxide: ↓ absorption
Lithium: ↓ thioridazine levels
Drug classifications
Anesthetics (barbiturate, general): ↑ CNS depression
Antacids: ↓ absorption
Anticholinergics: ↑ anticholinergic effects
Barbiturates: ↓ thioridazine effect
Centrally acting antihypertensives: ↓ antihypertensive effect
CNS depressants: Oversedation
◪ Herb/drug
Betel palm, kava: ↑ EPS
Cola tree, hops, nettle, nutmeg: ↑ effect
Kava: ↑ CNS depression
Lab test interferences
↑ Liver function tests, ↑ cardiac enzymes, ↑ cholesterol, ↑ blood glucose, ↑ prolactin, ↑ bilirubin, ↑ PBI, ↑ cholinesterase, ↑ ^{131}I
↓ Hormones (blood and urine)
False positive: Pregnancy tests, PKU
False negative: Urinary steroids, pregnancy test

NURSING CONSIDERATIONS
Assessment
• Assess mental status: orientation, mood, behavior, presence of hallucinations, and type before initial administration and monthly; this drug should significantly reduce psychotic behavior
• Check for swallowing of PO medication; check for hoarding or giving of medication to other patients
• Monitor I&O ratio, palpate bladder if low
G urinary output occurs, especially in elderly; urinalysis recommended before, during prolonged therapy
• Monitor bilirubin, CBC, liver function studies monthly

- Assess affect, orientation, LOC, reflexes, gait, coordination, sleep pattern disturbances
- Monitor B/P sitting, standing, and lying, take pulse and respirations q4h during initial treatment; establish baseline before starting treatment; report drops of 30 mm Hg; obtain baseline ECG, monitor Q- and T-wave changes
- Check for dizziness, faintness, palpitations, tachycardia on rising; severe orthostatic hypotension is common
◆◆ • Identify for neuroleptic malignant syndrome: hyperpyrexia, muscle rigidity, increased CPK, altered mental status, dyspnea, fatigue; drug should be discontinued
- Assess for EPS including akathisia (inability to sit still, no pattern to movements), tardive dyskinesia (bizarre movements of the jaw, mouth, tongue, extremities), pseudoparkinsonism (ragged tremors, pill rolling, shuffling gate); an antiparkinsonian drug should be prescribed
- Assess for constipation, urinary retention daily; if these occur, increase bulk, water in diet

Nursing diagnoses
☑ Thought processes, disturbed (uses)
☑ Coping, ineffective (uses)
☑ Knowledge, deficient (teaching)
☑ Noncompliance (teaching)

Implementation
- Administer drug in liq form mixed in glass of juice or cola if hoarding is suspected; do not mix in caffeine drinks, tannics, pectins
🄖 • Decrease dose in elderly because metabolism is slowed
- Administer PO with full glass of water, milk; or give with food to decrease GI upset
- Store in airtight, light-resistant container, oral sol in amber bottle

Patient/family education
- Teach patient to use good oral hygiene; frequent rinsing of mouth, sugarless gum for dry mouth
- Advise patient to avoid hazardous activities until drug response is determined; dizziness, blurred vision are common
- Inform patient that orthostatic hypotension occurs often and to rise from sitting or lying position gradually; to avoid hot tubs, hot showers, tub baths because hypotension may occur
- Instruct patient that in hot weather, heat stroke may occur; take extra precautions to stay cool
- Caution patient to avoid abrupt withdrawal of this drug, or EPS may result; drug should be withdrawn slowly

- Teach patient to avoid OTC preparations (cough, hay fever, cold) unless approved by prescriber; serious drug interactions may occur; avoid use with alcohol, CNS depressants; increased drowsiness may occur
- Advise patient to use sunglasses and sunscreen to prevent burns
- Teach patient about EPS and necessity for meticulous oral hygiene because oral candidiasis may occur
- Advise patient to take antacids 2 hr before or after this drug
- Instruct patient to report sore throat, malaise, fever, bleeding, mouth sores; if these occur, CBC should be performed and drug discontinued

Evaluation
Positive therapeutic outcome
- Decrease in emotional excitement, hallucinations, delusions, paranoia
- Reorganization of patterns of thought, speech

Treatment of overdose: Lavage if orally ingested; provide airway; *do not induce vomiting or use epINEPHrine,* CV monitoring, continuous ECG

---

thyroid USP (desiccated) (Rx)
(thye′roid)
Armour Thyroid, Thyrar, Thyroid Strong, Westhroid
Func. class.: Thyroid hormone
Chem. class.: Active thyroid hormone in natural state and ratio
Pregnancy category A

Action: Increases metabolic rates; controls protein synthesis; increases cardiac output, renal blood flow, O_2 consumption, body temp, blood volume, growth, development at cellular level

⮕ **Therapeutic Outcome:** Correction of lack of thyroid hormone

🄟 *Uses:* Hypothyroidism, cretinism (juvenile hypothyroidism), myxedema

Dosage and routes
Hypothyroidism
Adult: PO 65 mg qd, increased by 65 mg q30 days until desired response; maintenance dose 65-195 mg qd

🄖 *Elderly:* PO 7.5-15 mg qd, double dose q6-8 wk until desired response

T

Cretinism/juvenile hypothyroidism
P *Child over 1 yr:* PO up to 180 mg qd titrated to response

P *Child 4-12 mo:* PO 30-60 mg qd

P *Child 1-4 mo:* PO 15-30 mg qd; may increase q2 wk; titrated to response; maintenance dose 30-45 mg qd

Myxedema
Adult: PO 16 mg qd, double dose q2 wk, maintenance 65-195 mg/day

Available forms: Tabs 16, 32, 65, 98, 130, 195, 260, 325 mg; enteric-coated tabs 32, 65, 130 mg; sugar-coated tabs 32, 65, 130, 195 mg; caps 65, 130, 195, 325 mg

Adverse effects
(*italic* = common; **bold** = life-threatening)
CNS: Insomnia, tremors, headache, thyroid storm
CV: Tachycardia, palpitations, angina, **dysrhythmias,** hypertension, **cardiac arrest**
GI: Nausea, diarrhea, increased or decreased appetite, cramps
MISC: Menstrual irregularities, weight loss, sweating, heat intolerance, fever

Contraindications: Adrenal insufficiency, MI, thyrotoxicosis

G **Precautions:** Elderly, angina pectoris, hypertension, ischemia, cardiac disease, pregnancy **A,** lactation

N **Do Not Confuse:**
Thyrar/Thyrolar

Pharmacokinetics	
Absorption	Well absorbed
Distribution	Widely distributed, does not cross placenta
Metabolism	Liver, tissues
Excretion	Feces via bile, breast milk
Half-life	T_3—2 days; T_4—1 wk

Pharmacodynamics	
Onset	1 hr
Peak	12-48 hr
Duration	Unknown

Interactions
Individual drugs
Digoxin: ↓ effect of digoxin
Insulin: ↑ requirement for insulin
Drug classifications
Amphetamines, decongestants, vasopressors: ↑ CNS, cardiac stimulation
Anticoagulants, oral: ↑ requirements for anticoagulants

Antidepressants (tricyclic): ↑ antidepressants (tricyclic) effect
Bile acid sequestrants: ↓ thyroid absorption
Estrogens: ↓ thyroid hormone effect
Hypoglycemics, sympathomimetics: ↓ effect of each specific drug
Herb/drug
Agar, bugleweed, carnitine, kelpware, soy, spirulina: ↓ thyroid effect
Lab test interferences
↑ CPK, ↑ LDH, ↑ AST, ↑ PBI, ↑ blood glucose
↓ Thyroid function tests

NURSING CONSIDERATIONS
Assessment
• Identify if the patient is taking anticoagulants, antidiabetic agents; document on chart
• Take B/P, pulse before each dose; monitor I&O ratio and weight every day in same clothing, using same scale, at same time of day
• Monitor height, weight, psychomotor development, and growth rate if given to a P child
• Monitor T_3, T_4, FTIs, which are decreased; radioimmunoassay of TSH, which is increased; radioactive iodine uptake (RAIU), which is increased if patient's dose of medication is too low
• Monitor Pro-time; patient may require decreased dosage of anticoagulant; check for bleeding, bruising
• Assess for increased nervousness, excitability, irritability, which may indicate that dose of medication is too high, usually after 1-3 wk of treatment
• Assess cardiac status: angina, palpitation, G chest pain, change in VS; the elderly patient may have undetected cardiac problems and baseline ECG should be completed before treatment

Nursing diagnoses
✓ Knowledge, deficient (teaching)
✓ Noncompliance (teaching)

Implementation
• Give in AM if possible as a single dose to decrease sleeplessness; at same time each day to maintain drug level
• Give only for hormone imbalances; not to be used for obesity, male infertility, menstrual conditions, lethargy; give lowest dose that G relieves symptoms; lower dose to the elderly and in cardiac diseases
• Store in airtight, light-resistant container
• Wean patient off medication 4 wk before RAIU test

Patient/family education
• Teach patient that drug is not a cure but

controls symptoms and that treatment is long-term
• Instruct patient to report excitability, irritability, anxiety, sweating, heat intolerance, chest pain, palpitations, which indicate overdose
• Advise patient not to switch brands unless approved by prescriber; bioavailability may differ; do not take with food; absorption will be decreased
• Teach patient that drug may be discontinued after giving birth; thyroid panel will be evaluated after 1-2 mo
P • Teach patient that hyperthyroid child will show almost immediate behavior/personality
P change; that hair loss will occur in child and is temporary
• Caution patient that drug is not to be taken to reduce weight
• Caution patient to avoid OTC preparations containing iodine; read labels; other medications should not be used unless approved by prescriber
• Teach patient to avoid iodine-containing food: iodized salt, soybeans, tofu, turnips, certain kinds of seafood and bread

Evaluation
Positive therapeutic outcome
• Absence of depression
• Weight loss, increased diuresis, pulse, appetite
• Absence of constipation, peripheral edema, cold intolerance, pale, cool dry skin, brittle nails, alopecia, coarse hair, menorrhagia, night blindness, paresthesias, syncope, stupor, coma, rosy cheeks
• Improved levels of T_3, T_4 by laboratory tests
P • Child: Age-appropriate weight, height, and psychomotor development

Treatment of overdose:
Withhold dose for up to 1 wk, acute overdose—gastric lavage or induce emesis, then activated charcoal; provide supportive treatment to control symptoms

tiagabine (Rx)
(tie-ah-ga'been)
Gabitril
Func. class.: Anticonvulsant

Pregnancy category C

Action: Mechanism unknown; may increase seizure threshold

Uses: Adjunct treatment of partial seizures

Dosage and routes
Adult: PO 4 mg qd, may increase by 4-8 mg qwk until desired response, max 56 mg/day

P *Child 12-18 yr:* PO 4 mg qd, may increase by 4 mg at beginning of wk 2, may increase by 4-8 mg qwk until desired response, max 32 mg/day

Available forms: Tabs 4, 12, 16, 20 mg

Adverse effects
(*italic* = common; **bold** = life-threatening)
CNS: Dizziness, anxiety, somnolence, ataxia, confusion, asthenia, unsteady gait, depression
CV: Vasodilatation
GI: Nausea, diarrhea, vomiting
INTEG: Pruritus, rash
RESP: Pharyngitis, coughing

Contraindications: Hypersensitivity to this drug

P **Precautions:** Hepatic disease, renal disease,
G pregnancy **C**, lactation, child <12 yr, elderly

Pharmacokinetics	
Absorption	>95%
Distribution	Unknown
Metabolism	Liver
Excretion	Kidneys
Half-life	7-9 hr

Pharmacodynamics	
Unknown	

Interactions
Individual drugs
Valproate: Lower dose of tiagabine may be required
Drug classifications
CNS depressants: ↑ CNS depression

NURSING CONSIDERATIONS
Assessment
• Monitor renal studies: urinalysis, BUN, urine creatinine q3 mo
• Monitor hepatic studies: ALT, AST, bilirubin
• Assess description of seizures: location, duration, presence of aura

T

• Assess mental status: mood, sensorium, affect, behavioral changes; if mental status changes, notify prescriber

Implementation
• Store at room temp away from heat and light
• Provide assistance with ambulation during early part of treatment; dizziness occurs
• Provide seizure precautions: padded side rails; move objects that may harm patient

Patient/family education
• Advise patient to carry/wear emergency ID stating patient's name, drugs taken, condition, prescriber's name and phone number
• Advise patient to avoid driving, other activities that require alertness
• Teach patient not to discontinue medication quickly after long-term use

Evaluation
Positive therapeutic outcome
• Decreased seizure activity; document on patient's chart

Treatment of overdose: Lavage, VS

---

ticarcillin (Rx)
(tye-kar-sill'in)
ticar
Func. class.: Broad-spectrum antiinfective
Chem. class.: Extended-spectrum penicillin
Pregnancy category B

Action: Interferes with cell wall replication of susceptible organisms; osmotically unstable cell wall swells, bursts from osmotic pressure

⮑ **Therapeutic Outcome:** Decreased symptoms of infection

Uses: Respiratory, soft tissue, urinary tract infections, bacterial septicemia; effective for gram-positive cocci *(Staphylococcus aureus, Streptococcus faecalis, Streptococcus pneumoniae),* gram-negative cocci *(Neisseria gonorrhoeae),* gram-positive bacilli *(Clostridium perfringens, Clostridium tetani),* gram-negative bacilli *(Bacteroides, Fusobacterium nucleatum, Escherichia coli, Proteus mirabilis, Salmonella, Morganella morganii, Proteus rettgeri, Enterobacter, Pseudomonas aeruginosa, Serratia;* and *Peptococcus, Peptostreptococcus, Eubacterium)*

Dosage and routes
Bacterial septicemia, respiratory, skin, soft tissue, intraabdominal, reproductive infections
Adult: **IV** INF 200-300 mg/kg/day in divided doses q4-6h

P *Child <40 kg:* **IV** INF 200-300 mg/kg/day in divided doses q4-6h

Urinary tract complicated infections
P *Adult/child:* **IV** INF 150-200 mg/kg/day in divided doses q4-6h

Uncomplicated urinary infections
Adult: **IV** direct/IM 1 g q6h

P *Child <40 kg:* **IV** direct/IM 50-100 mg/kg/day q6-8h

Severe infections (Pseudomonas, Proteus, E. coli)
P *Neonates:* IM/**IV** <2 kg: 75 mg/kg q8-12h; IM/**IV** >2 kg 75-100 mg/kg q8h

Renal dose/hepatic dose
Adult: CCr >60 ml/min 3 g q4h; CCr 10-30 ml/min 2 g q8h; CCr <10 ml/min 2 g q12h or 1 g q6h; CCr <10 ml/min and hepatic dysfunction 2 g q24h or 1 g q12h

Available forms: Inj 1, 3, 6, 20, 30 g

Adverse effects
(*italic* = common; **bold** = life-threatening)
CNS: Lethargy, hallucinations, anxiety, depression, twitching, **coma, seizures**
GI: Nausea, vomiting, diarrhea; increased AST, ALT, abdominal pain, glossitis, colitis
GU: Oliguria, proteinuria, hematuria, *vaginitis, moniliasis,* **glomerulonephritis**
HEMA: Anemia, increased bleeding time, **bone marrow depression, granulocytopenia**
INTEG: Rash
META: Hypokalemia
SYST: **Anaphylaxis**

Contraindications: Hypersensitivity to penicillins

Precautions: Hypersensitivity to cephalosporins, pregnancy **B**, lactation, renal disease

Pharmacokinetics	
Absorption	Unknown
Distribution	Widely, breast milk
Metabolism	Liver, small amount
Excretion	Kidneys
Half-life	70 min

Pharmacodynamics		
	IM	IV
Onset	Unknown	Unknown
Peak	1 hr	30-45 min
Duration	4-6 hr	4 hr

Interactions
Individual drugs
Aspirin, probenecid: ↑ ticarcillin concentration
Heparin: ↑ effect of heparin
Drug classifications
Aminoglycosides (**IV**), erythromycins, tetracyclines: ↓ effect of ticarcillin
Contraceptives (oral): ↓ effect of oral contraceptives
Neuromuscular blockers: ↑ effect of neuromuscular blockers
Herb/drug
Khat: ↓ absorption
Lab test interferences
False positive: Urine glucose, urine protein

NURSING CONSIDERATIONS
Assessment
• Monitor I&O ratio; report hematuria, oliguria, since penicillin in high doses is nephrotoxic
• Monitor any patient with compromised renal system, since drug is excreted slowly in poor renal system function; toxicity may occur rapidly
• Monitor liver function tests: AST, ALT
• Monitor blood studies: WBC, RBC, Hgb, Hct, bleeding time
• Monitor renal function studies: urinalysis, protein, blood, BUN, creatinine
• Monitor C&S before drug therapy; drug may be given as soon as culture is performed
• Assess bowel pattern before, during treatment
• Check for skin eruptions after administration of penicillin to 1 wk after discontinuing drug
• Assess for anaphylaxis: wheezing, rash, pruritus, laryngeal edema, keep emergency equipment nearby
• Assess allergies before initiation of treatment, reaction of each medication
Implementation
IM route
• Inject into well-developed muscle
• Reconstitute ticarcillin 1 g/2 ml sterile water for inj, NaCl inj, 1% lidocaine HCl without epINEPHrine (385 mg/ml)
IV route
• Give **IV** after diluting 1 g or less/4 ml of sterile H$_2$O for inj; dilute further with 10-20 ml or more D$_5$W, 0.9% NaCl, or sterile H$_2$O for inj sol; give 1 g or less/5 min or more or by intermittent inf over ½-2 hr or by continuous inf at prescribed rate

Y-site compatibilities: Acyclovir, allopurinol, amifostine, aztreonam, cyclophosphamide, diltiazem, famotidine, filgrastim, fludarabine, granisetron, hydromorphone, heparin, IL-2, insulin (regular), magnesium sulfate, melphalan, meperidine, morphine, ondansetron, perphenazine, propofol, sargramostim, teniposide, theophylline, thiotepa, verapamil, vinorelbine

Additive compatibilities: Ranitidine, verapamil
• Give drug after C&S has been completed
• Have adrenalin, suction, tracheostomy set, endotracheal intubation equipment
• Provide adequate fluid intake (2 L) during diarrhea episodes
• Provide scratch test to assess allergy on order from prescriber; usually done when penicillin is only drug of choice
• Store at room temp, reconstituted sol 72 hr at room temp

Evaluation
Positive therapeutic outcome
• Absence of fever, purulent drainage, redness, inflammation

Patient/family education
• Advise patient that culture may be done after completed course of medication
• Teach patient to report sore throat, fever, fatigue (may indicate superinfection)
• Teach patient to carry/wear emergency ID if allergic to penicillins
• Advise patient to notify nurse of diarrhea

Treatment of overdose: Withdraw drug, maintain airway, administer epINEPHrine, aminophylline, O$_2$, **IV** corticosteroids for anaphylaxis

ticarcillin/clavulanate (Rx)
(tye-kar-sill'in)
Chem. class: Antiinfective—broad-spectrum
Func. class.: Extended-spectrum penicillin
Pregnancy category B

Action: Interferes with cell wall replication of susceptible organisms; osmotically unstable cell wall swells, bursts from osmotic pressure

Therapeutic Outcome: Resolution of infection

Uses: Respiratory, soft tissue, urinary tract infections; bacterial septicemia; effective for gram-positive cocci *(Staphylococcus aureus, Streptococcus faecalis, Streptococcus pneumoniae)*, gram-negative cocci *(Neisseria*

gonorrhoeae), gram-positive bacilli *(Clostridium perfringens, Clostridium tetani)*, gram-negative bacilli *(Bacteroides, Fusobacterium nucleatum, Escherichia coli, Proteus mirabilis, Salmonella, Morganella morganii, Proteus rettgeri, Enterobacter, Pseudomonas aeruginosa, Serratia, Peptococcus, Peptostreptococcus, Eubacterium)*

Dosage and routes
Renal dose
Adult: CCr 60 ml/min 3.1 g q4h; CCr 30-60 ml/min 2 g q4h; CCr 10-30 ml/min 2g q8h; CCr <10 ml/min 2 g q12h; CCr <10 ml/min with hepatic dysfunction 2 g q24h

Systemic/urinary tract infections, serious infections
Adult ≥60 kg: **IV** inf 3.1 g q4-6h
Adult <60 kg: **IV** inf 200-300 mg/kg/day q4-6h
P *Child >60 kg:* **IV** inf 3.1 g q4h
P *Child <60 kg:* **IV** inf 300 mg/kg/day q4h
Mild/moderate infections
P *Child ≥60 kg:* **IV** inf 3.1 g q6h
P *Child <60 kg:* **IV** inf 200 mg/kg/day q6h

Available forms: Inj IM, **IV** 3 g ticarcillin and 0.1 g clavulanate; **IV** inf 3 g ticarcillin and 0.1 g clavulanate; powder for inj 3 g ticarcillin, 0.1 g clavulanate, 30 g ticarcillin, 1 g clavulanate

Adverse effects
(*italic* = common; **bold** = life-threatening)
CNS: Lethargy, hallucinations, anxiety, depression, twitching, **coma, seizures**
GI: Nausea, *vomiting, diarrhea,* increased AST, ALT, abdominal pain, glossitis, colitis
GU: Oliguria, proteinuria, hematuria, *vaginitis, moniliasis,* **glomerulonephritis**
HEMA: Anemia, increased bleeding time, **bone marrow depression, granulocytopenia**
META: Hypokalemia, hyperkalemia, alkalosis, hypernatremia
SYST: **Anaphylaxis**

Contraindications: Hypersensitivity to
P penicillins; neonates

Precautions: Hypersensitivity to cephalosporins, pregnancy **B**, renal disease

Pharmacokinetics
Absorption	Completely absorbed (**IV**)
Distribution	Widely distributed, crosses blood-brain barrier
Metabolism	Liver
Excretion	Kidneys
Half-life	64-68 min

Pharmacodynamics
	IV
Onset	Unknown
Peak	30-45 min
Duration	4 hr

Interactions
Individual drugs
Aspirin, probenecid: ↑ ticarcillin concentration
Heparin: ↑ effect of heparin
Drug classifications
Aminoglycosides (**IV**): ↓ antimicrobial effect of ticarcillin
Contraceptives (oral): ↓ effect of oral contraceptives
Erythromycins: ↓ absorption
Neuromuscular blockers: ↑ neuromuscular blocking
Tetracyclines: ↓ ticarcillin effect
☐ Herb/drug
Khat: ↓ absorption
Lab test interferences
False positive: Urine glucose, urine protein, Coombs' test

NURSING CONSIDERATIONS
Assessment
• Monitor I&O ratio; report hematuria, oliguria because penicillin in high doses is nephrotoxic
• Monitor any patient with compromised renal system because drug is excreted slowly in poor renal system function; toxicity may occur rapidly
• Monitor liver function tests: AST, ALT
• Monitor blood studies: WBC, RBC, Hgb, Hct, bleeding time
• Monitor renal function studies: urinalysis, protein, blood
• Obtain C&S test results before initiating drug therapy; drug may be given as soon as culture is performed
• Assess bowel pattern before, during treatment
• Assess skin eruptions after administration of penicillin to 1 wk after discontinuing drug
• Assess for anaphylaxis: wheezing, rash, laryngeal edema; have emergency equipment nearby
• Assess allergies before initiation of treatment, reaction of each medication

Nursing diagnoses
✓ Infection, risk for (uses)
✓ Knowledge, deficient (teaching)

Implementation
IV IV route
- Give **IV** after diluting 3.1 g or less/13 ml of sterile H_2O or NaCl (200 mg/ml), shake; may further dilute in 50-100 ml or more 0.9% NaCl, D_5W, or LR sol and run over ½ hr

Y-site compatibilities: Allopurinol, aztreonam, cefepime, cyclophosphamide, diltiazem, famotidine, filgrastim, fluconazole, fludarabine, foscarnet, heparin, insulin (regular), melphalan, meperidine, morphine, ondansetron, perphenazine, sargramostim, teniposide, theophylline, vinorelbine
- Give drug after C&S has been completed
- Have adrenalin, suction, tracheostomy set, endotracheal intubation equipment available
- Give adequate fluid intake (2 L) during diarrhea episodes
- Obtain scratch test results to assess allergy after securing order from prescriber; usually done when penicillin is only drug of choice
- Store at room temp, reconstituted sol for 12-24 hr or 3-7 days refrigerated

Patient/family education
- Advise patient that C&S may be performed after completed course of medication
- Instruct patient to report sore throat, fever, fatigue (may indicate superinfection)
- Advise patient to carry/wear emergency ID if allergic to penicillins

Evaluation
Positive therapeutic outcome
- Absence of fever, purulent drainage, redness, inflammation

Treatment of overdose: Withdraw drug, maintain airway, administer epINEPHrine, aminophylline, O_2, **IV** corticosteroids for anaphylaxis

---

ticlopidine (Rx)
(tye-cloe'pi-deen)
Ticlid
Func. class.: Platelet aggregation inhibitor
Pregnancy category B

Action: Inhibits first and second phases of ADP-induced effects in platelet aggregation

Therapeutic Outcome: Decreased stroke by decreasing platelet aggregation

Uses: Reducing the risk of stroke in high-risk patients

Investigational uses: Intermittent claudication, chronic arterial occlusion, subarachnoid hemorrhage, uremic patients with AV shunts/fistulas, open heart surgery, coronary artery bypass grafts, primary glomerulonephritis

Dosage and routes
Adult: PO 250 mg bid with food

Available forms: Tabs 250 mg

Adverse effects
(*italic* = common; **bold** = life-threatening)
CNS: Dizziness
GI: Nausea, vomiting, diarrhea, GI discomfort, **cholestatic jaundice, hepatitis,** increased cholesterol LDL, VLDL
HEMA: **Bleeding (epistaxis, hematuria, conjunctival hemorrhage, GI bleeding), agranulocytosis, neutropenia, thrombocytopenia**
INTEG: Rash, pruritus

Contraindications: Hypersensitivity, severe liver disease, blood dyscrasias, active bleeding

Precautions: Past liver disease, renal disease, elderly, pregnancy **B**, lactation, children, increased bleeding risk

Pharmacokinetics	
Absorption	Well absorbed
Distribution	Unknown
Metabolism	Liver—extensively
Excretion	Kidneys—unchanged drug
Half-life	Increased with repeat dosing; 4-5 days (multiple doses)

Pharmacodynamics	
Onset	Unknown
Peak	1-3 hr
Duration	Unknown

Interactions
Individual drugs
Cimetidine: ↑ effects of ticlopidine
Digoxin: ↓ plasma levels of ticlopidine
Theophylline: ↑ effects of theophylline
Drug classifications
Antacids: ↓ plasma levels of ticlopidine
Anticoagulants, salicylates, thrombolytics: ↑ bleeding risk

NURSING CONSIDERATIONS
Assessment
- Monitor liver function studies: AST, ALT, bilirubin, creatinine if patient is on long-term therapy (4 mo or more)
- Monitor blood studies: CBC, Hct, Hgb, Pro-time if patient is on long-term therapy; CBC q2 wk × 3 mo therapy; thrombocytopenia, neutropenia may occur

- Monitor bleeding time baseline and throughout therapy, levels may be 2-5 × normal limit

Nursing diagnoses
✓ Injury, risk for (uses)
✓ Knowledge, deficient (teaching)

Patient/family education
- Advise patient that blood studies will be necessary during treatment
- Advise patient to report any unusual bleeding to prescriber
- Instruct patient to take with food or just after eating to minimize GI discomfort
- Caution patient to report side effects such as diarrhea, skin rashes, subcutaneous bleeding, signs of cholestasis (yellow skin and sclera, dark urine, light-colored stools)

Evaluation
Positive therapeutic outcome
- Absence of stroke

---

tiludronate (Rx)
(till-oo'droe-nate)
Skelid
Func. class.: Bone resorption inhibitor
Chem. class.: Bisphosphonate

Pregnancy category C

Action: Decreases bone reabsorption and new bone development

➡ **Therapeutic Outcome:** Decreased bone reabsorption and reduced calcium levels WNL

Uses: Paget's disease

Dosage and routes
Adult: PO 400 mg qd, with 8 oz of water × 3 mo

Available forms: Tabs 240 mg (equivalent to 200 mg tiludronic acid)

Adverse effects
(*italic* = common; **bold** = life-threatening)
CNS: Headache, somnolence, dizziness, anxiety, vertigo, nervousness, involuntary movements
CV: Chest pain, edema, hypertension, peripheral edema
ENDO: Hyperparathyroidism
GI: *Nausea, diarrhea,* dry mouth, gastritis, vomiting, flatulence, gastric ulcers, dyspepsia
GU: **Nephrotoxicity,** UTI

INTEG: Rash, epidermal necrosis, pruritus, sweating
MS: *Bone pain,* decreased mineralization of nonaffected bones, pathologic fractures
RESP: Bronchitis, rhinitis, rales, sinusitis, upper respiratory tract infection

Contraindications: Hypersensitivity to bisphosphonates, severe renal disease with creatinine >5 mg/dl

Precautions: Pregnancy **C**, renal disease, lactation, restricted vit D/Ca, GI disease

Pharmacokinetics
Absorption	Rapid
Distribution	Unknown, steady state 10 days
Metabolism	Protein binding 90%
Excretion	Feces (unabsorbed), kidney (unchanged)
Half-life	150 hr

Pharmacodynamics
Onset	Unknown
Peak	Unknown
Duration	Unknown

Interactions
Individual drugs
Aspirin: ↓ effect of tiludronate
Indomethacin: ↑ effect of tiludronate
Drug classifications
Antacids, mineral supplements with magnesium, calcium, or aluminum: ↓ absorption of tiludronate

NURSING CONSIDERATIONS
Assessment
- Assess for GI symptoms, polyuria, flushing, head swelling, tingling, headache; may indicate hypercalcemia; nervousness, irritability, twitching, seizures, spasm, paresthesia indicates hypocalcemia at start of treatment
- Identify nutritional status; evaluate diet for sources of vit D (milk, some seafood), calcium (dairy products, dark green vegetables), phosphates
- Monitor BUN, creatinine, uric acid, chloride, electrolytes, urine pH, urinary calcium, magnesium, phosphate, urinalysis (calcium should be kept at 9-10 mg/dl), albumin, alkaline phosphatase baseline and q3-6 mo; check urine sediment for casts throughout treatment
- Assess for increased drug level; toxic reactions occur rapidly; have calcium chloride or gluconate on hand if calcium level drops too low; check for tetany

---

 Herb/drug   Do Not Crush   Alert   Key Drug   Geriatric   Pediatric

Nursing diagnoses
☑ Injury, risk for (adverse reactions)
☑ Pain, chronic (uses)
☑ Knowledge, deficient (teaching)

Implementation
• Administer on empty stomach to improve absorption (2 hr ac), with 6-8 oz of water; take calcium or mineral supplements 2 hr before or 2 hr after tiludronate; take aluminum or magnesium antacids ≥2 hr after tiludronate; do not take indomethacin within 2 hr

Patient/family education
• Caution patient to notify prescriber of hypercalcemic relapse: renal calculi, nausea, vomiting, thirst, lethargy, deep bone or flank pain
• Teach patient to follow a low-calcium diet as prescribed (Paget's disease, hypercalcemia)
• Advise patient to notify prescriber of diarrhea, nausea; dose may be divided to lessen these symptoms

Evaluation
Positive therapeutic outcome
• Calcium levels 9-10 mg/dl
• Decreasing symptoms of Paget's disease including pain

timolol (Rx)
(tye'moe-lole)
Apo-Timol ♣, Blocadren, Novo-Timol ♣, timolol maleate, Timoptic
Func. class.: Antihypertensive; antiglaucoma
Chem. class.: Nonselective β-blocker

Pregnancy category C

Action: Competitively blocks stimulation of β-adrenergic receptor within vascular smooth muscle (decreases rate of SA node discharge, increases recovery time), slows conduction of AV node, decreases heart rate, which decreases O_2 consumption in myocardium; also decreases renin-aldosterone-angiotensin system; at high doses inhibits $β_2$ receptors in bronchial system

→ **Therapeutic Outcome:** Decreased B/P, decreased arrhythmias, absence of death from MI, decreased aqueous humor in the eye, absence of migraine headaches

Uses: Mild to moderate hypertension

Investigational uses: Mitral valve prolapse, hypertrophic cardiomyopathy, thyrotoxicosis, tremors, anxiety, pheochromocytoma, tachyarrhythmias, angina pectoris

Dosage and routes
Hypertension
Adult: PO 10 mg bid, or 20 mg qd, may increase by 10 mg q 7 days, not to exceed 60 mg/day

Myocardial Infarction
Adult: 10 mg bid beginning 1-4 wk after MI

Glaucoma
Adult: Ophth ῐ gtt qd or bid
▣ **Child:** Ophth ῐ gtt qd or bid (0.25% sol only)

Migraine headache prevention
Adult: PO 10 mg bid, or 20 mg qd, may increase to 30 mg/day, 20 mg in AM, 10 mg in PM

Available forms: Tabs 5, 10, 20 mg; ophth sol 0.25%, 0.5%

Adverse effects
(*italic* = common; **bold** = life-threatening)
CNS: Insomnia, dizziness, hallucinations, anxiety, fatigue, depression
CV: Hypotension, bradycardia, **CHF**, edema, chest pain, bradycardia, claudication, angina, AV block, ventricular dysrhythmias
EENT: Visual changes, sore throat, *double vision,* dry burning eyes
GI: Nausea, vomiting, **ischemic colitis,** diarrhea, *abdominal pain,* **mesenteric arterial thrombosis,** flatulence, constipation
GU: Impotence, urinary frequency
HEMA: **Agranulocytosis, thrombocytopenia, purpura**
INTEG: Rash, alopecia, pruritus, fever
META: Hypoglycemia
MUSC: Joint pain, muscle pain
RESP: **Bronchospasm,** dyspnea, cough, rales, nasal stuffiness

Contraindications: Hypersensitivity to β-blockers, cardiogenic shock, heart block (2nd or 3rd degree), sinus bradycardia, CHF, cardiac failure, severe COPD

Precautions: Major surgery, pregnancy C, lactation, diabetes mellitus, renal disease, thyroid disease, COPD, well-compensated heart failure, CAD, nonallergic bronchospasm, peripheral vascular disease, hepatic disease

Do Not Confuse:
Timoptic/Viroptic

Pharmacokinetics
Absorption	Well absorbed (PO), ophth (minimal)
Distribution	Protein binding <10%
Metabolism	Liver—extensively
Excretion	Breast milk
Half-life	3 hr

Pharmacodynamics	
	PO
Onset	Unknown
Peak	2-4 hr
Duration	12-24 hr

Interactions
Individual drugs
Alcohol: ↑ hypotension (large amounts)
HydrALAZINE, methyldopa, prazosin, reserpine: ↑ hypotension, bradycardia
Insulin: ↓ hypoglycemia
Thyroid hormones: ↓ effect of timolol
Verapamil: ↑ myocardial depression
Drug classifications
Anticholinergics, antihypertensives, nitrates: ↑ hypotension
β_2-Adrenergic agonists: ↑ β-blocking effect
Calcium channel blockers: ↑ effects of calcium channel blockers
Anticholinergics, cardiac glycosides: ↑ bradycardia
NSAIDs, sympathomimetics: ↓ antihypertensive effect
Sulfonylureas: ↓ hypoglycemic effect
Theophyllines: ↓ bronchodilatation
⬚ Herb/drug
Aconite: ↑ toxicity, death
Astragalus, cola tree: ↑ or ↓ antihypertensive effect
Barberry, betony, black catechu, black cohosh, bloodroot, broom, burdock, cat's claw, dandelion, goldenseal, Irish moss, Jamaican dogwood, kelp, khella, mistletoe, parsley: ↑ antihypertensive effect
Coltsfoot, guarana, khat, licorice: ↓ antihypertensive effect
Lab test interferences
Interference: Glucose, insulin tolerance test, ↑ liver function tests, ↑ renal function tests, ↑ potassium, ↑ uric acid ↓ Hct, ↓ Hgb, ↓ HDL

NURSING CONSIDERATIONS
Assessment
- Assess for headaches: location, severity, duration, frequency baseline and throughout treatment
- Monitor B/P during beginning treatment, periodically thereafter; pulse q4h; note rate, rhythm, quality: apical/radial pulse before administration; notify prescriber of any significant changes (pulse <50 bpm)
- Check for baselines in renal, liver function tests before therapy begins
- Assess for edema in feet, legs daily, monitor I&O ratio, daily weight; check for jugular vein distention, rales, bilaterally, dyspnea (CHF)
- Monitor skin turgor, dryness of mucous membranes for hydration status, especially Ⓖ elderly

Nursing diagnoses
☑ Cardiac output, decreased (uses)
☑ Injury, risk for physical (side effects)
☑ Knowledge, deficient (teaching)
☑ Noncompliance (teaching)

Implementation
PO route
- Given ac, hs, tab may be crushed or swallowed whole; give with food to prevent GI upset; reduced dosage in renal dysfunction
- Store protected from light, moisture; place in cool environment

Patient/family education
- Teach patient not to discontinue drug abruptly; taper over 2 wk; may cause precipitate angina if stopped abruptly
- Advise patient not to use OTC products containing α-adrenergic stimulants (such as nasal decongestants, cold preparations); to avoid alcohol, smoking and to limit sodium intake as prescribed
- Teach patient how to take pulse and B/P at home; advise patient when to notify prescriber
- Instruct patient to comply with weight control, dietary adjustments, modified exercise program
- Advise patient to carry/wear emergency ID to identify drug being taken, any allergies; tell patient drug controls symptoms but does not cure
- Caution patient to avoid hazardous activities if dizziness, drowsiness is present
- Teach patient to report symptoms of CHF; difficult breathing, especially on exertion or when lying down; night cough; swelling of extremities or bradycardia; dizziness; confusion; depression; fever
- Teach patient to take drug as prescribed, not to double doses, skip doses; take any missed doses as soon as remembered if at least 4 hr until next dose

Evaluation
Positive therapeutic outcome
- Decreased B/P in hypertension (after 1-2 wk)
- Absence of dysrhythmias

Treatment of overdose: Lavage, **IV** atropine for bradycardia, **IV** theophylline for bronchospasm, digitalis, O_2, diuretic for cardiac failure, hemodialysis, **IV** glucose for hyperglycemia, **IV** diazepam (or phenytoin) for seizures

⚠ HIGH ALERT

tinzaparin (Rx)
(tin-zay-par'in)
Innohep
Func. class.: Anticoagulant
Chem. class.: Unfractionated porcine heparin

Pregnancy category C

Action: Prevents conversion of fibrinogen to fibrin and prothrombin to thrombin by enhancing inhibitory effects of antithrombin III; produces higher ratio of antifactor Xa to antifactor IIa

➔ **Therapeutic Outcome:** Resolution of deep vein thrombosis

Uses: Treatment of deep vein thrombosis, pulmonary emboli when given with warfarin

Dosage and routes
Adult: SC 175 anti-Xa international units/kg qd ≥6 days and until adequate anticoagulation with warfarin (INR ≥2 for 2 consecutive days)

Available forms: Inj 40,000 international units/2 ml

Adverse effects
(*italic* = common; **bold** = life-threatening)
CNS: Fever, confusion, dizziness, insomnia
CV: Angina, dysrhythmias, peripheral edema
GI: Nausea, constipation, flatulence, dyspepsia, **hepatitis**
GU: UTI, hematuria, urinary retention, dysuria
HEMA: Hemorrhage, **hypochromic anemia, thrombocytopenia,** bleeding
INTEG: Ecchymosis
MISC: Headache, chest pain

Contraindications: Hypersensitivity to this drug, heparin, pork or benzyl alcohol; hemophilia, leukemia with bleeding, peptic ulcer disease, thrombocytopenic purpura, heparin-induced thrombocytopenia

G Precautions: Alcoholism, elderly, pregnancy **C**, hepatic disease (severe), renal disease (severe), blood dyscrasias, severe uncontrolled hypertension, subacute bacterial **P** endocarditis, acute nephritis, lactation, children

Pharmacokinetics

Absorption	Unknown
Distribution	Unknown
Metabolism	Unknown
Excretion	Unknown
Half-life	4.5 hr

Pharmacodynamics

Onset	Unknown
Peak	3-5 hr (max antithrombin activity)
Duration	Unknown

Interactions
Individual drug
Ticlopidine: ↑ tinzaparin action
Drug classifications
Anticoagulants (oral), NSAIDs, platelet inhibitors, salicylates, thrombolytics: ↑ tinzaparin action
☑ *Herb/drug*
Agrimony, alfalfa, angelica, anise, basil, bay, bilberry, black haw, bogbean, bromelain, buchu, chondroitin, cinchona bark, dong quai, fenugreek, feverfew, garlic, ginger, ginkgo, ginseng, horse chestnut, Irish moss, kelp, kelpware, khella, lovage, lungwort, meadowsweet, motherwort, mugwort, nettle, papaya, parsley (large amounts), pau d'arco, pineapple, poplar, prickly ash, safflower, saw palmetto, tonka bean, turmeric, wintergreen, yarrow: ↑ risk of bleeding
Chamomile, coenzyme Q10, flax, glucomannan, goldenseal, guar gum: ↓ anticoagulant effect

NURSING CONSIDERATIONS
Assessment
• Monitor blood studies (Hct, platelets, occult blood in stools), anti-Xa; thrombocytopenia may occur
• Assess for bleeding gums, petechiae, ecchymosis, black tarry stools, hematuria

Nursing diagnoses
☑ Cardiac output, decreased (uses)
☑ Knowledge, deficient (teaching)

Implementation
• Give only after screening patient for bleeding disorders
• Give SC only; do not give IM
• Give SC to recumbent patient; rotate inj sites (left/right anterolateral, left/right posterolateral abdominal wall)
• Insert whole length of needle into skin fold held with thumb and forefinger
◆ • Use only this drug when ordered; not interchangeable with heparin or LMWHs
• Give at same time each day to maintain steady blood levels
• Do not massage area or aspirate when giving SC inj
• Avoid all IM inj that may cause bleeding
• Do not mix with other drugs or infusion fluids
• Store at 77° F (25° C); do not freeze

T

Patient/family education
- Advise patient to use soft-bristle toothbrush to avoid bleeding gums, to use electric razor
- Instruct patient to report any signs of bleeding: gums, under skin, urine, stools

Evaluation
Positive therapeutic outcome
- Resolution of deep vein thrombosis

Treatment of overdose: Protamine 1 mg/100 anti-Xa international units of tinzaparin

---

! HIGH ALERT

tirofiban (Rx)
(tie-roh-fee′ban)
Aggrastat
Func. class.: Antiplatelet
Chem. class.: Glycoprotein IIb/IIIa inhibitor

Pregnancy category B

Action: Antagonist of platelet glycoprotein (GP) IIb/IIIa receptor that leads to binding of fibrinogen and von Willebrand's factor, which inhibits platelet aggregation

➡ **Therapeutic Outcome:** Decreased platelet count

Uses: Acute coronary syndrome in combination with heparin

Dosage and routes
Adult: **IV** 0.4 mcg/kg/min × 30 min, then 0.1 mcg/kg/min

Renal dose
Adult: **IV** CCr <30 ml/min 0.2 mcg/kg/min × 30 min, then 0.05 mcg/kg/min, during angiography and for up to 24 hr after angioplasty

Available forms: Inj for sol 250 mcg/ml, inj 50 mcg/ml

Adverse effects
(*italic* = common; **bold** = life-threatening)
CNS: Dizziness
CV: Bradycardia
HEMA: Bleeding, **thrombocytopenia**
INTEG: Rash
MISC: Dissection, coronary artery edema, pain in legs/pelvis, sweating

Contraindications: Hypersensitivity, active internal bleeding, stroke, major surgery, severe trauma, intracranial neoplasm, aneurysm, hemorrhage, acute pericarditis, platelets <100,000/mm³, history of thrombocytopenia

Precautions: Pregnancy **B**, lactation, G elderly, renal disease, bleeding tendencies

Pharmacokinetics
Absorption	Unknown
Distribution	Plasma clearance 20%-25%
Metabolism	Liver
Excretion	Urine/feces
Half-life	2 hr

Pharmacodynamics
Onset	Unknown
Peak	Unknown
Duration	Unknown

Interactions
Individual drugs
Abciximab, aspirin, cefamandole, cefoperazone, cefotetan, clopidogrel, dipyridamole, eptifibatide, heparin, plicamycin, ticlopidine, valproic acid: ↑ bleeding risk
Drug classifications
NSAIDs: ↑ bleeding risk
⊘ *Herb/drug*
Agrimony, alfalfa, angelica, anise, basil, bay, bilberry, black haw, bogbean, bromelain, buchu, chondroitin, cinchona bark, dong quai, fenugreek, feverfew, garlic, ginger, ginkgo, ginseng, horse chestnut, Irish moss, kelp, kelpware, khella, lovage, lungwort, meadowsweet, motherwort, mugwort, nettle, papaya, parsley (large amounts), pau d'arco, pineapple, poplar, prickly ash, safflower, saw palmetto, tonka bean, turmeric, wintergreen, yarrow: ↑ risk of bleeding
Chamomile, coenzyme Q10, flax, glucomannan, goldenseal, guar gum: ↓ anticoagulant effect

NURSING CONSIDERATIONS
Assessment
- Monitor platelet counts, Hct, Hgb, before treatment, within 6 hr of loading dose and at least qd thereafter; watch for bleeding from puncture sites, catheters or in stools, urine

Nursing diagnoses
☑ Tissue perfusion, ineffective (uses)

Implementation
- **IV:** Give ½ dose in renal disease
- Dilute inj: withdraw and discard 100 ml from a 500 ml bag of sterile 0.9% NaCl or D₅ and replace this vol with 50 ml of tirofiban inj from one vial
- Tirofiban inj for sol is premixed in containers of 500 ml 0.9% NaCl (50 mg/ml)
- Minimize other arterial/venous punctures

 Herb/drug   Do Not Crush   ♦ Alert   🔑 Key Drug   G Geriatric   P Pediatric

IM inj, catheter use, intubation, to reduce bleeding risks

Y-site compatibility: Heparin

Patient/family education
• Advise patient that it is necessary to quit smoking to prevent excessive vasoconstriction

Evaluation
Positive therapeutic outcome
• Treatment of acute coronary syndrome

---

tizanidine (Rx)
(tye-za'na-deen)
Zanaflex
Func. class.: Skeletal muscle relaxant, central acting
Chem. class.: Imidazole

Pregnancy category C

Action: Unknown; possesses central α_2-adrenergic agonist properties; reduces excitation of spinal cord interneurons; also acts on the basal ganglia, producing muscle relaxation

⮕Therapeutic Outcome: Decreased spasticity of muscles

Uses: Spinal cord injury, spasticity in multiple sclerosis, tension headache

Dosage and routes
Adult: PO Reduce dose in renal failure; 4-36 mg qd in 3 divided doses

Spasticity
Adult: PO 4-8 mg as a single dose; may increase in 2-4 mg increments until desired response, may repeat q6-8h up to 3 doses/24 hr, max 36 mg/day

Tension headache
Adult: PO 2 mg tid, may increase by 4-6 mg tid after 2-wk interval

Available forms: Tabs 2, 4 mg

Adverse effects
(*italic* = common; **bold** = life-threatening)
CNS: *Dizziness,* somnolence, speech disorder, dyskinesia, nervousness, hallucination, psychosis
GI: *Constipation, vomiting,* diarrhea, **hepatotoxicity,** *dry mouth,* ↑ ALT, abnormal liver function tests
GU: Urinary frequency, UTI
OTHER: Blurred vision, flulike symptoms, pharyngitis, rhinitis

Contraindications: Hypersensitivity

Precautions: Renal disease, hepatic
G disease, pregnancy **C,** elderly, hypotension,
P lactation, children

Pharmacokinetics	
Absorption	Complete
Distribution	Widely
Metabolism	Liver, extensively
Excretion	Kidneys, feces
Half-life	2½ hr

Pharmacodynamics	
Onset	Unknown
Peak	1-2 hr
Duration	3-6 hr

Interactions
Individual drugs
Alcohol: CNS depression
Drug classifications
Contraceptives (oral): ↓ clearance of tizanidine

Lab test interferences
↑ AST, ↑ alkaline phosphatase

NURSING CONSIDERATIONS
Assessment
• Assess for muscle spasticity baseline and throughout treatment
• Monitor B/P, heart rate
• Perform neurologic exam in spasticity: deep tendon reflexes, muscle tone, clonus, sensory function
• Monitor liver, renal function tests, electrolytes, CBC with differential during long-term treatment
• Assess for allergic reactions: rash, fever, respiratory distress; severe weakness, numbness in extremities
• Assess CNS depression: dizziness, drowsiness, psychiatric symptoms
• Check dosage, as individual titration is required

Nursing diagnoses
☑ Mobility, impaired
☑ Injury, risk for (adverse reactions)
☑ Knowledge, deficient (teaching)

Implementation
• Give with meals for GI symptoms; gum, frequent sips of water for dry mouth
• Store in airtight container at room temp

Patient/family education
• Advise patient not to discontinue medication quickly; spasticity, will occur; drug should be tapered off over 1-2 wk

- Advise patient not to take with alcohol, other CNS depressants, take as directed, if dose is missed, take as soon as remembered, unless it is almost time for next dose
- Caution patient to avoid altering activities while taking this drug; to avoid hazardous activities if drowsiness or dizziness occurs; to rise from sitting or lying slowly to prevent fainting
- Advise patient to avoid using OTC medications (cough preparations, antihistamines) unless directed by prescriber
- Notify prescriber if fainting, hallucinations, dark urine, stomach pain, yellowing of skin/eyes occurs

Evaluation
Positive therapeutic outcome
- Decreased pain, spasticity

---

tobramycin (Rx)
(toe-bra-mye'sin)
Nebcin, tobramycin sulfate, TOBI
Func. class.: Antiinfective
Chem. class.: Aminoglycoside
Pregnancy category D

Action: Interferes with protein synthesis in bacterial cell by binding to ribosomal subunit, causing inaccurate peptide sequence to form in protein chain, causing bacterial death

➡ **Therapeutic Outcome:** Bactericidal effects for the following organisms: *Pseudomonas aeruginosa, Enterobacter, Escherichia coli, Providencia, Citrobacter, Staphylococcus, Proteus, Klebsiella, Serratia*

Uses: Severe systemic infections of CNS, respiratory, GI, urinary tract, bone, skin, soft tissues, eye, cystic fibrosis (nebulizer) for *P. aeruginosa*

Dosage and routes
Adult: IM/**IV** 3 mg/kg/day in divided doses q8h; may give up to 5 mg/kg/day in divided doses q6-8h; once qd dosing is an option

P *Child:* IM/**IV** 6-7.5 mg/kg/ day in 3-4 equal divided doses

P *Child ≥6 yr:* NEB 300 mg bid in repeating cycles of 28 days on/28 days off; give inh over 10-15 min using a hand-held PARI LC PLUS reusable nebulizer with a DeVilbiss Pulmo-Aid compressor

P *Neonates <1 wk:* IM up to 4 mg/kg/day in divided doses q12h; **IV** up to 4 mg/kg/day in divided doses q12h diluted in 50-100 mg NS or D₅W; give over 30-60 min

Renal dose
P *Adult:* IM/**IV** 1 mg/kg, then dose determined by blood levels

Available forms: Inj 10, 40 mg/ml; powder for inj 1.2 g; inj 20 mg/2 ml; 0.3% ophth, neb sol 300 mg/5 ml

Adverse effects
(*italic* = common; **bold** = life-threatening)
CNS: Confusion, depression, numbness, tremors, **seizures,** muscle twitching, **neurotoxicity,** dizziness, vertigo
CV: Hypotension, hypertension, palpitations
EENT: Ototoxicity, deafness, visual disturbances, tinnitus
GI: *Nausea, vomiting, anorexia,* increased ALT, AST, bilirubin, hepatomegaly, **hepatic necrosis,** splenomegaly
GU: **Oliguria, hematuria, renal damage, azotemia, renal failure, nephrotoxicity**
HEMA: **Agranulocytosis, thrombocytopenia, leukopenia, eosinophilia,** anemia
INTEG: *Rash,* burning, urticaria, dermatitis, alopecia

Contraindications: Severe renal disease, hypersensitivity to aminoglycosides, pregnancy **D**

P **Precautions:** Neonates, mild renal disease, myasthenia gravis, lactation, hearing deficits, **G** Parkinson's disease, elderly

🔖 **Do Not Confuse:**
Tobrex/Tobra Dex

Pharmacokinetics	
Absorption	Well absorbed (IM), completely absorbed (**IV**)
Distribution	Widely distributed in extracellular fluids
Metabolism	Minimal—liver
Excretion	Mostly unchanged (>90%) kidneys
P **Half-life**	2-3 hr, increased in renal disease, neonates

Pharmacodynamics			
	IM	IV	OPHTH
Onset	Rapid	Rapid	Rapid
Peak	1 hr	Inf end	Unknown

Interactions
Individual drugs

Acyclovir, amphotericin B, bacitracin, cisplatin, ethacrynic acid, furosemide, mannitol, methoxyflurane, polymyxin, vancomycin: ↑ ototoxicity, neurotoxicity, nephrotoxicity
Succinylcholine: ↑ neuromuscular blockade, respiratory depression

---

Drug classifications
Aminoglycosides, cephalosporins, penicillins: ↑ ototoxicity, neurotoxicity, nephrotoxicity

⊘ Herb/drug
Lysine (large amounts): ↑ toxicity

NURSING CONSIDERATIONS
Assessment
• Assess patient for previous sensitivity reaction

Systemic route
• Assess patient for signs and symptoms of infection including characteristics of wounds, sputum, urine, stool WBC >10,000/mm³, temp; baseline and during treatment
• Complete C&S testing before beginning drug therapy to identify if correct treatment has been initiated
• Assess for allergic reactions: rash, urticaria, pruritus, chills, fever, joint pain
• Identify urine output; if decreasing, notify prescriber (may indicate nephrotoxicity); also, obtain BUN, creatinine, urine CCr (<80 ml/min) values; urinalysis daily for proteinuria, cells, casts; report sudden change in urine output
• Monitor blood studies: AST, ALT, CBC, Hct, bilirubin, LDH, alkaline phosphatase, Coombs' test monthly if patient is on long-term therapy
• Monitor electrolytes: potassium, sodium, chloride, magnesium monthly if patient is on long-term therapy
• Monitor for bleeding: ecchymosis, bleeding gums, hematuria, stool guaiac daily if patient is on long-term therapy
• Assess for overgrowth of infection: perineal itching, fever, malaise, redness, pain, swelling, drainage, rash, diarrhea, change in cough, sputum
• Obtain weight before treatment; calculation of dosage is usually based on ideal body weight, but may be calculated on actual body weight
• Monitor VS during inf, watch for hypotension, change in pulse
• Assess **IV** site for thrombophlebitis including pain, redness, swelling q30 min, change site if needed; apply warm compresses to discontinue site
• Obtain serum peak, drawn at 30-60 min after **IV** inf or 60 min after IM inj, trough level drawn just before next dose; peak 4-12 mcg/ml, trough 1-2 mcg/ml
• Monitor for deafness by audiometric testing, ringing, roaring in ears, vertigo; assess hearing before, during, after treatment
• Monitor for dehydration: high sp gr, decrease in skin turgor, dry mucous membranes, dark urine
• Monitor for overgrowth of infection including increased temp, malaise, redness, pain, swelling, perineal itching, diarrhea, stomatitis, change in cough, sputum

Nursing diagnoses
☑ Infection, risk for (uses)
☑ Diarrhea (adverse reactions)
☑ Injury, risk for (adverse reactions)
☑ Knowledge, deficient (teaching)
☑ Noncompliance (teaching)

Implementation
IM route
• Give inj deeply in large muscle mass
IV IV route
• Give **IV** diluted in 50-100 ml of 0.9% NaCl, $D_{10}W$, D_5/0.9% NaCl, 0.9% NaCl, Ringer's, LR, D_5W (adult), infuse over 20-60 min
• Flush after inf with D_5W, 0.9% NaCl
• Separate aminoglycosides and penicillins by ≥1 hr

Syringe compatibilities: Doxapram

Syringe incompatibilities: Cefamandole, clindamycin, heparin, sargramostim

Y-site compatibilities: Acyclovir, amifostine, amiodarone, amsacrine, aztreonam, ciprofloxacin, cyclophosphamide, diltiazem, enalaprilat, esmolol, filgrastim, fluconazole, fludarabine, foscarnet, furosemide, granisetron, hydromorphone, IL-2, insulin (regular), labetalol, magnesium sulfate, melphalan, meperidine, midazolam, morphine, perphenazine, tacrolimus, teniposide, theophylline, thiotepa, tolazoline, vinorelbine, zidovudine

Additive compatibilities: Aztreonam, bleomycin, calcium gluconate, cefoxitin, ciprofloxacin, clindamycin, furosemide, metronidazole, ofloxacin, ranitidine, verapamil

Additive incompatibilities: Cefamandole, floxacillin
Nebulizer route
• Give as close to q12h apart as possible; do not use <6 hr apart
• Do not mix with dornase alfa in the nebulizer

Patient/family education
Nebulizer
• Have patient inhale sitting or standing, breathe normally through the mouthpiece, may use nose clips

T

• Advise patient to use multiple therapies first, then tobramycin

Systemic route

• Teach patient to report sore throat, bruising, bleeding, joint pain; may indicate blood dyscrasias (rare)

• Advise patient to contact prescriber if vaginal itching, loose foul-smelling stools, furry tongue occur; may indicate superinfection

• Advise patient to notify prescriber of diarrhea with blood or pus; may indicate pseudomembranous colitis

Evaluation

Positive therapeutic outcome

• Absence of signs/symptoms of infection (WBC <10,000/mm^3, temp WNL, absence of red, draining wounds)

• Reported improvement in symptoms of infection

Treatment of overdose: Withdraw drug, hemodialysis, exchange transfusion in P the newborn, monitor serum levels of drug, may give ticarcillin or carbenicillin

---

tocainide (Rx)
(toe-kay'nide)
Tonocard
Func. class.: Antidysrhythmic (class IB)
Chem. class.: Lidocaine analog

Pregnancy category C

Action: Produces dose-dependent decreases in sodium and potassium conduction, thereby decreasing the excitability of myocardial cells; does not affect heart rate or B/P

➡ **Therapeutic Outcome:** Decreased ventricular dysrhythmia

Uses: Life-threatening ventricular dysrhythmias (multifocal/unifocal premature ventricular contractions [PVCs]), ventricular tachycardia

Dosage and routes
Adult: PO 400 mg q8h, may increase to 1.2-1.8 g/day in divided doses q8-12h

Available forms: Tabs 400, 600 mg

Adverse effects
(*italic* = common; **bold** = life-threatening)
CNS: Headache, dizziness, involuntary movement, confusion, psychosis, restlessness, irritability, paresthesias, tremors, **seizures**
CV: Hypotension, bradycardia, angina, PVCs, **heart block, CV collapse, sinus arrest, CHF,** chest pain, tachycardia, prodysrhythmias

EENT: Tinnitus, blurred vision, hearing loss
GI: Nausea, vomiting, anorexia, diarrhea, hepatitis
HEMA: **Blood dyscrasias: leukopenia, agranulocytosis, hypoplastic anemia, thrombocytopenia,** bone marrow depression
INTEG: Rash, urticaria, lupus, alopecia, sweating
RESP: Dyspnea, **respiratory depression, pulmonary fibrosis,** pulmonary edema, interstitial pneumonitis pneumonia

Contraindications: Hypersensitivity to amides, severe heart block

Precautions: Pregnancy C, lactation, P children, renal disease, liver disease, CHF, myasthenia gravis, blood dyscrasias, pulmonary disease, hypokalemia, atrial flutter/fibrillation

Pharmacokinetics

Absorption	Well absorbed
Distribution	Widely distributed, crossed blood-brain barrier
Metabolism	Liver
Excretion	Kidney (up to 40% unchanged)
Half-life	10-17 hr

Pharmacodynamics

Onset	1 hr
Peak	½-2 hr
Duration	8-12 hr

Interactions
Individual drugs
Cimetidine, rifampin: ↓ effects of tocainide
Propranolol: ↑ effects of propranolol
Quinidine: ↑ effects of quinidine
Drug classifications
Antidysrhythmics: ↑ effects of antidysrhythmics
Herb/drug
Aconite: ↑ toxicity, death
Aloe, broom, buckthorn (chronic use), cascara sagrada (chronic use), Chinese rhubarb, figwort, fumitory, goldenseal, kudzu, licorice: ↑ effect
Coltsfoot: ↓ effect
Horehound: ↑ serotonin effect
Lab test interferences
↑ CPK
False positive: ANA titer

NURSING CONSIDERATIONS
Assessment
• Assess for oxygenation or perfusion deficit: decreased B/P, chest pain, dizziness, loss of consciousness

---

- Assess respiratory status: auscultate lung fields for bibasilar crackles in patients with advanced CHF
- Assess for urinary retention: check for pain, abdominal absorption, palpate bladder; check males with benign prostatic hypertrophy; anticholinergic reaction may cause retention
- Monitor I&O ratio; electrolytes: (potassium, sodium, chloride); watch for decreasing urinary output, possible retention
- Monitor liver function studies: AST, ALT, bilirubin, alkaline phosphatase
- Monitor ECG to determine drug effectiveness; measure PR, QRS, QT intervals; check for PVCs, other dysrhythmias; monitor B/P for hypotension, hypertension; for rebound hypertension after 1-2 hr
- Monitor patient for CNS symptoms: confusion, psychosis, numbness, depression, involuntary movements; if these occur, drug should be discontinued
- Assess pulmonary toxicity: dyspnea, fatigue, cough, fever, chest pain; drug should be discontinued if these occur
- Assess cardiac rate, respiration (rate, rhythm, character), chest pain, ventricular tachycardia, supraventricular tachycardia or fibrillation

Nursing diagnoses
☑ Cardiac output, decreased (uses)
☑ Gas exchange, impaired (adverse reactions)
☑ Knowledge, deficient (teaching)

Implementation
- Give with meals to decrease GI upset

Patient/family education
- Inform patient or family of reason for medication and expected results
- Teach patient method for taking pulse at home and what to report to prescriber
- Advise patient to avoid hazardous activities until drug response is known; dizziness, confusion, sedation may occur
- Advise patient to carry/wear emergency ID indicating medications taken, condition, and prescriber's name and phone number
- Instruct patient to report bleeding, bruising, respiratory symptoms, chills, fever, sore throat to prescriber

Evaluation
Positive therapeutic outcome
- Decreased dysrhythmias

Treatment of overdose: Defibrillation, vasopressor for hypotension

tolcapone (Rx)
(toll'cah-pone)
Tasmar
Func. class.: Antiparkinson agent
Chem. class.: Catecholamine inhibitor (COMT)
Pregnancy category C

Action: Selective, reversible inhibitor of catecholamine; used as adjunct to levodopa/carbidopa therapy

➡ **Therapeutic Outcome:** Increased ability to move and speak

Uses: Parkinsonism

Dosage and routes
Adult: PO 100-200 mg tid, with levodopa/carbidopa therapy; max 600 mg/day; discontinue if no benefit in 3 wk

Renal dose
Adult: PO 100 mg tid or less

Available forms: Tabs 100, 200 mg

Adverse effects
(*italic* = common; **bold** = life-threatening)
CNS: Dystonia, dyskinesia, dreaming, *fatigue, headache, confusion,* psychosis, hallucination, dizziness
CV: Orthostatic hypotension, chest pain, hypotension
EENT: Cataract, eye inflammation
GI: Nausea, vomiting, abdominal distress, diarrhea, constipation, **fatal liver failure,** elevated liver function tests
GU: UTI, urine discoloration, uterine tumor, micturition disorder, hematuria
HEMA: **Hemolytic anemia, leukopenia, agranulocytosis**
INTEG: Sweating, alopecia

Contraindications: Hypersensitivity

Precautions: Renal disease, cardiac disease, hepatic disease, hypertension, pregnancy **C**, asthma, lactation

Pharmacokinetics
Absorption	Rapidly
Distribution	Protein binding 99%
Metabolism	Liver (extensively)
Excretion	Urine (60%), feces (40%)
Half-life	2-3 hr

Pharmacodynamics
Onset	Unknown
Peak	2 hr
Duration	Unknown

Interactions
Individual drugs
Apomorphine, DOBUTamine, isoproterenol, α-methyldopa: May influence pharmacokinetics
Drug classifications
MAOIs: ↓ normal catecholamine metabolism; MAO-B inhibitor may be used
 Herb/drug
Kava: ↓ effect

NURSING CONSIDERATIONS
Assessment
- Monitor liver function enzymes: AST, ALT, alkaline phosphatase, LDH, bilirubin, CBC
- Assess involuntary movements in parkinsonism: akinesia, tremors, staggering gait, muscle rigidity, drooling
- Monitor B/P, respiration during initial treatment; hypo/hypertension should be reported
- Monitor mental status: affect, mood, behavioral changes

Nursing diagnoses
☑ Mobility, impaired physical (uses)
☑ Injury, risk for (uses)
☑ Knowledge, deficient (teaching)

Implementation
PO route
- Administer tid with levodopa/carbidopa therapy
- Provide assistance with ambulation during beginning therapy

Patient/family education
- Advise patient to change positions slowly to prevent orthostatic hypotension
- Advise patient that urine, sweat may change color
- Teach patient that food taken within 1 hr ac or 2 hr pc increases action of drug by 20%
- Teach patient to report nausea, vomiting, anorexia

Evaluation
Positive therapeutic outcome
- Decrease in akathisia, increased mood

---

tolterodine (Rx)
(tol-tehr'oh-deen)
Detrol, Detrol LA
Func. class.: Overactive bladder product
Chem. class.: Muscarinic receptor antagonist

Pregnancy category C

Action: Relaxes smooth muscles in urinary tract by inhibiting acetylcholine at postganglionic sites

⇒ **Therapeutic Outcome:** Decreased symptoms of overactive bladder

Uses: Overactive bladder, (frequency, urgency)

Dosage and routes
Adult: **PO** 2 mg bid, hepatic disease 1 mg bid; 4 mg qd, may decrease to 2 mg if needed

Available forms: Tabs 1, 2 mg; ext rel caps 2, 4 mg

Adverse effects
(*italic* = common; **bold** = life-threatening)
CNS: *Anxiety,* paresthesia, fatigue, *dizziness,* headache
CV: Chest pain, hypertension
EENT: Vision abnormalities, xerophthalmia
GI: *Nausea, vomiting, anorexia,* abdominal pain constipation, dry mouth, dyspepsia
GU: Dysuria, retention, frequency, UTI
INTEG: Rash, pruritus
RESP: Bronchitis, cough, pharyngitis, upper respiratory tract infection

Contraindications: Hypersensitivity, uncontrolled narrow-angle glaucoma, urinary retention, gastric retention

Precautions: Pregnancy **C**, lactation, children, renal/hepatic disease, controlled narrow-angle glaucoma

Pharmacokinetics	
Absorption	Rapidly
Distribution	Highly protein bound
Metabolism	Liver (extensively)
Excretion	Urine/feces
Half-life	Unknown

Pharmacodynamics	
Onset	Unknown
Peak	Unknown
Duration	Unknown

Interactions
Drug classifications
Antibiotics (macrolide), antifungal agents:
↑ action of tolterodine
Food/drug
↑ Bioavailability of tolterodine

NURSING CONSIDERATIONS
Assessment
• Assess urinary patterns: distension, nocturia, frequency, urgency, incontinence
• Assess allergic reactions: rash; if this occurs, drug should be discontinued

Nursing diagnoses
✓ Urinary elimination, impaired (uses)
✓ Incontinence, functional urinary (uses)
✓ Knowledge, deficient (teaching)
✓ Activity intolerance (uses)

Patient/family education
• Advise patient to avoid hazardous activities; dizziness may occur

Evaluation
Positive therapeutic outcome
• Decreased urinary frequency, urgency

---

topiramate (Rx)
(to-pi-ra′mate)
Topamax
Func. class.: Anticonvulsant—misc
Chem. class.: Monosaccharide derivative

Pregnancy category C

Action: Mechanism of action unknown; may prevent seizure spread as opposed to an elevation of seizure threshold

➔ **Therapeutic Outcome:** Absence of seizures

P **Uses:** Partial seizures in adults and children 2-16 yr old; tonic-clonic seizures; seizures in Lennox-Gastaut syndrome

Investigational uses: Bipolar disorder,
P cluster headache, infantile spasms

Dosage and routes
Adjunctive therapy
Adult: PO 25-50 mg/day initially, titrate by 25-50 mg/wk, up to 400 mg/day in 2 divided doses

Renal dose
Adult: PO CCr <70 ml/min ½ dose

Bipolar disorder (off-label)
Adult: PO 50-200 mg/day, max 400 mg/day

Available forms: Tabs 25, 100, 200 mg; sprinkle caps 15, 25 mg

Adverse effects
(*italic* = common; **bold** = life-threatening)
CNS: Dizziness, fatigue, cognitive disorder, *insomnia,* anxiety, depression, paresthesia
EENT: Diplopia, vision abnormality
GI: *Diarrhea, anorexia,* nausea, dyspepsia, abdominal pain, constipation, dry mouth
GU: Breast pain, dysmenorrhea, menstrual disorder
INTEG: Rash
MISC: Weight loss, leukopenia
RESP: Upper respiratory tract infection, pharyngitis

Contraindications: Hypersensitivity

Precautions: Hepatic disease, renal dis-
P ease, lactation, children, pregnancy **C**, acute myopia, secondary angle closure glaucoma

Pharmacokinetics
Absorption	Well absorbed
Distribution	Crosses placenta, plasma protein binding (9%-17%); steady state 4 days
Metabolism	Unknown
Excretion	Kidneys unchanged 55%-97%
Half-life	21 hr

Pharmacodynamics
Onset	Unknown
Peak	2-4 hr
Duration	Unknown

Interactions
Individual drugs
Alcohol: ↑ CNS depression
Carbamazepine, phenytoin, valproic acid:
↓ levels of topiramate
Digoxin: ↓ levels of digoxin
Drug classifications
Carbonic anhydrase inhibitors: ↑ kidney stone formation
Contraceptives, oral: ↓ level of oral contraceptives
CNS depressants: ↑ CNS depression
Food/drug
↓ Levels of topiramate
⊘ *Herb/drug*
Ginkgo: ↑ effect
Ginseng, santonica: ↓ effect

NURSING CONSIDERATIONS
Assessment
• Assess mental status: mood, sensorium, affect, memory (long, short), especially in
G elderly
• Assess for blood dyscrasias: fever, sore

T

throat, bruising, rash, jaundice, epistaxis (long-term treatment only)
• Assess seizure activity including type, location, duration, and character; provide seizure precaution
• Monitor CBC during long-term therapy
• Assess body weight and evidence of cognitive disorder

Nursing diagnoses
☑ Injury, risk for (side effects)
☑ Knowledge, deficient (teaching)

Implementation
• May take without regard to meals
🚫• Do not crush, or break tabs; very bitter
• Sprinkle cap can be given whole or opened and sprinkled on soft food; do not chew

Patient/family education
• Teach patient to carry/wear emergency ID stating name, drugs taken, condition, prescriber's name and phone number
• Advise patient to avoid driving, other activities that require alertness
• Teach patient not to discontinue medication abruptly after long-term use

Evaluation
Positive therapeutic outcome
• Decreased seizure activity

Treatment of overdose: Lavage, VS

⚠ HIGH ALERT

topotecan (Rx)
(to-poe′ti-kan)
Hycamtin
Func. class: Antineoplastic hormone
Chem. class: Semisynthetic derivative of camptothecin (topoisomerase inhibitor)

Pregnancy category D

Action: Antitumor drug with topoisomerase I–inhibitory activity; topoisomerase I relieves torsional strain in DNA by causing single-strand breaks; causes double-strand DNA damage

➔ **Therapeutic Outcome:** Decreased tumor size

Uses: Metastatic carcinoma of the ovary after failure of traditional chemotherapy

Dosage and routes
Adult: **IV** inf 1.5 mg/m^2 over 30 min qd × 5 days starting on day 1 of a 21-day course × 4 courses; may be reduced to 0.25 mg/m^2 for subsequent courses if severe neutropenia occurs

Renal dose
Adult: **IV** CCr 20-39 ml/min 0.75 mg/m^2/day × 5 days on day 1 of a 21-day course

Available forms: Lyophilized powder for inj 4 mg

Adverse effects
(*italic* = common; **bold** = life-threatening)
CNS: Arthralgia, asthenia, headache, myalgia, pain
GI: Abdominal pain, constipation, diarrhea, obstruction, nausea, stomatitis, vomiting, increased ALT, AST, anorexia
HEMA: **Neutropenia, leukopenia, thrombocytopenia, anemia, sepsis**
INTEG: Total alopecia
RESP: Dyspnea

Contraindications: Hypersensitivity, lactation, severe bone marrow depression, pregnancy **D**

P Precautions: Children

Pharmacokinetics	
Absorption	Rapidly/completely
Distribution	Unknown
Metabolism	Liver
Excretion	Urine, feces to metabolites
Half-life	8 hr

Pharmacodynamics
Unknown

Interactions
Individual drugs
Cisplatin: ↑ myelosuppression
Granulocyte colony-stimulating factor: ↑ duration of neutropenia

NURSING CONSIDERATIONS
Assessment
• Monitor liver function studies: AST, ALT, alkaline phosphatase, which may be elevated
• Monitor for CNS symptoms: drowsiness, confusion, depression, anxiety
• Monitor CBC, differential, platelet count weekly; withhold drug if WBC <3500/mm^3 or platelet count is <100,000/mm^3; notify prescriber of these results; drug should be discontinued
• Assess buccal cavity q8h for dryness, sores or ulceration, white patches, oral pain, bleeding, dysphagia
• Assess GI symptoms: frequency of stools, cramping
• Assess signs of dehydration: rapid respiration, poor skin turgor, decreased urine output, dry skin, restlessness, weakness

---

 Herb/drug   Do Not Crush   Alert   Key Drug   Geriatric   **P** Pediatric

Nursing diagnoses
✓ Infection, risk for (adverse reactions)
✓ Knowledge, deficient (teaching)

Implementation
• Provide increased fluid intake to 2-3 L/day to prevent dehydration, unless contraindicated
• Change **IV** site q48h
• Rinse mouth tid-qid with water, club soda; brush teeth bid-tid with soft brush or cotton-tipped applicator for stomatitis; use unwaxed dental floss
• Provide nutritious diet with iron, vit K supplements, low fiber, few dairy products

Patient/family education
• Advise patient to avoid foods with citric acid or hot or rough texture if stomatitis is present; to drink adequate fluids
• Advise patient to report stomatitis; any bleeding, white spots, ulcerations in mouth; tell patient to examine mouth qd; report symptoms
• Assess patient to report signs of anemia; fatigue, headache, faintness, shortness of breath, irritability
• Teach patient to use contraception during therapy

Evaluation
Positive therapeutic outcome
• Decreased tumor size, spread of malignancy

---

toremifene (Rx)
(tore′me-feen)
Fareston
Func. class.: Antineoplastic
Chem. class.: Antiestrogen hormone

Pregnancy category D

Action: Inhibits cell division by binding to cytoplasmic estrogen receptors; resembles normal cell complex but inhibits DNA synthesis and estrogen response of target tissue

⇨ **Therapeutic Outcome:** Prevention of rapidly growing malignant cells

Uses: Advanced breast carcinoma that has not responded to other therapy in estrogen-receptor-positive patients (usually postmenopausal)

Dosage and routes
Adult: PO 60 mg qd

Available forms: Tabs 60 mg

Adverse effects
(*italic* = common; **bold** = life-threatening)
CNS: *Hot flashes, headache, lightheadedness,* depression
CV: Chest pain, **CHF, MI, pulmonary embolism**
EENT: Ocular lesions, retinopathy, corneal opacity, blurred vision (high doses)
GI: *Nausea, vomiting,* altered taste (anorexia)
GU: Vaginal bleeding, pruritus vulvae
HEMA: **Thrombocytopenia, leukopenia**
INTEG: *Rash,* alopecia
META: Hypercalcemia

Contraindications: Hypersensitivity, pregnancy **D,** history of thromboembolism

Precautions: Leukopenia, thrombocytopenia, lactation, cataracts

Pharmacokinetics
Absorption	Adequately absorbed
Distribution	Unknown
Metabolism	Liver, extensively
Excretion	Feces, slowly, small amounts (kidneys)
Half-life	Unknown

Pharmacodynamics
Onset	Unknown
Peak	3 hr
Duration	Unknown

Interactions
Individual drugs
Warfarin: ↑ warfarin effect
Lab test interferences
↑ Serum Ca

NURSING CONSIDERATIONS
Assessment
• Monitor CBC, differential, platelet count weekly; withhold drug if WBC is <4000/mm³ or platelet count is <75,000/mm³; notify prescriber of results; monitor calcium levels (hypercalcemia is common)
• Assess for tumor flare: increase in bone, tumor pain during beginning treatment; give analgesics as ordered to decrease pain
• Assess for bleeding: hematuria, guaiac, bruising or petechiae, mucosa or orifices q8h, no rectal temp

Nursing diagnoses
✓ Injury, risk for (adverse reactions)
✓ Knowledge, deficient (teaching)

T

Implementation

• Give with food or fluids to decrease GI upset; do not break, crush, or chew enteric products; repeat dose may be needed if vomiting occurs
• Store in light-resistant container at room temp

Patient/family education
• Instruct patient to report any complaints, side effects to prescriber; if dose is missed, do not double next dose
• Advise patient that vaginal bleeding, pruritus, hot flashes, can occur, and are reversible after discontinuing treatment
• Instruct patient to report immediately decreased visual acuity, which may be irreversible; stress need for routine eye exams
• Inform patient about who should be told about toremifene therapy
• Advise patient to report vaginal bleeding immediately; that tumor flare (increase in size of tumor, increased bone pain) may occur and will subside rapidly; may take analgesics for pain; that premenopausal women must use mechanical birth control method because ovulation may be induced (teratogenic drug)
• Caution patient to use sunscreen and protective clothing to prevent burns because photosensitivity is common
• Teach patient that hair loss may occur during treatment; a wig or hairpiece may make patient feel better; new hair may be different in color, texture
• Inform patient rash or lesions are temporary and may become large during beginning therapy

Evaluation
Positive therapeutic outcome
• Decreased spread of malignant cells in breast cancer

---

trace elements (chromium, copper, iodide, manganese, selenium, zinc) (Rx)
Concentrated Multiple Trace Elements, ConTE-PAK-4, M.T.E.-4 Concentrated, M.T.E.-5, M.T.E.-5 Concentrated, M.T.E.-6, M.T.E.-6 Concentrated, M.T.E.-7, MulTE-PAK-4, MulTE-PAK-5, Multiple Trace Element, Multiple Trace Element Neonatal, Multiple Trace Element Pediatric, Neotrace 4, Ped TE-PAK-4, Pedtrice-4, P.T.E.-4, P.T.E.-5
Func. class.: Mineral supplement

Pregnancy category C

Action: Needed for adequate absorption and synthesis of amino acids

⮕**Therapeutic Outcome:** Replacement for mineral deficiencies

Uses: Prevention of trace element deficiency, a component of TPN

Dosage and routes
Usual dosage may be given in TPN sol

Chromium
Adult: **IV** 10-15 mcg qd
P *Child:* **IV** 0.14-0.20 mcg/ kg/day

Copper
Adult: **IV** 0.5-1.5 mg/day
P *Child:* **IV** .05-0.2 mg/kg/day

Iodide
Adult: **IV** 1 mcg/kg/day

Manganese
Adult: **IV** 1-3 mg/day

Selenium
Adult: 40-120 mcg/day
P *Child:* 3 mcg/kg/day

Zinc
Adult: **IV** 2-4 mg/day
P *Child:* **IV** 0.05 mg/kg/day

Available forms: Many forms available; see particular elements

Adverse effects
(*italic* = common; **bold** = life-threatening)
CHROMIUM: **Seizures, coma,** nausea, vomiting, ulcers, **renal/hepatic toxicity**
COPPER: Personality changes, diarrhea, weakness, photophobia, muscle weakness
IODINE: Headache, edema of eyelids, acne, metallic taste, sore mouth, runny nose
MANGANESE: Incoordination, headache, irritability, lability, slurred speech, impotence

---

SELENIUM: Alopecia, depression, vomiting, GI cramping, nervousness, garlic smell
ZINC: Vomiting, oliguria, **hypothermia,** vision changes, **tachycardia,** jaundice, **coma**

Precautions: Liver, biliary disease, pregnancy **C,** lactation, vomiting or diarrhea

Pharmacokinetics	
Absorption	Completely absorbed
Distribution	Widely distributed
Metabolism	Unknown
Excretion	Depends on element
Half-life	Unknown

Pharmacodynamics
Unknown

Interactions: None

NURSING CONSIDERATIONS
Assessment
• Assess trace element levels; notify prescriber if low copper 0.07-0.15 mg/ml, zinc 0.05-0.15 mg/100 ml, manganese 4-20 mcg/100 ml, selenium 0.1-0.19 mcg/ml
• Assess trace element deficiency if patient is receiving TPN for extended period
• Obtain calorie count to identify nutritional deficiencies
• Assess for toxicity to individual element (see Adverse effects)

Nursing diagnoses
✓ Nutrition: less than body requirements, imbalanced (uses)
✓ Knowledge, deficient (teaching)

Implementation
• Give by **IV** inf, often mixed with TPN sol
• Discard unused portions
• Give by continuous inf diluted in 1 L or more **IV** sol; give at prescribed rate

Patient/family education
• Explain reason for and expected results of medication

Evaluation
Positive therapeutic outcome
• Absence of element deficiency

---

tramadol (Rx)
(trah'mah-dol)
Ultram
Func. class.: Central analgesic

Pregnancy category C

Action: Not completely understood, binds to opioid receptors and inhibits reuptake of norepinephrine, serotonin; does not cause histamine release or affect heart rate

➡ **Therapeutic Outcome:** Relief of pain

Uses: Management of moderate to severe pain

Dosage and routes
Adult: PO 50-100 mg prn q4-6h, max 400 mg/day

🄖 *Elderly >75 yr:* PO <300 mg/day in divided dose

Hepatic dose
PO 50 mg q12h

Renal dose
Adult: PO CCr <30 ml/min q12h, max 200 mg/day

Available forms: Tabs 50 mg

Adverse effects
(*italic* = common; **bold** = life-threatening)
CNS: Dizziness, CNS stimulation, somnolence, headache, anxiety, confusion, euphoria, **seizures,** hallucinations
CV: Vasodilatation, orthostatic hypotension, tachycardia, hypertension, abnormal ECG
GI: Nausea, constipation, vomiting, dry mouth, diarrhea, abdominal pain, anorexia, flatulence, GI bleeding
GU: Urinary retention/frequency, menopausal symptoms, dysuria, menstrual disorder
INTEG: Pruritus, rash, urticaria, vesicles

Contraindications: Hypersensitivity, acute intoxication with any CNS depressant

Precautions: Seizure disorder, pregnancy 🄿 C, lactation, children, elderly, renal, hepatic 🄖 disease, respiratory depression, head trauma, increased ICP, acute abdominal condition, drug abuse

🅽 **Do Not Confuse:**
tramadol/Toradol

Pharmacokinetics	
Absorption	Rapidly, almost completely absorbed
Distribution	Steady state 2 days
Metabolism	Extensively in liver, may cross blood-brain barrier
Excretion	Unchanged drug 30% in urine
Half-life	Unknown

Pharmacodynamics
Unknown

T

Interactions
Individual drugs
Alcohol: ↑ CNS depression
Carbamazepine: ↓ tramadol level
Drug classifications
MAOIs: Inhibition of norepinephrine and serotonin reuptake; use together with caution
Opiates, sedative/hypnotics: ↑ CNS depression
☑ *Herb/drug*
Chamomile, hops, kava, skullcap, valerian: ↑ CNS depression
Lab test interferences
↑ Creatinine, ↑ liver enzymes
↓ Hgb

NURSING CONSIDERATIONS
Assessment
- Assess pain: location, type, character; give before pain becomes extreme
- Monitor I&O ratio: check for decreasing output; may indicate urinary retention
- Assess need for drug
- Assess for constipation and bowel pattern; increase fluids, bulk in diet
- Monitor CNS changes: dizziness, drowsiness, hallucinations, euphoria, LOC, pupil reaction
- Determine allergic reactions: rash, urticaria

Nursing diagnoses
☑ Pain, acute (uses)
☑ Pain, chronic (uses)
☑ Sensory perception, disturbed: visual, auditory (adverse reactions)
☑ Injury, risk for (adverse reactions)
☑ Knowledge, deficient (teaching)

Implementation
- Give with antiemetic for nausea, vomiting
- Administer when pain is beginning to return; determine dosage interval by patient response
- Store in cool environment, protect from sunlight

Patient/family education
- Teach patient to report any symptoms of CNS changes, allergic reactions
- Teach patient that drowsiness, dizziness, and confusion may occur; to call for assistance
- Instruct patient to make position changes slowly; orthostatic hypotension may occur
- Tell patient to avoid OTC medication and alcohol unless approved by prescriber

Evaluation
Positive therapeutic outcome
- Decreased pain

---

trandolapril (Rx)
(tran-doe'la-prill)
Mavik
Func. class.: Antihypertensive
Chem. class.: Angiotensin-converting enzyme (ACE) inhibitor

Pregnancy category
D (2nd/3rd trimesters);
C (1st trimester)

Action: Selectively suppresses renin-angiotensin-aldosterone system; inhibits ACE; prevents conversion of angiotensin I to angiotensin II, resulting in dilatation of arterial and venous vessels and lowered B/P

➡ **Therapeutic Outcome:** Decreased B/P in hypertension

Uses: Hypertension alone or in combination, heart failure, after MI/left ventricular dysfunction after MI

Dosage and routes
Hypertension
Adult: PO 1 mg/day, 2 mg/day in African Americans, make dosage adjustment ≥wk; up to 8 mg/day

Heart failure (after MI/left ventricular dysfunction)
Adult: PO 1 mg/day, titrate upward to 4 mg/day if tolerated

Renal dose/hepatic dose
Adult: PO CCr <30 ml/min 0.5 mg/day, may increase gradually up to 4 mg/day

Available forms: Tabs 1, 2, 4 mg

Adverse effects
(*italic* = common; **bold** = life-threatening)
CNS: Dizziness, paresthesias, headache, fatigue, drowsiness, depression, sleep disturbances, anxiety
CV: Hypotension, MI, palpitations, angina, TIAs, stroke, bradycardia, dysrhythmias
GI: Nausea, vomiting, cramps, diarrhea, constipation, pancreatitis, *dyspepsia*
GU: **Proteinuria, renal failure**
HEMA: **Agranulocytosis, neutropenia, leukopenia,** anemia
INTEG: Rash, purpura, pruritus
MISC: Hyperkalemia, hyponatremia, impotence, *myalgia,* **angioedema,** muscle cramps, asthenia, hypocalcemia, gout
RESP: Dyspnea, cough

Contraindications: Hypersensitivity, history of angioedema, pregnancy **D** (2nd/3rd trimesters)

Precautions: Hyperkalemia, hepatic

---

disease, bilateral renal stenosis, post kidney transplant, aortal/mitral valve stenosis, cirrhosis, severe renal disease, untreated CHF, autoimmune diseases, severe hypertension, pregnancy **C** (1st trimester)

Pharmacokinetics

Absorption	40-60%
Distribution	Unknown
Metabolism	Liver
Excretion	Kidneys, feces
Half-life	0.6-1.1 hr, 16-24 hr

Pharmacodynamics

Onset	½ hr
Peak	4-10 hr
Duration	>8 days

Interactions

Individual drugs
Levodopa, reserpine: ↑ effect of each specific drug

Drug classifications
Antacids: ↓ absorption
Antihypertensives, diuretics: ↑ severe hypotension
Barbiturates, ergots, hypoglycemics, neuromuscular blocking agents: ↑ effects of each specific drug
Diuretics (potassium-sparing): ↑ toxicity
Phenothiazines: ↑ antihypertensive effects
Potassium supplements: ↑ toxicity of potassium
Salt substitutes: ↑ potassium levels

Herb/drug
Aconite: ↑ toxicity, death
Astragalus, cola tree: ↑ or ↓ antihypertensive effect
Barberry, betony, black catechu, black cohosh, bloodroot, broom, burdock, cat's claw, dandelion, goldenseal, Irish moss, Jamaican dogwood, kelp, khella, mistletoe, parsley: ↑ antihypertensive effect
Coltsfoot, guarana, khat, licorice: ↓ antihypertensive effect

NURSING CONSIDERATIONS
Assessment
• Monitor blood studies: neutrophils, decreased platelets
• Monitor B/P, orthostatic hypotension, syncope; if changes occur dosage change may be required
• Monitor renal studies: protein, BUN,

creatinine; increased levels may indicate nephrotic syndrome and renal failure
• Monitor renal symptoms: polyuria, oliguria, frequency, dysuria
• Establish baselines in renal, liver function tests before therapy begins
• Check potassium levels throughout treatment, although hyperkalemia rarely occurs
• Check for edema in feet, legs daily
• Assess for allergic reactions: rash, fever, pruritus, urticaria; drug should be discontinued if antihistamines fail to help

Nursing diagnoses
☑ Cardiac output, decreased (uses)
☑ Injury, risk for (adverse reactions)
☑ Knowledge, deficient (teaching)
☑ Noncompliance (teaching)

Implementation
• Store in airtight container at 86° F (36° C) or less

Patient/family education
• Advise patient not to discontinue drug abruptly; advise patient to tell all persons associated with health care
• Teach patient not to use OTC products (cough, cold, allergy medications) unless directed by physician; serious side effects can occur; xanthines, such as coffee, tea, chocolate, cola, can prevent action of drug
• Instruct patient on the importance of complying with dosage schedule, even if feeling better; to continue with medical regimen to decrease B/P: exercise, cessation of smoking, decreasing stress, diet modifications
• Emphasize the need to rise slowly to sitting or standing position to minimize orthostatic hypotension; not to exercise in hot weather, which can cause increased hypotension
• Advise patient to notify prescriber of mouth sores, sore throat, fever, swelling of hands or feet, irregular heartbeat, chest pain, coughing, shortness of breath
• Caution patient to report excessive perspiration, dehydration, vomiting, diarrhea; may lead to fall in B/P
• Caution patient that drug may cause dizziness, fainting, light-headedness; may occur during 1st few days of therapy; to avoid activities that may be hazardous
• Teach patient how to take B/P, and normal readings for age group

Evaluation
Positive therapeutic outcome
• Decreased B/P in hypertension

Treatment of overdose: Lavage, **IV** atropine for bradycardia, **IV** theophylline for

T

bronchospasm, digitalis, O$_2$, diuretic for cardiac failure, hemodialysis

tranylcypromine (Rx)
(tran-ill-sip'roe-meen)
Parnate
Func. class: Antidepressant—MAOI
Chem. class: Nonhydrazine

Pregnancy category C

Action: Increases concentrations of endogenous epinephrine, norepinephrine, serotonin, dopamine in storage sites in CNS by inhibition of MAO; increased concentration reduces depression

→ **Therapeutic Outcome:** Decreased symptoms of depression after 2-3 wk

Uses: Depression, when uncontrolled by other means

Investigational uses: Bulimia, cocaine addiction, migraines, seasonal affective disorder, panic disorder

Dosages and routes
Adult: PO 10 mg bid; may increase to 30 mg/day after 2 wk; up to 60 mg/day

Available forms: Tabs 10 mg

Adverse effects
(*italic* = common; **bold** = life-threatening)
CNS: Dizziness, drowsiness, confusion, headache, anxiety, tremors, stimulation, weakness, hyperreflexia, mania, insomnia, fatigue
CV: Orthostatic hypotension, hypertension, **dysrhythmias, hypertensive crisis**
EENT: Blurred vision
ENDO: **Syndrome of inappropriate antidiuretic hormone-like symptoms**
GI: Constipation, dry mouth, nausea, vomiting, *anorexia,* diarrhea, weight gain
GU: Change in libido, frequency
HEMA: Anemia
INTEG: Rash, flushing, increased perspiration

Contraindications: Hypersensitivity to
🅖 MAOIs, elderly, uncontrolled hypertension, CHF, severe hepatic disease, pheochromocytoma, severe renal disease, severe cardiac disease

Precautions: Suicidal patients, seizure disorders, severe depression, schizophrenia, hyperactivity, diabetes mellitus, pregnancy **C**,
🅟 child <16 yr, lactation

Pharmacokinetics
Absorption	Well absorbed
Distribution	Crosses placenta
Metabolism	Liver, extensively
Excretion	Kidneys, breast milk
Half-life	Unknown

Pharmacodynamics
Unknown

Interactions
Individual drugs
Alcohol: ↑ CNS depression
Buspirone, clonidine: ↑ pressor effect
Dextromethorphan, meperidine, methylphenidate: ↑ hypertensive crisis
Fluoxetine, fluvoxamine, paroxetine, sertraline: Serotonin syndrome, do not use together
Guanethidine: Hypertensive crisis
Levodopa, methyldopa, sumatriptan: ↑ effects of each specific drug
Drug classifications
Antidepressants (tricyclic), appetite suppressants, asthma inhalants, decongestants, sinus medications: ↑ hypertensive crisis
Antidiabetics, β-adrenergics blockers, rauwolfia alkaloids, sulfonamides: ↑ effects
Barbiturates, benzodiazepines, diuretics (thiazides): ↑ effects of each specific drug
Dibenzazepine agents: Hypertensive crisis
Opiates: ↑ CNS depression
Sympathomimetics (direct-acting— epINEPHrine): ↑ effects of sympathomimetics (direct-acting)
Sympathomimetics (indirect-acting— epINEPHrine): ↑ pressor effects
Food/drug
Foods containing tyramine: ↑ hypertensive crisis; avoid all
🗹 *Herb/drug*
Betel palm, butcher's broom, capsicum peppers, galanthamine, green tea (large amounts), guarana (large amounts), night-blooming cereus: Hypertensive crisis
Ginseng: Mania
Parsley: Serotonin syndrome

NURSING CONSIDERATIONS
Assessment
• Monitor B/P (lying, standing), pulse q4h; if systolic B/P drops 20 mm Hg hold drug, notify prescriber; take vital signs q4h in patients with CV disease

---

- Monitor hepatic studies: AST, ALT, bilirubin
- Check weight qwk; appetite may increase with drug
- Assess mental status: mood, sensorium, affect, suicidal tendencies; increase in psychiatric symptoms: depression, panic
- Monitor urinary retention, constipation; **P** constipation is more likely to occur in children **G** or elderly
◑● • Assess for withdrawal symptoms: headache, nausea, vomiting, muscle pain, weakness; do not usually occur unless drug was discontinued abruptly
- Identify alcohol consumption; if alcohol is consumed, hold dose until AM

Nursing diagnoses
☑ Coping, ineffective (uses)
☑ Injury, risk for (side effects)
☑ Knowledge, deficient (teaching)
☑ Noncompliance (teaching)

Implementation
- Give with food or milk for GI symptoms; crush if patient is unable to swallow medication whole
- Store at room temp; do not freeze

Patient/family education
- Advise patient that therapeutic effects may take 48 hr-3 wk
- Teach patient to use caution in driving or other activities requiring alertness because of drowsiness, dizziness, blurred vision; to avoid rising quickly from sitting to standing, espe-**G** cially elderly
- Caution patient to avoid alcohol ingestion, other CNS depressants
- Advise patient not to discontinue medication quickly after long-term use: may cause nausea, headache, malaise
- Advise patient to increase fluids, bulk in diet if constipation, urinary retention occur, espe-**G** cially elderly
- Teach patient to take gum, hard sugarless candy, or frequent sips of water for dry mouth
- Teach patient to avoid high-tyramine foods; cheese (aged), sour cream, beer, wine, pickled products, liver, raisins, bananas, figs, avocados, meat tenderizers, chocolate, yogurt; increased caffeine, ginseng
- Teach patient to report headache, palpitation, neck stiffness
- Instruct patient to carry/wear emergency ID with medications taken, condition treated, and prescriber's name and phone number
- Advise patient to rise slowly to prevent postural hypotension

Evaluation
Positive therapeutic outcome
- Decrease in depression
- Absence of suicidal thoughts

Treatment of overdose: Lavage, activated charcoal, monitor electrolytes, VS, diazepam **IV**, NaHCO₃

⚠ HIGH ALERT

trastuzumab (Rx)
(tras-tuz′uh-mab)
Herceptin
Func. class.: Antineoplastic—misc.
Chem. class.: Humanized monoclonal antibody

Pregnancy category B

Action: DNA-derived monoclonal antibody selectively binds to extracellular portion of human epidermal growth factor receptor 2 (HER2); it inhibits proliferation of cancer cells

⇒ Therapeutic Outcome: Decreasing symptoms of breast cancer

Uses: Breast cancer; metastatic with overexpression of HER2

Dosage and routes
Adult: **IV** 4 mg/kg given over 90 min, then maintenance 2 mg/kg given over 30 min; do not give as **IV** push or bol

Available forms: Lyophilized powder 440 mg

Adverse effects
(*italic* = common; **bold** = life-threatening)
CNS: *Dizziness, numbness, paresthesias,* depression, insomnia, neuropathy, peripheral neuritis
CV: **Tachycardia, CHF**
GI: Nausea, vomiting, anorexia, diarrhea
HEMA: Anemia, **leukopenia**
INTEG: *Rash,* acne, herpes simplex
META: Edema, peripheral edema
MISC: *Flulike syndrome; fever, headache, chills*
MS: Arthralgia, bone pain
RESP: Cough, dyspnea, pharyngitis, rhinitis, sinusitis
SYST: **Anaphylaxis, angioedema**

Contraindications: Hypersensitivity to this drug, Chinese hamster ovary cell protein

P **Precautions:** Pregnancy **B**, lactation, **G** children, elderly, cardiac disease, anemia, leukopenia

T

Pharmacokinetics	
Absorption	Unknown
Distribution	Unknown
Metabolism	Unknown
Excretion	Unknown
Half-life	1.7-12 days

Pharmacodynamics	
Onset	Unknown
Peak	Unknown
Duration	Unknown

Interactions
Individual drugs
Cyclophosphamide: ↑ cardiomyopathy risk; avoid use

Drug classifications
Anthracyclines: ↑ cardiomyopathy risk

NURSING CONSIDERATIONS
Assessment
• Assess for symptoms of infection; may be masked by drug
• Assess CNS reaction: LOC, mental status, dizziness, confusion
• Assess for CHF and other cardiac symptoms: dyspnea, coughing, gallop; obtain a full cardiac workup including ECG, echocardiogram, multigated angiogram
• Assess for hypersensitivity reactions, anaphylaxis
• Monitor for potentially fatal infusion reactions: fever, chills, nausea, vomiting, pain, headache, dizziness, hypotension; discontinue drug

Nursing diagnoses
✓ Infection, risk for (side effects)
✓ Nutrition: less than body requirements, imbalanced (side effects)
✓ Knowledge, deficient (teaching)

Implementation
• Give acetaminophen as ordered to alleviate fever and headache
• Increase fluid intake to 2-3 L/day
IV IV route
• Administer after reconstituting vial with 20 ml of bacteriostatic water for inj, 1.1% benzyl alcohol preserved (supplied) to yield 21 mg/ml, mark date on vial 28 days from reconstitution date, if patient is allergic to benzyl alcohol, reconstitute with sterile water for inj; use immediately
• Do not mix or dilute with other drugs or dextrose sol

Patient/family education
• Advise patient to take acetaminophen for fever
• Teach patient to avoid hazardous tasks, since confusion, dizziness may occur
• Teach patient to report signs of infection: sore throat, fever, diarrhea, vomiting
• Inform patient that emotional lability is common; instruct patient to notify prescriber if severe or incapacitating

Evaluation
Positive therapeutic outcome
• Decrease in size of tumors

---

trazodone (Rx)
(tray'zoe-done)
Desyrel, Desyrel Dividose, trazodone HCl, Trazon, Trialodine
Func. class.: Antidepressant—misc.
Chem. class.: Triazolopyridine
Pregnancy category C

Action: Selectively inhibits serotonin, norepinephrine uptake by brain, potentiates behavioral changes

➔ **Therapeutic Outcome:** Decreased symptoms of depression after 2-3 wk

Uses: Depression

Investigational uses: Chronic pain syndromes

Dosage and routes:
Adult: PO 150 mg/day in divided doses; may increase by 50 mg/day q3-4d, not to exceed 600 mg/day

G *Elderly:* PO 25-50 hs, increase by 25-50 mg q3-7 days, to desired dose, usual 75-150 mg/day

P *Child 6-18 yr:* PO 1.5-2 mg/kg/day in divided doses, may increase q3-4 days up to 6 mg/kg/day

Available forms: Tabs 50, 100, 150, 300 mg

Adverse effects
(*italic* = common; **bold** = life-threatening)
CNS: Dizziness, drowsiness, confusion, headache, anxiety, tremors, stimulation, weakness, insomnia, nightmares, extrapyramidal symptoms (EPS) (elderly), increase in psychiatric symptoms
CV: Orthostatic hypotension, ECG changes, tachycardia, **hypertension,** palpitations
EENT: Blurred vision, tinnitus, mydriasis
GI: Diarrhea, dry mouth, nausea, vomiting,

---

paralytic ileus, increased appetite, cramps, epigastric distress, jaundice, **hepatitis,** stomatitis, constipation
GU: Retention, **acute renal failure, priapism**
HEMA: **Agranulocytosis, thrombocytopenia, eosinophilia, leukopenia**
INTEG: Rash, urticaria, sweating, pruritus, photosensitivity

Contraindications: Hypersensitivity to tricyclic antidepressants, recovery phase of MI, seizure disorders, prostatic hypertrophy

Precautions: Suicidal patients, severe depression, increased intraocular pressure, narrow-angle glaucoma, urinary retention, cardiac disease, hepatic disease, hyperthyroidism, electroshock therapy, elective surgery, pregnancy **C**

Pharmacokinetics

Absorption	Well absorbed
Distribution	Widely distributed
Metabolism	Liver, extensively
Excretion	Kidneys—unchanged minimally
Half-life	4½-7½ hr

Pharmacodynamics
Unknown

Interactions
Individual drugs
Alcohol: ↑ CNS depression
Clonidine: Severe hypotension, avoid use
Disulfiram: Organic brain syndrome
Fluoxetine: ↑ levels, ↑ toxicity
Guanethidine: ↓ effects
Drug classifications
Analgesics, antihistamines:↑ CNS depression
Anticholinergics: ↑ side effects
Antihypertensives: May block antihypertensive effect
Barbiturates, benzodiazepines, CNS depressants: ↑ effects
MAOIs: ↑ hypertensive crisis, seizures
Phenothiazines: ↑ toxicity
Sympathomimetics (direct-acting): ↑ sympathomimetic effects
Sympathomimetics (indirect-acting): ↓ effects
Herb/drug
Chamomile, hops, kava, lavender, skullcap, valerian: ↑ CNS depression
Corkwood, jimsonweed: ↑ anticholinergic effect
SAM-e, St. John's wort: ↑ serotonin syndrome
Lab test interferences
↑ Serum bilirubin, ↑ blood glucose, ↑ alkaline phosphatase

↓ VMA, ↓ 5-HIAA, ↓ blood glucose
False: ↑ urinary catecholamines

NURSING CONSIDERATIONS
Assessment
• Assess for pain: location, duration, intensity before and 1-2 hr after medication
• Monitor B/P (lying, standing), pulse q4h; if systolic B/P drops 20 mm Hg hold drug, notify prescriber; take vital signs q4h in patients with CV disease
• Monitor blood studies: CBC, leukocytes, differential, cardiac enzymes if patient is receiving long-term therapy
• Monitor hepatic function studies: AST, ALT, bilirubin
• Check weight qwk; appetite may increase with drug
• Assess ECG for flattening of T wave, bundle branch block, AV block, dysrhythmias in cardiac patients
G • Assess for EPS primarily in elderly: rigidity, dystonia, akathisia
• Assess mental status: mood, sensorium, affect, suicidal tendencies; increase in psychiatric symptoms: depression, panic
• Monitor urinary retention, constipation;
P constipation is more likely to occur in children
G or elderly
• Assess for withdrawal symptoms: headache, nausea, vomiting, muscle pain, weakness; do not usually occur unless drug was discontinued abruptly
• Identify alcohol consumption; if alcohol is consumed, hold dose until AM

Nursing diagnoses
✓ Coping, ineffective (uses)
✓ Injury, risk for (adverse reactions)
✓ Knowledge, deficient (teaching)
✓ Noncompliance (teaching)

Implementation
• Give with food or milk for GI symptoms; crush if patient is unable to swallow medication whole
• Give dosage hs if oversedation occurs
G during day; may take entire dose hs; elderly may not tolerate once/day dosing
• Store at room temp; do not freeze

Patient/family education
• Teach patient that therapeutic effects may take 2-3 wk
• Teach patient to use caution in driving or other activities requiring alertness because of drowsiness, dizziness, blurred vision; to avoid rising quickly from sitting to standing, especially elderly

T

• Caution patient to avoid alcohol ingestion, other CNS depressants

• Teach patient not to discontinue medication quickly after long-term use: may cause nausea, headache, malaise

• Advise patient to wear sunscreen or large hat because photosensitivity occurs

• Teach patient to increase fluids, bulk in diet if constipation, urinary retention occur,
G especially elderly

• Advise patient to take gum, hard sugarless candy, or frequent sips of water for dry mouth

• Teach family to watch for suicidal ideation or tendencies

Evaluation
Positive therapeutic outcome
• Decrease in depression
• Absence of suicidal thoughts

Treatment of overdose: ECG monitoring, induce emesis, lavage, activated charcoal, administer anticonvulsant

---

treprostinil (Rx)
(treh-prah′stin-ill)
Remodulin
Func. class.: Antiplatelet agent

Pregnancy category B

Action: Direct vasodilatation of pulmonary, systemic arterial vascular beds, inhibition of platelet aggregation

➡ **Therapeutic Outcome:** Decreased pulmonary arterial hypertension (PAH)

Uses: Pulmonary arterial hypertension (PAH) NYHA class II through IV

Dosage and routes
Adult: **SC INF** 1.25 ng/kg/min by **CONT INF,** may reduce to 0.625 mg if not tolerated

Hepatic dose
Adult: **SC INF** 0.625 ng/kg/min and increase cautiously

Available forms: Inj 1, 2.5, 5, 10 mg/ml

Adverse effects
(*italic* = common; **bold** = life-threatening)
CNS: Dizziness, headache
CV: Vasodilatation, hypotension, edema
GI: Nausea, *diarrhea*
INTEG: Rash, pruritus
SYST: Infusion site reactions, infusion site pain
OTHER: Jaw pain

Contraindications: Hypersensitivity

Precautions: Past liver disease, renal
G disease, elderly, pregnancy (B), lactation,
P children

Pharmacokinetics
Absorption	Unknown
Distribution	Unknown
Metabolism	Liver
Excretion	Urine, feces
Half-life	2-4 hr, terminal

Pharmacodynamics
Unknown

Interactions
Individual drug
Aspirin: ↑ risk of bleeding
Drug classifications
Anticoagulants: ↑ risk of bleeding
Antihypertensives, diuretics, vasodilators: ↑ hypotension

NURSING CONSIDERATIONS
Assessment
• Monitor liver function tests: AST, ALT, bilirubin, creatinine (long-term therapy)
⬥• Monitor blood studies: CBC; CBC q2 wk × 3 mo, Hct, Hgb, PT (long-term therapy)
⬥• Monitor bleed time baseline and throughout; levels may be 2-5 × normal limit

Nursing diagnoses
☑ Tissue perfusion, ineffective: cardiovascular/pulmonary (uses)
☑ Knowledge, deficient (teaching)

Implementation
• Give by continuous SC infusion

Patient/family education
• Teach patient that blood work will be necessary during treatment
• Teach patient to report side effects such as diarrhea, skin rashes

Evaluation
Positive therapeutic outcome
• Decreased pulmonary arterial hypertension (PAH)

---

tretinoin (vitamin A acid, retinoic acid) (Rx)

(tret'i-noyn)

Retin-A, Stievaa ✤, Tretinoin LF IV, Vesanoid

Func. class.: Vitamin A acid/acne product, antineoplastic—misc.

Chem. class.: Tretinoin derivative

Pregnancy category
C (top), **D** (PO)

Action: Decreases cohesiveness of follicular epithelium, decreases microcomedone formation (top); induces maturation of acute promyelocytic leukemia, exact action is unknown (PO)

➡**Therapeutic Outcome:** Decreased signs/symptoms of leukemia

Uses: Acne vulgaris (grades 1-3) (top); acute promylocytic leukemia (PO)

Investigational uses: Skin cancer

Dosage and routes

P *Adult and child:* Top cleanse area, apply hs; cover lightly

Promyelocytic leukemia

Adult: PO 45 mg/m²/day given as 2 evenly divided doses until remission, discontinue treatment 30 days after remission or after 90 days of treatment, whichever is first

Available forms: Top cream 0.05%, 0.01%; top gel 0.025%, 0.01%; top liq 0.05%; caps 10 mg

Adverse effects

(*italic* = common; **bold** = life-threatening)

Topical route

INTEG: Rash, stinging, warmth, redness, erythema, blistering, crusting, peeling, contact dermatitis, hypopigmentation, hyperpigmentation

PO route

CNS: Headache, fever, sweating

GI: Nausea, vomiting, **hemorrhage,** abdominal pain, diarrhea, constipation, dyspepsia, distention, **hepatitis**

Contraindications: Hypersensitivity to retinoids or sensitive to parabens, pregnancy **D** (PO)

Precautions: Pregnancy **C** (top), lactation, eczema, sunburn

Pharmacokinetics

Absorption	Small amounts
Distribution	Unknown
Metabolism	Unknown
Excretion	Kidneys
Half-life	Unknown

Pharmacodynamics

Unknown

Interactions

Individual drugs

Benzoyl peroxide, resorcinol, salicylic acid (top), sulfur: ↑ peeling

Ketoconazole: ↑ plasma concentrations of tretinoin (oral)

Drug classifications

Abrasive soaps, alcohol, astringents, cleansers with drying effect: use with caution

NURSING CONSIDERATIONS

Assessment

Topical route

• Assess part of body involved, including time involved, what helps or aggravates condition, cysts, dryness, itching; lesions may become worse at beginning of treatment

Nursing diagnoses

☑ Skin integrity, impaired (uses)

☑ Body image, disturbed (uses)

☑ Knowledge, deficient (teaching)

Implementation

Topical route

• Apply using gloves, once daily before bedtime; cover area lightly using gauze

• Store at room temp

• Wash hands after application

Liquid

• Apply with gloves or cotton; apply only to affected areas

Patient/family education

Topical route

• Instruct patient to avoid application on normal skin, and to avoid getting cream in eyes, nose, other mucous membranes

• Advise patient to avoid sunlight, sunlamps or to use protective clothing or sunscreen to prevent burns

• Advise patient that treatment may cause warmth, stinging; dryness; peeling will occur

• Inform patient that cosmetics may be used over drug; not to use shaving lotions

• Inform patient that rash may occur during first 1-3 wk of therapy

• Caution patient that drug does not cure condition; only relieves symptoms; that thera-

T

peutic results may be seen in 2-3 wk but may not be optimal until after 6 wk

Evaluation
Positive therapeutic outcome
- Decrease in size and number of lesions

triamcinolone (Rx)
(trye-am-sin'oh-lone)
Amcort, Aristocort, Aristocort Forte, Aristocort Intralesional, Aristospan Intra-Articular, Aristospan Intralesional, Articulose L.A., Atolone, Azmacort, Cenocort A-40, Cenocort Forte, Kenacort, Kenaject-40, Kenalog, Kenalog-10, Kenalog-40, Tac-3, Tac-40, Triam-A, triamcinolone, triamcinolone acetonide, Triam Forte, Triamolone 40, Triamonide 40, Tri-Kort, Trilog, Trilone, Trisoject
Func. class.: Corticosteroid; antiinflammatory
Chem. class.: Glucocorticoid, intermediate-acting

Pregnancy category C

Action: Decreases inflammation by suppression of migration of polymorphonuclear leukocytes, fibroblasts, reversal to increase capillary permeability and lysosomal stabilization

➡ **Therapeutic Outcome:** Decreased inflammation, normal immune response

Uses: Severe inflammation, immunosuppression, neoplasms, asthma (steroid dependent), collagen, respiratory, dermatologic disorders

Dosage and routes
Adult: PO 4-12 mg/day in divided doses qd-qid; IM 40 mg qwk (acetonide, or diacetate), 5-48 mg into neoplasms (diacetate, acetonide), 2-40 mg into joint or soft tissue (diacetate, acetonide), 0.5 mg/sq in of affected intralesional skin (hexacetonide), 2-20 mg into joint or soft tissue (hexacetonide)

P *Child:* PO 117 mcg/kg/day as a single dose or divided doses

Asthma
Adult: INH 2 tid-qid, max 16 inh/day

P *Child 6-12 yr:* INH 1-2 tid-qid, max 12 inh/day

Available forms: Tabs 1, 2, 4, 8 mg; syr 2, 4.85 mg/5 ml; inj 25, 40 mg/ml diacetate; inj 3, 10, 40 mg/ml acetonide; inj 5, 20 mg/ml hexacetonide; inh 100 mcg/spray; intranasal 55 mcg/spray

Adverse effects
(*italic* = common; **bold** = life-threatening)
CNS: *Depression, flushing, sweating,* headache, mood changes
CV: *Hypertension,* **circulatory collapse, thrombophlebitis, embolism,** tachycardia, edema
EENT: Fungal infections, increased intraocular pressure, blurred vision
GI: *Diarrhea, nausea, abdominal distention,* **GI hemorrhage,** *increased appetite,* **pancreatitis**
HEMA: **Thrombocytopenia**
INTEG: Acne, poor wound healing, ecchymosis, petechiae
MS: Fractures, osteoporosis, weakness

Contraindications: Psychosis, hypersensitivity, idiopathic thrombocytopenia, acute glomerulonephritis, amebiasis, fungal infecP tions, nonasthmatic bronchial disease, child <2 yr, AIDS, TB, adrenal insufficiency

Precautions: Pregnancy **C**, diabetes mellitus, glaucoma, osteoporosis, seizure disorders, ulcerative colitis, CHF, myasthenia gravis, renal disease, esophagitis, peptic ulcer, lactation

Interactions
Individual drugs
Alcohol, amphotericin B, cycloSPORINE, digitalis, indomethacin: ↑ side effects
Ambenonium, isoniazid, neostigmine, somatrem: ↓ effects of each specific drug
Cholestyramine, colestipol, epHEDrine, phenytoin, rifampin, theophylline: ↓ action of triamcinolone
Indomethacin, ketoconazole: ↑ action of triamcinolone
Insulin: ↑ need for insulin
Drug classifications
Anticholinesterases, anticoagulants, anticonvulsants, antidiabetics, salicylates: ↓ effects of each specific drug
Antiinfectives (macrolide), contraceptives (oral), estrogens, salicylates: ↑ action of triamcinolone
Barbiturates: ↓ action of triamcinolone
Diuretics, salicylates: ↑ side effects
Hypoglycemic agents: ↑ need for hypoglycemic agents
Toxoids, vaccines: ↓ effects of toxoids, vaccines

Herb/drug
Aloe, buckthorn, cascara sagrada, Chinese
rhubarb, senna: ↑ hypokalemia
Lab test interferences
↑ Cholesterol, ↑ sodium, ↑ blood glucose, ↑
uric acid, ↑ calcium, ↑ urine glucose
↓ Calcium, ↓ potassium, ↓ T₄, ↓ T₃, ↓ thyroid
¹³¹I uptake test, ↓ urine 17-OHCS, ↓ 17-KS, ↓
PBI
False negative: Skin allergy tests

Pharmacokinetics

Absorption	Well absorbed (PO, IM)
Distribution	Crosses placenta, widely distributed
Metabolism	Liver—extensively
Excretion	Kidney, breast milk
Half-life	2-5 hr, adrenal suppression 3-4 days

NURSING CONSIDERATIONS
Assessment
- Monitor potassium, blood glucose, urine glucose while on long-term therapy; hypokalemia and hyperglycemia
- Monitor weight daily; notify prescriber of weekly gain >5 lb; I&O ratio; be alert for decreasing urinary output and increasing edema
- Monitor B/P q4h, pulse; notify prescriber if chest pain occurs
- Monitor plasma cortisol levels during long-term therapy (normal level; 138-635 nmol/L [SI units] when measured at 8 AM); adrenal function periodically for hypothalamic-pituitary-adrenal axis suppression
- Assess for infection: increased temp, WBC even after withdrawal of medication; drug masks infection symptoms
- Assess for potassium depletion: paresthesias, fatigue, nausea, vomiting, depression, polyuria, dysrhythmias, weakness
- Assess mental status: affect, mood, behavioral changes, aggression
- Assess nasal passages during long-term treatment for changes in mucus (nasal)
- Monitor temp; if fever develops, drug should be discontinued

- Assess for systemic absorption: increased temp, inflammation, irritation (top)

Nursing diagnoses
☑ Infection, risk for (adverse reactions)
☑ Knowledge, deficient (teaching)
☑ Noncompliance (teaching)

Implementation
PO route
- Give with food or milk to decrease GI symptoms, tablet may be crushed
IM route
- Give IM inj deeply in large muscle mass, rotate sites, avoid deltoid, use 21-G needle
- Give in one dose in AM to prevent adrenal suppression; avoid SC administration; may damage tissue
Inhalation route
🅖 • Use spacer device for elderly
- Give inh with water to decrease possibility of fungal infections; titrated dose, use lowest effective dose
- Give after cleaning aerosol top daily with warm water, dry thoroughly
- Store in cool environment; do not puncture or incinerate container
Topical route
- Apply only to affected areas; do not get in eyes
- Apply medication, then cover with occlusive dressing (only if prescribed), seal to normal skin, change q12h; systemic absorption may occur
- Apply only to dermatoses; do not use on weeping, denuded, or infected areas
- Cleanse skin before applying drug
- Continue treatment for a few days after area has cleared
- Store at room temp
Nasal route
- Have patient clear nasal passages before administration; use decongestant if needed; shake inhaler, invert, tilt head backward, insert nozzle into nostril, away from septum; hold other nostril closed and depress activator, inhale through nose, exhale through mouth

Patient/family education
- Advise patient that emergency ID as steroid user should be carried/worn

T

Pharmacodynamics

	PO	IM	TOP	INH	INTRANASAL
Onset	Unknown	Unknown	Min to hr	1-2 wk	Unknown
Peak	1-2 hr	1-2 hr	Hr to days	Unknown	2-3 wk
Duration	3 days	Unknown	Hr to days	Unknown	Unknown

• Instruct patient to notify prescriber if therapeutic response decreases; dosage adjustment may be needed; not to discontinue abruptly; adrenal crisis can result

• Caution patient to avoid OTC products: salicylates, alcohol in cough products, cold preparations unless directed by prescriber

• Advise patient on all aspects of drug usage including cushingoid symptoms

• Teach patient symptoms of adrenal insufficiency: nausea, anorexia, fatigue, dizziness, dyspnea, weakness, joint pain

• Teach patient that long-term therapy may be needed to clear infection (1-2 mo depending on type of infection)

Nasal route

• Instruct patient to clear nasal passages if sneezing attack occurs, repeat dose

• Advise patient to continue using product even if mild nasal bleeding occurs; is usually transient

• Teach patient method of instillation after providing written instruction from manufacturer

Inhalation route

• Teach patient proper administration technique; to wash inhaler with warm water and dry after each use

• Teach patient all aspects of drug usage including cushingoid symptoms

Topical route

• Instruct patient to avoid sunlight on affected area; burns may occur

Evaluation
Positive therapeutic outcome

• Decrease in runny nose (nasal)

• Decreased dyspnea, wheezing, dry rales on auscultation (inh)

• Ease of respirations, decreased inflammation

• Absence of severe itching, patches on skin, flaking (top)

---

triamterene (Rx)
(try-am′ter-een)
Dyrenium
Func. class.: Potassium-sparing diuretic
Chem. class.: Pteridine derivative

Pregnancy category B

Action: Acts primarily on distal tubule to inhibit reabsorption of sodium, chloride; increase potassium retention and conserve hydrogen ions

➔**Therapeutic Outcome:** Diuretic and

antihypertensive effect while retaining potassium

Uses: Edema, hypertension, diuretic-induced hypokalemia

Dosage and routes
Adult: PO 100 mg bid pc, max 300 mg/day

G *Elderly:* PO 50 mg qd, max 100 mg/day

Available forms: Caps 50, 100 mg

Adverse effects
(*italic* = common; **bold** = life-threatening)
CNS: Weakness, headache, dizziness, fatigue
ELECT: Hyperkalemia, hyponatremia, hypochloremia
GI: Nausea, diarrhea, vomiting, dry mouth, jaundice, liver disease
GU: **Azotemia, interstitial nephritis,** increased BUN, creatinine, renal stones, bluish discoloration of urine
HEMA: **Thrombocytopenia, megaloblastic anemia,** low folic acid levels
INTEG: Photosensitivity, rash

Contraindications: Hypersensitivity, anuria, severe renal, hepatic disease; hyperkalemia, lactation

Precautions: Dehydration, hepatic disease, CHF, renal disease, cirrhosis, pregnancy **B**

Pharmacokinetics	
Absorption	GI tract; well absorbed
Distribution	Crosses placenta
Metabolism	Liver
Excretion	Renal; breast milk
Half-life	3 hr

Pharmacodynamics	
Onset	2 hr
Peak	6-8 hr
Duration	12-16 hr

Interactions
Individual drugs
Amantadine: ↑ amantadine toxicity
Cimetidine: ↓ renal clearance of triamterene
Indomethacin: ↑ nephrotoxicity
Drug classifications
Angiotensin-converting enzyme inhibitors, diuretics (potassium-sparing), potassium products, salt substitutes: ↑ hyperkalemia
Antihypertensives: ↑ action
NSAIDs: ↓ nephrotoxicity
Herb/drug
Arginine: Fatal hypokalemia
Bearberry, gossypol: ↑ hypokalemia
Cucumber, dandelion, horsetail, licorice,

nettle, pumpkin, Queen Anne's lace: ↑ diuretic effect

St. John's wort: Severe photosensitivity

Lab test interferences

Interference: Quinidine serum levels, LDH

NURSING CONSIDERATIONS
Assessment

• Monitor for manifestations of hyperkalemia: *RENAL:* acidic urine, reduced urine osmolality, nocturia, polyuria, polydipsia; *CV:* hypotension, broad T wave, U wave, ectopy, tachycardia, weak pulse; *NEURO:* muscle weakness, altered LOC, drowsiness, apathy, lethargy, confusion, depression, anorexia, nausea, cramps, constipation, distention, paralytic ileus, hypoventilation, respiratory muscle weakness

• Monitor for manifestations of hyponatremia: *CV:* ↑ B/P, cold, clammy skin, hypo/hypervolemia; *GI:* anorexia, nausea, vomiting, diarrhea, abdominal cramps; *NEURO:* lethargy, increased ICP, confusion, headache, seizures, coma, fatigue, tremors, hyperreflexia

• Monitor for manifestations of hyperchloremia: *NEURO:* weakness, lethargy, coma; *RESP:* deep rapid breathing

• Assess fluid volume status: I&O ratios and record, weight, distended red veins, crackles in lung, color, quality, and sp gr of urine, skin turgor, adequacy of pulses, moist mucous membranes, bilateral lung sounds, peripheral pitting edema; dehydration symptoms of decreasing output, thirst, hypotension, dry mouth and mucous membranes should be reported

• Monitor electrolytes: potassium, sodium, calcium, magnesium; also include BUN, ABGs, uric acid, CBC, blood glucose

Nursing diagnoses

☑ Urinary elmination, impaired (adverse reactions)

☑ Fluid volume, deficient (adverse reactions)

☑ Fluid volume, excess (uses)

☑ Knowledge, deficient (teaching)

Implementation

• Give in AM to avoid interference with sleep

• With food, if nausea occurs

Patient/family education

• Teach patient to take medication early in the day to prevent nocturia

• Instruct the patient to take with food or milk if GI symptoms of nausea and anorexia occur

• Teach patient to maintain a record of weight on a weekly basis and notify prescriber of weight loss of 5 lb

• Caution the patient that this drug causes an increase in potassium levels, that foods high in potassium should be avoided; refer to dietitian for assistance planning

• Caution the patient not to exercise in hot weather, stand for prolonged periods of time because orthostatic hypotension will be enhanced

• Advise patient to wear protective clothing and sunscreen in the sun to prevent photosensitivity

• Teach patient not to use alcohol or any OTC medications without prescriber's approval because serious drug reactions may occur

• Emphasize the need to contact prescriber immediately if muscle cramps, weakness, nausea, dizziness, or numbness occur

• Teach patient to take own B/P and pulse and record

• Advise patient that dizziness and confusion may occur; avoid driving or other hazardous activities if alertness is decreased

• Teach patient to continue taking medication even if feeling better; this drug controls symptoms but does not cure the condition

• Advise the patient with hypertension to continue other medical treatment (exercise, weight loss, relaxation techniques, cessation of smoking)

Evaluation
Positive therapeutic outcome

• Prevention of hypokalemia (diuretic use)

• Decreased edema

• Decreased B/P

• Increased diuresis

Treatment of overdose: Lavage if taken orally; monitor electrolytes; administer sodium bicarbonate for potassium 6.5 mEq/L; monitor hydration, CV, renal status

---

triazolam (Rx)
(trye-az'oh-lam)

Apo-Triazo ✦, Gen-Triazolam ✦, Halcion, Novotriolam ✦, Nu-Triazol ✦

Func. class.: Sedative-hypnotic, antianxiety

Chem. class.: Benzodiazepine

Pregnancy category X

Controlled substance schedule IV (USA), schedule F (Canada)

T

Action: Produces CNS depression at limbic, thalamic, hypothalamic levels of CNS; may be mediated by neurotransmitter; γ-aminobutyric acid (GABA); results are sedation, hypnosis, skeletal muscle relaxation, anticonvulsant activity, anxiolytic action

→ **Therapeutic Outcome:** Decreased anxiety, insomnia

Uses: Insomnia (short-term), sedative/hypnotic

Dosage and routes
Adult: PO 0.125-0.5 mg hs

G *Elderly:* PO 0.625-0.125 mg hs

Available forms: Tabs 0.125, 0.25 mg

Adverse effects
(*italic* = common; **bold** = life-threatening)
CNS: Headache, lethargy, drowsiness, daytime sedation, dizziness, confusion, lightheadedness, anxiety, irritability, amnesia, poor coordination
CV: Chest pain, pulse changes
GI: Nausea, vomiting, diarrhea, heartburn, abdominal pain, constipation
HEMA: Leukopenia, granulocytopenia (rare)

Contraindications: Hypersensitivity to benzodiazepines, pregnancy **X**, lactation, intermittent porphyria

Precautions: Anemia, hepatic disease,
G renal disease, suicidal individuals, drug
P abuse, elderly, psychosis, child <15 yr, acute narrow-angle glaucoma, seizure disorders

Pharmacokinetics	
Absorption	Well absorbed
Distribution	Widely distributed, crosses placenta, crosses blood-brain barrier
Metabolism	Liver
Excretion	Kidneys, breast milk
Half-life	2-3 hr

Pharmacodynamics	
Onset	½ hr
Peak	Unknown
Duration	6-8 hr

Interactions
Individual drugs
Alcohol: ↑ action of both drugs
Cimetidine, disulfiram, isoniazid: ↑ action
Erythromycin, probenecid: ↑ effects
Rifampin: ↓ action of rifampin
Theophylline: ↓ effects of theophylline
Drug classifications
Antacids: ↓ effects of antacids
Antiinfectives (macrolide): ↑ effects
CNS depressants: ↑ effects of both drugs

Contraceptives (oral): ↑ effects; do not use concurrently
Smoking: ↓ effects
☑ *Herb/drug*
Black cohosh: ↑ hypotension
Chamomile, hops, kava, lavender, mistletoe, nettle, pokeweed, poppy, Queen Anne's lace, senega, skullcap, valerian: ↑ CNS depression
Lab test interferences
↑ AST, ↑ ALT, ↑ serum bilirubin
False: ↑ 17-OHCS
↓ radioactive iodine uptake

NURSING CONSIDERATIONS
Assessment
• Assess patient's mental status: mood, sensorium, anxiety, affect, sleeping pattern,
G drowsiness, dizziness, especially elderly; physical dependency, withdrawal symptoms: anxiety, panic attacks, agitation, seizures, headache, nausea, vomiting, muscle pain, weakness; suicidal tendencies; for indications of increasing tolerance and abuse
• Monitor patient's B/P (lying, standing), pulse; if systolic B/P drops 20 mm Hg, hold drug, notify prescriber
• Monitor blood studies: CBC during longterm therapy; blood dycrasias have occurred rarely; decreased hematocrit, neutropenia may occur
• Monitor hepatic function studies: AST, ALT, bilirubin, creatinine LDH, alkaline phosphatase
• Monitor I&O ratio; indicate renal dysfunction

Nursing diagnoses
☑ Anxiety (uses)
☑ Depression (uses)
☑ Injury, risk for (adverse reactions)
☑ Knowledge, deficient (teaching)

Implementation
• Give with food or milk to decrease GI symptoms; if patient is unable to swallow medication whole, tab may be crushed and mixed with foods or fluids
• Give sugarless gum, hard candy, frequent sips of water for dry mouth

Patient/family education
• Advise patient that drug may be taken with food or fluids, and tab may be crushed or swallowed whole
• Caution patient not to use for everyday stress or longer than 3 mo unless directed by prescriber; not to take more than prescribed amount; may be habit forming; not to double doses or skip doses
• Instruct patient to avoid OTC preparations

☑ Herb/drug   **Ⓢ** Do Not Crush   **◆** Alert   **◆ₚ** Key Drug   **G** Geriatric   **P** Pediatric

unless approved by prescriber; alcohol and CNS depressants will increase CNS depression
• Caution patient to avoid driving, activities that require alertness because drowsiness may occur; to avoid alcohol ingestion or other psychotropic medications; to rise slowly or
🅖 fainting may occur, especially elderly; that drowsiness may worsen at beginning of treatment
• Advise patient not to discontinue medication abruptly after long-term use; withdrawal symptoms include vomiting, cramping, tremors, seizures

Evaluation
Positive therapeutic outcome
• Decreased anxiety, restlessness, sleeplessness (short-term treatment only)

Treatment of overdose: Lavage, VS, supportive care

---

trifluoperazine (Rx)
(trye-floo-oh-per'a-zeen)
Apo-Trifluoperazine ✤, Novoflurazine ✤, Solazine ✤, Stelazine, Suprazine, Terfluzine, trifluoperazine HCl, Triflurin
Func. class.: Antipsychotic/neuroleptic
Chem. class.: Phenothiazine, piperazine

Pregnancy category C

Action: Depresses cerebral cortex, hypothalamus, limbic system, which control activity, aggression; blocks neurotransmission produced by DOPamine at synapse; exhibits strong α-adrenergic, anticholinergic blocking action; mechanism for antipsychotic effects is unclear

⮕**Therapeutic Outcome:** Decreased signs and symptoms of psychosis

Uses: Psychotic disorders, nonpsychotic anxiety, schizophrenia

Dosage and routes
Psychotic disorders
Adult: PO 2-5 mg bid, usual range 15-20 mg/day, may require 40 mg/day or more; IM 1-2 mg q4-6h

🅖 *Elderly:* PO 0.5-1 mg qd-bid, increase q4-7 days by 0.5-1 mg/day to desired dose

🅟 *Child >6 yr:* PO 1 mg qd or bid; IM *not recommended for children,* but 1 mg may be given qd or bid

Nonpsychotic anxiety
Adult: PO 1-2 mg bid, not to exceed 6 mg/day; do not give longer than 12 wk

Available forms: Tabs 1, 2, 5, 10 mg; conc 10 mg/ml; inj 2 mg/ml

Adverse effects
(*italic* = common; **bold** = life-threatening)
CNS: *EPS (pseudoparkinsonism, akathisia, dystonia, tardive dyskinesia),* **seizures,** *headache,* **neuroleptic malignant syndrome,** dizziness
CV: *Orthostatic hypotension,* hypertension, **cardiac arrest,** ECG changes, **tachycardia**
EENT: Blurred vision, glaucoma, dry eyes
GI: *Dry mouth, nausea, vomiting, anorexia, constipation,* diarrhea, jaundice, weight gain
GU: Urinary retention, urinary frequency, enuresis, impotence, amenorrhea, gynecomastia
HEMA: Anemia, **leukopenia, leukocytosis, agranulocytosis**
INTEG: *Rash,* photosensitivity, dermatitis
RESP: **Laryngospasm,** dyspnea, **respiratory depression**

Contraindications: Hypersensitivity, CV disease, coma, blood dyscrasias, severe
🅟 hepatic disease, child <6 yr, narrow-angle glaucoma

Precautions: Breast cancer, seizure disorders, pregnancy **C,** lactation, diabetes mellitus, respiratory conditions, prostatic hypertrophy,
🅖 elderly

◼ **Do Not Confuse:**
trifluoperazine/trihexyphenidyl

Pharmacokinetics
Absorption	Variably absorbed (PO), well absorbed (IM)
Distribution	Widely distributed, high concentrations in CNS, crosses placenta
Metabolism	Liver—extensively
Excretion	Kidneys, breast milk
Half-life	Unknown

Pharmacodynamics
	PO	IM
Onset	Rapid	Immediate
Peak	2-3 hr	1 hr
Duration	12 hr	12 hr

Interactions
Individual drugs
Alcohol: ↑ effects of both drugs, oversedation
Aluminum hydroxide, magnesium hydroxide: ↓ absorption
Levodopa: ↓ antiparkinson activity
Lithium: ↓ effects of lithium
Drug classifications
Anesthetics (barbiturate): Oversedation

T

Anesthetics (general), MAOIs, opiates, sedative/hypnotics: ↑ CNS depression
Antacids: ↓ absorption
Anticholinergics: ↑ anticholinergic effects
Anticonvulsants: ↓ effects of anticonvulsants
β-Adrenergic blockers: ↑ effects of both drugs

☑ Herb/drug
Chamomile, hops, kava, skullcap, valerian: ↑ CNS depression
Betel palm, kava: ↑ Extrapyramidal symptoms (EPS)
Cola tree, hops, nettle, nutmeg: ↑ action

Lab test interferences
↑ Liver function tests, ↑ cardiac enzymes, ↑ cholesterol, ↑ blood glucose, ↑ prolactin, ↑ bilirubin, ↑ PBI, ↓ cholinesterase, ↑ alkaline phosphatase, ↑ leukocytes, ↑ granulocytes, ↑ platelets
↓ Hormones (blood and urine)
False positive: Pregnancy tests, PKU, urine bilirubin
False negative: Urinary steroids, 17-OHCS

NURSING CONSIDERATIONS
Assessment
• Assess mental status: orientation, mood, behavior, presence of hallucinations and type before initial administration and monthly; drug should significantly reduce psychotic behavior
• Check for swallowing of PO medication; check for hoarding or giving of medication to other patients
• Monitor I&O ratio, palpate bladder if low 🅖 urinary output occurs, especially in elderly; urinalysis recommended before, during prolonged therapy
• Monitor bilirubin, CBC, liver function studies monthly
• Assess affect, orientation, LOC, reflexes, gait, coordination, sleep pattern disturbances
• Monitor B/P sitting, standing, and lying, take pulse and respirations q4h during initial treatment; establish baseline before starting treatment; report drops of 30 mm Hg; obtain baseline ECG, monitor Q- and T-wave changes
• Check for dizziness, faintness, palpitations, tachycardia on rising; severe orthostatic hypotension is common
🔶• Identify for neuroleptic malignant syndrome: hyperpyrexia, muscle rigidity, increased CPK, altered mental status; drug should be discontinued
• Assess for EPS including akathisia (inability to sit still, no pattern to movements), tardive dyskinesia (bizarre movements of the jaw, mouth, tongue, extremities), pseudoparkinsonism (ragged tremors, pill rolling, shuffling

gait); an antiparkinson drug should be prescribed
• Assess for constipation, urinary retention daily; if these occur, increase bulk, water in diet
• Assess for hypo/hyperglycemia; appetite patterns

Nursing diagnoses
☑ Thought processes, disturbed (uses)
☑ Coping, ineffective (uses)
☑ Knowledge, deficient (teaching)
☑ Noncompliance (teaching)

Implementation
PO route
• Give drug in liq form mixed in glass of juice if hoarding is suspected; do not mix in caffeine drinks, tannics, pectins
🅖• Give decreased dose in elderly; metabolism is slowed in the elderly
• Give PO with full glass of water, milk; or give with food to decrease GI upset
• Store in airtight, light-resistant container, oral sol in amber bottle

IM route
• Inj in deep muscle mass, do not give SC; do not administer sol with a precipitate

🅸🅥 IV route
• Give **IV** after diluting 10 mg/9 ml of 0.9% NaCl; give 1 mg or less/2 min

Syringe compatibilities: Glycopyrrolate

Additive compatibilities: Meperidine, netilmicin

Patient/family education
• Teach patient to use good oral hygiene; frequent rinsing of mouth, sugarless gum for dry mouth
• Caution patient to avoid hazardous activities until drug response is determined; dizziness, blurred vision is common
• Inform patient that orthostatic hypotension occurs often; to rise from sitting or lying position gradually and to remain lying down after IM inj for at least 30 min
• Caution patient to avoid tubs, hot showers, tub baths because hypotension may occur
• Instruct patient that heat stroke may occur in hot weather, so take extra precautions to stay cool
• Advise patient to avoid abrupt withdrawal of this drug, or EPS may result; drug should be withdrawn slowly
• Teach patient to avoid OTC preparations (cough, hay fever, cold) unless approved by prescriber because serious drug interactions may occur; avoid use with alcohol, CNS de-

---

pressants because increased drowsiness may occur

- Advise patient to use sunglasses and sunscreen to prevent burns
- Teach patient about EPS and necessity of meticulous oral hygiene because oral candidiasis may occur
- Advise patient to take antacids 2 hr before or after this drug
- Instruct patient to report sore throat, malaise, fever, bleeding, mouth sores; if these occur, CBC should be performed and drug discontinued

Evaluation
Positive therapeutic outcome
- Decrease in emotional excitement, hallucinations, delusions, paranoia
- Reorganization of patterns of thought, speech

Treatment of overdose: Lavage if orally ingested; provide airway; *do not induce vomiting or use epINEPHrine*

trihexyphenidyl (Rx)
(trye-hex-ee-fen′i-dill)
Apo-Trihex ✤, Artane, Artane Sequels, Novohexidyl ✤, PMS-Trihexyphenidyl ✤, Trihexy-2, Trihexy-5, trihexyphenidyl HCl, Trihexane
Func. class.: Cholinergic blocker; antiparkinson
Chem. class.: Synthetic tertiary amine

Pregnancy category C

Action: Blocks central muscarinic receptors, which decreases involuntary movements, sweating, salivation

➔**Therapeutic Outcome:** Decreased involuntary movements

Uses: parkinsonian symptoms, drug-induced extrapyramidal symptoms (EPS)

Dosage and routes
Parkinsonian symptoms
Adult: PO 1 mg, increased by 2 mg q3-5 days to a total of 6-10 mg/day, given in 3-4 divided doses; give ext rel cap q12h

Drug-induced EPS
Adult: PO 1 mg/day; usual dose 5-15 mg/day, given in 3-4 divided doses, give ext rel q12h

Available forms: Tabs 2, 5 mg; ext rel caps 5 mg; elixir 2 mg/5 ml

Adverse effects
(*italic* = common; **bold** = life-threatening)
CNS: Confusion, anxiety, restlessness, irritability, delusions, hallucinations, headache, sedation, depression, incoherence, dizziness, flushing, weakness
CV: Palpitations, tachycardia, postural hypotension
EENT: Blurred vision, photophobia, dilated pupils, difficulty swallowing, dry eyes, increased intraocular tension, angle-closure glaucoma
GI: *Dryness of mouth, constipation,* nausea, vomiting, abdominal distress, **paralytic ileus**
GU: Urinary hesitancy, urinary retention, dysuria
INTEG: Urticaria, rash
MISC: Suppression of lactation, nasal congestion, decreased sweating, increased temp, hyperthermia, heat stroke, numbness of fingers
MS: Weakness, cramping

Contraindications: Hypersensitivity, narrow-angle glaucoma, myasthenia gravis, GI/GU obstruction, myocardial ischemia, unstable CV disease, prostatic hypertrophy

Precautions: Pregnancy **C**, elderly, lactation, tachycardia, abdominal obstruction, infection, children, gastric ulcer

Do Not Confuse:
Artane/Altace, trihexyphenidyl/trifluoperazine

Pharmacokinetics	
Absorption	Well absorbed
Distribution	Unknown
Metabolism	Unknown
Excretion	Unknown
Half-life	5-10 hr

Pharmacodynamics		
	PO	PO-EXT REL
Onset	1 hr	Unknown
Peak	2-3 hr	Unknown
Duration	6-12 hr	Up to 24 hr

Interactions
Individual drugs
Alcohol: ↑ CNS depression
Amantadine: ↑ cholinergic effects
Digoxin: ↑ levels of digoxin
Haloperidol: ↓ action of haloperidol
Drug classifications
Analgesics, antihistamines, opioids, sedative/hypnotics: ↑ CNS depression
Antihistamines, phenothiazines: ↑ anticholinergic effects

NURSING CONSIDERATIONS
Assessment
• Monitor I&O ratio; retention commonly causes decreased urinary output, distention, frequency, incontinence
• Assess for parkinsonism, EPS: shuffling gait, muscle rigidity, involuntary movements, pill rolling, muscle spasms, drooling before and during treatment
• Monitor for urinary hesitancy, retention; palpate bladder if retention occurs
• Monitor for constipation, cramping, pain in abdomen, abdominal distention; increase fluids, bulk, exercise if this occurs
• Assess for tolerance over long-term therapy; dose may have to be increased or changed
• Assess for mental status: affect, mood, CNS depression, worsening of mental symptoms during early therapy

Nursing diagnoses
✓ Mobility, impaired physical (uses)
✓ Knowledge, deficient (teaching)

Implementation
• Give with or after meals to prevent GI upset; may give with fluids other than water; offer hard candy, frequent drinks, gum to relieve dry mouth
• Give hs to avoid daytime drowsiness in patient with parkinsonism
• Store at room temp

Patient/family education
• Teach patient to use caution in hot weather; drug may increase susceptibility to stroke because perspiration is decreased; patient should remain indoors
• Teach patient not to discontinue this drug abruptly; to taper off over 1 wk to prevent withdrawal symptoms (insomnia, involuntary movements, anxiety, tachycardias)
• Caution patient to avoid driving or other hazardous activities; drowsiness, dizziness may occur
• Advise patient to avoid OTC medications (cough, cold preparations with alcohol, antihistamines) unless directed by prescriber; increased CNS depression may occur
• Instruct patient to rise from sitting or recumbent position slowly to minimize orthostatic hypotension
• Advise patient to use gum, hard candy, frequent sips of water to decrease dry mouth; if dry mouth continues, saliva substitutes may be prescribed
• Instruct patient that doses should not be doubled, but missed dose may be taken up to 2 hr before next dose

Evaluation
Positive therapeutic outcome
• Absence of involuntary movements (pill rolling, tremors, muscle spasms)

---

trimethobenzamide (Rx)
(trye-meth-oh-ben'za-mide)
Arrestin, Benzacot, Brogan, Stemetic, T-Gen, Tebamide, Ticon, Tigan, Tijet-20, Triban, Trimazide, trimethobenzamide, trimethobenzamide HCl
Func. class.: Antiemetic, anticholinergic
Chem. class.: Ethanolamine derivative
Pregnancy category C

Action: Acts centrally by blocking chemoreceptor trigger zone, which in turn acts on vomiting center

→**Therapeutic Outcome:** Absence of nausea and vomiting

Uses: Nausea, vomiting, prevention of postoperative vomiting

Dosage and routes
Postoperative vomiting
Adult: IM/rec 200 mg before or during surgery; may repeat 3 hr after

Discontinuing anesthesia
P *Child 13-40 kg:* PO/rec 100-200 mg tid-qid
P *Child <13 kg:* PO/rec 100 mg tid-qid

Nausea/vomiting
Adult: PO 250-300 mg tid-qid; IM/rec 200 mg tid-qid

Available forms: Caps 100, 250, 300, mg; supp 100, 200 mg; inj 100 mg/ml

Adverse effects
(*italic* = common; **bold** = life-threatening)
CNS: Drowsiness, restlessness, headache, dizziness, insomnia, confusion, nervousness, tingling, *vertigo,* extrapyramidal symptoms (EPS)
CV: Hypertension, hypotension, palpitations
EENT: Dry mouth, blurred vision, diplopia, nasal congestion, photosensitivity
GI: Nausea, anorexia, diarrhea, vomiting, constipation
INTEG: Rash, urticaria, fever, chills, flushing

Contraindications: Hypersensitivity to
P opioids, shock, children (parenterally)

P **Precautions:** Children, cardiac dysrhyth-
G mias, elderly, asthma, pregnancy C, prostatic hypertrophy, bladder-neck obstruction, narrow-angle glaucoma, stenosing peptic ulcer, pyloroduodenal obstruction

---

Pharmacokinetics

Absorption	Unknown
Distribution	Unknown
Metabolism	Liver, extensively
Excretion	Kidneys
Half-life	Unknown

Pharmacodynamics

	PO	IM	REC
Onset	20-40 min	15 min	10-40 min
Peak	Unknown	Unknown	Unknown
Duration	3-4 hr	2-3 hr	3-4 hr

Interactions
Individual drugs
Alcohol: ↑ CNS depression
Drug classifications
Analgesics, antidepressants, antihistamines, CNS depressants, sedative/hypnotics: ↑ CNS effect
Antibiotics: May mask ototoxic symptoms

NURSING CONSIDERATIONS
Assessment
• Monitor VS, B/P; check patients with cardiac disease more often
• Assess for signs of toxicity of other drugs or masking of symptoms of disease: brain tumor, intestinal obstructions
• Observe for drowsiness, dizziness
• Assess for nausea, vomiting before and after treatment

Nursing diagnoses
☑ Knowledge, deficient (teaching)

Implementation
PO route
• Cap may be swallowed whole or opened and mixed with food or fluids
IM route
• Administer IM inj in large muscle mass; aspirate to avoid **IV** administration

Syringe compatibilities: Glycopyrrolate, hydromorphone, midazolam, nalbuphine

Y-site compatibilities: Heparin, hydrocortisone, potassium chloride, vit B/C

Patient/family education
• Teach patient to use good oral hygiene; frequent rinsing of mouth, sugarless gum for dry mouth
• Caution patient to avoid hazardous activities until drug response is determined, drowsiness may occur

• Inform patient that orthostatic hypotension occurs often and to rise from sitting or lying position gradually and to remain lying down after IM inj for at least 30 min
• Advise patient to avoid hot tubs, hot showers, tub baths because hypotension may occur
• Inform patient that in hot weather, heat stroke may occur; take extra precautions to stay cool
• Teach patient to avoid OTC preparations (cough, hayfever, cold) unless approved by prescriber because serious drug interactions may occur; avoid use with alcohol, CNS depressants because increased drowsiness may occur
• Teach patient about EPS
• Instruct patient to report sore throat, malaise, fever, bleeding, mouth sores; if these occur, CBC should be performed and drug discontinued

Evaluation
Positive therapeutic outcome
• Decreased nausea, vomiting

trimethoprim/ sulfamethoxazole (cotrimoxazole) (Rx)
(trye-meth′oh-prim/sul-fa-meth-ox′a-zole [ko-trye-mox′a-zole])
Apo-Sulfatrim*, Apo-Sulfatrim DS ♣, Bactrim, Bactrim IV, **Bethaprim**, Comoxol, Cotrim, Novo-Trimel ♣, Novo-Trimel DS ♣, Nu-Cotrimox ♣, Nu-Cotrimox DS ♣, Roubac ♣, Septra, Septra DS, SMZ/TMP, Sulfatrim
Func. class.: Antiinfective
Chem. class.: Sulfonamide—misc.

Pregnancy category C

Action: Sulfamethoxazole (SMZ) interferes with bacterial biosynthesis of proteins by competitive antagonism of PABA when adequate levels are maintained; trimethoprim (TMP) blocks synthesis of tetrahydrofolic acid; combination blocks two consecutive steps in bacterial synthesis of essential nucleic acids, protein

Therapeutic Outcome: Absence of infection, based on C&S

Uses: UTI, otitis media, acute and chronic prostatitis, shigellosis, *Pneumocystis carinii* pneumonitis, chronic bronchitis, chancroid, traveler's diarrhea

T

Dosage and routes
UTI
Adult: PO 160 mg TMP/800 mg SMZ q12h × 10-14 days

P *Child:* PO 8 mg/kg TMP/40 mg/kg SMZ qd in 2 divided doses q12h

Otitis media
P *Child:* PO 8 mg/kg TMP/40 mg/kg SMZ qd in 2 divided doses q12h × 10 days

Chronic bronchitis
Adult: PO 160 mg TMP/800 mg SMZ q12h × 14 days

Pneumocystis carinii pneumonitis
P *Adult and child:* PO 20 mg/kg TMP qd in 4 divided doses q6h × 14 days; **IV** 15-20 mg/kg/day (based on TMP) in 3-4 divided doses for up to 14 days
Renal dose
• Dosage reduction necessary in moderate to severe renal impairment (CCr <30 ml/min)

Available forms: Tabs 80 mg trimethoprim (TMP)/400 mg sulfamethoxazole (SMZ), 160 mg TMP/800 mg SMZ; susp 40 mg/200 mg/5 ml; **IV** 16 mg/80 mg/ml

Adverse effects
(*italic* = common; **bold** = life-threatening)
CNS: Headache, insomnia, hallucinations, depression, vertigo, fatigue, anxiety, seizures, drug fever, chills, aseptic meningitis
CV: **Allergic myocarditis**
GI: *Nausea, vomiting, abdominal pain,* stomatitis, **hepatitis**, glossitis, pancreatitis, diarrhea, **enterocolitis**, anorexia
GU: **Renal failure, toxic nephrosis;** increased BUN, creatinine; crystalluria
HEMA: **Leukopenia, neutropenia, thrombocytopenia, agranulocytosis, hemolytic anemia, hypoprothrombinemia, Henoch-Schönlein purpura, methemoglobinemia, eosinophilia I**
INTEG: Rash, dermatitis, urticaria, erythema, photosensitivity, pain, inflammation at injection site, **toxic epidermal necrolysis, erythema multiforme**
RESP: Cough, shortness of breath
SYST: **Anaphylaxis, systemic lupus erythematosus, Stevens-Johnson syndrome**

Contraindications: Hypersensitivity to trimethoprim or sulfonamides, pregnancy at
P term, megaloblastic anemia, infants <2 mo, CCr <15 ml/min, lactation, porphyria

Precautions: Pregnancy **C**, renal disease,
G elderly, glucose-6-phosphate dehydrogenase deficiency, impaired hepatic/renal function, possible folate deficiency, severe allergy, bronchial asthma

Pharmacokinetics
Absorption	Rapid
Distribution	Breast milk, crosses placenta, 68% protein bound
Metabolism	Liver
Excretion	Kidneys
Half-life	8-13 hr

Pharmacodynamics
Onset	Unknown
Peak	1-4 hr
Duration	Unknown

Interactions
Individual drugs
CycloSPORINE: ↓ response
Methotrexate: ↑ bone marrow depression
Phenytoin: ↓ hepatic clearance of phenytoin
Drug classifications
Anticoagulants (oral): ↑ anticoagulant effect
Diuretics (thiazide): ↑ thrombocytopenia
Sulfonylureas: ↑ hypoglycemic response
Lab test interferences
↑ Alkaline phosphatase, ↑ creatinine, ↑ bilirubin
False positive: Urinary glucose test

NURSING CONSIDERATIONS
Assessment
• Assess allergic reactions: rash, fever (AIDS patients more susceptible)
• Monitor I&O ratio; note color, character, pH of urine if drug administered for UTI; output should be 800 ml less than intake; if urine is highly acidic, alkalization may be needed
• Monitor kidney function studies: BUN, creatinine, urinalysis (long-term therapy)
• Assess type of infection; obtain C&S before starting therapy
• Assess blood dyscrasias, skin rash, fever, sore throat, bruising, bleeding, fatigue, joint pain
• Assess allergic reaction: rash, dermatitis, urticaria, pruritus, dyspnea, bronchospasm

Nursing diagnoses
☑ Infection, risk for (uses)
☑ Knowledge, deficient (teaching)
☑ Noncompliance (teaching)

Implementation
• Give with full glass of water to maintain adequate hydration; increase fluids to 2 L/day to decrease crystallization in kidneys

---

- Give medication after C&S; repeat C&S after full course of medication
- Store in airtight, light-resistant container at room temp
- Dilute 5 ml ampule/100-125 ml of D_5W, stable for 6 hr, give over 1½ hr, do not refrigerate

IV IV route

Syringe compatibilities: Heparin

Y-site compatibilities: Acyclovir, aldesleukin, allopurinol, amifostine, atracurium, aztreonam, cefepime, cyclophosphamide, diltiazem, enalaprilat, esmolol, filgrastim, fludarabine, gallium, granisetron, hydromorphone, labetalol, lorazepam, magnesium sulfate, melphalan, meperidine, morphine, pancuronium, perphenazine, piperacillin/tazobactam, sargramostim, tacrolimus, teniposide, thiotepa, vecuronium, zidovudine

Patient family education
- Teach patient to take each oral dose with full glass of water to prevent crystalluria; drink 8-10 glasses of water/day
- Teach patient to complete course of full treatment to prevent superinfection
- Teach patient to avoid sunlight or use sunscreen to prevent burns
- Teach patient to avoid OTC medications (aspirin, vit C) unless directed by prescriber
- If diabetic, teach patient to use Clinistix or Tes-Tape
- Teach patient to use alternative contraceptive measures; decreased effectiveness of oral contraceptives may result
- Teach patient to notify prescriber if skin rash, sore throat, fever, mouth sores, unusual bruising, bleeding occur

Evaluation
Positive therapeutic outcome
Absence of pain, fever, C&S negative

---

triptorelin (Rx)
(trip-toe′rel-in)
Trelstar Depot
Func. class.: Gonadotropin-releasing hormone antagonist
Chem. class.: Synthetic decapeptide analog of LHRH

Pregnancy category X

Action: Inhibitor of pituitary gonadotropin secretion; initially increases LH and FSH, with increases in testosterone, reduction in sex steroid levels

→**Therapeutic Outcome:** Decreased signs/symptoms of advanced prostate cancer

Uses: Advanced prostate cancer

Dosage and routes
Adult: IM 3.75 mg qmo

Available forms: Microgranules, depot inj 3.75 mg

Adverse effects
(*italic* = common; **bold** = life-threatening)
CNS: Headache, insomnia, dizziness, lability, fatigue
CV: Hypertension
ENDO: Gynecomastia, breast tenderness, hot flashes
GI: Nausea, vomiting, diarrhea
GU: Impotence, urinary retention, UTI
INTEG: Rash, pain on injection, pruritus, hypersensitivity
MISC: **Anaphylaxis, angioedema**
MS: Osteoneuralgia

Contraindications: Hypersensitivity to this product or other LHRH agonists or LHRH, pregnancy **X**, lactation

Pharmacokinetics	
Absorption	Unknown
Distribution	Unknown
Metabolism	CYP/450
Excretion	Liver, kidneys
Half-life	3 hr

Pharmacodynamics	
Unknown	

Interactions: None known

Lab test interferences
↑ Alkaline phosphatase, ↑ estradiol, ↑ FSH, ↑ LH, ↑ testosterone levels
↓ Testosterone levels, ↓ progesterone

NURSING CONSIDERATIONS
Assessment
- Assess for severe hypersensitivity: discontinue drug and give antihistamines, have emergency equipment nearby
- Monitor I&O ratios; palpate bladder for distention in urinary obstruction
- Monitor for relief of bone pain (back pain)
- Assess levels of testosterone and prostate-specific antigen (PSA)

Nursing diagnoses
✓Diarrhea (adverse reactions)
✓Knowledge, deficient (teaching)

T

Implementation
- Give IM using implant, inserted by qualified person
- Use syringe with 20-G needle, withdraw 2 ml of sterile water for inj, inject into vial, shake well, withdraw vial contents, inject immediately

Patient/family education
- Teach patient that gynecomastia may occur but will decrease after treatment is discontinued
- Teach patient that disease flare may occur at beginning of therapy

Evaluation
Positive therapeutic outcome
- More normal levels of PSA, acid phosphatase, alkaline phosphatase; testosterone level of <25 ng/dl

---

! HIGH ALERT

tubocurarine ⊙π (Rx)
(too-boh-cure′a-reen)
Tubarine ✤, Tubocuraine
Func. class.: Neuromuscular blocker
Chem. class.: Synthetic curariform

Pregnancy category C

Action: Inhibits transmission of nerve impulses by binding with cholinergic receptor sites, antagonizing action of acetylcholine; no analgesic response

⊃**Therapeutic Outcome:** Skeletal muscle paralysis during anesthesia

Uses: Facilitation of endotracheal intubation, skeletal muscle relaxation during mechanical ventilation, surgery, or general anesthesia

Dosage and routes
Adult: **IV** bol 0.4-0.5 mg/kg, then 0.08-0.10 mg/kg 20-45 min after 1st dose if needed for prolonged procedures

Available forms: Inj 3 mg/ml (20 U/ml)

Adverse effects
(*italic* = common; **bold** = life-threatening)
CV: Bradycardia, tachycardia, increased, decreased B/P
EENT: Increased secretions
INTEG: Rash, flushing, pruritus, urticaria
RESP: **Prolonged apnea, bronchospasm, cyanosis, respiratory depression**

Contraindications: Hypersensitivity

Precautions: Pregnancy C, cardiac disease, ▣ lactation, children <2 yr, electrolyte imbalances, dehydration, neuromuscular disease, respiratory disease

---

Pharmacokinetics

Absorption	Complete bioavailability
Distribution	Extensive, crosses placenta
Metabolism	Liver, small amount
Excretion	Kidneys—unchanged (30%-75%), bile (11%)
Half-life	1-3 hr

Pharmacodynamics

	IV	IM
Onset	3-5 min, dose dependent	15-30 min
Peak	2-3 min	Unknown
Duration	½-1½ hr	Unknown

Interactions
Individual drugs
Clindamycin, lidocaine, lithium, magnesium, polymyxin B, quindine: ↑ paralysis, length and intensity
Enflurane, isoflurane, lincomycin, trimethoprim: ↑ neuromuscular blockade
Drug classifications
Aminoglycosides: ↑ paralysis, length and intensity
Analgesics (opioid), anesthetics (local), antiinfectives (polymyxin), thiazides: ↑ neuromuscular blockade

NURSING CONSIDERATIONS
Assessment
- Monitor for electrolyte imbalances (potassium, magnesium) before drug is used; electrolyte imbalances may lead to increased action of this drug
- Monitor VS (B/P, pulse, respirations, airway) until fully recovered; rate, depth, pattern of respirations, strength of hand grip; patient should be intubated before use
- Monitor recovery: decreased paralysis of face, diaphragm, leg, arm, rest of body; residual weakness and respiratory problems may occur during recovery period
- Monitor allergic reactions: rash, fever, respiratory distress, pruritus; drug should be discontinued

Nursing diagnoses
✓ Breathing pattern, ineffective (uses)
✓ Communication, impaired verbal (adverse reactions)
✓ Fear (adverse reactions)
✓ Knowledge, deficient (teaching)

Implementation
- Use peripheral nerve stimulator by anesthesiologist to determine neuromuscular blockade; deep tendon reflexes should be monitored during extended periods

---

 Herb/drug   Do Not Crush   Alert   Key Drug   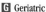 Geriatric   ▣ Pediatric

- Give **IV** undiluted by direct **IV** over 1-1½ min (only by qualified person, usually an anesthesiologist)

Syringe compatibilities: Pentobarbital, thiopental

Additive incompatibilities: Barbiturates, sodium bicarbonate

Solution compatibilities: D₅, D₁₀W, 0.9% NaCl, 0.45% NaCl, Ringer's, LR, dextrose/Ringer's or dextrose/LR combinations

Patient/family education
- Provide reassurance if communication is difficult during recovery from neuromuscular blockade
- Provide explanation to patient regarding all procedures or treatments; patient will remain conscious if anesthesia is not given also

Evaluation
Positive therapeutic outcome
- Paralysis of jaw, eyelid, head, neck, rest of body as evaluated by peripheral nerve stimulator

Treatment of overdose: Edrophonium or neostigmine, atropine, monitor VS; patient may require mechanical ventilation

---

! HIGH ALERT

urokinase (Rx)
(yoor-oh-kin′ase)
Abbokinase, Abbokinase Open-Cath
Func. class.: Thrombolytic enzyme
Chem. class.: β-Hemolytic *Streptococcus* filtrate (purified)

Pregnancy category B

Action: Promotes thrombolysis by directly converting plasminogen to plasmin

➡ **Therapeutic Outcome:** Lysis of emboli, or thrombosis in various parts of the body

Uses: Venous thrombosis, pulmonary embolism, arterial thrombosis, arterial embolism, arteriovenous cannula occlusion, lysis of coronary artery thrombi after MI

Dosage and routes
Lysis of pulmonary emboli
P **Adult and child: IV** 4400 international units/kg/hr × 12-24 hr, not to exceed 200 ml; then **IV** heparin, then anticoagulants

Coronary artery thrombosis
Adult: Instill 6000 international units/min

into occluded artery for 1-2 hr after giving **IV** bol of heparin 2500-10,000 units; may also give as **IV** inf of 2-3 million units over 45-90 min

Venous catheter occlusion
P **Adult and child:** Instill 5000 international units into line, wait 5 min, then aspirate; repeat aspiration attempts q5 min × ½ hr; if occlusion has not been removed, then cap line and wait ½-1 hr, then aspirate; may need 2nd dose if still occluded

Available forms: Powder for inj, lyophilized: 250,000 international units/vial; powder for catheter clearance

Adverse effects
(*italic* = common; **bold** = life-threatening)
CNS: Headache, fever
CV: Hypotension, dysrhythmias
GI: Nausea, vomiting
HEMA: Decreased Hct, **bleeding**
INTEG: Rash, urticaria, phlebitis at **IV** inf site, itching, flushing
MS: Low back pain
RESP: Altered respirations, cyanosis, shortness of breath, **bronchospasm**
SYST: **GI, GU, intracranial, retroperitoneal bleeding;** surface bleeding; **anaphylaxis** (rare)

Contraindications: Hypersensitivity, internal active bleeding, intraspinal surgery, neoplasms of CNS, ulcerative colitis/enteritis, severe uncontrolled hypertension, renal disease, hepatic disease, hypocoagulation, COPD, subacute bacterial endocarditis, rheumatic valvular disease, cerebral embolism/thrombosis/hemorrhage, intraarterial diagnostic procedure or surgery (10 days), recent major surgery/trauma, aneurysm, AV malformation

Precautions: Arterial emboli from left side of heart, pregnancy **B,** hepatic disease

Pharmacokinetics
Absorption	Completely
Distribution	Unknown
Metabolism	Liver
Excretion	Kidneys
Half-life	10-20 min

Pharmacodynamics
Onset	Rapid
Peak	Rapid
Duration	12 hr

U

Interactions
Individual drugs
Abciximab, aspirin, clopidogrel, dipyridamole, eptifibatide, heparin, indomethacin, phenylbutazone, plicamycin, ticlopidine, tirofiban, valproic acid: ↑ bleeding potential
Drug classifications
Anticoagulants (oral), cephalosporins (some), NSAIDs: ↑ bleeding potential
Glycoprotein IIb, IIIa inhibitors: ↑ bleeding risk
Lab test interferences
↑ Pro-time, ↑ APTT, ↑ TT

NURSING CONSIDERATIONS
Assessment
• Monitor VS, B/P, pulse, respirations (including peripheral), neurologic signs, temp at least q4h; temp >104° F (40° C) indicates internal bleeding; monitor rhythm closely; ventricular dysrhythmias may occur with hyperfusion; monitor heart, breath sounds, neurologic status, peripheral pulses
• Assess for bleeding during 1st hr of treatment: hematuria, hematemesis, bleeding from mucous membranes, epistaxis, ecchymosis; guaiac, all body fluids, stools; blood studies (Hct, platelets, PTT, Pro-time, TT, APTT) before starting therapy (Pro-time or APTT must be less than 2 × control); TT or PT q3-4h during treatment
• Assess hypersensitivity: fever, rash, itching, chills, facial swelling, dyspnea; mild reaction may be treated with antihistamines; notify prescriber of severe reactions, stop drug, keep resuscitative equipment nearby
• Monitor ECG on monitor, watch for segment changes, changes in rhythm; sinus bradycardia, ventricular tachycardia, accelerated idioventricular rhythm may occur because of reperfusion

Nursing diagnoses
✓ Tissue perfusion, ineffective (uses)
✓ Injury, risk for (adverse reactions)
✓ Gas exchange, impaired (uses)

Implementation
Ⅳ **Intermittent IV route**
• Give **IV** loading dose over 30 min to avoid hypotension
• **IV** after dilution with 4-5 g/250 ml of 0.9% NaCl, D₅W, LR, give over 1 hr; may give by continuous inf after loading dose(s) of 1 g/hr diluted in 50-100 ml of compatible sol; use infusion pump; do not give by direct **IV**
• Give heparin therapy after thrombolytic

therapy is discontinued, TT, ACT, or APTT less than 2 × control (about 3-4 hr)
• Avoid invasive procedures, inj, rectal temp
• Apply pressure for 30 sec to minor bleeding sites, 30 min to sites of atrial puncture, followed by pressure dressing; inform prescriber if this does not attain hemostasis
• Store powder at room temp or refrigerate; protect from excessive light

Additive incompatibilities: Do not mix with other medications

Patient/family education
• Teach patient reason for medication, signs and symptoms of bleeding, allergic reactions, when to notify health care prescriber

Evaluation
Positive therapeutic outcome
• Lysis of thrombi or emboli

---

valacyclovir (Rx)
(val-a-sye'kloh-vir)
Valtrex
Func. class.: Antiviral
Chem. class.: Acyclic purine nucleoside analog

Pregnancy category B

Action: Interferes with DNA synthesis by conversion to acyclovir, causing decreased viral replication, time of lesional healing

➡ **Therapeutic Outcome:** Absence of itching, painful lesions; crusting and healing of lesions

Uses: Treatment or suppression of herpes zoster, recurrent genital herpes, herpes labialis

Investigational uses: Prevention of cytomegalovirus infection, in advanced HIV posttransplant patients

Dosage and routes
Genital herpes
Adult: PO 1 g bid × 10 days initially; 1 g qd or 500 mg bid in those with <10 recurrences/yr

Herpes zoster
Adult: PO 1 g tid × 1 wk

Recurrent episodes
Adult: PO 500 mg bid × 3 days

Suppressive therapy
Adult: PO 1 g qd if ≤10 recurrences/yr

Herpes labialis
Adult: PO 2 g bid × 1 day

Renal dose
Adult: PO CCr 30-49 ml/min 1g q12h (herpes zoster); CCr 10-29 ml/min 1 g q24h (genital herpes); 500 mg q24h (recurrent genital herpes); CCr <10 ml/min 500 mg q24h (genital herpes), 500 mg q24h (recurrent genital herpes)

Available forms: Tabs 500, 1000 mg

Adverse effects
(*italic* = common; **bold** = life-threatening)
CNS: Tremors, lethargy, *dizziness, headache, weakness*
GI: *Nausea, vomiting, diarrhea, abdominal pain, constipation*
INTEG: *Rash*
HEMA: **Thrombocytopenic purpura, hemolytic uremic syndrome**

Contraindications: Hypersensitivity to this drug or acyclovir

Precautions: Lactation, hepatic disease, renal disease, electrolyte imbalance, dehydration, pregnancy **B**

Pharmacokinetics

Absorption	Unknown
Distribution	Crosses placenta, enters breast milk
Metabolism	Converts to acyclovir
Excretion	Unknown
Half-life	2½-3½ hr

Pharmacodynamics

Onset	Unknown
Peak	Unknown
Duration	Unknown

Interactions
Individual drugs
Cimetidine, probenecid: ↑ blood levels of valacyclovir

NURSING CONSIDERATIONS
Assessment
• Assess for signs of infection; characteristics of lesions
• Assess C&S before drug therapy; drug may be performed as soon as culture is performed; repeat C&S after treatment; determine the presence of other sexually transmitted diseases
• Assess bowel pattern before, during treatment
• Assess for skin eruptions: rash
• Assess allergies before treatment, reaction of each medication
◆• Assess for thrombocytopenic purpura, hemolytic uremic syndrome, may be fatal

Nursing diagnoses
✓ Infection, risk for (uses)

Patient/family education
• Advise patient to take as prescribed; if dose is missed, take as soon as remembered up to 1 hr before next dose; do not double dose
• Instruct patient to take drug orally before infection occurs; drug should be taken when itching or pain occurs, usually before eruptions
• Inform patient that partners need to be told that patient has herpes; they can become infected; condoms must be worn to prevent reinfections
• Tell patient that drug does not cure infection, just controls symptoms and does not prevent infection to others
• Advise women they must use a reliable form of contraception during treatment and for 90 days following; men should use barrier contraceptive during treatment and for 90 days following

Evaluation
Positive therapeutic outcome
• Absence of itching, painful lesions; crusting and healed lesions

Treatment of overdose:
• Discontinue drug
• Provide hemodialysis, resuscitation if needed

/ HIGH ALERT

valdecoxib (Rx)
(val-deh-cock'sib)
Bextra
Func. class.: Nonsteroidal antiinflammatory
Chem. class.: COX-2 inhibitor

Pregnancy category
C (1st/2nd trimester),
D (3rd trimester)

Action: Inhibits prostaglandin synthesis by decreasing COX-2 enzyme needed for biosynthesis; analgesic, antiinflammatory, antipyretic properties

→**Therapeutic Outcome:** Decreased pain, inflammation

Uses: Acute, chronic rheumatoid arthritis, osteoarthritis, primary dysmenorrhea

Dosage and routes
Do not exceed recommended dose, deaths have occurred

WITHDRAWN from market

V

Osteoarthritis/adult rheumatoid arthritis
Adult: PO 10 mg qd

Primary dysmenorrhea
Adult: PO 20 mg bid, prn

Available forms: Tabs 10, 20 mg

Adverse effects
(italic = common; **bold** = life-threatening)
CNS: *Fatigue, anxiety, depression, nervousness, paresthesia,* dizziness, insomnia
CV: **Tachycardia,** angina, **MI,** palpitations, dysrhythmias, hypertension, fluid retention
EENT: Tinnitus, hearing loss, blurred vision, glaucoma, cataract, conjunctivitis, eye pain
GI: *Nausea, anorexia, vomiting, constipation, dry mouth,* diverticulitis, gastritis, gastroenteritis, hemorrhoids, hiatal hernia, stomatitis, **GI bleeding**
GU: **Nephrotoxicity:** *dysuria,* **hematuria, oliguria, azotemia,** cystitis, UTI
HEMA: **Blood dyscrasias:** epistaxis, bruising, anemia
INTEG: Purpura, rash, pruritus, sweating, erythema, petechiae, photosensitivity, alopecia
RESP: Pharyngitis, shortness of breath, pneumonia, coughing
SYST: **Stevens-Johnson syndrome, anaphylaxis**

Contraindications: Hypersensitivity to this drug, aspirin, iodides, other NSAIDs, sulfonamides; asthma triad, asthma, pregnancy **D** 3rd trimester

Precautions: Pregnancy **C** 1st and 2nd trimester, lactation; bleeding, GI, cardiac, renal, hepatic disorders, hypersensitivity to other antiinflammatory agents, glucocorticoids, **G** anticoagulants, hypertension, severe **P** dehydration, elderly, children <18 yr

Pharmacokinetics

Absorption	Well absorbed (83%)
Distribution	Plasma protein binding 98%
Metabolism	Liver (CYP450 and non-CYP450 systems)
Excretion	Urine (metabolites, 70%)
Half-life	8-11 hr

Pharmacodynamics

Onset	Unknown
Peak	3 hr, delayed 1-2 hr by high-fat meal
Duration	Unknown

Interactions
Individual drugs
Aspirin: ↓ effect of aspirin, ↑ adverse reactions of valdecoxib

Fluconazole, ketoconazole: ↑ valdecoxib blood level
Furosemide: ↓ furosemide effect
Lithium: ↑ lithium toxicity
Drug classifications
ACE inhibitors: ↓ effect of ACE inhibitors
Anticoagulants: ↑ anticoagulant effect
Antineoplastics: ↑ antineoplastic toxicity
Diuretics (thiazide): ↓ effect of diuretics (thiazide)
Glucocorticoids, NSAIDs: ↑ adverse reactions
Herb/drug
Arginine, gossypol: ↑ gastric irritation
Bearberry, bilberry: ↑ NSAIDs effect
Bogbean, chondroitin: ↑ bleeding risk

NURSING CONSIDERATIONS
Assessment
- Assess for pain of rheumatoid arthritis, osteoarthritis; check ROM, inflammation of joints, characteristics of pain
- Assess blood counts during therapy; watch for decreasing platelets; if low, therapy may need to be discontinued, restarted after hematologic recovery
- Assess for blood dyscrasias (thrombocytopenia): bruising, fatigue, bleeding, poor healing

Nursing diagnoses
✓ Pain, acute (uses)
✓ Pain, chronic (uses)
✓ Mobility, impaired physical (uses)
✓ Injury, risk for (side effects)
✓ Knowledge, deficient (teaching)

Implementation
PO route
- Give with food or milk to decrease gastric symptoms, do not increase dose

Patient/family education
- Instruct patient to check with prescriber to determine when drug should be discontinued before surgery
- Advise patient that drug must be continued for prescribed time to be effective; to avoid other NSAIDs, aspirin, sulfonamides
- Advise patient to notify prescriber if pregnancy is planned or suspected
- Caution patient to notify prescriber of GI symptoms: black, tarry stools; cramping or rash; edema of extremities; weight gain
- Caution patient to report bleeding, bruising, fatigue, malaise since blood dyscrasias do occur
- Instruct patient to take with a full glass of water to enhance absorption

---

Evaluation
Positive therapeutic outcome
- Decreased pain, inflammation in arthritic conditions
- Decreased dysmenorrhea

Treatment of anaphylaxis: EpINEPHrine, antihistamines; resuscitate if needed

---

valganciclovir (Rx)
(val-gan-sy'kloh-veer)
Valcyte
Func. class: Antiviral
Chem. class: Synthetic nucleoside analog

Pregnancy category C

Action: Valganciclovir is metabolized to ganciclovir; inhibits replication of human cytomegalovirus in vivo and in vitro by selectively inhibiting viral DNA synthesis

▶ **Therapeutic Outcome:** Decreased proliferation of virus responsible for CMV retinitis

Uses: Cytomegalovirus (CMV) retinitis in immunocompromised persons, including those with AIDS, after indirect ophthalmoscopy confirms diagnosis

Dosage and routes
Adult: PO induction 900 mg bid × 21 days with food; maintenance 900 mg qd with food

Renal Dose
Reduce dose; CCr ≥60 ml/min same dosage as above; CCr 40-59 ml/min 450 mg bid, then 450 mg qd; CCr 25-39 ml/min 450 mg qd, then 450 mg q2 days; CCr 10-24 ml/min 450 mg q2 days, then 450 mg 2×/ week

Available forms: Tab 450 mg

Adverse effects
(*italic* = common; **bold** = life-threatening)
CNS: *Fever*, chills, **coma**, *confusion*, abnormal thoughts, dizziness, bizarre dreams, *headache*, psychosis, tremors, somnolence, *paresthesia, weakness*, **seizures**
EENT: Retinal detachment in CMV retinitis
GI: *Abnormal liver function tests, nausea, vomiting, anorexia, diarrhea, abdominal pain*, **hemorrhage**
GU: **Hematuria**, increased creatinine, BUN
HEMA: **Granulocytopenia, thrombocytopenia, irreversible neutropenia, anemia, eosinophilia**
INTEG: *Rash*, alopecia, *pruritus*, urticaria, pain at inj site, phlebitis
MISC: Local and systemic infections and sepsis

Contraindications: Hypersensitivity to acyclovir or ganciclovir, absolute neutrophil count <500/mm³, platelet count <25,000/ mm³, hemodialysis

Precautions: Preexisting cytopenias, renal
P function impairment, pregnancy **C,** lactation,
G children <6 mo, elderly

Pharmacokinetics

Absorption	Well absorbed from GI tract
Distribution	Plasma protein binding unknown; crosses blood-brain barrier, CSF
Metabolism	Rapidly metabolized in intestinal wall and liver to ganciclovir
Excretion	Kidneys (ganciclovir)
Half-life	3-4½ hr

Pharmacodynamics

Onset	Unknown
Peak	1-3 hr
Duration	Unknown

Interactions
Individual drugs
Adriamycin, amphotericin B, cycloSPORINE, dapsone, DOXOrubicin, flucytosine, pentamidine, trimethoprim/sulfamethoxazole, vinBLAStine, vinCRIStine: ↑ toxicity
Imipenem/cilastatin: ↑ seizures
Probenecid: ↓ renal clearance of valganciclovir
Radiation, zidovudine: Severe granulocytopenia; do not coadminister
Drug classifications
Antineoplastics: Severe granulocytopenia; do not coadminister
Nucleoside analogs, other: ↑ toxicity

NURSING CONSIDERATIONS
Assessment
- Assess for leukopenia/neutropenia/ thrombocytopenia: WBCs, platelets q2d during 2×/day dosing and then qwk
- Assess for leukopenia qd with WBC count in patients with prior leukopenia using other nucleoside analogs or for whom leukopenia counts are <1000 cells/mm³ at start of treatment
- Assess serum creatinine or CCr ≥q2 wk

Nursing diagnoses
☑Infection, risk for (uses)
☑Injury, risk for (uses, adverse reactions)
☑Knowledge, deficient (teaching)

Implementation
PO route
- Give with food

V

Patient/family education
- Inform patient that drug does not cure condition, that regular ophthalmologic examinations are necessary
- Caution patient that major toxicities may necessitate discontinuing drug
- Caution patient to use contraception during treatment and that infertility may occur; men should use barrier contraception for 90 days after treatment
- Instruct patient to take with food
- Instruct patient to report infection: fever, chills, sore throat; blood dyscrasias: bruising, bleeding, petechiae
- Advise patient to avoid crowds, persons with respiratory infections
- Caution patient to use sunscreen to prevent burns

Evaluation
Positive therapeutic outcome
- Decreased symptoms of CMV

Treatment of overdose: Maintain adequate hydration; dialysis may help reduce serum concentrations; consider use of hematopoietic growth factors

---

valproate (Rx)
(val-proh'ate)
Depacon
valproic acid (Rx)
Depakene, Myproic acid
divalproex sodium (Rx)
Depakote, Depakote ER, Epival
Func. class.: Anticonvulsant
Chem. class.: Carboxylic acid derivative

Pregnancy category D

Action: Increases levels of γ-aminobutyric acid (GABA) in brain, which decreases seizure activity

➔**Therapeutic Outcome:** Decreased symptoms of epilepsy, bipolar disorder

Uses: Simple (petit mal), complex (petit mal), absence, mixed seizures, manic episode associated with bipolar disorder, prophylaxis of migraine, adjunct in schizophrenia, tardive dyskinesia, aggression in children with ADHD, organic brain syndrome

Investigational uses: Tonic-clonic (grand mal), myoclonic seizures; rectal (valproic acid) for seizures

Dosage and routes
Epilepsy
Adult and child: PO 10-15 mg/kg/day divided in 2-3 doses, may increase by 5-10 mg/kg/day qwk, max 60 mg/kg/day in 2-3 divided doses; **IV** ≤20 mg/min over 1 hr

Mania (divalproex sodium)
Adult: PO 750 mg qd in divided doses, max 60 mg/kg/day

Migraine (divalproex sodium)
Adult: PO 250 mg bid, may increase to 1000 mg/day; or 500 mg (Depakote ER) qd × 7 days, then 1000 mg qd

Available forms: *Valproic acid:* caps 250 mg; *divalproex:* delayed rel tabs 125, 250, 500 mg; ext rel tabs 250, 500 mg; *sprinkle caps:* 125 mg; *valproate:* inj 100 mg/ml; syr 250 mg/5 ml

Adverse effects
(*italic* = common; **bold** = life-threatening)
CNS: Sedation, drowsiness, dizziness, headache, incoordination, depression, hallucinations, behavioral changes, tremors, aggression, weakness
EENT: Visual disturbances, taste perversion
GI: Nausea, vomiting, constipation, diarrhea, dyspepsia, anorexia, cramps, **hepatic failure, pancreatitis, toxic hepatitis,** stomatitis
GU: Enuresis, irregular menses
HEMA: **Thrombocytopenia, leukopenia, lymphocytosis,** increased Pro-time, bruising, epistaxis
INTEG: Rash, alopecia, photosensitivity, dry skin

Contraindications: Hypersensitivity, pregnancy **D**, hepatic disease

Precautions: Lactation, child <2 yr, elderly

Pharmacokinetics
Absorption	Unknown
Distribution	Breast milk, crosses placenta, widely distributed
Metabolism	Liver
Excretion	Kidneys
Half-life	9-16 hr

Pharmacodynamics
Onset	15-30 min
Peak	1-4 hr
Duration	4-6 hr

 Herb/drug   Do Not Crush   Alert   Key Drug   Geriatric   Pediatric

Interactions
Individual drugs
Abciximab, cefamandole, cefoperazone, cefotetan, eptifibatide, heparin, tirofiban: ↑ bleeding risk
Alcohol: ↑ CNS depression
Cimetidine: ↓ metabolism of valproic acid
Chlorpromazine, erythromycin, felbamate: ↑ valproic acid
Phenytoin: ↑ action of phenytoin
Warfarin: ↑ warfarin effect
Drug classifications
Antihistamnes, barbiturates, MAOIs, opioids: ↑ CNS depression
Antiplatelets, NSAIDs, thrombolytics: ↑ bleeding risk
Salicylates: ↑ valproic acid effect
Lab test interferences
False positive: Ketones
Interference: Thyroid function tests

NURSING CONSIDERATIONS
Assessment
- Monitor blood studies: Hct, Hgb, RBC, serum folate, platelets, Pro-time, vit D if on long-term therapy
- Monitor hepatic studies: AST, ALT, bilirubin, creatinine, failure
- Monitor blood levels: therapeutic level 50-100 mcg/ml
- Assess mental status: mood, sensorium, affect, memory (long, short)
- Assess respiratory dysfunction: respiratory depression, character, rate, rhythm; hold drug if respirations are <12/min or if pupils are dilated

Implementation
- ⊘ Give tablets or capsules whole
- Give elixir alone; do not dilute with carbonated beverage; do not give syrup to patients on sodium restriction
- Give with food or milk to decrease GI symptoms

Patient/family education
- Teach patient that physical dependency may result from extended use
- Instruct patient to avoid driving, other activities that require alertness
- Advise patient not to discontinue medication quickly after long-term use; seizures may result
- Advise patient to report visual disturbances, rash, diarrhea, light-colored stools, jaundice, protracted vomiting to prescriber

Evaluation
Positive therapeutic outcome
- Decreased seizures

---

valrubicin (Rx)
(val-roo'bih-sin)
Valstar
Func. class.: Antineoplastic, antibiotic
Chem. class.: Anthracycline glycoside

Pregnancy category C

Action: A semisynthetic analog of DOXOrubicin that inhibits DNA synthesis primarily; replication is decreased by binding to DNA, which causes strand splitting; active throughout entire cell cycle; a vesicant

⮕ **Therapeutic Outcome:** Decreased symptoms of breast cancer

Uses: Bladder cancer

Dosage and routes
Adult: Intravesically 800 mg qwk × 6 wk, delay administration ≥2 wk after transurethral resection or fulguration

Available forms: Sol for intravesical instillation 40 mg/ml

Adverse effects
(*italic* = common; **bold** = life-threatening)
CV: Chest pain
GI: Nausea, vomiting, anorexia, diarrhea
GU: UTI, urinary retention, hematuria
HEMA: Thrombocytopenia, leukopenia, *anemia*
INTEG: Rash

Contraindications: Hypersensitivity to anthracyclines or Cremophor EL, urinary tract infection, small bladder

Precautions: Pregnancy C, lactation, 🅿 children

Pharmacokinetics	
Absorption	Unknown
Distribution	Penetrates bladder wall
Metabolism	Unknown
Excretion	Unknown
Half-life	Unknown

Pharmacodynamics	
Onset	Unknown
Peak	Unknown
Duration	Unknown

V

Interactions: Unknown

NURSING CONSIDERATIONS
Assessment
- Monitor I&O ratio; report fall in urine output of <30 ml/hr

---

• Monitor temp q4h; fever may indicate beginning of infection
• Monitor local irritation, pain, burning at injection site

Nursing diagnoses
☑ Infection, risk for (side effects)
☑ Nutrition: less than body requirements, imbalanced (side effects)
☑ Knowledge, deficient (teaching)

Implementation
• Administer after urinary catheter is inserted under aseptic conditions, drain bladder and instill the diluted 75 ml of valrubicin by gravity for several min, withdraw catheter; drug should be retained for 2 hr, then void
• Use procedure for handling and disposal of cytotoxic agents
IV • Do not use polyvinyl chloride (PVC) **IV** tubing
• Prepare/store valrubicin sol in glass, polypropylene, or polyolefin tubing/containers
• For instillation, 5-ml vials (200 mg valrubicin/5-ml vial) should be warmed to room temp, withdraw 20 ml from the 4 vials and dilute with 55 ml of 0.9% NaCl inj to 75 ml of diluted valrubicin sol
• Valrubicin sol is clear red, at lower temps a waxy precipitate may form, warm in hand until sol is clear
• Perform strict hand-washing technique; use gloves, protective clothing
• Provide increased fluid intake to 2 L/day to prevent urate, calculi formation
• Store at room temp for 12 hr after reconstituting

Patient/family education
• Advise patient to report any complaints, side effects to nurse or prescriber
• Advise patient to consume fluids to 2 L/day unless contraindicated
• Teach patient that urine and other body fluids may be red-orange for 48 hr
• Teach patient that contraceptive measures are recommended during therapy

Evaluation
Positive therapeutic outcome
• Decreased tumor size, spread of malignancy

---

valsartan (Rx)
(val-zar′tan)
Diovan
Func. class.: Antihypertensive
Chem. class.: Angiotensin II receptor antagonist (type AT₁)

Pregnancy category UK

Action: Blocks the vasoconstrictor and aldosterone-secreting effects of angiotensin II; selectively blocks the binding of angiotensin II to the AT₁ receptor found in tissues

➡ **Therapeutic Outcome:** Decreased B/P

Uses: Hypertension, alone or in combination

Dosage and routes
Adult: PO 80-160 mg qd alone or in combination with other antihypertensives, may increase to 320 mg

Available forms: Tabs 80, 160, 320 mg

Adverse effects
(*italic* = common; **bold** = life-threatening)
CNS: *Dizziness, insomnia,* drowsiness, vertigo, headache, fatigue
CV: Angina pectoris, 2nd-degree AV block, **cerebrovascular accident,** hypotension, **MI, dysrhythmias**
EENT: Conjunctivitis
GI: Diarrhea, abdominal pain, nausea, **hepatotoxicity**
GU: Impotence, **nephrotoxicity**
HEMA: *Anemia,* neutropenia
MS: Cramps, myalgia, pain, stiffness
RESP: *Cough*

Contraindications: Hypersensitivity, pregnancy **UK,** severe hepatic disease, bilateral renal artery stenosis, pregnancy **D** 2nd/3rd trimester

Precautions: Hypersensitivity to angiotensin-converting enzyme inhibitors, CHF, hypertrophic cardiomyopathy, aortic/mitral **P** valve stenosis, CAD; lactation, children, **G** elderly

Pharmacokinetics	
Absorption	Well
Distribution	Bound to plasma proteins
Metabolism	Extensive
Excretion	Feces, urine, breast milk
Half-life	9 hr

Pharmacodynamics	
Onset	Unknown
Peak	2 hr
Duration	24 hr

Interactions: None significant

☑ *Herb/drug*

Aconite: ↑ toxicity, death

Astragalus, cola tree: ↑ or ↓ antihypertensive effect

Barberry, betony, black catechu, black cohosh, bloodroot, broom, burdock, cat's claw, dandelion, goldenseal, Irish moss, Jamaican dogwood, kelp, khella, mistletoe, parsley: ↑ antihypertensive effect

Coltsfoot, guarana, khat, licorice: ↓ antihypertensive effect

NURSING CONSIDERATIONS
Assessment

- Assess B/P, pulse q4h; note rate, rhythm, quality
- Monitor electrolytes: potassium, sodium, chloride; total CO_2
- Obtain baselines in renal, liver function tests before therapy begins
- Assess blood studies: BUN, creatinine, before treatment
- Monitor for edema in feet, legs daily
- Assess for skin turgor, dryness of mucous membranes for hydration status

Nursing diagnoses

✓ Fluid volume, deficient (side effects)

✓ Noncompliance (teaching)

✓ Knowledge, deficient (teaching)

Implementation

- Administer without regard to meals

Patient/family education

- Teach patient not to take this drug if breastfeeding or pregnant, or have had an allergic reaction to this drug
- If a dose is missed, instruct patient to take as soon as possible, unless it is within an hour before next dose
- Advise patient to comply with dosage schedule, even if feeling better
- Teach patient to notify prescriber of fever, swelling of hands or feet, irregular heartbeat, chest pain
- Advise patient excessive perspiration, dehydration, diarrhea may lead to fall in blood pressure; consult prescriber if these occur
- Inform patient that drug may cause dizziness, fainting; light-headedness may occur
- Caution patient to rise slowly to sitting or standing position to minimize orthostatic hypotension

Evaluation
Positive therapeutic outcome

- Decreased B/P

---

vancomycin
(van-koe-mye'sin)

Lyphocin, Vancocin, Vancoled, vancomycin HCl

Func. clas.: Antiinfective—misc.

Chem. clas.: Tricyclic glycopeptide

Pregnancy category C

Action: Inhibits bacterial cell wall synthesis

➥ **Therapeutic Outcome:** Bactericidal for the following organisms: staphylococci, streptococci, *Corynebacterium, Clostridium*

Uses: Resistant staphylococcal infections, pseudomembranous colitis, staphylococcal enterocolitis, group A β-hemolytic streptococci, endocarditis prophylaxis for dental procedures, diphtheroid endocarditis

Dosage and routes
Serious staphylococcal infections

Adult: **IV** 500 mg (7.5 mg/kg) q6-8h or 1 g (15 mg/kg) q12h

P *Child:* **IV** 40 mg/kg/day divided q6-8h

P *Neonates:* **IV** 15 mg/kg initially followed by 10 mg/kg q8-24h

Pseudomembranous/staphylococcal enterocolitis

Adult: PO 500 mg-2 g/day in 3-4 divided doses for 7-10 days

P *Child:* PO 40 mg/kg/day divided q6h, max 2 g/day

Endocarditis prophylaxis for dental procedure

Adult: **IV** 1 g over 1 hr, 1 hr before dental procedure

P *Child:* **IV** 20 mg/kg over 1 hr, 1 hr before procedure

Available forms: Pulvules 125, 250 mg; powder for oral sol 1, 10 g; powder for inj **IV** 500 mg; vials 1, 5, 10 g

Adverse effects
(*italic* = common; **bold** = life-threatening)

CV: **Cardiac arrest, vascular collapse** (rare)

EENT: Ototoxicity, permanent deafness, tinnitus

GI: **Nausea, pseudomembranous colitis**

GU: **Nephrotoxicity: increased BUN, creatinine, albumin, fatal uremia**

HEMA: **Leukopenia, eosinophilia, neutropenia**

INTEG: Chills, fever, rash, thrombophlebitis at inj site, urticaria, pruritus, necrosis (red man's syndrome)

V

RESP: Wheezing, dyspnea
SYST: **Anaphylaxis**

Contraindications: Hypersensitivity, previous hearing loss

G **Precautions:** Renal disease, pregnancy **C**,
P lactation, elderly, neonates

Pharmacokinetics

Absorption	Poorly absorbed (PO), completely absorbed (**IV**)
Distribution	Widely distributed, crosses placenta
Metabolism	Liver
Excretion	PO—feces, **IV**—kidneys
Half-life	4-8 hr

Pharmacodynamics

	IV
Onset	Immediate
Peak	Inf end

Interactions
Individual drugs
Amphotericin B, bacitracin, cisplatin, colistin, polymyxin B: ↑ ototoxicity or nephrotoxicity
Drug classifications
Aminoglycosides, cephalosporins, nondepolarizing muscle relaxants: ↑ ototoxicity or nephrotoxicity

NURSING CONSIDERATIONS
Assessment
• Monitor I&O ratio; report hematuria, oliguria because nephrotoxicity may occur
• Monitor any patient with compromised renal system (BUN, creatinine); drug is excreted slowly in poor renal system function; toxicity may occur rapidly
• Monitor blood studies: WBC; serum levels; peak 1 hr after 1-hr inf 25-40 mg/ml; trough before next dose 5-10 mg/ml
• Obtain C&S before drug therapy; drug may be given as soon as culture is performed
• Assess auditory function during, after treatment; hearing loss, ringing, roaring in ears; drug should be discontinued
• Monitor B/P during administration; sudden drop may indicate Red man's syndrome
• Assess for signs of infection
• Assess respiratory status: rate, character, wheezing, tightness in chest
• Identify allergies before treatment, reaction of each medication

Nursing diagnoses
✓ Infection, risk for (uses)
✓ Knowledge, deficient (teaching)

Implementation
IV **IV route**
• Give after reconstitution with 10 ml of sterile water for inj (500 mg/10 ml); further dilution is needed for **IV**, 500 mg/100 ml of 0.9% NaCl, D$_5$W given as intermittent inf over 1 hr; decrease rate of infusion if red man's syndrome occurs

Y-site compatibilities: Acyclovir, allopurinol, amiodarone, amsacrine, atracurium, cyclophosphamide, diltiazem, enalaprilat, esmolol, filgrastim, fluconazole, fludarabine, gallium, granisetron, hydromorphone, insulin (regular), labetalol, lorazepam, magnesium sulfate, melphalan, meperidine, meropenem, midazolam, morphine, ondansetron, paclitaxel, pancuronium, perphenazine, propofol, sodium bicarbonate, tacrolimus, teniposide, theophylline, thiotepa, tolazoline, vecuronium, vinorelbine, warfarin, zidovudine

Additive compatibilities: Amikacin, atracurium, calcium gluconate, cefepime, cimetidine, corticotropin, dimenhyDRINATE, hydrocortisone, meropenem, ofloxacin, potassium chloride, ranitidine, verapamil, vit B/C
• Give antihistamine if red man's syndrome occurs: decreased B/P, flushing of neck, face
• Give dose based on serum concentration
• Store at room temp for up to 2 wk after reconstitution
• Have adrenalin, suction, tracheostomy set, endotracheal intubation equipment on unit; anaphylaxis may occur
• Provide adequate intake of fluids (2 L) to prevent nephrotoxicity

Patient/family education
• Teach patient aspects of drug therapy: need to complete entire course of medication to ensure organism death (7-10 days); culture may be performed after completed course of medication
• Advise patient to report sore throat, fever, fatigue; could indicate superinfection
• Instruct patient that drug must be taken in equal intervals around clock to maintain blood levels

Evaluation
Positive therapeutic outcome
• Absence of fever, sore throat
• Negative culture after treatment

 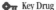

vardenafil
Levitra
See Appendix A, Selected New Drugs

---

vasopressin ⛐ (Rx)
(vay-soe-press'in)
Pitressin Synthetic, Pressyn ♥
Func. class.: Pituitary hormone
Chem. class.: Lysine vasopressin

Pregnancy category C

Action: Promotes reabsorption of water by action on renal tubular epithelium, causes vasoconstriction on muscles in the GI system

➔ **Therapeutic Outcome:** Increased osmolality, decreased urine output in diabetes insipidus

Uses: Diabetes insipidus (nonnephrogenic/nonpsychogenic), abdominal distention postoperatively, bleeding esophageal varices

Dosage and routes
Diabetes insipidus
Adult: IM/SC 5-10 units bid-qid prn; IM/SC 2.5-5 units q2-3 days (Pitressin Tannate) for chronic therapy

🄿 *Child:* IM/SC 2.5-10 units bid-qid prn; IM/SC 1.25-2.5 units q2-3 days (Pitressin Tannate) for chronic therapy

Abdominal distention
Adult: IM 5 units, then q3-4, increasing to 10 units if needed (aqueous)

Available forms: Inj 20, 5 units/ml (tannate), spray, cotton pledgets

Adverse effects
(*italic* = common; **bold** = life-threatening)
CNS: Drowsiness, headache, lethargy, flushing
CV: Increased B/P
EENT: Nasal irritation, congestion, rhinitis
GI: Nausea, heartburn, cramps
GU: Vulval pain, uterine cramping
MISC: Tremor, sweating, vertigo, urticaria, bronchial constriction

Contraindications: Hypersensitivity, chronic nephritis

Precautions: CAD, pregnancy **C**

Pharmacokinetics
Absorption	Erratically absorbed (IM)
Distribution	Widely distributed extracellular fluid
Metabolism	Liver—rapidly
Excretion	Kidneys—unchanged
Half-life	10-20 min

Pharmacodynamics
	IV	IM
Onset	Unknown	1 hr
Peak	Unknown	Unknown
Duration	3-8 hr	3-8 hr

Interactions
Individual drugs
Alcohol, demeclocycline, epINEPHrine (large doses), heparin, lithium: ↓ response
Carbamazepine, chlorpropamide, clofibrate: ↑ response
Drug classifications
Ganglionic blockers: ↑ vasopressor response

NURSING CONSIDERATIONS
Assessment
• Monitor nasal mucosa for irritation if given by intranasal spray
• Assess intranasal use: nausea, congestion, cramps, headache; usually decreased with decreased dose
• Monitor pulse, B/P when giving drug **IV** or SC
• Monitor I&O ratio, weight daily; check for edema in extremities; if water retention is severe, diuretic may be prescribed; check for water intoxication: lethargy, behavioral changes, disorientation, neuromuscular excitability

Nursing diagnoses
☑ Fluid volume, excess (side effects)
☑ Fluid volume, deficit (uses)
☑ Knowledge, deficient (teaching)

Implementation
IM route
• May be given IM/SC for diagnosis of diabetes insipidus
• Give patient 16 oz water at administration to prevent nausea, vomiting, cramping

Patient/family education
• Teach patient technique for nasal instillation: to insert tube into nasal cavity to instill drug
• Caution patient to avoid OTC products for cough, hay fever because these preparations may contain epinephrine, decrease drug response; do not use with alcohol
• Advise patient to carry/wear emergency ID specifying therapy, disease process (diabetes insipidus)

Evaluation
Positive therapeutic outcome
• Absence of severe thirst
• Decreased urine output, osmolality

V.

! HIGH ALERT

vecuronium (Rx)
(ve-kure-oh'nee-yum)
Norcuron
Func. class.: Neuromuscular blocker
Chem. class.: Synthetic curariform

Pregnancy category C

Action: Inhibits transmission of nerve impulses by binding with cholinergic receptor sites, antagonizing action of acetylcholine; no analgesic response

→ Therapeutic Outcome: Skeletal muscle paralysis during anesthesia

Uses: Facilitation of endotracheal intubation; skeletal muscle relaxation during mechanical ventilation, surgery, or general anesthesia

Dosage and routes
P *Adult and child >9 yr:* **IV** bol 0.08-0.10 mg/kg, then 0.010-0.015 mg/kg for prolonged procedures

Available forms: 10 mg/5 ml vial

Adverse effects
(*italic* = common; **bold** = life-threatening)
CNS: Skeletal muscle weakness or paralysis (rarely)
***RESP:* Prolonged apnea, possible respiratory paralysis**

Contraindications: Hypersensitivity

Precautions: Pregnancy **C**, cardiac disease,
P lactation, children <2 yr, electrolyte imbalances, dehydration, neuromuscular disease, respiratory, hepatic disease

▧ Do Not Confuse:
Nocuron/Narcan

Pharmacokinetics

Absorption	Completely absorbed
Distribution	Rapid—to extracellular fluids
Metabolism	Liver (20%)
Excretion	Kidneys—unchanged (35%)
Half-life	1½ hr, increased in liver disease

Pharmacodynamics

Onset	1 min
Peak	3-5 min
Duration	15-25 min (recovery index)

Interactions
Individual drugs
Clindamycin, lithium, polymyxin B, quinidine, succinylcholine: ↑ paralysis, length and intensity

Enflurane, isoflurane, lincomycin: ↑ neuromuscular blockade
Drug classifications
Aminoglycosides: ↑ paralysis, length and intensity
Analgesics (opioid), local anesthetics, thiazides: ↑ neuromuscular blockade

NURSING CONSIDERATIONS
Assessment
• Monitor for electrolyte imbalances (potassium, magnesium) before drug is used; electrolyte imbalances may lead to increased action of this drug
• Monitor patient's vital signs (B/P, pulse, respirations, airway) until fully recovered; rate, depth, pattern of respirations, strength of hand grip; patient should be intubated before use
• Monitor patient's recovery: decreased paralysis of face, diaphragm, leg, arm, rest of body; residual weakness and respiratory problems may occur during recovery period
• Monitor allergic reactions: rash, fever, respiratory distress, pruritus; drug should be discontinued

Nursing diagnoses
☑ Breathing pattern, ineffective (uses)
☑ Communication, impaired verbal (adverse reactions)
☑ Fear (adverse reactions)
☑ Knowledge, deficient (teaching)

Implementation
• Use peripheral nerve stimulator by anesthesiologist to determine neuromuscular blockade; deep tendon reflexes should be monitored during extended periods
IV • Give by direct **IV** after reconstituting with bacteriostatic water, over 5 min, D₅W, 0.9% NaCl or LR
• Give by direct **IV** after reconstituting dose in 5-10 ml of provided diluent; give by titrating to patient response
• Give by continuous inf after diluting to 10-20 mg/100 ml and by titrating to patient response (only by qualified person, usually an anesthesiologist); do not administer IM
• Store in light-resistant area

Syringe incompatibilities: Barbiturates

Y-site compatibilities: Aminophylline, cefazolin, cefuroxime, cimetidine, diltiazem, DOBUTamine, DOPamine, epINEPHrine, esmolol, fentanyl, fluconazole, gentamicin, heparin, hydrocortisone, hydromorphone, isoproterenol, labetalol, lorazepam, midazolam, milrinone, morphine, niCARdipine, nitroglycerin, nitroprusside, norepinephrine,

---

propofol, ranitidine, trimethoprim/sulfamethoxazole, vancomycin

Y-site incompatibilities: Barbiturates

Patient/family education
• Provide reassurance if communication is difficult during recovery from neuromuscular blockade
• Provide explanation to patients regarding all procedures or treatments; patient will remain conscious if anesthesia is not given also

Evaluation
Positive therapeutic outcome
• Paralysis of jaw, eyelid, head, neck, rest of body as evaluated by peripheral nerve stimulator

Treatment of overdose: Edrophonium or neostigmine, atropine, monitor VS; may require mechanical ventilation

---

venlafaxine (Rx)
(ven-la-fax′een)
Effexor, Effexor XR
Func. class.: Second-generation antidepressant—misc.

Pregnancy category C

Action: Potent inhibitor of neuronal serotonin and norepinephrine uptake, weak inhibitor of dopamine; no muscarinic, histaminergic, or α-adrenergic receptors in vitro

Therapeutic Outcome: Relief of depression

Uses: Prevention/treatment of depression, to treat depression at end of life, long-term treatment of generalized anxiety disorder (Effexor XR)

Investigational uses: Hot flashes, obsessive-compulsive disorder (OCD)

Dosage and routes
Depression
Adult: PO 75 mg/day in 2 or 3 divided doses; taken with food, may be increased to 150 mg/day; if needed may be further increased to 225 mg/day; increments of 75 mg/day should be made at intervals of no less than 4 days; some hospitalized patients may require up to 375 mg/day in 3 divided doses; ext rel 37.5-75 mg PO qd, max 225 mg/day; give Effexor XR qd

Hepatic dose
Moderate impairment 50% of dose

Renal dose
Mild to moderate impairment 75% of dose

Hot flashes (Investigational)
Adult: PO 12.5 mg bid × 4 wk or ext rel cap 37.5 mg × 4 wk

Available forms: Tabs scored 25, 37.5, 50, 75, 100 mg; ext rel caps 37.5, 75, 150 mg

Adverse effects
(*italic* = common; **bold** = life-threatening)
CNS: Emotional lability, vertigo, apathy, ataxia, CNS stimulation, euphoria, hallucinations, hostility, increased libido, hypertonia, hypotonia, psychosis, insomnia, anxiety
CV: Migraine, angina pectoris, extrasystoles, postural hypotension, syncope, thrombophlebitis, hypertension
EENT: Abnormal vision, taste, *ear pain,* cataract, conjunctivitis, corneal lesions, dry eyes, otitis media, photophobia
GI: Dysphagia, eructation, colitis, gastritis, gingivitis, **rectal hemorrhage,** stomatitis, stomach and mouth ulceration, nausea, anorexia, dry mouth
GU: Anorgasmia, abnormal ejaculation, *dysuria, hematuria, metrorrhagia, vaginitis, impaired urination,* albuminuria, amenorrhea, kidney calculus, cystitis, nocturia, breast and bladder pain, polyuria, **uterine hemorrhage, vaginal hemorrhage,** moniliasis
INTEG: Ecchymosis, acne, alopecia, brittle nails, dry skin, photosensitivity
META: Peripheral edema, weight loss or gain, diabetes mellitus, edema, glycosuria, hyperlipemia, hypokalemia
MS: Arthritis, bone pain, bursitis, myasthenia tenosynovitis, arthralgia
RESP: Bronchitis, dyspnea, asthma, chest congestion, epistaxis, hyperventilation, laryngitis
SYST: Accidental injury, malaise, neck pain, enlarged abdomen, cyst, facial edema, hangover effect, hernia

Contraindications: Hypersensitivity

Precautions: Mania, pregnancy **C,** lactation, children, elderly, recent MI, cardiac disease, seizure disorder, hypertension

Pharmacokinetics	
Absorption	Well absorbed
Distribution	Widely distributed, 27% protein binding
Metabolism	Liver—extensively
Excretion	Kidneys, 87%
Half-life	5-7 hr, 11-13 hr (active metabolite)

Pharmacodynamics
Unknown

V

Interactions
Individual drugs
Alcohol: ↑ CNS depression
Cimetidine, fluoxetine, sertraline: ↑ toxicity
Lithium: ↑ serotonin effect
Drug classifications
Antihistamines, opioids, sedative/hypnotics:
↑ CNS depression
MAOIs: Hypertensive crisis, seizures
Phenothiazines: ↑ toxicity
Herb/drug
Chamomile, hops, kava, lavender, skullcap,
valerian: ↑ CNS depression
Corkwood, jimsonweed: ↑ anticholinergic
effect
SAM-e, St. John's wort: serotonin syndrome

NURSING CONSIDERATIONS
Assessment
• Monitor B/P (lying, standing), pulse q4h; if
systolic B/P drops 20 mm Hg hold drug, notify
prescriber; take vital signs q4h in patients with
CV disease
• Monitor blood studies: CBC, leukocytes,
differential, cardiac enzymes if patient is
receiving long-term therapy
• Monitor hepatic studies: AST, ALT, bilirubin
• Check weight qwk; weight loss or gain;
appetite may increase, peripheral edema may
occur
• Assess mental status: mood, sensorium,
affect, suicidal tendencies; increase in psychi-
atric symptoms: depression, panic
• Monitor urinary retention, constipation;
P constipation is more likely to occur in children
G or elderly
• Assess for withdrawal symptoms: headache,
nausea, vomiting, muscle pain, weakness; do
not usually occur unless drug was discontin-
ued abruptly
• Identify alcohol consumption; if alcohol is
consumed, hold dose
Nursing diagnoses
✓ Coping, ineffective (uses)
✓ Injury, risk for physical (side effects)
✓ Knowledge, deficient (teaching)
✓ Noncompliance (teaching)
Implementation
• Give with food or milk for GI symptoms
• Crush if patient is unable to swallow medi-
cation whole
• Store at room temp; do not freeze
Patient/family education
• Teach patient that therapeutic effects may
take 2-3 wk
• Teach patient to use caution in driving or
other activities requiring alertness because of

drowsiness, dizziness, blurred vision; to avoid
rising quickly from sitting to standing, espe-
G cially elderly
• Teach patient to avoid alcohol ingestion,
other CNS depressants
Evaluation
Positive therapeutic outcome
• Decreased depression
• Absence of suicidal thoughts
Treatment of overdose: ECG monitor-
ing, induce emesis, lavage, activated charcoal,
administer anticonvulsant

---

verapamil ⬥π (Rx)
(ver-ap'a-mil)
Apo-Verap, Calan, Calan SR, Covera-HS,
Isoptin, Isoptin SR, verapamil HCl,
verapamil HCl SR, Verelan
Func. class.: Calcium-channel blocker;
antihypertensive; antianginal
Chem. class.: Diphenylalkylamine
Pregnancy category C

Action: Inhibits calcium ion influx across
cell membrane during cardiac depolarization;
produces relaxation of coronary vascular
smooth muscle; peripheral vascular smooth
muscle; dilates coronary vascular arteries;
increases myocardial oxygen delivery in
patients with vasospastic angina

➔ **Therapeutic Outcome:** Decreased
angina pectoris, dysrhythmias, B/P

Uses: Chronic stable vasospastic, unstable
angina; dysrhythmias, hypertension, supraventricular tachycardia, atrial flutter or fibrillation

Investigational uses: Prevention of
migraine headaches, ventricular outflow
obstruction in hypertrophic cardiomyopathy

Dosage and routes
Angina
Adult: PO 80-120 mg tid, increase qwk

Dysrhythmias
Adult: PO 240-320 mg/day in 3-4 divided
doses in digitalized patients

Hypertension
Adult: PO 80 mg tid, may titrate upward; ext
rel 120-240 mg/day as a single dose, may
increase to 240-480 mg/day

Adult: IV bol 5-10 mg (0.075-0.15 mg/kg)
over 2 min, may repeat 10 mg (0.15 mg/kg)
½ hr after first dose

P *Child 1-15 yr:* **IV** bol 0.1-0.3 mg/kg over >2 min, repeat in 30 min, not to exceed 5 mg in a single dose

P *Child 0-1 yr:* **IV** bol 0.1-0.2 mg/kg over ≥2 min

Available forms: Tabs 40, 80, 120 mg; sus rel tabs, 120, 180, 240 mg; inj 2.5 mg/ml; sus rel caps 120, 180, 240, 360 mg; sus rel tabs 120, 180, 240 mg; ext rel caps: 100, 120, 180, 200, 240, 300 mg

Adverse effects
(*italic* = common; **bold** = life-threatening)
CNS: Headache, drowsiness, dizziness, anxiety, depression, weakness, asthenia, fatigue, insomnia, confusion, light-headedness
CV: Edema, **CHF,** bradycardia, hypotension, palpitations, AV block
GI: Nausea, diarrhea, gastric upset, *constipation,* elevated liver function studies
GU: Impotence, nocturia, polyuria
INTEG: Rash
SYST: **Stevens-Johnson syndrome**

Contraindications: Sick sinus syndrome, 2nd- or 3rd-degree heart block, hypotension <90 mm Hg systolic, cardiogenic shock, severe CHF

Precautions: CHF, hypotension, hepatic
P injury, pregnancy **C,** lactation, children, renal disease, concomitant β-blocker therapy,
G elderly

Pharmacokinetics	
Absorption	Well absorbed (PO)
Distribution	Not known
Metabolism	Liver—extensively
Excretion	Kidneys, (70%)
Half-life	Biphasic 4 min, 3-7 hr

Pharmacodynamics			
	PO	PO-SUS REL	IV
Onset	1-2 hr	Unknown	1-5 min
Peak	½-1½ hr	5-7 hr	3-5 min
Duration	3-7 hr	24 hr	2 hr

Interactions
Individual drugs
Carbamazepine: ↑ toxicity
Cimetidine, cycloSPORINE, digoxin, theophylline: ↑ levels of each specific drug
Lithium: ↓ lithium levels
Prazosin, quinidine: ↑ hypotension
Drug classifications
Antihypertensives: ↑ hypotension

β-Adrenergic blockers: ↑ bradycardia, CHF
Nondepolarizing muscle relaxants: ↑ effect
Food/drug
Grapefruit juice: ↑ hypotension
Herb/drug
Barberry, betel palm, burdock, goldenseal, khat, lily of the valley, plantain, yohimbe: ↓ effect

NURSING CONSIDERATIONS
Assessment
• Assess fluid volume status: I&O ratio and record; weight; distended red veins; crackles in lung; color; quality, sp gr of urine; skin turgor; adequacy of pulses; moist mucous membranes; bilateral lung sounds; peripheral pitting edema; dehydration symptoms of decreasing output, thirst, hypotension, dry mouth, and mucous membranes should be reported
• Monitor B/P and pulse, pulmonary capillary wedge pressure (PCWP), central venous pressure, index, often during inf; if B/P drops 30 mm Hg, stop inf and call prescriber
• Monitor ALT, AST, bilirubin daily; if these are elevated, hepatotoxicity is suspected
• Monitor if platelets are <150,000/mm³, if so, drug is usually discontinued and another drug started
• Assess for extravasation; change site q48h
• Monitor cardiac status: B/P, pulse, respiration, ECG

Nursing diagnoses
✓ Cardiac output, decreased (uses)
✓ Knowledge, deficient (teaching)

Implementation
PO route
• Give once a day before meals hs; sus rel give with food to decrease GI symptoms
Ⓢ Do not crush, break, chew ext rel, sus rel products
Ⅳ **IV route**
• Give by direct **IV** undiluted (Y-site, 3-way stopcock) over at least 2 min, or 3 min
G elderly ; discard unused solution; to prevent serious hypotension, patient should be recumbent for 1 hr or more

Syringe compatibilities: Amrinone, heparin, milrinone

Y-site compatibilities: Amrinone, aprofloxacin, dobutamine, DOPamine, famotidine, hydrALAZINE, meperidine, methicillin, milrinone, penicillin G potassium, piperacillin, propofol, ticarcillin

V

Y-site incompatibilities: Albumin, ampicillin, mezlocillin, nafcillin, oxacillin, sodium bicarbonate

Additive compatibilities: Amikacin, amiodarone, ascorbic acid, atropine, bretylium, calcium chloride, calcium gluconate, cefamandole, cefazolin, cefotaxime, cefoxitin, cephapirin, chloramphenicol, cimetidine, clindamycin, dexamethasone, diazepam, digoxin, DOPamine, epINEPHrine, erythromycin, gentamicin, heparin, hydrocortisone, hydromorphone, hydrocortisone sodium phosphate, insulin (regular), isoproterenol, lidocaine, magnesium sulfate, mannitol, meperidine, metaraminol, methicillin, methyldopate, methylPREDNISolone, metoclopramide, mezlocillin, morphine, moxalactam, multivitamins, naloxone, nitroglycerin, norepinephrine, oxytocin, pancuronium, penicillin G potassium, penicillin G sodium, pentobarbital, phenobarbital, phentolamine, phenytoin, piperacillin, potassium chloride, potassium phosphates, procainamide, propranolol, protamine, quinidine, sodium bicarbonate, sodium nitroprusside, theophylline, ticarcillin, tobramycin, tolazoline, vancomycin, vasopressin, vit B/C

Patient/family education
- Advise patient to increase fluids/fiber to counteract constipation
- Caution patient to avoid hazardous activities until stabilized on drug and dizziness is no longer a problem
- Instruct patient to limit caffeine consumption; to avoid alcohol and OTC drugs unless directed by prescriber
- Advise patient to comply with medical regimen: diet, exercise, stress reduction, drug therapy; to notify prescriber of irregular heartbeat, shortness of breath, swelling of feet and hands, pronounced dizziness, constipation, nausea, hypotension
- Teach patient to use as directed even if feeling better; may be taken with other CV drugs (nitrates, β-blockers)

Evaluation
Positive therapeutic outcome
- Decreased anginal pain
- Decreased dysrhythmias
- Decreased B/P

Treatment of overdose: Defibrillation, atropine for AV block, vasopressor for hypotension

---

⚠ HIGH ALERT

*vinBLAStine (VLB) (Rx)
(vin-blast'een)
Velban, Velbe ✤, vinBLAStine sulfate
Func. class.: Antineoplastic
Chem. class.: Vinca rosea alkaloid

Pregnancy category D

Action: Inhibits mitotic activity, arrests cell cycle at metaphase; inhibits RNA synthesis, blocks cellular use of glutamic acid needed for purine synthesis; a vesicant

⇒Therapeutic Outcome: Prevention of rapid growth of malignant cells, immunosuppressive

Uses: Breast, testicular cancer; lymphomas; neuroblastoma; Hodgkin's, non-Hodgkin's lymphomas; mycosis fungoides; histiocytosis; Kaposi's sarcoma

Dosage and routes
Adult: **IV** 0.1 mg/kg or 3.7 mg/m² qwk or q2 wk, max 0.5 mg/kg or 18.5 mg/m² qwk
P *Child:* 2.5 mg/m² then dose of 3.75, 5.0, 6.25, and 7.5 at 7-day intervals

Available forms: Inj powder 10 mg for 10 ml **IV** inj

Adverse effects
(*italic* = common; **bold** = life-threatening)
CNS: Paresthesias, peripheral neuropathy, depression, headache, **seizures**
CV: Tachycardia, orthostatic hypotension
GI: Nausea, *vomiting,* ileus, *anorexia, stomatitis,* constipation, abdominal pain, GI and rectal bleeding, **hepatotoxicity,** pharyngitis
GU: Urinary retention, **renal failure**
HEMA: **Thrombocytopenia, leukopenia, myelosuppression**
INTEG: *Rash,* alopecia, photosensitivity
META: syndrome of inappropriate diuretic hormone
RESP: **Fibrosis, pulmonary infiltrate, bronchospasm**

Contraindications: Hypersensitivity,
P infants, pregnancy **D**, leukopenia, granulocytopenia, lactation

Precautions: Renal disease, hepatic disease

▧ Do Not Confuse:
vinBLAStine/vinCRIStine

🗹 Herb/drug   🅢 Do Not Crush   ◆ Alert   ◆⚏ Key Drug   🅖 Geriatric   🅟 Pediatric

Pharmacokinetics

Absorption	Complete bioavailability
Distribution	Crosses blood-brain barrier slightly
Metabolism	Liver—active antineoplastic
Excretion	Biliary, kidneys
Half-life	Triphasic—35 min, 53 min, 19 hr

Pharmacodynamics
Unknown

Interactions
Individual drugs
Bleomycin: ↑ synergism
Methotrexate: ↑ methotrexate action
Mitomycin: ↑ bronchospasm
Phenytoin: ↓ Phenytoin level
Radiation: ↑ toxicity, bone marrow suppression

Drug classifications
Antineoplastics: ↑ toxicity, bone marrow suppression
Live virus vaccines: ↑ adverse reactions

NURSING CONSIDERATIONS
Assessment
• Monitor B/P (baseline and q15 min) during administration
• Monitor CBC, differential, platelet count weekly; withhold drug if WBC is <2000/mm³ or platelet count is <75,000/mm³; notify prescriber of results, recovery will take 3 wk
• Assess for dyspnea, rales, unproductive cough, chest pain, tachypnea
• Monitor renal function studies: BUN, serum uric acid, urine CCr before, during therapy; I&O ratio; report fall in urine output of 30 ml/hr; for decreased hyperuricemia
• Monitor for cold, fever, sore throat (may indicate beginning of infection); notify prescriber if these occur
• Assess for bleeding: hematuria, guaiac, bruising or petechiae, mucosa or orifices q8h, no rectal temp; avoid IM inj; use pressure to venipuncture sites
• Identify nutritional status: an antiemetic may need to be prescribed
• Assess for symptoms indicating severe allergic reactions: rash, pruritus, urticaria, itching, flushing, bronchospasm, hypotension; epINEPHrine and resuscitative equipment should be nearby

Nursing diagnoses
☑ Injury, risk for (adverse reactions)
☑ Body image, disturbed (adverse reactions)
☑ Infection, risk for (adverse reactions)
☑ Knowledge, deficient (teaching)

Implementation
• Give by intermittent inf
• Sol should be prepared by qualified personnel only under controlled conditions
• Use Luer-LoK tubing to prevent leakage; do not let sol come in contact with skin; if contact occurs, wash well with soap and water
IV • Administer **IV** after diluting 10 mg/10 ml NaCl; give through Y-tube or 3-way stopcock or directly over 1 min
• Give hyaluronidase 150 units/ml in 1 ml of NaCl, warm compress for extravasation for vesicant activity treatment

Syringe compatibilities: Bleomycin, cisplatin, cyclophosphamide, droperidol, fluorouracil, leucovorin, methotrexate, metoclopramide, mitomycin, vinCRIStine

Y-site compatibilities: Allopurinol, amifostine, aztreonam, bleomycin, cisplatin, cyclophosphamide, DOXOrubicin, droperidol, filgrastim, fludarabine, fluorouracil, granisetron, heparin, leucovorin, melphalan, methotrexate, metoclopramide, mitomycin, ondansetron, paclitaxel, piperacillin/tazobactam, sargramostim, teniposide, thiotepa, vinCRIStine, vinorelbine

Y-site incompatibilities: Furosemide

Additive compatibilities: Bleomycin

Patient/family education
• Teach patient to avoid use of products containing aspirin or NSAIDs, razors, commercial mouthwash because bleeding may occur; to report symptoms of bleeding (hematuria, tarry stools)
• Instruct patient to report signs of anemia, (fatigue, headache, irritability, faintness, shortness of breath)
• Caution patient to report any changes in breathing or coughing even several mo after treatment
• Advise patient that contraception will be necessary during treatment; teratogenesis may occur
• Advise patient to use sunscreen, wear protective clothing, and sunglasses
• Inform patient that hair may be lost during treatment; a wig or hairpiece may make patient feel better; new hair will be different in color, texture
• Advise patient to avoid vaccinations during treatment; serious reactions may occur
• Teach patient to report signs/symptoms of infection: fever, chills, sore throat; patient

V

should avoid crowds and persons with known infections

Evaluation
Positive therapeutic outcome
- Decreased spread of malignant cells

! HIGH ALERT

*vinCRIStine (VCR) 🔑 (Rx)
(vin-kris′teen)
Oncovin, Vincasar PFS, vinCRIStine sulfate
Func. class.: Antineoplastic—misc
Chem. class.: Vinca alkaloid

Pregnancy category D

Action: Inhibits mitotic activity, arrests cell cycle at metaphase; inhibits RNA synthesis, blocks cellular use of glutamic acid needed for purine synthesis; a vesicant

➡ **Therapeutic Outcome:** Prevention of rapid growth of malignant cells, immunosuppression

Uses: Breast, lung cancer; lymphomas; neuroblastomas; Hodgkin's disease; acute lymphoblastic and other leukemias; rhabdomyosarcoma, Wilms' tumor; osteogenic and other sarcomas

Dosage and routes
Adult: **IV** 1-2 mg/m²/wk, max 2 mg

P *Child:* **IV** 1.5-2 mg/m²/wk, max 2 mg

Available forms: Inj 1 mg/ml; powder for inj 5 mg/vial

Adverse effects
(*italic* = common; **bold** = life-threatening)
CNS: Decreased reflexes, numbness, weakness, motor difficulties, CNS depression, cranial nerve paralysis, **seizures**
CV: Orthostatic hypotension
GI: Nausea, vomiting, anorexia, stomatitis, constipation, **paralytic ileus, abdominal pain, hepatotoxicity**
HEMA: **Thrombocytopenia, leukopenia, myelosuppression, anemia**
INTEG: Alopecia

Contraindications: Hypersensitivity,
P infants, pregnancy **D**, radiation therapy, lactation

Precautions: Renal disease, hepatic disease, hypertension, neuromuscular disease

⚊ Do Not Confuse:
vinCRIStine/vinBLAStine

Pharmacokinetics
Absorption	Complete bioavailability
Distribution	Rapidly, widely distributed; blood-brain barrier
Metabolism	Liver
Excretion	Biliary, in feces, crosses placenta
Half-life	Triphasic 0.85 min, 7.4 min, 1.64 min

Pharmacodynamics
Onset	Unknown
Peak	Unknown
Duration	1 wk

Interactions
Individual drugs
L-Asparaginase: ↓ action of vinCRIStine
Digoxin: ↓ digoxin level
Methotrexate: ↑ action of methotrexate
Mitomycin: ↑ acute pulmonary reactions
Radiation: ↑ toxicity, bone marrow suppression; do not use together
Drug classifications
Anticoagulants: ↑ action of anticoagulants
Antineoplastics: ↑ toxicity, bone marrow suppression
Live virus vaccines: ↓ antibody response
Peripheral nervous system drugs: Neurotoxicity

NURSING CONSIDERATIONS
Assessment
- Monitor CBC, differential, platelet count weekly; withhold drug if WBC is <4000/mm³ or platelet count is <75,000/mm³; notify prescriber of results; platelets may increase or decrease
- Assess neurologic status: paresthesia, weakness, cranial nerve palsies, orthostatic hypotension, lethargy, agitation, psychosis; notify prescriber
- Monitor renal function studies: BUN, serum uric acid, urine CCr before, during therapy; I&O ratio; report fall in urine output of 30 ml/hr; for decreased hyperuricemia, hyponatremia, and increased fluid retention (syndrome of inappropriate antidiuretic hormone)
- Monitor for cold, fever, sore throat (may indicate beginning of infection)
- Identify for increased uric acid levels, joint pain in extremities; increase fluid intake to 2-3 L/day unless contraindicated

Nursing diagnoses
☑ Injury, risk for (adverse reactions)
☑ Body image, disturbed (adverse reactions)
☑ Infection, risk for (adverse reactions)
☑ Knowledge, deficient (teaching)

 Herb/drug   Do Not Crush   Alert   Key Drug   G Geriatric   P Pediatric

Implementation

IV • Administer **IV** after diluting with diluent provided or 1 mg/10 ml of sterile water or 0.9% NaCl; give through Y-tube or 3-way stopcock or directly over 1 min
• Hyaluronidase 150 units/ml in 1 ml of NaCl; apply warm compress for extravasation

Syringe compatibilities: Bleomycin, cisplatin, cyclophosphamide, doxapram, DOXOrubicin, droperidol, fluorouracil, heparin, leucovorin, methotrexate, metoclopramide, mitomycin, ondansetron, vinCRIStine

Syringe incompatibilities: Furosemide

Y-site compatibilities: Allopurinol, amifostine, aztreonam, bleomycin, cisplatin, cladribine, cyclophosphamide, DOXOrubicin, droperidol, filgrastim, fludarabine, fluorouracil, granisetron, heparin, leucovorin, methotrexate, metoclopramide, mitomycin, ondansetron, paclitaxel, sargramostim, teniposide, thiotepa, vinCRIStine, vinorelbine

Y-site incompatibilities: Furosemide

Patient/family education

• Teach patient to avoid use of products containing aspirin or NSAIDs, razors, commercial mouthwash because bleeding may occur; to report symptoms of bleeding (hematuria, tarry stools)
• Instruct patient to report signs of anemia (fatigue, headache, irritability, faintness, shortness of breath)
• Caution patient to report any changes in breathing or coughing, even several mo after treatment
• Advise patient that contraception will be necessary during treatment; teratogenesis may occur
• Inform patient that hair may be lost during treatment; a wig or hairpiece may make patient feel better; new hair will be different in color, texture
• Advise patient to avoid vaccinations during treatment; serious reactions may occur
• Teach patient to report signs/symptoms of infection: fever, chills, sore throat; patient should avoid crowds or persons with known infections
• Advise patient to increase fluids, bulk in diet, exercise to prevent constipation

Evaluation

Positive therapeutic outcome
• Decreased spread of malignancies

⚠ HIGH ALERT

vinorelbine (Rx)
(vi-nor'el-bine)
Navelbine
Func. class.: Antineoplastic—misc.
Chem. class.: Semisynthetic vinca alkaloid

Pregnancy category D

Action: Inhibits mitotic activity, arrests cell cycle at metaphase; inhibits RNA synthesis, blocks cellular use of glutamic acid needed for purine synthesis; a vesicant

➡Therapeutic Outcome: Decreased spread of malignancy

Uses: Breast cancer; unresectable, advanced non–small-cell lung cancer (NSCLC) stage IV; may be used alone or in combination with cisplatin for stage III or IV NSCLC

Dosage and routes
Adult: **IV** 30 mg/m^2 qwk

Hepatic dose
Adult: **IV** total bilirubin 2.1-3 mg/dl 15 mg/m^2 qwk; total bilirubin ≥3 mg/dl 7.5 mg/m^2 qd

Available forms: Inj 10 mg/ml

Adverse effects
(*italic* = common; **bold** = life-threatening)
CNS: Paresthesias, peripheral neuropathy, depression, headache, **seizures,** weakness, jaw pain
CV: Chest pain
RESP: Shortness of breath
GI: *Nausea, vomiting,* ileus, *anorexia, stomatitis,* constipation, abdominal pain, GI, diarrhea, **hepatotoxicity**
HEMA: **Neutropenia, anemia, thrombocytopenia, granulocytopenia**
INTEG: *Rash,* alopecia, photosensitivity
META: Syndrome of inappropriate diuretic hormone
MS: Myalgia

Contraindications: Hypersensitivity, **P** infants, pregnancy **D**, granulocyte count <1000 cells/mm^3 pretreatment

G Precautions: Renal disease, hepatic **P** disease, elderly, lactation, children

Pharmacokinetics	
Absorption	Poor bioavailability (<50%)
Distribution	Unknown
Metabolism	Liver—to metabolite
Excretion	Bile
Half-life	43 hr

V

Pharmacodynamics	
Onset	Unknown
Peak	1-2 hr
Duration	Unknown

Interactions
Individual drugs
Fluorouracil: ↑ toxicity a possibility

NURSING CONSIDERATIONS
Assessment
• Monitor B/P (baseline and q15 min) during administration
• Monitor CBC, differential, platelet count weekly; withhold drug if WBC is <4000/mm³ or platelet count is <75,000/mm³; notify prescriber of results, recovery will take 3 wk
• Assess for dyspnea, rales, unproductive cough, chest pain, tachypnea
• Monitor renal function studies: BUN, serum uric acid, urine CCr before, during therapy, I&O ratio; report fall in urine output of 30 ml/hr; for decreased hyperuricemia
• Monitor for cold, fever, sore throat (may indicate beginning infection); notify health care prescriber if these occur
• Assess for bleeding: hematuria, guaiac, bruising or petechiae, mucosa or orifices q8h; no rectal temp; avoid IM inj; use pressure on venipuncture sites
• Identify nutritional status: an antiemetic may need to be prescribed
• Assess for symptoms indicating severe allergic reactions: rash, pruritus, urticaria, itching, flushing, bronchospasm, hypotension; epINEPHrine and resuscitative equipment should be nearby

Nursing diagnoses
☑ Injury, risk for (adverse reactions)
☑ Body image, disturbed (adverse reactions)
☑ Infection, risk for (adverse reactions)
☑ Knowledge, deficient (teaching)

Implementation
• Hyaluronidase 150 units/ml in 1 ml of NaCl, warm compress for extravasation for vesicant activity treatment
• Antacid before oral agent; give drug after evening meal before bedtime
• Antiemetic 30-60 min before giving drug and prn to prevent vomiting
Continuous infusion
IV • Give 40 mg/m² q3 wk after **IV** bol of 8 mg/m²; may be given in combination with DOXOrubicin, fluorouracil, cisplatin

Y-site compatibilities:
Amikacin, aztreonam, bleomycin, buprenor-phine, butorphanol, calcium gluconate, carboplatin, cefotaxime, cisplatin, cimetidine, clindamycin, dexamethasone, enalaprilat, etoposide, famotidine, filgrastim, fluconazole, fludarabine, gentamicin, hydrocortisone, lorazepam, meperidine, morphine, netilmicin, ondansetron, plicamycin, streptozocin, tenipo-side, ticarcillin, tobramycin, vancomycin, vinBLAStine, vincristine, zidovudine

Patient/family education
• Teach patient to use liq diet: cola, Jell-O; dry toast or crackers may be added if patient is not nauseated or vomiting
• Advise patient to rinse mouth 3-4 ×/day with water and brush teeth 2-3 ×/day with soft brush or cotton-tipped applicators for stomatitis; use unwaxed dental floss
• Inform patient that a nutritious diet with iron, vitamin supplements is necessary
• Advise patient to avoid crowds, people with infections, vaccinations

Evaluation
Positive therapeutic outcome
• Decreased spread of malignant cells

---

vitamin A (PO, OTC; IM, Rx)
Aquasol A, Del-Vi-A, Vitamin A
Func. class.: Vitamin, fat-soluble
Chem. class.: Retinol
Pregnancy category C

Action: Needed for normal bone and tooth development, visual dark adaptation, skin disease, mucosa tissue repair, assists in pro-duction of adrenal steroids, cholesterol, RNA

⇨ **Therapeutic Outcome:** Prevention, absence of vit A deficiency

Uses: Vit A deficiency

Dosage and routes
P *Adult and child >8 yr:* PO 100,000-500,000 international units qd × 3 days, then 50,000 qd × 2 wk; dose based on severity of deficiency; maintenance 10,000-20,000 international units for 2 mo

P *Child 1-8 yr:* IM 5000-15,000 international units qd × 10 days

P *Infants <1 yr:* IM 5000-15,000 interna-tional units × 10 days

Maintenance
P *Child 4-8 yr:* IM 15,000 international units qd × 2 mo

P *Child <4 yr:* IM 10,000 international units qd × 2 mo

Available forms: Caps 10,000, 25,000, 50,000 international units; drops 5000 international units; inj 50,000 international units/ml; tabs 10,000, 25,000, 50,000 international units

Adverse effects
(*italic* = common; **bold** = life-threatening)
CNS: Headache, increased ICP, intracranial hypertension, lethargy, malaise
EENT: Gingivitis, papilledema, exophthalmos, inflammation of tongue and lips
GI: Nausea, vomiting, anorexia, abdominal pain, *jaundice*
INTEG: Drying of skin, pruritus, increased pigmentation, night sweats, alopecia
MS: Arthralgia, retarded growth, hard areas on bone
META: Hypomenorrhea, hypercalcemia

Contraindications: Hypersensitivity to vit A, malabsorption syndrome (PO)

Precautions: Lactation, impaired renal function, pregnancy **C**

Pharmacokinetics
Absorption	Rapidly absorbed
Distribution	Stored in liver, kidneys, lungs
Metabolism	Liver
Excretion	Breast milk
Half-life	Unknown

Pharmacodynamics
Unknown

Interactions
Individual drugs
Cholestyramine, colestipol, mineral oil: ↓ absorption of vit A
Drug classifications
Contraceptives (oral), corticosteroids: ↑ levels of vit A
Lab test interferences
False: ↑ Bilirubin, ↑ serum cholesterol

NURSING CONSIDERATIONS
Assessment
• Assess nutritional status: increase intake of yellow and dark green vegetables, yellow/orange fruits, vit A–fortified foods, liver, egg yolks
• Assess vit A deficiency: decreased growth; night blindness; dry, brittle nails; hair loss; urinary stones; increased infection; hyperkeratosis of skin; drying of cornea
• Identify vit A deficiency by plasma vit A, carotene level
• Assess for chronic vit A toxicity: increased

calcium, BUN, glucose, cholesterol, triglyceride level

Nursing diagnoses
☑ Nutrition: less than body requirements (uses)
☑ Knowledge, deficient (teaching)

Implementation
PO route
• Give with food (PO) for better absorption; do not give **IV** because anaphylaxis may occur, IM only
• Oral preparations are not indicated for vit A deficiency in those with malabsorption syndrome
• Store in airtight, light-resistant container

Patient/family education
• Instruct patient that if dose is missed, it should be omitted
• Inform patient that ophth exams may be required periodically throughout therapy
• Instruct patient not to use mineral oil while taking this drug because absorption will be decreased
• Advise patient to notify prescriber of nausea, vomiting, lip cracking, loss of hair, headache
• Caution patient not to take more than the prescribed amount

Evaluation
Positive therapeutic outcome
• Increase in growth rate, weight
• Absence of dry skin and mucous membranes, night blindness

Treatment of overdose: Discontinue drug

---

vitamin A acid
See tretinoin

---

vitamin B₁
See thiamine

V

(vitamin B₁₂) cyanocobalamin (PO, OTC; IM/SC, Rx)

(sye-an-oh-koe-bal'a-min)

Acti-B₁₂ ✤, Alphamine, Anacobin ✤, Bedoz ✤, B₁₂, Resin, Cobex, Crystamine, Crysti-12, Cyanoject, Cyomin, Hydrobexan, Hydro Cobex, Rubesol-1000, Rubion ✤, Rubramin PC, Vitamin B₁₂

Func. class.: Vitamin B₁₂, water-soluble vitamin

(vitamin B₁₂a) hydroxocobalamin (vit B₁₂) (Rx)

(hye-drox'-o-ko-bal'-a-min)

Acti-B₁₂ ✤, Alphamin, Hydro-Crysti12, Hydroxo-12, Hydroxycobalamin, LA-12

Pregnancy category A

Action: Needed for adequate nerve functioning, protein and carbohydrate metabolism, normal growth, RBC development and cell reproduction

➡ **Therapeutic Outcome:** Prevention, correction of vit B₁₂ deficiency

Uses: Vit B₁₂ deficiency; pernicious anemia; vit B₁₂ malabsorption syndrome; Schilling test; increased requirements with pregnancy, thyrotoxicosis, hemolytic anemia, hemorrhage, renal and hepatic disease

Dosage and routes

Adult: PO 25 mcg qd × 5-10 days, maintenance 100-200 mg IM qmo; IM/SC 30-100 mcg qd × 5-10 days, maintenance 100-200 mcg IM qmo

P *Child:* PO 1 mcg qd × 5-10 days, maintenance 60 mcg IM qmo or more; IM/SC 1-30 mcg qd × 5-10 days, maintenance 60 mcg IM qmo or more

Pernicious anemia/malabsorption syndrome

Adult: IM 100-1000 mcg qd × 2 wk, then 100-1000 mcg IM qmo

P *Child:* IM 100-500 mcg over 2 wk or more given in 100-500 mcg doses, then 60 mcg IM/SC monthly

Schilling test

P *Adult and child:* IM 1000 mcg in one dose

Available forms: Tabs 25, 50, 100, 250, 500, 1000 mcg; inj 100, 120, 1000 mcg/ml

Adverse effects

(*italic* = common; **bold** = life-threatening)

CNS: Flushing, optic nerve atrophy

CV: **CHF,** peripheral vascular thrombosis, **pulmonary edema**

GI: *Diarrhea*

INTEG: Itching, rash, pain at site

META: Hypokalemia

SYST: **Anaphylactic shock**

Contraindications: Hypersensitivity, optic nerve atrophy

P **Precautions:** Pregnancy **A,** lactation, children, cardiac disease, uremia, iron deficiency, folic acid deficiency

Pharmacokinetics

Absorption	Well absorbed (IM, SC)
Distribution	Crosses placenta
Metabolism	Stored in liver, kidney, stomach
Excretion	50%-90% (urine), breast milk
Half-life	Unknown

Pharmacodynamics

Unknown

Interactions

Individual drugs

Alcohol, aminosalicylic acid, chloramphenicol, cimetidine, colchicine: ↓ absorption

Drug classifications

Aminoglycosides, anticonvulsants, potassium products: ↓ absorption

Lab test interferences

False positive: Intrinsic factor

NURSING CONSIDERATIONS

Assessment

• Assess for deficiency: anorexia, dyspepsia on exertion, palpitations, paresthesias, psychosis, visual disturbances, pallor, red inflamed tongue, neuropathy, edema of legs

• Monitor potassium levels during beginning treatment in patients with megaloblastic anemia

• Monitor CBC for increase in reticulocyte count during 1st wk of therapy, then increase in RBC and hemoglobin; folic acid levels, vit B₁₂ levels

• Assess nutritional status: egg yolks, fish, organ meats, dairy products, clams, oysters, which are good sources for vit B₁₂

• Monitor for pulmonary edema or worsening of CHF in cardiac patients

Nursing diagnoses

✓ Nutrition: less than body requirements, imbalanced (uses)

✓ Knowledge, deficient (teaching)
✓ Noncompliance (teaching) (overuse)

Implementation
PO route
- Give with fruit juice to disguise taste; administer immediately after mixing
- Give with meals if possible for better absorption

IM route
- Give by IM inj for pernicious anemia for life unless contraindicated

IV IV route
- May be mixed with TPN sol, but **IV** route is not recommended

Y-site compatibilities: Heparin, hydrocortisone sodium succinate, potassium chloride

Solution compatibilities: Dextrose/Ringer's or lactated Ringer's combinations, dextrose/saline combinations, D_5W, $D_{10}W$, 0.45% NaCl, Ringer's or lactated Ringer's sol, ascorbic acid

Patient/family education
- Instruct patient that treatment must continue for life if diagnosed as having pernicious anemia
- Advise patient to eat well-balanced diet from the food pyramid and comply with dietary recommendation
- Caution patient not to exceed the RDA of vit B_{12} because adverse reactions may occur

Evaluation
Positive therapeutic outcome
- Decreased anorexia, dyspnea on exertion, palpitations, paresthesias, psychosis, visual disturbances, edema of legs
- Prevention or correction of vit B_{12} deficiency

Treatment of overdose: Discontinue drug

---

vitamin D (cholecalciferol, vitamin D₃ or ergocalciferol, vitamin D₂) (Rx, OTC)
Calciferol, Delta-D, Drisdol, Radiostol ♣, Radiostol Forte ♣, vitamin D, vitamin D₃
Func. class.: Vitamin D
Chem. class: Fat-soluble vitamin

Pregnancy category C

Action: Needed for regulation of calcium, phosphate levels; normal bone development;
parathyroid activity; neuromuscular functioning

➡ **Therapeutic Outcome:** Prevention of rickets, osteomalacia, normal calcium/phosphate levels

Uses: Vit D deficiency, rickets, renal osteodystrophy, hypoparathyroidism, hypophosphatemia, psoriasis, rheumatoid arthritis

Dosage and routes
Deficiency
Adult: PO/IM 12,000 international units qd, then increased to 500,000 international units/day

P *Child:* PO/IM 1500/5000 international units qd × 2-4 wk, may repeat after 2 wk or 600,000 international units as single dose

Hypoparathyroidism
P *Adult and child:* PO/IM 200,000 international units given with 4 g calcium tab

Available forms: Tabs 400, 1000, 50,000 international units; caps 25,000, 50,000; oral sol 8000 international units/ml; inj 500,000 international units/ml, 500,000 international units/5 ml

Adverse effects
(*italic* = common; **bold** = life-threatening)
CNS: Fatigue, weakness, drowsiness, **seizures,** headache, psychosis
CV: Hypertension, dysrhythmias
GI: Nausea, vomiting, anorexia, cramps, diarrhea, constipation, metallic taste, dry mouth
GU: Polyuria, nocturia, **hematuria, albuminuria, renal failure,** decreased libido
INTEG: Pruritus, photophobia
MS: Decreased bone growth, early joint pain, early muscle pain

Contraindications: Hypersensitivity, hypercalcemia, renal dysfunction, hyperphosphatemia

Precautions: CV disease, renal calculi, pregnancy **C**

🔃 **Do Not Confuse:**
Calciferol/calcitriol

Pharmacokinetics

Absorption	Well absorbed
Distribution	Stored in liver
Metabolism	Liver, sun
Excretion	Bile, kidney
Half-life	12-22 hr

V

Pharmacodynamics

	PO	IM
Onset	Unknown	Unknown
Peak	4 hr	Unknown
Duration	15-20 days	Unknown

Interactions
Individual drugs
Cholestyramine, colestipol, phenobarbital, phenytoin: ↓ effects of vit D
Verapamil: ↑ toxicity
Drug classifications
Antacids, diuretics (thiazide): ↑ toxicity

NURSING CONSIDERATIONS
Assessment
• Monitor BUN, urinary calcium, AST, ALT, cholesterol, creatinine, uric acid, chloride, magnesium, electrolytes, urine pH, phosphate—may increase; calcium should be kept at 9-10 mg/dl; vit D at 50-135 international units/dl, phosphate at 70 mg/dl; alkaline phosphatase may be decreased
• Monitor for increased blood level; toxic reactions may occur rapidly
• Assess for dry mouth, metallic taste, polyuria, bone pain, muscle weakness, headache, fatigue, tinnitus, change in LOC, irregular pulse, dysrhythmias, increased respirations, anorexia, nausea, vomiting, cramps, diarrhea, constipation; may indicate hypercalcemia
• Assess renal status: decreased urinary output (oliguria, anuria), edema in extremities, weight gain 5 lb, periorbital edema
• Assess nutritional status, diet for sources of vit D (milk, cod, halibut, salmon, sardines, egg yolk) calcium (dairy products, dark green vegetables), phosphates (dairy products)

Nursing diagnoses
☑ Nutrition, less than body requirements, imbalanced (uses)
☑ Knowledge, deficient (teaching)

Implementation
PO route
• PO may be increased q4 wk depending on blood level
• Store in airtight, light-resistant container at room temp
IM route
• Give inj deeply in large muscle mass, administer slowly, aspirate to avoid **IV** administration, rotate inj site

Patient/family education
• Advise patient to omit dose if missed; to avoid vitamin supplements unless directed by prescriber
• Inform patient of necessary foods to be included in diet
• Advise patient to keep appointments for evaluation because therapeutic and toxic levels are narrow
• Instruct patient to report weakness, lethargy, headache, anorexia, loss of weight; to report nausea, vomiting, abdominal cramps, diarrhea, constipation, excessive thirst, polyuria, muscle and bone pain
• Caution patient to decrease intake of antacids and laxatives containing magnesium

Evaluation
Positive therapeutic outcome
• Calcium levels 9-10 ml/dl
• Decreasing symptoms of bone disease

---

vitamin E (OTC)
Amino-Opti-E, Aquasol E, Daltose ✦, E-Complex-600, E-Ferol, E-Vitamin Succinate, E-200 I.U. Softgels, Gordo-Vite E, Tocopherol, vitamin E, Vita-Plus E Softgells, Vitec
Func. class.: Vitamin E
Chem. class.: Fat-soluble vitamin
Pregnancy category A

Action: Needed for digestion and metabolism of polyunsaturated fats, decreases platelet aggregation, decreases blood clot formation, promotes normal growth and development of muscle tissue, prostaglandin synthesis

⮕ **Therapeutic Outcome:** Prevention and treatment of vit E deficiency

Uses: Vit E deficiency, impaired fat absorption, hemolytic anemia in premature neonates, prevention of retrolental fibroplasia, sickle cell anemia, supplement in malabsorption syndrome

Dosage and routes
Deficiency
Adult: PO 60-75 international units qd
P *Child:* PO 1 mg/0.6 g of dietary fat

Prevention of deficiency
Adult: PO 30 units/day
P *Infant:* PO 5 international units/day

Topical route
P *Adult and child:* TOP apply to affected areas as needed

Available forms: Caps 100, 200, 400, 500, 600, 800 ✦, 1000 international units; tabs 100, 200, 400 international units; drops

---

 Herb/drug   Do Not Crush   Alert   Key Drug   Geriatric   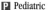 Pediatric

50 mg/ml; chew tabs 400 units; ointment, cream, lotion, oil

Adverse effects
(*italic* = common; **bold** = life-threatening)
CNS: Headache, fatigue
CV: Increased risk of thrombophlebitis
EENT: Blurred vision
GI: Nausea, cramps, diarrhea
GU: Gonadal dysfunction
INTEG: Sterile abscess, contact dermatitis
META: Altered metabolism of hormones, thyroid, pituitary, adrenal, altered immunity
MS: Weakness

P **Contraindications:** **IV** use in infants

Precautions: Pregnancy **A**

Pharmacokinetics	
Absorption	20%-80% (PO)
Distribution	Widely distributed, stored in fat
Metabolism	Liver
Excretion	Bile
Half-life	Unknown

Pharmacodynamics
Unknown

Interactions
Individual drugs
Cholestyramine, colestipol, mineral oil, sucralfate: ↓ absorption
Drug classification
Anticoagulants (oral): ↑ action of anticoagulants

NURSING CONSIDERATIONS
Assessment
- Monitor vit E levels during treatment
- Assess nutritional status: intake of wheat germ, dark green leafy vegetables, nuts, eggs, liver, vegetable oils, dairy products, cereals
- Assess for vit E deficiency (usually in **P** neonates): irritability, restlessness, hemolytic anemia

Nursing diagnoses
☑ Nutrition: less than body requirements, imbalanced (uses)
☑ Knowledge, deficient (teaching)

Implementation
PO route
- Chewable tab: chew well
- Sol: may be dropped in mouth or mixed with food
- Store in airtight, light-resistant container
Topical route
- Apply top to moisturize dry skin

Patient/family education
- Inform patient necessary foods to be included in diet high in vit E
- Instruct patient to omit if dose missed
- Instruct patient to avoid vit supplements unless directed by prescriber because overdose may occur

Evaluation
Positive therapeutic outcome
- Absence of hemolytic anemia
- Adequate vit E levels
- Improvement in skin lesions
- Decrease in edema

---

voriconazole (Rx)
(vohr-i-kahn'a-zol)
Vfend
Func. class: Antifungal
Pregnancy category D

Action: Inhibits fungal CYP450-mediation demethylation, needed for biosynthesis

➡ **Therapeutic Outcome:** Decreasing signs, symptoms of infection

Uses: Invasive aspergillosis, serious fungal infections (*Scedosporium apiospermum, Fusarium* sp.)

Dosage and routes
Adult: **PO** Give 1 hr ac or pc; ≥40 kg: 200 mg q12h; <40 kg: 100 mg q12h
Adult: **IV** Loading dose 6 mg/kg q12h × 2 dose, then 4 mg/kg q12h; may switch to oral dosing

Available forms: Tabs 50, 200 mg; powder for inj, lyophilized 200 mg voriconazole, 3200 mg sulfobutyl ester β-cyclodextrin sodium (SBECD)

Adverse effects
(*italic* = common; **bold** = life-threatening)
CNS: *Headache,* paresthesias, peripheral neuropathy, hallucinations, psychosis, extrapyramidal sysmptoms (EPS), depression, Guillain-Barré syndrome, insomnia, suicidal ideation, dizziness
CV: *Tachycardia,* hyper/hypotension, vasodilatation, **atrial dysrhythmias, atrial fibrillation, AV block, bradycardia, CHF, MI**
EENT: Blurred vision, eye hemorrhage
INTEG: *Burning, irritation,* pain, necrosis at inj site with extravasation, dermatitis, rash, photosensitivity
GI: *Nausea, vomiting, anorexia,* diarrhea, cramps, **hemorrhagic gastroenteritis,**

V

acute liver failure, hepatitis, intestinal perforation, pancreatitis
GU: *Hypokalemia,* azotemia, **renal tubular necrosis, permanent renal impairment, anuria, oliguria**
HEMA: Anemia, **eosinophilia,** hypomagnesemia, **thrombocytopenia, leukopenia, pancytopenia**
MISC: Respiratory disorder
SYST: **Stevens-Johnson syndrome, toxic epidermal necrolysis, sepsis**

Contraindications: Hypersensitivity, severe bone marrow depression, pregnancy **D,** **P** lactation, children

Precautions: Renal disease

Pharmacokinetics

Absorption	Unknown
Distribution	Protein binding 58%
Metabolism	By CYP45 enzyme
Excretion	Via hepatic metabolism
Half-life	Unknown

Pharmacodynamics

Onset	Unknown
Peak	1-2 hr
Duration	Unknown

Interactions
Individual drugs
Cisplatin, cycloSPORINE, digoxin, polymyxin B, vancomycin: ↑ nephrotoxicity
Phenytoin, pimozide, prednisolone, quinidine, rifabutin, sirolimus, tacrolimus, warfarin: ↑ effects of each specific drug
Drug classifications
Aminoglycosides: ↑ nephrotoxicity
Benzodiazepines, calcium channel blockers, ergots, HMG-CoA reductase inhibitors, non-nucleoside reverse transcriptase inhibitors, protease inhibitors, sulfonylureas, vinca alkaloids: ↑ effects of each specific drug
Corticosteroids, diuretics (thiazide), skeletal muscle relaxants: ↑ hypokalemia
Food/drug
High-fat foods: Avoid use with high-fat meals
🗹 *Herb/drug*
Gossypol: ↑ nephrotoxicity

NURSING CONSIDERATIONS
Assessment
• Monitor VS q15-30 min during first infusion; note changes in pulse, B/P

• Monitor I&O ratio; watch for decreasing urinary output, change in specific gravity; discontinue drug to prevent permanent damage to renal tubules
• Monitor blood studies: CBC, K, Na, Ca, Mg q2 wk; BUN, creatinine weekly
• Monitor weight weekly; if weight increases over 2 lb/wk, edema is present; renal damage should be considered
◆• Assess for renal toxicity: increasing BUN, serum creatinine; if BUN is >40 mg/dl or if serum creatinine >3 mg/dl, drug may be discontinued or dosage reduced
◆• Assess for hepatotoxicity: increasing AST, ALT, alkaline phosphatase, bilirubin
• Assess for allergic reaction: dermatitis, rash; drug should be discontinued, antihistamines (mild reaction) or epinephrine (severe reaction) administered
• Assess for hypokalemia: anorexia, drowsiness, weakness, decreased reflexes, dizziness, increased urinary output, increased thirst, paresthesias
• Assess for ototoxicity: tinnitus (ringing, roaring in ears), vertigo, loss of hearing (rare)

Nursing diagnoses
☑ Infection, risk (uses)
☑ Injury, risk of (uses, adverse reactions)
☑ Knowledge, deficient (teaching)

Implementation
• Store at room temp (powder, tabs)
IV **IV route**
• Give drug only after C&S confirms organism, drug needed to treat condition; make sure drug is used in life-threatening infections
• Reconstitute powder with 19 ml water for inj to 10 mg/ml, shake until dissolved; infuse over 1-2 hr at a conc of 5 mg/ml or less; do not admix with other drugs, 4.2% sodium bicarbonate inf

Patient/family education
• Teach that long-term therapy may be needed to clear infection (2 wk-3 mo depending on type of infection)
• Advise patient to notify prescriber of bleeding, bruising, or soft tissue swelling
• Teach to take 1 hr before or after meal
• Advise patient not to drive at night because of vision changes
• Advise to avoid strong, direct sunlight
• Advise that women of childbearing age should use effective contraceptive

---

🗹 Herb/drug   ⓢ Do Not Crush   ◆ Alert   ◆ₙ Key Drug   **G** Geriatric   **P** Pediatric

Evaluation
Positive therapeutic outcome
- Decreased fever, malaise, rash, negative C&S for infecting organism

---

! HIGH ALERT

warfarin ⊙ₙ (Rx)
(war'far-in)
Coumadin, Sofarin, warfarin sodium, Warfilone Sodium ✦
Func. class.: Anticoagulant

Pregnancy category X

Action: Interferes with blood clotting by indirect means; depresses hepatic synthesis of vit K–dependent coagulation factors (II, VII, IX, X)

➡ **Therapeutic Outcome:** Prevention of clotting

Uses: Pulmonary emboli, deep vein thrombosis, prevention or treatment of venous thrombosis, pulmonary embolism, thromboembolic complications associated with atrial fibrillation or cardiac valve replacement, after MI to reduce risk of death

Dosage and routes
Adult: PO/**IV** 2.5-10 mg/day × 3 days, then titrated to Pro-time or INR qd

G *Elderly:* PO/**IV** 2-10 mg/day

P *Child:* PO 0.1 mg/kg/day titrated to INR

Available forms: Tabs 1, 2, 2.5, 3, 4, 5, 6, 7.5, 10 mg; 5.4 mg powder for inj

Adverse effects
(*italic* = common; **bold** = life-threatening)
CNS: Fever
GI: Diarrhea, nausea, vomiting, anorexia, stomatitis, cramps, **hepatitis**
GU: **Hematuria**
HEMA: **Hemorrhage, agranulocytosis, leukopenia, eosinophilia**
INTEG: Rash, dermatitis, urticaria, alopecia, pruritus

Contraindications: Hypersensitivity, hemophilia, leukemia with bleeding, peptic ulcer disease, thrombocytopenic purpura, hepatic disease (severe), malignant hypertension, subacute bacterial endocarditis, acute nephritis, blood dyscrasias, pregnancy **X**, eclampsia, preeclampsia, lactation

G **Precautions:** Alcoholism, elderly , CHF

ℕ Do Not Confuse:
Coumadin/Cardura, Coumadin/Compazine

Pharmacokinetics	
Absorption	Well absorbed (PO), completely absorbed
Distribution	Crosses placenta, 99% plasma protein binding
Metabolism	Liver
Excretion	Kidney, feces (active, inactive metabolites)
Half-life	effective ½-2½ days

Pharmacodynamics	
	PO
Onset	12-24 hr
Peak	½-4 days
Duration	3-5 days

Interactions
Individual drugs
Allopurinol, amiodarone, cefamandole, chloral hydrate, chloramphenicol, cimetidine, clofibrate, clotrimoxazole, diflunisal, disulfiram, erythromycin, furosemide, glucagon, heparin, indomethacin, isoniazid, mefenamic acid, metronidazole, phenylbutazone, quinidine, sulfinpyrazone, sulindac, thyroid, valproate: ↑ warfarin action
Carbamazepine, dicloxicillin, griseofulvin, nafcillin, phenytoin, rifampin, sucralfate, vitamin K, vitamin supplements: ↓ warfarin action

Drug classifications
Antidepressants (tricyclic), ethacrynic acids, HMG-CoA reductase inhibitors, NSAIDs, penicillins, quinolones, salicylates, SSRIs, steroids, sulfonamides, thrombolytics: ↑ warfarin action
Barbiturates, contraceptives (oral), estrogens: ↓ warfarin action
Sulfonylureas (oral): ↑ toxicity

Food/drug
Vit K foods: ↓ warfarin action

▱ Herb/drug
Agrimony, alfalfa, angelica, anise, basil, bay, bilberry, black haw, bogbean, bromelain, buchu, chondroitin, cinchona bark, dong quai, fenugreek, feverfew, garlic, ginger, ginkgo, ginseng, horse chestnut, Irish moss, kelp, kelpware, khella, lovage, lungwort, meadowsweet, motherwort, mugwort, nettle, papaya, parsley (large amounts), pau d'arco, pine-

W

---

apple, poplar, prickly ash, safflower, saw palmetto, tonka bean, turmeric, wintergreen, yarrow: ↑ risk of bleeding
Chamomile, coenzyme Q10, flax, glucomannan, goldenseal, guar gum: ↓ anticoagulant effect

Lab test interferences
↑ T_3 uptake
↓ Uric acid

NURSING CONSIDERATIONS
Assessment
• Monitor blood studies (Hct, occult blood in stools) q3 mo; partial Pro-time, which should be 1½-2 × control, PTT; often done qd, APTT, ACT; platelet count q2-3 days; thrombocytopenia may occur
• Monitor B/P, watch for increasing signs of hypertension
• Assess for bleeding: bleeding gums, petechiae, ecchymosis, black tarry stools, hematuria, epistaxis; decreased B/P may indicate bleeding and possible hemorrhage
• Assess for fever, skin rash, urticaria
• Assess for needed dosage change q1-2 wk
◆Assess patients carefully for symptoms of Churg-Strauss syndrome (rare): eosinophilia, vasculitis, rash, worsening pulmonary symptoms, cardiac complications, neuropathy

Nursing diagnoses
✓ Injury, risk for (uses, adverse reactions)
✓ Tissue perfusion, ineffective (uses)
✓ Knowledge, deficient (teaching)

Implementation
PO route
• Warfarin is usually given with **IV** heparin for 3 or more days, warfarin blood level may take several days
Ⓥ IV route
• Reconstitute with 2.7 ml of sterile water for inj; do not use solution that is discolored or has particulates
• Give over 1-2 min into peripheral vein

Y-site compatibilities: Cefazolin, ceftriaxone, DOPamine, heparin, lidocaine, morphine, nitroglycerin, potassium chloride, ranitidine

Patient/family education
• Caution patient to avoid OTC preparations unless directed by prescriber; may cause serious drug interactions
• Advise patient that drug may be withheld during active bleeding (menstruation), depending on condition
• Advise patient to use soft-bristle toothbrush to avoid bleeding gums, avoid contact sports, use electric razor, avoid IM inj
• Instruct patient to carry/wear emergency ID identifying drug taken
• Advise patient to report any signs of bleeding: gums, under skin, urine, stools
• Teach patient to read food labels; limited intake of vit K foods (green leafy vegetables) is necessary to maintain consistent prothrombin levels

Evaluation
Positive therapeutic outcome
• Decrease of deep vein thrombosis
• Pro-time (1.3-2.0 × control)

---

zafirlukast (Rx)
(za-feer'loo-cast)
Accolate
Func. class.: Bronchodilator
Chem. class.: Leukotriene receptor antagonist

Pregnancy category B

Action: Antagonizes the contractile action of leukotrienes (LTC_4, LTD_4, LTE_4) in airway smooth muscle; inhibits bronchoconstriction caused by antigens

⟶**Therapeutic Outcome:** Ability to breathe more easily

Uses: Prophylaxis and chronic
Ⓟ treatment of asthma in adults/children >12 yr

Investigational uses: Chronic urticaria

Dosage and routes
Ⓟ *Adult/child ≥12 yr:* PO 20 mg bid, take 1 hr ac or 2 hr pc
Ⓟ *Child 5-11 yr:* PO 10 mg bid

Available forms: Tabs 10, 20 mg

Adverse effects
(*italic* = common; **bold** = life-threatening)
CNS: Headache, dizziness
GI: Nausea, diarrhea, abdominal pain, vomiting, dyspepsia
MISC: Infections, pain, asthenia, myalgia, fever, increased ALT, urticaria, rash, ***angioedema***

Contraindications: Hypersensitivity

Ⓖ **Precautions:** Pregnancy **B**, elderly, lactation,
Ⓟ children, hepatic disease

Pharmacokinetics

Absorption	Rapidly
Distribution	Unknown
Metabolism	Extensively by CYP450 2C9, 3A4 enzyme systems, protein binding (99%)
Excretion	Feces
Half-life	10 hr

Pharmacodynamics

Onset	Unknown
Peak	3 hr
Duration	Unknown

Interactions
Individual drugs
Aspirin: ↑ plasma levels of zafirlukast
Erythromycin, theophylline: ↓ plasma levels of zafirlukast
Warfarin: ↑ Pro-time
Food/drug
↓ Bioavailability of zafirlukast
Herb/drug
Green tea (large amounts), guarana: ↑ effect

NURSING CONSIDERATIONS
Assessment
• Assess respiratory rate, rhythm, depth; auscultate lung fields bilaterally; notify prescriber of abnormalities

Nursing diagnoses
☑ Breathing pattern, ineffective (uses)
☑ Knowledge, deficient (teaching)
☑ Noncompliance (teaching)

Implementation
• Give PO 1 hr ac or 2 hr pc; absorption may be decreased if given with food

Patient/family education
• Advise patient to check OTC medications, current prescription medications, which will increase stimulation
• Advise patient to avoid hazardous activities; dizziness may occur
• Advise patient that if GI upset occurs, to take drug with 8 oz of water; avoid food if possible, absorption may be decreased
• Advise to take even if symptom free
• Advise patient to notify prescriber of nausea, vomiting, diarrhea, abdominal pain, fatigue, jaundice, anorexia, flulike symptoms (hepatic dysfunction)
• Advise patient not to use for acute asthma episodes, or to use while breastfeeding

Evaluation
Positive therapeutic outcome
• Ability to breathe more easily

zalcitabine (Rx)
(zal-sit'a-bin)
ddC, dideoxycitidine, HIVID
Func. class.: Antiretroviral
Chem. class.: (NRTI) Nucleoside reverse transcriptase inhibitor
Pregnancy category C

Action: Inhibits HIV replication by the conversion of this drug by cellular enzymes to an active antiviral metabolite; a chain terminator

➔**Therapeutic Outcome:** Improved symptoms of HIV infection

Uses: HIV infections in combination in adults and children >13 yr

Dosage and routes
Adult: PO 0.75 mg q8h in combination with other antiretrovirals; in presence of peripheral neuropathy initiate dose at 0.375 mg q8h of zalcitabine
Renal dose
Adult: PO CCr 10-40 ml/min 0.75 mg q12h; CCr <10 ml/min 0.75 mg q24h

Available forms: Tabs 0.375, 0.75 mg

Adverse effects
(*italic* = common; **bold** = life-threatening)
CNS: Headache, peripheral neuropathy, **seizures,** confusion, anxiety, hypertonia, abnormal thinking, asthenia, insomnia, CNS depression, pain, *dizziness,* chills, *fever*
CV: Hypertension, vasodilatation, dysrhythmia, syncope, palpitation, tachycardia, **cardiomyopathy, CHF**
EENT: Ear pain, otitis, photophobia, visual impairment
ENDO: Hypoglycemia, hyponatremia, hyperbilirubinemia, hyperglycemia
GI: **Pancreatitis,** *diarrhea, nausea, vomiting,* abdominal pain, constipation, stomatitis, dysplasia, liver abnormalities, *oral ulcers,* flatulence, taste perversion, dry mouth, oral thrush, melena, *increased ALT, AST, alkaline phosphatase, amylase,* increased bilirubin
GU: Uric acid, **toxic nephropathy,** polyuria
HEMA: **Leukopenia, granulocytopenia, thrombocytopenia,** anemia
INTEG: Rash, *pruritus,* alopecia, sweating, acne
MS: Myalgia, arthritis, myopathy, muscular atrophy
RESP: Cough, pneumonia, dyspnea, asthma, hypoventilation
SYST: **Lactic acidosis**

Contraindications: Hypersensitivity

Precautions: Renal, hepatic, disease, pregnancy **C**, lactation, children <13 yr, patients with peripheral neuropathy, heart failure

Pharmacokinetics

Absorption	Minimally absorbed
Distribution	Unknown
Metabolism	Liver
Excretion	Kidneys
Half-life	1-3 hr, increased in renal disease

Pharmacodynamics

Onset	Unknown
Peak	1½-2½ hr
Duration	Unknown

Interactions
Individual drugs
Amphotericin B, chloramphenicol, cimetidine, cisplatin, dapsone, disulfiram, ethionamide, foscarnet, glutethimide, gold, hydralazine, iodoquinol, isoniazid, metronidazole, nitrofurantoin, phenytoin, probenecid, ribavirin, vinCRIStine: ↑ peripheral neuropathy
ddI, d4T: ↑ pancreatitis risk
Ketoconazole, metoclopramide: ↓ absorption
Drug classifications
Aminoglycosides: ↑ peripheral neuropathy
Antacids: ↓ absorption
Nucleoside analogs: ↑ peripheral neuropathy risk

NURSING CONSIDERATIONS
Assessment
• Assess for peripheral neuropathy: tingling or pain in hands and feet, distal numbness; if these occur during therapy, drug may be decreased or discontinued
• Assess for lactic acidosis; severe hepatomegaly with steatosis, which can be fatal; drug should be discontinued
• Assess for pancreatitis: abdominal pain, nausea, vomiting, elevated liver enzymes; drug should be discontinued because condition can be fatal
P • Assess children by dilated retinal examination q6 mo to rule out retinal depigmentation
• Monitor CBC, differential, platelet count qmo; withhold drug if WBC is <4000/mm³ or platelet count is <75,000/mm³; notify prescriber of results
• Monitor renal function studies (BUN, serum uric acid, urine CCr) before, during therapy; these may be elevated throughout treatment
• Monitor temp q4h, may indicate beginning of infection

• Monitor liver function tests (bilirubin, AST, ALT, amylase, alkaline phosphatase, triglycerides) before, during therapy as needed or qmo
• Monitor viral load, CD4 baseline and throughout treatment

Nursing diagnoses
☑ Infection, risk for (uses)
☑ Injury, risk for (adverse reactions)
☑ Knowledge, deficient (teaching)

Implementation
• Give on empty stomach, q8h around the clock

Patient/family education
• Advise patient to take on empty stomach; not to take dapsone at same time as ddC; to use exactly as prescribed
• Instruct patient to report signs of infection: increased temp, sore throat, flu-like symptoms; to avoid crowds and those with known infections
• Caution patient to report signs of anemia: fatigue, headache, faintness, shortness of breath, irritability
• Advise patient to report bleeding; avoid use of razors or commercial mouthwash
• Inform patient that hair may be lost during therapy (rare); a wig or hairpiece may make patient feel better
• Caution patient to avoid OTC products or other medications without approval of prescriber
• Caution patient not to have any sexual contact without use of a condom, that needles should not be shared, that blood from infected individual should not come in contact with another's mucous membranes

Evaluation
Positive therapeutic outcome
• Absence of infection; symptoms of HIV infection

---

zaleplon (Rx)
(zale′plon)
Sonata
Func. class.: Sedative-hypnotic, antianxiety
Chem. class.: Pyrazolopyrimidine

Pregnancy category C
Controlled substance schedule IV

Action: Binds selectively to ω-1 receptor of the γ-aminobutyric acid type A ($GABA_A$) receptor complex; results are sedation, hypnosis, skeletal muscle relaxation, anticonvulsant activity, anxiolytic action

---

 Herb/drug   Do Not Crush   Alert   Key Drug   Geriatric   Pediatric

➡️ **Therapeutic Outcome:** Ability to sleep

Uses: Insomnia

Dosage and routes
Adult: PO 10 mg hs; may increase dose to 20 mg hs if needed; 5 mg may be used in low weight persons

🅖 *Elderly:* PO 15 mg hs; may increase if needed

Available forms: Caps 5, 10 mg

Adverse effects
(*italic* = common; **bold** = life-threatening)
CNS: Drowsiness, amnesia, depersonalization, hallucinations, hypesthesia, paresthesia, somnolence, tremor, vertigo, dizziness, anxiety, *lethargy, daytime sedation,* confusion
EENT: Vision changes, ear/eye pain, hyperacusis, parosmia
GI: Nausea, anorexia, colitis, dyspepsia, dry mouth, constipation, abdominal pain
MISC: Asthenia, fever, headache, myalgia, dysmenorrhea

Contraindications: Hypersensitivity

Precautions: Hepatic disease, renal disease, elderly, psychosis, child <15 yr, pregnancy **C**, lactation

Pharmacokinetics

Absorption	Rapidly absorbed
Distribution	Extravascular tissues, crosses blood-brain barrier; crosses placenta
Metabolism	Extensively, liver to inactive metabolites
Excretion	Kidneys
Half-life	1 hr

Pharmacodynamics

Onset	Rapid
Peak	1 hr
Duration	Unknown

Interactions
Individual drugs
Cimetidine: ↑ action of zaleplon
Rifampin: ↓ zaleplon levels
Food/drug
Prolonged absorption
High-fat/heavy meal: Sleep onset reduced
🖋 *Herb/drug*
Black cohosh: ↑ hypotension
Catnip, chamomile, clary, cowslip, hops, kava, lavender, mistletoe, nettle, pokeweed, poppy, Queen Anne's lace, senega, skullcap, valerian: ↑ CNS depression

NURSING CONSIDERATIONS
Assessment
• Assess for previous drug dependence or tolerance; if drug dependent or tolerant, amount of medication should be restricted
• Monitor patient's mental status: mood, sensorium, affect, sleeping patterns, drowsiness, dizziness, suicidal tendencies

Nursing diagnoses
✓ Sleep pattern, disturbed (uses)
✓ Knowledge, deficient (teaching)
✓ Noncompliance (teaching)

Implementation
• Give ½-1 hr before bedtime for sleeplessness; give on empty stomach
• Advise patient that drug may cause memory problems, dependence (if used for longer periods of time), changes in behavior/thinking

Patient/family education
• Inform patient that drug is for short-term use only
• Teach patient to take immediately before going to bed
• Advise patient not to ingest a high-fat/heavy meal before taking
• Advise patient to avoid OTC preparations unless approved by a physician, to avoid alcohol ingestion or other psychotropic medications unless prescribed by a health care provider, that 1-2 wk of therapy may be required before therapeutic effects occur
• Caution patient to avoid driving, activities requiring alertness; drowsiness may occur; until medication response is known, tell patient that drowsiness may worsen at beginning of treatment
• Instruct patient not to discontinue medication abruptly after long-term use

Evaluation
Positive therapeutic outcome
• Decreased sleeplessness

zanamivir (Rx)
(zan-a-mee'veer)
Relenza
Func. class.: Antiviral
Chem class.: Nevramidase inhibitor

Pregnancy category B

Action: Inhibits the enzyme needed for influenza virus replication

➡️ **Therapeutic Outcome:** Decreased symptoms of influenza type A for those who have been symptomatic for no more than 2 days

Uses: Treatment of influenza type A

Dosage and routes

🅟 *Adult and child >12 yr:* INH 2 inhalations (two 5 mg blisters) q12h × 5 days, on the 1st day 2 doses should be taken with at least 2 hr between doses

Available forms: Blisters of powder for inhalation 5 mg

Adverse effects

(*italic* = common; **bold** = life-threatening)
CNS: Headache, dizziness, fatigue
EENT: Ear, nose, throat infections
GI: Nausea, vomiting, diarrhea
RESP: Nasal symptoms, cough, sinusitis, bronchitis

Contraindications: Hypersensitivity

🅖 **Precautions:** Elderly, lactation, children
🅟 <12 yr, respiratory disease, pregnancy **B**

Pharmacokinetics	
Absorption	4%-17% absorbed
Distribution	<10% protein binding
Metabolism	Not metabolized
Excretion	Kidneys unchanged
Half-life	2½-5 hr

Pharmacodynamics
Unknown

Interactions: None known

NURSING CONSIDERATIONS
Assessment
• Assess for symptoms of influenza A: increased temp, malaise, aches and pains
• Assess for skin eruptions, photosensitivity after administration of drug
• Monitor respiratory status: rate, character, wheezing, tightness in chest
• Assess for allergies before initiation of treatment, reaction of each medication

Nursing diagnoses
✓ Infection, risk for (uses)
✓ Knowledge, deficient (teaching)

Implementation
• Give before exposure to influenza; continue for 5 days after contact
• Store in airtight, dry container

Patient/family education
• Give patient "Patient's instruction for use" and review all points before using delivery system

• Teach patient to avoid hazardous activities if dizziness occurs
• Teach patient to take drug exactly as prescribed; to use for the entire 5 days
• Inform patient that this drug does not reduce transmission risk of influenza to others
• Advise patients with asthma or COPD to carry a fast-acting inhaled bronchodilator since bronchospasm may occur; to use scheduled inhaled bronchodilators before using this drug

Evaluation
Positive therapeutic outcome
• Absence of fever, malaise, cough, dyspnea in influenza A

---

zidovudine 🔑 **(Rx)**
(zye-doe′vue-deen)
Apo-Zidovudine ✦, Azidothymidine, AZT, Novo-AZT ✦, Retrovir
Func. class.: Antiretroviral
Chem. class.: (NRTI) Nucleoside reverse transcriptase inhibitor
Pregnancy category C

Action: Inhibits replication of HIV by incorporating into cellular DNA by viral reverse transcriptase, thereby terminating the cellular DNA chain

➔ **Therapeutic Outcome:** Decreased symptoms of HIV infection

Uses: Used in combination with other antiretrovirals for HIV infection

Dosage and routes
Adult: PO 600 mg qd in divided doses, either 200 mg tid or 300 mg bid in combination with other antiretrovirals; **IV** 1-2 mg/kg q4h, initiate PO as soon as possible

🅟 *Child 6 wk-12 yr:* PO 160 mg/m² q8h (480 mg/m²/day, max 200 mg q8h) in combination with other antiretrovirals; **IV** same as adult

🅟 *Neonates:* PO 2-3 mg/kg/dose q6h; **IV** 1.5 mg/kg infused over 30 min q6h

Prevention of maternal-fetal HIV transmission
🅟 *Neonatal:* PO 2 mg/kg/dose q6h × 6 wk beginning 8-12 hr after birth; **IV** 1.5 mg/kg/dose over 30 min q6h until able to take PO

Maternal (>14 wk gestation): PO 100 mg 5 ×/day until start of labor, then during labor/delivery **IV** 2 mg/kg over 1 hr followed

---

by **IV** inf 1 mg/kg/hr until umbilical cord clamped

Symptomatic HIV infection

P **Child 3 mo-12 yr:** PO 90-180 mg/m² q6h, max 200 mg q6h; **IV** 1-2 mg/kg over 1 hr q4h

Adult: PO 100 mg q4h; **IV** 1-2 mg/kg over 1 hr q4h

Prevention of HIV after needlestick

Adult: PO 200 mg tid plus lamivudine 150 mg bid, plus a protease inhibitor for high-risk exposure; begin within 2 hr of exposure

Available forms: Caps 100 mg; tabs 300 mg; inj 200 mg/20 ml; oral syr 50 mg/5 ml

Adverse effects

(*italic* = common; **bold** = life-threatening)

CNS: *Fever, headache, malaise,* diaphoresis, *dizziness, insomnia,* paresthesia, somnolence, chills, tremor, twitching, anxiety, confusion, depression, lability, vertigo, loss of mental acuity, **seizures**

EENT: Taste change, hearing loss, photophobia

GI: *Nausea, vomiting, diarrhea,* anorexia, cramps, *dyspepsia,* constipation, dysphagia, *flatulence,* rectal bleeding, mouth ulcer

GU: Dysuria, polyuria, frequency, hesitancy

HEMA: **Granulocytopenia, anemia**

INTEG: Rash, acne, pruritus, urticaria

MS: Myalgia, arthralgia, muscle spasm

RESP: Dyspnea

Contraindications: Hypersensitivity

Precautions: Granulocyte count <1000/mm³ or Hgb <9.5 g/dl, pregnancy **C**, lactation, P children, severe renal disease, severe hepatic function

Pharmacokinetics

Absorption	Well absorbed (PO), completely absorbed (**IV**)
Distribution	Widely distributed—crosses placenta, CSF
Metabolism	Liver—mostly
Excretion	Kidneys
Half-life	1 hr

Pharmacodynamics

	PO	IV
Onset	Unknown	Rapid
Peak	½-1½ hr	Inf end
Duration	Unknown	Unknown

Interactions

Individual drugs

Fluconazole, probenecid: ↑ toxicity

Ganciclovir, radiation: ↑ bone marrow suppression

Drug classifications

Antineoplastics: ↑ bone marrow suppression

NURSING CONSIDERATIONS

Assessment

• Assess for peripheral neuropathy: tingling or pain in hands and feet, distal numbness; if these occur, drug may be decreased or discontinued

• Assess for pancreatitis: abdominal pain, nausea, vomiting, elevated liver enzymes; drug should be discontinued because condition can be fatal

P• Assess children by dilated retinal examination q6 mo to rule out retinal depigmentation

• Monitor CBC, differential, platelet count qmo; withhold drug if WBC is <4000/mm³ or platelet count is <75,000/mm³; notify prescriber of results; monitor viral load, CD4 counts baseline and throughout treatment

• Monitor renal function studies: BUN, serum uric acid, urine CCr before, during therapy; these may be elevated throughout treatment

• Monitor temp q4h, may indicate beginning of infection

• Monitor liver function tests before, during therapy (bilirubin, AST, ALT amylase, alkaline phosphatase) prn or qmo

Nursing diagnoses

✓Infection, risk for (uses)

✓Injury, risk for physical (adverse reactions)

✓Knowledge, deficient (teaching)

Implementation

PO route

• Give on empty stomach, bid or tid

Ⓜ**IV route**

• Give by intermittent inf after diluting with D₅W; give over 1 hr (<4 mg/ml), do not give by direct **IV**

Y-site compatibilities: Acyclovir, allopurinol, amikacin, amphotericin B, aztreonam, ceftazidime, ceftriaxone, cimetidine, clindamycin, dexamethasone, DOBUTamine, DOPamine, erythromycin, fluconazole, fludarabine, gentamicin, heparin, imipenem/cilastatin, lorazepam, metoclopramide, morphine, nafcillin, ondansetron, oxacillin, pentamidine, phenylephrine, piperacillin, potassium chloride, ranitidine, sargramostim, tobramycin, trimethoprim/sulfamethoxazole, vancomycin

Additive incompatibilities: Blood products or protein solutions

Patient/family education

- Caution patient to take on empty stomach; not to take dapsone at same time as didanosine; to use exactly as prescribed
- Advise patient to report signs of infection: increased temp, sore throat, flu-like symptoms; to avoid crowds and those with known infections
- Instruct patient to report signs of anemia: fatigue, headache, faintness, shortness of breath, irritability
- Advise patient to report bleeding; avoid use of razors or commercial mouthwash
- Inform patient that hair may be lost during therapy (rare); a wig or hairpiece may make patient feel better
- Caution patient to avoid OTC products or other medications without approval of prescriber
- Caution patient not to have any sexual contact without use of a condom, needles should not be shared, blood from infected individual should not come in contact with another's mucous membranes

Evaluation

Positive therapeutic outcome

- Decreased infection; symptoms of HIV infection

---

zileuton (Rx)

(zye-loo'tahn)

Zyflo

Func. class.: Bronchodilator

Chem. class.: 5-Lipoxygenase inhibitor, leukotriene pathway inhibitor

Pregnancy category C

Action: Inhibits leukotriene (LT) formation; leukotrienes exert their effects by increasing neutrophil, eosinophil migration; aggregation of neutrophils, monocytes; smooth muscle contraction, capillary permeability; these actions further lead to bronchoconstriction, inflammation, edema

⇒**Therapeutic Outcome:** Ability to breathe more easily

Uses: Asthma

Investigational uses: Ulcerative colitis, rheumatoid arthritis

Dosage and routes

Asthma

P *Adult and child >12 yr:* PO 600 mg qid, may be given with meal and hs

Ulcerative colitis (off-label)

Adult: PO 600 mg bid

Available forms: Tabs 600 mg

Adverse effects

(*italic* = common; **bold** = life-threatening)

CNS: Dizziness, insomnia, fatigue, paresthesias, headache

GI: Nausea, abdominal pain, dyspepsia, diarrhea, liver function test abnormalities

INTEG: Hives

MS: Myalgia, asthenia

Contraindications: Active hepatic disease, elevations in liver function tests 3 × upper limits, hypersensitivity

Precautions: Acute attacks of asthma, alcohol consumption, pregnancy **C**, lactation, history of hepatic disease

Pharmacokinetics

Absorption	Rapid
Distribution	Protein binding 93%
Metabolism	Liver
Excretion	Urine
Half-life	2.1-2.5 hr

Pharmacodynamics

Onset	Unknown
Peak	1-3 hr
Duration	Unknown

Interactions

Individual drugs

Propranolol: ↑ propranolol effects

Theophylline: ↑ theophylline effects

Warfarin: ↑ warfarin effect

⊘ *Herb/drug*

Green tea (large amounts), guarana: ↑ effect

NURSING CONSIDERATIONS

Assessment

- Assess CBC, blood chemistry, during treatment
- Assess liver function tests before and qmo × 3 mo, then q2-3 mo during first year treatment
- Assess respiratory rate, rhythm, depth; auscultate lung fields bilaterally; notify prescriber of abnormalities
- Assess allergic reactions: rash, urticaria; drug should be discontinued

Nursing diagnoses

☑ Breathing pattern, ineffective (uses)

☑ Knowledge, deficient (teaching)

☑ Noncompliance (teaching)

Implementation
- Give PO after meals to decrease GI symptoms

Patient/family education
- Advise patient to check OTC medications, current prescription medications for epHEDrine, which will increase stimulation; to avoid alcohol
- Advise patient to avoid hazardous activities; dizziness may occur
- Advise patient that if GI upset occurs, to take drug with 8 oz of water or food
- Advise patient to notify prescriber of nausea, vomiting, anxiety, insomnia
- Advise to take even without symptoms
- Advise not to use for acute asthma attack

Evaluation
Positive therapeutic outcome
- Ability to breathe more easily

zinc sulfate
(PO, OTC; IV, Rx)
(zink sul'fate)
Orazinc, PMS Egozine ♣, Verazinc, Zinca-Pak, Zincate, Zinc 15, Zinc-220, zinc sulfate
Func. class.: Trace element; nutritional supplement

Pregnancy category A

Action: Needed for adequate healing, bone and joint development, taste and smell (23% zinc)

⇒ **Therapeutic Outcome:** Replacement of zinc

Uses: Prevention of zinc deficiency, adjunct to vit A therapy

Investigational uses: Wound healing

Dosage and routes
Dietary supplement
Adult: PO 25-50 mg/day

Nutritional supplement (**IV**)
Adult: 2.5-4 mg/day, may increase by 2 mg/day if needed

P *Child to 5 yr:* **IV** 100 mcg/kg/day

P *Infants: <1500 g-3 kg:* **IV** 300 mcg/kg/day

Available forms: Tabs 66, 110 mg; caps 220 mg; inj 1, 5 mg/ml

Adverse effects
(*italic* = common; **bold** = life-threatening)
GI: Nausea, vomiting, cramps, heartburn, ulcer formation

OVERDOSE: Diarrhea, rash, dehydration, restlessness
Precautions: Pregnancy **A**

Pharmacokinetics
Absorption	Poorly absorbed (PO), completely absorbed (**IV**)
Distribution	Widely distributed
Metabolism	Liver
Excretion	90%—feces, 10%—kidneys
Half-life	Unknown

Pharmacodynamics
Unknown

Interactions
Drug classification
Other covalent cations: ↓ absorption
⬚ *Herb/drug*
Allspice: ↓ zinc absorption
Black catechu: Forms insoluble complex

NURSING CONSIDERATIONS
Assessment
- Monitor zinc levels during treatment

Nursing diagnoses
☑ Nutrition: less than body requirements, imbalanced (uses)
☑ Knowledge, deficient (teaching)

Implementation
PO route
- Give with meals to decrease gastric upset; restrict dairy products, caffeine, which decrease absorption
IV **IV route**
- Part of TPN

Patient/family education
- Inform patient that element must be taken for 2 mo to be effective
- Advise patient to report immediately nausea, diarrhea, rash, severe vomiting, restlessness, abdominal pain, tarry stools

Evaluation
Positive therapeutic outcome
- Absence of zinc deficiency
- Improved wound healing

ziprasidone (Rx)

(zi-praz'ih-dohn)

Geodon

Func. class.: Antipsychotic/neuroleptic
Chem. class.: Benzisoxazole derivative

Pregnancy category C

Action: Unknown; may be mediated through both dopamine type 2 (D_2) and serotonin type 2 (5-HT_2) antagonism

➔ **Therapeutic Outcome:** Decreased signs/symptoms of psychosis

Uses: Schizophrenia, acute agitation

Dosage and routes

Adult: PO 20 mg bid with food, adjust dosage every 2 days upward to max of 80 mg bid; IM 10-20 mg; may give 10 mg q2h, doses of 20 mg may be given q4h, max 40 mg/day

Available forms: Tabs 20, 40, 60, 80 mg; inj 20 mg/ml

Adverse effects

(*italic* = common; **bold** = life-threatening)

CNS: EPS (*pseudoparkinsonism, akathisia, dystonia, tardive dyskinesia*), *drowsiness, insomnia, agitation, anxiety, headache,* **seizures, neuroleptic malignant syndrome,** dizziness, tremor

CV: Orthostatic hypotension, ***tachycardia, prolonged QT/QTc, sudden death,*** hypertension

EENT: Blurred vision

GI: Nausea, vomiting, *anorexia, constipation,* jaundice, weight gain, diarrhea, dry mouth, abdominal pain

RESP: Rhinitis, dyspnea

Contraindications: Hypersensitivity, lactation, seizure disorders

🅿 **Precautions:** Children, renal disease,
🅖 pregnancy **C**, hepatic disease, elderly, breast cancer

Pharmacokinetics	
Absorption	Unknown
Distribution	Protein binding 90%
Metabolism	Liver—extensively to metabolite
Excretion	Unknown
Half-life	Unknown

Pharmacodynamics	
Unknown	

Interactions

Individual drugs

Alcohol: ↑ sedation
Carbamazepine: ↑ excretion of ziprasidone
Ketoconazole: ↑ ziprasidone
Lithium: ↑ extrapyramidal symptoms (EPS)

Drug classifications

Antihypertensives: ↑ hypotension
Antipsychotics: ↑ EPS
CNS depressants: ↑ sedation

�herb/drug

Betel palm, kava: ↑ EPS
Chamomile, hops, kava, skullcap, valerian: ↑ CNS depression
Cola tree, hops, nettle, nutmeg: ↑ action

NURSING CONSIDERATIONS

Assessment

• Assess mental status before initial administration

• Check swallowing of PO medication; check for hoarding or giving of medication to other patients

• Monitor I&O ratio; palpate bladder if urinary output is low

• Monitor bilirubin, CBC, liver function studies qmo

• Monitor urinalysis before, during prolonged therapy

• Assess affect, orientation, LOC, reflexes, gait, coordination, sleep pattern disturbances

• Monitor B/P standing and lying; also pulse, respirations; take these q4h during initial treatment; establish baseline before starting treatment; report drops of 30 mm Hg; watch for ECG changes

• Assess dizziness, faintness, palpitations, tachycardia on rising

• Assess EPS, including akathisia (inability to sit still, no pattern to movements), tardive dyskinesia (bizarre movements of the jaw, mouth, tongue, extremities), pseudoparkinsonism (rigidity, tremors, pill rolling, shuffling gait)

🔷 Assess for neuroleptic malignant syndrome: hyperthermia, increased CPK, altered mental status, muscle rigidity

• Assess skin turgor qd

• Assess constipation, urinary retention qd; if these occur, increase bulk and water in diet

Nursing diagnoses

☑ Thought processes, disturbed (uses)
☑ Coping, ineffective (uses)
☑ Knowledge, deficient (teaching)
☑ Noncompliance (teaching)

Implementation

G • Give reduced dose in elderly
• Give antiparkinsonian agent on order from prescriber, to be used for EPS
• Provide decreased stimulus by dimming lights, avoiding loud noises
• Provide supervised ambulation until patient is stabilized on medication; do not involve in strenuous exercise program because fainting is possible; patient should not stand still for a long time
• Provide increased fluids to prevent constipation
• Provide sips of water, candy, gum for dry mouth
• Store in airtight, light-resistant container

IM route
• Add 1.2 ml sterile water for inj to vial, shake vigorously until drug is dissolved, do not admix

Patient/family education

• Advise patient that orthostatic hypotension may occur and to rise from sitting or lying position gradually
• Advise patient to avoid hot tubs, hot showers, tub baths; hypotension may occur
• Advise patient to avoid abrupt withdrawal of this drug; EPS may result; drug should be withdrawn slowly
• Advise patient to avoid OTC preparations (cough, hay fever, cold) unless approved by prescriber, since serious drug interactions may occur; avoid use with alcohol, CNS depressants; increased drowsiness may occur
• Teach patient to avoid hazardous activities if drowsy or dizzy
• Teach patient compliance with drug regimen
• Teach patient to report impaired vision, tremors, muscle twitching
• Teach patient that in hot weather, heat stroke may occur; take extra precautions to stay cool

Evaluation

Positive therapeutic outcome
• Decrease in emotional excitement, hallucinations, delusions, paranoia; reorganization of patterns of thought, speech

Treatment of overdose: Lavage if orally ingested; provide airway; *do not induce vomiting*

---

zoledronic acid (Rx)
(zoh'leh-drah'nick ass'id))
Zometa
Func. class.: Bone-resorption inhibitor
Chem. class.: Bisphosphonate

Pregnancy category D

Action: Inhibits normal and abnormal bone resorption; potent inhibitor of osteoclastic bone resorption; inhibits osteoclastic activity, reduces bone resorption and inhibits skeletal calcium release caused by stimulating factors released by tumors; reduction of abnormal bone resorption is responsible for therapeutic effect in hypercalcemia; may directly block dissolution of hydroxyapatite bone crystals

➡ **Therapeutic Outcome:** Serum calcium at normal level

Uses: Moderate to severe hypercalcemia associated with malignancy; multiple myeloma; bone metastases from solid tumors (used with antineoplastics)

Dosage and routes
Hypercalemia of malignancy
Adult: **IV** inf 4 mg, given as a single inf over ≥15 min, may re-treat with 4 mg if serum calcium does not return to normal within 1 wk

Multiple myeloma/metastatic bone lesions
Adult: **IV** inf 4 mg, given over 15 min q3-4 wk; may continue treatment for 9-15 months, depending on condition

Available forms: Powder for inj 4 mg

Adverse effects
(*italic* = common; **bold** = life-threatening)
CV: Hypotension
GI: Abdominal pain, anorexia, constipation, nausea, diarrhea, vomiting
GU: UTI, possible reduced renal function
META: Anemia, hypokalemia, hypomagnesemia, hypophosphatemia
MISC: Fever, chills, flu-like symptoms
MS: Bone pain, *arthralgias, myalgias*

Contraindications: Hypersensitivity to bisphosphonates, pregnancy **D**

P **Precautions:** Children, nursing mothers, renal dysfunction, asthma-sensitive asthmatic patients

---

Pharmacokinetics

Absorption	Rapidly cleared from circulation
Distribution	Taken up mainly by bones; plasma protein binding ~22%
Metabolism	Not metabolized
Excretion	Kidneys (~50% eliminated in urine within 24 hr)
Half-life	146 hr

Pharmacodynamics

Onset	Unknown
Peak	15 min
Duration	Unknown

Interactions
Individual drugs
Calcium, vitamin D: ↓ zoledronic acid effect
Digoxin: Hypomagnesemia, hypokalemia
Infusion solutions (calcium-containing): Do not mix with Ca-containing infusion sol such as Ringer's sol
Drug classifications
Aminoglycosides, loop diuretics: ↓ serum calcium

NURSING CONSIDERATIONS
Assessment
• Assess renal studies and Ca, P, Mg, K, creatinine, if creatinine is elevated hold treatment
• Assess for hypercalcemia: paresthesia, twitching, laryngospasm; Chvostek's, Trousseau's signs

Nursing diagnoses
☑ Injury, risk for (uses, adverse reactions)
☑ Fluid, volume excess (side effects)
☑ Knowledge, deficient (teaching)

Implementation
• Saline hydration must be performed before administration; urine output should be 2 L/day during treatment, do not overhydrate
• Sol reconstituted with sterile water may be stored under refrigeration for up to 24 hr **IV**
• Administer after reconstituting by adding 5 ml of sterile water for inj to each vial, then add up to ≥100 ml of sterile 0.9% NaCl, D₅, run over ≥5 min
IV• Administer in separate **IV** line from all other drugs

Patient/family education
• Instruct patient to report hypercalcemic relapse: nausea, vomiting, bone pain, thirst
• Advise patient to continue with dietary recommendations including calcium and vit D; take a multiple vitamin daily, 500 mg of cal-

cium 400 international units vit D in multiple myeloma

Evaluation
Positive therapeutic outcome
• Calcium levels decreased to normal

Treatment of overdose: Correct clinically relevant reductions in serum calcium by administering **IV** calcium gluconate; in serum phosphorus, with potassium or sodium phosphate; in serum magnesium, with magnesium sulfate

---

zolmitriptan (Rx)
(zole-mih-trip'tan)
Zomig, Zomig-ZMT
Func. class.: Migraine agent
Chem. class.: 5-HT₁ receptor agonist
Pregnancy category C

Action: Binds selectively to the vascular serotonin type 1 (5-HT₁) receptor subtype, exerts antimigraine effect; causes vasoconstriction in cranial arteries

→**Therapeutic Outcome:** Decreased severity, frequency of headache

Uses: Acute treatment of migraine with or without aura

Dosage and routes:
Adult: PO Start at 2.5 mg or lower (tab may be broken), may repeat after 2 hr, max 10 mg/24 hr

Available forms: Tabs 2.5, 5 mg; orally disintegrating tabs 2.5 mg

Adverse effects
(*italic* = common; **bold** = life-threatening)
CV: Palpitations
GI: Abdominal discomfort, nausea
MS: Weakness, neck stiffness, myalgia
CNS: Tingling, hot sensation, burning, feeling of pressure, tightness, numbness, dizziness, sedation
RESP: Chest tightness, pressure

Contraindications: Angina pectoris, history of MI, documented silent ischemia, ischemic heart disease, concurrent ergotamine-containing preparations, uncontrolled hypertension, hypersensitivity, basilar or hemiplegic migraine, risk of CV events

Precautions: Postmenopausal women, men >40 yr, risk factors for CAD, hypercholesterolemia, obesity, diabetes, impaired hepatic or **P** renal function, pregnancy **C**, lactation, **G** children, elderly

---

Pharmacokinetics

Absorption	Unknown
Distribution	25% plasma protein binding
Metabolism	Liver
Excretion	Urine, feces
Half-life	3-3½ hr

Pharmacodynamics

Onset	Unknown
Peak	Unknown
Duration	2-3½ hr

Interactions
Individual drugs
Cimetidine: ↑ half-life of zolmitriptan
Ergot: ↑ vasospastic effects
Drug classifications
Contraceptives (oral): ↑ half-life of zolmitriptan
Ergot derivatives: ↑ vasospastic effects
MAOIs: Do not use within 2 wk
Selective serotonin reuptake inhibitors (SSRIs): ↑ weakness, hyperreflexia, incoordination
☑ Herb/drug
Butterbur: ↑ effect
SAM-e, St. John's Wort: serotonin syndrome

NURSING CONSIDERATIONS
Assessment
• Assess tingling, hot sensation, burning, feeling of pressure, numbness, flushing
• Assess for stress level, activity, recreation, coping mechanisms
• Assess neurologic status: LOC, blurring vision, nausea, vomiting, tingling in extremities preceding headache
• Monitor ingestion of tyramine foods (pickled products, beer, wine, aged cheese), food additives, preservatives, colorings, artifical sweeteners, chocolate, caffeine, which may precipitate these types of headaches
• Assess for serotonin syndrome, if also taking an SSRI

Nursing diagnoses
☑ Pain, acute (uses)
☑ Noncompliance (teaching)
☑ Knowledge, deficient (teaching)

Implementation
• Give with fluids as soon as symptoms of migraine occur
• Provide quiet, calm environment with decreased stimulation for noise, bright light, excessive talking

Patient/family education
• Teach patient to report any side effects to prescriber
• Advise patient to use contraception while taking drug

Evaluation
Positive therapeutic outcome
• Decrease in frequency, severity of headache

---

zolpidem (Rx)
(zole-pi′dem)
Ambien
Func. class.: Sedative-hypnotic
Chem. class.: Nonbenzodiazepine of imidazopyridine class

Pregnancy category B
Controlled substance schedule IV

Action: Produces CNS depression at limbic, thalamic, hypothalamic levels of CNS; may be mediated by neurotransmitter γ-aminobutyric acid (GABA); results are sedation, hypnosis, skeletal muscle relaxation, anticonvulsant activity, anxiolytic action

➡ Therapeutic Outcome: Ability to sleep, sedation

Uses: Insomnia, short-term treatment

Dosage and routes
Adult: PO 10 mg hs × 7-10 days only; total dose should not exceed 10 mg
G *Elderly:* PO 5 mg hs

Available forms: Tabs 5, 10 mg

Adverse effects
(*italic* = common; **bold** = life-threatening)
CNS: Headache, lethargy, drowsiness, daytime sedation, dizziness, confusion, lightheadedness, anxiety, irritability, amnesia, poor coordination
CV: Chest pain, palpitation
GI: Nausea, vomiting, diarrhea, heartburn, abdominal pain, constipation
***HEMA:* Leukopenia, granulocytopenia** (rare)

Contraindications: Hypersensitivity to benzodiazepines

Precautions: Anemia, hepatic disease, renal disease, suicidal individuals, drug abuse, **G** elderly, psychosis, child <18 yr, seizure disor- **P** ders, pregnancy **B**, lactation

---

Pharmacokinetics

Absorption	Rapidly absorbed
Distribution	Unknown
Metabolism	Liver—inactive metabolite
Excretion	Kidneys, breast milk
Half-life	2½ hr, increased in elderly

Pharmacodynamics

Unknown

Interactions
Individual drugs
Alcohol: ↑ action of both drugs
Drug classifications
CNS depressants: ↑ action of both drugs
Food/drug
↓ Absorption
 Herb/drug
Chamomile, hops, kava, skullcap, valerian:
↑ CNS depression
Lab test interferences
↑ ALT, ↑ AST, ↑ serum bilirubin
↓ Radioactive iodine uptake
False: ↑ Urinary 17-OHCS

NURSING CONSIDERATIONS
Assessment
• Assess mental status: mood, sensorium, anxiety, affect, sleeping pattern, drowsiness, dizziness, especially elderly; physical dependency, withdrawal symptoms: anxiety, panic attacks, agitation, seizures, headache, nausea, vomiting, muscle pain, weakness; suicidal tendencies; for indications of increasing tolerance and abuse
• Monitor B/P (lying, standing), pulse; if systolic B/P drops 20 mm Hg, hold drug, notify prescriber
• Monitor blood studies: CBC during long-term therapy; blood dycrasias have occurred rarely; decreased hematocrit, neutropenia may occur
• Monitor hepatic studies: AST, ALT, bilirubin, creatinine LDH, alkaline phosphatase
• Monitor I&O ratio for renal dysfunction

Nursing diagnoses
☑ Anxiety (uses)
☑ Depression (uses)
☑ Injury, risk for (adverse reactions)
☑ Knowledge, deficient (teaching)

Implementation
• Give ½-1 hr before bedtime for sleeplessness; give several hr before patient is to arise (to avoid hangover)
• Store in airtight container in cool environment

Patient/family education
• Instruct patient that drug may be taken with food, or fluids and tab may be crushed or swallowed whole
• Caution patient not to use for everyday stress or longer than 3 mo unless directed by prescriber; not to take more than prescribed amount; may be habit forming; not to double or skip doses
• Caution patient to avoid OTC preparations unless approved by prescriber; alcohol and CNS depressants will increase CNS depression
• Advise patient to avoid driving, activities that require alertness, because drowsiness may occur; to avoid alcohol ingestion or other psychotropic medications; to rise slowly or fainting may occur, especially elderly; that drowsiness may worsen at beginning of treatment
• Instruct patient not to discontinue medication abruptly after long-term use; withdrawal symptoms include vomiting, cramping, tremors, seizures

Evaluation
Positive therapeutic outcome
• Ability to sleep at night
• Decreased amount of early morning awakening if taking drug for insomnia

Treatment of overdose: Lavage, VS, supportive care

---

zonisamide (Rx)
(zone-is'a-mide)
Zonegran
Func. class.: Anticonvulsant
Chem. class.: Sulfonamides
Pregnancy category C

Action: May act through sodium and calcium channels, but exact action is unknown

⇒ **Therapeutic Outcome:** Decreased seizures

Uses: Epilepsy, adjunctive therapy of partial seizures

Dosage and routes
P *Adults and child >16 yr:* PO 100 mg qd, may increase after 2 wk to 200 mg/day, may increase q2 wk, max dose 600 mg/day

Available forms: Caps 100 mg

Adverse effects
(*italic* = common; **bold** = life-threatening)
CNS: Dizziness, insomnia, paresthesias, depression, fatigue, headache, confusion, somnolence, agitation, irritability

---

EENT: Diplopia, verbal difficulty, speech abnormalities, taste perversion
GI: Nausea, constipation, anorexia, weight loss, diarrhea, dyspepsia
INTEG: Rash

Contraindications: Hypersensitivity to this drug or sulfonamides

Precautions: Allergies, hepatic disease, **G** renal disease, elderly, pregnancy **C**, lactation, **P** child <16 yr

Pharmacokinetics

Absorption	Unknown
Distribution	Unknown
Metabolism	Liver
Excretion	Kidneys
Half-life	63 hr

Pharmacodynamics

Onset	Unknown
Peak	2-6 hr
Duration	Unknown

Interactions
Drugs inducing CYP450 enzyme (carbamazepine, phenytoin, phenobarbital): ↑ half-life of zonisamide

NURSING CONSIDERATIONS
Assessment
• Assess for seizures: duration, type, intensity, precipitating factors
• Renal function: albumin conc
• Assess mental status: mood, sensorium, affect, memory (long, short)

Nursing diagnoses
☑ Injury, risk for (uses, adverse reactions)
☑ Knowledge, deficient (teaching)
☑ Noncompliance (teaching)

Patient/family education
• Advise patient not to discontinue drug abruptly; seizures may occur
• Advise patient to avoid hazardous activities until stabilized on drug
• Advise patient to carry/wear emergency ID stating drug use

Evaluation
Positive therapeutic outcome
• Decrease in severity of seizures

ALPHA-ADRENERGIC BLOCKERS

Action: Binds to α-adrenergic receptors, causing dilatation of peripheral blood vessels; lowers peripheral resistance, resulting in decreased blood pressure.

Uses: Used for pheochromocytoma, prevention of tissue necrosis, and sloughing associated with extravasation of IV vasopressors.

Adverse effects: The most common side effects are hypotension, tachycardia, nasal stuffiness, nausea, vomiting, and diarrhea.

Contraindications: Hypersensitive reactions may occur, and allergies should be identified before these products are given. Patients with myocardial infarction, coronary insufficiency, angina, or other evidence of coronary artery disease should not use these products.

Pharmacokinetics: Onset, peak, and duration vary among products.

Interactions: Vasoconstrictive and hypertensive effects of epinephrine are antagonized by α-adrenergic blockers.

NURSING CONSIDERATIONS
Assessment
- Monitor electrolytes: potassium, sodium chloride, carbon dioxide
- Monitor weight daily, I&O
- Monitor B/P with patient lying, standing before starting treatment, q4h thereafter
- Assess for nausea, vomiting, diarrhea
- Assess for skin turgor, dryness of mucous membranes for hydration status

Nursing diagnoses
- ✓ Altered tissue perfusion (uses)
- ✓ Risk for injury (adverse reactions)
- ✓ Disturbed sleep pattern (adverse reactions)

Implementation
PO Route
- Start with low dose, gradually increasing to prevent side effects
- Give with food or milk for GI symptoms

Evaluation
- Therapeutic response: decreased B/P, increased peripheral pulses

Patient/family education
- Caution patient to avoid alcoholic beverages
- Advise patient to report dizziness, palpitations, fainting
- Instruct patient to change position slowly or fainting may occur
- Teach patient to take drug exactly as prescribed; to avoid all OTC products (cough, cold, allergy) unless directed by prescriber

Selected Generic Names
phentolamine

ANESTHETICS—GENERAL/LOCAL

Action: Anesthetics (general) act on the CNS to produce tranquilization and sleep before invasive procedures. Anesthetics (local) inhibit conduction of nerve impulses from sensory nerves.

Uses: General anesthetics are used to premedicate for surgery, and for induction and maintenance in general anesthesia. For local anesthetics, refer to individual product listing for indications.

Adverse effects: The most common side effects are dystonia, akathisia, flexion of arms, fine tremors, drowsiness, restlessness, and hypotension. Also common are chills, respiratory depression, and laryngospasm.

Contraindications: Persons with CVA, increased intracranial pressure, severe hypertension, cardiac decompensation should not use these products, since severe adverse reactions can occur.

G Precautions: Anesthetics (general) should be used with caution in the elderly, cardiovascular disease (hypotension, bradydysrhythmias), renal disease, liver disease, Parkinson's disease, **P** children <2 yr. The precaution for anesthetics (local) is pregnancy.

Pharmacokinetics: Onset, peak, and duration vary widely among products. Most products are metabolized in the liver and excreted in urine.

Interactions: MAOIs, tricyclics, phenothiazines may cause severe hypotension or hypertension when used with local anesthetics. CNS depressants will potentiate general and local anesthetics.

NURSING CONSIDERATIONS
Assessment
- Monitor VS q10 min during **IV** administration, q30 min after IM dose

Nursing diagnoses
General
✓Risk for injury (adverse reactions)
✓Deficient knowledge (teaching)
Local
✓Acute, pain (uses)
✓Deficient knowledge (teaching)

Implementation
- Give anticholinergic preoperatively to decrease secretions
- Administer only with resuscitative equipment nearby
- Provide quiet environment for recovery to decrease psychotic symptoms

Evaluation
- Therapeutic response: maintenance of anesthesia, decreased pain

---

Selected Generic Names

General anesthetics:
droperidol
etomidate
fentanyl citrate (high alert)
fentanyl citrate/droperidol (high alert)
ketamine (high alert)
methohexital
midazolam
procaine
thiopental (high alert)

Local anesthetics:
◆ᴛ**lidocaine HCl** (high alert)
propofol (high alert)
ropivacaine
tetracaine

 Herb/drug   Do Not Crush   Alert   Key Drug   Geriatric   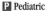 Pediatric

ANTACIDS

Action: Antacids are basic compounds that neutralize gastric acidity and decrease the rate of gastric emptying. Products are divided into those containing aluminum, magnesium, calcium, or a combination of these.

Uses: Hyperacidity is decreased by antacids in conditions such as peptic ulcer disease, reflux esophagitis, gastritis, or hiatal hernia.

Adverse effects: The most common side effect caused by aluminum-containing antacids is constipation, which may lead to fecal impaction and bowel obstruction. Diarrhea occurs often when magnesium products are given. Alkalosis may occur when systemic products are used. Constipation occurs more frequently than laxation with calcium carbonate. The release of CO_2 from carbonate-containing antacids causes belching, abdominal distention, and flatulence. Sodium bicarbonate may act as a systemic antacid and produce systemic electrolyte disturbances and alkalosis. Calcium carbonate and sodium bicarbonate may cause rebound hyperacidity and milk-alkali syndrome. Alkaluria may occur when products are used on a long-term basis, particularly in persons with abnormal renal function.

Contraindications: Sensitivity to aluminum or magnesium products may cause hypersensitive reactions. Aluminum products should not be used by persons sensitive to aluminum; magnesium products should not be used by persons sensitive to magnesium. Check for sensitivity before administering.

Precautions: Magnesium products should be given cautiously to patients with renal insufficiency, during pregnancy, or lactation. Sodium content of antacids may be significant; use with caution for patients with hypertension, CHF, or those on a low-sodium diet.

Pharmacokinetics: Duration is 20-40 min. If ingested 1 hr pc, acidity is reduced for at least 3 hr.

Interactions: Drugs whose effects may be increased by some antacids: quinidine, amphetamines, pseudoephedrine, levodopa, valproic acid, dicumarol. Drugs whose effects may be decreased by some antacids: cimetidine, corticosteroids, ranitidine, iron salts, phenothiazines, phenytoin, digoxin, tetracyclines, ketoconazole, salicylates, isoniazid.

NURSING CONSIDERATIONS

Assessment
- Assess for aggravating and alleviating factors of epigastric pain or hyperacidity; identify the location, duration, and characteristics of epigastric pain
- Assess GI symptoms, including constipation, diarrhea, abdominal pain; if severe abdominal pain with fever occurs, these drugs should not be given
- Assess renal symptoms, including increasing urinary pH, electrolytes

Nursing diagnoses
☑Chronic pain (uses)
☑Constipation (adverse reactions)
☑Diarrhea (adverse reactions)

Implementation
- Give all products with an 8-oz glass of water to ensure absorption in the stomach
- Give another antacid if constipation occurs with aluminum products

Evaluation
- Therapeutic response: absence of epigastric pain, decreased acidity

Patient/family education

- Advise patient not to take other drugs within 1-2 hr of antacid administration, since antacids may impair absorption of other drugs

Selected Generic Names

aluminum hydroxide

bismuth subsalicylate

calcium carbonate

magaldrate

magnesium oxide

sodium bicarbonate

ANTIANGINALS

Action: The antianginals are divided into the nitrates, calcium channel blockers, and β-adrenergic blockers. The nitrates dilate coronary arteries, causing decreased preload, and dilate systemic arteries, causing decreased afterload. Calcium channel blockers dilate coronary arteries, decrease SA/AV node conduction. β-Adrenergic blockers decrease heart rate so that myocardial O_2 use is decreased. Dipyridamole selectively dilates coronary arteries to increase coronary blood flow.

Uses: Antianginals are used in chronic stable angina pectoris, unstable angina, vasospastic angina. Some (i.e., calcium channel blockers and β-blockers) may be used as dysrhythmias and in hypertension.

Adverse effects: The most common side effects are postural hypotension, headache, flushing, dizziness, nausea, edema, and drowsiness. Also common are rash, dysrhythmias, and fatigue.

Contraindications: Persons with known hypersensitivity, increased intracranial pressure, or cerebral hemorrhage should not use some of these products.

Precautions: Antianginals should be used with caution in postural hypotension, pregnancy, **P** lactation, children, renal disease, and hepatic injury.

Pharmacokinetics: Onset, peak, and duration vary widely among coronary products. Most products are metabolized in the liver and excreted in urine.

Interactions: Please check individual monographs, since interactions vary widely among products.

NURSING CONSIDERATIONS

Assessment

- Orthostatic B/P, pulse
- Assess for pain: duration, time started, activity being performed, character
- Assess for tolerance if taken over long period
- Assess for headache, lightheadedness, decreased B/P; may indicate a need for decreased dosage

Nursing diagnoses

☑ Altered tissue perfusion: cardiopulmonary (uses)

☑ Chronic pain (uses)

☑ Risk for injury (uses)

☑ Deficient knowledge (teaching)

☑ Decreased cardiac output (adverse reactions)

Implementation

- Store protected from light, moisture; place in cool environment

Evaluation

- Therapeutic response: decreased, prevention of anginal pain

☑ Herb/drug   Ⓢ Do Not Crush   ◆ Alert   ◆ℼ Key Drug   Ⓖ Geriatric   Ⓟ Pediatric

Patient/family education
- Instruct patient to keep tabs in original container
- Instruct patient not to use OTC products unless directed by prescriber
- Advise patient to report bradycardia, dizziness, confusion, depression, fever
- Teach patient to take pulse at home; advise when to notify prescriber
- Advise patient to avoid alcohol, smoking, sodium intake
- Advise patient to comply with weight control, dietary adjustments, modified exercise program
- Teach patient to carry/wear emergency ID to identify drug being taken, allergies
- Caution patient to make position changes slowly to prevent fainting

Selected Generic Names

Nitrates:
amyl nitrite
isosorbide
♦π nitroglycerin

β-*Adrenergic blockers:*
atenolol
metoprolol
nadolol
propranolol

Calcium channel blockers:
amlodipine
bepridil
diltiazem (high alert)
nicardipine
nifedipine
♦π verapamil

ANTICHOLINERGICS

Action: Anticholinergics inhibit the muscarinic actions of acetylcholine at receptor sites in the autonomic nervous system; anticholinergics are also known as antimuscarinic drugs.

Uses: Anticholinergics are used for a variety of conditions: gastrointestinal anticholinergics are used to decrease motility (smooth muscle tone) in the GI, biliary, and urinary tracts and for their ability to decrease gastric secretions (propantheline, glycopyrrolate); decreasing involuntary movements in parkinsonism (benztropine, trihexyphenidyl); bradydysrhythmias (atropine); nausea and vomiting (scopolamine); and as cycloplegic mydriatics (atropine, hematropine, scopalamine, cyclopentolate, tropicamide).

Adverse effects: The most common side effects are dry mouth, constipation, urinary retention, urinary hesitancy, headache, and dizziness. Also common is paralytic ileus.

Contraindications: Persons with narrow-angle glaucoma, myasthenia gravis, or GI/GU obstruction should not use some of these products.

G Precautions: Anticholinergics should be used with caution in patients who are elderly, pregnant, or lactating or in those with prostatic hypertrophy, CHF, or hypertension; use with caution in presence of high environmental temp.

Pharmacokinetics: Onset, peak, and duration vary widely among products. Most products are metabolized in the liver and excreted in urine.

Interactions: Increased anticholinergic effects may occur when used with MAOIs and tricyclic antidepressants and amantadine. Anticholinergics may cause a decreased effect of phenothiazines and levodopa.

NURSING CONSIDERATIONS
Assessment
- Assess I&O ratio; retention commonly causes decreased urinary output
- Assess for urinary hesitancy, retention; palpate bladder if retention occurs
- Assess for constipation; increase fluids, bulk, exercise if this occurs
- Identify tolerance over long-term therapy; dosage may need to be increased or changed

♣ Canada Only   N Do Not Confuse   * "Tall Man" lettering (See Preface)

- Assess mental status: affect, mood, CNS depression, worsening of mental symptoms during early therapy

Nursing diagnoses
✓ Decreased cardiac output (uses)
✓ Constipation (adverse reactions)
✓ Deficient knowledge (teaching)

Implementation
IV IM/IV Routes
- Give parenteral dose with patient recumbent to prevent postural hypotension
- Give parenteral dose slowly; keep in bed for at least 1 hr after dose; monitor VS
- Give after checking dose carefully; even slight overdose could lead to toxicity

PO Route
- Give with or after meals to prevent GI upset; may give with fluids other than water
- Store at room temp
- Give hard candy, frequent drinks, sugarless gum to relieve dry mouth

Evaluation
- Therapeutic response: decreased secretions, absence of nausea and vomiting

Patient/family education
- Caution patient to avoid driving and other hazardous activities; drowsiness may occur
- Advise patient to avoid OTC medication: cough, cold preparations with alcohol, antihistamines unless directed by prescriber

---

Selected Generic Names

◆π atropine (high alert)
◆π benztropine
biperiden
glycopyrrolate

propantheline
scopolamine (transdermal)
trihexyphenidyl

ANTICOAGULANTS

Action: Anticoagulants interfere with blood clotting by preventing clot formation.

Uses: Anticoagulants are used for deep vein thrombosis, pulmonary emboli, myocardial infarction, open heart surgery, disseminated intravascular clotting syndrome, atrial fibrillation with embolization, and in transfusion and dialysis.

Adverse effects: The most serious adverse reactions are hemorrhage, agranulocytosis, leukopenia, eosinophilia, and thrombocytopenia, depending on the specific product. The most common side effects are diarrhea, rash, and fever.

Contraindications: Persons with hemophilia, leukemia with bleeding, peptic ulcer disease, thrombocytopenic purpura, blood dyscrasias, acute nephritis, and subacute bacterial endocarditis should not use these products.

G Precautions: Anticoagulants should be used with caution in alcoholism, elderly, and pregnancy.

Pharmacokinetics: Onset, peak, and duration vary widely among products. Most products are metabolized in the liver and excreted in urine.

Interactions: Salicylates, steroids, and nonsteroidal antiinflammatories will potentiate the action of anticoagulants. Anticoagulants may cause serious effects; please check individual monographs.

 Herb/drug   Do Not Crush   Alert   Key Drug   G Geriatric   P Pediatric

NURSING CONSIDERATIONS
Assessment
- Monitor blood studies (Hct, platelets, occult blood in stools) q3 mo
- Monitor partial prothrombin time, which should be 1½-2 × control, PPT; often qd, APTT, ACT, INR
- Monitor B/P; watch for increasing signs of hypertension
- Monitor for bleeding gums, petechiae, ecchymosis, black tarry stools, hematuria
- Monitor for fever, skin rash, urticaria
- Monitor for needed dosage change q1-2 wk

Nursing diagnoses
✓ Altered tissue perfusion (uses)
✓ Risk for injury (side effects)
✓ Deficient knowledge (teaching)

Implementation
SC Route
- Give at same time each day to maintain steady blood levels
- Do not massage area or aspirate when giving SC inj; give in abdomen between pelvic bones; rotate sites; do not pull back on plunger, leave in for 10 sec; apply gentle pressure for 1 min
- Do not change needles
- Avoid all IM inj that may cause bleeding
- Store in tight container (PO dose)

Evaluation
- Therapeutic response: decrease of deep vein thrombosis

Patient/family education
- Advise patient to avoid OTC preparations that may cause serious drug interactions unless directed by prescriber
- Inform patient that drug may be held during active bleeding (menstruation), depending on condition
- Caution patient to use soft-bristle toothbrush to avoid bleeding gums; avoid contact sports; use electric razor
- Instruct patient to carry/wear emergency ID identifying drug taken
- Instruct patient to report any signs of bleeding: gums, under skin, urine, stools

---

Selected Generic Names

ardeparin (high alert)
argatroban
dalteparin (high alert)
danaparoid (high alert)
desirudin (Appx A)
enoxaparin (high alert)

fondaparinux
◆π heparin (high alert)
lepirudin (high alert)
tinzaparin (high alert)
◆π warfarin (high alert)

ANTICONVULSANTS

Action: Anticonvulsants are divided into the barbiturates (p. 948), benzodiazepines (p. 950), hydantoins, succinimides, and miscellaneous products. Barbiturates and benzodiazepines are discussed in separate sections. Hydantoins act by inhibiting the spread of seizure activity in the motor cortex. Succinimides act by inhibiting spike and wave formation; they also decrease amplitude, frequency, duration, and spread of discharge in seizures.

Uses: Hydantoins are used in generalized tonic-clonic seizures, status epilepticus, and psychomotor seizures. Succinimides are used for absence of (petit mal) seizures. Barbiturates are used in generalized tonic-clonic and cortical focal seizures.

Adverse effects: Bone marrow depression is the most life-threatening adverse reaction associated with hydantoins or succinimides. The most common side effects are GI symptoms. Other common side effects for hydantoins are gingival hyperplasia and CNS effects such as nystagmus, ataxia, slurred speech, and confusion.

Contraindications: Hypersensitive reactions may occur, and allergies should be identified before these products are given.

Precautions: Persons with renal or hepatic disease should be watched closely.

Pharmacokinetics: Onset, peak, and duration vary widely among products. Most products are metabolized in the liver and excreted in urine, bile, and feces.

Interactions: Decreased effects of estrogens, oral contraceptives (hydantoins).

NURSING CONSIDERATIONS
Assessment
- Monitor renal function studies, including BUN, creatinine, serum uric acid, urine CCr before and during therapy
- Monitor blood studies: RBC, Hct, Hgb, reticulocyte counts weekly for 4 wk then monthly
- Monitor hepatic studies: AST, ALT, bilirubin, creatinine
- Assess mental status, including mood, sensorium, affect, behavioral changes; if mental status changes, notify prescriber
- Assess for eye problems, including need for ophth examinations before, during, and after treatment (slit lamp, fundoscopy, tonometry)
- Assess for allergic reaction, including red, raised rash; if this occurs, drug should be discontinued
- Assess for blood dyscrasias, including fever, sore throat, bruising, rash, jaundice
- Monitor toxicity, including bone marrow depression, nausea, vomiting, ataxia, diplopia, cardiovascular collapse, Stevens-Johnson syndrome

Nursing diagnoses
✓ Risk for injury (uses)
✓ Noncompliance (teaching)
✓ Disturbed sleep pattern (adverse reactions)

Implementation
PO Route
- Give with food, milk to decrease GI symptoms
- Good oral hygiene is important for patients taking hydantoins

Evaluation
- Therapeutic response, including decreased seizure activity; document on patient's chart

Patient/family education
- Advise patient to carry/wear emergency ID stating drugs taken, condition, prescriber's name, phone number
- Advise patient to avoid driving, other activities that require alertness

 Herb/drug   Do Not Crush   Alert   ◆π Key Drug   **G** Geriatric   **P** Pediatric

Selected Generic Names

Hydantoins:
fosphenytoin
♦π phenytoin

Miscellaneous:
acetazolamide
carbamazepine
clonazepam
♦π diazepam
felbamate
gabapentin
lamotrigine

magnesium sulfate (high alert)
tiagabine
topiramate
valproate/valproic acid/
   divalproex sodium
zonisamide

Barbiturates:
amobarbital
♦π phenobarbital (high alert)
primidone
thiopental (high alert)

ANTIDEPRESSANTS

Action: Antidepressants are divided into the tricyclics, MAOIs, and miscellaneous antidepressants. The tricyclics work by blocking reuptake of norepinephrine and serotonin into nerve endings and increasing action of norepinephrine and serotonin in nerve cells. MAOIs act by increasing concentrations of endogenous epinephrine, norepinephrine, serotonin, dopamine in storage sites in CNS by inhibition of MAO; increased concentration reduces depression.

P Uses: Antidepressants are used for depression and in some cases enuresis in children.

Adverse effects: The most serious adverse reactions are paralytic ileus, acute renal failure, hypertension, and hypertensive crisis, depending on the specific product. Common side effects are dizziness, drowsiness, diarrhea, dry mouth, urinary retention, and orthostatic hypotension.

Contraindications: The contraindications for antidepressants are convulsive disorders, prostatic hypertrophy, severe renal, hepatic, cardiac disease depending on the type of medication.

Precautions: Antidepressants should be used cautiously in suicidal patients, severe depression, **G** schizophrenia, hyperactivity, diabetes mellitus, pregnancy, and the elderly.

Pharmacokinetics: Onset, peak, and duration vary widely among products. Most products are metabolized in the liver and excreted in urine.

Interactions: Please check individual monographs, since interactions vary widely among products.

NURSING CONSIDERATIONS
Assessment

- Monitor B/P (lying, standing), pulse q4h; if systolic B/P drops 20 mm Hg, hold drug, notify prescriber; take VS q4h in patients with cardiovascular disease
- Monitor blood studies: CBC, leukocytes, differential, cardiac enzymes if patient is receiving long-term therapy
- Monitor hepatic studies: AST, ALT, bilirubin, creatinine
- Monitor weight weekly; appetite may increase with drug
- **G** Monitor for extrapyramidal symptoms (EPS) primarily in elderly: rigidity, dystonia, akathisia
- Assess mental status: mood, sensorium, affect, suicidal tendencies, increase in psychiatric symptoms (depression, panic)
- **P G** Check for urinary retention, constipation; constipation is more likely to occur in children, elderly
- Assess for withdrawal symptoms: headache, nausea, vomiting, muscle pain, weakness; do not usually occur unless drug was discontinued abruptly
- Identify alcohol consumption; if alcohol is consumed, hold dose until AM

Nursing diagnoses
✓ Ineffective coping (uses)
✓ Risk for injury (uses/adverse reactions)
✓ Deficient knowledge (teaching)

Implementation
PO Route
- Give increased fluids, bulk in diet if constipation, urinary retention occur
- Give with food or milk for GI symptoms
- Give gum, hard candy, or frequent sips of water for dry mouth
- Store in airtight container at room temp; do not refreeze
- Provide assistance with ambulation during beginning therapy, since drowsiness/dizziness occurs

Evaluation
- Therapeutic response: decreased depression

Patient/family education
- Teach patient that therapeutic effects may take 2-3 wk
- Advise patient to use caution in driving or other activities requiring alertness because of drowsiness, dizziness, blurred vision
- Caution patient to avoid alcohol ingestion, other CNS depressants
- Instruct patient not to discontinue medication quickly after long-term use; may cause nausea, headache, malaise
- Instruct patient to wear sunscreen or large hat, since photosensitivity may occur

---

Selected Generic Names

Tetracyclic:
mirtazapine

Tricyclics:
amitriptyline
amoxapine
clomipramine
desipramine
doxepin
🗝 imipramine
nortriptyline
trimipramine

Miscellaneous:
bupropion

maprotiline
nefazodone
trazodone
venlafaxine

MAOIs:
phenelzine
tranylcypromine

SSRIs
citalopram
fluoxetine
paroxetine
sertraline

ANTIDIABETICS

Action: Antidiabetics are divided into the insulins that decrease blood glucose, phosphate, and potassium and increase blood pyruvate and lactate; and oral antidiabetics that cause functioning β-cells in the pancreas to release insulin, improves the effect of endogenous and exogenous insulin.
Uses: Insulins are used for ketoacidosis and diabetes mellitus types 1 and 2; oral antidiabetics are used for stable adult-onset diabetes mellitus type 2.
Adverse effects: The most common side effect of insulin and oral antidiabetics is hypoglycemia. Other adverse reactions for oral antidiabetics include blood dyscrasias, hepatotoxicity, and,

---

 Herb/drug　　 Do Not Crush　　 Alert　　 Key Drug　　 Geriatric　　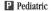 Pediatric rarely, cholestatic jaundice. Adverse reactions for insulin products include allergic responses and, more rarely, anaphylaxis.

Contraindications: Hypersensitive reactions may occur, and allergies should be identified before these products are given. Oral antidiabetics should not be used in juvenile or brittle diabetes, diabetic ketoacidosis, severe renal disease, or severe hepatic disease.

G Precautions: Oral antidiabetics should be used with caution in the elderly, in cardiac disease, pregnancy, lactation, and in the presence of alcohol.

Pharmacokinetics: Onset, peak, and duration vary widely among products. Oral antidiabetics are metabolized in the liver, with metabolites excreted in urine, bile, and feces.

Interactions: Interactions vary widely among products. Check individual monograph for specific information.

NURSING CONSIDERATIONS
Assessment
- Monitor blood, urine glucose levels during treatment to determine diabetes control (oral products)
- Monitor fasting blood glucose, 2 hr PP (60-100 mg/dl normal fasting level) (70-130 mg/dl—normal 2-hr level)
- Assess for hypoglycemic reaction that can occur during peak time

Nursing diagnoses
☑ Imbalanced nutrition: more than body requirements (uses)

Implementation
SC Route
- Give insulin after warming to room temp by rotating in palms to prevent lipodystrophy from injecting cold insulin
- Give human insulin to those allergic to beef or pork
- Rotate inj sites when giving insulin; use abdomen, upper back, thighs, upper arm, buttocks; keep a record of sites

PO Route
- Give oral antidiabetic 30 min ac

Evaluation
- Therapeutic response, including decrease in polyuria, polydipsia, polyphagia, clear sensorium, absence of dizziness, stable gait

Patient/family education
- Advise patient to avoid alcohol and salicylates except on advice of prescriber
- Teach patient symptoms of ketoacidosis: nausea, thirst, polyuria, dry mouth, decreased B/P, dry, flushed skin, acetone breath, drowsiness, Kussmaul respirations
- Teach patient symptoms of hypoglycemia: headache, tremors, fatigue, weakness; and that candy or sugar should be carried to treat hypoglycemia
- Advise patient to test urine for glucose/ketones tid if this drug is replacing insulin
- Advise patient to continue weight control, dietary restrictions, exercise, hygiene

Selected Generic Names

acetohexamide
chlorpropamide
glipizide
glyburide
◆π insulin, isophane suspension (high alert)
insulin, lispro (high alert)
◆π insulin, regular (high alert)
◆π insulin, regular concentrated (high alert)
insulin, zinc suspension (Ultralente) (high alert)

insulin, zinc suspension (Lente) (high alert)
metformin
miglitol
pioglitazone
repaglinide
rosiglitazone
tolazamide
tolbutamide

ANTIDIARRHEALS

Action: Antidiarrheals work by various actions including direct action on intestinal muscles to decrease GI peristalsis; or by inhibiting prostaglandin synthesis responsible for GI hypermotility; acting on mucosal receptors responsible for peristalsis; or decreasing water content of stools.

Uses: Antidiarrheals are used for diarrhea of undetermined causes.

Adverse effects: The most serious adverse reactions of some products are paralytic ileus, toxic megacolon, and angioneurotic edema. The most common side effects are constipation, nausea, dry mouth, and abdominal pain.

Contraindications: Persons with severe ulcerative colitis, pseudomembranous colitis with some products.

G P Precautions: Antidiarrheal should be used with caution in the elderly, pregnancy, lactation, children, dehydration.

Pharmacokinetics: Onset, peak, and duration vary widely among products. Most products are metabolized in the liver and excreted in urine.

Interactions: Please check individual monographs, since interactions vary widely among products.

NURSING CONSIDERATIONS
Assessment
- Monitor electrolytes (potassium, sodium, chloride) if on long-term therapy
- Monitor bowel pattern before; for rebound constipation after termination of medication
- Assess response after 48 hr; if no response, drug should be discontinued
- **P** Identify dehydration in children

Nursing diagnoses
✓ Diarrhea (uses)
✓ Constipation (adverse reactions)
✓ Deficient fluid volume (adverse reactions)
✓ Deficient knowledge (teaching)

Implementation
PO Route
- Give for 48 hr only

Evaluation
- Therapeutic response: decreased diarrhea

 Herb/drug   Do Not Crush   Alert   Key Drug   Geriatric   Pediatric

Patient/family education
- Advise patient to avoid OTC products
- Caution patient not to exceed recommended dose

Selected Generic Names
bismuth subsalicylate

difenoxin

kaolin/pectin

loperamide

ANTIDYSRHYTHMICS

Action: Antidysrhythmics are divided into four classes and miscellaneous antidysrhythmics:
- Class I increases the action potential duration and the effective refractory period and reduces disparity in the refractory period between a normal and infarcted myocardium; further subclasses include Ia, Ib, Ic
- Class II decreases the rate of SA node discharge, increases recovery time, slows conduction through the AV node, and decreases heart rate, which decreases O_2 consumption in the myocardium
- Class III increases the action potential duration and the effective refractory period
- Class IV inhibits calcium ion influx across the cell membrane during cardiac depolarization; decreases SA node discharge, decreases conduction velocity through the AV node
- Miscellaneous antidysrhythmics include those such as adenosine, which slows conduction through the AV node, and digoxin, which decreases conduction velocity and prolongs the effective refractory period in the AV node

Uses: These products are used for PVCs, tachycardia, hypertension, atrial fibrillation, angina pectoris.

Adverse effects: Side effects and adverse reactions vary widely among products.

Contraindications: Contraindications vary widely among products.

Precautions: Precautions vary widely among products.

Pharmacokinetics: Onset, peak, and duration vary widely among products.

Interactions: Interactions vary widely among products; check individual monograph for specific information.

NURSING CONSIDERATIONS
Assessment
- Monitor ECG continuously to determine drug effectiveness, PVCs, or other dysrhythmias
- Assess for dehydration or hypovolemia
- Monitor B/P continuously for hypotension, hypertension
- Monitor I&O ratio
- Monitor serum potassium
- Assess for edema in feet and legs daily

Nursing diagnoses
☑ Altered tissue perfusion: cardiopulmonary (uses)
☑ Decreased cardiac output (uses)
☑ Diarrhea (adverse reactions)
☑ Impaired gas exchange (adverse reactions)

Evaluation
- Therapeutic response, including decrease in B/P in hypertension, decreased B/P, edema, moist rales in CHF

Patient/family education

- Advise patient to comply with dosage schedule, even if patient is feeling better
- Instruct patient to report bradycardia, dizziness, confusion, depression, fever

---

Selected Generic Names

Class I:
moricizine

Class Ia:
disopyramide
◆π procainamide
◆π quinidine

Class Ib:
lidocaine (high alert)
mexiletine
◆π phenytoin
tocainide

Class Ic:
flecainide
indecainide

Class II:
acebutolol
esmolol
◆π **propranolol**
sotalol

Class III:
amiodarone (high alert)
◆π **bretylium** (high alert)
ibutilide (high alert)

Class IV:
◆π verapamil

Miscellaneous:
adenosine (high alert)
atropine (high alert)
◆π **digoxin** (high alert)

ANTIFUNGALS (SYSTEMIC)

Action: Antifungals act by increasing cell membrane permeability in susceptible organisms by binding sterols and decreasing potassium, sodium, and nutrients in the cell.

Uses: Antifungals are used for infections of histoplasmosis, blastomycosis, coccidioidomycosis, cryptococcosis, aspergillosis, phycomycosis, candidiasis, sporotrichosis causing severe meningitis, septicemia, and skin infections.

Adverse effects: The most serious adverse reactions include renal tubular acidosis, permanent renal impairment, anuria, oliguria, hemorrhagic gastroenteritis, acute liver failure, and blood dyscrasias. Some common side effects include hypokalemia, nausea, vomiting, anorexia, headache, fever, and chills.

Contraindications: Persons with severe bone depression or hypersensitivity should not use these products.

Precautions: Antifungals should be used with caution in renal disease, pregnancy, and hepatic disease.

Pharmacokinetics: Onset, peak, and duration vary widely among products. Most products are metabolized in the liver and excreted in urine.

Interactions: Please check individual monographs, since interactions vary widely among products.

NURSING CONSIDERATIONS
Assessment

- Monitor VS q15-30 min during first inf; note changes in pulse, B/P
- Monitor I&O ratio; watch for decreasing urinary output, change in sp gr; discontinue drug to prevent permanent damage to renal tubules
- Monitor blood studies; CBC, potassium, sodium, calcium, magnesium q2 wk
- Monitor weight weekly; if weight increases over 2 lb/wk, edema is present; renal damage should be considered

---

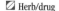 Herb/drug   Ⓢ Do Not Crush   ◆ Alert   ◆π Key Drug   Ⓖ Geriatric   Ⓟ Pediatric

- Assess for renal toxicity: increasing BUN, is >40 mg/dl or if serum creatinine >3 mg/dl; drug may be discontinued or dosage reduced
- Assess for hepatotoxicity: increasing AST, ALT, alkaline phosphatase, bilirubin
- Assess for allergic reaction: dermatitis, rash; drug should be discontinued; antihistamines (mild reaction) or epinephrine (severe reaction) administered
- Assess for hypokalemia: anorexia, drowsiness, weakness, decreased reflexes, dizziness, increased urinary output, increased thirst, paresthesias
- Assess for ototoxicity: tinnitus (ringing, roaring in ears), vertigo, loss of hearing (rare)

Nursing diagnoses
☑ Risk for infection (uses)
☑ Risk for injury (adverse reactions)
☑ Deficient knowledge (teaching)

Implementation
IV IV Route
- Give by **IV** using in-line filter (mean pore diameter >1 μm) using distal veins; check for extravasation, necrosis q8h
- Give drug only after C&S confirms organism, drug needed to treat condition; make sure drug is used in life-threatening infections
- Provide protection from light during inf; cover with foil
- Give symptomatic treatment as ordered for adverse reactions: aspirin, antihistamines, antiemetics, antispasmodics
- Store protected from moisture and light; diluted sol is stable for 24 hr

Evaluation
- Therapeutic response: decreased fever, malaise, rash, negative C&S for infecting organism

Patient/family education
- Teach patient that long-term therapy may be needed to clear infection (2 wk-3 mo depending on type of infection)

Selected Generic Names

amphotericin B
fluconazole
griseofulvin
itraconazole

ketoconazole
nystatin
voriconazole

ANTIHISTAMINES

Action: Antihistamines compete with histamines for H_1 receptor sites. They antagonize in varying degrees most of the pharmacologic effects of histamines.

Uses: Products are used to control the symptoms of allergies, rhinitis, and pruritus.

Adverse effects: Most products cause drowsiness; however, two of the newer products, loratadine and fexofenadine, produce little, if any, drowsiness. Other common side effects are headache and thickening of bronchial secretions. Serious blood dyscrasias may occur, but are rare. Urinary retention, GI effects occur with many of these products.

Contraindications: Hypersensitivity to H_1-receptor antagonists occurs rarely. Patients with acute asthma and lower respiratory tract disease should not use these products, since thick secretions may result. Other contraindications include narrow-angle glaucoma, bladder neck P obstruction, stenosing peptic ulcer, symptomatic prostatic hypertrophy, newborn, lactation.

Precautions: These products must be used cautiously in conjunction with intraocular pressure, since they increase intraocular pressure. Caution should also be used in patients with renal and **G** cardiac disease, hypertension, and seizure disorders, pregnancy, lactation, and in the elderly.

Pharmacokinetics: Onset varies from 20-60 min, with duration lasting 4-12 hr. In general, pharmacokinetics vary widely among products.

Interactions: Barbiturates, opioids, hypnotics, tricyclic antidepressants, and alcohol can increase CNS depression when taken with antihistamines.

NURSING CONSIDERATIONS
Assessment

- Check I&O ratio; be alert for urinary retention, frequency, dysuria; drug should be discontinued if these occur
- Assess for blood dyscrasias: thrombocytopenia, agranulocytosis (rare)
- Assess for respiratory status, including rate rhythm, increase in bronchial secretions, wheezing, chest tightness
- Assess for cardiac status, including palpitations, increased pulse, hypotension
- Assess CBC during long-term therapy, since hemolytic anemia, although rare, may occur
- Administer with food or milk to decrease GI symptoms; absorption may be decreased slightly
- Administer whole (sus rel tab)
- Provide hard candy, gum, frequent rinsing of mouth for dryness

Nursing diagnoses
☑ Ineffective airway clearance (uses)

Evaluation
- Therapeutic response: absence of allergy symptoms, itching

Patient/family education
- Advise patient to notify prescriber if confusion, sedation, hypotension occur
- Caution patient to avoid driving and other hazardous activity if drowsiness occurs
- Instruct patient to avoid concurrent use of alcohol and other CNS depressants
- Inform patient to discontinue a few days before skin testing

---

Selected Generic Names

azatadine	desloratadine
brompheniramine	✆ℼ diphenhydramine
cetirizine	fexofenadine
chlorpheniramine	loratadine
cyproheptadine	promethazine

ANTIHYPERTENSIVES

Action: Antihypertensives are divided into angiotensin converting enzyme (ACE) inhibitors, β-adrenergic blockers, calcium channel blockers, centrally acting adrenergics, diuretics, peripherally acting antiadrenergics, and vasodilators. β-Blockers, calcium channel blockers, and diuretics are discussed in separate sections. ACE inhibitors selectively suppress conversion of renin-angiotensin I to angiotensin II; dilatation of arterial and venous vessels occurs. Centrally acting adrenergics act by inhibiting the sympathetic vasomotor center in the CNS, which reduces impulses in the sympathetic nervous system; blood pressure, pulse rate, and cardiac output decrease. Peripherally acting antiadrenergics inhibit sympathetic vasoconstriction by inhibiting release of norepinephrine and/or depleting norepinephrine stores in adrenergic nerve endings.

☑ Herb/drug   ⊘ Do Not Crush   ✦ Alert   ✆ℼ Key Drug   **G** Geriatric   **P** Pediatric

Vasodilators act on arteriolar smooth muscle by producing direct relaxation or vasodilatation; a reduction in blood pressure, with concomitant increases in heart rate and cardiac output, occurs.

Uses: Used for hypertension and for heart failure not responsive to conventional therapy. Some products are used in hypertensive crisis, angina, and for some cardiac dysrhythmias.

Adverse effects: The most common side effects are marked hypotension, bradycardia, tachycardia, headache, nausea, and vomiting. Side effects and adverse reactions may vary widely between classes and specific products.

Contraindications: Hypersensitive reactions may occur, and allergies should be identified before these products are given. Antihypertensives should not be used in patients with heart block **P** or in children.

G **Precautions:** Antihypertensives should be used with caution in the elderly, in dialysis patients, and in the presence of hypovolemia, leukemia, and electrolyte imbalances.

Pharmacokinetics: Onset, peak, and duration vary widely among products. Most products are metabolized in the liver, with metabolites excreted in urine, bile, and feces.

Interactions: Interactions vary widely among products; check individual monograph for specific information.

NURSING CONSIDERATIONS
Assessment
- Monitor blood studies: neutrophil; decreased platelets occur with many of the products
- Monitor renal studies: protein, BUN, creatinine; watch for increased levels, which may indicate nephrotic syndrome; obtain baselines in renal and liver function studies before beginning treatment
- Assess for edema in feet and legs daily
- Identify allergic reaction, including rash, fever, pruritus, urticaria: drug should be discontinued if antihistamines fail to help
- Identify symptoms of CHF: edema, dyspnea, wet rales, B/P
- Assess for renal symptoms: polyuria, oliguria, frequency

Nursing diagnoses
☑ Altered tissue perfusion (uses)
☑ Decreased cardiac output (uses)
☑ Diarrhea (adverse reactions)
☑ Impaired gas exchange (adverse reactions)

Implementation
- Place patient in supine or Trendelenburg position for severe hypotension

Evaluation
- Therapeutic response: decrease in B/P in hypotension; decreased B/P, edema, moist rales in CHF

Patient/family education
- Instruct patient to comply with dosage schedule, even if feeling better
- Advise patient to rise slowly to sitting or standing position to minimize orthostatic hypotension

Selected Generic Names

ACE inhibitors:
benazepril
captopril
enalapril
esoprostenol
fosinopril
lisinopril
quinapril
ramipril
spirapril
trandolapril

Angiotension II receptors:
candesartan
eprosartan
irbesartan
losartan
telmisartan
valsartan

*Centrally acting
adrenergics:*
◆π clonidine
methyldopa

Peripherally acting antiadrenergics:
doxazosin
◆π prazosin
reserpine
terazosin

Vasodilators:
diazoxide
fenoldopam
hydralazine
minoxidil
nitroprusside (high alert)

Antidrenergic:
Combined α/β-blocker: labetalol

ANTIINFECTIVES

Action: Antiinfectives are divided into several groups, which include but are not limited to penicillins, cephalosporins, aminoglycosides, sulfonamides, tetracyclines, monobactam, erythromycins, and quinolones. These drugs inhibit the growth and replication of susceptible bacterial organisms.

Uses: Used for infections of susceptible organisms. These products are effective against bacterial, rickettsial, and spirochete infections.

Adverse effects: The most common side effects are nausea, vomiting, and diarrhea. Adverse reactions include bone marrow depression and anaphylaxis.

Contraindications: Hypersensitive reactions may occur, and allergies should be identified before these products are given. Cross-sensitivity can occur between products of different classes (penicillins or cephalosporins). Often persons allergic to penicillins are also allergic to cephalosporins.

Precautions: Antiinfectives should be used with caution in persons with renal and liver disease.

Pharmacokinetics: Onset, peak, and duration vary widely among products. Most products are metabolized in the liver, and metabolites are excreted in urine, bile, and feces.

Interactions: Interactions vary widely among products; check individual monograph for specific information.

NURSING CONSIDERATIONS
Assessment

* Assess for nephrotoxicity, including increased BUN, creatinine
* Monitor blood studies: AST, ALT, CBC, Hct, bilirubin; test monthly if patient is on long-term therapy
* Monitor bowel pattern qd; if severe diarrhea occurs, drug should be discontinued
* Monitor urine output; if decreasing, notify prescriber; may indicate nephrotoxicity
* Assess for allergic reaction, including rash, fever, pruritus, urticaria; drug should be discontinued

 Herb/drug   Do Not Crush   Alert   Key Drug   Geriatric   P Pediatric

- Assess for bleeding: ecchymosis, bleeding gums, hematuria, stool guaiac daily
- Assess for overgrowth of infection: perineal itching, fever, malaise, redness, pain, swelling, drainage, rash, diarrhea, change in cough, sputum

Nursing diagnoses
☑ Risk for infection (uses)
☑ Diarrhea (adverse reactions)

Implementation
- Give for 10-14 days to ensure organism death, prevention of superinfection
- Give after C&S completed; drug may be taken as soon as culture is obtained

Evaluation
- Therapeutic response: absence of fever, fatigue, malaise, draining wounds

Patient/family education
- Teach patient to comply with dosage schedule, even if feeling better
- Advise patient to report sore throat, bruising, bleeding, joint pain; may indicate blood dyscrasias (rare)

Selected Generic Names

Aminoglycosides:
amikacin
gentamicin
kanamycin
neomycin
netilmicin
tobramycin

Cephalosporins:
cefaclor
cefadroxil
cefamandole
cefazolin
cefdinir
cefditoren
cefepime
cefixime
cefmetazole
cefonicid
cefoperazone
ceforanide
cefotaxime
cefprozil
ceftibuten
cefuroximine
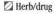 cephalexin
cephalothin
cephapirin
cephradine
moxalactam

Fluoroquinolones:
alatrofloxacin
ciprofloxacin
gemifloxacin (Appx A)
levofloxacin
lomefloxacin
norfloxacin
ofloxacin
sparfloxacin
trovafloxacin

Macrolides:
azithromycin
clarithromycin
erythromycin

Miscellaneous:
daptomycin (Appx A)
ertapenem
meropenem

Penicillins:
amoxicillin/clavulanate
ampicillin/sulbactam
cloxacillin
dicloxacillin
imipenem/cilastatin
methicillin
mezlocillin
nafcillin
oxacillin
penicillin G benzathine
penicillin G potassium
penicillin G procaine
penicillin V
piperacillin
ticarcillin/clavulanate

Sulfonamides:
sulfasalazine
sulfisoxazole

Tetracyclines:
doxycycline
minocycline
tetracycline

ANTINEOPLASTICS

Action: Antineoplastics are divided into alkylating agents, antimetabolites, antibiotic agents, hormonal agents, and miscellaneous agents. Alkylating agents act by cross-linking strands of DNA. Antimetabolites act by inhibiting DNA synthesis. Antibiotic agents act by inhibiting RNA synthesis and by delaying or inhibiting mitosis. Hormones alter the effect of androgens, luteinizing hormone, follicle-stimulating hormone, or estrogen by changing the hormonal environment.

Uses: Uses vary widely among products and classes of drugs. They are used to treat leukemia, Hodgkin's disease, lymphomas, and other tumors throughout the body.

▨ Herb/drug   Ⓢ Do Not Crush   ◆ Alert   ◆ᴛᴛ Key Drug   Ⓖ Geriatric   Ⓟ Pediatric

Adverse effects: Most products cause thrombocytopenia, leukopenia, and anemia, and, if these reactions occur, the drug may need to be stopped until the problem is corrected. Other side effects include nausea, vomiting, glossitis, and hair loss. Some products also cause hepatotoxicity, nephrotoxicity, and cardiotoxicity.

Contraindications: Hypersensitive reactions may occur, and allergies should be identified before these products are given. Also, persons with severe liver and kidney disease should not use these products unless the benefits outweigh the risks.

Precautions: Persons with bleeding, severe bone marrow depression, or renal or hepatic disease should be watched closely.

Pharmacokinetics: Onset, peak, and duration vary widely among products. Most products cross the placenta and are excreted in breast milk and in urine.

Interactions: Toxicity may occur when used with other antineoplastics or radiation.

NURSING CONSIDERATIONS
Assessment
- Monitor CBC, differential, platelet count weekly; withhold drug if WBC is <4000 or platelet count is <75,000; notify prescriber of results
- Monitor renal function studies, including BUN, creatinine, serum uric acid, and urine creatinine clearance before and during therapy
- Monitor I&O ratio; report fall in urine output of 30 ml/hr
- Monitor temp q4h (may indicate beginning infection)
- Monitor liver function tests before and during therapy (bilirubin, AST, ALT, LDH) prn or monthly
- Assess for bleeding, including hematuria, guaiac, bruising or petechiae, mucosa, or orifices q8h; obtain prescription for viscous lidocaine (Xylocaine)
- Identify jaundice of skin, sclera, dark urine, clay-colored stools, itchy skin, abdominal pain, fever, diarrhea
- Assess for edema in feet, joint pain, stomach pain, shaking
- Assess for inflammation of mucosa, breaks in skin

Nursing diagnoses
☑Risk for infection (adverse reactions)
☑Imbalanced nutrition: less than body requirements (adverse reactions)
☑Altered oral mucous membrane (adverse reactions)

Implementation
- Check **IV** site for irritation; phlebitis
- Have epinephrine available for hypersensitivity reaction
- Give antibiotics for prophylaxis of infection
- Provide strict medical asepsis, protective isolation if WBC levels are low
- Provide comprehensive oral hygiene, using careful technique and soft-bristle brush

Evaluation
- Therapeutic response: decreased tumor size

Patient/family education
- Advise patient to report signs of infection, including increased temp, sore throat, malaise
- Instruct patient to report signs of anemia, including fatigue, headache, faintness, shortness of breath, irritability
- Instruct patient to report bleeding and to avoid use of razors and commercial mouthwash

Selected Generic Names

Alkylating agents:
busulfan (high alert)
carboplatin (high alert)
carmustine (high alert)
chlorambucil
cisplatin (high alert)
◆π cyclophosphamide (high alert)
dacarbazine (high alert)
lomustine
mechlorethamine
melphalan (high alert)
thiotepa

Antimetabolites:
capecitabine
cytarabine (high alert)
etoposide (high alert)
fludarabine
fluorouracil (high alert)
mercaptopurine
thioguanine (6-TG)

Antibiotic agents:
◆π bleomycin (high alert)
dactinomycin (high alert)
daunorubicin (high alert)
◆π doxorubicin (high alert)
epirubicin (high alert)
◆π methotrexate (high alert)
mitomycin (high alert)
mitoxantrone (high alert)
plicamycin (high alert)

Hormonal agents:
flutamide
goserelin acetate
irinotecan (high alert)
leuprolide (high alert)
megestrol
mitotane
nilutamide
tamoxifen
testolactone
topotecan (high alert)

Miscellaneous agents:
alemtuzumab
altretamine
anastrozole
arsenic trioxide
asparaginase (high alert)
bortezomib (Appx A)
cladribine
gefitinib (Appx A)
gemcitabine
imatinib
interferon alfa-2A,
interferon alfa-2B
irinotecan (high alert)
pentostatin (high alert)
porfimer
procarbazine
rituximab
vinblastine (high alert)
◆π vincristine (high alert)

ANTIPARKINSONIAN AGENTS

Action: Antiparkinsonian agents are divided into cholinergics and dopamine agonists. Cholinergics work by the blocking or competing at central acetylcholine receptors; dopamine agonists work by decarboxylation to dopamine or by activation of dopamine receptors; monoamine oxidase type B inhibitors increase dopamine activity by inhibiting MAO type B activity.

Uses: These agents are used alone or in combination for patients with Parkinson's disease.

Adverse effects: Side effects and adverse reactions vary widely among products. The most common side effects include involuntary movements, headache, numbness, insomnia, nightmares, nausea, vomiting, dry mouth, and orthostatic hypotension.

Contraindications: Persons with hypersensitivity, narrow-angle glaucoma, and undiagnosed skin lesions should not use these products.

Precautions: Antiparkinsonian agents should be used with caution in pregnancy, lactation, P children, renal, cardiac, hepatic disease, and affective disorder.

Pharmacokinetics: Onset, peak, and duration vary widely among products. Most products are metabolized in the liver and excreted in urine.

☑ Herb/drug   Ⓢ Do Not Crush   ◆ Alert   ◆π Key Drug   Ⓖ Geriatric   P Pediatric

Interactions: Please check individual monographs, since interactions vary widely among products.

NURSING CONSIDERATIONS
Assessment
- Monitor B/P, respiration
- Assess mental status: affect, behavioral changes, depression, complete suicide assessment

Nursing diagnoses
☑ Risk for injury (uses)
☑ Risk for impaired mobility (uses)
☑ Deficient knowledge (teaching)

Implementation
- Give drug up until NPO before surgery
- Adjust dosage depending on patient response
- Give with meals; limit protein taken with drug
- Give only after MAOIs have been discontinued for 2 wk
- Assist with ambulation, during beginning therapy if needed
- Test for diabetes mellitus and acromegaly if on long-term therapy

Evaluation
- Therapeutic response: decrease in akathisia, improvement in mood

Patient/family education
- Advise patient to change positions slowly to prevent orthostatic hypotension
- Instruct patient to report side effects: twitching, eye spasm; indicate overdose
- Advise patient to use drug exactly as prescribed; if drug is discontinued abruptly, parkinsonian crisis may occur

Selected Generic Names

benztropine
biperiden
bromocriptine
cabergoline
carbidopa-levodopa

levodopa
pramipexole
procyclidine
selegiline
tolcapone
trihexyphenidyl

ANTIPSYCHOTICS

Action: Antipsychotics/neuroleptics are divided into several subgroups: phenothiazines, thioxanthenes, butyrophenones, dibenzoxazepines, dibenzodiazepines, and indolones and other heterocyclic compounds. Although chemically different, these subgroups share many pharmacologic and clinical properties. All antipsychotics work to block postsynaptic dopamine receptors in the brain that are responsible for psychotic behavior, including hallucinations, delusions, and paranoia.

Uses: Antipsychotic behavior is decreased in conditions such as schizophrenia, paranoia, and mania. These agents are also effective for severe anxiety, intractable hiccups, nausea, vomiting, behavioral problems in children, and before surgery for relaxation.

Adverse effects: The most common side effects include extrapyramidal symptoms (EPS) such as pseudoparkinsonism, akathisia, dystonia, and tardive dyskinesia, which may be controlled by use of antiparkinsonian agents. Serious adverse reactions such as hypotension, agranulocytosis, cardiac arrest, and laryngospasm have occurred. Other common side effects include dry mouth and photosensitivity.

Contraindications: Persons with liver damage, severe hypertension or coronary disease, cerebral arteriosclerosis, blood dyscrasias, bone marrow depression, parkinsonism, severe **P** depression, or narrow-angle glaucoma, children <12 yr, or persons withdrawing from alcohol or barbiturates should not use antipsychotics until these conditions are corrected.

G **Precautions:** Caution must be used when antipsychotics are given to the elderly, since metabolism is slowed and adverse reactions can occur rapidly. Hepatic and renal disease may cause poor metabolism and excretion of the drug. Seizure threshold is decreased with these products; increases in the dose of anticonvulsants may be required. Persons with diabetes mellitus, prostatic hypertrophy, chronic respiratory disease, and peptic ulcer disease should be monitored closely.

Pharmacokinetics: Onset, peak, and duration vary widely with different products and routes. Products are metabolized by the liver, are excreted in urine as metabolites, are highly bound to plasma proteins, cross the placenta, and enter breast milk. Half-life can be extended over 3 days.

Interactions: Because other CNS depressants can cause oversedation, these combinations should be used carefully. Anticholinergics may decrease the therapeutic actions of phenothiazines and also cause increased anticholinergic effects.

NURSING CONSIDERATIONS
Assessment
- Monitor bilirubin, CBC, liver function studies monthly, since these drugs are metabolized in the liver and excreted in urine
- Monitor I&O ratio: palpate bladder if low urinary output occurs, since urinary retention occurs with many of these products
- Assess affect, orientation, LOC, reflexes, gait, coordination, sleep pattern disturbances
- Assess dizziness, faintness, palpitations, tachycardia on rising
- Check B/P with patient lying and standing; wide fluctuations between lying and standing B/P may require dosage or product change, since orthostatic hypotension is occurring
- Assess for EPS, including akathisia, tardive dyskinesia, pseudoparkinsonism

Nursing diagnoses
☑ Altered thought processes (uses)
☑ Disturbed sensory perception (uses)

Implementation
- Give antiparkinsonian agent if EPS occur
- Administer liq conc mixed in glass of juice or cola, since taste is unpleasant; avoid contact with skin when preparing liq conc or parenteral medications
- Supervise ambulation until stabilized on medication; do not involve in strenuous exercise program, since fainting is possible; patient should not stand still for long periods
- Increase fluids to prevent constipation
- Give sips of water, candy, gum for dry mouth

Evaluation
- Therapeutic response: decrease in excitement, hallucinations, delusions, paranoia, reorganization of thought patterns, speech

Patient/family education
- Advise patient to rise from sitting or lying position gradually, since fainting may occur
- Instruct patient to remain lying down for at least 30 min after IM inj
- Caution patient to avoid hot tubs, hot showers, or tub baths, since hypotension may occur

---

 Herb/drug   ⊘ Do Not Crush   ◆ Alert   ◆ₜₜ Key Drug   **G** Geriatric   **P** Pediatric

- Advise patient to wear sunscreen or protective clothing to prevent burns
- Advise patient to take extra precautions during hot weather to stay cool; heat stroke can occur
- Caution patient to avoid driving and other activities requiring alertness until response to medication is known
- Inform patient that drowsiness or impaired mental/motor activity is evident the first 2 wk, but tends to decrease over time

Selected Generic Names

Phenothiazines:
◆π chlorpromazine
fluphenazine
perphenazine
prochlorperazine
thioridazine
thiothixene
trifluoperazine

Butyrophenone:
◆π haloperidol

Miscellaneous:
loxapine
molindone
olanzapine
quetiapine
risperidone

ANTITUBERCULARS

Action: Antituberculars act by inhibiting RNA or DNA, or interfering with lipid and protein synthesis, thereby decreasing tubercle bacilli replication.

Uses: Antituberculars are used for pulmonary tuberculosis.

Adverse effects: They vary widely among products. Most products can cause nausea, vomiting, anorexia, and rash. Serious adverse reactions include renal failure, nephrotoxicity, ototoxicity, and hepatic necrosis.

Contraindications: Persons with severe renal disease or hypersensitivity should not use these products.

Precautions: Antituberculars should be used with caution in pregnancy, lactation, and hepatic disease.

Pharmacokinetics: Onset, peak, and duration vary widely among products. Most products are metabolized in the liver and excreted in urine.

Interactions: Please check individual monographs, since interactions vary widely among products.

NURSING CONSIDERATIONS
Assessment
- Assess for signs of anemia: Hct, Hgb, fatigue
- Monitor liver studies weekly: ALT, AST, bilirubin
- Monitor renal status before treatment and monthly thereafter: BUN, creatinine, output, sp gr, urinalysis
- Monitor hepatic status: decreased appetite, jaundice, dark urine, fatigue

Nursing diagnoses
✓ Risk for infection (uses)
✓ Risk for injury (adverse reactions)
✓ Deficient knowledge (teaching)
✓ Noncompliance (teaching)

Implementation
- Give some of these agents on empty stomach, 1 hr ac (only for isoniazid and rifampin) or 2 hr pc
- Give antiemetic if vomiting occurs
- Give after C&S is completed; monthly to detect resistance

Evaluation
- Therapeutic response: decreased symptoms of TB, culture negative

Patient/family education
- Teach patient that compliance with dosage schedule, duration is necessary
- Teach patient that scheduled appointments must be kept; relapse may occur
- Advise patient to avoid alcohol while taking drug
- Advise patient to report flulike symptoms: excessive fatigue, anorexia, vomiting, sore throat; unusual bleeding, yellowish discoloration of skin/eyes

---

Selected Generic Names

ethambutol

⚷ isoniazid

pyrazinamide

rifabutin

rifampin

streptomycin

ANTITUSSIVES/EXPECTORANTS

Action: Antitussives suppress the cough reflex by direct action on the cough center in the medulla. Expectorants act by liquefying and reducing the viscosity of thick, tenacious secretions.

Uses: Antitussives/expectorants are used to treat cough occurring in pneumonia, bronchitis, TB, cystic fibrosis, and emphysema; as an adjunct in atelectasis (expectorants); and for nonproductive cough (antitussives).

Adverse effects: The most common side effects are drowsiness, dizziness, and nausea.

Contraindications: Some products are contraindicated in hypothyroidism, iodine sensitivity, pregnancy, and lactation.

G Precautions: Some products should be used cautiously in asthma, elderly, and debilitated patients.

Pharmacokinetics: Onset, peak, and duration vary widely among products. Some products are metabolized in the liver and excreted in urine.

Interactions: Please check individual monographs, since interactions vary widely among products.

NURSING CONSIDERATIONS
Assessment
- Assess cough: type, frequency, character including sputum

Nursing diagnoses:
- ✓ Ineffective breathing pattern (uses)
- ✓ Ineffective airway clearance (uses)
- ✓ Deficient knowledge (teaching)

 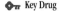

Implementation

G • Give decreased dosage to elderly patients; their metabolism may be slowed
- Increase fluids to liquefy secretions
- Humidify patient's room

Evaluation
- Therapeutic response: absence of cough

Patient/family education
- Advise patient to avoid driving and other hazardous activities until stabilized on this medication
- Caution patient to avoid smoking, smoke-filled rooms, perfumes, dust, environmental pollutants, cleaners that increase cough

---

Selected Generic Names

◆π acetylcysteine   guaifenesin
◆π codeine   hydrocodone
   dextromethorphan   potassium iodide
◆π diphenhydramine

ANTIVIRALS/ANTIRETROVIRALS

Action: Antivirals/antiretrovirals act by interfering with DNA synthesis that is needed for viral replication.

Uses: Antivirals/antiretrovirals are used for mucocutaneous herpes simplex virus, herpes genitalis (HSV_1, HSV_2), advanced HIV infections, herpes simplex virus encephalitis, varicella-zoster encephalomyelitis.

Adverse effects: Serious adverse reactions are fatal metabolic encephalopathy, blood dyscrasias, and acute renal failure. Common side effects are nausea, vomiting, anorexia, diarrhea, headache, vaginitis, and moniliasis.

Contraindications: Persons with hypersensitivity and immunosuppressed individuals with herpes zoster should not use these products.

Precautions: Antivirals/antiretrovirals should be used with caution in renal disease, liver disease, lactation, pregnancy, and dehydration.

Pharmacokinetics: Onset, peak, and duration vary widely among products. Most products are metabolized in the liver and excreted in urine.

Interactions: Please check individual monographs, since interactions vary widely among products.

NURSING CONSIDERATIONS
Assessment
- Assess for signs of infection, anemia
- Monitor I&O ratio; report hematuria, oliguria, fatigue, weakness; may indicate nephrotoxicity; check for protein in urine during treatment
- Monitor any patient with compromised renal system, since drug is excreted slowly in poor renal system function; toxicity may occur rapidly
- Check liver studies: AST, ALT
- Check blood studies: WBC, RBC, Hct, Hgb, bleeding time; blood dyscrasias may occur; drug should be discontinued
- Check renal studies: urinalysis, protein, BUN, creatinine, CCr

---

- Obtain C&S before drug therapy; drug may be taken as soon as culture is obtained; repeat C&S after treatment
- Assess bowel pattern before, during treatment; if severe abdominal pain with bleeding occurs, drug should be discontinued
- Identify skin eruptions: rash, urticaria, itching
- Assess for allergies before treatment, reaction of each medication; place allergies on chart

Nursing diagnoses
✓Risk for infection (uses)
✓Risk for injury (adverse reactions)
✓Deficient knowledge (teaching)

Implementation
- Give increased fluids to 3 L/day to decrease crystalluria when given IB
- Store at room temp for up to 12 hr after reconstitution
- Give adequate intake of fluids (2000 ml) to prevent deposit in kidneys

Evaluation
- Therapeutic response: absence of or control of infection

Patient/family education
- Inform patient that drug does not cure infection, just controls symptoms
- Instruct patient to report sore throat, fever, fatigue; could indicate superinfection
- Advise patient that drug must be taken in equal intervals around the clock to maintain blood levels for duration of therapy
- Advise patient to notify prescriber of side effects of bruising, bleeding, fatigue, malaise; may indicate blood dyscrasias

---

Selected Generic Names

abacavir
◆π acyclovir
atazanvir (Appx A)
cidofovir
delavirdine
didanosine
emtricitabine (Appx A)
enfuvirtide (Appx A)
famciclovir
fosamprenavir (Appx A)
foscarnet
ganciclovir
idoxuridine

indinavir
nelfinavir
nevirapine
rimantadine
ritonavir
saquinavir
stavudine
tenofovir
valganciclovir
vidarabine
zalcitabine
◆π zidovudine

BARBITURATES

Action: Barbiturates act by decreasing impulse transmission to the cerebral cortex.
Uses: All forms of epilepsy can be controlled, since the seizure threshold is increased. Uses also
P include febrile seizures in children, sedation, insomnia, hyperbilirubinemia, chronic cholestasis with some of these products. Ultra–short-acting barbiturates are used as anesthetics.

 Herb/drug   Do Not Crush   ◆ Alert   ◆π Key Drug   **G** Geriatric   **P** Pediatric

Adverse effects: The most common side effects are drowsiness and nausea. Serious adverse reactions such as Stevens-Johnson syndrome and blood dyscrasias may occur with high doses and long-term treatment.

Contraindications: Hypersensitivity may occur, and allergies should be identified before administering. Barbiturates are identified as pregnancy category **D** and should not be used in pregnancy. Other contraindications include porphyria and marked impairment of liver function.

Precautions: Caution must be used when these products are given to the elderly or debilitated; usually smaller doses are needed, since metabolism is slowed. Persons with renal and hepatic disease may show delayed excretion. Barbiturates may produce excitability in children.

Pharmacokinetics: Onset of action can be slow, up to 1 hr, with a peak of 8 hr and a duration of 3-10 hr. These drugs are metabolized by the liver, excreted by the kidneys, cross the placenta, and enter breast milk.

Interactions: Increased CNS depressant effect may occur with alcohol, MAOIs, sedatives, or opioids. These products should be used together cautiously. Oral anticoagulants, corticosteroids, griseofulvin, quinidine, oral contraceptives, and theophylline may show a decreased effect when used with barbiturates.

NURSING CONSIDERATIONS
Assessment
- Monitor hepatic and renal studies: AST, ALT, bilirubin, creatinine, LDH, alkaline phosphatase, BUN if patient is on long-term therapy, since these products are metabolized and excreted by the liver and kidney
- Monitor blood studies: CBC, hematocrit, hemoglobin, and prothrombin time if patient is on long-term therapy, since these products increase the possibility of bleeding and blood dyscrasias
- Identify barbiturate toxicity: hypotension, pulmonary constriction, cold, clammy skin, cyanosis of lips, insomnia, nausea, vomiting, hallucinations, delirium, weakness

Nursing diagnoses
☑Disturbed sleep pattern (uses)
☑Risk for injury (adverse reactions)

Evaluation
- Therapeutic response: appropriate sedation or seizure control

Patient/family education
- Inform patient that physical dependency may result when used for extended periods (45-90 days, depending on dosage)
- Advise patient to avoid driving and activities that require alertness, since drowsiness and dizziness may occur
- Caution patient to abstain from alcohol and other psychotropic medications unless prescribed by prescriber
- Instruct patient not to discontinue medication abruptly after long-term use; withdrawal symptoms will occur

---

Selected Generic Names
amobarbital

pentobarbital (high alert)

✦π phenobarbital

secobarbital (high alert)

thiopental (high alert)

BENZODIAZEPINES

Action: Benzodiazepines potentiate the effects of GABA, including any other inhibitory transmitters in the CNS, resulting in decreased anxiety.

Uses: Anxiety is relieved in conditions such as phobic disorders. Benzodiazepines are also used for acute alcohol withdrawal to relieve the possibility of delirium tremens, and some products are used before surgery for relaxation.

Adverse effects: The most common side effects are dizziness, drowsiness, blurred vision, and orthostatic hypotension. Most adverse effects are mediated through the CNS. There is a risk for physical dependence and abuse.

P Contraindications: Hypersensitivity, acute narrow-angle glaucoma, children <6 months, liver disease (clonazepam), lactation (diazepam).

G Precautions: Caution must be used when these products are given to the elderly or debilitated; usually smaller dosages are needed, since metabolism is slowed. Persons with renal and hepatic disease may show delayed excretion. Clonazepam may increase incidence of seizures.

Pharmacokinetics: Onset of action is ½-1 hr, with a peak of 1-2 hr and a duration of 4-6 hr. These drugs are metabolized by the liver, excreted by the kidneys, cross the placenta, and enter breast milk.

Interactions: Increased CNS depressant effect may occur with other CNS depressants. These products should be used together cautiously. Alcohol should not be used; fatal reactions can occur. The serum concentration and toxicity of digoxin may be increased.

NURSING CONSIDERATIONS
Assessment
- Monitor B/P (with patient lying, standing), pulse; if systolic B/P drops 20 mm Hg, hold drug, notify prescriber; orthostatic hypotension is severe
- Monitor hepatic and renal studies: AST, ALT, bilirubin, creatinine, LDH, alkaline phosphatase
- Assess for physical dependency, withdrawal symptoms, including headache, nausea, vomiting, muscle pain, weakness after long-term use

Nursing diagnoses
☑ Anxiety (uses)
☑ Risk for injury (adverse reactions)

Implementation
- Give with food or milk for GI symptoms; may give crushed if patient is unable to swallow medication whole

Evaluation
- Therapeutic response: relaxation or decreased anxiety

Patient/family education
- Teach patient that drug should not be used for everyday stress or long term; not to take more than prescribed amount, since drug is habit forming
- Caution patient to avoid driving and activities that require alertness, since drowsiness and dizziness occur
- Caution patient to abstain from alcohol and other psychotropic medications except on advice of prescriber
- Advise patient not to discontinue medication abruptly after long-term use; withdrawal symptoms will occur

 Herb/drug   Do Not Crush   Alert   Key Drug   Geriatric   Pediatric

Selected Generic Names

alprazolam	midazolam
chlordiazepoxide	oxazepam
clonazepam	prazepam
✚πdiazepam	quazepam
flurazepam	temazepam
halazepam	triazolam
lorazepam	

β-ADRENERGIC BLOCKERS

Action: β-Blockers are divided into selective and nonselective blockers. Nonselective blockers produce a fall in blood pressure without reflex tachycardia or reduction in heart rate through a mixture of β-blocking effects; elevated plasma renins are reduced. Selective β-blockers competitively block stimulation of $β_1$-receptors in cardiac smooth muscle; these drugs produce chronotropic and inotropic effects.

Uses: β-Blockers are used for hypertension, ventricular dysrhythmias, and prophylaxis of angina pectoris.

Adverse effects: The most common side effects are orthostatic hypotension, bradycardia, diarrhea, nausea, vomiting. Serious adverse reactions include blood dyscrasias, bronchospasm, and CHF.

Contraindications: Hypersensitive reactions may occur, and allergies should be identified before these products are given. β-Adrenergic blockers should not be used in heart block, CHF, or cardiogenic shock.

G **Precautions:** β-Blockers should be used with caution in the elderly or in renal and thyroid disease, COPD, CAD, diabetes mellitus, pregnancy, or asthma.

Pharmacokinetics: Onset, peak, and duration vary widely among products. Most products are metabolized in the liver, with metabolites excreted in urine, bile, and feces.

Interactions: Interactions vary widely among products; check individual monograph for specific information.

NURSING CONSIDERATIONS
Assessment
- Monitor renal studies, including protein, BUN, creatinine; watch for increased levels that may indicate nephrotic syndrome; obtain baselines in renal and liver function studies before beginning treatment
- Monitor I&O ratio, weight daily
- Monitor B/P during beginning treatment and periodically thereafter, pulse q4h; note rate, rhythm, quality
- Monitor apical/radial pulse before administration; notify prescriber of significant changes
- Check for edema in feet and legs daily

Nursing diagnoses
✓Altered tissue perfusion (uses)
✓Decreased cardiac output (uses)
✓Diarrhea (adverse reactions)
✓Impaired gas exchange (adverse reactions)

Implementation
- Give PO ac, hs; tab may be crushed or swallowed whole
- Give reduced dosage in renal dysfunction

✚ Canada Only ◼ Do Not Confuse * "Tall Man" lettering (See Preface)

Evaluation
- Therapeutic response: decrease in B/P in hypertension; decreased B/P, edema, moist rales in CHF

Patient/family education
- Instruct patient to comply with dosage schedule, even if feeling better
- Caution patient to rise slowly to sitting or standing position to minimize orthostatic hypotension
- Advise patient to report bradycardia, dizziness, confusion, depression, fever
- Teach patient to take pulse at home; advise when to notify prescriber
- Instruct patient to comply with weight control, dietary adjustment, modified exercise program
- Advise patient to wear support hose to minimize effects of orthostatic hypotension
- Advise patient not to discontinue drug abruptly; taper over 2 wk; may precipitate angina

---

Selected Generic Names

Selective β_1-receptor blockers:
acebutolol
atenolol
esmolol
metoprolol

Nonselective β_1 and β_2-blockers:
carteolol

nadolol
pindolol
⬥π propranolol
timolol

Combined α_1, β_1, and β_2-receptor blocker:
labetalol

BRONCHODILATORS

Action: Bronchodilators are divided into anticholinergics, α/β-adrenergic agonists, β-adrenergic agonists, and phosphodiesterase inhibitors. Anticholinergics act by inhibiting interaction of acetylcholine at receptor sites on bronchial smooth muscle; α/β-adrenergic agonists by relaxing bronchial smooth muscle and increasing diameter of nasal passages; β-adrenergic agonists by action on β_2-receptors, which relaxes bronchial smooth muscle; phosphodiesterase inhibitors by blocking phosphodiesterase and increasing cAMP, which mediates smooth muscle relaxation in the respiratory system.

Uses: Bronchodilators are used for bronchial asthma, bronchospasm associated with bronchitis, emphysema, other obstructive pulmonary diseases, and Cheyne-Stokes respirations, as well as prevention of exercise-induced asthma.

Adverse effects: The most common side effects are tremors, anxiety, nausea, vomiting, and irritation in the throat. The most serious adverse reactions include bronchospasm and dyspnea.

Contraindications: Persons with hypersensitivity, narrow-angle glaucoma, tachydysrhythmias, and severe cardiac disease should not use some of these products.

Precautions: Bronchodilators should be used with caution in lactation, pregnancy, hyperthyroidism, hypertension, prostatic hypertrophy, and seizure disorders.

Pharmacokinetics: Onset, peak, and duration vary widely among products. Most products are metabolized in the liver and excreted in urine.

Interactions: Please check individual monographs, since interactions vary widely among products.

NURSING CONSIDERATIONS
Assessment
- Monitor respiratory function: vital capacity, FEV, ABGs, lung sounds, heart rate and rhythm

---

🗹 Herb/drug   🅢 Do Not Crush   ⬥ Alert   ⬥π Key Drug   🅖 Geriatric   🅟 Pediatric

Nursing diagnoses
- ✓Ineffective airway clearance (uses)
- ✓Activity intolerance (uses)
- ✓Risk for injury (adverse reactions)
- ✓Deficient knowledge (teaching)

Implementation
- Give after shaking; exhale, place mouthpiece in mouth, inhale slowly, hold breath, remove, exhale slowly
- Give gum, sips of water for dry mouth
- Give PO with meals to decrease gastric irritation
- Store in light-resistant container; do not expose to temp over 86° F

Evaluation
- Therapeutic response: absence of dyspnea, wheezing

Patient/family education
- Advise patient not to use OTC medications; extra stimulation may occur
- Teach patient use of inhaler; review package insert with patient; to wash inhaler in warm water qd and dry
- Advise patient to avoid getting aerosol in eyes
- Caution patient to avoid smoking, smoke-filled rooms, persons with respiratory tract infections

---

Selected Generic Names

⬥ℼalbuterol
aminophylline
⬥ℼatropine
dyphylline
ephedrine (high alert)
⬥ℼepinephrine (high alert)
formoterol
ipratropium

isoproterenol
levalbuterol
metaproterenol
mibefradil
oxtriphylline
pirbuterol
terbutaline
⬥ℼtheophylline

CALCIUM CHANNEL BLOCKERS

Action: These products inhibit calcium ion influx across the cell membrane in cardiac and vascular smooth muscle. This action produces relaxation of coronary vascular smooth muscle, dilates coronary arteries, slows SA/AV node conduction, and dilates peripheral arteries.

Uses: These products are used for chronic stable angina pectoris, vasospastic angina, dysrhythmias, hypertension, and unstable angina.

Adverse effects: The most common side effects are dysrhythmias and edema. Also common are headache, fatigue, drowsiness, and flushing.

Contraindications: Persons with 2nd- or 3rd-degree heart block, sick sinus syndrome, hypotension of <90 mm Hg systolic, Wolff-Parkinson-White syndrome, or cardiogenic shock should not use these products, since worsening of those conditions may occur.

Precautions: CHF may worsen, since edema may be increased. Hypotension may worsen, since B/P is decreased. Patients with renal and liver disease should use these products cautiously, since they are metabolized in the liver and excreted by the kidneys.

♣ Canada Only   ◩ Do Not Confuse   * "Tall Man" lettering (See Preface)

Pharmacokinetics: Onset, peak, and duration vary widely with route of administration. Drugs are metabolized by the liver and excreted in the urine primarily as metabolites.

Interactions: Increased levels of digoxin and theophylline may occur when used with these products. Increased effects of β-blockers and antihypertensives may occur with calcium channel blockers.

NURSING CONSIDERATIONS
Assessment
• Monitor cardiac system, including B/P, pulse, respirations, ECG intervals (PR, QRS, QT)

Nursing diagnoses
☑Altered tissue perfusion: cardiopulmonary (uses)
☑Decreased cardiac output (adverse reactions)

Implementation
• Give PO ac and hs

Evaluation
• Therapeutic response: decreased anginal pain, decreased B/P, dysrhythmias

Patient/family education
• Teach patient how to take pulse before taking drug; patient should record or graph pulses to identify changes
• Advise patient to avoid hazardous activities until stabilized on this drug, since dizziness occurs frequently
• Inform patient of need for compliance to all areas of medical regimen, including diet, exercise, stress reduction, drug therapy

---

Selected Generic Names
amlodipine	isradipine
bepridil	nicardipine
diltiazem (high alert)	nifedipine
felodipine	◆π verapamil

CARDIAC GLYCOSIDES

Action: Products act by inhibiting sodium and potassium ATPase and then making more calcium available to activate contracted proteins. Cardiac contractility and cardiac output are increased.

Uses: These products are used for CHF, atrial fibrillation, atrial flutter, atrial tachycardia, and rapid digitalization in these disorders.

Adverse effects: The most common side effects are cardiac disturbances, headache, hypotension, GI symptoms. Also common are blurred vision and yellow-green halos.

Contraindications: Hypersensitive reactions may occur, and allergies should be identified before these products are given. Also, persons with ventricular tachycardia, ventricular fibrillation, and carotid sinus syndrome should not use these products.

Precautions: Persons with acute MI and those who have or may develop serum potassium, calcium, or magnesium imbalances should use these products cautiously. Also, persons with AV ⏹ block, severe respiratory disease, hypothyroidism, renal and liver disease, and the elderly should exercise caution when these drugs are prescribed.

Pharmacokinetics: Onset, peak, and duration vary widely with the route of administration.

Digitoxin is inactivated by the liver, and inactive metabolites are excreted in urine. Digoxin is excreted in urine mainly as the parent drug and metabolites.

Interactions: Toxicity may occur when used with diuretics, succinylcholine, quinidine, and thioamines. Increased blood levels may occur with propantheline bromide, spironolactone, quinidine, verapamil, aminoglycosides (PO), amiodarone, anticholinergics, and quinine. Diuretics may increase toxicity.

NURSING CONSIDERATIONS
Assessment
- Montior cardiac system, including B/P, pulse, respirations, and increased urine output
- Monitor apical pulse for 1 min before giving drug; if pulse <60, take again in 1 hr; if <60 notify prescriber
- Monitor electrolytes, including potassium, sodium, chloride, calcium, magnesium; renal function studies, including BUN and creatinine; and blood studies, including AST, ALT, bilirubin
- Monitor I&O ratio, daily weights
- Monitor therapeutic drug levels

Nursing diagnoses
☑ Altered tissue perfusion: cardiopulmonary (uses)
☑ Decreased cardiac output (adverse reactions)

Implementation
- Give potassium supplements if ordered for potassium levels <3

Evaluation
- Therapeutic response: decreased weight, edema, pulse, respiration, and increased urine output

Patient/family education
- Teach patient how to take pulse before taking drug; patient should record or graph pulse to identify changes
- Advise patient to avoid hazardous activities until stabilized on this drug, since dizziness occurs frequently
- Inform patient of need for compliance to all areas of medical regimen, including diet, exercise, stress reduction, drug therapy

---

Selected Generic Names
◆π digoxin (high alert)

CHOLINERGICS

Action: Cholinergics act by preventing destruction of acetylcholine, which increases concentration at sites where acetylcholine is released; this exaggerates the effects of acetylcholine and facilitates transmission of impulses across myoneural junction. Cholinergics may also act by stimulating receptors for acetylcholine.

Uses: Cholinergics are used for myasthenia gravis, as antagonists of nondepolarizing neuromuscular blockade, postoperative bladder distention and urinary distention, postoperative ileus.

Adverse effects: The most serious adverse reactions are respiratory depression, bronchospasm, constriction, laryngospasm, respiratory arrest, convulsions, and paralysis. The most common side effects are nausea, diarrhea, and vomiting.

Contraindications: Persons with obstruction of the intestine or renal system should not use these products.

Precautions: Caution should be used in patients with bradycardia, hypotension, seizure 🅿 disorders, bronchial asthma, coronary occlusion, hyperthyroidism, and in lactation and children.

Pharmacokinetics: Onset, peak, and duration vary widely among products. Most products are metabolized in the liver and excreted in urine.

Interactions: Please check individual monographs since interactions vary widely among products.

NURSING CONSIDERATIONS
Assessment
- Monitor VS, respiration q8h
- Monitor I&O ratio; check for urinary retention or incontinence
- Assess for bradycardia, hypotension, bronchospasm, headache, dizziness, convulsions, respiratory depression; drug should be discontinued if toxicity occurs

Nursing diagnoses
☑ Impaired urinary elimination (uses)
☑ Ineffective breathing pattern (uses)
☑ Deficient knowledge (teaching)
☑ Noncompliance (teaching)

Implementation
- Give only with atropine sulfate available for cholinergic crisis
- Give only after all other cholinergics have been discontinued
- Give increased dosages if tolerance occurs
- Give larger doses after exercise or fatigue
- Give on empty stomach for better absorption
- Store at room temp

Evaluation
- Therapeutic response: increased muscle strength, hand grasp, improved muscle gait, absence of labored breathing (if severe)

Patient/family education
- Inform patient that drug is not a cure; it only relieves symptoms (myasthenia gravis)
- Advise patient to carry/wear emergency ID specifying myasthenia gravis, drugs taken

---

Selected Generic Names

♦🇹 bethanechol
edrophonium
neostigmine

physostigmine
pyridostigmine

CHOLINERGIC BLOCKERS

Action: Cholinergic blockers inhibit or block acetylcholine at receptor sites in the autonomic nervous system.

Uses: Many products are used to decrease secretions before surgery, to reverse neuromuscular blockade, and to decrease motility of GI, biliary, urinary tracts. Other products are used for parkinsonian symptoms, including dystonia associated with neuroleptic drugs.

Adverse effects: The most common side effects are dryness of the mouth and constipation, which can be prevented by frequent rinsing of the mouth and increasing water and bulk in the diet.

☑ Herb/drug   🚫 Do Not Crush   ♦ Alert   ♦🇹 Key Drug   🇬 Geriatric   🅿 Pediatric

Contraindications: Hypersensitivity can occur, and allergies should be identified before administering these products. Persons with GI and GU obstruction should not use these products, since constipation and urinary retention may occur. They are also contraindicated in angle closure glaucoma and myasthenia gravis.

G Precautions: Caution must be used when these products are given to the elderly, since metabolism is slowed. Also, persons with tachycardia or prostatic hypertrophy should use these products with caution.

Pharmacokinetics: Onset, peak, and duration vary with route.

Interactions: Increase in anticholinergic effect occurs when used with opioids, barbiturates, antihistamines, MAOIs, phenothiazines, amantadine.

NURSING CONSIDERATIONS

Assessment

- Assess I&O ratio; be alert for urinary retention, frequency, dysuria; drug should be discontinued if these occur
- Assess urinary hesitancy, retention; palpate bladder if retention occurs
- Assess constipation; increase fluids, bulk, exercise
- Assess for tolerance over long-term therapy; dosage may need to be changed
- Assess mental status: affect, mood, CNS depression, worsening of mental symptoms during early therapy

Nursing diagnoses

✓ Impaired physical mobility (uses)
✓ Acute pain (uses)
✓ Chronic pain (uses)

Implementation

- Give with food or milk to decrease GI symptoms
- Give parenteral dose with patient recumbent to prevent postural hypotension; give dose slowly, monitoring VS
- Give hard candy, gum, frequent rinsing of mouth for dryness

Evaluation

- Therapeutic response: absence of cramps, absence of extrapyramidal symptoms (EPS)

Patient/family education

- Caution patient to avoid driving and other hazardous activity if drowsiness occurs
- Advise patient to avoid concurrent use of cough, cold preparations with alcohol, antihistamines unless directed by prescriber
- Caution patient to use with caution in hot weather, since medication may increase susceptibility to heat stroke

---

Selected Generic Names

◆π atropine (high alert)
◆π benztropine
biperiden

glycopyrrolate
scopolamine
trihexyphenidyl

CORTICOSTEROIDS

Action: Corticosteroids are divided into glucocorticoids and mineralocorticoids. Glucocorticoids decrease inflammation by the suppression of migration of polymorphonuclear leukocytes, fibroblasts, increased capillary permeability, and lysosomal stabilization. They also have varied metabolic effects and modify the body's immune responses to many different stimuli. Mineralocorticoids act by increasing resorption of sodium by increasing hydrogen and potassium excretion in the distal tubule.

Uses: Glucocorticoids are used to decrease inflammation and for immunosuppression. In addition, some products may be given for allergy, adrenal insufficiency, or cerebral edema. Mineralocorticoids are given for adrenal insufficiency or adrenogenital syndrome.

Adverse effects: The most common side effects include change in behavior, including insomnia and euphoria; GI irritation, including peptic ulcer; metabolic reactions, including hypokalemia, hyperglycemia, and carbohydrate intolerance; and sodium and fluid retention. Most adverse reactions are dose dependent.

Contraindications: Hypersensitivity may occur and should be identified before administering. Since these products mask infection, they should not be used in systemic fungal infections or amebiasis. Mothers taking pharmacologic doses of corticosteroids should not nurse.

Precautions: Caution must be used when these products are prescribed for diabetic patients, since hyperglycemia may occur. Also, patients with glaucoma, seizure disorders, peptic ulcer, **P** impaired renal function, CHF, hypertension, ulcerative colitis, or myasthenia gravis should be **G** monitored closely if corticosteroids are given. Use with caution in children and the elderly and during pregnancy.

Pharmacokinetics: For oral preparations the onset of action occurs between 1-2 hr, and duration can be up to 2 days, with a half-life of 2-4 days. Pharmacokinetics vary widely among products. These products cross the placenta and appear in breast milk.

Interactions: Decreased corticosteroid effect may occur with barbiturates, rifampin, phenytoin; corticosteroid dosage may need to be increased. There is a possibility of GI bleeding when used with salicylates, indomethacin. Steroids may reduce salicylate levels. When using with digitalis glycosides, potassium-depleting diuretics, and amphotericin, serum potassium levels should be monitored.

NURSING CONSIDERATIONS
Assessment
- Monitor potassium, blood glucose, urine glucose while on long-term therapy; hypokalemia and hyperglycemia are common
- Monitor weight daily; notify prescriber if weekly gain of >5 lb, since these products alter fluid and electrolyte balance
- Assess for potassium depletion, including paresthesias, fatigue, nausea, vomiting, depression, polyuria, dysrhythmias, weakness
- Assess for mental status, including affect, mood, behavioral changes, aggression; if severe personality changes occur, including depression, drug may need to be tapered and then discontinued
- Monitor I&O ratio; be alert for decreasing urinary output and increasing edema
- Monitor plasma cortisol levels during long-term therapy (normal level is 138-635 nmol/L when drawn at 8 AM)
- Assess for infection, including increased temp, WBC, even after withdrawal of medication; drug masks symptoms of infection
- Assess for adrenal insufficiency: nausea, anorexia, fatigue, dizziness, dyspnea, weakness, joint pain

Nursing diagnoses
☑ Risk for infection (adverse reactions)
☑ Disturbed body image (adverse reactions)
☑ Risk for violence: self-directed (suicide) (adverse reactions)

Implementation
- Give with food or milk to decrease GI symptoms

Evaluation
- Therapeutic response: decreased inflammation

Patient/family education
- Advise patient that emergency ID as steroid user should be carried/worn
- Advise patient not to discontinue this medication abruptly or adrenal crisis can result
- Teach patient all aspects of drug use, including cushingoid symptoms
- Instruct patient that single daily or alternate-day doses should be taken in the morning before 9 AM (for replacement therapy)
- Instruct patient to take with meals or a snack

Selected Generic Names

Glucocorticoids:
beclomethasone
betamethasone
◆π cortisone
hydrocortisone
methylprednisolone

prednisolone
◆π prednisone
triamcinolone

Mineralocorticoid:
fludrocortisone

DIURETICS

Action: Diuretics are divided into subgroups: thiazides and thiazide-like diuretics, loop diuretics, carbonic anhydrase inhibitors, osmotic diuretics, and potassium-sparing diuretics. Each one of these subgroups differs in its mechanism of action. Thiazides and thiazide-like diuretics increase excretion of water and sodium by inhibiting resorption in the early distal tubule. Loop diuretics inhibit resorption of sodium and chloride in the thick ascending limb of the loop of Henle. Carbonic anhydrase inhibitors increase sodium excretion by decreasing sodium-hydrogen ion exchange throughout the renal tubule. Carbonic anhydrase inhibitors also decrease secretion of aqueous humor in the eye and thus decrease intraocular pressure. Osmotic diuretics increase the osmotic pressure of glomerular filtrate, thus decreasing net absorption of sodium. The potassium-sparing diuretics interfere with sodium resorption at the distal tubule, thus decreasing potassium excretion.
Uses: Blood pressure is reduced in hypertension; edema is reduced in CHF; intraocular pressure is decreased in glaucoma.
Adverse effects: Hypokalemia, hyperuricemia, and hyperglycemia occur most frequently with thiazide diuretics. Aplastic anemia, blood dyscrasias, volume depletion, and dehydration may occur when thiazide-like diuretics, loop diuretics, or carbonic anhydrase inhibitors are given. Side effects and adverse reactions vary widely for the miscellaneous products.
Contraindications: Persons with electrolyte imbalances (sodium, chloride, potassium), dehydration, or anuria should not be given these products until the problem is corrected.
G Precautions: Caution must be used when diuretics are given to the elderly, since electrolyte disturbances and dehydration can occur rapidly. Hepatic and renal disorders may cause poor metabolism and excretion of the drug.
Pharmacokinetics: Onset, peak, and duration vary widely among the different subgroups of these drugs.
Interactions: Cholestyramine and colestipol decrease the absorption of thiazide diuretics. Concurrent use of thiazides with diazoxide may increase hyperuricemia, hyperglycemia, and antihypertensive effects of thiazides. Ototoxicity may occur when loop diuretics are used with aminoglycosides. Thiazide and loop diuretics may increase therapeutic and toxic effects of lithium.

NURSING CONSIDERATIONS
Assessment
- Monitor weight, I&O ratio daily to determine fluid loss; check skin turgor for dehydration
- Monitor electrolytes: potassium, sodium, chloride: include BUN, blood glucose, CBC, serum creatinine, blood pH, ABGs, uric acid, calcium; electrolyte imbalances may occur quickly
- Monitor B/P with patient lying, standing; postural hypotension may occur, since fluid loss occurs from intravascular spaces first
- Assess for signs of metabolic alkalosis, including drowsiness and restlessness
- Assess for signs of hypokalemia with some products, including postural hypotension, malaise, fatigue, tachycardia, leg cramps, weakness

Nursing diagnoses
☑ Excess fluid volume (uses)
☑ Decreased cardiac output (adverse reactions)

Implementation
- Give in AM to avoid interference with sleep if using drug as a diuretic
- Give potassium replacement if potassium is less than 3 mg/dl

Evaluation
- Therapeutic reponse: improvement in edema of feet, legs, sacral area daily if medication is being used in CHF; improvement in B/P if medication is being used as a diuretic; improvement in intraocular pressure if medication is being used to decrease aqueous humor in the eye

Patient/family education
- Teach patient to take drug early in the day (diuretic) to prevent nocturia

---

Selected Generic Names

Thiazides:
✆π hydrochlorothiazide

Thiazide-like:
chlorthalidone
indapamide
metolazone

Loop:
bumetanide
✆π furosemide
torsemide

Carbonic anhydrase inhibitors:
acetazolamide

Potassium-sparing:
amiloride
spironolactone
triamterene

Osmotic:
mannitol

HISTAMINE H$_2$ ANTAGONISTS

Action: Histamine H$_2$ antagonists act by inhibiting histamine at H$_2$ receptor site in parietal cells, which inhibits gastric acid secretion.

Uses: Histamine H$_2$ antagonists are used for short-term treatment of duodenal and gastric ulcers and maintenance therapy for duodenal ulcer; and for gastroesophageal reflux disease.

Adverse effects: The most serious adverse reactions are agranulocytosis, thrombocytopenia, neutropenia, aplastic anemia, and exfoliative dermatitis. The most common side effects are confusion (not with rantidine), headache and diarrhea.

☑ Herb/drug   🚫 Do Not Crush   ◆ Alert   ✆π Key Drug   G Geriatric   P Pediatric

Contraindications: Persons with hypersensitivity should not use these products.

P Precautions: Caution should be used in pregnancy, lactation, children <16 yr, organic brain syndrome, hepatic disease, renal disease.

Pharmacokinetics: Onset, peak, and duration vary widely among products. Most products are metabolized in the liver and excreted in urine.

Interactions: Antacids interfere with absorption of histamine H_2 antagonists. Check individual monographs for other interactions.

NURSING CONSIDERATIONS
Assessment
- Monitor gastric pH (>5 should be maintained)
- Monitor I&O ratio, BUN, creatinine

Nursing diagnoses
✓ Chronic pain (uses)
✓ Risk for injury (bleeding)
✓ Deficient knowledge (teaching)

Implementation
- Give with meals for prolonged drug effect
- Give antacids 1 hr before or 1 hr after cimetidine
- Give **IV** slowly; bradycardia may occur; give over 30 min
- Store diluted sol at room temp for up to 48 hr

Evaluation
- Therapeutic response: decreased pain in abdomen

Patient/family education
- Advise patient that gynecomastia, impotence may occur, but is reversible
- Caution patient to avoid driving and other hazardous activities until patient is stabilized on this medication
- Caution patient to avoid black pepper, caffeine, alcohol, harsh spices, extremes in temp of food
- Caution patient to avoid OTC preparations: aspirin, cough, cold preparations
- Inform patient that drug must be continued for prescribed time to be effective
- Advise patient to report bruising, fatigue, malaise; blood dyscrasias may occur

---

Selected Generic Names

⚮ cimetidine   ranitidine
famotidine

IMMUNOSUPPRESSANTS

Action: Immunosuppressants produce immunosuppression by inhibiting T lymphocytes.

Uses: Most products are used for organ transplants to prevent rejection.

Adverse effects: The most serious adverse reactions are albuminuria, hematuria, proteinuria, renal failure, and hepatotoxicity. The most common side effects are oral *Candida* infection, gum hyperplasia, tremors, and headache. The most serious adverse reactions for azathioprine are hematologic (leukopenia and thrombocytopenia) and GI (nausea and vomiting). There is a risk of secondary infection.

Contraindications: Products are contraindicated in hypersensitivity.

Precautions: Caution should be used in severe renal disease, severe hepatic disease, and pregnancy.

Pharmacokinetics: Onset, peak, and duration vary widely among products. Most products are metabolized in the liver and excreted in urine.

Interactions: Please check individual monographs, since interactions vary widely among products.

NURSING CONSIDERATIONS
Assessment
- Monitor renal studies: BUN, creatinine at least monthly during treatment, 3 mo after treatment
- Monitor liver function studies: alkaline phosphatase, AST, ALT, bilirubin
- Monitor drug blood levels during treatment
- Assess for hepatotoxicity: dark urine, jaundice, itching, light-colored stools; drug should be discontinued

Nursing diagnoses
☑Risk for infection (adverse reactions)
☑Risk for injury (uses)
☑Deficient knowledge (teaching)

Implementation
- Give for several days before transplant surgery
- Give with meals for GI upset or place drug in chocolate milk
- Give with oral antifungal for *Candida* infections

Evaluation
- Therapeutic response: absence of rejection

Patient/family education
- Advise patient to report fever, chills, sore throat, fatigue, since serious infections may occur
- Caution patient to use contraceptive measures during treatment and for 12 wk after ending therapy

Selected Generic Names

☞ azathioprine
basiliximab (high alert)
cyclosporine

muromonab-CD3
sirolimus
tacrolimus

LAXATIVES

Action: Laxatives are divided into bulk products, lubricants, osmotics, saline laxative stimulants, and stool softeners. Bulks work by absorbing water and expanding to increase moisture content and bulk in the stool. Lubricants increase water retention in the stool, causing reabsorption of water in the bowel. Stimulants act by increasing peristalsis by direct effect on the intestine. Saline draws water into the intestinal lumen. Osmotics increase distention and promote peristalsis. Stool softeners reduce surface tension of liq in the bowel.

Uses: Laxatives are used as a preparation for bowel, rectal examination, constipation, or as stool softeners.

Adverse effects: The most common side effects are nausea, abdominal cramps, and diarrhea.

☑ Herb/drug   ⊘ Do Not Crush   ◆ Alert   ☞ Key Drug   🄶 Geriatric   🄿 Pediatric

Contraindications: Persons with GI obstruction, perforation, gastric retention, toxic colitis, megacolon, abdominal pain, nausea, vomiting, and fecal impaction should not use these products.

Precautions: Caution should be used in rectal bleeding, large hemorrhoids, and anal excoriation.

Pharmacokinetics: Onset, peak, and duration vary among products.

Interactions: Please check individual monographs, since interactions vary widely among products.

NURSING CONSIDERATIONS

Assessment

- Monitor blood, urine electrolytes if drug is used often by patient
- Monitor I&O ratio to identify fluid loss
- Determine cause of constipation; identify whether fluids, bulk, or exercise is missing from lifestyle
- Assess for cramping, rectal bleeding, nausea, vomiting; if these symptoms occur, drug should be discontinued

Nursing diagnoses

✓Constipation (uses)

✓Diarrhea (adverse reactions)

✓Deficient knowledge (teaching)

Implementation

- Give alone only with water for better absorption; do not take within 1 hr of antacids, milk, or cimetidine

Evaluation

- Therapeutic response: decrease in constipation

Patient/family education

⊘• Teach patient to swallow tab whole; do not chew
- Caution patient not to use laxatives for long-term therapy; bowel tone will be lost; that normal bowel movements do not always occur daily
- Caution patient not to use in presence of abdominal pain, nausea, vomiting
- Advise patient to notify prescriber of abdominal pain, nausea, vomiting
- Advise patient to notify prescriber if constipation is unrelieved or if symptoms of electrolyte imbalance occur: muscle cramps, pain, weakness, dizziness

---

Selected Generic Names

Bulk laxative:
psyllium

Osmotic agents:
glycerin
lactulose

Saline:
magnesium salts
sodium phosphate/biphosphate

Stimulants:
bisacodyl
cascara
phenolphthalein
senna

Stool softeners:
docusate

NEUROMUSCULAR BLOCKING AGENTS

Action: Neuromuscular blocking agents are divided into depolarizing and nondepolarizing blockers. They act by inhibiting transmission of nerve impulses by binding with cholinergic receptor sites.

Uses: Neuromuscular blocking agents are used to facilitate endotracheal intubation and skeletal muscle relaxation during mechanical ventilation, surgery, or general anesthesia.

Adverse effects: The most serious adverse reactions are prolonged apnea, bronchospasm, cyanosis, respiratory depression, and malignant hyperthermia. The most common side effects are bradycardia and decreased motility.

Contraindications: Persons that are hypersensitive should not be given this product.

Precautions: Caution should be used in pregnancy, thyroid disease, collagen disease, cardiac **P** disease, lactation, children <2 yr, electrolyte imbalances, dehydration, neuromuscular disease (myasthenia gravis), and respiratory disease.

Pharmacokinetics: Onset, peak, and duration vary widely among products. Most products are metabolized in the liver and excreted in urine.

Interactions: Aminoglycosides potentiate neuromuscular blockade. See individual monographs.

NURSING CONSIDERATIONS
Assessment

- Monitor for electrolyte imbalances (potassium, magnesium); may lead to increased action of this drug
- Monitor VS (B/P, pulse, respirations, airway) q15 min until fully recovered; rate, depth, pattern of respirations, strength of hand grip
- Monitor I&O ratio; check for urinary retention, frequency, hesitancy
- Assess for recovery: decreased paralysis of face, diaphragm, leg, arm, rest of body
- Assess for allergic reactions: rash, fever, respiratory distress, pruritus; drug should be discontinued

Nursing diagnoses
✓ Ineffective breathing pattern (uses)
✓ Risk for injury (adverse reactions)
✓ Deficient knowledge (teaching)

Implementation

- Administer using nerve stimulator by anesthesiologist to determine neuromuscular blockade
- Administer anticholinesterase to reverse neuromuscular blockade
- Administer **IV** undiluted over 1-2 min (only by qualified person, usually an anesthesiologist)
- Store in light-resistant, cool area
- Reassure if communication is difficult during recovery from neuromuscular blockade

Evaluation

- Therapeutic response: paralysis of jaw, eyelid, head, neck, rest of body

Selected Generic Names

atracurium
doxacurium (high alert)
gallamine (high alert)
metocurine
mivacurium (high alert)

pancuronium (high alert)
pipecuronium (high alert)
succinylcholine (high alert)
◆π tubocurarine (high alert)
vecuronium (high alert)

⊘ Herb/drug   ⊗ Do Not Crush   ◆ Alert   ◆π Key Drug   G Geriatric   P Pediatric

NONSTEROIDAL ANTIINFLAMMATORIES

Action: Nonsteroidal antiinflammatories decrease prostaglandin synthesis by inhibiting an enzyme needed for biosynthesis.

Uses: Nonsteroidal antiinflammatories are used to treat mild to moderate pain, osteoarthritis, rheumatoid arthritis, and dysmenorrhea.

Adverse effects: The most serious adverse reactions are nephrotoxicity (dysuria, hematuria, oliguria, azotemia), blood dyscrasias, and cholestatic hepatitis. The most common side effects are nausea, abdominal pain, anorexia, dizziness, and drowsiness.

Contraindications: Persons with hypersensitivity, asthma, severe renal disease, and severe hepatic disease should not use these products.

P G Precautions: Caution should be used in pregnancy, lactation, children, bleeding disorders, GI disorders, cardiac disorders, hypersensitivity to other antiinflammatory agents, and the elderly.

Pharmacokinetics: Onset, peak, and duration vary widely among products. Most products are metabolized in the liver and excreted in urine.

Interactions: Please check individual monographs, since interactions vary widely among products.

NURSING CONSIDERATIONS
Assessment
- Monitor renal, liver, blood studies: BUN, creatinine, AST, ALT, Hgb, before treatment, periodically thereafter
- Monitor audiometric, ophth examination before, during, and after treatment.
- Check for eye, ear problems: blurred vision, tinnitus, may indicate toxicity

Nursing diagnoses
- ✓ Chronic pain (uses)
- ✓ Impaired physical mobility (uses)
- ✓ Deficient knowledge (teaching)
- ✓ Noncompliance (teaching)

Implementation
- Give with food to decrease GI symptoms; however, best to take on empty stomach to facilitate absorption
- Store at room temp

Evaluation
- Therapeutic response: decreased pain, stiffness in joints, decreased swelling in joints, ability to move more easily

Patient/family education
- Advise patient to report blurred vision, ringing, roaring in ears; may indicate toxicity
- Caution patient to avoid driving, other hazardous activities if dizziness, drowsiness occurs, **G** especially elderly
- Advise patient to report change in urine pattern, increased weight, edema, increased pain in joints, fever, blood in urine; indicate nephrotoxicity
- Inform patient that therapeutic effects may take up to 1 mo

Selected Generic Names

celecoxib
diclofenac
etodolac
ibuprofen
indomethacin
ketoprofen
ketorolac

meclofenamate
nabumetone
naproxen
piroxicam
rofecoxib
sulindac
valdecoxib

OPIOID ANALGESICS

Action: These agents depress pain impulse transmission at the spinal cord level by interacting with opioid receptors. Products are divided into opiates and nonopiates.

Uses: Most products are used to control moderate to severe pain and are used before and after surgery.

Adverse effects: GI symptoms, including nausea, vomiting, anorexia, constipation, and cramps are the most common side effects. Other common side effects include lightheadedness, dizziness, sedation. Serious adverse reactions such as respiratory depression, respiratory arrest, circulatory depression, and increased intracranial pressure may result, but are less common and usually dose dependent.

Contraindications: Hypersensitive reactions occur frequently. Check for sensitivity before administering. These drugs should not be used if opioid addiction is suspected, and they are also contraindicated in acute bronchial asthma and upper airway obstruction.

Precautions: Caution must be used when these products are given to persons with an addictive personality, since the possibility of addiction is so great. Also, persons with increased intracranial pressure may experience an even greater increase in intracranial pressure. Persons with severe heart disease, hepatic or renal disease, respiratory conditions, and seizure disorders should be monitored closely for worsening condition.

Pharmacokinetics: Onset of action is immediate by **IV** route and rapid by IM and PO routes. Peak occurs from 1-2 hr, depending on route, with a duration of 2-8 hr. These agents cross the placenta and appear in breast milk.

Interactions: Barbiturates, other opioids, hypnotics, antipsychotics, or alcohol can increase CNS depression when taken with opioids.

NURSING CONSIDERATIONS
Assessment

- Monitor I&O ratio; be alert for urinary retention, frequency, dysuria; drug should be discontinued if these occur
- Assess for respiratory dysfunction, including respiratory depression, rate, rhythm, character; notify prescriber if respirations are <12/min
- Assess for CNS changes: dizziness, drowsiness, hallucinations, euphoria, LOC, pupil reaction
- Assess for allergic reactions: rash, urticaria
- Assess for need for pain medication, use pain scoring

Nursing diagnoses
☑Acute pain (uses)
☑Impaired gas exchange (adverse reactions)

Implementation
- Give with antiemetic if nausea or vomiting occurs

 Herb/drug   Do Not Crush   Alert   Key Drug   Geriatric   **P** Pediatric

- Give when pain is beginning to return; determine dosage interval by patient response
- Provide assistance with ambulation; patient should not be ambulating during drug peak

Evaluation
- Therapeutic response: decrease in pain

Patient/family education
- Advise patient to report any symptoms of CNS changes, allergic reactions, or shortness of breath
- Caution patient that physical dependency may result when used for extended periods
- Teach patient that withdrawal symptoms may occur, including nausea, vomiting, cramps, fever, faintness, anorexia
- Advise patient to avoid alcohol and other CNS depressants

Selected Generic Names

buprenorphine
butorphanol
✤π codeine
fentanyl (high alert)
fentanyl transdermal
hydromorphone (high alert)
✤π meperidine (high alert)

methadone HCl (high alert)
✤π morphine (high alert)
oxycodone (high alert)
oxymorphone (high alert)
pentazocine (high alert)
propoxyphene (high alert)
remifentanil (high alert)

SALICYLATES

Action: Salicylates have analgesic, antipyretic, and antiinflammatory effects. The antiinflammatory and analgesic activities may be mediated through the inhibition of prostaglandin synthesis. Antipyretic action results from inhibition of the hypothalamic heat-regulating center.

Uses: The primary uses of salicylates are relief of mild to moderate pain and fever and in inflammatory conditions such as arthritis, thromboembolic disorders, and rheumatic fever.

Adverse effects: The most common side effects are GI symptoms and rash. Serious blood dyscrasias and hepatotoxicity may result when used for long periods at high doses. Tinnitus or impaired hearing may indicate that blood salicylate levels are reaching or exceeding the upper limit of the therapeutic range.

Contraindications: Hypersensitivity to salicylates is common. Check for sensitivity before administering. Persons with bleeding disorders, GI bleeding, and vit K deficiency should not use these products, since salicylates increase prothrombin time. Children should not use these products, since salicylates have been associated with Reye's syndrome.

Precautions: Caution is needed when salicylates are given to patients with anemia, hepatic or renal disease, or Hodgkin's disease. Caution should also be exercised in pregnancy and lactation.

Pharmacokinetics: Onset of action occurs in 15-30 min, with a peak of 1-2 hr and a duration up to 6 hr. These drugs are metabolized by the liver and excreted by the kidneys.

Interactions: Increased effects of anticoagulants, insulin, methotrexate, heparin, valproic acid, and oral sulfonylureas may occur when used with salicylates. Aspirin may decrease serum concentrations of nonsteroidal antiinflammatory agents.

NURSING CONSIDERATIONS
Assessment
- Monitor hepatic and renal studies: AST, ALT, bilirubin, creatinine, LDH, alkaline phosphatase, BUN if patient is on long-term therapy, since these products are metabolized and excreted by the liver and kidney
- Monitor blood studies: CBC, Hct, Hgb, and prothrombin time if patient is on long-term therapy, since these products increase the possibility of bleeding and blood dyscrasias
- Assess for hepatotoxicity: dark urine, clay-colored stools, jaundiced skin and sclera, itching, abdominal pain, fever, diarrhea, which may occur with long-term use
- Assess for ototoxicity: tinnitus, ringing, roaring in ears; audiometric testing is needed before and after long-term therapy

Nursing diagnoses
- ✓ Acute pain (uses)
- ✓ Chronic pain (uses)
- ✓ Impaired physical mobility (uses)
- ✓ Activity intolerance (uses)
- ✓ Disturbed sensory perception: auditory (adverse reactions)
- ✓ Ineffective thermoregulation (uses)

Implementation
- Give with food or milk to decrease gastric irritation; give 30 min ac or 1 hr pc with a full glass of water

Evaluation
- Therapeutic response: decreased pain, fever

Patient/family education
- Advise patient that blood sugar levels should be monitored closely, if patient is diabetic
- Caution patient not to exceed recommended dosage; acute poisoning may result
- Inform patient that therapeutic response takes 2 wk in arthritis
- Caution patient to avoid use of alcohol, since GI bleeding may result
- Advise patient to notify prescriber if ringing in the ears or persistent GI pain occurs
- Advise patient to take with full glass of water to reduce risk of lodging in esophagus

---

Selected Generic Names

♦π aspirin
choline salicylate

magnesium salicylate
salsalate

THROMBOLYTICS

Action: Thrombolytics activate conversion of plasminogen to plasmin (fibrinolysin): plasmin is able to break down clots (fibrin).

Uses: Thrombolytics are used to treat deep vein thrombosis, pulmonary embolism, arterial thrombosis, arterial embolism, arteriovenous cannula occlusion, lysis of coronary artery thrombi after MI, acute evolving transmural MI.

Adverse effects: Serious adverse reactions include GI, GU, intracranial, and retroperitoneal bleeding, and anaphylaxis. The most common side effects are decreased Hct, urticaria, headache, and nausea.

Contraindications: Persons with hypersensitivity, active bleeding, intraspinal surgery, neoplasms of the CNS, ulcerative colitis/enteritis, severe hypertension, renal disease, hepatic disease,

---

🖉 Herb/drug   🅢 Do Not Crush   ◆ Alert   ◆π Key Drug   🄶 Geriatric   🄿 Pediatric hypocoagulation, COPD, subacute bacterial endocarditis, rheumatic valvular disease, cerebral embolism/thrombosis/hemorrhage, intraarterial diagnostic procedure or surgery (10 days), and recent major surgery should not use these products.

Precautions: Caution should be used in arterial emboli from left side of heart and pregnancy.

Pharmacokinetics: Onset, peak, and duration vary widely among products. Most products are metabolized in the liver and excreted in urine.

Interactions: Please check individual monographs, since interactions vary widely among products.

NURSING CONSIDERATIONS
Assessment
- Monitor VS, B/P, pulse, respirations, neurologic signs, temp at least q4h, temp is an indicator of internal bleeding, cardiac rhythm following intracoronary administration; systolic pressure increase of >25 mm Hg should be reported to prescriber
- Assess for neurologic changes that may indicate intracranial bleeding
- Assess retroperitoneal bleeding: back pain, leg weakness, diminished pulses
- Assess for allergy: fever, rash, itching, chills; mild reaction may be treated with antihistamines
- Assess for bleeding during 1st hr of treatment: hematuria, hematemesis, bleeding from mucous membranes, epistaxis, ecchymosis
- Monitor blood studies (Hct, platelets, PTT, PT, TT, APTT) before starting therapy; PT or APTT must be less than 2 times control before starting therapy TT or PT q3-4h during treatment

Nursing diagnoses
✓ Risk for injury (uses)

Implementation
- Administer as soon as thrombi identified; not useful for thrombi over 1 wk old
- Administer cryoprecipitate or fresh, frozen plasma if bleeding occurs
- Administer loading dose at beginning of therapy; may require increased loading doses
- Give heparin after fibrinogen level is over 100 mg/dl; heparin inf to increase PTT to 1.5-2 times baseline for 3-7 days
- About 10% of patients have high streptococcal antibody titers requiring increased loading doses
- Give **IV** therapy using 0.8-μm filter
- Store reconstituted sol in refrigerator; discard after 24 hr
- Provide bed rest during entire course of treatment
- Avoid venous or arterial puncture, injection, rec temp
- Provide treatment of fever with acetaminophen or aspirin
- Apply pressure for 30 sec to minor bleeding sites; inform prescriber if this does not attain hemostasis; apply pressure dressing

Evaluation
- Therapeutic response: resolution of thrombosis, embolism

Selected Generic Names

alteplase (high alert)
anistreplase (high alert)
drotrecogin alfa

❖π streptokinase (high alert)
tenecteplase
urokinase (high alert)

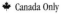 ❦ Canada Only   ⓝ Do Not Confuse   * "Tall Man" lettering (See Preface)

THYROID HORMONES

Action: Increase metabolic rates, resulting in increased cardiac output, O_2 consumption, body temp, blood volume, growth, development at cellular level, respiratory rate, enzyme system activity

Uses: Products are used for thyroid replacement.

Adverse effects: The most common side effects include insomnia, tremors, tachycardia, palpitations, angina, dysrhythmias, weight loss, and changes in appetite. Serious adverse reactions include thyroid storm.

Contraindications: Persons with adrenal insufficiency, myocardial infarction, or thyrotoxicosis should not use these products.

G Precautions: The elderly and patients with angina pectoris, hypertension, ischemia, cardiac disease, or diabetes mellitus or insipidus should be watched closely when using these products. Caution should be used in pregnancy and lactation.

Pharmacokinetics: Pharmacokinetics vary widely among products; check specific monographs.

Interactions

- Impaired absorption of thyroid products may occur when administered with cholestyramine (separate by 4-5 hr)
- Increased effects of anticoagulants, sympathomimetics, tricyclic antidepressants, catecholamines may occur
- Decreased effects of digitalis, glycosides, insulin, hypoglycemics may occur
- Decreased effects of thyroid products may occur with estrogens

NURSING CONSIDERATIONS
Assessment

- Monitor B/P, pulse before each dose
- Monitor I&O ratio
- Monitor weight qd in same clothing, using same scale, at same time of day
- **P** Monitor height, growth rate if given to a child
- Monitor T_3, T_4, which are decreased; radioimmunoassay of TSH, which is increased; ratio uptake, which is decreased if patient is on too low a dosage of medication
- Assess for increased nervousness, excitability, irritability; may indicate too high a dosage of medication usually after 1-3 wk of treatment
- Assess for cardiac status: angina, palpitation, chest pain, change in VS

Nursing diagnoses
- ✓ Deficient knowledge (teaching)
- ✓ Noncompliance (teaching)
- ✓ Disturbed body image (adverse reactions)

Implementation

- Give at same time each day to maintain drug level
- Give only for hormone imbalances; not to be used for obesity, male infertility, menstrual conditions, lethargy
- Remove medication 4 wk before RAIU test

Evaluation

- Therapeutic response: absence of depression; increased weight loss, diuresis, pulse, appetite; absence of constipation, peripheral edema, cold intolerance, pale, cool, dry skin, brittle nails, alopecia, coarse hair, menorrhagia, night blindness, paresthesias, syncope, stupor, coma, rosy cheeks

Patient/family education
- **P**• Advise patient that hair loss will occur in child and is temporary
- Advise patient to report excitability, irritability, anxiety; indicates overdose
- Caution patient not to switch brands unless directed by prescriber
- **P**• Caution patient that hypothyroid child will show almost immediate behavior/personality change
- Advise patient that treatment drug is not to be taken to reduce weight
- Advise patient to avoid OTC preparations with iodine; read labels; to avoid iodine-containing food, iodinized salt, soybeans, tofu, turnips, some seafood, some bread

---

Selected Generic Names

◆☊levothyroxine (T_4)   liotrix
liothyronine (T_3)   thyroid USP

VASODILATORS

Action: Vasodilators act in various ways. Please check individual monograph for specific action.
Uses: Vasodilators are used to treat intermittent claudication, arteriosclerosis obliterans, vasospasm and muscular ischemia, ischemic cerebral vascular disease, hypertension, and angina.
Adverse effects: The most common side effects are headache, nausea, hypotension or hypertension, and ECG changes.
Contraindications: Some drugs are contraindicated in acute MI, paroxysmal tachycardia, and thyrotoxicosis.
Precautions: Caution should be used in uncompensated heart disease or peptic ulcer disease.
Pharmacokinetics: Onset, peak, and duration vary widely among products. Most products are metabolized in the liver and excreted in urine.
Interactions: Please check individual monographs, since interactions vary widely among products.

NURSING CONSIDERATIONS
Assessment
- Assess bleeding time in individuals with bleeding disorders
- Assess cardiac status: B/P, pulse, rate, rhythm, character; watch for increasing pulse

Nursing diagnoses
- ☑Decreased cardiac output (uses)
- ☑Altered tissue perfusion: cardiovascular/pulmonary (uses)
- ☑Deficient knowledge (teaching)

Implementation
- Give with meals to reduce GI symptoms
- Store in tight container at room temp

Evaluation
- Therapeutic response: ability to walk without pain, increased temp in extremities, increased pulse volume

Patient/family education
- Inform patient that medication is not cure, may need to be taken continuously
- Advise patient that it is necessary to quit smoking to prevent excessive vasoconstriction

---

- Advise patient that improvement may be sudden, but usually occurs gradually over several wk
- Instruct patient to report headache, weakness, increased pulse, since drug may need to be decreased or discontinued
- Instruct patient to avoid hazardous activities until stabilized on medication; dizziness may occur

---

Selected Generic Names

amyl nitrite
bosentan
dipyridamole
hydralazine

minoxidil
nesiritide
papaverine

VITAMINS

Action: Action varies widely among products and classes; check specific monographs.
Uses: Vitamins are used to correct and prevent vitamin deficiencies.
Adverse effects: There is an absence of side effects or adverse reactions with the water-soluble vitamins (C, B). However, fat-soluble vitamins (A, D, E, K) may accumulate in the body and cause adverse reactions (refer to specific monographs).
Contraindications: Hypersensitive reactions may occur, and allergies should be identified before these products are given.
Pharmacokinetics: Onset, peak, and duration vary widely among products; check individual monograph for specific information.

NURSING CONSIDERATIONS
Nursing diagnoses
✓Imbalanced nutrition, less than body requirements (uses)

Implementation
- Give PO with food for better absorption
- Store in tight, light-resistant container

Evaluation
- Therapeutic response: absence of vitamin deficiency

Patient/family education
- Advise patient not to take more than prescribed amount

Selected Generic Names

Fat-soluble:
phytonadione
vit A
vit D
vit E

Water-soluble:
ascorbic acid (C)

pyridoxine (B_6)
riboflavin (B_2)
thiamine (B_1)

Miscellaneous:
multivitamins

 Herb/drug   Do Not Crush   Alert   Key Drug   Geriatric   Pediatric

Appendix A

Selected New Drugs

⚠ RARELY USED

agalsidase beta
See Appendix F

⚠ RARELY USED

alefacept
See Appendix F

alfuzosin (Rx)
(al-fyoo'zoe-sin)
Uroxatral
Func. class.: Antiadrenergic
Chem. class.: Quinazolone

Pregnancy category B

Action: Binds preferentially to α_{1A}-adrenoceptor subtype located mainly in the prostate

➡ **Therapeutic Outcome:** Resolution of symptoms of benign prostatic hyperplasia

Uses: Symptoms of benign prostatic hyperplasia; has not been studied for and is not indicated for the treatment of high blood pressure

Dosage and routes
Adult: PO ext rel 10 mg qd, taken after same meal each day

Available forms: Tabs, ext rel 10 mg

Adverse effects
(*italic* = common; **bold** = life-threatening)
CNS: Dizziness, headache, fatigue
CV: Postural hypotension (dizziness, lightheadedness, fainting) within a few hours of administration, chest pain, tachycardia
GI: Nausea, abdominal pain, dyspepsia, constipation
GU: Impotence, priaprism
MISC: Body pain in general, rash
RESP: Upper respiratory tract infection, pharyngitis, bronchitis, sinusitis

Contraindications: Hypersensitivity, moderate to severe hepatic impairment

Precautions: Not indicated for use in women or children, pregnancy **B**, lactation, coronary artery disease, coronary insufficiency, mild hepatic disease, mild/moderate/severe renal disease, history of QT prolongation or coadministration with medications known to prolong QT interval

Pharmacokinetics
Absorption	Unknown
Distribution	Moderately protein bound (82%-90%)
Metabolism	Liver (by CYP3A4 enzyme)
Excretion	Urine
Half-life	10 hr

Pharmacodynamics
Onset	Unknown
Peak	Unknown
Duration	Unknown

Interactions
Individual drugs
Doxazosin, itraconazole, ketoconazole, prazosin, ritonavir, terazosin: Do not take concurrently
Umetadine: possible ↑ side effects
Drug classifications
CYP3A4 inhibitors: Do not take concurrently

NURSING CONSIDERATIONS
Assessment
• Assess for prostatic hyperplasia: change in urinary patterns, baseline and throughout treatment
• Monitor CBC with differential and liver function tests; B/P and heart rate
• Monitor BUN, uric acid, urodynamic studies (urinary flow rates, residual volume)
• Monitor I&O ratios, weight qd, edema; report weight gain or edema

Nursing diagnoses
☑ Urinary elimination, impaired (uses)
☑ Knowledge, deficient (teaching)

Implementation
PO route
🚫• Give whole; do not chew or crush tablets
• Store in tight container in cool environment

Patient/family education
- Advise not to drive or operate machinery for 4 hr after first dose or after dosage increase

Evaluation
Therapeutic response
- Decreased symptoms of benign prostatic hyperplasia

---

aprepitant (Rx)
(ap-re′pi-tant)
Emend
Func. class.: Antiemetic—misc

Pregnancy category B

Action: Selective antagonist of human substance P/neurokinin 1 (NK$_1$) receptors

⇒ **Therapeutic Outcome:** Decreased nausea, vomiting during chemotherapy

Uses: Prevention of nausea, vomiting associated with cancer chemotherapy including high-dose cisplatin; used in combination with other antiemetics

Dosage and routes
Adult: PO day 1 (1 hr prior to chemotherapy) aprepitant 125 mg with 12 mg dexamethasone PO, with 32 mg ondansetron **IV**; day 2 aprepitant 80 mg with 8 mg dexamethasone PO; day 3 aprepitant 80 mg with 8 mg dexamethasone PO; day 4 only dexamethasone 8 mg PO

Available forms: Caps 80, 125 mg

Adverse effects
(*italic* = common; **bold** = life-threatening)
CNS: *Headache, dizziness,* insomnia, anxiety, depression, confusion, peripheral neuropathy
CV: Bradycardia, DVT, hypertension
GI: *Diarrhea, constipation,* abdominal pain, anorexia, gastritis, ↑ AST, ALT, *nausea,* vomiting, heartburn
GU: ↑ BUN, serum creatine, proteinuria, dysuria
HEMA: Anemia, **thrombocytopenia, neutropenia**
MISC: Asthenia, fatigue, dehydration, fever, hiccups, tinnitus

Contraindications: Hypersensitivity

Precautions: Pregnancy **B**, lactation, ☐ children

Pharmacokinetics
Absorption	Unknown
Distribution	95% protein bound
Metabolism	Liver (CYP3A4 enzymes to an active metabolite)
Excretion	Not in kidneys
Half-life	10-12 hr

Pharmacodynamics
Onset	Unknown
Peak	Unknown
Duration	Unknown

Interactions
Individual drugs
Paroxetine: ↓ action of both drugs
Drug classifications
CYP2C9 substrates, phenytoin, TOLBUTamide, warfarin: ↓ action of oral contraceptives
CYP3A4 inhibitors (clarithromycin, diltiazem, itraconazole, ketoconazole, nefazodone, nelfinavir, ritonavir, troleandomycin): ↑ aprepitant action
CYP3A4 inducers (carbamazepine, phenytoin, rifampin): ↓ aprepitant action
CYP3A4 substrates (alprazolam, cisapride, dexamethasone, docetaxel, etoposide, ifosfamide, imatinib, irinotecan, methylPREDNISolone, midazolam, paclitaxel, pimozide, triazolam, vinBLAStine, vinCRIStine, vinorelbine): ↑ action

NURSING CONSIDERATIONS
Assessment
- Assess for absence of nausea, vomiting during chemotherapy

Nursing diagnoses
☑ Knowledge, deficient (teaching)

Implementation
- Give PO on 3-day schedule
- Store at room temperature

Patient/family education
- Teach to report diarrhea, constipation
- Advise to take only as prescribed, take 1st dose 1 hr prior to chemotherapy
- Advise to report all medication to prescriber prior to taking this medication
- Instruct to use nonhormonal form of contraception while taking this agent
- Advise those on warfarin to have clotting monitored closely during 2-wk period following administration of aprepitant

Evaluation
Therapeutic response
- Absence of nausea, vomiting during cancer chemotherapy

▨ Herb/drug	Ⓢ Do Not Crush	◆ Alert	✆ Key Drug	Ⓖ Geriatric	Ⓟ Pediatric

atazanavir (Rx)
(at-a-za-na'veer)
Reyataz
Func. class.: Antiretroviral
Chem. class.: Protease inhibitor

Pregnancy category B

Action: Inhibits human immunodeficiency virus (HIV-1) protease, which prevents maturation of the infectious virus

→ Therapeutic Outcome: Decreasing symptoms of HIV

Uses: HIV-1 infection in combination with other antiretroviral agents

Dosage and routes
Adult: PO 400 mg qd

Hepatic dose
Adult: PO (Child-Pugh B) 300 mg qd; (Child-Pugh C) do not use

Available forms: Caps 100, 150, 200 mg

Adverse effects
(*italic* = common; **bold** = life-threatening)
CNS: Headache, depression, dizziness, insomnia, peripheral neuropathy
GI: Diarrhea, abdominal pain, nausea, **hepatotoxicity**
INTEG: Rash, **Stevens-Johnson syndrome**, *photosensitivity*
MISC: Fatigue, fever, arthralgia, back pain, cough, lipodystrophy, pain

Contraindications: Hypersensitivity

P Precautions: Liver disease, pregnancy **B**, **G** lactation, children, elderly

Pharmacokinetics	
Absorption	Rapid, ↑ with food
Distribution	86% protein bound
Metabolism	Liver extensively
Excretion	27% excreted unchanged in urine/feces (minimal)
Half-life	7 hr

Pharmacodynamics	
Onset	Unknown
Peak	2 hr
Duration	Unknown

Interactions
Individual drugs
CycloSPORINE, irinotecan, sildenafil, sirolimus, tacrolimus, warfarin: ↑ levels resulting in ↑ toxicity

Didanosine, efavirenz, rifampin: ↓ atazanavir levels
Indinavir: ↑ hyperbilirubinemia
Drug classifications
Antacids, H$_2$-receptor antagonists, proton pump inhibitors: ↓ atazanavir levels
Antidepressants (tricyclics), antidysrhythmics, calcium channel blockers, HMG-CoA reductase inhibitors: ↑ levels resulting in ↑ toxicity
Contraceptives (oral): ↑ effects
☑ Herb/drug
St. John's wort: ↓ atazanavir levels
Lab test interferences
↑ AST, ALT, total bilirubin, amylase, lipase

NURSING CONSIDERATIONS
Assessment
◆• Assess for hepatic failure
• Assess for signs of infection, anemia
• Monitor liver function studies: ALT, AST, bilirubin
• Monitor bowel pattern before, during treatment; if severe abdominal pain with bleeding occurs, drug should be discontinued; monitor hydration
• Monitor viral load, CD4 count throughout treatment
• Assess skin eruptions, rash, urticaria, itching
• Identify allergies before treatment, reaction of each medication; place allergies on chart

Nursing diagnoses
☑ Injury, risk for (uses, adverse reactions)
☑ Knowledge, deficient (teaching)

Implementation
• Administer with food

Patient/family education
• Advise to take as prescribed with other antiretrovirals as prescribed; if dose is missed, take as soon as remembered up to 1 hr before next dose; do not double dose; do not share with others
• Teach that drug must be taken daily to maintain blood levels for duration of therapy
• Teach that photosensitivity may occur; use protective clothing or stay out of the sun
• Instruct to notify prescriber if diarrhea, nausea, vomiting, rash occur; dizziness, light-headedness, ECG may be altered
• Inform that drug interacts with many drugs and St. John's wort; advise prescriber of all drugs, herbal products used
• Advise that redistribution of body fat may occur; the effect is not known
• Teach that drug does not cure HIV-1 infection or prevent transmission to others, only controls symptoms

• Advise that if taking sildenafil with atazanavir, there may be an increased risk of sildenafil-associated adverse events, including hypotension and prolonged penile erection; notify physician promptly of these symptoms

Evaluation
Therapeutic response
• Increasing CD4 counts; decreased viral load, resolution of symptoms of HIV-1 infection

---

bortezomib (Rx)
(bor-tez'oh-mib)
Velcade
Func. class.: Antineoplastic—misc.
Chem. class.: Proteasome inhibitor

Pregnancy category D

Action: Reversible inhibitor of chymotrypsin-like activity in mammalian cells; causes a delay in tumor growth

➔ **Therapeutic Outcome:** Decreased growth and spread of malignant cells.

Uses: Multiple myeloma when at least two other treatments have failed.

Dosage and routes
Adult: **IV** BOL 1.3 mg/m²/dose 2×/wk for 2 weeks (days 1, 4, 8, 11) followed by 10-day rest period (days 12 to 21)
Grade 1 with pain or grade 2: Reduce to 1 mg/m²
Withhold use at onset of grade 3 nonhematologic or grade 4 hematologic toxicities

Available forms: Lyophilized powder for inj 3.5 mg

Adverse effects
(*italic* = common; **bold** = life-threatening)
CNS: Anxiety, insomnia, dizziness, headache, peripheral neuropathy, rigors, paresthesia
CV: Hypotension, edema
GI: Abdominal pain, constipation, diarrhea, dyspepsia, nausea, vomiting, anorexia
HEMA: Anemia, **neutropenia, thrombocytopenia,**
MISC: Dehydration, weight loss, herpes zoster, rash, pruritus, blurred vision
MS: Fatigue, malaise, weakness, arthralgia, bone pain, muscle cramps, myalgia, back pain
RESP: Cough, pneumonia, dyspnea, URI

Contraindications: Hypersensitivity to this drug, boron, or mannitol, pregnancy **D**

Precautions: Peripheral neuropathy, **G** elderly, hepatic, renal disease, hypotension, **P** lactation, children

Pharmacokinetics
Absorption	Unknown
Distribution	Protein binding 83%
Metabolism	P450 enzymes (3A4, 2D6, 2C19, 2C9, 1A2)
Excretion	Unknown
Half-life	9-15 hr

Pharmacodynamics
Onset	Unknown
Peak	Unknown
Duration	Unknown

Interactions
Individual drugs
Bortezomib: ↑ exposure to CYP450 2C19 substrates
Drug classifications
Oral hypoglycemics: ↑ hypo/hyperglycemia
Drugs that induce or inhibit cytochrome P450 3A4: ↑ toxicity or ↓ efficacy

NURSING CONSIDERATIONS
Assessment
• Assess hematologic status: platelets, CBC throughout treatment
• Monitor for extravasation at inj site

Nursing diagnoses
✓ Injury, physical (uses, adverse reactions)
✓ Knowledge, deficient (teaching)

Implementation
• Reconstitute each vial with 3.5 ml 0.9% NaCl
• Use protective clothing during handling, preparation; avoid contact with skin

Patient/family education
• Teach to use contraception while on this drug, pregnancy **D**, avoid breastfeeding
• Advise to monitor blood glucose levels if diabetic
• Instruct to contact prescriber if new or worsening peripheral neuropathy, severe vomiting, diarrhea
• Advise to avoid driving, operating machinery until effect is known
• Advise to avoid using other medications unless approved by prescriber

Evaluation
Therapeutic response
• Improvement of multiple myeloma symptoms

 Herb/drug   Do Not Crush   Alert   Key Drug   Geriatric   Pediatric

daptomycin (Rx)
(dap'toe-mye-sin)
Cubicin
Func. class.: Antiinfective—misc.
Chem. class.: Lipopeptides

Pregnancy category B

Action: New class of antiinfective; binds to the bacterial membrane and results in a rapid depolarization of the membrane potential, leading to inhibition of DNA, RNA, and protein synthesis

➲ **Therapeutic Outcome:** Absence of infections

Uses: Complicated skin, skin structure infections caused by *Staphylococcus aureus,* including methicillin-resistant strains, *Streptococcus pyogenes, S. agalactiae, S. dysgalactiae, Enterococcus faecalis* (vancomycin-susceptible strains only)

Dosage and routes
Adult: **IV** INF 4 mg/kg over ½ hr diluted in 0.9% NaCl, give q24h ×7-14 days

Renal dose
Adult: **IV** INF CCr >30 ml/min 4 mg/kg q24h; CCr <30 ml/min; hemodialysis, CAPD 4 mg/kg q48h

Available forms: lyophilized powder for inj 250, 500 mg

Adverse effects
(*italic* = common; **bold** = life-threatening)
CNS: Headache, insomnia, dizziness
CV: Hypotension, hypertension, ↑ CPK
GI: Nausea, constipation, diarrhea, vomiting, dyspepsia, **pseudomembranous colitis**
GU: **Nephrotoxicity:** ↑ **BUN, creatinine, albumin**
INTEG: Rash, pruritus
MISC: Fungal infections, UTI, anemia
MS: Muscle pain or weakness, arthralgia, pain

Contraindications: Hypersensitivity

P **Precautions:** Renal disease, pregnancy **B**,
G children, lactation, elderly

Pharmacokinetics	
Absorption	Unknown
Distribution	Protein binding 92%
Metabolism	Unknown
Excretion	Unknown
Half-life	Unknown *

Pharmacodynamics	
Onset	Unknown
Peak	Unknown
Duration	Unknown

Interactions
Drug classifications
Myopathy: HMG-CoA reductase inhibitors

NURSING CONSIDERATIONS
Assessment
• Monitor I&O ratio: report hematuria, oliguria; nephrotoxicity may occur
◆• Monitor any patient with compromised renal system, toxicity may occur; BUN, creatinine
• Monitor blood studies: CBC
• Monitor C&S, drug may be given as soon as culture is taken
• Monitor B/P during administration; hypo/hypertension may occur
• Assess signs of infection
• Assess respiratory status: rate, character, wheezing
• Identify allergies before treatment, reaction of each medication

Nursing diagnoses
✓ Infection, risk for (uses)
✓ Knowledge, deficient (teaching)

Implementation
IV **IV route**
• Give after reconstitution with 5 ml 0.9% NaCl (250 mg/5 ml) or 10 ml 0.9% NaCl (500 mg/10 ml), further dilution is needed with 0.9% NaCl, infuse over ½ hr

Solution compatibilities: 0.9% NaCl, LR

Patient/family education
• Identify allergies before treatment, reaction of each medication
• Teach all aspects of drug therapy
• Advise to report sore throat, fever, fatigue; could indicate superinfection

Evaluation
Therapeutic response
• Negative culture

desirudin (Rx)
(des-i-'rude'in)
Iprivask
Func. class.: Anticoagulant
Chem. class.: Thrombin inhibitor

Pregnancy category C

Action: Inhibits thrombin resulting in prolongation of clotting time

→ **Therapeutic Outcome:** Absence of deep vein thrombosis

Uses: Prophylaxis for deep vein thrombosis in those undergoing hip replacement

Dosage and routes
Adult: **SC** 15 mg, 1st dose 5-15 min before surgery, but after regional block anesthesia, then 15 mg q12h, up to 12 days

Available forms: Lyophilized powder 15 mg

Adverse effects
(*italic* = common; **bold** = life-threatening)
MISC: Inj site mass, nausea, deep thrombophlebitis, anemia, hypersensitivity
SYST: Bleeding, hemorrhage

Contraindications: Hypersensitivity to natural or synthetic hirudins, active bleeding, irreversible coagulation disorders

P **Precautions:** Pregnancy C, lactation, children, elderly, hepatic and renal impairment, patients with ↑ risks of hemorrhage

Pharmacokinetics

Absorption	Unknown
Distribution	Unknown
Metabolism	Kidney (40%-50% unchanged)
Excretion	Kidney
Half-life	Unknown

Pharmacodynamics

Onset	Unknown
Peak	Unknown
Duration	Unknown

Interactions
Drug classifications
Anticoagulants: ↑ anticoagulant effect
Antiplatelets (abciximab, clopidogrel, ketorolac, NSAIDs, salicylates, sulfinpyrazone, triclopidine): ↑ anticoagulant effect
Thrombolytics: ↑ anticoagulant effect

NURSING CONSIDERATIONS
Assessment
• Monitor APTT qd in those with increased risk for bleeding
◆ • Assess for neurologic changes that may indicate intracranial bleeding
◆ • Assess for retroperitoneal bleeding: back pain, leg weakness, diminished pulses
• Assess for bleeding: gums, petechiae, ecchymosis, black tarry stool, hematuria; notify prescriber

Nursing diagnoses
☑ Tissue perfusion, altered (uses)
☑ Injury, risk for (uses, adverse reactions)
☑ Knowledge, deficient (teaching)

Implementation
• Give alone, do not mix with other drugs or solutions
• Give for 9-12 days
• Give only after screening patient for bleeding disorders
• Give SC only, do not give IM
• Give with patient recumbent, rotate inj sites (left/right anterolateral, left/right posterolateral abdominal wall)
• Insert whole length of needle into skin fold held with thumb and forefinger
• Give at same time of day to maintain blood level
• Administer only this drug when ordered, not interchangeable with heparin
• Bed rest during entire course of treatment
• Avoidance of venous or arterial puncture, inj, rectal temp
• Treatment of fever with acetaminophen

Patient/family education
• Teach about drug use and expected results; to report adverse reactions; bleeding, bruising
• Advise to avoid all OTC drugs unless prescribed
• Instruct to use soft-bristle toothbrush to avoid bleeding gums, to use electric razor

Evaluation
Therapeutic response
• Absence of DVT

❗RARELY USED

efalizumab
See Appendix F

 Herb/drug   Do Not Crush   Alert   Key Drug   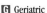 Geriatric   P Pediatric

emtricitabine (Rx)
(em-tri-sit'uh-bean)
Emtriva
Func. class.: Antiretroviral
Chem. class.: Nucleoside reverse transcriptase inhibitor (NRTI)
Pregnancy category B

Action: Synthetic nucleoside analog of cytosine; inhibits replication of HIV virus by competing with the natural substrate and then becoming incorporated into cellular DNA by viral reverse transcriptase, thereby terminating cellular DNA chain

➡ **Therapeutic Outcome:** Decreasing symptoms of HIV

Uses: HIV-1 infection with other antiretrovirals.

Dosage and routes
Adult: PO 200 mg qd

Renal dose
Adult: PO CCr 30-49 ml/min 200 mg q48h; 15-29 ml/min 200 mg q72h; <15 ml/min 200 mg q96h

Available forms: Cap 200 mg

Adverse effects
(*italic* = common; **bold** = life-threatening)
CNS: Headache, abnormal dreams, depression, dizziness, insomnia, neuropathy, paresthesia
GI: Nausea, vomiting, diarrhea, anorexia, abdominal pain, dyspepsia
INTEG: Rash, skin discoloration
MS: Arthralgia, myalgia
RESP: Cough
SYST: Change in body fat distribution

Contraindications: Hypersensitivity

P Precautions: Pregnancy **B**, lactation, **G** children, elderly, renal disease, hepatic insufficiency, chronic hepatitis B

Pharmacokinetics

Absorption	Rapidly, extensively absorbed
Distribution	Protein binding <4%
Metabolism	Unknown
Excretion	Excreted unchanged in urine (86%), feces (14%)
Half-life	10 hr

Pharmacodynamics

Onset	Unknown
Peak	1-2 hr
Duration	Unknown

Interactions: None known

NURSING CONSIDERATIONS
Assessment
• Monitor liver, renal function tests: AST, ALT, bilirubin, amylase, lipase, triglycerides periodically during treatment
• Assess for lactic acidosis, severe hepatomegaly with steatosis; if lab reports confirm these conditions, discontinue treatment

Nursing diagnoses
✓ Infection, risk for (uses)
✓ Injury, risk for (adverse reactions)
✓ Knowledge, deficient (teaching)

Implementation
PO route
• Give without regard to meals
• Store at 25° C (77° F)

Patient/family education
• Teach that GI complaints resolve after 3-4 wk of treatment
• Advise not to breastfeed while taking this drug
• Instruct that drug must be taken at same time of day to maintain blood level
• Advise that drug will control symptoms, but is not a cure for HIV; patient is still infectious, may pass HIV virus on to others
• Instruct that other drugs may be necessary to prevent other infections
• Advise that changes in body fat distribution may occur

Evaluation
Therapeutic response
• ↓ in signs/symptoms of HIV

enfuvirtide (Rx)
(en-fyoo'vir-tide)
Fuzeon
Func. class.: Antiretroviral
Chem. class.: Fusion inhibitor
Pregnancy category B

Action: Inhibitor of the fusion of HIV-1 with CD4+ cells

➡ **Therapeutic Outcome:** Decreasing symptoms of HIV

Uses: Treatment of HIV-1 infection in combination with other antiretrovirals

Dosage and routes
Adult: SC 90 mg (1 ml) bid
P *Child 6-16 yr:* SC 2 mg/kg bid, max 90 mg bid

Available forms: Powder for inj, lyophilized 108 mg (90 mg/ml when reconstituted)

Adverse effects
(*italic* = common; **bold** = life-threatening)
CNS: Anxiety, peripheral neuropathy, taste disturbance, **Guillain-Barré syndrome,** insomnia, depression
GI: Abdominal pain, anorexia, constipation, pancreatitis
GU: **Glomerulonephritis, renal failure**
HEMA: **Thrombocytopenia, neutropenia**
INTEG: Inj site reaction
MISC: Influenza, cough, conjunctivitis, lymphadenopathy, myalgias, hyperglycemia, pneumonia

Contraindications: Hypersensitivity

Precautions: Liver disease, pregnancy **B**, lactation, children <6 yr, myelosuppression, infections

Pharmacokinetics	
Absorption	Well
Distribution	92% protein binding
Metabolism	Undergoes catabolism
Excretion	Unknown
Half-life	Unknown

Pharmacodynamics	
Onset	Unknown
Peak	Unknown
Duration	Unknown

Interactions
None known

NURSING CONSIDERATIONS
Assessment
• Assess for signs of infection, inj site reactions
• Monitor renal studies: BUN, creatinine, renal failure may occur
• Monitor bowel pattern before, during treatment; if severe abdominal pain or constipation occurs, notify prescriber; monitor hydration
• Assess skin eruptions, rash, urticaria, itching
• Identify allergies before treatment, reaction to each medication
• CBC, blood chemistry, plasma HIV RNA, absolute CD4+/CD8+ cell counts/%, serum β_2 microglobulin, serum ICD+24 antigen levels, cholesterol

Nursing diagnoses
☑ Infection, risk for (uses)
☑ Injury, risk for (adverse reactions)
☑ Knowledge, deficient (teaching)

Implementation
• Give SC, bid, rotate sites

Patient/family education
• Instruct to notify prescriber if pregnancy is suspected, or if breastfeeding
• Advise that pneumonia may occur, to contact prescriber if cough, fever occur
• Teach that hypersensitive reactions may occur, rash, pruritus; stop drug, contact prescriber
• Teach that this drug is not a cure for HIV-1 infection but controls symptoms, HIV-1 can still be transmitted to others
• Teach that this drug is to be used in combination only with other antiretrovirals

Evaluation
Therapeutic response
• Increased CD4 cell counts; decreased viral load; slowing progression of HIV-1 infection

---

fosamprenavir (Rx)
(fos-am-pren'a-veer)
Lexiva
Func. class.: Antiretroviral
Chem. class.: Protease inhibitor
Pregnancy category C

Action: Prodrug of amprenavir; inhibits human immunodeficiency virus (HIV) protease, which prevents maturation of the infectious virus

⇒ **Therapeutic Outcome:** Decreasing symptoms of HIV

Uses: HIV-1 infection in combination with antiretrovirals

Dosage and routes
Therapy-naïve patients
Adult: PO 1400 mg bid without ritonavir, or fosamprenavir 1400 mg qd and ritonavir 200 mg qd, or fosamprenavir 700 mg bid and ritonavir 100 mg bid

Protease experienced patients (PI)
Adult: PO 700 mg bid and ritonavir 100 mg bid

Combination with efavirenz
Adult: PO add another 100 mg/day of ritonavir for a total of 300 mg/day when all three drugs are given

---

Hepatic dose
Adult (Child-Pugh 5-8): PO 700 mg bid; do not use in Child-Pugh 9-12

Available forms: Tabs 700 mg (equivalent to 600 mg amprenavir)

Adverse effects
(*italic* = common; **bold** = life-threatening)
CNS: Headache, fatigue, depression, oral paresthesia
GI: *Nausea, diarrhea, vomiting, abdominal pain*
INTEG: Rash, pruritus
MISC: Redistribution or accumulation of body fat

Contraindications: Hypersensitivity to protease inhibitors

Precautions: Liver disease, hemolytic anemia,diabetes, sulfa sensitivity, pregnancy **C**, G lactation, elderly

Pharmacokinetics	
Absorption	Unknown
Distribution	90% protein binding
Metabolism	In the liver by CYP4503AY (CYP3A4)
Excretion	Excretion of unchanged drug is minimal
Half-life	Unknown

Pharmacodynamics	
Onset	Unknown
Peak	1-4 hr
Duration	Unknown

Interactions
Individual drugs
⬦Amiodarone, antacids, lidocaine: Serious dysrhythmias
⬦Calcium channel blockers: Serious dysrhythmias
Contraceptives (oral), methadone: ↓ effect
Efavirenz, nevirapine, ranitidine, saquinavir: ↓ fosamprenavir levels
HMG-CoA reductase inhibitors: ↑ toxicity; do not use with pimozide, ergots, midazolam, triazolam, flecainide, propafenone
Itraconazole, ketoconazole, rifbutin, sildenafil, vardenafil: ↑ effect
Avoid use with rifampin, delavirdine, carbamazepine, phenobarbital, phenytoin because may lose virologic response and possibly lead to resistance to fosamprenavir
Warfarin: May affect coagulation
Drug classifications
Avoid use with H2 receptor antagonists, proton pump inhibitors because may lose virologic response and possibly lead to resistance of fosamprenavir
🗌 *Herb/drug*
Avoid use with St. John's wort because may lose virologic response and possibly lead to resistance of fosamprenavir

NURSING CONSIDERATIONS
Assessment
• Assess bowel pattern before, during treatment; monitor hydration
• Assess skin eruptions, rash, urticaria, itching
• Monitor viral load, CD4 cell counts baseline and throughout treatment

Nursing diagnoses
☑ Infection, risk for (uses)
☑ Injury, risk for (adverse reactions)
☑ Knowledge, deficient (teaching)

Implementation
• Administer without regard to food

Patient/family education
• Advise to avoid taking with other medications unless directed by provider
• Teach that drug does not cure, but does manage symptoms; that drug does not prevent transmission of HIV to others
• Advise to use nonhormonal form of birth control while taking this drug
• Instruct if dose is missed, take as soon as remembered up to 1 hr before next dose; do not double dose
• Instruct not to alter dose or stop therapy without talking to physician
• Advise physician if patient has a sulfa allergy
• Advise to report all medications, including herbal supplements, to physician
• Advise that patients receiving phosphodiesterase type 5 inhibitors may be at ↑ risk for PDE5 inhibitor adverse effects

Evaluation
Positive therapeutic response
• Decreasing symptoms of HIV

gefitinib (Rx)
(ge-fi'tye-nib)
Iressa
Func. class.: Antineoplastic—misc.
Chem. class.: Epidermal growth factor receptor inhibitor
Pregnancy category D

Action: Not fully understood; inhibits intracellular phosphorylation of cell surface receptors associated with epidermal growth factor receptors

→ **Therapeutic Outcome:** Decreased growth and spread of malignant cells

Uses: Non–small cell lung cancer (NSCLC)

Dosage and routes
Adult: PO 250 mg qd
CYP3A4 inducers concurrently (such as rifampin or phenytoin)
Adult: PO 500 mg qd

Available forms: Tabs 250 mg

Adverse effects
(*italic* = common; **bold** = life-threatening)
GI: Nausea, diarrhea, vomiting, anorexia, **pancreatitis,** mouth ulceration
INTEG: Rash, pruritus, acne, dry skin, **toxic epidermal neurolysis, angioedema**
MISC: Peripheral edema, amblyopia, conjunctivitis, eye pain, corneal erosion/ulcer
RESP: **Interstitial lung disease,** cough, dyspnea

Contraindications: Hypersensitivity, pregnancy **D**

Precautions: Renal, hepatic, ocular, **P** pulmonary disorders, lactation, children, **G** elderly

Pharmacokinetics	
Absorption	Slowly
Distribution	Unknown
Metabolism	Unknown
Excretion	In feces (86%), urine (<4%)
Half-life	Unknown

Pharmacodynamics	
Onset	Unknown
Peak	3-7 hr
Duration	Unknown

Interactions
Individual drugs
Cimetidine, phenytoin, ranitidine, rifampin, sodium bicarbonate: ↓ levels
Clarithromycin, erythromycin, itraconazole, ketoconazole: ↑ concentration
Metoprolol, warfarin: ↑ plasma concentration

NURSING CONSIDERATIONS
Assessment
◆• Assess pulmonary changes: lung sounds, cough, dyspnea; interstitial lung disease may occur, may be fatal; discontinue therapy if confirmed
• Assess ocular changes: eye irritation, corneal erosion/ulcer, aberrant eyelash growth
◆• Assess for pancreatitis: abdominal pain, levels of amylase, lipase
◆• Assess for toxic epidermal necrosis, angioedema
• Monitor GI symptoms: frequency of stools; if diarrhea is poorly tolerated, therapy may be discontinued for up to 14 days

Nursing diagnoses
✓ Injury, risk for (adverse reactions)
✓ Body image, disturbed (adverse reactions)
✓ Infection, risk for (adverse reactions)
✓ Knowledge, deficient (teaching)

Implementation
• Give PO, without regard to food

Patient/family education
• Teach to report adverse reactions immediately: SOB, severe abdominal pain, occular changes, skin eruptions
• Advise of reason for treatment, expected results
• Advise to use contraception during treatment, pregnancy **D**

Evaluation
Positive therapeutic outcome
• ↓ Non–small cell lung cancer cells

---

gemifloxacin (Rx)
(gem-ah-flox'a-sin)
Factive
Func. class.: Antiinfective
Chem. class.: Fluoroquinolone

Pregnancy category C

Action: Inhibits DNA gyrase, which is an enzyme involved in replication, transcription, and repair of bacterial DNA

→ **Therapeutic Outcome:** Negative C&S, decreasing symptoms of infection

Uses: Acute bacterial exacerbation of chronic bronchitis caused by *Streptococcus pneumoniae, Haemophilus influenzae, H. parainfluenzae, Moraxella catarrhalis;* community-acquired pneumonia caused by *Streptococcus pneumoniae* including multidrug-resistant strains, *H. influenzae, M. catarrhalis, Mycoplasma pneumoniae, Chlamydia pneumoniae, Klebsiella pneumoniae*

Dosage and routes
Adult: PO 320 mg/day × 5-7 days depending on type of infection

---

 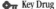

Renal dose
Adult: PO CCr ≤40 ml/min 160 mg q24hr

Available forms: Tabs 320 mg

Adverse effects
(*italic* = common; **bold** = life-threatening)
CNS: Dizziness, headache, somnolence, depression, insomnia, nervousness, confusion, agitation, ***seizures***
EENT: Visual disturbances
GI: Diarrhea, *nausea,* vomiting, anorexia, flatulence, heartburn, dry mouth; ↑ AST, ALT; constipation, abdominal pain, oral thrush, glossitis, stomatitis, pseudomembranous colitis
INTEG: Rash, pruritus, urticaria, *photosensitivity*
SYST: **Anaphylaxis, Stevens-Johnson syndrome**

Contraindications: Hypersensitivity to quinolones

Precautions: Hypokalemia, hypomagnesemia, pregnancy **C**, lactation, children, elderly, renal disease, seizure disorders, excessive exposure to sunlight, psychosis, increased intracranial pressure, history of dysrhythmias, history of QT interval prolongation

Pharmacokinetics	
Absorption	Unknown
Distribution	Unknown
Metabolism	Unknown
Excretion	In urine as active drug, metabolites
Half-life	6-8 hr

Pharmacodynamics	
Onset	Unknown
Peak	1-2 hr
Duration	Unknown

Interactions
Individual drugs
Cimetidine, probenecid: May ↑ toxicity
CycloSPORINE, warfarin: ↑ levels, watch for toxicity
Theophylline: May ↓ clearance, watch for toxicity
Drug classifications
Antacids containing aluminum, magnesium, sucralfate, zinc, iron: ↓ absorption, give 4 hr ac or 2 hr pc
Antiarrhythmics (amiodarone, bretylium, procainamide, quinidine, sotalol, disopyramide): May ↓ effect, resulting in life-threatening dysrhythmias
NSAIDs: May ↑ CNS stimulation, seizures

NURSING CONSIDERATIONS
Assessment
• Monitor kidney, liver function tests: BUN, creatinine, AST, ALT
• Monitor I&O ratio; urine pH, <5.5 is ideal
• Assess CNS symptoms: insomnia, vertigo, headache, agitation, confusion
• Assess allergic reactions and anaphylaxis: rash, flushing, urticaria, pruritus, chills, fever, joint pain; may occur a few days after therapy begins; epINEPHrine and resuscitation equipment should be available for anaphylactic reaction
• Monitor bowel pattern qd, if severe diarrhea occurs, drug should be discontinued
• Assess for overgrowth of infection: perineal itching, fever, malaise, redness, pain, swelling, drainage, rash, diarrhea, change in cough, sputum

Nursing diagnoses
✓ Infection, risk for (uses)
✓ Knowledge, deficient (teaching)
✓ Noncompliance (teaching)

Implementation
• Administer 4 hr before or 2 hr after antacids, iron, calcium, zinc products

Patient/family education
• Advise that patient may take with or without food
• Advise that fluids must be increased to 2 L/day to avoid crystallization in kidneys
• Instruct that if dizziness or light-headedness occurs, to ambulate, perform activities with assistance
• Instruct to complete full course of drug therapy
• Teach to contact prescriber if adverse reactions occur
• Teach to avoid iron- or mineral-containing supplements or antacids within 4 hr before and 2 hr after dosing
• Advise that photosensitivity may occur and sunscreen should be used
• Advise to use frequent rinsing of mouth, sugarless candy or gum for dry mouth
• Teach to avoid other medication unless approved by prescriber
• Teach not to use theophylline with this product, toxicity may result; contact prescriber if taking theophylline

Evaluation
Therapeutic response
• Negative C&S, absence of signs/symptoms of infection

! RARELY USED

laronidase
See Appendix F

memantine (Rx)
(me-man'teen)
Namenda
Func. class.: Anti-Alzheimer's disease agent
Chem. class.: NMDA receptor antagonist

Pregnancy category B

Action: Antagonist action of CNS NMDA receptors that may contribute to the symptoms of Alzheimer's disease

➡ **Therapeutic Outcome:** Improved mood, orientation, decreasing confusion

Uses: Treatment of moderate to severe dementia in Alzheimer's disease

Investigational uses: Vascular dementia

Dosage and routes
Adult: PO 5 mg qd, may increase dose in 5-mg increments ≥1-wk intervals

Available forms: Tabs 5, 10 mg

Adverse effects
(*italic* = common; **bold** = life-threatening)
CNS: Dizziness, confusion, somnolence, headache, hallucinations
CV: Hypertension
GI: Vomiting, constipation
INTEG: Rash
MISC: Back pain, fatigue, pain
RESP: Coughing, dyspnea

Contraindications: Hypersensitivity

Precautions: Renal disease, GU conditions, which raise urine pH; pregnancy **B**, lactation, **P** children

Pharmacokinetics	
Absorption	Rapidly absorbed PO
Distribution	44% protein binding
Metabolism	Very little
Excretion	57%-82% excreted unchanged in urine
Half-life	Terminal elimination half-life 60-80 hr

Pharmacodynamics	
Onset	Unknown
Peak	Unknown
Duration	Unknown

Interactions
Individual drugs
Cimetidine, hydrochlorothiazide, nicotine, quinidine, ranitidine, triamterene: May alter levels of both drugs
Drug classifications
Drugs that make the urine alkaline (sodium bicarbonate, carbonic anhydrase inhibitors): ↓ clearance

NURSING CONSIDERATIONS
Assessment
• Monitor B/P: hypertension
• Assess mental status: affect, mood, behavioral changes; hallucinations, confusion
• Assess GI status: vomiting, constipation, add bulk, increase fluids for constipation
• Assess GU status: urinary frequency

Nursing diagnoses
☑ Thought processes, altered (uses)
☑ Injury, risk for (uses)
☑ Knowledge, deficient (teaching)
☑ Noncompliance (teaching)

Implementation
• Give twice a day if dose >5 mg
• Dosage is adjusted to response no more than q1 wk
• Provide assistance with ambulation during beginning therapy; dizziness may occur

Patient/family education
• Advise to report side effects: restlessness, psychosis, visual hallucinations, stupor, loss of consciousness; indicate overdose
• Advise to use drug exactly as prescribed; drug is not a cure

Evaluation
Therapeutic response
• Decrease in confusion, improved mood

! RARELY USED

miglustat
See Appendix F

omalizumab (Rx)
(oh-mah-lye-zoo'mab)
Xolair
Func. class.: Monoclonal antibody

Pregnancy category B

Action: Recombinant DNA-derived humanized IgG murine monoclonal antibody that selectively binds to IgE to limit the release of mediators in the allergic response

---

 Herb/drug   Do Not Crush   Alert   Key Drug   Geriatric   **P** Pediatric

⇥ **Therapeutic Outcome:** Ability to breathe more easily

Uses: Moderate to severe persistent asthma

Investigational uses: Seasonal allergic rhinitis

Dosage and routes
Adult: **SC** 150-375 mg × 2-4 wk, divide inj into 2 sites, if dose is >150 mg

Available forms: Powder for inj, lyophilized 202.5 mg (150 mg/1.2 ml after reconstitution)

Adverse effects
(*italic* = common; **bold** = life-threatening)
INTEG: Pruritus, dermatitis, inj site reactions
MISC: Earache, dizziness, fatigue, pain, **malignancies,** viral infections
MS: Arthralgia, fracture, leg, arm pain
RESP: Sinusitis, upper respiratory tract infections, pharyngitis

Contraindications: Hypersensitivity

Precautions: Acute attacks of asthma, ▣ lactation, children <12 yr, pregnancy **B**

Pharmacokinetics	
Absorption	Slow
Distribution	Unknown
Metabolism	Degradation by liver
Excretion	In bile
Half-life	26 days

Pharmacodynamics	
Onset	Unknown
Peak	7-8 days
Duration	Unknown

Interactions
None known

NURSING CONSIDERATIONS
Assessment
• Monitor respiratory rate, rhythm, depth; auscultate lung fields bilaterally; notify prescriber of abnormalities
• Assess for allergic reactions: rash, urticaria; drug should be discontinued

Nursing diagnoses
☑ Impaired gas exchange (uses)
☑ Knowledge, deficient (teaching)

Implementation
SC route
• Given q2-4 wk; product is viscous; if >150 mg is given, divide into two sites; the inj may take 5-10 sec to administer
• Do not give more than 150 mg/inj site

Patient/family education
• Advise that improvement will not be immediate
• Teach not to stop taking or decrease current asthma medications unless instructed by prescriber

Evaluation
Therapeutic response
• Ability to breathe more easily

---

palonosetron (Rx)
(pa-lone-o′se-tron)
Aloxi
Func. class.: Antiemetic
Chem. class.: 5-HT₃ receptor antagonist
Pregnancy category B

Action: Prevents nausea, vomiting by blocking serotonin peripherally, centrally, and in the small intestine at the 5-HT₃ receptor

⇥ **Therapeutic Outcome:** Decreased nausea, vomiting during chemotherapy

Uses: Prevention of nausea, vomiting associated with cancer chemotherapy

Dosage and routes
Adult: **IV** 0.25 mg as a single dose over 30 sec, 30 min prior to chemotherapy

Available forms: Inj 0.25 mg/5 ml

Adverse effects
(*italic* = common; **bold** = life-threatening)
CNS: *Headache, dizziness, drowsiness, fatigue, insomnia*
GI: *Diarrhea, constipation,* abdominal pain
MISC: Weakness, hyperkalemia, anxiety, rash, **bronchospasm** (rare), arthralgia, *fever, urinary retention*

Contraindications: Hypersensitivity

Precautions: Pregnancy **B**, lactation, ▣ children, elderly, prolongation of QT interval ▣ or other cardiac conduction intervals (patients with hypokalemia, hypomagnesemia, taking diuretics, with congenital QT syndrome, and taking antidysrhythmics or other drugs that may prolong QT interval and cumulative high-dose antithramycline therapy)

Pharmacokinetics	
Absorption	Unknown
Distribution	62% protein bound
Metabolism	Liver
Excretion	Unchanged drug and metabolites excreted by kidney
Half-life	40 hr

Pharmacodynamics

Onset	Unknown
Peak	Unknown
Duration	Unknown

Interactions
None known

NURSING CONSIDERATIONS
Assessment
- Monitor for absence of nausea, vomiting during chemotherapy
- Assess hypersensitivity reaction: rash, bronchospasm

Nursing diagnoses
☑ Knowledge, deficient (teaching)

Implementation
IV **IV route**
- Give as a single dose over 30 sec
- Do not mix with other drugs, flush **IV** line before and after administration
- Store at room temp

Patient/family education
- Teach to report diarrhea, constipation, rash, or changes in respirations or discomfort at insertion site

Evaluation
Positive therapeutic outcome
- Absence of nausea, vomiting during cancer chemotherapy

⚠ RARELY USED

pegvisomant
See Appendix F

---

rosuvastatin (Rx)
(roe-soo′va-sta-tin)
Crestor
Func. class.: Antilipemic
Chem. class.: HMG-CoA reductase inhibitor

Pregnancy category X

Action: Inhibits HMG-CoA reductase enzyme, which reduces cholesterol synthesis

➡ **Therapeutic Outcome:** Decreasing cholesterol levels

Uses: As an adjunct in primary hypercholesterolemia (types IIa, IIb), mixed dyslipidemia elevated serum triglycerides, homozygous familial hypercholesterolemia (FH)

Dosage and routes
Patient should first be placed on a cholesterol-lowering diet

Hypercholesterolemia
Adult: PO 5-40 mg qd; initial dose 10 mg qd, reanalyze lipid levels at 2-4 wk and adjust dosage accordingly

Homozygous FH
Adult: PO 20 mg qd, max 40 mg

Dose in patients taking cycloSPORINE
Adult: 5 mg qd

Dose when taken with gemfibrozil
Adult: 10 mg qd

Available forms: Tabs 5, 10, 20, 40 mg

Adverse effects
(*italic* = common; **bold** = life-threatening)
CNS: Headache, dizziness, insomnia, paresthesia
GI: Nausea, constipation, abdominal pain, flatus, diarrhea, dyspepsia, heartburn, **liver dysfunction,** vomiting
HEMA: **Thrombocytopenia, hemolytic anemia, leukopenia**
INTEG: Rash, pruritus, photosensitivity
MS: Asthenia, muscle cramps, arthritis, arthralgia, myalgia, **myositis, rhabdomyolysis,** leg, shoulder or localized pain
RESP: Rhinitis, sinusitis, *pharyngitis,* bronchitis, ↑ cough

Contraindications: Hypersensitivity, pregnancy **X**, lactation, active liver disease

Precautions: Past liver disease, alcoholism, severe acute infections, trauma, hypotension, uncontrolled seizure disorders, severe metabolic disorders, electrolyte imbalances, **P** children, severe renal impairment, elderly, **G** hypothyroidism

Pharmacokinetics

Absorption	Unknown
Distribution	88% protein bound, crosses placenta
Metabolism	Minimal liver metabolism (about 10%)
Excretion	Primarily in feces (90%)
Half-life	19 hr

Pharmacodynamics

Onset	Unknown
Peak	3-5 hr
Duration	Unknown

 Herb/drug   Do Not Crush   Alert   Key Drug   Geriatric   **P** Pediatric

Interactions
Individual drugs
Clofibrate, cycloSPORINE, gemfibrozil, niacin: ↑ myalgia, myositis
Warfarin: ↑ bleeding
Drug classifications
Antifungals (azole): ↑ myalgia, myositis
Bile acid sequestrants: ↑ effects
Food/drug
Grapefruit juice: Possible toxicity

NURSING CONSIDERATIONS
Assessment
• Assess diet: obtain diet history including fat, cholesterol in diet
• Monitor fasting cholesterol, LDL, HDL, triglycerides periodically during treatment
• Monitor liver function tests q1-2 mo during the first 1½ yr of treatment; AST, ALT, liver function tests may increase
• Monitor renal function in patients with compromised renal system: BUN, creatinine, I&O ratio
• Obtain ophthalmic exam before, 1 mo after treatment begins, annually; lens opacities may occur
◆• Assess for muscle pain, tenderness, obtain CPK; if these occur, drug may need to be discontinued

Nursing diagnoses
☑ Knowledge, deficient (teaching)
☑ Noncompliance (teaching)

Implementation
• May be taken at any time of day, with or without food
• Store in cool environment in airtight, light-resistant container

Patient/family education
• Advise to report suspected pregnancy
• Advise that blood work and ophthalmic exam will be necessary during treatment
• Teach to report blurred vision, severe GI symptoms, dizziness, headache, muscle pain, weakness
• Teach to use sunscreen or stay out of the sun to prevent photosensitivity
• Teach that previously prescribed regimen will continue: low-cholesterol diet, exercise program, smoking cessation

Evaluation
Positive therapeutic outcome
• Cholesterol at desired level after 8 wk

tadalafil (Rx)
(tah-dal′a-fil)
Cialis
Func. class.: Impotence agent
Chem. class.: Phosphodiesterase type 5 inhibitor

Action: Inhibits phosphodiesterase type 5 (PDE5); enhances erectile function by increasing the amount of cGMP, which causes smooth muscle relaxation and increased blood flow into the corpus cavernosum; improves erectile function for up to 36 hr

⇥**Therapeutic Outcome:** Erection

Uses: Treatment of erectile dysfunction

Dosage and routes
Adult: PO 10 mg, taken prior to sexual activity, dose may be reduced to 5 mg or increased to a max of 20 mg; usual max dosing frequency is once per day
Renal dose
Adult (CCr 31-50 ml/min): PO 5 mg/qd, max 10 mg q48hr; CCr <30 ml/min, max 5 mg
Hepatic dose
Adult (Child-Pugh class A, B): PO max 10 mg qd; Child-Pugh class C, not recommended
Concomitant medications
Ketoconazole, ritonavir, max 10 mg q72hr

Available forms: Tabs 5, 10, 20 mg
Adverse effects
(*italic* = common; **bold** = life-threatening)
CV: **MI, sudden death, CV collapse**
CNS: *Headache, flushing, dizziness*
MISC: Back pain/myalgia, *dyspepsia, nasal congestion, UTI,* blurred vision, changes in color vision, *diarrhea,* pruritus

Contraindications: Hypersensitivity, patients taking organic nitrates regularly or intermittently, patients taking any α-adrenergic antagonist other than 0.4 mg once daily tamsulosin

Precautions: Anatomic penile deformities, sickle cell anemia, leukemia, multiple myeloma; tadalafil is not indicated for use in
Ⓟ newborns, children, or women

Pharmacokinetics

Absorption	Rapid; rate and extent of absorption of tadalafil are not influenced by food
Distribution	94% protein bound
Metabolism	Liver
Excretion	Excreted primarily as metabolites, feces, urine; plasma concentration 61% in feces, 36% in urine
Half-life	17.5 hr

Pharmacodynamics

Onset	Rapid
Peak	6 hr
Duration	Unknown

Interactions
Individual drugs
Ketoconazole, ritonavir: ↑ levels (although not studied, may also include other HIV protease inhibitors)
Drug classifications
◆• Do not use with nitrates because of unsafe drop in B/P that could result in heart attack or stroke
• Antihypertensive medications: ↓ B/P

NURSING CONSIDERATIONS
Assessment
• Use of organic nitrates that should not be used with this drug

Nursing diagnoses
☑ Sexual dysfunction (uses)
☑ Knowledge, deficient (teaching)

Implementation
PO route
• Before sexual activity; do not use more than once a day

Patient/family education
• Advise that drug does not protect against STDs, including HIV
• Instruct to tell physician if patient has a bleeding problem
• Advise that drug should not be used with nitrates in any form
• Advise that drug has no effect in the absence of sexual stimulation
• Instruct to seek medical help if an erection lasts more than 4 hr
• Advise to tell physician of all medicines, vitamins, and herbs patient is taking, especially α-blockers, erythromycin, indinavir, itraconazole, ketoconozole, nitrates, ritonavir
• Advise that tadalafil is contraindicated for use with α-blockers except 0.4 mg/daily tamsulosin

Evaluation
Positive therapeutic outcome
• Sustainable erection

---

vardenafil (Rx)
(var-den'a-fil)
Levitra
Func. class.: Impotence agent
Chem. class.: Phosphodiesterase type 5 inhibitor

Pregnancy category B

Action: Inhibits phosphodiesterase type 5 (PDE5); enhances erectile function by increasing the amount of cGMP, which causes smooth muscle relaxation and increased blood flow into the corpus cavernosum

▶ **Therapeutic Outcome:** Erection

Uses: Treatment of erectile dysfunction

Dosage and routes
Adult: PO 10 mg, taken 1 hr before sexual activity, dose may be reduced to 5 mg or increased to a max of 20 mg; max dosing frequency is once daily

G *Elderly >65 yr:* PO 5 mg initially

Hepatic dose (Child-Pugh B)
Adult: PO 5 mg, max 10 mg

Concomitant medications
Ritonavir, max 2.5 mg q72 h; for indinavir, ketoconazole 400 mg/day and itraconazole 400 mg/day, max 2.5 mg/day; for ketoconazole 200 mg/day, itraconazole 200 mg/day and erythromycin max 5 mg/day

Available forms: Tabs 2.5, 5, 10, 20 mg

Adverse effects
(*italic* = common; **bold** = life-threatening)
CNS: Headache, flushing, dizziness, insomnia
CV: Hypertension, **MI, CV collapse**
EENT: Conjunctivitis, tinnitus, photophobia, diminished vision, glaucoma
GU: Abnormal ejaculation, priapism
MISC: Rash, GERD, GGTP ↑
MS: Myalgia, arthralgia, neck pain
RESP: Rhinitis, sinusitis, dyspnea, pharyngitis, epistaxis

Contraindications: Hypersensitivity, coadministration of α-blockers or nitrates

Precautions: Hepatic impairment, retinitis pigmentosa, cardiovascular disease including congenital or acquired QT prolongation, anatomic penile deformities, sickle cell anemia, leukemia, multiple myeloma, pregnancy

---

 Herb/drug   Do Not Crush   ◆ Alert   Key Drug   **G** Geriatric   **P** Pediatric

P **B**, not indicated for women, children, or newborns

Pharmacokinetics

Absorption	Rapid; reduced absorption with high-fat meal
Distribution	Bioavailability 15%; protein binding 95%
Metabolism	Liver
Excretion	Primarily in feces (91%-95%)
Half-life	4-5 hr

Pharmacodynamics

Onset	20 min
Peak	½-1½
Duration	<5 hr

Interactions
Individual drugs
Cimetidine, erythromycin, itraconazole, ketoconazole: ↑ levels
Indinavir, ritonavir: ↓ protease inhibitor effect
Nifedipine: ↓ B/P
Drug classifications
α-Blockers, protease inhibitors: Do not use concurrently
◆ Do not use with nitrates because of unsafe ↓ in B/P that could result in heart attack or stroke

NURSING CONSIDERATIONS
Assessment
• Assess for use of organic nitrates that should not be used with this drug

Nursing diagnoses
☑ Sexual dysfunction (uses)
☑ Knowledge, deficient (teaching)
Implementation
PO route
• Give approximately 1 hr before sexual activity, do not use more than once a day
Patient/family education
• Advise that drug does not protect against sexually transmitted diseases, including HIV
• Teach that drug absorption is reduced with a high-fat meal
• Instruct that drug should not be used with nitrates in any form
• Inform that drug has no effect in the absence of sexual stimulation
• Teach that patient should seek immediate medical attention if erections last for more than 4 hr
• Advise to inform physician of all medications being taken
Evaluation
Positive therapeutic outcome
• Sustainable erection

Appendix B

Recent FDA Drug Approvals

GENERIC NAME	TRADE NAME	USE
abarelix	Plenaxis	Prostate cancer
bevacizumab	Avastin	Metastatic colorectal carcinoma
botulism immune globulin IV (Human) (BIG-IV)	BabyBIG	Infant botulism
cetuximab	Erbitux	Metastatic colorectal cancer
cinacalet	Sensipar	Parathyroid carcinoma
ibandronate	Boniva	Osteoporosis
pemetrexed	Alimta	Mesothelioma
sertaconazole	Ertaczo	*Tinea pedis*
tiotropium	Spiriva	COPD

Appendix C

High Alert Drugs

The Institute for Safe Medication Practices (ISMP) recently compiled a list of the medications with the greatest potential for patient harm if they are used in error. These high alert medications include drugs in the 19 classes listed below, as well as the specific drugs listed below. To help nurses identify these drugs, in this book each specific drug monograph is highlighted with a light color screen. Although care should be taken in giving any medication, nurses are advised to exercise extra precautions when administering these high-risk drugs.

Class/Category of Medications

adrenergic agonists, IV (e.g., epINEPHrine)
adrenergic antagonists, IV (e.g., propranolol)
anesthetic agents, general, inhaled, and IV (e.g., propofol)
cardioplegic solutions
chemotherapeutic agents, parenteral and oral
dextrose, hypertonic, 20% or greater
dialysis solutions, peritoneal and hemodialysis
epidural or intrathecal medications
glycoprotein IIb/IIIa inhibitors (e.g., eptifibatide)
hypoglycemics, oral
inotropic medications, IV (e.g., digoxin, milrinone)

liposomal forms of drugs (e.g., liposomal amphotericin B)
moderate sedation agents, IV (e.g., midazolam)
moderate sedation agents, oral, for children (e.g., chloral hydrate)
neuromuscular blocking agents (e.g., succinylcholine)
opioids, IV and oral (including liquid concentrates and immediate- and sustained-release)
radiocontrast agents, IV
thrombolytics/fibrinolytics, IV (e.g., tenecteplase)
total perenteral nutrition solutions

Individual Medications

abciximab
adenosine
aldesleukin
alteplase
amiodarone
anistreplase
antihemophilic factor
antithrombin III
ardeparin
argatroban
arsenic trioxide
asparaginase
atropine
basiliximab
bivalirudin
bleomycin
bretylium
busulfan
calfactant
carboplatin
carmustine
cisplatin
coagulation factor VIIa, recombinant
colchicine
cyclophosphamide
cytarabine
dacarbazine
daclizumab
dactinomycin
dalteparin
danaparoid
DAUNOrubicin

dezocine
digoxin
diltiazem
DOPamine
doxacurium
DOXOrubicin
droperidol
enoxaparin
epHEDrine
epINEPHrine
epirubicin
eptifibatide
etoposide
factor IX complex/factor IV
fentanyl
fentanyl/droperidol
fluorouracil
gallamine
gemtuzumab
heparin
hydromorphone
ibutilide
idarubicin
ifosfamide
inamrinone
insulin
irinotecan
ketamine
lepirudin
leuprolide
lidocaine
magnesium sulfate

melphalan
meperidine
methadone
methotrexate
milrinone
mitomycin
mitoxantrone
mivacurium
morphine
nalbuphine
nesiritide
nitroprusside
norepinephrine
oxycodone
oxymorphone
oxytocin
pancuronium
pegaspargase
pentazocine
pentobarbital IV
pentostatin
phenobarbital IV
pipecuronium
plicamycin

poractant alfa
potassium chloride inj concentrate
potassium phosphates inj
propofol
propoxyphene
remifentanil
rocuronium
secobarbital IV
sodium chloride inj, hypertonic
streptokinase
succinylcholine
sufentanil
tenecteplase
thiopental
tinzaparin
topotecan
trastuzumab
tubocurarine
urokinase
vecuronium
vinBLAStine
vinCRIStine
vinorelbine
warfarin

1. Cohen MR, Kilo CM: High-alert medications: safeguarding against errors. In Cohen MR, editor: *Medication Errors,* Washington, D.C., 1999, American Pharmaceutical Association.
2. Joint Commission on Accreditation of Healthcare Organizations: High-alert medications and patient safety, *Sentinel Event Alert,* Nov, 1999. Available at www.jcaho.org/edu_pub/sealert/sea11.html [Accessed on 4/30/02].
3. ISMP's List of High-Alert Medications, accessed on 2/13/04 at http: //www.ismp.org/msaarticles/highalert.htm.

Appendix D

Ophthalmic, Nasal, Topical, and Otic Products

OPHTHALMIC PRODUCTS

α-ADRENERGIC BLOCKER
dapiprazole (Rx)
(da-pip'ra-zole)
Rev-Eyes

ANESTHETICS
proparacaine (Rx)
(proe-par'a-kane)
Alcaine, Diocaine ♣, Ophthaine, Ophthestic
tetracaine
(tet'ra-kane)
Pontocaine, Tetracaine

ANTIHISTAMINES
azelastine (Rx)
(ay-zell'ah-steen)
Optivar
emedastine
(ee-med'-a-steen)
Emadine
epinastine (Rx)
(ep-een-as'teen)
Elestat
ketotifen (Rx)
(kee-toh-tif'en)
Zaditor
olopatadine (Rx)
(oh-loh-pat'ah-deen)
Patanol

ANTIINFECTIVES
bacitracin (Rx)
(bass-i-tray'sin)
AK-Tracin, Bacitracin Ophthalmic
chloramphenicol (Rx)
(klor-am-fen'i-kole)
AK-Chlor, Chloramphenicol, Chloromycetin Ophthalmic, Chloroptic, Chloroptic S.O.P., Fenicol ♣, Isopto Fenical ♣, Pentamycin ♣
ciprofloxacin (Rx)
(sip-ro-floks'a-sin)
Ciloxan

erythromycin (Rx)
(er-ith-roe-mye'sin)
Erythromycin, Ilotycin
fomivirsen (Rx)
(foh-muh-vir'sun)
Vitravene
ganciclovir (Rx)
(gan-sye'kloe-vir)
Vitrasert
gatifloxacin (Rx)
(gat-ih-floks'ah-sin)
Zymar
gentamicin (Rx)
(jen-ta-mye'sin)
Garamycin Ophthalmic, Genoptic Ophthalmic, Genoptic S.O.P., Gentacidin, Gentamicin Ophthalmic, Gentak
idoxuridine-IDU (Rx)
(eye-dox-yoor'i-deen)
Herplex
levofloxacin (Rx)
(lee-voh-flock'sah-sin)
Quixin
moxifloxacin (Rx)
Vigamox
natamycin (Rx)
(nat-a-mye'sin)
Natacyn
norfloxacin (Rx)
(nor-floks'a-sin)
Chibroxin
ofloxacin (Rx)
(oh-floks'a-sin)
Ocuflox
polymyxin B (Rx)
(pol-ee-mix'in)
Polymyxin B Sulfate Sterile

silver nitrate 1% (Rx)
silver nitrate
sulfacetamide sodium (Rx)
(sul-fa-seet'a-mide)
AK-Sulf, Bleph-10, Bleph-10 S.O.P.,
Cetamide, Isopto Cetamide, Ocusulf-10,
Sodium Sulamyd, sodium sulfacetamide,
Storz-Sulf, Sulf-10, Sulster
sulfisoxazole diolamine (Rx)
Gantrisin
tetracycline (Rx)
(tet-ra-sye'kleen)
Achromycin Ophthalmic
tobramycin (Rx)
(toe-bra-mye'sin)
AKTob, Defy, Tobrex
trifluridine (Rx)
(trye-floor'i-deen)
Viroptic
vidarabine (Rx)
(vye-dare'a-been)
Vira-A

β-ADRENERGIC BLOCKERS
betaxolol (Rx)
(beh-tax'oh-lole)
Betoptic, Betoptic S
carteolol (Rx)
(kar-tee'oh-lole)
Carteolol HCl, Ocupress
levobetaxolol (Rx)
(lee-voh-beh-tax'oh-lohl)
Betaxon
levobunolol (Rx)
(lee-voe-byoo'no-lole)
AK Beta, Betagen
metipranolol (Rx)
(met-ee-pran'oh-lole)
OptiPranolol
timolol (Rx)
(tym'-moe-lole)
Apo-Timop ✿, Betimol, Timoptic,
Timoptic-XE[3]

CARBONIC ANHYDRASE
INHIBITORS
brinzolamide (Rx)
(brin-zoh'la-mide)
Azopt
dorzolamide (Rx)
(dor-zol'a-mide)
Trusopt

CHOLINERGICS
(Direct-acting)
acetylcholine (Rx)
(ah-see-til-koe'leen)
Miochol-E
carbachol (Rx)
(kar'ba-kole)
Carbastat, Carboptic, Isopto Carbachol,
Miostat
pilocarpine (Rx)
(pye-loe-kar'peen)
Adsorbocarpine, Akarpine, Isopto Carpine,
Ocu-Carpine, Ocusert Pilo-20, Ocusert Pilo-
40, Pilagan, Pilocar, pilocarpine, Pilopine
HS, Piloptic-½, Piloptic-1, Piloptic-2,
Piloptic-3, Piloptic-4, Piloptic-6, Pilostat,
Pilopto-Carpine

CHOLINESTERASE INHIBITORS
demecarium (Rx)
(dem-e-kare'ee-um)
Humorsol
ecothiophate (Rx)
(ek-oh-thye'oh-fate)
Phospholine Iodide

CORTICOSTEROIDS
dexamethasone
(dex-a-meth'a-sone)
AK-Dex, Decadron Phosphate,
Dexamethasone Ophthalmic Suspension,
Maxidex
fluorometholone (Rx)
(flure-oh-meth'oh-lone)
Flarex, Fluor-Op, FML, FML Forte, FML
S.O.P.
loteprednol (Rx)
(loe-tee-pred-nole)
Alrex, Lotemax
medrysone (Rx)
(me'dri-sone)
HMS
prednisolone (Rx)
(pred-niss'oh-lone)
Econopred, Econopred Plus, AK-Pred,
Inflamase Forte, Inflamase Mild, PredForte
rimexolone (Rx)
(ri-mex'a-lone)
Vexol

 Herb/drug   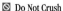 Do Not Crush   ✦ Alert   ⚭ Key Drug   G Geriatric   P Pediatric

MYDRIATICS
atropine (Rx)
(a'troe-peen)
Atropine-1, Atropine Care, Atropine Sulfate
Ophthalmic, Atropisol, Isopto Atropine
cyclopentolate (Rx)
(sye-kloe-pen'toe-late)
AK-Pentolate, Cyclogyl, Cyclopentolate HCl
homatropine (Rx)
(home-a'troe-peen)
Isopto Homatropine, Minims
Homatropine ✦, Homatropine HBr,
Hydroxyamphetamine HBr (Rx), Paredrine
scopolamine (Rx)
(skoe-pol'a-meen)
Isopto Hyoscine
tropicamide (Rx)
(troe-pik'a-mide)
Mydriacyl, Opticyl, Tropicacyl, Tropicamide

NONSTEROIDAL ANTIINFLAMMATORIES
diclofenac (Rx)
(dye-kloe'fen-ak)
Voltaran
flurbiprofen (Rx)
(flure-bi'-pro-fen)
Ocufen
ketorolac (Rx)
(kee-toe'role-ak)
Acular
suprofen
(soo-proe'fen)
Profenal

SYMPATHOMIMETICS
apraclonidine
(a-pra-klon'i-deen)
Iopidine
brimonidine (Rx)
(brem-on'-i-dine)
Alphagan, Alphagan P
dipivefrin
(dye-pi'vef-rin)
Propine, AKPro
*epINEPHrine/epinephryl borate (Rx)
(ep-i-nef'rin)
Epifrin, Glaucon/Epinal, Eppy ✦

OPHTHALMIC DECONGESTANTS/ VASOCONSTRICTORS
levocabastine (Rx)
(lee-voh-cab'ah-steen)
Livostin
lodoxamide
(loe-dox'ah-mide)
Alomide
naphazoline (OTC, Rx)
(naf-az'oh-leen)
20/20 Eye Drops, AK-Con Allergy Drops,
Albalon, Allerest Eye Drops, Clear Eyes,
Clear Eyes ACR, Comfort Eye Drops, Degest
2 Maximum Strength Allergy Drops,
Nafazair, naphazoline HCl, Naphcon,
Naphcon Forte, Opcon, Vasoclear, Vasocon
Regular, Estivin II
oxymetazoline (Rx, OTC)
(ox-i-met-ah-zoh'leen)
OcuClear, Visine L.R.
phenylephrine (OTC)
(fen-ill-ef'rin)
AK-Dilate, AK-Nefrin, Isopto Frin, Neo-
Synephrine 2.5%, Neo-Synephrine 10%,
phenylephrine HCl, 2.5% Mydfrin,
Phenoptic, Relief, Prefrin
tetrahydrozoline (OTC)
(tet-ra-hye-dro'zoe-leen)
Collyrium Fresh, Eyesine, Geneye, Geneye
Extra, Mallazine Eye Drops, Murine Plus,
Optigene 3, tetrahydrozoline HCl,
Tetrasine, Tetrasine Extra, Visine
Moisturizing

MISCELLANEOUS OPHTHALMICS
bimatoprost (Rx)
(by-mat'oh-prahst)
Lumigan
brinzolamide (Rx)
(brin-zole'aa-mide)
Azopt
dorzolamide (Rx)
(dor-zol'a-mid)
Trusopt
ketotifen
(ke-toe-tie'fen)
Zaditor
latanoprost (Rx)
(la-tan'oh-proest)
Xalatan

travoprost (Rx)
(trav'oh-prahst)
Travatan
unoprostone (Rx)
(yoo-noh-prahs'tohn)
Rescula

Pregnancy category:
demecarium, isoflurophate
X; apraclonidine, cyclo-
pentolate, ecothiopate,
glucocorticoids, levobunalol,
metipranolol, pilocarpine,
proparacaine, suprofen, tetracaine
C; dapiprazole, dipivefrin B

β-Adrenergic blockers
Action: Reduces production of aqueous humor by unknown mechanism

Uses: Ocular hypertension, chronic open-angle glaucoma

Anesthetics
Action: Decreases ion permeability by stabilizing neuronal membrane

Uses: Cataract extraction, tonometry, gonioscopy, removal of foreign objects, corneal suture removal, glaucoma surgery (ophth); pruritus, sunburn, toothache, sore throat, cold sores, oral pain, rectal pain and irritation, control of gagging (top)

Antiinfectives
Action: Inhibits folic acid synthesis by preventing PABA use, which is necessary for bacterial growth

Uses: Conjunctivitis, superficial eye infections, corneal ulcers, prophylaxis against infection after removal of foreign matter from the eye

Antiinflammatories
Action: Decreases inflammation, resulting in decreased pain, photophobia, hyperemia, cellular infiltration

Uses: Inflammation of eye, eyelids, conjunctiva, cornea; uveitis, iridocyclitis, allergic conditions, burns, foreign bodies, postoperatively in cataract

Carbonic anhydrase inhibitor
Action: Converted to epinephrine, which decreases aqueous production and increases outflow

Uses: Open-angle glaucoma, ocular hypertension

Direct-acting miotic
Action: Acts directly on cholinergic receptor sites; induces miosis, spasm of accommodation, fall in intraocular pressure, caused by stimulation of ciliary, pupillary sphincter muscles, which leads to pulling away of iris from filtration angle, resulting in increased outflow of aqueous humor

Uses: Primary glaucoma, early stages of wide-angle glaucoma (less useful in advanced stages), chronic open-angle glaucoma, acute narrow-angle glaucoma before emergency surgery; also neutralizes mydriatics used during eye exam; may be used alternately with mydriatics to break adhesions between iris and lens

Adverse effects
(*italic* = common; **bold** = life-threatening)
CNS: Headache
CV: Hypertension, tachycardia, dysrhythmias
EENT: Burning, stinging
GI: Bitter taste

Contraindications: Hypersensitivity

Precautions: Pregnancy, lactation, children, aphakia, hypersensitivity to carbonic anhydrase inhibitors, sulfonamides, thiazide diuretics, ocular inhibitors, hepatic and renal insufficiency

NURSING CONSIDERATIONS
Assessment
- Monitor ophthalmic exams and intraocular pressure readings
- Monitor blood counts; liver, renal function tests and serum electrolytes during long-term treatment

Nursing diagnoses
☑ Sensory perception, disturbed: visual (uses)
☑ Knowledge, deficient (teaching)

Implementation
- Storage at room temp away from light

Patient/family education
- Teach how to instill drops
- Advise patient that drug may cause burning, itching, blurring, dryness of eye area

Evaluation
Positive therapeutic outcome
- Absence of increased intraocular pressure

 Herb/drug   Do Not Crush   Alert   Key Drug   Geriatric   Pediatric

NASAL AGENTS

NASAL DECONGESTANTS
azelastine (Rx)
(ay-zell'ah-steen)
Astelin
desoxyephedrine (OTC)
(des-oxy-e-fed'rin)
Vicks Inhaler
*__epHEDrine__ (OTC)
(e-fed'rin)
Pretz-D
*__epINEPHrine__ (OTC)
(ep-i-neff'rin)
Adrenalin
naphazoline (OTC)
(naff-a-zoe'leen)
Privine
oxymetazoline (OTC)
(ox-i-met-az'oh-leen)
12 Hour Nasal, Afrin 12 Hour Original, Afrin 12-Hour Original Pump Mist, Afrin Severe Congestion With Menthol, Afrin Sinus With Vapornase, Afrin No-Drip 12-Hour, Afrin No-Drip 12-Hour Extra Moisturizing, Dristan, Duramist Plus, Duration, Genasal, Nafrine ✤, Neo-Synephrine 12 Hour, Nostrilla, oxymetazoline HCl, Nasal Relief, Nasal Decongestant, Maximum Strength, Vicks Sinex 12 Hour Long-Acting, Vicks Sinex 12-Hour Ultra Fine Mist for Sinus Relief
phenylephrine (OTC)
(fen-ill-eff'rin)
Alconefrin 12, Children's Nostril, Neo-Synephrine, Sinex
propylhexadrine (OTC)
(proe-pil-hex'a-dreen)
Benzedrex Inhaler
tetrahydrozoline (OTC)
(tet-ra-hye-dro'zoe-leen)
Tyzine, Tyzine Pediatric
xylometazoline (OTC)
(zye-loh-meh-tazz'oh-leen)
Otrivin, Otrivin Pediatric Nasal

NASAL STEROIDS
beclomethasone (Rx)
(be-kloe-meth'a-sone)
Beconase AQ Nasal, Beconase Inhalation, Vancenase AQ Nasal, Vancenase Nasal
budesonide (Rx)
Flonase, Flunisolide (Rx), Fluticasone (Rx), Memetasone (Rx), Nasacort, Nasacort AQ, Nasalide, Nasaret, Nasonex, Rhinocort, Rhinocort Aqua, Triamcinolone (Rx)

Pregnancy category C

Action: Produces vasoconstriction (rapid, long acting) of arterioles, thereby decreasing fluid exudation, mucosal engorgement by stimulation of α-adrenergic receptors in vascular smooth muscle

➡ **Therapeutic Outcome:** Absence of nasal congestion

Uses: Nasal congestion

Dosage and routes
Desoxyephedrine
▣ *Adult and child >6 yr:* 1-2 INH in each nostril q2h or less
EpHEDrine
Adult: Fill dropper to the level marked, then use in each nostril q4h or less
EpINEPHrine
▣ *Adult and child >6 yr:* Apply with swab, drops, spray prn
Naphazoline
▣ *Adult and child >6 yr:* 1-2 drops/spray q6h or less
Oxymetazoline
▣ *Adult and child >6 yr:* INSTILL 2-3 gtt or sprays to each nostril bid
▣ *Child 2-6 yr:* INSTILL 2-3 gtt or sprays 0.025 sol bid, not to exceed 3 days
Phenylephrine
▣ *Adult and child >12 yr:* 2-3 drops/spray (0.25-0.5) in each nostril: q3-4h or less; or 2-3 drops/spray (1%) in each nostril q4h or less
▣ *Child 6-12 yr:* 2-3 drops/spray (0.25%) in each nostril q3-4h
▣ *Infant >6 mo:* 1-2 drops (0.16%) in each nostril q3h
Propylhexadrine
▣ *Adult and child >6 yr:* 1-2 INH in each nostril q2h or less

Tetrahydrozoline

P *Adult and child >6 yr:* 2-4 drops (0.1%) q3-4h prn or 3-4 sprays in each nostril q4h prn

P *Child 2-6 yr:* 2-3 drops (0.05%) in each nostril q4-6h prn

Xylometazoline

P *Adult and child >12 yr:* 2-3 drops/spray (0.1%) in each nostril q8-10h

P *Child 2-12 yr:* 2-3 drops (0.05%) in each nostril q8-10h

Available forms: Nasal sol 0.025%, 0.05%

Adverse effects

(*italic* = common; **bold** = life-threatening)

CNS: Anxiety, restlessness, tremors, weakness, insomnia, dizziness, fever, headache

EENT: Irritation, burning, sneezing, stinging, dryness, rebound congestion

GI: Nausea, vomiting, anorexia

INTEG: Contact dermatitis

Contraindications: Hypersensitivity to sympathomimetic amines

P **Precautions:** Children <6 yr, elderly,

G diabetes, cardiovascular disease, hypertension, hyperthyroidism, increased intracranial pressure, prostatic hypertrophy, pregnancy **C**, glaucoma

NURSING CONSIDERATIONS
Assessment

• Assess for redness, swelling, pain in nasal passages before and during treatment

• Assess for syst absorption: hypertension, tachycardia; notify prescriber; syst absorption occurs at high doses or after prolonged use

Nursing diagnoses

✓ Airway clearance, ineffective (uses)

✓ Knowledge, deficient (teaching)

✓ Noncompliance (teaching)

Implementation

• Have patient tilt head back, squeeze bulb to create a vacuum, and draw correct amount of sol into dropper; insert 2 gtt of sol into nostril; repeat in other nostril

• Store in light-resistant container; do not expose to high temp or let sol come into contact with aluminum

• Give for <4 consecutive days

• Provide environmental humidification to decrease nasal congestion, dryness

Patient/family education

• Advise patient that stinging may occur for several applications; drying of mucosa may be decreased by environmental humidification

• Caution patient to notify prescriber if irregular pulse, insomnia, dizziness, or tremors occur

• Teach patient proper administration to avoid syst absorption

• Advise patient to rinse dropper with very hot water to prevent contamination

Evaluation

Positive therapeutic outcome

• Decreased nasal congestion

TOPICAL GLUCOCORTICOIDS

alclometasone (Rx)
(al-kloe-met'a-sone)
Adovate

amcinonide (Rx)
(am-sin'oh-nide)
Cyclocort

**augmental
betamethasone (Rx)**
(bay-ta-meth'a-sone)
Diprolene, Diprolene AF

betamethasone (Rx)
(bay-ta-meth'a-sone)
Alphatrex, Beben ✦, Betacort ✦, Betatrex, Beta-Val, Bethovate ✦, Celestoderm ✦, Dermabet, Diprosone, Ectosonel ✦, Luxiq, Maxivate, Metaderm ✦, Psorion, Valisone

clobetasol (Rx)
(kloe-bay'ta-sol)
Dermovate ✦, Temovate

clocortolone (Rx)
(kloe-kore'toe-lone)
Cormax, Cloderm, Embeline E 0.05%

desonide (Rx)
(dess'oh-nide)
Desonide, Des Owen, Tridesilon

desoximetasone (Rx)
(dess-ox-i-met'a-sone)
Topicort, Topicort LP

dexamethasone (Rx)
(dex-a-meth'a-sone)
Aeroseb-Dex, Decaderm, Decaspray

diflorasone (Rx)
(dye-flor'a-sone)
Florone, Maxiflor, Psorcon

fluocinolone (Rx)
(floo-oh-sin'oh-lone)
Fluocin, Licon, Lidemol ✦, Lidex, Lyderm ✦, Topsyn ✦, Vasoderm

---

 Herb/drug   Do Not Crush   Alert   Key Drug   Geriatric   Pediatric

flurandrenolide (Rx)
(flure-an-dren'oh-lide)
Cordran, Cordran SP, Cordran Tape, Drenison 1/4 ♣, Drenison Tape ♣

fluticasone (Rx)
(floo-tik'a-sone)
Cutivate

halcinonide (Rx)
(hal-sin'oh-nide)
Halog, Halog-E

halobetasol (Rx)
(hal-oh-bay'ta-sol)
Ultravate

hydrocortisone (Rx)
(hye-droe-kor'ti-sone)
Actiocort, Aeroseb-HC, Ala-Cort, Allercort, Alphaderm, Anusol HC, Bactine, Barriere-HC ♣, CaldeCORT Anti-Itch, Carmol HC, Cetacort, Cortacet ♣, Cortaid, Cortate ♣, Cort-Dome, Cortef ♣, Corticaine, Corticreme ♣, Cortifair, Cortizone, Cortoderm ♣, Cortril, Delcort, Dermacort, DemiCort, Dermtex HC, Emo-Cort, Epifoam, FoilleCort, Gly-Cort, Gynecort, Hi-Cor, Hycort, Hyderm ♣, Hydro-Tex, Hytone, Lacti-Care-HC, Lanacort, Lemoderm, Locoid, My Cort, Novoehydrocort ♣, Nutracort Pharm, Pharmacort, Pentacort, Rederm, Rhulicort S-T Cort, Synacort, Sarna HC ♣, Texa-Cort, Unicort ♣, Westcort

mometasone (Rx)
(moe-met'a-sone)
Elocon

prednicarbate (Rx)
(pred-ni-kar'bate)
Dermatop

triamcinolone (Rx)
(trye-am-sin'oh-lone)
Aristocort, Delta-Tritex, Flutex, Kenac, Kenalog, Kenonel, Triaderm, Trianide ♣, Triderm, Trymex

Pregnancy category C

Action: Antipruritic, antiinflammatory

⊐**Therapeutic Outcome:** Decreased itching, inflammation

Uses: Psoriasis, eczema, contact dermatitis, pruritus; usually reserved for severe dermatoses that have not responded to less potent formulation

Dosage and routes
P *Adult and child:* Apply to affected area

Adverse effects
(*italic* = common; **bold** = life-threatening)
INTEG: *Acne, atrophy, epidermal thinning, purpura, striae*

Contraindications: Hypersensitivity, viral infections, fungal infections

Precautions: Pregnancy C

NURSING CONSIDERATIONS
Assessment
• Temp; if fever develops, drug should be discontinued
• For systemic absorption, increased temp, inflammation, irritation

Nursing diagnoses
☑ Pain, chronic (uses)
☑ Knowledge, deficient (teaching)
☑ Skin integrity, impaired (uses)

Implementation
• Apply only to affected areas; do not get in eyes
• Apply and leave site uncovered or lightly covered; occlusive dressing is not recommended—systemic absorption may occur
• Use only on dermatoses; do not use on weeping, denuded, or infected area
• Cleanse area before application of drug
• Continue treatment for a few days after area has cleared
• Store at room temp

Patient/family education
• Teach patient to avoid sunlight on affected area, burns may occur
• Teach patient to limit treatment to 14 days

Evaluation
Positive therapeutic outcome
• Absence of severe itching, patches on skin, flaking

TOPICAL ANTIFUNGALS

amphotericin B (OTC)
(am-foe-ter'i-sin)
Fungizone

butenafine (Rx)
(byoo-tin'a-feen)
Lotrimin Ultra, Mentex

ciclopirox (OTC)
(sye-kloe-peer'ox)
Loprox, Penlac Nail Lacquer

clioquinol (OTC)
(klye-oh-kwin'ole)
Vioforim

clotrimazole (OTC)
(kloe-trye′ma-zole)
Canestew ✤, Clotrimaderm ✤,
Clotrimazole, Cruex, Desenex, Lotrimin AF,
Myclo ✤, Neozol ✤

econazole (OTC)
(ee-kon′a-zole)
Spectazole

haloprogin (OTC)
(hal-oh-proe′jin)
Halotex

ketoconazole (OTC)
(kee-toe-kon′a-zole)
Nizoral

miconazole (OTC)
(mye-kon′a-zole)
Absorbine Antifungal Foot Powder, Breeze
Mist Antifungal, Fungoid Tincture, Lotrimin
AF, Maximum Strength Desenex
Antifungal, Micatin, Monistat-Derm, Ony-
Clear Tetterine, ZeaSob-AF

naftifine (OTC)
(naff′ti-feen)
Naftin

nystatin (OTC)
(nye-stat′in)
Mycostatin, Nodostine ✤, Nilstat,
Nyoderm ✤, Nystex

oxiconazole (OTC)
(ox-i-kon′a-zole)
Oxistat

selenium (OTC)
(see-leen′ee-um)
Exsel, Head and Shoulders Intensive
Treatment, Selenium Sulfide, Selsun, Selsun
Blue

terbinafine (OTC)
(ter-bin′a-feen)
Lamisil

tolnaftate (OTC)
(tole-naf′tate)
Absorbine Athlete's Foot Cream, Aftate For
Athlete's Foot, Aftate for Jock Itch,
Genaspor, Quinsana Plus, Tinactin, Ting,
tolnaftate

undecylenic acid (OTC)
(un-deh-sih-len′ik)
Blis-To-Sol, Breeze Mist, Caldesene, Cruex,
Decylenes, Desenex, Pedi-Pro, Phicon

Pregnancy category B

Action: Interferes with fungal cell membrane permeability

➦ Therapeutic Outcome: Absence of
itching and white patches of the skin

Uses: Tinea cruris, tinea pedis, diaper rash,
minor skin irritations; amphotericin B is used
for *Candida* infections

Dosage and routes
Massage into affected area, surrounding area
qd or bid, continue for 7-14 days, not to
exceed 4 wk

Adverse effects
(*italic* = common; **bold** = life-threatening)
INTEG: Burning, stinging, dryness, itching,
local irritation

Contraindications: Hypersensitivity

Precautions: Pregnancy **B**, lactation,
P children

Interactions: None

NURSING CONSIDERATIONS
Assessment
• Assess skin for fungal infections; peeling,
dryness, itching before and throughout treatment
• Assess for continuing infection; increased
size, number of lesions

Nursing diagnoses
☑ Skin integrity, impaired (uses)
☑ Infection, risk for (uses)
☑ Knowledge, deficient (teaching)

Implementation
• Apply to affected area, surrounding area; do
not cover with occlusive dressings
• Store below 30° C (86° F)

Teach patient/family
• Instruct to apply with glove to prevent
further infection; not to cover with occlusive
dressings
• Teach patient that long-term therapy may be
needed to clear infection (2 wk-6 mo depending on organism); compliance is needed even
after feeling better
• Teach patient proper hygiene; hand-washing
technique, nail care, use of concomitant top
agents if prescribed
• Caution patient to avoid use of OTC creams,
ointments, lotions unless directed by prescriber
• Instruct patient to use medical asepsis
(hand washing) before, after each
application; to change socks and shoes once
a day during treatment of tinea pedis
• Advise patient to report to health care
prescriber if infection persists or recurs; if
blisters, burning, oozing, swelling occur
• Caution patient to avoid alcohol because
nausea, vomiting, hypertension may occur

 Herb/drug   Do Not Crush   Alert   Key Drug   Geriatric   **P** Pediatric

- Caution patient to use sunscreen or avoid direct sunlight to prevent photosensitivity
- Advise patient to notify prescriber of sore throat, fever, skin rash, which may indicate overgrowth of organisms

Evaluation
Positive therapeutic outcome
- Decrease in size, number of lesions

TOPICAL ANTIINFECTIVES

azelaic acid (Rx)
(a-zuh-lay'ic)
Azelex, Finacea
bacitracin (OTC)
(bass-i-tray'sin)
Bacitin ✤, Bacitracin
clindamycin (Rx)
(klin-da-my'sin)
Cleocin T, Clindets, Clindagel, ClindaMax
erythromycin (OTC, Rx)
(er-ith-roe-mye'sin)
A/T/S, Akne-Mycin, Eryderm, Erygel, Erythromycin, Staticin, T-Statd
gentamicin (Rx)
(jen-ta-mye'sin)
Gentamicin
mafenide (Rx)
(ma'fe-nide)
Sulfamylon
metronidazole (Rx)
MetroGel, MetroCream, MetroLotion, Noritate
mupirocin (Rx)
(myoo-peer'oh-sin)
Bactroban
neomycin (OTC)
(nee-oh-mye'sin)
Myciguent, Neomycin Sulfate
nitrofurazone (Rx)
(nye-troe-fyoor'a-zone)
Furacin, Nitrofurazone
silver sulfadiazine (Rx)
(sul-fa-dye'a-zeen)
Flamazine ✤, Silvadene, SSD, SSD AF, Thermazene

Action: Interferes with bacterial protein synthesis

▷ **Therapeutic Outcome:** Resolution of infection

Uses: Skin infections, minor burns, wounds, skin grafts, primary pyodermas, otitis externa

Adverse effects
(*italic* = common; **bold** = life-threatening)
INTEG: Rash, urticaria, scaling, redness

Contraindications: Hypersensitivity, large areas, burns, ulcerations

Precautions: Pregnancy C, lactation, impaired renal function, external ear or perforated eardrum

NURSING CONSIDERATIONS
Assessment
- Assess for allergic reaction: burning, stinging, swelling, redness
- Assess for signs of nephrotoxicity or ototoxicity

Nursing diagnoses
☑ Infection, risk for (uses)
☑ Skin integrity (uses)
☑ Knowledge, deficient (teaching)

Implementation
- Apply enough medication to cover lesions completely
- Apply after cleansing with soap, water before each application; dry well
- Apply to less than 20% of body surface area when patient has impaired renal function
- Store at room temp in dry place

Evaluation
Positive therapeutic outcome
- Decrease in size, number of lesions

TOPICAL ANTIVIRALS

acyclovir (Rx)
(ay-sye'kloe-ver)
Zovirax
penciclovir (Rx)
(pen-sye'kloe-ver)
Denavir
Pregnancy category C

Action: Interferes with viral DNA replication

▷ **Therapeutic Outcome:** Resolution of infection

Uses: Simple mucocutaneous herpes simplex, in immunocompromised clients with initial herpes genitalis

Adverse effects
(*italic* = common; **bold** = life-threatening)
INTEG: Rash, urticaria, stinging, burning, pruritus, vulvitis

Contraindications: Hypersensitivity

Precautions: Pregnancy C, lactation

NURSING CONSIDERATIONS
Assessment
- Assess for allergic reaction: burning, stinging, swelling, redness, rash, vulvitis, pruritus
- Assess for signs of nephrotoxicity or ototoxicity

Nursing diagnoses
☑ Infection, risk for (uses)
☑ Skin integrity (uses)
☑ Knowledge, deficient (teaching)

Implementation
- Apply with finger cot or rubber glove to prevent further infection
- Apply enough medication to cover lesions completely
- Apply after cleansing with soap, water before each application; dry well
- Storage at room temp in dry place

Patient/family education
- Teach patient not to use in eyes or when there is no evidence of infection
- Advise patient to apply with glove to prevent further infection
- Advise patient to avoid use of OTC creams, ointments, lotions unless directed by prescriber
- Advise patient to use medical asepsis (hand washing) before, after each application and avoid contact with eyes
- Advise patient to adhere strictly to prescribed regimen to maximize successful treatment outcome
- Advise patient to begin taking drug when symptoms arise

Evaluation
Positive therapeutic outcome
- Decrease in size, number of lesions

TOPICAL ANESTHETICS

benzocaine (OTC)
(ben'zoe-kane)
Americaine Anesthetic, Anbesol Maximum Strength, Baby Anbesol, Biozene, Boil-Ease, Children's Chloraseptic, Dermoplast, Foille, Foille Plus, Hurricaine, Lanacaine, Medamint, Orabase, Oracin, Ora-Jel
dibucaine (OTC)
(dye'byoo-kane)
dibucaine, Nupercainal

lidocaine (OTC, Rx)
(lye'doe-kane)
Anestacon, Burn-O-Jel, Dentipatch, Derma Flex, ELA-Max, Lidocaine HCl Topical, Lidocaine viscous, Noe Extra Burn Relief, Numby Staff, Solarcaine, Xylocaine, Xylocaine 10% Oral, Xylocaine Viscous, Zilactin-L
pramoxine (OTC)
(pra-mox'een)
Fleet Relief, Itch-X, PrameGel, Prax, Tronothane
tetracaine (OTC, Rx)
(tet'ra-cane)
Pontocaine, Viractin
Pregnancy category C

Action: Inhibits conduction of nerve impulses from sensory nerves

▸**Therapeutic Outcome:** Decreasing inflammation, itching, pain

Uses: Oral irritation, sore throat, toothache, cold sore, canker sore, sunburn, minor cuts, insect bites, pain, itching

Dosage and routes
P *Adult and child:* Top apply qid as needed; RECT insert tid and after each BM

Adverse effects
(*italic* = common; **bold** = life-threatening)
INTEG: Rash, irritation, sensitization

Contraindications: Hypersensitivity,
P infants <1 yr, application to large areas

P Precautions: Child <6 yr, sepsis, pregnancy **C**, denuded skin

NURSING CONSIDERATIONS
Assessment
- Assess pain: location, duration, characteristics before and after administration
- Assess for infection: redness, drainage, inflammation; this drug should not be used until infection is treated

Implementation
- Store in tight, light-resistant container; do not freeze, puncture, or incinerate aerosol container

Patient/family education
- Teach patient to avoid contact with eyes
- Teach patient not to use for prolonged periods: use for <1 wk; if condition remains, prescriber should be contacted

Evaluation
Positive therapeutic outcome
- Decreased redness, swelling, pain

☑ Herb/drug   ⊗ Do Not Crush   ◆ Alert   ◆ Key Drug   **G** Geriatric   **P** Pediatric

TOPICAL MISCELLANEOUS

docosanol (OTC)
(doh-koh'sah-nohl)
Abreva
pimecrolimus (Rx)
(pim-eh-kroh-ly'mus)
Elidel

Pregnancy category C

Action: Docosanol unknown; pimecrolimus may bind with macrophilin and inhibit calcium-dependent phosphatase

➡ **Therapeutic Outcome:** Decreased redness, swelling, pain

Uses: Docosanol applied to fever blisters to promote more rapid healing; pimecrolimus used to treat mild to moderate atopic dermatitis in nonimmunocompromised patients ≥2 yr who are unresponsive to other treatment

Dosage and routes
Docosanol
Adult: Top rub into blisters 5×/day until healing occurs

Pimecrolimus
P *Adult and child ≥2 yr:* Top apply thin layer 2×/day and rub in, use as long as needed

Adverse effects
(*italic* = common; **bold** = life-threatening)
Docosanol
None known

Pimecrolimus
INTEG: Burning

Contraindications: Hypersensitivity

Precautions: Lactation, pregnancy **C**, dermal infections

NURSING CONSIDERATIONS
Assessment
• Assess skin condition (color, pain, inflammation) before and after administration
• Assess for signs and symptoms of skin infections (redness, draining lesions); if present, avoid use of product (pimecrolimus)

Nursing diagnoses
✓ Skin integrity, impaired (uses)
✓ Infection, risk for (uses)
✓ Knowledge, deficient (teaching)

Implementation
• Apply to skin, rub in gently

Patient/family education
• Advise patient to avoid contact between medication and eyes

• Instruct patient to discontinue use of product when condition clears

Evaluation
Positive therapeutic outcome
• Decreased inflammation, redness

VAGINAL ANTIFUNGALS

butoconazole (OTC)
(byoo-toh-kone'ah-zole)
Femstat
clotrimazole (OTC)
(kloe-trye'ma-zole)
Canesten ✦, Clotriamazole, Gyne-Lotrimin 3, Gyne-Lotrimin 7, Mycelex G, Mycelex Twin Pak, Myclo ✦
miconazole (OTC)
(mye-kon'a-zole)
Femizole-M, Monistat, Monistat 3, Monistat 7, Monistat Dual Pak, M-Zole 3
nystatin (OTC)
(nye-stat'in)
mycostatin, Nadostine ✦, Nilstat, Nyoderm ✦, O-V Statin
terconazole (OTC)
(ter-kone'ah-zole)
Terazol
tioconazole (OTC)
(tye-oh-kone'ah-zole)
Gyne-Trosyd ✦, Vagistat

Pregnancy category:
Nystatin A;
clotrimazole B;
butoconazole, terconazole, tioconazole C

Action: Interferes with fungal DNA replication; binds sterols in fungal cell membranes, which increases permeability, leaking of nutrients

➡ **Therapeutic Outcome:** Fungistatic/fungicidal against susceptible organisms: *Candida* only

Uses: Vaginal, vulval, vulvovaginal candidiasis (moniliasis)

Dosage and routes
Butoconazole
Adult: VAG 5 g (1 applicator) hs × 3-6 days

Clotrimazole
Adult: 100 mg (1 vag tab, 100 mg) hs × 1 wk, or 200 mg (2 vag tab, 100 mg) hs × 3 nights, or 500 mg (1 vag tab, 500 mg); or 5 g (1 applicator) hs × 1-2 wks

Miconazole
Adult: 200 mg supp hs × 3 days or 100 mg supp × 1 wk

Nystatin
Adult: 100,000 units qd × 2 wk

Terconazole
Adult: VAG 5 g (1 applicator) hs × 7 days

Tioconazole
Adult: 1 applicator hs × 1 wk

Adverse effects
(*italic* = common; **bold** = life-threatening)
GU: Vulvovaginal burning, itching, pelvic cramps
INTEG: Rash, urticaria, stinging, burning
MISC: *Headache,* body pain

Contraindications: Hypersensitivity

P **Precautions:** Children <2 yr, pregnancy, lactation

Interactions: None

NURSING CONSIDERATIONS
Assessment
• Assess for allergic reaction: burning, stinging, itching, discharge, soreness

Nursing diagnoses
✓ Skin integrity, impaired (uses)
✓ Infection, risk for (uses)
✓ Knowledge, deficient (teaching)

Implementation
Topical route
• Administer one full applicator every night high into the vagina
• Store at room temp in dry place

Teach patient/family
• Instruct patient in asepsis (hand washing) before, after each application
• Teach patient to apply with applicator only; to avoid use of any other vaginal product unless directed by prescriber; sanitary napkin may prevent soiling of undergarments
• Instruct patient to abstain from sexual intercourse until treatment is completed; reinfection and irritation may occur
• Advise patient to notify prescriber if symptoms persist

Evaluation
Positive therapeutic outcome
• Decrease in itching or white discharge (vaginal)

OTIC ANTIINFECTIVES

ofloxacin (Rx)
(o-flox'a-sin)
Floxin, Floxin Otic, Ocuflox
Pregnancy category C

Action: Interferes with conversion of intermediate DNA fragments into high-molecular-weight DNA in bacteria

➡ **Therapeutic Outcome:** Bactericidal action against gram-positive pathogens *Staphylococcus epidermidis,* methicillin-resistant strains of *Staphylococcus aureus, Streptococcus pyogenes, Streptococcus pneumoniae;* gram-negative pathogens *Escherichia coli, Klebsiella* species, *Enterobacter, Salmonella, Shigella, Proteus vulgaris, Proteus rettgeri, Providencia stuartii, Morganella morganii, Pseudomonas aeruginosa, Serratia, Haemophilus* species, *Acinetobacter, Neisseria gonorrhoeae, Neisseria meningitidis, Yersinia, Vibrio, Brucella, Campylobacter,* and *Aeromonas* species; anaerobic pathogens *Bacteroides fragilis intermedius, Clostridium perfringens, Gardnerella vaginalis, Peptococcus niger, Peptostreptococcus* species; *Chlamydia pneumoniae, Chlamydia trachomatis, Legionella pneumoniae, Mycobacterium tuberculosis, Mycoplasma pneumoniae*

Uses: Treatment of lower respiratory tract infections (pneumonia, bronchitis), genitourinary infections (prostatitis, UTIs), skin and skin structure infections, conjunctivitis (ophth)

Dosage and routes
Lower respiratory tract infection/ skin and skin structure infections
Adult: PO/**IV** 400 mg q12h × 10 days

Cervicitis, urethritis
Adult: PO/**IV** 300 mg q12h × 7 days

Prostatitis
Adult: PO 300 mg q12h × 6 wk

Acute, uncomplicated gonorrhea
Adult: PO/**IV** 400 mg as a single dose

Urinary tract infection
Adult: PO/**IV** 200-400 mg q12h × 3-10 days

Conjunctivitis
P *Adult and child:* Ophth 1-2 gtt q2-4h × 2 days, then qid × 5 days

Renal dose
Adult: PO CCr 10-50 ml/min give q24h; CCr <10 ml/min give ½ of dose q24h

Available forms: Tabs 200, 300, 400 mg; inj 20, 40 mg/ml; ophth sol 0.3%

Adverse effects

(*italic* = common; **bold** = life-threatening)

CNS: Dizziness, headache, fatigue, somnolence, depression, insomnia, lethargy, malaise, **seizures**

EENT: Visual disturbances

GI: Diarrhea, nausea, vomiting, anorexia, flatulence, heartburn, dry mouth, increased AST, ALT, abdominal pain, constipation, **pseudomembranous colitis**

INTEG: Rash, pruritus

SYST: **Anaphylaxis, Stevens-Johnson syndrome**

Contraindication: Hypersensitivity to quinolones

Precautions: Pregnancy **C,** lactation, P children, elderly, renal disease, seizure G disorders, excessive sunlight

NURSING CONSIDERATIONS

Assessment

• Assess patient for previous sensitivity reaction

• Assess patient for signs and symptoms of infection including characteristics of wounds, sputum, urine, stool, WBC >10,000/mm³, fever; obtain baselines and monitor during treatment

• Obtain C&S before beginning drug therapy to identify if correct treatment has been initiated

• Assess for allergic reactions: rash, urticaria, pruritus

• Monitor blood studies: AST, ALT, CBC, serum glucose monthly if patient is on long-term therapy

• Assess bowel pattern qd; if severe diarrhea occurs, drug should be discontinued

• Assess for overgrowth of infection: perineal itching, fever, malaise, redness, pain, swelling, drainage, rash, diarrhea, change in cough, sputum

• Assess for CNS symptoms: seizures, vertigo, drowsiness, agitation, confusion, tremors

Nursing diagnoses

☑ Infection, risk for (uses)

☑ Diarrhea (adverse reactions)

☑ Injury, risk for (adverse reactions)

☑ Knowledge, deficient (teaching)

☑ Noncompliance (teaching)

Implementation

PO route

• Give in equal intervals q12h around the clock to maintain proper blood levels; do not give within 2 hr of other agents, since drug interactions are possible: give with 8 oz of water

• Do not give with iron, aluminum, zinc products or antacids, which decrease absorption and form insoluble chelate

IV IV route

• For intermittent inf, dilute to 4 mg/ml with D₅W, D₅/0.9% NaCl, 0.9% NaCl, D₅/LR, sodium bicarbonate, sodium lactate, D₅/Plasmalyte 56; give over 1 hr or more

Syringe compatibilities:
cefotaxime

Y-site compatibilities:
Ampicillin, cisatracurium, docetaxel, etoposide, gemcitabine, granisetron, linezolid, propofol, remifentanil, thiotepa

Additive compatibilities:
Amoxicillin, ceftazidime, clindamycin, gentamicin, piperacillin, tobramycin, vancomycin

Patient/family education

• Store for 2 wk refrigerated or 6 mo frozen, after reconstitution

• Instruct patient to take all medication prescribed for the length of time ordered; drug must be taken around the clock to maintain blood levels; do not give medication to others

• Teach patient to use sunscreen when outdoors to decrease phototoxicity

• Advise patient to increase fluids to 2 L/day to prevent crystalluria

• Caution patient to avoid driving and other hazardous activities until response is known; dizziness, confusion, drowsiness may occur

Evaluation

Positive therapeutic outcome

• Absence of signs/symptoms of infection

• Reported improvement in symptoms of infection

• Absence of red or itching eyes (ophth)

Appendix E

Combination Products

✚222:
aspirin 375 mg
codeine 8 mg
caffeine 30 mg
Uses: Opioid analgesic
✚282 MEP:
aspirin 375 mg
codeine 15 mg
caffeine 30 mg
Uses: Opioid analgesic
✚292:
aspirin 375 mg
codeine 30 mg
caffeine 30 mg
Uses: Opioid analgesic
✚692:
aspirin 375 mg
propoxyphene 65 mg
caffeine 30 mg
Uses: Opioid analgesic
A-200 Shampoo:
0.33% pyrethrins
4% piperonyl butoxide
Uses: Scabicide, pediculicide
Aceta w/Codeine:
acetaminophen 300 mg
codeine 30 mg
Uses: Opioid analgesic
Aceta-Gesic:
325 mg acetaminophen
30 mg phenyltoloxamine
Uses: Nonopioid analgesic
Acid-X:
acetaminophen 500 mg
calcium carbonate 250 mg
Uses: Analgesic, antacid
Actifed:
pseudoephedrine 60 mg
triprolidine 2.5 mg
Uses: Decongestant
Actifed, Allergy, Nighttime:
pseudoephedrine 30 mg
diphenhydramine 25 mg
Uses: Decongestant, antihistamine
Actifed Plus:
pseudoephedrine 30 mg
triprolidine 1.25 mg
acetaminophen 500 mg
Uses: Decongestant, antihistamine
Actifed Sinus Daytime:
pseudoephedrine 30 mg
acetaminophen 500 mg
Uses: Decongestant

Actifed Sinus Nighttime:
pseudoephedrine 30 mg
diphenhydramine 25 mg
acetaminophen 500 mg
Uses: Decongestant, antihistamine
Activella:
estradiol 1 mg
norethindrone 0.5 mg
Uses: Menopause
Adderall 5 mg:
dextroamphetamine sulfate 1.25 mg
dextroamphetamine saccharate 1.25 mg
amphetamine sulfate 1.25 mg
amphetamine aspartate 1.25 mg
Uses: CNS stimulant
Adderall 10 mg:
dextroamphetamine sulfate 5 mg
dextroamphetamine saccharate 2.5 mg
amphetamine sulfate 2.5 mg
amphetamine aspartate 2.5 mg
Uses: CNS stimulant
Adderall 20 mg:
dextroamphetamine sulfate 5 mg
dextroamphetamine saccharate 5 mg
amphetamine sulfate 5 mg
amphetamine aspartate 5 mg
Uses: CNS stimulant
Adderall 30 mg:
dextroamphetamine sulfate 7.5 mg
dextroamphetamine saccharate 7.5 mg
amphetamine sulfate 7.5 mg
amphetamine aspartate 7.5 mg
Uses: CNS stimulant
Advicor 500:
niacin 500 mg
lovastatin 20 mg
Uses: Hyperlipidemia
Advicor 750:
niacin 750 mg
lovastatin 20 mg
Uses: Hyperlipidemia
Advicor 1000:
niacin 1000 mg
lovastatin 20 mg
Uses: Hyperlipidemia
Advil Cold & Sinus Caplets:
pseudoephedrine 30 mg
ibuprofen 200 mg
Uses: Decongestant
Aggrenox:
200 mg ext rel dipyridamole
25 mg aspirin
Uses: Antiplatelet

AK-Cide Ophthalmic Suspension/Ointment:
10% sulfacetamide sodium
0.5% prednisolone acetate
Uses: Ophthalmic antiinfective, antiinflammatory
Alamast:
0.005% lauralkonium
glycerin
dibasic/monobasic sodium phosphate
phosphoric acid
Uses: Allergic conjunctivitis
Aldactazide 25/25:
spironolactone 25 mg
hydrochlorothiazide 25 mg
Uses: Diuretic
Aldactazide 50/50:
spironolactone 50 mg
hydrochlorothiazide 50 mg
Uses: Diuretic
Aldoclor-150:
methyldopa 250 mg
chlorothiazide 150 mg
Uses: Antihypertensive
Aldoclor-250:
methyldopa 250 mg
chlorothiazide 250 mg
Uses: Antihypertensive
Aldoril-15:
methyldopa 250 mg
hydrochlorothiazide 15 mg
Uses: Antihypertensive
Aldoril-25:
methyldopa 250 mg
hydrochlorothiazide 25 mg
Uses: Antihypertensive
Aldoril D30:
hydrochlorothiazide 30 mg
methyldopa 500 mg
Uses: Hypertension
Aldoril D50:
hydrochlorothiazide 50 mg
methyldopa 500 mg
Uses: Hypertension
Aleve Cold & Sinus Tablets:
pseudoephedrine 120 mg
Naproxen 200 mg
Uses: Colds, sinus
Alka-Seltzer Effervescent, Original:
sodium bicarbonate 1916 mg
citric acid 1000 mg
aspirin 325 mg
Uses: Antacid, adsorbent, antiflatulent
Alka-Seltzer Cold:
sodium bicarbonate 958 mg
citric acid 832 mg
potassium bicarbonate 312 mg
Uses: Antacid, adsorbent
Alka-Seltzer Plus Allergy Liqui-Gels:
pseudoephedrine 30 mg
chlorpheniramine 2 mg
acetaminophen 325 mg
Uses: Decongestant, antihistamine

Alka-Seltzer Plus Night-Time Cold Liqui-Gels:
doxylamine 6.25 mg
dextromethorphan 10 mg
pseudoephedrine 30 mg
acetaminophen 250 mg
Uses: Antitussive, decongestant
Alka-Seltzer Plus Cold & Cough Liqui-Gels:
pseudoephedrine 30 mg
chlorpheniramine 2 mg
dextromethorphan 10 mg
acetaminophen 250 mg
Uses: Antitussive, decongestant
Alka-Seltzer Plus Cold Liqui-Gels:
pseudoephedrine 30 mg
chlorpheniramine 2 mg
acetaminophen 250 mg
Uses: Decongestant, antihistamine
**Alka-Seltzer Plus Flu & Body Aches
  Non-Drowsy Liqui-Gels:**
pseudoephedrine 30 mg
dextromethorphan 10 mg
acetaminophen 250 mg
Uses: Decongestant, antitussive, analgesic
**Allerest Headache Strength Advanced
  Formula:**
pseudoephedrine 30 mg
chlorpheniramine 2 mg
acetaminophen 325 mg
Uses: Decongestant, antihistamine
Allerest Maximum Strength Tablets:
pseudoephedrine 30 mg
chlorpheniramine 2 mg
Uses: Decongestant, antihistamine
Allerest No-Drowsiness:
pseudoephedrine 30 mg
acetaminophen 325 mg
Uses: Decongestant, analgesic
Allerest Sinus Pain Formula:
pseudoephedrine 30 mg
chlorpheniramine 2 mg
acetaminophen 500 mg
Uses: Decongestant, antihistamine, analgesic
All-Nite Cold Formula Liquid:
Per 5 ml:
pseudoephedrine 10 mg
doxylamine 1.25 mg
dextromethorphan 5 mg
acetaminophen 167 mg
Uses: Decongestant, antihistamine, analgesic
Alor 5/500:
hydrocodone 5 mg
aspirin 500 mg
Uses: Analgesic
Amaphen:
acetaminophen 325 mg
butalbital 50 mg
caffeine 40 mg
Uses: Analgesic, barbiturates
Ambenyl Cough Syrup:
Per 5 ml:
bromodiphenhydramine 12.5 mg
codeine 10 mg
5% alcohol
Uses: Antihistamine, opioid analgesic

Anacin:
aspirin 400 mg
caffeine 32 mg
Uses: Analgesic
Anacin Maximum Strength:
aspirin 500 mg
caffeine 32 mg
Uses: Analgesic
Anacin PM (Aspirin Free):
diphenhydramine 25 mg
acetaminophen 500 mg
Uses: Analgesic
Anacin w/Codeine:
aspirin 325 mg
codeine 8 mg
caffeine 32 mg
Uses: Opioid analgesic
Anaplex HD Syrup:
Per 5 ml:
hydrocodone 1.7 mg
phenylephrine 5 mg
chlorpheniramine 2 mg
Uses: Analgesic, adrenergic, antihistamine
Anaplex Liquid:
Per 5 ml:
chlorpheniramine 2 mg
pseudoephedrine 30 mg
Uses: Antihistamine, decongestant
Anatuss DM:
guaifenesin 400 mg
pseudoephedrine 60 mg
dextromethorphan 20 mg
Uses: Expectorant, adrenergic, antitussive
Anatuss DM Syrup:
Per 5 ml:
guaifenesin 100 mg
pseudoephedrine 30 mg
dextromethorphan 10 mg
Uses: Expectorant, adrenergic, antitussive
Anatuss LA:
pseudoephedrine 120 mg
guaifenesin 400 mg
Uses: Adrenergic, expectorant
Anexsia 5/500:
hydrocodone 5 mg
acetaminophen 500 mg
Uses: Analgesic
Anexsia 5/500:
hydrocodone 5 mg
acetaminophen 500 mg
Uses: Opioid analgesic
Anexsia 7.5/650:
hydrocodone 7.5 mg
acetaminophen 650 mg
Uses: Analgesic
Anexsia 10/660:
hydrocodone 10 mg
acetaminophen 660 mg
Uses: Analgesic
Anoquan:
acetaminophen 325 mg
caffeine 40 mg
butalbital 50 mg
Uses: Nonopioid analgesic, antipyretic

Antrocol Elixir:
Per 5 ml:
atropine 0.195 mg
phenobarbital 16 mg
alcohol 20%
Uses: Anticholinergic, barbiturate
Apresazide 25/25:
hydralazine 25 mg
hydrochlorothiazide 25 mg
Uses: Antihypertensive
Apresazide 50/50:
hydralazine 50 mg
hydrochlorothiazide 50 mg
Uses: Antihypertensive
Aprodine w/Codeine Syrup:
Per 5 ml:
pseudoephedrine 30 mg
triprolidine 1.25 mg
codeine 10 mg
Uses: Adrenergic, analgesic
Aprodine Syrup:
Per 5 ml:
pseudoephedrine 30 mg
triprolidine 1.25 mg
Uses: Adrenergic, analgesic
Arthritis Pain Formula:
aspirin 500 mg
aluminum hydroxide 27 mg
magnesium hydroxide 100 mg
Uses: Analgesic, antacid
Arthrotec:
diclofenac 50 or 75 mg
misoprostol 200 mcg
Uses: NSAID, gastric protectant
Asbron G Elixir:
theophylline 150 mg
guaifenesin 100 mg
alcohol 15%
Uses: Bronchodilator, expectorant
Asbron G Inlay:
theophylline 150 mg
guaifenesin 100 mg
sucrose
Uses: Bronchodilator, expectorant
Ascriptin:
aspirin 325 mg
magnesium hydroxide 50 mg
aluminum hydroxide 50 mg
calcium carbonate 50 mg
Uses: Nonopioid analgesic, antipyretic
Ascriptin A/D:
aspirin 325 mg
aluminum hydroxide 75 mg
magnesium hydroxide 75 mg
calcium carbonate 75 mg
Uses: Analgesic
Aspirin-Free Bayer Select Allergy Sinus:
pseudoephedrine 30 mg
chlorpheniramine 2 mg
acetaminophen 500 mg
Uses: Adrenergic, antihistamine, analgesic

Aspirin-Free Bayer Select Head & Chest Cold:
pseudoephedrine 30 mg
guaifenesin 100 mg
dextromethorphan 10 mg
acetaminophen 325 mg
Uses: Adrenergic, antitussive, expectorant, analgesic

Aspirin Free Excedrin:
acetaminophen 500 mg
caffeine 65 mg
Uses: Analgesic

Aspirin Free Excedrin Dual:
acetaminophen 500 mg
calcium carbonate 111 mg
magnesium carbonate 64 mg
magnesium oxide 30 mg
Uses: Analgesic, antacid

Augmentin 250:
amoxicillin 250 mg
clavulanic acid 125 mg
Uses: Antiinfective

Augmentin 500:
amoxicillin 500 mg
clavulanic acid 125 mg
Uses: Antiinfective

Augmentin 875:
amoxicillin 875 mg
clavulanic acid 125 mg
Uses: Antiinfective

Augmentin 125 Chewable:
amoxicillin 125 mg
clavulanic acid 31.25 mg
Uses: Antiinfective

Augmentin 250 Chewable:
amoxicillin 250 mg
clavulanic acid 62.5 mg
Uses: Antiinfective

Augmentin 125 mg/5 ml Suspension:
Per 5 ml:
amoxicillin 125 mg
clavulanic acid 31.25 mg
Uses: Antiinfective

Augmentin 250 mg/5 ml Suspension:
Per 5 ml:
amoxicillin 250 mg
clavulanic acid 62.5 mg
Uses: Antiinfective

Auralgan Otic Solution:
5.4% antipyrine
1.4% benzocaine
Uses: Otic analgesic

Avalide:
hydrochlorothiazide 12.5 mg
irbesartan 150 mg
Uses: Hypertension

Avalide 300:
hydrochlorothiazide 12.5 mg
irbesartan 300 mg
Uses: Hypertension

Azo-Gantanol:
sulfamethoxazole 500 mg
phenazopyridine 100 mg
Uses: Sulfonamide

Azo-Gantrisin:
sulfisoxazole 500 mg
phenazopyridine 50 mg
Uses: Sulfonamide

Azo-Sulfamethoxazole:
sulfamethoxazole 500 mg
phenazopyridine 100 mg
Uses: Sulfonamide

Azo-Sulfisoxazole:
sulfisoxazole 500 mg
phenazopyridine 50 mg
Uses: Sulfonamide

B&O Supprettes No. 15A Supps:
belladonna extract 15 mg
opium 30 mg
Uses: Anticholinergic, opioid analgesic

B&O Supprettes No. 16A Supps:
belladonna extract 16.2 mg
opium 60 mg
Uses: Anticholinergic, opioid analgesic

Bactrim:
trimethoprim 80 mg
sulfamethoxazole 400 mg
Uses: Antiinfective

Bactrim DS:
trimethoprim 160 mg
sulfamethoxazole 800 mg
Uses: Antiinfective

Bactrim I.V.:
trimethoprim 80 mg
sulfamethoxazole 400 mg
Uses: Antiinfective

Bancap HC:
acetaminophen 500 mg
hydrocodone 5 mg
Uses: Analgesic

Bayer Plus, Extra Strength:
aspirin 500 mg
calcium carbonate
magnesium carbonate
magnesium oxide
Uses: Analgesic, antacid

Bayer Select Chest Cold:
dextromethorphan 15 mg
acetaminophen 500 mg
Uses: Antitussive, analgesic

Bayer Select Flu Relief:
acetaminophen 500 mg
pseudoephedrine 30 mg
dextromethorphan 15 mg
chlorpheniramine 2 mg
Uses: Analgesic, adrenergic, antitussive, antihistamine

Bayer Select Head & Chest Cold, Aspirin Free Caplets:
pseudoephedrine 30 mg
dextromethorphan 10 mg
guaifenesin 100 mg
acetaminophen 325 mg
Uses: Adrenergic, antitussive, expectorant, analgesic

Bayer Select Head Cold:
pseudoephedrine 30 mg
acetaminophen 500 mg
Uses: Adrenergic, analgesic

Bayer Select Maximum Strength Headache:
acetaminophen 500 mg
caffeine 65 mg
Uses: Nonopioid analgesic
Bayer Select Maximum Strength Menstrual:
acetaminophen 500 mg
pamabrom 25 mg
Uses: Nonopioid analgesic
Bayer Select Maximum Strength Night-Time Pain Relief:
acetaminophen 500 mg
diphenhydramine 25 mg
Uses: Analgesic, antihistamine
Bayer Select Maximum Strength Sinus Pain Relief:
acetaminophen 500 mg
pseudoephedrine 30 mg
Uses: Analgesic, adrenergic
Bayer Select Night Time Cold:
acetaminophen 500 mg
pseudoephedrine 30 mg
dextromethorphan 15 mg
triprolidine 1.25 mg
Uses: Analgesic, adrenergic, antitussive, antihistamine
BC Powder Original Formula:
aspirin 650 mg
salicylamide 195 mg
caffeine 33.3 mg
Uses: Nonopioid analgesic
BC Powder Arthritis Strength:
aspirin 742 mg
salicylamide 222 mg
caffeine 38 mg
Uses: Nonopioid analgesic
Bellatal:
phenobarbital 16.2 mg
hyoscyamine sulfate 0.1037 mg
atropine sulfate 0.0194 mg
scopolamine hydrobromide 0.0065 mg
Uses: Barbiturate, anticholinergic
Bellergal-S:
ergotamine 0.6 mg
belladonna alkaloids 0.2 mg
phenobarbital 40 mg
Uses: α-Adrenergic blocker, anticholinergic, barbiturate
Bel-Phen-Ergot-SR:
phenobarbital 40 mg
ergotamine tartrate 0.6 mg
belladonna alkaloids 0.2 mg
Uses: α-Adrenergic blocker, anticholinergic, barbiturate
Benadryl Allergy Decongestant Liquid:
Per 5 ml:
diphenhydramine 12.5 mg
pseudoephedrine 30 mg
Uses: Antihistamine, adrenergic
Benadryl Allergy/Sinus Headache Caplets:
diphenhydramine 12.5 mg
pseudoephedrine 30 mg
acetaminophen 500 mg
Uses: Antihistamine, adrenergic, analgesic

Benadryl Decongestant Allergy:
pseudoephedrine 60 mg
diphenhydramine 25 mg
Uses: Adrenergic, antihistamine
Benylin Expectorant Liquid:
Per 5 ml:
dextromethorphan 5 mg
guaifenesin 100 mg
5% alcohol
Uses: Expectorant, antitussive
Benylin Multi-Symptom Liquid:
Per 5 ml:
dextromethorphan 5 mg
pseudoephedrine 15 mg
guaifenesin 100 mg
Uses: Antitussive, adrenergic, expectorant
Betoptic-Pilo:
0.25% betaxolol
1.75% pilocarpine
Uses: Ophthalmic
Biohist-LA Tablets:
pseudoephedrine 120 mg
carbinoxamine 8 mg
Uses: Adrenergic
Blephamide Ophthalmic Suspension/Ointment:
0.2% prednisolone
10% sodium sulfacetamide
Uses: Ophthalmic antiinfective, antiinflammatory
Bromfed Capsules:
pseudoephedrine 120 mg
brompheniramine 12 mg
Uses: Antihistamine, adrenergic
Bromfed-PD Capsules:
pseudoephedrine 60 mg
brompheniramine 6 mg
Uses: Adrenergic, antihistamine
Bromfed Tablets:
pseudoephedrine 60 mg
brompheniramine 4 mg
Uses: Antihistamine, adrenergic
Bromfenex:
brompheniramine 12 mg
pseudoephedrine 120 mg
Uses: Antihistamine, adrenergic
Bromfenex PD:
brompheniramine 6 mg
pseudoephedrine 60 mg
Uses: Antihistamine, adrenergic
Bromo-Seltzer:
sodium bicarb 2781 mg
acetaminophen 325 mg
citric acid 2224 mg
Uses: Antacid, analgesic
Brondelate Elixir:
theophylline 192 mg
guaifenesin 150 mg
Uses: Bronchodilator, expectorant
Brontex:
codeine 10 mg
guaifenesin 300 mg
Uses: Analgesic, expectorant

Bufferin:
aspirin 325 mg
calcium carbonate 158 mg
magnesium oxide 63 mg
magnesium carbonate 34 mg
Uses: Analgesic, antacid
Bufferin AF Nite-Time:
acetaminophen 500 mg
diphenhydramine 38 mg
Uses: Analgesic, antihistamine
Butace:
acetaminophen 325 mg
caffeine 40 mg
butalbital 50 mg
Uses: Nonopioid analgesic
Butibel:
belladonna extract 15 mg
butabarbital 15 mg
Uses: Anticholinergic, barbiturate
Cafatine PB:
ergotamine 1 mg
caffeine 100 mg
belladonna alkaloids 0.125 mg
pentobarbital 30 mg
Uses: Migraine agent
Cafergot:
ergotamine 1 mg
caffeine 100 mg
Uses: Adrenergic blocker
Cafergot Suppositories:
ergotamine 2 mg
caffeine 100 mg
Uses: Adrenergic blocker
Caladryl:
8% calamine, camphor
2.2% alcohol
1% pramoxine
Uses: Topical antihistamine
Caladryl Clear:
1% pramoxine
0.1% zinc acetate
2% alcohol
camphor
Uses: Topical antihistamine
Calcet:
calcium 152.8 mg
vitamin D 100 international units
Uses: Supplement
Calcidrine Syrup:
Per 5 ml:
codeine 8.4 mg
calcium iodide 152 mg
Uses: Analgesic
Caltrate 600+D:
vitamin D 200 international units
calcium 600 mg
Uses: Supplement
Cama Arthritis Pain Reliever:
aspirin 500 mg
magnesium oxide 150 mg
aluminum hydroxide 125 mg
Uses: Nonopioid analgesic, antacid

Capital w/Codeine:
Per 5 ml:
acetaminophen 120 mg
codeine 12 mg
Uses: Opioid analgesic
Capozide 25/15:
captopril 25 mg
hydrochlorothiazide 15 mg
Uses: Antihypertensive
Capozide 25/25:
captopril 25 mg
hydrochorothiazide 25 mg
Uses: Antihypertensive
Capozide 50/15:
captopril 50 mg
hydrochlorothiazide 15 mg
Uses: Antihypertensive
Capozide 50/25:
captopril 50 mg
hydrochlorothiazide 25 mg
Uses: Antihypertensive
Cardec DM Syrup:
Per 5 ml:
pseudoephedrine 60 mg
carbinoxamine 4 mg
dextromethorphan 15 mg
Uses: Adrenergic, antitussive
Cetacaine Topical:
14% benzocaine
2% tetracaine
0.5% benzalkonium chloride
0.005% cetyl dimethyl ethyl ammonium bromide
Uses: Local analgesic
Ceta Plus:
hydrocodone 5 mg
acetaminophen 500 mg
Uses: Analgesic
Cetapred Ointment:
0.25% prednisolone
10% sodium sulfacetamide
Uses: Ophthalmic antiinfective, antiinflammatory
Cheracol Syrup:
Per 5 ml:
codeine 10 mg
guaifenesin 100 mg
Uses: Analgesic, expectorant
Children's Cepacol Liquid:
Per 5 ml:
acetaminophen 160 mg
pseudoephedrine 15 mg
Uses: Analgesic, adrenergic
Chlor-Trimeton Allergy 4 Hour Decongestant:
pseudoephedrine 60 mg
chlorpheniramine 4 mg
Uses: Antihistamine, adrenergic
Chlor-Trimeton 12 Hour Relief Tablets:
pseudoephedrine 120 mg
chlorpheniramine 8 mg
Uses: Antihistamine, adrenergic
Chromagen:
ferrous fumarate 66 mg
vitamin B_{12} 10 mcg
vitamin C 250 mg
intrinsic factor 100 mg
Uses: Supplement

Claritin-D:
loratidine 5 mg
pseudoephedrine 120 mg
Uses: Antihistamine, adrenergic
Claritin-D 24-Hour:
loratidine 10 mg
pseudoephedrine 240 mg
Uses: Antihistamine, adrenergic
Clindex:
chlordiazepoxide 5 mg
clidinium 2.5 mg
Uses: Antianxiety, anticholinergic
Clomycin Ointment:
bacitracin 500 units
neomycin sulfate 3.5 g
polymyxin B sulfate 500 units
lidocaine 40 mg
Uses: Antiinfective, local anesthetic
Co-Apap:
pseudoephedrine 30 mg
chlorpheniramine 2 mg
dextromethorphan 15 mg
acetaminophen 325 mg
Uses: Adrenergic, antihistamine, antitussive,
    analgesic
Co-Gesic:
acetaminophen 500 mg
hydrocodone 5 mg
Uses: Analgesic
Codehist DH Elixir:
Per 5 ml:
pseudoephedrine 30 mg
chlorpheniramine 2 mg
codeine 10 mg
Uses: Adrenergic, antihistamine, analgesic
Codiclear DH Syrup:
Per 5 ml:
hydrocodone 5 mg
guaifenesin 100 mg
Uses: Analgesic, expectorant
Codimal:
pseudoephedrine 30 mg
chlorpheniramine 2 mg
acetaminophen 500 mg
Uses: Adrenergic, antihistamine, analgesic
Codimal DH Syrup:
Per 5 ml:
hydrocodone 1.66 mg
phenylephrine 5 mg
pyrilamine 8.33 mg
Uses: Analgesic, adrenergic
Codimal DM Syrup:
Per 5 ml:
phenylephrine 5 mg
pyrilamine 8.33 mg
dextromethorphan 10 mg
Uses: Adrenergic, antitussive
Codimal-LA:
chlorpheniramine 8 mg
pseudoephedrine 120 mg
Uses: Antihistamine, adrenergic

Codimal PH Syrup:
Per 5 ml:
codeine 10 mg
phenylephrine 5 mg
pyrilamine 8.33 mg
Uses: Analgesic, adrenergic
Col-Probenecid:
probenecid 500 mg
colchicine 0.5 mg
Uses: Antigout agent
ColBenemid:
probenecid 500 mg
colchicine 0.5 mg
Uses: Antigout agent
Coldrine:
pseudoephedrine 30 mg
acetaminophen 500 mg
Uses: Decongestant, nonopioid analgesic
Coly-Mycin S Otic Suspension:
1% hydrocortisone
neomycin base 3.3 mg/ml
colistin 3 mg/ml
0.05% thonzonium bromide
Uses: Otic antiinfective
CombiPatch:
estradiol 0.05 mg
norethindone 0.14 mg
Uses: Menopause
CombiPatch:
estradiol 0.05 mg
norethindone 0.25 mg
Uses: Menopause
Combipres 0.1:
chlorthalidone 15 mg
clonidine 0.1 mg
Uses: Antihypertensive
Combipres 0.2:
chlorthalidone 15 mg
clonidine 0.2 mg
Uses: Antihypertensive
Combipres 0.3:
chlorthalidone 15 mg
clonidine 0.3 mg
Uses: Antihypertensive
Combivent:
ipratropium bromide 18 mcg
albuterol 103 mcg/actuation
Uses: Bronchodilator
Combivir:
lamivudine 150 mg
zidovudine 300 mg
Uses: Antiviral
Comhist Tablets:
phenylephrine 10 mg
chlorpheniramine 2 mg
phenyltoloxamine 25 mg
Uses: Adrenergic, antihistamine
Comhist LA:
phenylephrine 20 mg
chlorpheniramine 4 mg
phenyltoloxamine 50 mg
Uses: Adrenergic, antihistamine

Comtrex Liquid:
Per 5 ml:
chlorpheniramine 0.67 mg
acetaminophen 108.3 mg
dextromethorphan 3.3 mg
pseudoephedrine 10 mg
Uses: Antihistamine, analgesic, antitussive,
decongestant
Comtrex Allergy-Sinus:
chlorpheniramine 2 mg
acetaminophen 500 mg
pseudoephedrine 30 mg
Uses: Antihistamine, analgesic, decongestant
Comtrex Maximum Strength Caplets:
acetaminophen 500 mg
pseudoephedrine 30 mg
chlorpheniramine 2 mg
dextromethorphan 15 mg
Uses: Analgesic, decongestant, antihistamine,
antitussive
**Comtrex Maximum Strength Multi-Symptom
Cold, Flu Relief:**
pseudoephedrine 30 mg
dextromethorphan 15 mg
chlorpheniramine 2 mg
acetaminophen 500 mg
Uses: Analgesic, decongestant, antihistamine,
antitussive
**Comtrex Maximum Strength Non-Drowsy
Caplets:**
acetaminophen 500 mg
pseudoephedrine 30 mg
dextromethorphan 15 mg
Uses: Analgesic, decongestant, antitussive
Congess SR:
guaifenesin 250 mg
pseudoephedrine 120 mg
Uses: Expectorant, decongestant
Congestac:
guaifenesin 400 mg
pseudoephedrine 60 mg
Uses: Expectorant, decongestant
Contac Cough & Chest Cold Liquid:
Per 5 ml:
pseudoephedrine 15 mg
dextromethorphan 5 mg
guaifenesin 50 mg
acetaminophen 125 mg
Uses: Decongestant, antitussive, expectorant,
analgesic
Contac Cough & Sore Throat Liquid:
Per 5 ml:
dextromethorphan 5 mg
acetaminophen 125 mg
Uses: Antitussive, analgesic
Contac Day Allergy/Sinus:
pseudoephedrine 60 mg
acetaminophen 650 mg
Uses: Decongestant, analgesic
Contac Day Cold and Flu:
pseudoephedrine 60 mg
dextromethorphan 30 mg
acetaminophen 650 mg
Uses: Decongestant, antitussive, analgesic

Contac Night Allergy Sinus:
pseudoephedrine 60 mg
diphenhydramine 50 mg
acetaminophen 650 mg
Uses: Decongestant, antihistamine, analgesic
Contac Night Cold and Flu Caplets:
pseudoephedrine 60 mg
diphenhydramine 50 mg
acetaminophen 650 mg
Uses: Decongestant, antihistamine, antitussive,
analgesic
Contac Severe Cold & Flu Nighttime Liquid:
Per 5 ml:
pseudoephedrine 10 mg
chlorpheniramine 0.67 mg
dextromethorphan 5 mg
acetaminophen 167 mg
18.5% alcohol
Uses: Decongestant, antihistamine, antitussive,
analgesic
Coricidin:
chlorpheniramine 2 mg
acetaminophen 325 mg
Uses: Antihistamine, analgesic
Coricidin D Tablets:
chlorpheniramine 2 mg
acetaminophen 325 mg
Uses: Antihistamine, analgesic
Coricidin D Cold, Flu & Sinus:
chlorpheniramine 2 mg
acetaminophen 325 mg
pseudoephedrine sulfate 30 mg
Uses: Antihistamine, analgesic, decongestant
Cortisporin Ophthalmic/Otic Suspension:
0.35% neomycin polymyxin B 10,000 units/ml
1% hydrocortisone
Uses: Ophthalmic antiinfective, antiinflammatory
Cortisporin Ophthalmic Ointment:
0.35% neomycin base
bacitracin 400 units
polymyxin B 10,000 units
hydrocortisone 1%
Uses: Ophthalmic antiinfective
Cortisporin Topical Cream:
0.5% neomycin sulfate
polymyxin B 10,000 units
0.5% hydrocortisone
Uses: Topical antiinfective
Cortisporin Topical Ointment:
0.5% neomycin sulfate
bacitracin 400 units
polymyxin B 5000 units
1% hydrocortisone
Uses: Topical antiinfective
Corzide 40/5:
nadolol 40 mg
bendroflumethiazide 5 mg
Uses: Antihypertensive
Corzide 80/5:
nadolol 80 mg
bendroflumethiazide 5 mg
Uses: Antihypertensive

Cough-X:
dextromethorphan 5 mg
benzocaine 2 mg
Uses: Antitussive, local anesthetic
Creon:
lipase 8000 units
amylase 30,000 units
protease 13,000 units
pancreatin 300 mg
Uses: Digestive enzyme
Cyclomydril Ophthalmic Solution:
0.2% cyclopentolate
1% phenylephrine
Uses: Mydriatic
Dallergy Caplets:
chlorpheniramine 8 mg
phenylephrine 20 mg
methscopolamine 2.5 mg
Uses: Antihistamine, adrenergic
Dallergy Syrup:
Per 5 ml:
chlorpheniramine 2 mg
phenylephrine 10 mg
methscopolamine 0.625 mg
Uses: Antihistamine, adrenergic
Dallergy Tablets:
chlorpheniramine 4 mg
phenylephrine 10 mg
methscopolamine 1.25 mg
Uses: Antihistamine, adrenergic
Dallergy-D Syrup:
Per 5 ml:
phenylephrine 5 mg
chlorpheniramine 2 mg
Uses: Antihistamine, adrenergic
Damason-P:
hydrocodone 5 mg
aspirin 500 mg
Uses: Analgesic
Darvocet-N 50:
acetaminophen 325 mg
propoxyphene 50 mg
Uses: Analgesic
Darvocet-N 100:
propoxyphene-N 100 mg
acetaminophen 650 mg
Uses: Analgesic
Darvon Compound-65:
propoxyphene 65 mg
aspirin 389 mg
caffeine 32.4 mg
Uses: Analgesic
♣Darvon-N Compound:
aspirin 375 mg
propoxyphene 100 mg
caffeine 30 mg
Uses: Analgesic
♣Darvon-N w/A.S.A.:
aspirin 325 mg
propoxyphene 100 mg
Uses: Analgesic
Deconamine:
pseudoephedrine 60 mg
chlorpheniramine 4 mg
Uses: Antihistamine, decongestant

Deconamine CX:
hydrocodone 5 mg
pseudoephedrine 30 mg
guaifenesin 300 mg
Uses: Analgesic, decongestant, expectorant
Deconamine SR:
pseudoephedrine 120 mg
chlorpheniramine 8 mg
Uses: Antihistamine, decongestant
Deconamine Syrup:
Per 5 ml:
pseudoephedrine 30 mg
chlorpheniramine 2 mg
Uses: Antihistamine, decongestant
Defen-LA:
pseudoephedrine 60 mg
guaifenesin 600 mg
Uses: Decongestant, expectorant
Demi-Regroton:
chlorthalidone 25 mg
reserpine 0.125 mg
Uses: Antihypertensive
Demulen 1/50:
ethinyl estradiol 50 mcg
ethynodiol diacetate 1 mg
Uses: Oral contraceptive
Depo-Testadiol:
estradiol cypionate 2 mg
testosterone cypionate 50 mg/ml
Uses: Menopause
Dexacidin Ophthalmic Ointment/Suspension:
Per ml:
0.1% dexamethasone
0.35% neomycin
polymyxin B 10,000 units/g
Uses: Ophthalmic antiinfective/antiinflammatory
Dexasporin Ophthalmic Ointment:
Per gram:
0.1% dexamethasone
0.35% neomycin
polymyxin B 10,000 units
Uses: Ophthalmic antiinfective/antiinflammatory
DHC Plus:
dihydrocodeine 16 mg
acetaminophen 356.4 mg
caffeine 30 mg
Uses: Analgesic
Dialose Plus:
docusate sodium 100 mg
yellow phenolphthalein 65 mg
Uses: Laxative
Di-Gel Advanced Formula:
magnesium hydroxide 128 mg
calcium carbonate 280 mg
simethicone 20 mg
Uses: Antacid, adsorbent, antiflatulent
Di-Gel Liquid:
Per 5 ml:
aluminum hydroxide 200 mg
magnesium hydroxide 200 mg
simethicone 20 mg
Uses: Antacid, adsorbent, antiflatulent

Dihistine DH Liquid:
Per 5 ml:
pseudoephedrine 30 mg
chlorpheniramine 2 mg
codeine 10 mg
Uses: Decongestant, antihistamine, analgesic
Dilaudid Cough Syrup:
Per 5 ml:
guaifenesin 100 mg
hydromorphone 1 mg
5% alcohol
Uses: Expectorant, analgesic
Dilor-G Liquid:
dyphylline 300 mg
guaifenesin 300 mg
Uses: Bronchodilator, expectorant
Dilor-G Tablets:
dyphylline 200 mg
guaifenesin 200 mg
Uses: Bronchodilator, expectorant
Dimetane Decongestant:
brompheniramine 4 mg
phenylephrine 10 mg
Uses: Antihistamine, adrenergic
Dimetane-DX Cough Syrup:
Per 5 ml:
brompheniramine 2 mg
pseudoephedrine 30 mg
dextromethorphan 10 mg
Uses: Antihistamine, decongestant, antitussive
Dimetapp Sinus:
pseudoephedrine 30 mg
ibuprofen 200 mg
Uses: Decongestant, analgesic
Diurigen w/Reserpine:
chlorothiazide 250 mg
reserpine 0.125 mg
Uses: Antihypertensive
Diutensin-R:
methylclothiazide 2.5 mg
reserpine 0.1 mg
Uses: Antihypertensive
Doan's PM Extra Strength:
magnesium salicylate 500 mg
diphenhydramine 25 mg
Uses: Analgesic, antihistamine
Dolacet:
hydrocodone 5 mg
acetaminophen 500 mg
Uses: Analgesic
Donnatal:
phenobarbital 16.2 mg
hyoscyamine 0.1037 mg
atropine 0.0194 mg
scopolamine 0.0065 mg
Uses: Anticholinergic, barbiturate
Donnatal Elixir:
Per 5 ml:
phenobarbital 16.2 mg
hyoscyamine 0.1037 mg
atropine 0.0194 mg
scopolamine 0.0065 mg
23% alcohol
Uses: Anticholinergic, barbiturate

Donnatal Extentabs:
phenobarbital 48.6 mg
hyoscyamine 0.3111 mg
atropine 0.0582 mg
scopolamine 0.0195 mg
Uses: Anticholinergic, barbiturate
Donnazyme:
pancreatin 500 mg
lipase 1000 units
protease 12,500 units
amylase 12,500 units
Uses: Pancreatic enzymes
Dorcol Children's Cold Formula Liquid:
Per 5 ml:
pseudoephedrine 15 mg
chlorpheniramine 1 mg
Uses: Decongestant, antihistamine
Doxidan:
docusate calcium 60 mg
phenolphthalein 65 mg
Uses: Stool softener
Dristan Cold:
pseudoephedrine 30 mg
acetaminophen 500 mg
Uses: Decongestant, analgesic
Dristan Cold Maximum Strength Caplets:
pseudoephedrine 30 mg
brompheniramine 2 mg
acetaminophen 500 mg
Uses: Decongestant, antihistamine, analgesic
Dristan Cold Multi-Symptom Formula:
acetaminophen 325 mg
phenylephrine 5 mg
chlorpheniramine 2 mg
Uses: Analgesic, adrenergic, antihistamine
Dristan Sinus:
pseudoephedrine 30 mg
ibuprofen 200 mg
Uses: Decongestant, analgesic
Drixoral Allergy Sinus:
pseudoephedrine 60 mg
dexbrompheniramine 3 mg
acetaminophen 500 mg
Uses: Decongestant, antihistamine, analgesic
Drixoral Cold & Allergy:
pseudoephedrine 120 mg
dexbrompheniramine 6 mg
Uses: Decongestant, antihistamine
Drixoral Cold & Flu:
pseudoephedrine 60 mg
dexbrompheniramine 3 mg
acetaminophen 500 mg
Uses: Decongestant, antihistamine, analgesic
Drixoral Cough & Congestion Liquid Caps:
pseudoephedrine 60 mg
dextromethorphan 30 mg
Uses: Decongestant, antitussive
Drixoral Cough & Sore Throat Liquid Caps:
dextromethorphan 15 mg
acetaminophen 325 mg
Uses: Antitussive, analgesic

Drixoral Plus:
pseudoephedrine 60 mg
dexbrompheniramine 3 mg
acetaminophen 500 mg
Uses: Decongestant, antihistamine, analgesic
DT:
Per 5 ml dose:
diphtheria toxoid 2LfU
tetanus toxoid 5LfU
Uses: Vaccine
DTP:
Per 0.5 ml dose:
diphtheria toxoid 6.5LfU
tetanus toxoid 5LfU
pertussis 4LfU
Uses: Vaccine
Dura-Vent/DA:
phenylephrine 20 mg
chlorpheniramine 8 mg
methscopolamine 2.5 mg
Uses: Adrenergic, antihistamine
Dyazide:
hydrochlorothiazide 25 mg
triamterene 37.5 mg
Uses: Diuretic
Dylline-GG Liquid:
dyphylline 300 mg
guaifenesin 300 mg
Uses: Bronchodilator, expectorant
Dynafed Asthma Relief:
ephedrine 25 mg
guaifenesin 200 mg
Uses: Adrenergic, expectorant
Dynafed Plus Maximum Strength:
pseudoephedrine 30 mg
acetaminophen 500 mg
Uses: Decongestant, analgesic
Dyphylline-GG Elixir:
Per 5 ml:
dyphylline 100 mg
guaifenesin 100 mg
Uses: Bronchodilator, expectorant
E-Lor:
acetaminophen 650 mg
propoxyphene 65 mg
Uses: Analgesic
E-Pilo-1 Ophthalmic Solution:
1% epinephrine bitartrate
1% pilocarpine
Uses: Miotic
E-Pilo-2 Ophthalmic Solution:
1% epinephrine bitartrate
2% pilocarpine
Uses: Miotic
E-Pilo-4 Ophthalmic Solution:
1% epinephrine bitartrate
4% pilocarpine
Uses: Miotic
Elase-Chloromycetin Ointment:
Per gram:
fibrinolysin 1 unit
desoxyribonuclease 666.6 units
chloramphenicol 10 mg
Uses: Enzyme, antiinfective

Elase Ointment:
Per gram:
fibrinolysin 1 unit
desoxyribonuclease 666.6 units
Uses: Enzyme
Elixophyllin GG Liquid:
Per 5 ml:
theophylline 100 mg
guaifenesin 100 mg
Uses: Expectorant, bronchodilator
EMLA Cream:
lidocaine 2.5 mg
prilocaine 2.5 mg
Uses: Local anesthetic
Empirin w/Codeine #3:
aspirin 325 mg
codeine phosphate 30 mg
Uses: Analgesic
Empirin w/Codeine #4:
aspirin 325 mg
codeine phosphate 60 mg
Uses: Analgesic
Empracet-60:
acetaminophen 300 mg
codeine 60 mg
Uses: Analgesic
Endocet:
acetaminophen 325 mg
oxycodone 5 mg
Uses: Analgesic
Endodan:
aspirin 325 mg
oxycodone 5 mg
Uses: Analgesic
Endolor:
acetaminophen 325 mg
caffeine 40 mg
butalbital 50 mg
Uses: Nonopioid analgesic
Enduronyl:
methyclothiazide 5 mg
deserpidine 0.25 mg
Uses: Antihypertensive
Enduronyl Forte:
methyclothiazide 5.0 mg
deserpidine 0.5 mg
Uses: Antihypertensive
Entex PSE:
pseudoephedrine 120 mg
guaifenesin 600 mg
Uses: Adrenergic, expectorant
Epifoam Aerosol Foam:
1% hydrocortisone
1% pramoxine
Uses: Topical corticosteroid
Equagesic:
meprobamate 200 mg
aspirin 325 mg
Uses: Antianxiety
Eryzole:
Per 5 ml:
erythromycin 200 mg
sulfisoxazole 600 mg
Uses: Macrolide antiinfective

Esgic-Plus:
butalbital 50 mg
acetaminophen 500 mg
caffeine 40 mg
Uses: Barbiturate, analgesic
Esimil:
guanethidine 10 mg
hydrochlorothiazide 25 mg
Uses: Antihypertensive
Estratest:
esterified estrogens 1.25 mg
methyltestosterone 2.5 mg
Uses: Menopause
Estratest H.S.:
esterified estrogens 0.625 mg
methyltestosterone 1.25 mg
Uses: Menopause
Etrafon:
perphenazine 2 mg
amitriptyline 25 mg
Uses: Antipsychotic, antidepressant
Etrafon 2-10:
perphenazine 2 mg
amitriptyline 10 mg
Uses: Antidepressant
Etrafon A:
perphenazine 4 mg
amitriptyline 10 mg
Uses: Antidepressant
Etrafon Forte:
perphenazine 4 mg
amitriptyline 25 mg
Uses: Antipsychotic, antidepressant
Excedrin Aspirin Free Caplets and Geltabs:
500 mg acetaminophen
65 mg caffeine
Uses: Nonopioid analgesic
Excedrin Extra Strength:
aspirin 250 mg
acetaminophen 250 mg
caffeine 65 mg
Uses: Nonopioid analgesic
Excedrin Migraine:
aspirin 250 mg
acetaminophen 250 mg
caffeine 65 mg
Uses: Migraine agent
Excedrin P.M.:
acetaminophen 500 mg
diphenhydramine citrate 38 mg
Uses: Analgesic, antihistamine
Excedrin P.M. Liquid:
Per 30 ml:
acetaminophen 1000 mg
diphenhydramine 50 mg
Uses: Analgesic, antihistamine
Excedrin P.M. Liquigels:
acetaminophen 500 mg
diphenhydramine 25 mg
Uses: Analgesic, antihistamine
Excedrin Sinus Extra Strength:
pseudoephedrine 30 mg
acetaminophen 500 mg
Uses: Decongestant, analgesic

Fansidar:
sulfidoxine 500 mg
pyrimethamine 25 mg
Uses: Antimalarial
Fedahist:
pseudoephedrine 60 mg
chlorpheniramine 4 mg
Uses: Decongestant, antihistamine
Fedahist Expectorant Syrup:
Per 5 ml:
guaifenesin 200 mg
pseudoephedrine 20 mg
Uses: Expectorant, decongestant
Fedahist Gyrocaps:
pseudoephedrine 65 mg
chlorpheniramine 10 mg
Uses: Decongestant, antihistamine
Fedahist Timecaps:
pseudoephedrine 120 mg
chlorpheniramine 8 mg
Uses: Decongestant, antihistamine
Feen-A-Mint Pills:
docusate sodium 100 mg
phenolphthalein 65 mg
Uses: Laxative
Fem-1:
acetaminophen 500 mg
pamabrom 25 mg
Uses: Nonopioid analgesic
FemBack Caplets:
150 mg acetaminophen
150 mg salicylamide
44 mg phenyltoloxamine
Uses: Nonopioid analgesic
Femcet:
acetaminophen 325 mg
caffeine 40 mg
butalbital 50 mg
Uses: Nonopioid analgesic
Femhrt:
ethinyl estradiol 5 mcg
norethindrone 1 mg
Uses: Menopause
Ferro-Sequels:
docusate sodium 100 mg
ferrous fumarate 150 mg
Uses: Laxative, hematinic
Fiorgen:
aspirin 325 mg
caffeine 40 mg
butalbital 50 mg
Uses: Nonopioid analgesic
Fioricet:
acetaminophen 325 mg
caffeine 40 mg
butalbital 50 mg
Uses: Analgesic, barbiturate
Fioricet w/Codeine:
acetaminophen 325 mg
caffeine 40 mg
butalbital 50 mg
codeine 30 mg
Uses: Analgesic, barbiturate

Fiorinal:
aspirin 325 mg
caffeine 40 mg
butalbital 50 mg
Uses: Analgesic, barbiturate
Fiorinal w/Codeine:
aspirin 325 mg
caffeine 40 mg
butalbital 50 mg
codeine 30 mg
Uses: Analgesic, barbiturate
FML-S Ophthalmic Suspension:
0.1% fluorometholone
10% sulfacetamide
Uses: Ophthalmic antiinfective/antiinflammatory
Gas-Ban:
calcium carbonate 500 mg
simethicone 40 mg
Uses: Antiflatulent, antacid
Gas-Ban DS Liquid:
Per 5 ml:
aluminum hydroxide 400 mg
magnesium hydroxide 400 mg
simethicone 40 mg
Uses: Antiflatulent, antacid
Gaviscon:
magnesium trisilicate 20 mg
aluminum hydroxide 80 mg
Uses: Antacid, adsorbent, antiflatulent
Gaviscon Liquid:
Per 5 ml:
aluminum hydroxide 31.7 mg
magnesium carbonate 119.3 mg
Uses: Antacid, adsorbent, antiflatulent
Gelprin:
acetaminophen 125 mg
aspirin 240 mg
caffeine 32 mg
Uses: Analgesic
Gelusil:
aluminum hydroxide 200 mg
magnesium hydroxide 200 mg
simethicone 25 mg
Uses: Antacid, adsorbent, antiflatulent
Genatuss DM Syrup:
Per 5 ml:
guaifenesin 100 mg
dextromethorphan 10 mg
Uses: Expectorant, antitussive
Glucovance:
glyburide: 1.25 mg
metformin: 250 mg
Uses: Antidiabetic
Glucovance:
glyburide: 2.5 mg
metformin: 500 mg
Uses: Antidiabetic
Glucovance:
glyburide: 5 mg
metformin: 500 mg
Uses: Antidiabetic

Goody's Extra Strength Headache Powder:
250 mg acetaminophen
520 mg aspirin
32.5 mg caffeine
Uses: Nonopiate analgesic
Goody's Body Pain Powder:
325 mg acetaminophen
500 mg aspirin
Granulex Aerosol:
Per 0.82 ml:
trypsin 0.1 mg
balsam peru 72.5 mg
castor oil 650 mg
Uses: Top enzyme
Guaifenex PSE 60:
pseudoephedrine 60 mg
guaifenesin 600 mg
Uses: Decongestant, expectorant
Guaifenex PSE 120:
pseudoephedrine 120 mg
guaifenesin 600 mg
Uses: Decongestant, expectorant
Haley's M-O Liquid:
Per 15 ml:
magnesium hydroxide 900 mg
mineral oil 3.75 ml
Uses: Laxative
Halotussin-DM Sugar Free Liquid:
Per 5 ml:
guaifenesin 100 mg
dextromethorphan 10 mg
Uses: Expectorant, antitussive
Helidac:
In a compliance package:
bismuth subsalicylate 262.4 mg tabs
metronidazole 250 mg tabs
tetracycline 500 mg caps
Uses: Antiinfective
Humibid DM Sprinkle Caps:
dextromethorphan 15 mg
guaifenesin 300 mg
Uses: Expectorant, antitussive
Humibid DM Tablets:
dextromethorphan 30 mg
guaifenesin 600 mg
Uses: Expectorant, antitussive
Hycodan:
hydrocodone 5 mg
homatropine 1.5 mg
Uses: Analgesic, mydriatic
Hycodan Syrup:
Per 5 ml:
hydrocodone 5 mg
homatropine 1.5 mg
Uses: Analgesic, mydriatic
Hycomine Compound:
chlorpheniramine 2 mg
acetaminophen 250 mg
phenylephrine 10 mg
hydrocodone 5 mg
caffeine 30 mg
Uses: Antihistamine, analgesic, adrenergic

Hycotuss Expectorant:
Per 5 ml:
guaifenesin 100 mg
hydrocodone 5 mg
10% alcohol
Uses: Expectorant
Hydergine:
dihydroergocornine 0.167 mg
dihydroergocristine 0.167 mg
dihydroergocryptine 0.167 mg
Uses: Adrenergic blocker
Hydro-Serp:
hydrochlorothiazide 50 mg
reserpine 0.125 mg
Uses: Antihypertensive
Hydrocet:
hydrocodone 5 mg
acetaminophen 500 mg
Uses: Opioid analgesic
Hydrogesic:
hydrocodone 5 mg
acetaminophen 500 mg
Uses: Opioid analgesic
Hydropres-50:
hydrochlorothiazide 50 mg
reserpine 0.125 mg
Uses: Antihypertensive
Hydroserpine:
hydrochlorothiazide 25 mg
reserpine 0.125 mg
Uses: Antihypertensive
Hydroserpine:
hydrochlorothiazide 50 mg
reserpine 0.125 mg
Uses: Antihypertensive
Hyzaar:
losartan potassium 50 mg
hydrochlorothiazide 12.5 mg
potassium 4.24 mg
Uses: Antihypertensive
Iberet Filmtab:
ferrous sulfate 105 mg
ascorbic acid 150 mg
B-complex vitamins
Uses: Supplement
Iberet Liquid:
Per 5 ml:
ferrous sulfate 78.75 mg
ascorbic acid 112.5 mg
B-complex vitamins
Uses: Supplement
Imodium Advanced:
loperamide 2 mg
simethicone 125 mg
Uses: Antidiarrheal, antiflatulent
Inderide 40/25:
propranolol 40 mg
hydrochlorothiazide 25 mg
Uses: Antihypertensive
Inderide 80/25:
propranolol 80 mg
hydrochlorothiazide 25 mg
Uses: Antihypertensive

Inderide LA 80/50:
propranolol 80 mg
hydrochlorothiazide 50 mg
Uses: Antihypertensive
Inderide LA 120/50:
propranolol 120 mg
hydrochlorothiazide 50 mg
Uses: Antihypertensive
Inderide LA 160/50:
propranolol 160 mg
hydrochlorothiazide 50 mg
Uses: Antihypertensive
Innovar:
Per ml:
droperidol 2.5 mg
fentanyl 0.05 mg
Uses: Opioid analgesic, general anesthetic
Iofed:
brompheniramine 12 mg
pseudoephedrine 120 mg
Uses: Antihistamine, adrenergic
Iofed PD:
brompheniramine 6 mg
pseudoephedrine 60 mg
Uses: Antihistamine, adrenergic
Iophen-C Liquid:
Per 5 ml:
iodinated glycerol 30 mg
codeine 10 mg
Uses: Expectorant, analgesic
Iophen-DM Liquid:
Per 5 ml:
iodinated glycerol 30 mg
dextromethorphan 10 mg
Uses: Expectorant, antitussive
Isollyl:
aspirin 325 mg
caffeine 40 mg
butalbital 50 mg
Uses: Nonopioid analgesic
Isopap:
isometheptene 65 mg
APAP 325 mg
dicloral-phenazone 100 mg
Uses: Migraine agent
Kaletra:
lopinavir 133.3 mg
ritonavir 33.3 mg
Uses: HIV
Kondremul w/Phenolphthalein:
Per 15 ml:
phenolphthalein 150 mg
55% mineral oil
Irish moss
Uses: Laxative
Lactinex:
Mixed culture of:
Lactobacillus acidophilus and
Lactobacillus bulgaricus
Uses: Supplement
Lanorinal:
aspirin 325 mg
caffeine 40 mg
butalbital 50 mg
Uses: Nonopioid analgesic

Lenoltec w/Codeine No. 1:
acetaminophen 650 mg
hydrocodone 10 mg
Uses: Analgesic
Levsin PB Drops:
Per ml:
hyoscyamine 0.125 mg
phenobarbital 15 mg
5% alcohol
Uses: Anticholinergic, barbiturate
Levsin w/Phenobarbital:
hyoscyamine 0.125 mg
phenobarbital 15 mg
Uses: Anticholinergic, barbiturate
Lexxel:
enalapril 5 mg
felodipine 5 mg
Uses: Antihypertensive
Librax:
chlordiazepoxide 5 mg
clidinium 2.5 mg
Uses: Antianxiety, anticholinergic
Lida-Mantel-HC-Cream:
0.5% hydrocortisone
3% lidocaine
Uses: Antiinflammatory, analgesic
Limbitrol DS:
chlordiazepoxide 10 mg
amitriptyline 25 mg
Uses: Antidepressant, antianxiety
Lobac:
salicylamide 200 mg
phenyltoloxamine 20 mg
acetaminophen 300 mg
Uses: Skeletal muscle relaxant, analgesic
Loestrin Fe 1.5/30:
norethindrone acetate 1.5 mg
ethinyl estradiol 30 mcg
Uses: Oral contraceptive
Lomotil:
diphenoxylate 2.5 mg
atropine 0.025 mg
Uses: Antidiarrheal, anticholinergic
Lomotil Liquid:
Per 5 ml:
diphenoxylate 2.5 mg
atropine 0.025 mg
Uses: Antidiarrheal, anticholinergic
Lo Ovral:
ethinyl estradiol 30 mcg
norgestrel 0.3 mg
Uses: Oral contraceptive
Lopressor HCT 50/25:
metoprolol 50 mg
hydrochlorothiazide 25 mg
Uses: Antihypertensive
Lopressor HCT 100/25:
metoprolol 100 mg
hydrochlorothiazide 25 mg
Uses: Antihypertensive
Lopressor HCT 100/50:
metoprolol 100 mg
hydrochlorothiazide 50 mg
Uses: Antihypertensive

Lorcet 10/650:
acetaminophen 650 mg
hydrocodone 10 mg
Uses: Analgesic
Lorcet Plus:
acetaminophen 650 mg
hydrocodone 7.5 mg
Uses: Analgesic
Lortab 2.5/500:
hydrocodone 2.5 mg
acetaminophen 500 mg
Uses: Analgesic
Lortab 5/500:
hydrocodone 5 mg
acetaminophen 500 mg
Uses: Analgesic
Lortab 7.5/500:
hydrocodone 7.5 mg
acetaminophen 500 mg
Uses: Analgesic
Lortab 10/500:
hydrocodone 10 mg
acetaminophen 500 mg
Uses: Analgesic
Lortab ASA:
aspirin 500 mg
hydrocodone 5 mg
Uses: Analgesic
Lortab Elixir:
Per 5 ml:
hydrocodone 2.5 mg
acetaminophen 167 mg
Uses: Analgesic
Lotensin HCT 5/6.25:
benazepril 5 mg
hydrochlorothiazide 6.25 mg
Uses: Antihypertensive
Lotensin HCT 10/12.5:
benazepril 10 mg
hydrochlorothiazide 12.5 mg
Uses: Antihypertensive
Lotensin HCT 20/12.5:
benazepril 20 mg
hydrochlorothiazide 12.5 mg
Uses: Antihypertensive
Lotensin HCT 20/25:
benazepril 20 mg
hydrochlorothiazide 25 mg
Uses: Antihypertensive
Lotrel 2.5/10:
amlopidine 2.5 mg
benazepril 10 mg
Uses: Antihypertensive
Lotrel 5/10:
amlodipine 5 mg
benazepril 10 mg
Uses: Antihypertensive
Lotrel 5/20:
amlodipine 5 mg
benazepril 20 mg
Uses: Antihypertensive
Lotrisone Topical:
0.05% betamethasone
1% clotrimazole
Uses: Local antiinfective, antiinflammatory

Lufyllin-EPG Elixir:
Per 5 ml:
dyphylline 150 mg
ephedrine 24 mg
guaifenesin 300 mg
phenobarbital 24 mg
Uses: Bronchodilator, expectorant
Lufyllin-EPG Tablets:
dyphylline 100 mg
ephedrine 16 mg
guaifenesin 200 mg
phenobarbital 16 mg
Uses: Bronchodilator, adrenergic, expectorant,
   barbiturate
Lufyllin-GG:
dyphylline 200 mg
guaifenesin 200 mg
Uses: Bronchodilator, expectorant
Lufyllin-GG Elixir:
dyphylline 100 mg
guaifenesin 100 mg
alcohol 17%
Uses: Bronchodilator, expectorant
Lunelle:
25 mg medroxyprogesterone
5 mg estradiol cypionate/0.5 ml
Uses: Contraceptive
M-M-R-II:
measles
mumps
rubella
Uses: Vaccine, toxoid
M-R Vax II:
measles
rubella
Uses: Vaccine, toxoid
Maalox:
aluminum hydroxide 200 mg
magnesium hydroxide 200 mg
Uses: Antacid, adsorbent, antiflatulent
Maalox Plus:
aluminum hydroxide 200 mg
magnesium hydroxide 200 mg
simethicone 25 mg
Uses: Antacid, adsorbent, antiflatulent
Maalox Plus Extra Strength Suspension:
Per 5 ml:
aluminum hydroxide 500 mg
magnesium hydroxide 450 mg
simethicone 40 mg
Uses: Antacid, adsorbent, antiflatulent
Maalox Suspension:
Per 5 ml:
aluminum hydroxide 225 mg
magnesium hydroxide 200 mg
Uses: Antacid, adsorbent, antiflatulent
Macrobid:
nitrofurantoin macrocrystals 25 mg
nitrofurantoin monohydrate 75 mg
Uses: Antiinfective

Magnaprin:
aspirin 325 mg
magnesium hydroxide 50 mg
aluminum hydroxide 50 mg
calcium carbonate 50 mg
Uses: Nonopioid analgesic
Magnaprin Arthritis Strength:
aspirin 325 mg
magnesium hydroxide 75 mg
aluminum hydroxide 75 mg
calcium carbonate 75 mg
Uses: Nonopioid analgesic
Malarone:
250 mg atovaquone
100 mg proguanil
Uses: Malaria
Malarone Pediatric:
62.5 mg atovaquone
25 mg proguanil
Uses: Malaria
Mapap Cold Formula:
acetaminophen 325 mg
chlorpheniramine 2 mg
pseudoephedrine 30 mg
dextromethorphan 15 mg
Uses: Bronchodilator, expectorant
Marax:
ephedrine 25 mg
theophylline 130 mg
hydroxyzine 10 mg
Uses: Bronchodilator, sedative/hypnotic
Marnal:
aspirin 325 mg
caffeine 40 mg
butalbital 50 mg
Uses: Nonopioid analgesic
Maxzide 1:
polythiazide 0.5 mg
prazosin 1 mg
Uses: Antihypertensive
Maxzide 2:
polythiazide 0.5 mg
prazosin 2 mg
Uses: Antihypertensive
Maxitrol Ophthalmic Suspension/Ointment:
Per ml:
0.35% neomycin
0.1% dexamethasone
polymyxin B 10,000 units
Uses: Ophthalmic antiinfective, antiinflammatory
Maxzide:
hydrochlorothiazide 50 mg
triamterene 75 mg
Uses: Antihypertensive, diuretic
Maxzide-25 MG:
hydrochlorothiazide 25 mg
triamterene 37.5 mg
Uses: Diuretic

Medi-Flu Liquid:
Per 5 ml:
pseudoephedrine 10 mg
chlorpheniramine 0.67 mg
dextromethorphan 5 mg
acetaminophen 167 mg
18.5% alcohol
Uses: Decongestant, antihistamine, antitussive,
   analgesic
Medigesic:
acetaminophen 325 mg
caffeine 40 mg
butalbital 50 mg
Uses: Nonopioid analgesic
Mepergan Fortis:
meperidine 50 mg
promethazine 25 mg
Uses: Analgesic, antihistamine
Mepergan Injection:
meperidine 25 mg
promethazine 25 mg
Uses: Analgesic
Metimyd Ophthalmic Suspension/Ointment:
0.5% prednisolone
10% sodium sulfacetamide
Uses: Ophthalmic antiinfective, antiinflammatory
**Midol Maximum Strength Multi-Symptom
   Menstrual Gelcaps:**
acetaminophen 500 mg
pyrilamine 15 mg
caffeine 60 mg
Uses: Analgesic
Midol PM:
acetaminophen 500 mg
diphenhydramine 25 mg
Uses: Analgesic, antihistamine
Midol PMS Maximum Strength Caplets:
acetaminophen 500 mg
pyrilamine 15 mg
pamabrom 25 mg
Uses: Analgesic
Midol, Teen:
acetaminophen 400 mg
pamabrom 25 mg
Uses: Analgesic
Midrin:
isometheptene 65 mg
acetaminophen 325 mg
dichloralphenazone 100 mg
Uses: Analgesic
Minizide 1:
prazosin 1 mg
polythiazide 0.5 mg
Uses: Antihypertensive
Minizide 2:
prazosin 2 mg
polythiazide 0.5 mg
Uses: Antihypertensive
Minizide 5:
prazosin 5 mg
polythiazide 0.5 mg
Uses: Antihypertensive

Modane Plus:
docusate sodium 100 mg
phenolphthalein 65 mg
Uses: Laxative
Moduretic:
hydrochlorothiazide 50 mg
amiloride 5 mg
Uses: Diuretic
Motrin IB Sinus:
pseudoephedrine 30 mg
ibuprofen 200 mg
Uses: Adrenergic, analgesic
Murocoll-2 Ophthalmic Drops:
0.3% scopolamine
10% phenylephrine
Uses: Ophthalmic anticholinergic, mydriatic
Mycolog II Topical:
Per gram:
0.1% triamcinolone acetonide
nystatin 100,000 units
Uses: Local antiinfective, antiinflammatory
Mylanta:
aluminum hydroxide 200 mg
magnesium hydroxide 200 mg
simethicone 20 mg
Uses: Antacid, adsorbent, antiflatulent
Mylanta Double Strength Liquid:
Per 5 ml:
aluminum hydroxide 400 mg
magnesium hydroxide 400 mg
simethicone 40 mg
Uses: Antacid, adsorbent, antiflatulent
Mylanta Gelcaps:
calcium carbonate 311 mg
magnesium carbonate 232 mg
Uses: Antacid, adsorbent, antiflatulent
Naldecon Tablets:
phenylpropanolamine 40 mg
phenylephrine 10 mg
phenyltoloxamine 15 mg
chlorpheniramine 5 mg
Uses: Antihistamine, decongestant
Naldecon Senior DX Liquid:
Per 5 ml:
dextromethorphan 10 mg
guaifenesin 200 mg
Uses: Expectorant, antitussive
Naphcon-A Ophthalmic Solution:
0.25% naphazoline
0.3% pheniramine
Uses: Ophthalmic vasoconstrictor
Nasatab LA:
guaifenesin 500 mg
pseudoephedrine 120 mg
Uses: Expectorant, decongestant
NeoDecadron Ophthalmic Ointment:
0.35% neomycin
0.05% dexamethasone
Uses: Ophthalmic antiinfective, antiinflammatory
NeoDecadron Ophthalmic Solution:
0.35% neomycin
0.1% dexamethasone
Uses: Ophthalmic antiinfective, antiinflammatory

NeoDecadron Topical:
neomycin 0.5%
dexamethasone 0.1%
Uses: Top antiinfective, antiinflammatory
Neosporin Cream:
Per gram:
polymyxin B 10,000 units
neomycin 3.5 mg
Uses: Top antiinfective
Neosporin G.U. Irrigant:
Per ml:
neomycin 40 mg
polymyxin B 200,000 units
Uses: Antiinfective
Neosporin Ointment:
Per gram:
polymyxin B 5000 units
bacitracin zinc 400 units
neomycin 3.5 mg
Uses: Top antiinfective
Neosporin Ophthalmic Solution:
Per ml:
neomycin 1.75 mg
polymyxin B 10,000 units
gramicidin 0.025 mg
Uses: Ophthalmic antiinfective
Neosporin Ophthalmic Ointment:
Per gram:
neomycin 3.5 mg
polymyxin B 10,000 units
bacitracin zinc 400 units
Uses: Ophthalmic antiinfective
Neosporin Plus Cream:
polymyxin B 10,000 units
neomycin 3.5 mg
lidocaine 40 mg
Uses: Top antiinfective
Niferex-150 Forte:
ferrous sulfate 150 mg
vitamin B_{12} 25 mcg
folic acid 1 mg
Uses: Supplement
Norgesic:
orphenadrine 25 mg
aspirin 385 mg
caffeine 30 mg
Uses: Skeletal muscle relaxant, analgesic
Norgesic Forte:
orphenadrine 50 mg
aspirin 770 mg
caffeine 60 mg
Uses: Skeletal muscle relaxant, analgesic
Novacet Lotion:
sodium sulfacetamine 10%
sulfur 5%
Uses: Acne agent
Novafed A:
pseudoephedrine 120 mg
chlorpheniramine 8 mg
Uses: Adrenergic, antihistamine

Novahistone Elixir:
Per 5 ml:
phenylephrine 5 mg
chlorpheniramine 2 mg
alcohol 5%
Uses: Antihistamine
✤**Novo-Gesic C8:**
acetaminophen 300 mg
codeine 8 mg
caffeine 15 mg
Uses: Analgesic
NuLytely:
PEG 3350/420 g
sodium bicarbonate 5.72 g
sodium chloride 11.2 g
potassium chloride 1.48 g
Uses: Laxative
NyQuil Hot Therapy:
Per packet:
acetaminophen 1000 mg
pseudoephedrine 60 mg
dextromethorphan 30 mg
doxylamine 12.5 mg
Uses: Analgesic, adrenergic, antitussive
NyQuil Nighttime Cold/Flu Medicine Liquid:
Per 5 ml:
pseudoephedrine 10 mg
doxylamine 1.25 mg
dextromethorphan 5 mg
acetaminophen 167 mg
25% alcohol
Uses: Adrenergic, antitussive, analgesic
Octicair Otic Suspension:
hydrocortisone 1%
neomycin 5 mg/ml
polymyxin B 10,000 units/ml
Uses: Otic antiinflammatory, antiinfective
Opcon-A Ophthalmic Solution:
0.027% naphazoline
0.315% pheniramine
Uses: Ophthalmic vasoconstrictor
Ornade Spansules:
phenylpropanolamine 75 mg
chlorpheniramine 12 mg
Uses: Antihistamine, decongestant
Ornex:
pseudoephedrine 30 mg
acetaminophen 500 mg
Uses: Adrenergic, analgesic
Ornex No Drowsiness Caplets:
acetaminophen 325 mg
pseudoephedrine 30 mg
Uses: Adrenergic, analgesic
Ortho-cept:
ethinyl estradiol 30 mcg
desogestrel 0.15 mg
Uses: Oral contraceptive

Ortho-Novum 7/7/7:
Phase I:
0.5 mg norethindrone
35 mcg ethinyl estradiol
Phase II:
0.75 mg norethindrone
35 mcg ethinyl estradiol
Phase III:
1 mg norethinidrone
35 mcg estradiol
Uses: Oral contraceptive
Ortho-Prefest:
estradiol 1 mg
norgestimate 0.09 mg
Uses: Menopause
Otocort Otic Suspension:
hydrocortisone 1%
neomycin 5 mg/ml
polymyxin B 10,000 units
Uses: Otic antiinflammatory, antiinfective
✤**Oxycocet:**
acetaminophen 325 mg
oxycodone 5 mg
Uses: Analgesic
P-A-C Analgesic:
aspirin 400 mg
caffeine 32 mg
Uses: Nonopioid analgesic
Pain-X Topical:
0.05% capsaicin
5% menthol
4% camphor
Uses: Topical analgesic
Pamprin Maximum Pain Relief:
acetaminophen 250 mg
pamabrom 25 mg
magnesium salicylate 250 mg
Uses: Analgesic
Pamprin Multi-Symptom:
acetaminophen 500 mg
pamabrom 25 mg
pyrilamine 15 mg
Uses: Analgesic
Panacet 5/500:
hydrocodone 5 mg
acetaminophen 500 mg
Uses: Analgesic
Panasal 5/500:
hydrocodone 5 mg
aspirin 500 mg
Uses: Analgesic
Pancrease Capsules:
amylase 20,000 units
protease 25,000 units
lipase 4500 units (microspheres)
Uses: Digestive enzyme
PediaCare Coid-Allergy Chewable:
pseudoephedrine 15 mg
chlorpheniramine 1 mg
Uses: Adrenergic, antihistamine

PediaCare Cough-Cold Liquid:
Per 5 ml:
pseudoephedrine 15 mg
chlorpheniramine 1 mg
dextromethorphan 5 mg
Uses: Adrenergic, antihistamine, antitussive
PediaCare NightRest Cough-Cold Liquid:
Per 5 ml:
pseudoephedrine 15 mg
chlorpheniramine 1 mg
dextromethorphan 7.5 mg
Uses: Adrenergic, antihistamine, antitussive
Pediacof Syrup:
Per 5 ml:
codeine 5 mg
phenylephrine 2.5 mg
chlorpheniramine 0.75 mg
potassium iodide 75 mg
5% alcohol
Uses: Narcotic analgesic, antihistamine
Pediazole Suspension:
Per 5 ml:
erythromycin 200 mg
sulfisoxazole 600 mg
Uses: Antiinfective
Percocet:
oxycodone 5 mg
acetaminophen 325 mg
Uses: Analgesic
Percodan:
oxycodone 4.88 mg
aspirin 325 mg
Uses: Analgesic
Percodan-Demi:
aspirin 325 mg
oxycodone HCl 2.25 mg
oxycodone terephthalate 0.19 mg
Uses: Analgesic
✤**Percodan-Demi:**
aspirin 325 mg
oxycodone 2.5 mg
Uses: Analgesic
Percogesic:
phenyltoloxamine 30 mg
acetaminophen 325 mg
Uses: Analgesic
Perdiem Granules:
Per teaspoon:
senna 0.74 g
psyllium 3.25 g
sodium 1.8 mg
potassium 35.5 mg
Uses: Laxative
Peri-Colace Capsules:
docusate sodium 100 mg
casanthranol 30 mg
Uses: Laxative
Peri-Colace Syrup:
Per 15 ml:
docusate sodium 60 mg
casanthranol 30 mg
Uses: Laxative

Phenaphen w/Codeine No. 3:
aspirin 325 mg
codeine 30 mg
Uses: Analgesic
Phenaphen w/Codeine No. 4:
aspirin 325 mg
codeine 60 mg
Uses: Analgesic
Phenerbel-S:
ergotamine tartrate 0.6 mg
belladonna alkaloids 0.2 mg
phenobarbital 40 mg
Uses: α-Adrenergic blocker, anticholinergic
Phenergan VC Syrup:
Per 5 ml:
phenylephrine 5 mg
promethazine 6.25 mg
Uses: Adrenergic, antihistamine
Phenergan VC w/Codeine Syrup:
Per 5 ml:
phenylephrine 5 mg
promethazine 6.25 mg
codeine 10 mg
Uses: Adrenergic, antihistamine, opioid analgesic
Phenergan w/Codeine Syrup:
Per 5 ml:
promethazine 6.25 mg
codeine 10 mg
Uses: Antihistamine, analgesic
Pherazine DM Syrup:
Per 5 ml:
dextromethorphan 15 mg
promethazine 6.25 mg
7% alcohol
Uses: Antitussive, antihistamine
Phillips' Laxative Gelcaps:
docusate sodium 83 mg
phenolphthalein 90 mg
Uses: Laxative
Phrenilin:
acetaminophen 325 mg
butalbital 50 mg
Uses: Nonopioid analgesic
Phrenilin Forte:
acetaminophen 650 mg
butalbital 50 mg
Uses: Nonopioid analgesic
PMB-400:
conjugated estrogens 0.45 mg
meprobamate 400 mg
Uses: Oral contraceptive
Polaramine Expectorant Liquid:
Per 5 ml:
guaifenesin 100 mg
dexchlorpheniramine 2 mg
pseudoephedrine 20 mg
7.5% alcohol
Uses: Expectorant
Polycillin-PRB Oral Suspension:
Per single dose:
ampicillin 3.5 g
probenecid 1 g
Uses: Antiinfective

Polycitra Syrup:
Per 5 ml:
potassium citrate 550 mg
sodium citrate 500 mg
citric acid 334 mg
Uses: Laxative
Poly-Histine Elixir:
Per 5 ml:
pheniramine 4 mg
pyrilamine 4 mg
phenyltoloxamine 4 mg
4% alcohol
Uses: Antihistamine
Poly-Pred Ophthalmic Suspension:
Per ml:
0.5% prednisolone acetate
0.35% neomycin
polymyxin B 10,000 units
Uses: Ophthalmic antiinflammatory, antiinfective
Polysporin Ointment:
Per gram:
polymyxin B 10,000 units
bacitracin zinc 500 units
Uses: Top antiinfective
Polysporin Ophthalmic Ointment:
Per gram:
polymyxin B 10,000 units
bacitracin zinc 500 units
Uses: Ophthalmic antiinfective
Polytrim Ophthalmic:
Per ml:
trimethoprim 1 mg
polymyxin B 10,000 units
Uses: Ophthalmic antiinfective
Premphase:
In a compliance package:
conjugated estrogens 0.625 mg
medroxyprogesterone 5 mg
Uses: Menopause
Prempro:
In a compliance package:
conjugated estrogens 0.625 mg
medroxyprogesterone 2.5 mg
Uses: Menopause
Premsyn PMS:
acetaminophen 500 mg
pamabrom 25 mg
pyrilamine 15 mg
Uses: Analgesic
Prevpac:
In a compliance package:
amoxicillin 500 mg caps
clarithromycin 500 mg tabs
lansoprazole 30 mg caps
Uses: Antiinfective
Primatene:
theophylline 130 mg
ephedrine 24 mg
phenobarbital 7.5 mg
Uses: Bronchodilator, barbiturate

Primatene Dual Action:
theophylline 60 mg
ephedrine 12.5 mg
guaifenesin 100 mg
Uses: Bronchodilator, expectorant, adrenergic
Primaxin 250 mg
IV for Injection:
imipenem 250 mg
cilastatin sodium 250 mg
Uses: Antiinfective
Primaxin 500 mg
IV for Injection:
imipenem 500 mg
cilastatin sodium 500 mg
Uses: Antiinfective
Prinzide 10-12.5:
lisinopril 10 mg
hydrochlorothiazide 12.5 mg
Uses: Antihypertensive
Prinzide 12.5:
lisinopril 20 mg
hydrochlorothiazide 12.5 mg
Uses: Antihypertensive
Prinzide 25:
lisinopril 20 mg
hydrochlorothiazide 25 mg
Uses: Antihypertensive
Probampacin Oral Suspension:
Per single dose:
ampicillin 3.5 g
probenecid 1 g
Uses: Antiinfective
Proben-C:
colchicine 0.5 mg
probenecid 500 mg
Uses: Antigout agent
Proctofoam-HC Aerosol Foam:
1% hydrocortisone
1% pramoxine
Uses: Topical corticosteroid
Propacet 100:
propoxyphene-N 100 mg
acetaminophen 650 mg
Uses: Analgesic
Pseudo-Chlor:
pseudoephedrine 120 mg
chlorpheniramine 8 mg
Uses: Antihistamine
Pseudo-Gest Plus:
pseudoephedrine 60 mg
chlorpheniramine 4 mg
Uses: Antihistamine
P-V-Tussin:
phenindamine 25 mg
guaifenesin 200 mg
hydrocodone 5 mg
Uses: Antihistamine, analgesic
P-V-Tussin Syrup:
Per 5 ml:
chlorpheniramine 2 mg
phenindamine 5 mg
phenylephrine 5 mg
pyrilamine 6 mg
Uses: Antihistamine, decongestant

Quadrinal:
ephedrine 24 mg
theophylline 65 mg
potassium iodide 320 mg
phenobarbital 24 mg
Uses: Adrenergic, bronchodilator, barbiturate
Quelidrine Cough Syrup:
Per 5 ml:
dextromethorphan 10 mg
phenylephrine 5 mg
ephedrine 5 mg
chlorpheniramine 2 mg
ammonium chloride 40 mg
ipecac 0.005 ml
Uses: Expectorant, adrenergic, antihistamine
Quibron-300:
theophylline 300 mg
guaifenesin 180 mg
Uses: Bronchodilator, expectorant
Quibron:
theophylline, 150 mg
guaifenesin 90 mg
Uses: Bronchodilator, expectorant
R&C Shampoo:
0.3% pyrethrins
3% piperonyl butoxide
Uses: Scabicide, pediculicide
Rauzide:
bendroflumethiazide 4 mg
powdered Rauwolfia serpentina 50 mg
Uses: Diuretic, antihypertensive
Regroton:
chlorthalidone 50 mg
reserpine 0.25 mg
Uses: Diuretic, antihypertensive
Regulace:
docusate sodium 100 mg
casanthranol 30 mg
Uses: Laxative
Renese-R:
polythiazide 2 mg
reserpine 0.25 mg
Uses: Diuretic, antihypertensive
Repan:
acetaminophen 325 mg
caffeine 40 mg
butalbital 50 mg
Uses: Nonopioid analgesic
Respahist:
pseudoephedrine 60 mg
brompheniramine 6 mg
Uses: Adrenergic, antihistamine
Respaire-60:
guaifenesin 200 mg
pseudoephedrine 60 mg
Uses: Expectorant, adrenergic
RID Shampoo:
0.3% pyrethrins
3% piperonyl butoxide
Uses: Scabicide, pediculicide
Rifamate:
isoniazid 150 mg
rifampin 300 mg
Uses: Antitubercular, antileprotic

Rifater:
rifampin 120 mg
isoniazid 50 mg
pyrazinamide 300 mg
Uses: Antitubercular
Rimactane/INH Dual Pack:
isoniazid 300 mg (30 tabs)
rifampin 300 mg (60 caps)
Uses: Antitubercular
Riopan Plus Suspension:
Per 5 ml:
magaldrate 540 mg
simethicone 40 mg
Uses: Antacid, adsorbent, antiflatulent
Robaxisal:
methocarbamol 400 mg
aspirin 325 mg
Uses: Skeletal muscle relaxant, analgesic
Robitussin A-C Syrup:
Per 5 ml:
codeine 10 mg
guaifenesin 100 mg
3.5% alcohol
Uses: Analgesic, expectorant
Robitussin Cold & Cough Liqui-Gels:
pseudoephedrine 30 mg
guaifenesin 200 mg
dextromethorphan 10 mg
Uses: Antitussive, expectorant
Robitussin-DAC Syrup:
Per 5 ml:
codeine 10 mg
guaifenesin 100 mg
pseudoephedrine 30 mg
1.4% alcohol
Uses: Analgesic, expectorant, adrenergic
Robitussin-DM Liquid:
Per 5 ml:
guaifenesin 100 mg
dextromethorphan 10 mg
Uses: Expectorant, antitussive
**Robitussin Maximum Strength Cough and
 Cold Liquid:**
dextromethorphan 15 mg
pseudoephedrine 30 mg
Uses: Antitussive, adrenergic
Robitussin Night Relief Liquid:
dextromethorphan 5 mg
pyrilamine 8.3 mg
pseudoephedrine 10 mg
acetaminophen 108.3 mg
Uses: Antitussive, adrenergic
Robitussin Pediatric Cough & Cold Liquid:
Per 5 ml:
pseudoephedrine 15 mg
dextromethorphan 7.5 mg
Uses: Antitussive, adrenergic
Robitussin-PE Syrup:
guaifenesin 100 mg
pseudoephedrine 30 mg
1.4% alcohol
Uses: Expectorant, adrenergic

Robitussin Severe Congestion Liqui-Gels:
guaifenesin 200 mg
pseudoephedrine 30 mg
Uses: Expectorant, adrenergic
Rolaids Calcium Rich:
magnesium hydroxide 80 mg
calcium carbonate 412 mg
Uses: Antacid, adsorbent, antiflatulent
Rondec:
pseudoephedrine 60 mg
carbinoxamine 4 mg
Uses: Adrenergic
Rondec DM Drops:
Per ml:
pseudoephedrine 25 mg
carbinoxamine 2 mg
dextromethorphan 4 mg
Uses: Adrenergic, antitussive
Rondec DM Syrup:
Per 5 ml:
pseudoephedrine 60 mg
carbinoxamine 4 mg
dextromethorphan 15 mg
Uses: Adrenergic, antitussive
Rondec Oral Drops:
Per 5 ml:
pseudoephedrine 25 mg
carbinoxamine 2 mg
Uses: Adrenergic
Roxicet:
Per 5 ml:
acetaminophen 325 mg
oxycodone 5 mg
Uses: Opioid analgesic
Roxicet 5/500:
oxycodone 5 mg
acetaminophen 500 mg
Uses: Opioid analgesic
Roxiprin:
aspirin 325 mg
oxycodone HCl 4.5 mg
oxycodone terephthalate 0.38 mg
Uses: Analgesic
Roxicet Oral Solution:
Per 5 ml:
acetaminophen 325 mg
oxycodone 5 mg
Uses: Analgesic
Ru-Tuss DE:
pseudoephedrine 120 mg
guaifenesin 600 mg
Uses: Adrenergic, expectorant
Ru-Tuss Expectorant Liquid:
Per 5 ml:
guaifenesin 100 mg
pseudoephedrine 30 mg
dextromethorphan 10 mg
10% alcohol
Uses: Adrenergic, expectorant, antitussive
Ryna-C Liquid:
Per 5 ml:
pseudoephedrine 30 mg
chlorpheniramine 2 mg
codeine 10 mg
Uses: Adrenergic, antihistamine, analgesic

Ryna Liquid:
Per 5 ml:
pseudoephedrine 30 mg
chlorpheniramine 2 mg
Uses: Adrenergic, antihistamine
Rynatan:
phenylephrine 25 mg
chlorpheniramine 8 mg
pyrilamine 25 mg
Uses: Adrenergic, antihistamine
Rynatan Pediatric Suspension:
Per 5 ml:
phenylephrine 5 mg
chlorpheniramine 2 mg
pyrilamine 12.5 mg
Uses: Adrenergic, antihistamine
Rynatuss:
ephedrine 10 mg
carbetapentane 60 mg
chlorpheniramine 5 mg
phenylephrine 10 mg
Uses: Adrenergic, antihistamine
Saleto Tablets:
115 mg acetaminophen
210 mg aspirin
65 mg salicylamide
16 mg caffeine
Uses: Nonopioid analgesic
Salutensin:
hydroflumethiazide 50 mg
reserpine 0.125 mg
Uses: Antihypertensive
Salutensin Demi:
hydroflumethiazide 25 mg
reserpine 0.125 mg
Uses: Antihypertensive
Scot-Tussin DM Liquid:
Per 5 ml:
chlorpheniramine 2 mg
dextromethorphan 15 mg
Uses: Antihistamine, antitussive
Scot-Tussin Original 5-Action Liquid:
phenylephrine 4.2 mg
pheniramine 13.3 mg
sodium citrate 83.3 mg
sodium salicylate 83.3 mg
caffeine citrate 25 mg
Uses: Adrenergic, analgesic
Scot-Tussin Senior Clear Liquid:
Per 5 ml:
guaifenesin 200 mg
dextromethorphan 15 mg
Uses: Antitussive, expectorant
Sedapap-10:
acetaminophen 650 mg
butalbital 50 mg
Uses: Analgesic, barbiturate
Semprex-D:
acrivastine 8 mg
pseudoephedrine 60 mg
Uses: Adrenergic, bronchodilator
Senokot-S:
docusate 50 mg
senna concentrate 187 mg
Uses: Laxative

Septra:
sulfamethoxazole 400 mg
trimethroprim 80 mg
Uses: Antiinfective
Septra DS:
sulfamethoxazole 800 mg
trimethroprim 160 mg
Uses: Antiinfective
Septra IV for Injection:
Per 5 ml:
trimethoprim 80 mg
sulfamethoxazole 400 mg
Uses: Antiinfective
Septra Suspension:
Per 5 ml:
trimethoprim 40 mg
sulfamethoxazole 200 mg
Uses: Antiinfective
Ser-A-Gen:
hydrochlorothiazide 15 mg
hydralazine 25 mg
reserpine 0.1 mg
Uses: Antihypertensive
Ser-Ap-Es:
hydrochlorothiazide 15 mg
reserpine 0.1 mg
hydralazine 25 mg
Uses: Diuretic, antihypertensive
Seralazide:
hydrochlorothiazide 15 mg
hydralazine 25 mg
reserpine 0.1 mg
Uses: Antihypertensive
Serpazide:
hydrochlorothiazide 15 mg
hydralazine 25 mg
reserpine 0.1 mg
Uses: Antihypertensive
Silafed Syrup:
Per 5 ml:
pseudoephedrine 30 mg
triprolidine 1.25 mg
Uses: Adrenergic, antihistamine
Sinarest Extra Strength:
pseudoephedrine 30 mg
chlorpheniramine 2 mg
acetaminophen 500 mg
Uses: Adrenergic, antihistamine, analgesic
Sinarest No Drowsiness:
pseudoephedrine 30 mg
acetaminophen 500 mg
Uses: Adrenergic, analgesic
Sinarest Sinus:
pseudoephedrine 30 mg
chlorpheniramine 2 mg
acetaminophen 325 mg
Uses: Adrenergic, antihistamine, analgesic
Sine-Aid IB:
pseudoephedrine 30 mg
ibuprofen 200 mg
Uses: Adrenergic, analgesic
Sine-Aid Maximum Strength:
pseudoephedrine 30 mg
acetaminophen 500 mg
Uses: Adrenergic, analgesic

Sinemet 10/100:
carbidopa 10 mg
levodopa 100 mg
Uses: Antiparkinsonian
Sinemet 25/100:
carbidopa 25 mg
levodopa 100 mg
Uses: Antiparkinsonian
Sinemet 25/250:
carbidopa 25 mg
levodopa 250 mg
Uses: Antiparkinsonian
Sinemet CR 25-100:
carbidopa 25 mg
levodopa 100 mg
Uses: Antiparkinsonian
Sinemet CR 50-200:
carbidopa 50 mg
levodopa 200 mg
Uses: Antiparkinsonian
**Sine-Off Maximum Strength No Drowsiness
    Formula Caplets:**
pseudoephedrine 30 mg
acetaminophen 500 mg
Uses: Adrenergic, analgesic
Sine-Off Sinus Medicine:
pseudoephedrine 30 mg
chlorpheniramine 2 mg
acetaminophen 500 mg
Uses: Adrenergic, antihistamine, analgesic
Sinus Excedrin Extra Strength:
acetaminophen 500 mg
pseudoephedrine 30 mg
Uses: Nonopioid analgesic
Sinus-Relief:
acetaminophen 325 mg
pseudoephedrine 30 mg
Uses: Nonopioid analgesic
Sinutab:
acetaminophen 325 mg
chlorpheniramine 2 mg
pseudoephedrine 30 mg
Uses: Nonopioid analgesic
Sinutab Without Drowsiness:
acetaminophen 325 mg
pseudoephedrine 30 mg
Uses: Nonopioid analgesic
Sinutab Maximum Strength Sinus Allergy:
acetaminophen 500 mg
pseudoephedrine 30 mg
chlorpheniramine 2 mg
Uses: Analgesic, adrenergic, antihistamine
**Sinutab Maximum Strength Without
    Drowsiness:**
acetaminophen 500 mg
pseudoephedrine 30 mg
Uses: Analgesic, adrenergic
Sinutab Non-Drying:
pseudoepedrine 30 mg
guaifenesin 200 mg
Uses: Adrenergic, expectorant
Slo-Phyllin GG Syrup:
theophylline 150 mg
guaifenesin 90 mg
Uses: Bronchodilator, expectorant

Soma Compound w/Codeine:
carisoprodol 200 mg
aspirin 325 mg
codeine 16 mg
Uses: Skeletal muscle relaxant
Soma Compound:
carisoprodol 200 mg
aspirin 325 mg
Uses: Skeletal muscle relaxant, analgesic
Spec-T Lozenge:
dextromethorphan 10 mg
benzocaine 10 mg
Uses: Antitussive, topical anesthetic
Stalevo 50:
carbidopa 12.5 mg
levodopa 50 mg
entacapone 200 mg
Uses: Parkinsonism
Stalevo 100:
carbidopa 25 mg
levodopa 100 mg
entacapone 200 mg
Uses: Parkinsonism
Stalevo 150:
carbidopa 37.5 mg
levodopa 150 mg
entacapone 200 mg
Uses: Parkinsonism
Sudafed Cold & Cough Liquicaps:
pseudoephedrine 30 mg
dextromethorphan 10 mg
guaifenesin 100 mg
acetaminophen 250 mg
Uses: Adrenergic, antitussive, expectorant,
    analgesic
Sudafed Plus:
pseudoephedrine 60 mg
chlorpheniramine 4 mg
Uses: Adrenergic, antihistamine
Sudafed Severe Cold:
pseudoephedrine 30 mg
dextromethorphan 15 mg
Uses: Adrenergic, antitussive
Sudafed Sinus Maximum Strength:
pseudoephedrine 30 mg
acetaminophen 500 mg
Uses: Adrenergic, analgesic
Sudal 60/500:
pseudoephedrine 60 mg
guaifenesin 500 mg
Uses: Adrenergic, expectorant
Sudal 120/600:
pseudoephedrine 120 mg
guaifenesin 600 mg
Uses: Adrenergic, expectorant
Sulfimycin:
Per 5 ml:
erythromycin 200 mg
sulfisoxazole 600 mg
Uses: Macrolide antiinfective
Sultrin Triple Sulfa Vaginal Cream:
3.42% sulfathiazole
2.86% sulfacetamine
3.7% sulfabenzamide
Uses: Antiinfective

Sultrin Triple Sulfa Vaginal Tablets:
sulfathiazole 172.5 mg
sulfacetamide 143.75
sulfabenzamide 184 mg
Uses: Antiinfective
Synalgos-DC:
aspirin 356.4 mg
caffeine 30 mg
dihydrocodeine 16 mg
Uses: Analgesic
Synercid:
quinupristin 150 mg
dalfopristin 350 mg
Uses: Antiinfective
Synophylate-GG Syrup:
theophylline 150 mg
guaifenesin 100 mg
alcohol 15%
Uses: Bronchodilator, expectorant
Syntest D.S.:
esterified estrogens 1.25 mg
methyltestosterone 2.5 mg
Uses: Menopause
Syntest H.S.:
esterified estrogens 0.625 mg
methyltestosterone 1.25 mg
Uses: Menopause
Talacen:
acetaminophen 650 mg
pentazocine 25 mg
Uses: Analgesic
Talwin Compound:
aspirin 325 mg
pentazocine 12.5 mg
Uses: Analgesic
Talwin NX:
pentazocine 50 mg
naloxone 0.5 mg
Uses: Analgesic, opioid antagonist
Tarka 182:
trandolapril 2 mg (immed rel)
verapamil 180 mg (sus rel)
Uses: Antihypertensive, calcium channel blocker
Tarka 241:
trandolapril 1 mg (immed rel)
verapamil 240 mg (sus rel)
Uses: Antihypertensive, calcium channel blocker
Tarka 242:
trandolapril 2 mg (immed rel)
verapamil 240 mg (sus rel)
Uses: Antihypertensive, calcium channel blocker
Tarka 244:
trandolapril 4 mg (immed rel)
verapamil 240 mg (sus rel)
Uses: Antihypertensive, calcium channel blocker
Tavist Sinus:
acetaminophen 500 mg
pseudoephedrine 30 mg
Uses: Analgesic, adrenergic
✤**Tecnal:**
aspirin 330 mg
caffeine 40 mg
butalbital 50 mg
Uses: Nonpioid analgesic

Teczem:
enalapril 5 mg (extended release)
diltiazem 180 mg (extended release)
Uses: Antihypertensive, calcium channel blocker
Tedrigen:
ephedrine 22.5 mg
theophylline 120 mg
phenobarbital 7.5 mg
Uses: Adrenergic, bronchodilator, barbiturate
Tegrin-LT Shampoo:
0.33% pyrethrins
3.15% piperonyl butoxide
Uses: Scabicide, pediculicide
Tencet:
acetaminophen 325 mg
caffeine 40 mg
butalbital 50 mg
Uses: Nonopioid analgesic
Tenoretic 50:
atenolol 50 mg
chlorthalidone 25 mg
Uses: Antihypertensive
Tenoretic 100:
atenolol 100 mg
chlorthalidone 25 mg
Uses: Antihypertensive
Terra-Cortril Ophthalmic Suspension:
1.5% hydrocortisone acetate
0.5% oxytetracycline
Uses: Ophthalmic antiinflammatory, antiinfective
**Terramycin w/Polymycin B Sulfate
    Ophthalmic Ointment:**
Per gram:
polymyxin B 10,000 units
oxytetracycline 5 mg
Uses: Ophthalmic antiinfective
T-Gesic:
hydrocodone 5 mg
acetaminophen 500 mg
Uses: Analgesic
Theodrine:
ephedrine 22.5 mg
theophylline 120 mg
Uses: Adrenergic, bronchodilator
Theolate Liquid:
theophylline 150 mg
guaifenesin 90 mg
Uses: Bronchodilator, expectorant
Theophylline Kl Elixir:
theophylline 80 mg
potassium iodide 130 mg
Uses: Bronchodilator, expectorant
Thera-Flu, Flu & Cold Medicine Powder:
Per packet:
pseudoephedrine 60 mg
chlorpheniramine 4 mg
acetaminophen 650 mg
Uses: Adrenergic, antihistamine, analgesic

Thera-Flu, Flu, Cold & Cough Powder:
Per packet:
pseudoephedrine 60 mg
chlorpheniramine 4 mg
dextromethorphan 20 mg
acetaminophen 650 mg
Uses: Adrenergic, antihistamine, antitussive,
analgesic
Thera-Flu NightTime Powder:
Per packet:
pseudoephedrine 60 mg
chlorpheniramine 4 mg
dextromethorphan 30 mg
acetaminophen 1000 mg
Uses: Adrenergic, antihistamine, antitussive,
analgesic
**Thera-Flu Non-Drowsy Flu, Cold & Cough
Maximum Strength Powder**
Per packet:
pseudoephedrine 60 mg
dextromethorphan 30 mg
acetaminophen 1000 mg
Uses: Adrenergic, antitussive, analgesic
**Thera-Flu Non-Drowsy Formula Maximum
Strength Caplets:**
pseudoephedrine 30 mg
dextromethorphan 15 mg
acetaminophen 500 mg
Uses: Adrenergic, antitussive, analgesic
Timentin for Injection:
Per 3.1-g vial:
ticarcillin 3 g
clavulanic acid 0.1 g
Uses: Antiinfective
Timolide 10/25:
timolol 10 mg
hydrochlorothiazide 25 mg
Uses: Antihypertensive
Titralac Plus:
calcium carbonate 420 mg
simethicone 21 mg
Uses: Antacid, adsorbent, antiflatulent
Tobra Dex Ophthalmic Suspension/Ointment:
tobramycin 0.3%
dexamethasone 0.1%
Uses: Ophthalmic antiinfective, antiinflammatory
Triacin-C Cough Syrup:
Per 5 ml:
codeine 10 mg
pseudoephedrine 30 mg
triprolidine 1.25 mg
Uses: Analgesic, adrenergic, antihistamine
Triad:
acetaminophen 325 mg
caffeine 40 mg
butalbital 50 mg
Uses: Nonopioid analgesic
Triaminic-12:
phenylpropanolamine 75 mg
chlorpheniramine 12 mg
Uses: Antihistamine

Tri-Hydroserpine:
hydralazine 25 mg
hydrochlorothiazide 15 mg
reserpine 0.1 mg
Uses: Antihypertensive
Tri-Levlen:
Phase I:
levonorgestrel 0.05 mg
ethinyl estradiol 30 mcg
Phase II:
levonorgestrel 0.075 mg
ethinyl estradiol 40 mcg
Phase III:
levonorgestrel 0.125 mg
ethinyl estradiol 30 mcg
Uses: Oral contraceptive
**Triaminic AM Cough & Decongestant
Formula Liquid:**
Per 5 ml:
pseudoephedrine 15 mg
dextromethorphan 7.5 mg
Uses: Adrenergic, antitussive
Triaminic Nite Light Liquid:
Per 5 ml:
pseudoephedrine 15 mg
chlorpheniramine 1 mg
dextromethorphan 7.5 mg
Uses: Adrenergic, antihistamine, antitussive
Triaminic Sore Throat Formula Liquid:
Per 5 ml:
pseudoephedrine 15 mg
dextromethorphan 7.5 mg
acetaminophen 160 mg
Uses: Adrenergic, antitussive
Triavil 2-10:
perphenazine 2 mg
amitriptyline 10 mg
Uses: Antidepressant, antipsychotic
Triavil 4-10:
perphenazine 4 mg
amitriptyline 10 mg
Uses: Antidepressant, antipsychotic
Triavil 2-25:
perphenazine 2 mg
amitriptyline 25 mg
Uses: Antidepressant, antipsychotic
Trinalin Repetabs:
azatadine maleate 1 mg
pseudoephedrine 120 mg
Uses: Antihistamine
Triphasil:
Phase I:
levonorgestrel 0.05 mg
ethinyl estradiol 30 mcg
Phase II:
levonorgestrel 0.075 mg
ethinyl estradiol 40 mcg
Phase III:
levonorgestrel 0.125 mg
ethinyl estradiol 30 mcg
Uses: Oral contraceptive

Triple Antibiotic Ophthalmic Ointment:
Per gram:
polymyxin B 10,000 units
neomycin 3.5 mg
bacitracin 400 units
Uses: Antiinfective
Trizivir:
300 mg abacavir
150 mg lamivudine
300 mg zidovudine
Uses: HIV
Tuinal 100 mg:
amobarbital 50 mg
secobarbital 50 mg
Uses: Sedative-hypnotic
Tuinal 200 mg:
amobarbital 100 mg
secobarbital 100 mg
Uses: Sedative-hypnotic
Tusibron-DM Syrup:
Per 5 ml:
guaifenesin 100 mg
dextromethorphan 15 mg
Uses: Expectorant, antitussive
Tussionex Pennkinetic Suspension:
Per 5 ml:
chlorpheniramine 8 mg
hydrocodone 10 mg
Uses: Antihistamine, analgesic
Tussi-Organidin NR Liquid:
Per 5 ml:
codeine 10 mg
guaifenesin 100 mg
Uses: Analgesic, expectorant
Tussi-Organidin DM NR Liquid:
Per 5 ml:
guaifenesin 100 mg
dextromethorphan 10 mg
Uses: Expectorant, antitussive
Two-Dyne:
acetaminophen 325 mg
caffeine 40 mg
butalbital 50 mg
Uses: Nonopioid analgesic
Tylenol Allergy Sinus, Maximum Strength Gelcaps:
acetaminophen 500 mg
chlorpheniramine 2 mg
pseudoephedrine 30 mg
Uses: Antihistamine, adrenergic, analgesic
Tylenol Children's Cold:
acetaminophen 80 mg
chlorpheniramine 0.5 mg
pseudoephedrine 7.5 mg
Uses: Antihistamine, adrenergic, analgesic
Tylenol Children's Cold Liquid:
Per 5 ml:
acetaminophen 160 mg
chlorpheniramine 1 mg
pseudoephedrine 15 mg
Uses: Antihistamine, adrenergic, analgesic

Tylenol Children's Cold Multi-Symptom Plus Cough Liquid:
Per 5 ml:
acetaminophen 160 mg
dextromethorphan 5 mg
chlorpheniramine 1 mg
pseudoephedrine 15 mg
Uses: Antihistamine, adrenergic, analgesic
Tylenol Children's Cold Plus Cough Chewable:
acetaminophen 80 mg
pseudoephedrine 7.5 mg
dextromethorphan 2.5 mg
chlorpheniramine 0.5 mg
Uses: Antihistamine, adrenergic, analgesic
Tylenol Cold Multi-Symptom:
acetaminophen 325 mg
chlorpheniramine 2 mg
pseudoephedrine 30 mg
dextromethorphan 15 mg
Uses: Antihistamine, adrenergic, analgesic
Tylenol Cold No Drowsiness:
acetaminophen 325 mg
pseudoephedrine 30 mg
dextromethorphan 15 mg
Uses: Analgesic, adrenergic, antitussive
Tylenol Flu Maximum Strength Gelcaps:
dextromethorphan 15 mg
pseudoephedrine 30 mg
acetaminophen 500 mg
Uses: Analgesic, adrenergic, antitussive
Tylenol Flu NightTime Maximum Strength Gelcaps:
pseudoephedrine 30 mg
chlorpheniramine 2 mg
acetaminophen 500 mg
Uses: Adrenergic, antihistamine, analgesic
Tylenol Flu NightTime Maximum Strength Powder:
pseudoephedrine 60 mg
diphenhydramine 50 mg
acetaminophen 1000 mg
Uses: Adrenergic, antihistamine, analgesic
Tylenol Headache Plus, Extra Strength:
acetaminophen 500 mg
calcium carbonate 250 mg
Uses: Analgesic, antacid
Tylenol Multi-Symptom Cough Liquid:
Per 5 ml:
dextromethorphan 10 mg
acetaminophen 216.7 mg
5% alcohol
Uses: Antitussive, analgesic
Tylenol Multi-Symptom Cough w/Decongestant Liquid:
Per 5 ml:
dextromethorphan 10 mg
acetaminophen 200 mg
pseudoephedrine 20 mg
Uses: Antitussive, analgesic, adrenergic

Tylenol Multi-Symptom Hot Medication:
Per packet:
acetaminophen 650 mg
chlorpheniramine 4 mg
pseudoephedrine 60 mg
dextromethorphan 30 mg
Uses: Analgesic, antihistamine, adrenergic,
  antitussive
Tylenol PM, Extra Strength:
acetaminophen 500 mg
diphenhydramine 25 mg
Uses: Analgesic, antihistamine
Tylenol Severe Allergy:
diphenhydramine 12.5 mg
acetaminophen 500 mg
Uses: Analgesic, antihistamine
Tylenol Sinus Maximum Strength:
pseudoephedrine 30 mg
acetaminophen 500 mg
Uses: Adrenergic, analgesic
Tylenol w/Codeine Elixir:
Per 5 ml:
acetaminophen 120 mg
codeine 12 mg
Uses: Analgesic
Tylenol w/Codeine No. 1:
acetaminophen 300 mg
codeine 7.5 mg
Uses: Analgesic
Tylenol w/Codeine No. 2:
acetaminophen 300 mg
codeine 15 mg
Uses: Analgesic
Tylenol w/Codeine No. 3:
acetaminophen 300 mg
codeine 30 mg
Uses: Analgesic
Tylenol w/Codeine No. 4:
acetaminophen 300 mg
codeine 60 mg
Uses: Analgesic
Tylox:
oxycodone 5 mg
acetaminophen 500 mg
Uses: Analgesic
Tyrodone Liquid:
Per 5 ml:
hydrocodone 5 mg
pseudoephedrine 60 mg
5% alcohol
Uses: Analgesic, adrenergic
Unasyn for Injection 1.5 g:
ampicillin 1 g
sulbactam 0.5 g
Uses: Antiinfective
Unasyn for Injection 3 g:
ampicillin 2 g
sulbactam 1 g
Uses: Antiinfective
Uniretic:
moexipril 7.5 mg
hydrochlorothiazide 12.5 mg
or moexipril 15 mg
hydrochlorothiazide 25 mg
Uses: Antihypertensive, diuretic

Unituss HC Syrup:
hydrocodone 2.5 mg
phenylephrine 5 mg
chlorpheniramine 2 mg
Uses: Analgesic, adrenergic, antihistamine
Urised:
methenamine 40.8 mg
phenylsalicylate 18.1 mg
atropine 0.03 mg
hyoscyamine 0.03 mg
benzoic acid 4.5 mg
methylene blue 5.4 mg
Uses: Antiinfective
Urobiotic 250:
oxytetracycline 250 mg
sulfamethizole 250 mg
phenazopyridine 50 mg
Uses: Antiinfective
Ursinus Inlay:
pseudoephedrine 30 mg
aspirin 325 mg
Uses: Adrenergic, analgesic
Vanquish:
aspirin 227 mg
acetaminophen 194 mg
caffeine 33 mg
aluminum hydroxide 25 mg
magnesium hydroxide 50 mg
Uses: Nonopioid analgesic
Vaseretic 10-25:
enalapril 10 mg
hydrochlorothiazide 25 mg
Uses: Antihypertensive, diuretic
Vasocidin Ophthalmic Ointment:
sulfacetamide 10%
prednisolone 0.5%
Uses: Ophthalmic antiinfective, antiinflammatory
Vasocidin Ophthalmic Solution:
sulfacetamide 10%
prednisolone 0.25%
Uses: Ophthalmic antiinfective, antiinflammatory
Vasocon-A Ophthalmic Solution:
naphazoline 0.05%
antazoline 0.5%
Uses: Ophthalmic vasoconstrictor
Vicks 44D Cough & Head Congestion Liquid:
Per 5 ml:
dextromethorphan 10 mg
pseudoephedrine 20 mg
Uses: Antitussive, adrenergic
Vicks 44E Liquid:
Per 5 ml:
dextromethorphan 6.7 mg
guaifenesin 66.7 mg
Uses: Antitussive, expectorant
Vicks 44M Cold, Flu, & Cough LiquiCaps:
dextromethorphan 10 mg
pseudoephedrine 30 mg
chlorpheniramine 2 mg
acetaminophen 250 mg
Uses: Antitussive, adrenergic, antihistamine,
  analgesic

Vicks 44 Non-Drowsy Cold & Cough LiquiCaps:
dextromethorphan 30 mg
pseudoephedrine 60 mg
Uses: Antitussive, adrenergic

Vicks Children's NyQuil Nighttime Cough/ Cold Liquid:
Per 5 ml:
pseudoephedrine 10 mg
chlorpheniramine 0.67 mg
dextromethorphan 5 mg
Uses: Adrenergic, antihistamine, antitussive

Vicks Cough Silencers:
dextromethorphan 2.5 mg
benzocaine 1 mg
Uses: Antitussive, top anesthetic

Vicks DayQuil Liquid:
Per 5 ml:
dextromethorphan 3.3 mg
pseudoephedrine 10 mg
acetaminophen 108.3 mg
guaifenesin 33.3 mg
Uses: Antitussive, adrenergic, analgesic, expectorant

Vicks DayQuil Sinus Pressure & Pain Relief:
pseudoephedrine 30 mg
acetaminophen 500 mg
Uses: Adrenergic, analgesic

Vicks NyQuil Liquicaps:
pseudoephedrine 30 mg
doxylamine 6.25 mg
dextromethorphan 10 mg
acetaminophen 250 mg
Uses: Adrenergic, antihistamine, antitussive, analgesic

Vicks NyQuil Multi-Symptom Cold Flu Relief Liquid:
pseudoephedrine 10 mg
doxylamine 2.1 mg
dextromethorphan 5 mg
acetaminophen 167 mg
Uses: Adrenergic, antihistamine, antitussive, analgesic

Vicks Pediatric Formula 44e Liquid:
Per 5 ml:
dextromethorphan 3.3 mg
guaifenesin 33.3 mg
Uses: Expectorant, antitussive

Vicks Pediatric Formula 44m Multi-Symptom Cough & Cold Liquid
pseudoephedrine 10 mg
chlorpheniramine 0.67 mg
dextromethorphan 5 mg
Uses: Adrenergic, antihistamine, antitussive

Vicodin:
acetaminophen 500 mg
hydrocodone 5 mg
Uses: Analgesic

Vicodin ES:
acetaminophen 750 mg
hydrocodone 7.5 mg
Uses: Analgesic

Vicodin HP:
acetaminophen 660 mg
hydrocodone 10 mg
Uses: Analgesic

VicodinTuss:
Per 5 ml:
hydrocodone 5 mg
guaifenesin 100 mg
Uses: Analgesic, expectorant

Vicoprofen:
hydrocodone 7.5 mg
ibuprofen 200 mg
Uses: Analgesic

Wigraine Suppositories:
ergotamine 2 mg
caffeine 100 mg
Uses: α-Adrenergic blocker

Yasmin:
ethinyl estradiol 30 mcg
dropirenone 3 mg
Uses: Oral contraceptive

Zestoretic 10/12.5:
lisinopril 10 mg
hydrochlorothiazide 12.5 mg
Uses: Antihypertensive

Zestoretic 20/12.5:
lisinopril 20 mg
hydrochlorothiazide 12.5 mg
Uses: Antihypertensive

Zestoretic 20/25:
lisinopril 20 mg
hydrochlorothiazide 25 mg
Uses: Antihypertensive

Ziac 2.5:
bisoprolol 2.5 mg
hydrochlorothiazide 6.25 mg
Uses: Antihypertensive

Ziac 5:
bisoprolol 5 mg
hydrochlorothiazide 6.25 mg
Uses: Antihypertensive

Ziac 10:
bisoprolol 10 mg
hydrochlorothiazide 6.25 mg
Uses: Antihypertensive

Zydone:
hydrocodone 5 mg
acetaminophen 500 mg
Uses: Analgesic

Appendix F

Rarely Used Drugs

⚠ HIGH ALERT

abciximab (Rx)
Func. class.: Platelet aggregation inhibitor

Dosage and routes
Adult: **IV** 250 mcg (0.25 mg)/kg bolus 10-60 min before percutaneous transluminal angioplasty (PTCA), followed by 10 mcg/min cont inf for 12 hr

Uses: Used with heparin and aspirin to prevent acute cardiac ischemia following PTCA in patients at high risk for reclosure of affected arteries

Contraindications: Hypersensitivity to this drug or murine protein; GI, GU bleeding; CVA within 2 yr, bleeding disorders, intracranial neoplasm, intracranial arteriovenous malformations, intracranial aneurysm, platelet count <100,000 cells/mm³, recent surgery, aneurysm, uncontrolled severe hypertension, vasculitis

---

agalsidase beta (Rx)
Func. class.: Drug—misc.

Dosage and routes
Adult: **IV** inf 1 mg/kg q2 wk, run at ≤0.25 mg/min (15 mg/hr), slow if infusion-associated reaction occurs

Uses: Fabry disease
Contraindications: Hypersensitivity

---

alefacept (Rx)
Func. class.: Immunosuppressive

Dosage and routes
Adult: **IV** BOL 7.5 mg q wk or IM 15 mg q wk, for 12 wk

Uses: Adults with moderate to severe plaque psoriasis
Contraindications: Hypersensitivity

---

alfentanil (Rx)
Func. class.: Opioid analgesic

Controlled Substance Schedule II

Dosage and routes
Anesthesia <30 min
Combination
Adult: **IV** 8-50 mcg/kg, may increase by 3-15 mcg/kg

Anesthetic induction
Adult: **IV** 3-5 mcg/kg, then 0.5-1.5 mcg/kg/min; total dose is 8-40 mcg/kg

Anesthesia 30-60 min
Induction
Adult: **IV** 20-50 mcg/kg

Maintenance
Adult: **IV** 5-15 mcg/kg; may give up to 75 mcg/kg total dose

Continuous anesthesia >45 min
Induction
Adult: **IV** 50-75 mcg/kg

Maintenance
Adult: **IV** 0.5-3.0 mcg/kg/min; rate should be decreased by 30%-50% after 1 hr maintenance inf; may be increased to 4 mcg/kg/min or bol doses of 7 mcg/kg

Induction of anesthesia >45 min
Adult: **IV** 130-245 mcg/kg, then 0.5-1.5 mcg/kg/min

MAC
Induction
Adult: **IV** duration ≤½ hr 3-8 mcg/kg

Maintenance
Adult: 3-5 mcg/kg q5-20min to 1 mcg/kg/min, total dose 3-40 mcg/kg

Uses: In combination with other drugs in general anesthesia, as a primary anesthetic in general surgery, monitored anesthesia care (MAC)

P Contraindications: Child <12 yr, hypersensitivity

---

alprostadil (Rx)
Func. class.: Hormone

Dosage and routes
Patent ductus arteriosus
P *Infants:* **IV** inf 0.1 mcg/kg/min, until desired response, then reduce to lowest effective amount, 0.4 mcg/kg/min not likely to produce greater beneficial effects

Erectile dysfunction of vasculogenic or mixed etiology, psychogenic
Men: Intracavernosal 2.5 mcg may increase by 2.5 mcg; may then increase by 5-10 mcg until adequate response occurs; intraurethral administer as needed to achieve erection

Uses: To maintain patent ductus arteriosus (temporary treatment), erectile dysfunction

Contraindications: Hypersensitivity, respiratory distress syndrome (RDS)

altretamine (Rx)
Func. class.: Antineoplastic—misc.

Dosage and routes
Adult: PO 260 mg/m^2 day for 14 or 21 days in a 28-day cycle; give in 4 divided doses pc and hs

Uses: Palliative treatment of recurrent, persistent ovarian cancer following first-line treatment with cisplatin or alkylating agent–based combination

Contraindications: Hypersensitivity, severe bone marrow depression, severe neurologic toxicity, pregnancy **D**

amantadine (Rx)
Func. class.: Antiviral, antiparkinsonian agent

Dosage and routes
Influenza type A
P *Adult and child >12 yr:* PO 200 mg/day in single dose or divided bid

P *Child 9-12 yr:* PO 100 mg bid

P *Child 1-9 yr:* PO 4.4-8.8 mg/kg/day divided bid-tid, not to exceed 200 mg/day

Extrapyramidal reaction/ parkinsonism
Adult: PO 100 mg bid, up to 400 mg/day in extrapyramidal symptoms (EPS); give for 1 wk, then 100 mg as needed up to 400 mg in parkinsonism; CCr 40-50 ml/min 100 mg/day; CCr 30 ml/min 200 mg 2×/wk; CCr 20 ml/min 100 mg 3×/wk; CCr <10 ml/min 100 mg alternating with 200 mg q7d

Uses: Prophylaxis or treatment of influenza type A, extrapyramidal symptoms (EPS), parkinsonism, respiratory tract infections

Contraindications: Hypersensitivity, **P** lactation, child <1 yr, eczematic rash

◼ Do not confuse
amantadine/ranitidine, amantadine/ rimantadine, Symmetrel/Synthroid

aminocaproic acid (Rx)
Func. class.: Hemostatic

Dosage and routes
Adult: PO/**IV** 5-g loading dose, then 1-1.25 g qh if needed, not to exceed 30 g/day

Uses: Hemorrhage from hyperfibrinolysis; adjunctive therapy in hemophilia, amegakaryocytic thrombocytopenia, hereditary angioneurotic edema

Investigational uses: Prevention of recurrent subarachnoid hemorrhage

Contraindications: Hypersensitivity, abnormal bleeding, postpartum bleeding, DIC, upper urinary tract bleeding, new burns

aminoglutethimide (Rx)
Func. class.: Antineoplastic, adrenal steroid inhibitor

Dosage and routes
Adult: PO 250 mg qid at 6-hr intervals, may increase by 250 mg/day q1-2 wk, not to exceed 2 g/day

Uses: Suppression of adrenal function in Cushing's syndrome, adrenal cancer

Contraindications: Hypersensitivity, hypothyroidism, pregnancy **D**

aminolevulinic acid (Rx)
Func. class.: Photochemotherapy

Dosage and routes
Adult: Top 1 application of solution and 1 dose of illumination/treatment site × 8 wk

Uses: Face/scalp nonhyperkeratotic actinic keratoses

Contraindications: Hypersensitivity to porphyrins

---

ammonium chloride (PO-OTC, IV-Rx)
Func. class.: Acidifier

Dosage and routes
Alkalosis
P *Adult and child:* **IV** Inf 0.9-1.3 ml/min of a 2.14% sol, not to exceed 5 ml/min

Acidifier
Adult: PO 4-12 g/day in divided doses
P *Child:* PO 75 mg/kg/day in divided doses

Expectorant
Adult: PO 250-500 mg q2-4h as needed

Uses: Alkalosis (metabolic), systemic and urinary acidifier, expectorant, diuretic

Contraindications: Hypersensitivity, severe hepatic disease, severe renal disease

amyl nitrite (Rx)
Func. class.: Coronary vasodilator (antianginal, antidote for cyanide)

Dosage and routes
Angina
Adult: INH 0.18-0.3 ml as needed, 1-6 puffs from 1 cap; may repeat in 3-5 min

Cyanide poisoning
Adult: INH 0.3-ml ampule 15 sec until preparation of sodium nitrite inf is ready

Uses: Acute angina pectoris

Contraindications: Hypersensitivity to nitrites, severe anemia, increased intracranial pressure, hypertension, pregnancy **X**

atracurium (Rx)
Func. class.: Neuromuscular blocker (nondepolarizing)

Dosage and routes
P *Adult and child >2 yr:* **IV** bol 0.3-0.5 mg/kg, then 0.08-0.10 mg/kg 20-45 min after first dose if needed for prolonged procedures
P *Child, 1 mo-2 yr:* **IV** bol 0.3-0.4 mg/kg

Uses: Facilitation of endotracheal intubation, skeletal muscle relaxation during mechanical ventilation, surgery, or general anesthesia

Contraindications: Hypersensitivity

auranofin (Rx)
Func. class.: Antiinflammatory

Dosage and routes
Adult: PO 6 mg qd or 3 mg bid; may increase to 9 mg/day after 3 mo

Uses: Rheumatoid arthritis; not for first-line therapy

Investigational uses: SLE, psoriatic arthritis, pemphigus

Contraindications: Hypersensitivity to gold, necrotizing enterocolitis, bone marrow
P aplasia, child <6 yr, lactation, pulmonary fibrosis, exfoliative dermatitis, blood dyscrasias, recent radiation therapy, renal/hepatic disease, marked hypertension, uncontrolled CHF

Do not confuse
Ridaura/Cardura

aurothioglucose/gold sodium thiomalate (Rx)
Func. class.: Antiinflammatory (gold)

Dosage and routes
Aurothioglucose
Adult: IM 10 mg; then 25 mg weekly × 2-3 wk; then 50 mg/wk until total of 1 g is administered; then 25-50 mg q3-4 wk if there is improvement without toxicity; total of 800 mg-1 g
P *Child 6-12 yr:* IM 1 mg/kg/wk × 20 wk, or ¼ of adult dosage
Gold sodium thiomalate
Adult: IM 10 mg, then 25 mg after 1 wk, then 50 mg weekly for total of 14-20 doses; then 50 mg q2 wk × 4; then 50 mg q3 wk × 4; then 50 mg monthly for maintenance
P *Child <6 yr:* IM 1 mg/kg/wk × 20 wk, then q3-4 wk if improvement without toxicity, not to exceed 2.5 mg

Uses: Rheumatoid arthritis resistant to other treatment, psoriatic arthritis

Contraindications: Hypersensitivity to gold, SLE, uncontrolled diabetes mellitus, marked hypertension, recent radiation therapy, CHF, lactation, renal disease, liver disease

aztreonam (Rx)
Func. class.: Antiinfective—misc.

Dosage and routes
Urinary tract infections
Adult: **IV**/IM 500 mg-1 g q8-12h

Systemic infections
Adult: **IV**/IM 1-2 g q8-12h

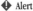 *Child:* **IV**/IM 90-120 mg/kg/day divided q6-8h

Severe systemic infections
Adult: **IV**/IM 2 g q6-8h; do not exceed 8 g/day
Continue treatment for 48 hr after negative culture or until patient is asymptomatic

Uses: Urinary tract infection; septicemia; skin, muscle, bone, lower respiratory tract, intraabdominal infections, and other infections caused by gram-negative organisms

Contraindications: Hypersensitivity

bacitracin (Rx)
Func. class.: Antiinfective—misc.

Dosage and routes
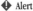 *Infant >2.5 kg:* IM 1000 units/kg/day in divided doses q8-12h

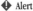 *Infant ≤2.5 kg:* IM 900 units/kg/day in divided doses q8-12h

Uses: Staphylococcal pneumonia, empyema

Contraindications: Hypersensitivity, severe renal disease (IM use)

benzonatate (Rx)
Func. class.: Antitussive, nonopioid

Dosage and routes
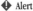 *Adult and child:* PO 100 mg tid, not to exceed 600 mg/day

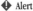 *Child <10 yr:* PO 8 mg/kg in 3-6 divided doses

Uses: Nonproductive cough

Contraindications: Hypersensitivity

benzoyl peroxide (OTC)
Func. class.: Antiacne medication

Dosage and routes
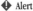 *Adult and child:* Top apply to affected area qd or bid

Uses: Mild to moderate acne

Contraindications: Hypersensitivity to benzoic acid derivatives

benzquinamide (Rx)
Func. class.: Antiemetic

Dosage and routes
Adult: IM 50 mg or 0.5-1 mg/kg; may be repeated in 1 hr, then q3-4h prn; **IV** 25 mg or 0.2-0.4 mg/kg as a one-time dose

Uses: To inhibit nausea, vomiting associated with anesthetic

Contraindications: Hypersensitivity, hypertension

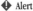 beractant (Rx)
Func. class.: Natural lung surfactant

Dosage and routes
Intratracheal instill: 4 doses can be
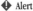 administered in the 1st 48 hr of life; give doses no more frequently than q6h; each dose is 100 mg of phospholipids/kg birth weight (4 ml/kg)

Uses: Prevention and treatment (rescue) of respiratory distress syndrome in premature 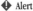 infants

bitolterol (Rx)
Func. class.: Bronchodilator, adrenergic β_2-agonist

Dosage and routes
Inhaler
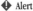 *Adult and child >12 yr:* INH 2 puffs, wait 1-3 min before 3rd puff if needed, not to exceed 3 INH q6h or 2 INH q4h

Nebulization
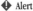 *Adult and child >12 yr:* INH 0.5 ml (1 mg) tid by intermittent flow or 1.25 mg tid by cont flow, max 8 mg (intermittent), 14 mg (cont)

Uses: Asthma, bronchospasm

Contraindications: Hypersensitivity to sympathomimetics

cabergoline (Rx)
Func. class.: Dopamine receptor/agonist

Dosage and routes
Hyperprolactinemic indications
Adult: PO 0.25 mg 2×/wk, may increase by 0.25 mg 2×/wk at 4 wk intervals, max 1 mg 2×/wk; maintenance therapy may be needed for 6 mo

Uses: Reduced prolactin/secretion in postpartum lactation

Investigational uses: Parkinson's disease, normalization of androgen levels and improved menstrual cycles in polycystic ovarian syndrome

Contraindications: Hypersensitivity to uncontrolled hypertension

*chlorproPAMIDE (Rx)
Func. class.: Antidiabetic, oral

Dosage and routes
Adult: PO 100-250 mg qd initially, then 100-500 mg maintenance according to response; not to exceed 750 mg/day

Uses: Stable adult-onset diabetes mellitus (type 2)

Contraindications: Hypersensitivity to sulfonylureas, juvenile or brittle diabetes, pregnancy **C,** renal failure

cladribine (CdA) (Rx)
Func. class.: Antineoplastic antiinfective

Dosage and routes
Adult: **IV** 0.09 mg/kg diluted with 0.9% NaCl qs to 100 ml; pass through 0.22-mcg microfilter, given for 1 wk

Uses: Treatment of active hairy cell leukemia; may be useful in chronic lymphocytic leukemia, non-Hodgkin's lymphomas, acute myeloid leukemia, autoimmune hemolytic anemia

Contraindications: Hypersensitivity, lactation

clioquinol (OTC)
Func. class.: Local antiinfective

Dosage and routes
Top apply to affected area bid-tid × 7 days only

Uses: Cutaneous infections: athlete's foot, eczema, and other fungal infections

Contraindications: Hypersensitivity to iodine, chloroxine

clobetasol (Rx)
Func. class.: Topical corticosteroid

Dosage and routes
P *Adult and child:* Top apply to affected area bid

Uses: Psoriasis, eczema, contact dermatitis, pruritus; usually reserved for severe dermatoses that have not responded to less potent formulation

Contraindications: Hypersensitivity to corticosteroids, fungal infections

clocortolone (Rx)
Func. class.: Topical corticosteroid

Dosage and routes
P *Adult and child:* Top apply to affected area tid-qid

Uses: Psoriasis, eczema, contact dermatitis, pruritus

Contraindications: Hypersensitivity to corticosteroids, fungal infections

clofazimine (Rx)
Func. class.: Leprostatic

Dosage and routes
Erythema nodosum leprosum
Adult: PO 100-200 mg qd × 3 mo, then taper dosage to 100 mg when disease is controlled; do not exceed 200 mg/day

Dapsone-resistant leprosy
Adult: PO 100 mg/day in combination with at least one other antileprosy drug × 3 yr, then 100 mg qd clofazimine (only)

Uses: Lepromatous leprosy, dapsone-resistant leprosy, lepromatous leprosy complicated by erythema nodosum leprosum

Contraindications: Hypersensitivity to this drug

clotrimazole (Rx) (OTC)
Func. class.: Local antiinfective

Dosage and routes
P *Adult and child:* Top rub into affected area bid × 1-4 wk; loz dissolve in mouth 5 times/day × 2 wk; intravag 1 applicator/1 tab × 1-2 wk hs; oral troches 10 mg 5 times/day × 14 days

Uses: Tinea pedis, tinea cruris, tinea corporis, tinea versicolor, *C. albicans* infection of the vagina, vulva, throat, mouth

Contraindications: Hypersensitivity

colfosceril (Rx)
Func. class.: Synthetic lung surfactant

Dosage and routes
Prophylactic treatment
Endotracheally: 5 ml/kg as soon as possible after birth and repeat doses 12 and 24 hr
P later to infants remaining on mechanical ventilation

Rescue treatment
Endotracheally: Administer in two half doses of 5 ml/kg doses; give initial dose after treatment of RDS, then second dose in 12 hr

P **Uses:** Treatment of RDS in premature infants

corticotropin (ACTH) (Rx)
Func. class.: Pituitary hormone

Dosage and routes
Testing of adrenocortical function
Adult: IM/SC up to 80 units in divided doses; **IV** 10-25 units in 500 ml D₅W given over 8 hr

Inflammation
Adult: SC/IM 40 units in 4 divided doses (aqueous) or 40 units q12-24h (gel/repository form)

Infantile spasms
Infant: IM Gel 20 units/day × 2 wks, increase if needed

Uses: Testing adrenocortical function, treatment of adrenal insufficiency caused by administration of corticosteroids (long term), multiple sclerosis, infantile spasms

Contraindications: Hypersensitivity, scleroderma, osteoporosis, CHF, peptic ulcer disease, hypertension, systemic fungal infections, smallpox vaccination, recent surgery,

ocular herpes simplex, primary adrenocortical insufficiency/hyperfunction

cosyntropin (Rx)
Func. class.: Pituitary hormone

Dosage and routes
P *Adult and child >2 yr:* IM/ **IV** 0.25-1 mg between blood sampling
P *Child <2 yr:* IM/**IV** 0.125 mg

Uses: Testing adrenocortical function

Contraindications: Hypersensitivity

crotamiton (Rx)
Func. class.: Scabicide

Dosage and routes
Scabies
Adult and child: Cream wash area with soap, water; remove visible crusts, apply cream, apply another coat in 24 hr, remove with soap, water in 48 hr

Pruritus: Massage into affected area, repeat as necessary

Uses: Scabies, pruritus

Contraindications: Hypersensitivity, skin inflammation, abrasions, breaks in skin, mucous membranes

dapsone (DDS) (Rx)
Func. class.: Leprostatic

Dosage and routes
Hansen's disease
Adult: PO 100 mg qd with rifampin 600 mg qd × 6 mo, then dapsone alone for 3-10 yr
P *Child:* PO 1-2 mg/kg/day

PCP
Adult: PO 50-100 mg/day usually given with trimethoprim 20 mg/kg/day in 4 divided doses for 3 wk
P *Child:* PO 2 mg/kg/day

Uses: Hansen's disease, PCP (*Pneumocystis carinii* pneumonia), malaria, dermatitis herpetiformis

Contraindications: Hypersensitivity to sulfones, severe anemia

deferoxamine (Rx)
Func. class.: Heavy metal antagonist

Dosage and routes
Acute iron toxicity
P *Adult and child:* IM/**IV** 1 g; then 500 mg q4h × 2 doses; then 500 mg q4-12h × 2 doses, not to exceed 15 mg/kg/hr or 6 g/24 hr

Chronic iron toxicity
P *Adult and child:* IM 500 mg-1 g/day plus **IV** inf 2 g given by separate line with each blood transfusion, not to exceed 15 mg/kg/hr or 6 g/24 hr; SC 1-2 g over 8-24 hr by SC infusion pump

Uses: Acute, chronic iron intoxication, hemochromatosis, hemosiderosis

Contraindications: Hypersensitivity, anuria, severe renal disease

demeclocycline (Rx)
Func. class.: Antiinfective
Chem. class.: Tetracycline

Dosage and routes
Adult: PO 150 mg q6h or 300 mg q12h
P *Child >8 yr:* PO 6-12 mg/kg/day in divided doses q6-12h

Gonorrhea
Adult: PO 600 mg, then 300 mg q12h × 4 days, total 3 g

Uses: Uncommon gram-positive/gram-negative bacteria, protozoa, *Rickettsia, Mycoplasma, Haemophilus ducreyi, Yersinia pestis, Campylobacter fetus, Chlamydia trachomatis,* psittacosis, granuloma inguinale

Contraindications: Hypersensitivity to
P tetracyclines, children <8 yr, pregnancy **D**

desipramine
Func. class.: Antidepressant, tricyclic

Dosage and routes
Adult: PO 75-150 mg/day in divided doses; may increase to 300 mg/day or may give daily dose hs

P *Adolescent and elderly:* PO 25-50
G mg/day, may increase to 100 mg/day

Uses: Depression

Contraindications: Hypersensitivity to tricyclics, recovery phase of myocardial infarction, narrow-angle glaucoma, seizure
P disorders, prostatic hypertrophy, child <12 yr

dicyclomine (Rx)
Func. class.: Gastrointestinal anticholinergic

Dosage and routes
Adult: PO 10-20 mg tid-qid; IM 20 mg q4-6h
P *Child >2 yr:* PO 10 mg tid-qid
P *Child 6 mo-2 yr:* PO 5 mg tid-qid

Uses: Treatment of peptic ulcer disease in
P combination with other drugs; infant colic, urinary incontinence

Contraindications: Hypersensitivity to anticholinergics, narrow-angle glaucoma, GI obstruction, myasthenia gravis, paralytic ileus, GI atony, toxic megacolon

dienestrol (Rx)
Func. class.: Estrogen

Dosage and routes
Adult: Vag cream 1-2 applications qd × 2 wk, then ½ dose × 2 wk, then 1 application

Uses: Atrophic vaginitis, kraurosis vulvae

Contraindications: Breast cancer, thromboembolic disorders, reproductive cancer, genital bleeding (abnormal, undiagnosed), pregnancy **X**

diflunisal (Rx)
Func. class.: Nonsteroidal antiinflammatory/analgesic (nonopioid)

Dosage and routes
Adult: PO loading dose 1 g; then 500-1000 mg/day in 2 divided doses, q12h, not to exceed 1500 mg/day

Geriatric: PO ½ adult dose

Uses: Mild to moderate pain or fever including arthritis; 3-4 × more potent than aspirin

Contraindications: Hypersensitivity to salicylates, GI bleeding, bleeding disorders,
P children <12 yr, vit K deficiency

dimercaprol (Rx)
Func. class.: Heavy metal antagonist

Dosage and routes
Severe gold/arsenic poisoning
Adult: IM 3 mg/kg q4h × 2 days; then qid × 1 day; then bid × 10 days

Mild gold/arsenic poisoning
Adult: IM 2.5 mg/kg qid × 2 days; then bid × 1 day; then qd × 10 days

Acute lead poisoning
Adult: IM 4 mg/kg; then q4 h with edetate calcium disodium 12.5 mg/kg IM; not to exceed 5 mg/kg/dose

Mercury poisoning
Adult: IM 5 mg/kg; then 2.5 mg/kg/day or bid × 10 days

Uses: Arsenic, gold, mercury, lead poisoning; adjunct in severe lead poisoning with encephalopathy

Contraindications: Hypersensitivity, anuria, hepatic insufficiency, poisoning with P other metals, severe renal disease, child <3 yr, pregnancy **D**

disulfiram (Rx)
Func. class.: Alcohol deterrent

Dosage and routes
Adult: PO 250-500 mg qd × 1-2 wk, then 125-500 mg qd until fully socially recovered

Uses: Chronic alcoholism (as adjunct)

Contraindications: Hypersensitivity, alcohol intoxication, psychoses, CV disease, pregnancy **X**

! HIGH ALERT

doxacurium (Rx)
Func. class.: Neuromuscular blocker (nondepolarizing)

Dosage and routes
Adult: **IV** 0.05 mg/kg; 0.08 mg/kg is used for prolonged neuromuscular blockade; maintenance 0.025 mg/kg

P *Child 2-12 yr:* **IV** 0.03-0.05 mg/kg; may decrease for maintenance dose

Uses: Facilitation of endotracheal intubation, skeletal muscle relaxation during mechanical ventilation, surgery, or general anesthesia

Contraindications: Hypersensitivity, P neonates

D-penicillamine (Rx)
Func. class.: Heavy metal antagonist
Chem. class.: Chelating agent

Dosage and routes
Cystinuria
Adult: PO 250 mg qid ac, not to exceed 5 g/day

P *Child:* PO 30 mg/kg/day in divided doses qid ac

Wilson's disease
Adult: PO 250 mg qid ac

P *Child:* PO 20 mg/kg/day in divided doses ac

Rheumatoid arthritis
Adult: PO 125-250 mg/day, then increase 250 mg q2-3 mo if needed, not to exceed 1 g/day

P *Child:* PO 3 mg/kg/day × 3 mo, then 6 mg/kg/day in divided doses × 3 mo, then increase to max 10 mg/kg/day

Uses: Wilson's disease, rheumatoid arthritis, cystinuria, heavy metal poisoning (lead, mercury, gold)

Contraindications: Hypersensitivity to penicillins, anuria, agranulocytosis, severe renal disease, pregnancy **D**, lactation

edetate calcium disodium (Rx)
Func. class.: Heavy metal antagonist; antidote

Dosage and routes
Acute lead encephalopathy
P *Adult and child:* 1.5 g/m^2/day × 3-5 days, with dimercaprol; may be given again after 4 days off drug

Lead poisoning
Adult: **IV** 1 g/250-500 ml D$_5$W or 0.9% NaCl over 1-2 hr or q12h × 3-5 days; may repeat after 2 days; not to exceed 50 mg/kg/day; may be given as a cont inf over 8-24 hr

Adult: IM 35 mg/kg bid

P *Child:* IM 35 mg/kg/day in divided doses q8-12h, not to exceed 50 mg/kg/day; may give for 3-5 days, off 4 days before next course

Uses: Lead poisoning, acute lead encephalopathy

Contraindications: Hypersensitivity, anuria, poisoning of other metals, severe renal P disease, child <3 yr

---

edetate disodium (Rx)
Func. class.: Metal antagonist

Dosage and routes
P *Adult and child:* **IV** inf 15-50 mg/kg/day in 2 divided doses, diluted in 500 ml D$_5$W or 0.9% NaCl, given over 3-4 hr, not to exceed 3 g/day (adult) or 70 mg/kg/day (child); allow 5 days between courses (child), 2 days (adult)

Uses: Hypercalcemic crisis, control of ventricular dysrhythmias associated with digitalis toxicity

Contraindications: Hypersensitivity, anuria, hepatic insufficiency, poisoning of
P other metals, severe renal disease, child <3 yr, seizure disorders, active/inactive TB

efalizumab (Rx)
Func. class.: Immunosuppressive

Dosage and routes
Adult: SC 0.7 mg/kg as a conditioning dose, then SC 1 mg/kg qwk, max single dose 200 mg

Uses: Adults 18 years of age and older with moderate to severe plaque psoriasis

Contraindications: Hypersensitivity

estramustine
Func. class.: Antineoplastic

Dosage and routes
Adult: PO 10-16 mg/kg in 3-4 divided doses/day; treatment may continue for ≥3 mo or 600 mg/m^2/day in 3 divided doses

Uses: Metastatic prostate cancer

Contraindications: Hypersensitivity to estradiol, thromboembolic disorders, pregnancy **D**

ethosuximide (Rx)
Func. class.: Anticonvulsant

Dosage and routes
P *Adult and child >6 yr:* PO 250 mg bid initially; may increase by 250 mg q4-7d, not to exceed 1.5 g/day

P *Child 3-6 yr:* PO 250 mg/day or 125 mg bid; may increase by 250 mg q4-7d, not to exceed 1.5 g/day

Uses: Absence seizures, partial seizures, tonic-clonic seizures

Contraindications: Hypersensitivity to succinimide derivatives

etomidate (Rx)
Func. class.: General anesthetic

Dosage and routes
P *Adult and child >10 yr:* **IV** 0.2-0.6 mg/kg over ½-1 min

Uses: Induction of general anesthesia

Contraindications: Hypersensitivity, labor/delivery

felbamate (Rx)
Func. class.: Anticonvulsant

Dosage and routes
Adjunctive therapy
Adult: PO add 1.2 g/day in 3-4 divided doses; reduce other anticonvulsants (valproic acid, phenytoin, carbamazepine, and derivatives) by 20% to control plasma concentrations; may increase felbamate in 1.2 g/day increments qwk, up to 3.6 g/day

Monotherapy
Adult: PO 1.2 g/day in 3-4 divided doses; titrate with close supervision; increase dose in 600-mg increments q2 wk to 3.6 g/day if needed

Lennox-Gastaut syndrome
P *Child (2-14 yr):* PO add 15 mg/kg/day in 3-4 divided doses; reduce other anticonvulsants (valproic acid, phenytoin, carbamazepine, and derivatives) by 20% to control plasma concentrations; may increase felbamate 15 mg/kg/day qwk up to 45 mg/day

Uses: Partial seizures, with or without generalization in adults; partial and general-
P ized seizures in children with Lennox-Gastaut syndrome

Contraindications: Hypersensitivity to this drug, other carbamates

fenoprofen (Rx)
Func. class.: Nonsteroidal antiinflammatory/ nonopioid analgesic

Dosage and routes
Pain
Adult: PO 200 mg q4-6h prn

♣ Canada Only   N Do Not Confuse   * "Tall Man" lettering (See Preface)

Arthritis
Adult: PO 300-600 mg qid, not to exceed 3.2 g/day

Uses: Mild to moderate pain, osteoarthritis, rheumatoid arthritis, acute gout, arthritis, ankylosing spondylitis, inflammation, dysmenorrhea

Contraindications: Hypersensitivity, asthma, severe renal disease, severe hepatic disease

---

flavoxate (Rx)
Func. class.: Spasmolytic

Dosage and routes
P *Adult and child >12 yr:* PO 100-200 mg tid-qid

Uses: Relief of nocturia, incontinence, suprapubic pain, dysuria, frequency associated with urologic conditions (symptomatic only)

Contraindications: Hypersensitivity, GI obstruction, GI hemorrhage, GU obstruction

---

floxuridine (Rx)
Func. class.: Antineoplastic, antimetabolite

Dosage and routes
Adult: Intraarterial by cont inf 0.1-0.6 mg/kg/day × 1-6 wk; hepatic artery inj 0.4-0.6 mg/kg/day × 1-6 wk

Uses: GI adenocarcinoma metastatic to liver; cancer of breast, head, neck, liver, brain, gallbladder, bile duct

Contraindications: Hypersensitivity, myelosuppression, pregnancy **D**, poor nutritional status, serious infections

---

fludarabine (Rx)
Func. class.: Antineoplastic, antimetabolite

Dosage and routes
Adult: **IV** 25 mg/m^2 over 30 min qd × 5 days, may repeat q28 days; reconstitute with 2 ml of sterile water for inj; dissolution should occur in <15 sec

Uses: Chronic lymphocytic leukemia; non-Hodgkin's lymphoma

Contraindications: Hypersensitivity, pregnancy **D**

---

flunisolide (Rx)
Func. class.: Steroid, intranasal

Dosage and routes
Adult: Instill 2 sprays in each nostril bid, then increase to tid if needed, not to exceed 8 sprays/day in each nostril

P *Child 6-14 yr:* Instill 1 spray in each nostril tid or 2 sprays bid, not to exceed 4 sprays/day in each nostril

P *Adult and child >6 yr:* Spray 2 puffs bid, not to exceed 4 puffs bid

Uses: Rhinitis (seasonal or perennial), nasal polyps; chronic steroid-dependent asthma (inh)

Contraindications: Hypersensitivity,
P child <12 yr; fungal, bacterial infection of nose

---

gallamine (Rx)
Func. class.: Neuromuscular blocker (nondepolarizing)

Dosage and routes
P *Adult and child >1 mo:* **IV** 1 mg/kg, not to exceed 100 mg, then 0.5-1 mg/kg q30-40 min

P *Child <1 mo, >5 kg:* **IV** 0.25-0.75 mg/kg, then 0.01-0.05 mg/kg q30-40 min

Uses: Facilitation of endotracheal intubation, skeletal muscle relaxation during mechanical ventilation, surgery, or general anesthesia

Contraindications: Hypersensitivity to iodides

---

glycerin, anhydrous (Rx)
Func. class.: Ophthalmic

Dosage and routes
Adult: Instill 1-2 gtt after local anesthetic

Uses: Reduce corneal edema

Contraindications: Hypersensitivity

---

griseofulvin microsize/ultramicrosize (Rx)
Func. class.: Antifungal

Dosage and routes
Adult: PO 500-1000 mg qd in single or divided doses (microsize), 125-165 mg bid (ultramicrosize), or 250-330 mg qd; may need

---

 Herb/drug   Do Not Crush   Alert   Key Drug   Geriatric   Pediatric

500-660 mg in divided doses for severe infections

P *Child:* PO 10 mg/kg/day or 30 mg/m²/day (microsize) or 5 mg/kg/day (ultramicrosize)

Uses: Mycotic infections: tinea corporis, tinea pedis, tinea cruris, tinea barbae, tinea capitis, tinea unguium if caused by *Epidermophyton, Microsporum, Trichophyton*

Contraindications: Hypersensitivity, porphyria, hepatic disease, lupus erythematosus

---

guanabenz (Rx)
Func. class.: Antihypertensive

Dosage and routes
Adult: PO 4 mg bid, increasing in increments of 4-8 mg/day q1-2 wk, not to exceed 32 mg bid

Uses: Hypertension

Contraindications: Hypersensitivity to guanabenz

---

guanadrel (Rx)
Func. class.: Antihypertensive

Dosage and routes
Adult: PO 5 mg bid, adjusted to desired response weekly or monthly; may need 20-75 mg/day in divided doses; higher doses are given tid or qid

G *Elderly:* PO 5 mg/day, titrate as needed

Renal dose
• CCr 10-50 ml/min dose q12-24h; CCr <10 ml/min dose q24-48h

Uses: Hypertension (moderate to severe as an adjunct)

Contraindications: Hypersensitivity,
P pheochromocytoma, lactation, CHF, child <18 yr

---

guanethidine (Rx)
Func. class.: Antihypertensive

Dosage and routes
Adult: PO 10-12.5 mg qd, increase by 10 mg qwk; may require 25-50 mg qd

Adult: (hospitalized) 25-50 mg; may increase by 25-50 mg/day or every other day

P *Child:* PO 0.2 mg/kg/day (6 mg/m²/day);

increase q7-10d, 0.2 mg/kg or 6 mg/m²/day, not to exceed 3000 mcg/kg/24 hr

Uses: Moderate to severe hypertension

Contraindications: Hypersensitivity, pheochromocytoma, recent MI, CHF, cardiac failure, sinus bradycardia

---

guanfacine (Rx)
Func. class.: Antihypertensive

Dosage and routes
Adult: PO 1 mg/day hs; may increase dose in 2-3 wk to 2-3 mg/day

Uses: Hypertension in individual using a thiazide diuretic

Investigational uses: ADHD

Contraindications: Hypersensitivity

---

halcinonide (Rx)
Func. class.: Corticosteroid, synthetic

Dosage and routes
Adult: Top apply to affected area bid-tid (not around eyes)

Uses: Inflammation of corticosteroid-responsive dermatoses

Contraindications: Hypersensitivity, viral infections, fungal infections

---

halofantrine (Rx)
Func. class.: Antimalarial

Dosage and routes
Adult: PO 500 mg q6h × 3 doses; may need to repeat after 1 wk

Uses: Mild to moderate malaria

Contraindications: Hypersensitivity, pregnancy, lactation, QT interval prolongation, AV conduction disorders, thiamine deficiency, ventricular dysrhythmias

---

hyaluronidase (Rx)
Func. class.: Enzyme

Dosage and routes
Adjunct
P *Adult and child:* Inj 150 units with other drug

Urography
 Adult and child: SC 75 units over scapula, then contrast medium injected at same site

Hypodermoclysis
 Adult and child >3 yr: SC 150 units/L of lysis sol

Uses: Hypodermoclysis, subcutaneous urography; adjunct to dispersion of other drugs

Contraindications: Hypersensitivity to bovine products, CHF, hypoproteinemia, around infected/inflamed or cancerous area

---

hydroquinone (Rx)
Func. class.: Depigmentating agent

Dosage and routes
 Adult and child: Top apply to affected area qd-bid

Uses: Bleaching skin, including age spots, freckles, lentigo, chloasma

Contraindications: Hypersensitivity, inflamed skin, prickly heat, sunburn

---

hydroxychloroquine (Rx)
Func. class.: Antimalarial, antiarthritic

Dosage and routes
Malaria
 Adult and child: PO 5 mg/kg/wk on same day of week, not to exceed 400 mg; treatment should begin 2 wk before entering endemic area; continue 8 wk after leaving; if treatment begins after exposure, 800 mg for adult, 10
 mg/kg for children in 2 divided doses 6 hr apart

Lupus erythematosus
Adult: PO 400 mg qd-bid; length depends on patient response; maintenance 200-400 mg qd

Rheumatoid arthritis
Adult: PO 400-600 mg qd, then 200-300 mg qd after good response

Uses: Malaria caused by *Plasmodium vivax*, *P. malariae*, *P. ovale*, *P. falciparum* (some strains); SLE, rheumatoid arthritis

Contraindications: Hypersensitivity,
 retinal field changes, porphyria, children (long-term)

---

hydroxyprogesterone (Rx)
Func. class.: Progestin, hormone

Dosage and routes
Menstrual disorders
Adult: IM 125-375 mg q4 wk; discontinue after 4 cycles

Uterine cancer
Adult: IM 1 g 5-7 times/wk

Uses: Uterine carcinoma, menstrual disorders (abnormal uterine bleeding, amenorrhea)

Contraindications: Breast cancer, hypersensitivity, thromboembolic disorders, reproductive cancer, genital bleeding (abnormal, undiagnosed), pregnancy

---

idoxuridine-IDU (Rx)
Func. class.: Antiviral

Dosage and routes
 Adult and child: Instill 1 gtt qh during day and q2h during night

Uses: Herpes simplex keratitis, CMV, varicella-zoster alone or with corticosteroids

Contraindications: Hypersensitivity

---

indecainide (Rx)
Func. class.: Antidysrhythmic (Class IC)

Dosage and routes
Adult: PO 100-200 mg/day in divided dose q12h; 50 mg q12h initially, then increase dose by 25 mg increments q4d, max 400 mg/day

Uses: Life-threatening dysrhythmias, sustained ventricular tachycardia

Contraindications: 2nd- or 3rd-degree AV block, right bundle branch block, cardiogenic shock, hypersensitivity

---

iodoquinol (Rx)
Func. class.: Amebicide

Dosage and routes
Adult: PO 630-650 mg tid × 20 days, not to exceed 2 g/day

 Child: PO 30-40 mg/kg/day in 2-3 divided doses × 20 days, not to exceed 1.95 g/24 hr × 20 days; do not repeat treatment before 2-3 wk

---

Uses: Intestinal amebiasis

Contraindications: Hypersensitivity to this drug or iodine, renal disease, hepatic disease, severe thyroid disease, preexisting optic neuropathy

---

isotretinoin (Rx)
Func. class.: Dermatologic antiacne agent

Dosage and routes
Adult: PO 0.5-2 mg/kg/day in 2 divided doses × 15-20 wk; if relapse occurs, repeat after 8 wk off drug

Uses: Severe recalcitrant cystic acne

Contraindications: Hypersensitivity, inflamed skin, pregnancy **X**

---

isoxsuprine (Rx)
Func. class.: Peripheral vasodilator

Dosage and routes
Adult: PO 10-20 mg tid or qid

Uses: Symptoms of cerebrovascular insufficiency, peripheral vascular disease including arteriosclerosis obliterans, thromboangiitis obliterans, Raynaud's disease

Contraindications: Hypersensitivity, postpartum, arterial bleeding

---

kanamycin (Rx)
Func. class.: Antiinfective

Dosage and routes
Severe systemic infections
P *Adult and child:* **IV** inf 15 mg/kg/day in divided doses q8-12h; diluted 500 mg/200 ml of 0.9% NaCl or D_5W given over 30-60 min, not to exceed 1.5 g/day; IM 15 mg/kg/day in divided doses q8-12h, not to exceed 1.5 g/day; irrigation not to exceed 1.5 g/day; inh 250 mg qid

Preoperative bowel sterilization
Adult: PO 1 g qh × 4 doses, then q6h × 36-72 hr

Renal dose
Adult: IM/**IV** 7.5 mg/kg, may increase or decrease dose based on renal status

Uses: Severe systemic infections of CNS, respiratory tract, GI tract, urinary tract, bone, skin, soft tissues; peritonitis, preoperatively to sterilize bowel; decreases ammonia-producing

bacteria in bowel and IP after fecal spill during surgery

Contraindications: Bowel obstruction, severe renal disease, hypersensitivity

---

! HIGH ALERT

ketamine (Rx)
Func. class.: General anesthetic

Dosage and routes
P *Adult and child:* **IV** 1-4.5 mg/kg over 1 min
P *Adult and child:* IM 6.5-13 mg/kg

Maintenance: ½ to full induction dose may be repeated

Uses: Short anesthesia for diagnostic/surgical procedures; as an adjunct with other anesthetics

Contraindications: Hypersensitivity, CVA, increased intracranial pressure, severe hypertension, cardiac decompensation, child <2 yr

---

laronidase (Rx)
Func. class.: Drug—misc.

Dosage and routes
Adult: **IV** inf 0.58 mg/kg qwk; pretreat with antipyretic and/or antihistamines 1 hr prior to **IV** inf

Uses: Mucopolysaccharidosis I (MPSI), patients with Hurler and Hurler-Scheie forms of MPSI

Contraindications: Hypersensitivity

---

levobupivacaine (Rx)
Func. class.: Local anesthetic

Dosage and routes
Varies with route of anesthesia

Uses: Local, regional anesthesia, surgical anesthesia, pain management, continuous epidural analgesia

Contraindications: Hypersensitivity, children <12 yr, elderly, severe liver disease

---

levorphanol (Rx)
Func. class.: Opioid analgesic (agonist)
Controlled Substance Schedule II

Dosage and routes
Adult: PO/SC/**IV** 2-3 mg q4-5h prn; PCA 0.1 mg/ml

Uses: Moderate to severe pain

Contraindications: Hypersensitivity, addiction (opioid)

lincomycin (Rx)
Func. class.: Antibacterial

Dosage and routes
Adult: PO 500 mg q6-8h, not to exceed 8 g/day; IM 600 mg/day or q12h; **IV** 600 mg-1 g q8-12h; dilute in 100 ml **IV** sol; infuse over 1 hr, not to exceed 8 g/day

P *Child >1 mo:* PO 30-60 mg/kg/day in divided doses q6-8h; IM 10 mg/kg/day q12h; **IV** 10-20 mg/kg/day in divided doses q8-12h; dilute to 100 ml **IV** sol; infuse over 1 hr

Uses: Infections caused by group A β-hemolytic streptococci, pneumococci, staphylococci (respiratory tract, skin, soft tissue, urinary tract infections, osteomyelitis, septicemia)

Contraindications: Hypersensitivity, **P** ulcerative colitis/enteritis, infants <1 mo

masoprocol (Rx)
Func. class.: Topical product—misc.

Dosage and routes
Adult: Top apply to lesion bid × 2-4 wk

Uses: Actinic keratoses

Contraindications: Hypersensitivity, **P** children

mazindol (Rx)
Func. class.: Anorexiant

Dosage and routes
Adult: PO 1 mg/hr ac, or 2 mg 1 hr ac lunch, or 1 mg tid 1 hr ac

Uses: Exogenous obesity

Contraindications: Hypersensitivity to sympathomimetic amine, glaucoma, drug **P** abuse, cardiovascular disease, children <12 yr, hypertension, severe arteriosclerosis, agitated states, hyperthyroidism, concurrent MAOI use or use within 14 days

mefenamic acid (Rx)
Func. class.: Nonsteroidal antiinflammatory

Dosage and routes
P *Adult and child >14 yr:* PO 500 mg, then 250 mg q6h, use not to exceed 1 wk

Uses: Mild to moderate pain, dysmenorrhea, inflammatory disease

Contraindications: Hypersensitivity, asthma, severe renal disease, severe hepatic disease, ulcer disease

mefloquine (Rx)
Func. class.: Antimalarial

Dosage and routes
Adult: PO 1250 mg as a single dose (treatment); 250 mg 1 wk before trip, then for 4 wk after returning, then 250 mg q2 wk (prevention)

Uses: Treatment and prevention of *Plasmodium falciparum, P. vivax,* malaria

Contraindications: Hypersensitivity

mepenzolate (Rx)
Func. class.: GI anticholinergic

Dosage and routes
Adult: PO 25-50 mg qid with meals, hs; titrate to patient response

Uses: Treatment of peptic ulcer disease, irritable bowel syndrome in combination with other drugs; for other GI disorders

Contraindications: Hypersensitivity to anticholinergics, narrow-angle glaucoma, GI obstruction, myasthenia gravis, paralytic ileus, GI atony, toxic megacolon

meprobamate (Rx)
Func. class.: Sedative/hypnotic; antianxiety

Dosage and routes
Adult: PO 1.2-1.6 g/day in 2-3 divided doses, not to exceed 2.4 g/day or 800-1600 mg/day in 2 divided doses (sus rel); max 2.4 g/day

G *Elderly:* PO 200 mg bid-tid, adjust to lowest possible dose

 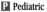

P *Child 6-12 yr:* PO 100-200 mg bid-tid or 200 mg (sus rel) bid

Uses: Anxiety, sedation

Contraindications: Hypersensitivity, renal failure, porphyria, pregnancy **D**, history of drug abuse or dependence

---

methohexital (Rx)
Func. class.: General anesthetic

Dosage and routes
Induction
P *Adult and child:* **IV** 50-120 mg given 1 ml/5 sec

Maintenance
P *Adult and child:* **IV** 20-40 mg q4-7 min of a 0.1% sol

Uses: General anesthesia for electroshock therapy, reduction of fractures, adjunct with other anesthetics, balanced anesthesia

Contraindications: Hypersensitivity, status asthmaticus, hepatic/intermittent porphyrias

---

methoxsalen (Rx)
Func. class.: Pigmentating agent

Dosage and routes
Vitiligo
P *Adult and child >12 yr:* PO 20 mg qd2-4 hr before exposure to therapeutic ultraviolet rays; administer on alternate days; Top apply 1-2 hr before exposure to UVA light; treatment intervals regulated by erythema response

Psoriasis
Adult: PO dosage individualized to weight; taken 2 hr before exposure to therapeutic ultraviolet rays

Uses: Vitiligo, psoriasis

Contraindications: Hypersensitivity, melanoma, LE, albinism, sunburn, cataracts,
P squamous cell cancer, child ≤12 yr, diseases associated with photosensitivity

---

methscopolamine (Rx)
Func. class.: GI anticholinergic

Dosage and routes
Adult: PO 2.5-5 mg ½ hr ac, hs

Uses: Peptic ulcer disease, preoperatively

Contraindications: Hypersensitivity to

anticholinergics, narrow-angle glaucoma, GI obstruction, myasthenia gravis, paralytic ileus, GI atony, toxic megacolon

---

methsuximide (Rx)
Func. class.: Anticonvulsant

Dosage and routes
P *Adult and child:* PO 300 mg/day; may increase by 300 mg/wk, not to exceed 1.2 g/day in divided doses

Uses: Refractory absence seizures (petit mal)

Contraindications: Hypersensitivity to succinimide derivatives

---

miglustat (Rx)
Func. class.: Agent—misc.

Dosage and routes
Adult: PO 100 mg tid, without regard to food

Uses: Adults with mild to moderate type 1 Gaucher disease

Contraindications: Hypersensitivity, pregnancy **X**

---

mitotane (Rx)
Func. class.: Antineoplastic

Dosage and routes
Adult: PO 9-10 g/day in divided doses tid or qid; may have to decrease dosage if severe reactions occur

Uses: Adrenocortical carcinoma

Investigational uses: Pituitary disorders with cushingoid symptoms

Contraindications: Hypersensitivity

---

modafinil (Rx)
Func. class.: Cerebral stimulant

Dosage and routes
Adult: PO 200 mg qd in the AM, may increase to 400 mg qd if needed

Hepatic dose
Reduce dose by 50%

Uses: Narcolepsy

Contraindications: Hypersensitivity, hyperthyroidism, hypertension, glaucoma, severe arteriosclerosis, drug abuse, CV disease, anxiety

---

molindone (Rx)
Func. class.: Antipsychotic/neuroleptic

Dosage and routes
Adult: PO 50-75 mg/day increasing to 225 mg/day if needed

Uses: Psychotic disorders

Contraindications: Hypersensitivity, **P** coma, child

papaverine (Rx)
Func. class.: Peripheral vasodilator

Dosage and routes
Adult: PO 100-300 mg 3-5 × day; sus rel cap 150-300 mg q8-12h; IM/IV 30-120 mg q3h prn; intracavernosal (IC) 30 mg/0.5-1 mg phentolamine or 60 mg alone

Uses: Arterial spasm resulting in cerebral and peripheral ischemia, myocardial ischemia associated with vascular spasm or dysrhythmias, angina pectoris, peripheral pulmonary embolism, visceral spasm as in ureteral, biliary, GI colic, peripheral vascular disease

Contraindications: Hypersensitivity, complete AV heart block

paraldehyde (Rx)
Func. class.: Anticonvulsant

Dosage and routes
Seizures
Adult: IM 5-10 ml; divide 10 ml into 2 inj; IV 0.2-0.4 ml/kg in NS inj
P *Child:* IM 0.15 ml/kg; rect 0.3 ml/kg q4-6h or 1 ml/yr of age, not to exceed 5 ml; may repeat in 1 hr prn; IV 5 ml/90 ml NS inj; begin infusion at 5 ml/hr; titrate to patient response

Alcohol withdrawal
Adult: PO/rect 5-10 ml, not to exceed 60 ml; IM 5 ml q4-6h × 24 hr, then q6h on following days, not to exceed 30 ml

Sedation
Adult: PO/rec 4-10 ml; IM 5 ml; IV 3-5 ml in emergency only
P *Child:* PO/rec/IM 0.15 ml/kg

Tetanus
Adult: IV 4-5 ml or 12 ml by gastric tube q4h diluted with water; IM 5-10 ml prn

Uses: Refractory seizures, status epilepticus, sedation, insomnia, alcohol withdrawal, tetanus, eclampsia

Contraindications: Hypersensitivity, gastroenteritis with ulceration

paramethadione (Rx)
Func. class.: Anticonvulsant

Dosage and routes
Adult: PO 300 mg tid; may increase by 300 mg/wk, not to exceed 600 mg qid
P *Child >6 yr:* PO 0.9 g/day in divided doses tid or qid
P *Child 2-6 yr:* PO 0.6 g/day in divided doses tid or qid
P *Child <2 yr:* PO 0.3 g/day in divided doses tid or qid

Uses: Refractory absence (petit mal) seizures

Contraindications: Hypersensitivity, blood dyscrasias, pregnancy **D**, lactation

paromomycin (Rx)
Func. class.: Amebicide

Dosage and routes
Intestinal amebiasis
P *Adult and child:* PO 25-35 mg/kg/day in 3 divided doses × 5-10 day pc
Hepatic coma
Adult: 4 g in divided doses × 5-6 day

Uses: Intestinal amebiasis, adjunct in hepatic coma

Contraindications: Hypersensitivity, renal disease, GI obstruction

pegvisomant (Rx)
Func. class.: Agent—misc.

Dosage and routes
Adult: SC loading dose of 40 mg, under supervision of prescriber, then SC 10 mg qd; measure IGF-I levels q4-6 wk

Uses: Acromegaly, in those patients who have an inadequate response to other treatment

Contraindications: Hypersensitivity, latex allergy

☑ Herb/drug   ◎ Do Not Crush   ◆ Alert   ◆〒 Key Drug   **G** Geriatric   **P** Pediatric

perflutren lipid microsphere (Rx)
Func. class.: Diagnostic drug

Dosage and routes: Use only after activation in the Vialmix apparatus

Adult: **IV** bol 10 mcg/kg of the activated product within 30-60 sec, followed by 10-ml saline flush, may repeat

Adult: **IV** inf 1.3 ml/50 ml preservative-free saline, give at 4 ml/min, not to exceed 10 ml/min

Uses: Contrast enhancement during echocardiographic procedures

Contraindications: Hypersensitivity to octafluoropropane, known cardiac shunts, administration by direct intraarterial inj

permethrin (OTC, Rx)
Func. class.: Pediculicide

Dosage and routes
Lice (head)
P *Adult and child:* Wash hair, towel dry; apply liberally to hair, leave on 10 min, rinse with water

Scabies
P *Adult and child:* Top 5% cream applied and massaged into all skin surfaces; leave cream on 8-14 hr, then wash

Uses: Lice, nits, ticks, flea nits

Contraindications: Hypersensitivity

phenacemide (Rx)
Func. class.: Anticonvulsant

Dosage and routes
Adult: PO 500 mg tid, may increase by 500 mg/wk, not to exceed 5 g/day

P *Child 5-10 yr:* PO 250 mg tid, may increase by 250 mg/wk, not to exceed 1.5 g/day prn

Uses: Refractory, generalized tonic-clonic (grand mal), complex-partial (psychomotor), absence (petit mal), atypical seizures

Contraindications: Hypersensitivity, psychiatric condition, pregnancy **D**, lactation

phendimetrazine (Rx)
Func. class.: Anorexiant

Dosage and routes
Adult: PO 35 mg bid-tid 1 hr ac, not to exceed 70 mg tid; sus rel 105 mg qd ac AM

Uses: Exogenous obesity

Contraindications: Hypersensitivity, hyperthyroidism, hypertension, glaucoma, severe arteriosclerosis, severe cardiovascular P disease, children <12 yr, agitated states, drug abuse, MAOI use within 14 days

phenoxybenzamine (Rx)
Func. class.: Antihypertensive

Dosage and routes
Adult: PO 10 mg qd; increase by 10 mg qod; usual range 20-40 mg bid-tid

P *Child:* PO 0.2 mg/kg or 6 mg/m²/day, max 10 mg, may increase at 4-day intervals; maintenance dosage 0.4-1.2 mg/kg/day or 12-36 mg/m²/day given in divided doses tid or qid

Uses: Pheochromocytoma

Contraindications: Hypersensitivity, CHF, angina, cerebral vascular insufficiency, coronary arteriosclerosis

phentermine (Rx)
Func. class.: Cerebral stimulant

Dosage and routes
Adult: PO 8 mg tid 30 min before meals or 15-37.5 mg qd before breakfast

Uses: Exogenous obesity

Contraindications: Hypersensitivity, hyperthyroidism, hypertension, glaucoma, severe arteriosclerosis, angina pectoris, P cardiovascular disease, pregnancy **C**, child <12 yr

physostigmine (Rx)
Func. class.: Antidote, reversible anticholinesterase

Dosage and routes
Overdose of anticholinergics
Adult: IM/**IV** 2 mg; give no more than 1 mg/min; may repeat

P *Child:* IM/**IV** inj 0.02 mg/kg, not more than 0.5 mg/min; may repeat at 5-10 min intervals until max dose of 2 mg

Postanesthesia
Adult: IM/**IV** 0.5-1 mg; give no more than 1 mg/min (**IV**); can repeat at 10-30 min intervals

Uses: To reverse CNS effects of diazepam, anticholinergics, tricyclics, Alzheimer's disease, hereditary ataxia

Contraindications: Hypotension, obstruction of intestine or renal system, asthma, gangrene, CV disease, choline esters, depolarizing neuromuscular blocking agents, diabetes

---

pinacidil (Rx)
Func. class.: Antihypertensive

Dosage and routes
Adult: PO 12.5-25 mg bid

Uses: Severe hypertension not responsive to other therapy

Contraindications: Acute MI, dissecting aortic aneurysm, hypersensitivity, pheochromocytoma

---

! HIGH ALERT

poractant alfa (Rx)
Func. class.: Lung surfactant

Dosage and routes
P *Intratracheal instill:* Premature infant 2.5 ml/kg birth weight, up to 2 subsequent doses of 1.25 ml/kg birth weight can be administered at 12-hr intervals, max 5 ml/kg

Uses: Treatment (rescue) of respiratory
P distress syndrome (RDS) in premature infants

---

pralidoxime (Rx)
Func. class.: Cholinesterase reactivator

Dosage and routes
Anticholinesterase overdose
Adult: **IV** 1-2 g, then 250 mg q5 min until desired response

Organophosphate poisoning
Adult: **IV** inf 1-2 g/100 ml 0.9% NaCl over 15-30 min; may repeat in 1 hr; PO 1-3 g q5h

P *Child:* **IV** inf 20-40 mg/kg/dose diluted in 100 ml 0.9% NaCl over 15-30 min

Uses: Cholinergic crisis in myasthenia gravis, organophosphate poisoning antidote, early relief of paralysis of respiratory muscles; used as an adjunct to systemic atropine administration

Contraindications: Hypersensitivity, carbamate insecticide poisoning

---

prazepam (Rx)
Func. class.: Sedative/hypnotic; antianxiety agent

Dosage and routes
Adult: PO 10 mg tid; 20-60 mg in divided doses or 20 mg at hs

G *Elderly:* PO 10-15 mg/day in divided doses

Uses: Anxiety

Contraindications: Hypersensitivity to benzodiazepines, narrow-angle glaucoma,
P psychosis, pregnancy **D**, child <18 yr

---

reserpine (Rx)
Func. class.: Antihypertensive, antiadrenergic agent (peripherally acting)

Dosage and routes
Hypertension
Adult: PO 0.25-0.5 mg qd × 1-2 wk, then 0.1-0.25 mg qd for maintenance

G *Elderly:* PO 0.05 mg qd, increase by 0.05 weekly to desired dose

Psychiatric disorders
Adult: PO 0.5 mg qd, range 0.1-1 mg

Uses: Hypertension

Contraindications: Hypersensitivity, depression, suicidal patients, active peptic ulcer disease, ulcerative colitis, pregnancy **D**, Parkinson's disease

Do Not Confuse:
reserpine/Risperdal

---

respiratory syncytial virus immune globulin (RSV-IGIV) (Rx)
Func. class.: Immune serums

Dosage and routes
P *Child <2 yr:* **IV** inf 1.5 ml/kg/hr × 15 min, then 3 ml/kg/hr 15-30 min; then 6 ml/kg/hr from 30 min to end of inf given monthly

---

 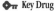

Uses: Prevention of serious lower respiratory ℗ tract infection caused by RSV in children <2 yr with bronchopulmonary dysplasia or premature birth

Contraindications: Hypersensitivity to this drug or other human immunoglobulin preparations; IgA deficiency

---

⚠ HIGH ALERT

secobarbital (Rx)
Func. class.: Sedative/hypnotic-barbiturate

Controlled substance schedule II (USA), schedule G (Canada)

Dosage and routes
Insomnia
Adult: PO/IM 100-200 mg hs
℗ *Child:* IM 3-5 mg/kg, max 100 mg, do not inject >5 ml in one site

Sedation/preoperatively
Adult: PO 200-300 mg 1-2 hr preoperatively
℗ *Child:* PO 50-100 mg 1-2 hr preoperatively

Status epilepticus
℗ *Adult and child:* IM/IV 250-350 mg

Acute psychotic agitation
℗ *Adult and child:* IM/IV 5.5 mg/kg q3-4h

Uses: Insomnia, sedation, preoperative medication, status epilepticus, acute tetanus seizures

Contraindications: Hypersensitivity to barbiturates, respiratory depression, pregnancy **D**, addiction to barbiturates, severe liver impairment, porphyria, uncontrolled severe pain

---

sevelamer (Rx)
Func. class.: Polymeric phosphate binder

Dosage and routes
Reduction of serum phosphorus in adults not taking phosphate binders

Adult: PO initially 800-1600 mg tid with meals based on serum phosphorus level (see below); adjust dose gradually at 2-wk intervals until serum phosphorus 6 mg/dl

Adult, serum phosphorus 9 mg/dl: 1600 mg tid with meals

Adult, serum phosphorus 7.5 and <9 mg/dl: 1200-1600 mg tid with meals

Adult, serum phosphorus >6 and <7.5 mg/dl: 800 mg tid with meals

Uses: End-stage renal disease (ESRD)

Contraindications: Hypophosphatemia, bowel obstruction, hypersensitivity

---

sibutramine (Rx)
Func. class.: Appetite suppressant

Controlled substance schedule IV

Dosage and routes
Adult: PO 10 mg qd; may be increased to 15 mg qd after 4 wk, or lowered to 5 mg qd depending on response

Uses: Obesity in conjunction with other treatments

Contraindications: Hypersensitivity, hypothyroidism, anorexia nervosa, severe hepatic/renal disease, uncontrolled hypertension, history of CAD, CHF, dysrhythmias, lactation

---

streptozocin (Rx)
Func. class.: Antineoplastic alkylating agent

Dosage and routes
Adult: IV 500 mg/m^2 × 5 days q6 wk until desired response; or 1 g/m^2 qwk × 2 wk, not to exceed 1.5 g/m^2 in 1 dose

Uses: Metastatic islet cell carcinoma of pancreas

Investigational uses: Prevention of spread of Hodgkin's disease, metastatic carcinoid tumor, pancreatic adenocarcinoma, colon malignancies

Contraindications: Hypersensitivity

---

teniposide (Rx)
Func. class.: Antineoplastic

Dosage and routes
℗ *Child:* IV inf Combo teniposide 165 mg/m^2 and cytarabine 300 mg/m^2 2×/wk × 8-9 doses or combo teniposide 250 mg/m^2 and vinCRIStine 1.5 mg/m^2 qwk × 4-8 wk and predniSONE 40 mg/m^2 PO × 28 days

℗ **Uses:** Childhood acute lymphoblastic leukemia (ALL), refractory childhood acute lymphocytic leukemia

---

Contraindications: Hypersensitivity, bone marrow depression, severe hepatic disease, severe renal disease, bacterial infection, pregnancy **D**

thioguanine (6-TG) (Rx)
Func. class.: Antineoplastic-antimetabolite

Dosage and routes
P *Adult and child:* PO 2 mg/kg/day, then increase slowly to 3 mg/kg/day after 4 wk

Uses: Acute leukemias, chronic granulocytic leukemia, lymphomas, multiple myeloma, solid tumors

Contraindications: Prior drug resistance, leukopenia (WBC 2500/mm³), thrombocytopenia (platelets <100,000/mm³), anemia, pregnancy **D**

! HIGH ALERT
thiopental (Rx)
Func. class.: General anesthetic

Dosage and routes
Induction
Adult: **IV** 210-280 mg or 3-5 mg/kg

General anesthetic
Adult: **IV** 50-75 mg given at 20-40 sec intervals

Narcoanalysis
Adult: **IV** 100 mg/min, not to exceed 50 ml/min

Sedation or narcosis
Adult: Rec 12-20 mg/lb

Increased intracranial pressure
Adult: 1.5-3.5 mg/kg

Uses: Short general anesthesia, narcoanalysis, induction anesthesia before other anesthetics

Investigational uses: Increased intracranial pressure

Contraindications: Hypersensitivity, status asthmaticus, hepatic/intermittent porphyrias

thiotepa (Rx)
Func. class.: Antineoplastic

Dosage and routes
Adult: **IV** 0.3-0.4 mg/kg at 1-4 wk intervals

Neoplastic effusions
Adult: Intracavity 0.6-0.8 mg/kg

Bladder cancer
Adult: Instill 60 mg/30-60 ml water for inj in bladder for 2 hr once/wk × 4 wk

Uses: Hodgkin's disease, lymphomas; breast, ovarian, lung, bladder cancer; neoplastic effusions

Contraindications: Hypersensitivity, pregnancy **D**

thiothixene (Rx)
Func. class.: Antipsychotic/neuroleptic

Dosage and routes
Adult: PO 2-5 mg bid-qid depending on severity of condition; dose gradually increased to 15-30 mg if needed; IM 4 mg bid-qid; max dose 30 mg qd; administer PO dose as soon as possible

G *Elderly:* PO 1-2 mg qd-bid, increase by 1-2 mg q4-7 days to desired dose

Uses: Psychotic disorders, schizophrenia, acute agitation

Contraindications: Hypersensitivity, **P** blood dyscrasias, child <12 yr, bone marrow depression, circulatory collapse, CNS depression, coma, alcoholism, CV disease, hepatic disease, Reye's syndrome, narrow-angle glaucoma

*TOLAZamide (Rx)
Func. class.: Antidiabetic, oral

Dosage and routes
Adult: PO 100 mg/day for FBS <200 mg/dl or 250 mg/day for FBS >200 mg/dl; dose should be titrated to patient response (1 g or less/day)

Uses: Type 2 diabetes mellitus

Contraindications: Hypersensitivity to **P** sulfonylureas, juvenile or brittle diabetes

*TOLBUTamide ⚷π (Rx)
Func. class.: Antidiabetic

Dosage and routes
Adult: PO 1-2 g/day in divided doses, titrated to patient response; **IV** 1 g (Fajan's test)

Uses: Type 2 diabetes mellitus

Contraindications: Hypersensitivity to
P sulfonylureas, juvenile or brittle diabetes

trientine (Rx)
Func. class.: Heavy metal antagonist

Dosage and routes
Adult: PO 750-1250 mg in divided doses bid-qid, max 2000 mg/day
P *Child:* PO 500-1500 mg in divided doses bid-qid

Uses: Wilson's disease, chelating agent if other agents are not tolerated

Contraindications: Hypersensitivity, cystinuria, rheumatoid arthritis, biliary cirrhosis

xylometazoline (OTC)
Func. class.: Nasal decongestant

Dosage and routes
P *Adult and child >12 yr:* Instill 2-3 gtt or 2 sprays q8-10h (0.1%)
P *Child <12 yr:* Instill 2-3 gtt or 1% spray q8-10h (0.05%)

Uses: Nasal congestion; adjunct in otitis media

Contraindications: Hypersensitivity to sympathomimetic amines

Appendix G   Less Frequently Used Antihistamines

GENERIC NAME	TRADE NAME(S)	USES	DOSAGES AND ROUTES	AVAILABLE FORMS	INTERACTIONS	CONTRAINDICATIONS
acrivastine/ pseudoephedrine (Rx)	Semprex-D	• Rhinitis • Allergy symptoms • Chronic idiopathic urticaria	**P** Adult, child >12 yr: PO 8 mg q4-6h	• Caps 8 mg/60 mg	• Increased CNS depression: alcohol, opioids, sedatives, hypnotics • Hypertensive crisis: MAOIs ☒ May increase CNS depression: kava ☒ May increase anticholinergic effect: henbane leaf	• Hypersensitivity to this drug or triprolidine • Severe hypertension • Cardiac disease
azatadine (Rx)	Optimine	• Allergy symptoms • Rhinitis • Chronic urticaria	• Adult: PO 1-2 mg bid, not to exceed 4 mg/ day **G** Elderly: PO 1 mg qd-bid	• Tabs 1 mg	• Increased CNS depression: barbiturates, opioids, hypnotics, tricyclic antidepressants, alcohol • Decreased effect of: oral anticoagulants ☒ Increased effect of azatadine: MAOIs ☒ Increased CNS depression: kava ☒ Increased anticholinergic effect: henbane leaf	• Hypersensitivity to H_1-receptor antagonists • Acute asthma attack • Lower respiratory tract disease **P** Child <12 yr
buclizine (Rx)	Bucladin-S, Softabs	• Motion sickness • Dizziness • Nausea • Vomiting • Antihistamine	• Adult: PO 25-50 mg prn ½ hr before travel; may be repeated q4-6h prn	• Tabs 50 mg	☒ Increased anticholinergic effect: henbane leaf ☒ Increased CNS depression: kava	• Hypersensitivity to cyclizines • Shock

					Contraindications
cyclizine (OTC, **Rx**)	Marezine	• Motion sickness • Prevention of post-operative vomiting • Antihistamine	*Vomiting* • Adult: IM 25-50 mg ½ hr before termination of surgery, then q4-6h prn (lactate) **P** Child: IM 3 mg/kg divided in 3 equal doses *Motion sickness* • Adult: PO 50 mg then q4-6h prn, not to exceed 200 mg/day (HCl) **P** Child: PO 25 mg q4-6h prn	• Tabs (HCl) 50 mg • Inj (lactate) 50 mg/ml	• May increase CNS effect: alcohol, tranquilizers, opioids ☑ Increased CNS depression: kava	• Hypersensitivity to cyclizines • Shock
dexchlorpheniramine (**Rx**)	Dexchlor, dexchlorpheniramine maleate, Poladex, Polaramine	• Allergy symptoms • Rhinitis • Pruritus • Contact dermatitis	• Adult: PO 1-2 mg tid-qid; repeat action 4-6 mg bid-tid **P** Child 6-11 yr: PO 1 mg q4-6h, or time rel 4 mg hs **P** Child 2-5 yr: PO 0.5 mg q4-6h; do not use repeat action form	• Tabs 2 mg • Repeat action tabs 4, 6 mg • Syr 2 mg/ 5 ml	• Increased CNS depression: barbiturates, opioids, hypnotics, tricyclic antidepressants, alcohol • Decreased effect: oral anticoagulants, heparin • Increased effect of dexchlorpheniramine: MAOIs ☑ Increased anticholinergic effect: henbane leaf	• Hypersensitivity to H_1-receptor antagonists • Acute asthma attack • Lower respiratory tract disease

Continued

KEY: ☑ = Herb/drug interaction, **G** = Geriatric, **P** = Pediatric

Appendix G Less frequently used antihistamines—cont'd

GENERIC NAME	TRADE NAME(S)	USES	DOSAGES AND ROUTES	AVAILABLE FORMS	INTERACTIONS	CONTRAINDICATIONS
trimeprazine (Rx)	Panectyl ✦, Temaril	• Pruritus	• Adult: PO 2.5 mg qid; time-rel 5 mg bid **G** Elderly: PO 2.5 mg bid **P** Child 3-12 yr: PO 2.5 mg tid or hs **P** Child 6 mo-1 yr: PO 1.25 mg tid or hs	• Tabs 2.5 mg • Time rel spanules 5 mg • Syr 2.5 mg/ 5 ml	• Increased CNS depression: barbiturates, opioids, hypnotics, tricyclic antidepressants, alcohol • Decreased effect of oral anticoagulants, heparin • Increased effect of trimeprazine: MAOIs ⊠ Increased anticholinergic effect: henbane leaf	• Hypersensitivity to H_1-receptor antagonists • Acute asthma attack • Lower respiratory tract disease
tripelennamine (Rx)	PBZ, PBZ-SR, Pelamine, tripelennamine HCl	• Rhinitis • Allergy symptoms	• Adults: PO 25-50 mg q4-6h, not to exceed 600 mg/day; time-rel 100 mg bid-tid, not to exceed 600 mg/day **P** Child >5 yr: PO time-rel 50 mg q8-12h, not to exceed 300 mg/day **P** Child <5 yr: PO 5 mg/kg/day in 4-6 divided doses, not to exceed 300 mg/day	• Tabs 25, 50 mg • Time-rel tabs 100 mg • Elix 37.5 mg/5 ml	• Increased CNS depression: barbiturates, opioids, hypnotics, tricyclic antidepressants, alcohol • Decreased effect of oral anticoagulants, heparin • Increased effect of tripelennamine: MAOIs ⊠ Increased anticholinergic effect: henbane leaf	• Hypersensitivity to H_1-receptor antagonists • Acute asthma attack • Lower respiratory tract disease

KEY: ✦ = Canada only

Appendix H Vaccines and Toxoids

GENERIC NAME	TRADE NAME	USES	DOSAGES AND ROUTES	CONTRAINDICATIONS
BCG vaccine	TICE BCG	TB exposure	**P** Adult/child >1 mo: 0.2-0.3 ml **P** Child <1 mo: Reduce dose by 50% using 2 ml of sterile water after reconstituting	Hypersensitivity, hypogamma-globulinemia, positive TB test, burns
cholera vaccine	No trade name	Immunization for cholera in other countries	**P** Adult/child >10 yr: IM/SC 2× of 0.5 ml, 7-30 days before traveling to areas with cholera Booster is used q6 mo 0.5 ml prn	Hypersensitivity, acute febrile illness
diphtheria and tetanus toxoids, adsorbed	No trade name	Induces antitoxins to provide immunity to diphtheria, tetanus	**P** Adult/child ≥7 yr: IM (adult strength) 0.5 ml q4-8 wk × 2 doses, then 3rd dose 6-12 mo after 2nd dose, booster IM 0.5 ml q10 yr **P** Child 1-6 yr: IM (pediatric strength) 0.5 ml q4 wk × 2 doses, booster 6-12 mo after 2nd dose **P** Infant 6 wk-1 yr: IM (pediatric strength) 0.5 ml q4 wk × 3 doses, booster 6-12 mo after 3rd dose	Hypersensitivity to mercury, thi-merosal, immunocompromised patients, radiation, corticoste-roids, acute illness
diphtheria and tetanus toxoids and whole-cell pertussis vaccine (DPT, DTP)	DTwP, Tr-Immunol	Prevention of diphtheria, tetanus, pertussis	Adult: booster dose q10 yr **P** Child >6 wk-6 yr: IM 0.5 ml at 2, 4, 6 mo, 1-½ yr; booster needed 0.5 ml at age 6	Hypersensitivity, active infection, poliomyelitis outbreak, immu-nosuppression, febrile illness
diphtheria and tetanus toxoids and acellular pertussis vaccine	Acel-Imune, DTaP, Tri-pedia			

TB, Tuberculosis; *DPT,* diphtheria-pertussis-tetanus (vaccine); *DTP,* diphtheria and tetanus toxoids and pertussis vaccine.
KEY: **P** = Pediatric

Continued

GENERIC NAME	TRADE NAME	USES	DOSAGES AND ROUTES	CONTRAINDICATIONS
haemophilus b conjugate vaccine, diphtheria CRM$_{197}$ protein conjugate (HbOC) haemophilus b conjugate vaccine, meningococcal protein conjugate (PRP-OMP)	HibTITER PedvaxHIB	**P** Polysaccharide immunization of children 2-6 yr against *H. influenzae b*, conjugate immunization of child 2, 4, 6 mo	**HibTITER (IM only)** **P** Child: IM 0.5 ml **P** Child 2-6 mo: 0.5 ml q2 mo × 3 inj **P** Child 7-11 mo: Previously unvaccinated 0.5 ml q2mo inj **P** Child 12-14 mo: previously unvaccinated 0.5 ml × 1 inj **PEDVAXHIB (IM only)** **P** Child 2-14 mo: 0.5 ml × 2 inj at 2, 4 mo of age (6 mo dose not needed), then booster at 12-18 mo against invasive disease **P** Child ≥15 mo: Previously unvaccinated 0.5 ml inj	Hypersensitivity, febrile illness, active infection
hepatitis A vaccine, inactivated	Havrix, Vaqta	Active immunization against hepatitis A virus	Adults: IM 1, 440 EL. units (Havrix) or 50 units (Vaqta) as a single dose, booster dose is the same given at 6, 12 mo **P** Child 2-18 yr: IM 720 EL. units (Havrix) or 25 units (Vaqta) as a single dose, booster dose is the same given at 6, 12 mo	Hypersensitivity
hepatitis B vaccine, recombinant	Engerix-B, Recombivax HB	Immunization against all subtypes of hepatitis B virus	Varies widely	Hypersensitivity to this vaccine or yeast

influenza virus vaccine, trivalent A and B (whole virus/split virus)	Fluogen, FluShield, Fluviral ♦ Fluvirin, Fluzone, influenza virus vaccine, trivalent	Prevention of Russian, Chilean, Philippine influenza	**P** Adult/child >12 yr: IM 0.5 ml in 1 dose **P** Child 3-12 yr: IM 0.5 ml, repeat in 1 mo (split) unless 1978-1985 vaccine was given **P** Child 6 mo to 3 yr: IM 0.25 ml, repeat in 1 mo (split) unless 1978-1985 vaccine was given	Hypersensitivity, active infection, chicken egg allergy, Guillain-Barré syndrome, active neurologic disorders
Japanese encephalitis virus vaccine, inactivated	JE-VAX	Active immunity against Japanese encephalitis (JE)	**P** Adult/child ≥3 yr: SC 1 ml, days 0, 7, 30; booster SC 1 ml 2 yr after last dose **P** Child 1-3 yr: SC 0.5 ml, days 0, 7, 30; booster SC 0.5 ml 2 yr after last dose	Hypersensitivity to murine, thimerosal; allergic reactions to previous dose
Lyme disease vaccine (recombinant OspA)	LYMErix	Immunization against Lyme disease	Adult and adolescent 15-70: IM 30 mcg in deltoid, repeat at 1, 12 mo after first dose	Hypersensitivity, antibiotic refractory Lyme arthritis
measles and rubella virus vaccine, live attenuated	M-R-Vax II	Immunity to measles and rubella by antibody production	**P** Adult/child ≥15 mo: SC 0.5 ml (1000 units)	Hypersensitivity, immunocompromised patients, active untreated TB, cancer, blood dyscrasias, radiation, corticosteroids, pregnancy; allergic reactions to neomycin, eggs
measles, mumps, and rubella vaccine, live	M-M-R-II	Prevention of measles, mumps, rubella	Adult: SC 1 vial; 2 vials separated by 1 mo, in person born after 1957 **P** Child >15 mo and adult: SC 0.5 ml	Hypersensitivity, blood dyscrasias, anemia, active infection, immunosuppression; egg, chicken allergy; pregnancy; febrile illness, neomycin allergy; neoplasms

Continued

♦ Canada only; **P** = Pediatric

GENERIC NAME	TRADE NAME	USES	DOSAGES AND ROUTES	CONTRAINDICATIONS
measles virus vaccine, live attenuated	Attenuvax	Immunity to measles by antibody production	**P** Adult/child ≥15 mo: SC 0.5 ml (1000 units), one dose 15 mo, 2nd dose age 4-6 or 11, or 12	Hypersensitivity to eggs, neomycin; cancer, radiation, corticosteroids, pregnancy, immunocompromised patients, blood dyscrasias, active untreated TB
meningococcal polysaccharide vaccine	Menomune-A/C/Y/W-135	Prophylaxis to meningococcal meningitis	**P** Adult/child >2 yr: SC 0.5 ml	Hypersensitivity to thimerosal, pregnancy, acute illness
mumps virus vaccine, live	Mumpsvax	Active immunity to mumps	**P** Adult/child ≥1 yr: SC 0.5 ml (20,000 units)	Hypersensitivity to eggs, neomycin; cancer, radiation, corticosteroids, pregnancy, immunocompromised patients, blood dyscrasias, active untreated TB
plague vaccine	No trade name	Active immunity to *Yersinia pestis* plague	Adult: IM 1 ml, then 0.2 ml in 4-12 wk, then 0.2 ml 5-6 mo after 2nd dose; booster 0.1-0.2 ml q6 mo when in area where plague is present	Hypersensitivity to phenol, sulfites, formaldehyde, beef, soy, casein; pregnancy, coagulation disorders
pneumococcal 7-valent conjugate vaccine	Prevnar	Immunity against *Streptococcus pneumoniae*	**P** Child: IM 0.5 ml × 3 doses (7-11 mo); × 2 doses (12-23 mo); × 1 dose >2-9 yr	Hypersensitivity to diphtheria toxoid or this product
pneumococcal vaccine, polyvalent	Pneumovax 23, Pnu-Imune 23	Pneumococcal immunization	**P** Adult/child >2 yr: IM/SC 0.5 ml	Hypersensitivity, Hodgkin's disease, ARDS
poliovirus vaccine, live, oral, trivalent (TOPV) poliovirus vaccine (IPV)	Orimune, IPOL	Prevention of polio	**P** Adult/child >2 yr: PO 0.5 ml, given q8 wk × 2 doses, then 0.5 ml ½-1 yr after dose 2 **P** Infant: PO 0.5 at 2, 4, 18 mo; booster at 4-6 yr; may also be given IPV at 2, 4 mo, then TOPV at 12-18 mo, booster at 4-6 yr	Hypersensitivity, active infection, allergy to neomycin/streptomycin, immunosuppression, vomiting, diarrhea

rabies vaccine, adsorbed	No trade name	Active immunity to rabies	**Preexposure** **P** Adult/child: IM 1 ml day 0, 7, 21, or 28 days (total 3 doses); booster IM 1 ml prn q2-5 yr **Postexposure** **P** Adult/child not vaccinated: IM 20 international units/kg of HRIG and 5 1 ml inj of rabies vaccine on days 0, 7, 14, 28	Severe hypersensitivity to previous inj of vaccine, thimerosal
rabies vaccine, HDCV	IMOVax Rabies, IM-OVax Rabies I.D.	Active immunity to rabies	**Preexposure** **P** Adult/child: IM 1 ml day 0, 7, 21 or 28 **Postexposure** **P** Adult/child: IM 1 ml on day 0, 3, 7, 14, 28	No contraindications
rubella and mumps virus vaccine, live	Biavax II	Immunity to rubella and mumps by antibody production	**P** Adult/child ≥1 yr: SC 0.5 ml	Hypersensitivity to eggs, neomycin; cancer, radiation, corticosteroids, pregnancy, immunocompromised patients, blood dyscrasias, active untreated TB
rubella virus vaccine, live attenuated (RA 27/3)	Meruvax II	Immunity to rubella by antibody production	**P** Adult/child ≥1 yr: SC 0.5 ml (1000 units)	Hypersensitivity to eggs, neomycin; cancer, radiation, corticosteroids
tetanus toxoid, adsorbed/tetanus toxoid	No trade name	Tetanus toxoid: used for prophylactic treatment of wounds	**P** Adult/child: IM 0.5 ml q4-6 wk × 2 doses, then 0.5 ml 1 yr after dose 2 (adsorbed); SC/IM 0.5 ml q4-8 wk × 3 doses, then 0.5 ml 1/2-1 yr after dose 3, booster dose 0.5 ml q10 yr	Hypersensitivity, active infection, poliomyelitis outbreak, immunosuppression

Continued

ARDS, Acute respiratory distress syndrome; *HRIG,* human rabies immune globulin; *HDCV,* human diploid cell vaccine.

GENERIC NAME	TRADE NAME	USES	DOSAGES AND ROUTES	CONTRAINDICATIONS
typhoid vaccine, parenteral typhoid vaccine, oral	No trade name Vivotif Berna Vaccine	Active immunity to typhoid fever	Adult: PO 1 cap 1 hr before meals × 4 doses, booster q5 yr **P** Adult/child >10 yr: SC 0.5 ml, repeat in 4 wk, booster q3 yr **P** Child 6 mo-10 yr: SC 0.25 ml, repeat in 4 wk, booster q3 yr	Parenteral: systemic or allergic reaction, acute respiratory or other acute infection, intensive physical exercise in high temp Oral: hypersensitivity, acute febrile illness, suppressive or antibiotic drugs
typhoid Vi polysaccharide vaccine	Typhim Vi	Active immunity to typhoid fever	**P** Adult/child ≥2 yr: IM 0.5 ml as a single dose, reimmunize q2 yr 0.5 ml IM, if needed	Hypersensitivity, chronic typhoid carriers
varicella virus vaccine	Varivax	Prevention of varicella-zoster (chickenpox)	**P** Adult/child ≥13 yr: SC 0.5 ml, 2nd dose SC 0.5 ml 4-8 wk later	Hypersensitivity to neomycin; blood dyscrasias, immunosuppression, active untreated TB, acute illness, pregnancy, diseases of lymphatic system
yellow fever vaccine	YF-Vax	Active immunity to yellow fever	**P** Adult/child ≥9 mo: SC 0.5 ml deeply, booster q10 yr **P** Child 6-9 mo: same as above if exposed	Hypersensitivity to egg or chicken embryo protein, pregnancy, **P** child <6 mo, immunodeficiency

Appendix I

Herbal Products

agrimony

Uses: Mild diarrhea, gastroenteritis, intestinal mucous secretion, inflammation of the mouth and throat, cuts and scrapes, amenorrhea

alfalfa

Uses: Poor appetite, hay fever and asthma, high cholesterol, nutrient source

aloe

Uses of aloe vera gel:
External: Minor burns, skin irritations, minor wounds, frostbite, radiation-caused injuries
Internal: To heal intestinal inflammation and ulcers, as a digestive aid to stimulate bile secretion

angelica

Uses: Heartburn, indigestion, gas, colic, poor blood flow to the extremities, bronchitis, poor appetite, psoriasis, vitiligo, as an antiseptic

arnica

Uses: Topical application for muscle and joint inflammation and swelling; in homeopathic preparations as a remedy for shock, injury, pain

astragalus

Uses: Immune stimulant, viral infections, HIV/AIDS, cancer, vascular disorders, improve circulation, lower blood pressure, possible efficacy in myasthenia gravis

bilberry

Uses: Diabetic retinopathy, macular degeneration, glaucoma, cataract, capillary fragility, varicose veins, hemorrhoids, mild diarrhea

black cohosh

Uses:
Menopause: Hot flashes, nervous conditions associated with menopause
Dysmenorrhea: Menstrual cramps, pain, inflammation

black haw (cramp bark)

Uses: Dysmenorrhea, menstrual cramps and pain, menopausal metrorrhagia, hysteria, asthma, lower blood pressure, heart palpitations

blessed thistle

Uses: Loss of appetite, indigestion, intestinal gas

blue cohosh

Uses: Menopausal symptoms, uterine and ovarian pain, improve flow of menstrual blood, antiinflammatory, antirheumatic, popular remedy in black ethnic medicine

borage

Uses: Antiinflammatory for premenstrual syndrome, rheumatoid arthritis, Raynaud's disease, other inflammatory conditions, atopic dermatitis, infant cradle cap, cystic fibrosis, high blood pressure, diabetes

Adapted from: Dubusk, Ruth, and Treadwell, Phillip. *Serious Drug/Herb Interactions.* Skidmore-Roth Publishing, Inc. 1999.

burdock root

Uses: Skin diseases, inflammation, rashes, cold and fever, cancer, gout, arthritis

calendula

Uses:
External: Minor skin ailments
Internal: Inflammation throughout the gastrointestinal tract, toxic liver and gallbladder, menstrual bleeding and pain, yeast infections

capsicum (cayenne)

Uses: Muscle spasms, pain of inflammation, neuromas, psoriasis, dry mouth, as an antioxidant food, as a food seasoning

cascara

Uses: Chronic constipation, hepatitis, gallstones

cat's claw

Uses: Cancer, herpes, HIV/AIDS, rheumatoid arthritis, gastritis, gout, wounds, gastric ulcers

chamomile

Uses:
External: As an antiseptic and soothing agent for inflamed skin and minor wounds
Internal: As an antispasmodic, gas-relieving, and antiinflammatory agent for the treatment of digestive problems; light sleep aid and sedative for adults and children; possible anticancer agent

chaparral

Uses: Not recommended—potentially toxic to the liver and kidneys

chicory

Uses: Coffee substitute, source of fructo-oligosaccharides, mild laxative for children, gout, rheumatism, loss of appetite, digestive distress

comfrey

Uses: Bruises, sprains, broken bones, acne, boils

cranberry

Uses: UTIs; susceptibility to kidney stones

dong quai

Uses: To restore vitality to tired women; for a variety of gynecologic, menstrual, and menopausal symptoms; cirrhosis of the liver

echinacea

Uses: Low immune status, hard-to-heal superficial wounds, sun protection

elder (elderberry)

Uses: Susceptibility to colds, flu, yeast infections; nasal and chest congestion; earache associated with chronic congestion; hay fever

eleuthero (See siberian ginseng)

evening primrose

Uses: Premenstrual syndrome, arthritis and inflammatory disorders in general, dry skin, eczema, asthma, diabetes, migraines, chronic fatigue syndrome, heart disease and stroke, circulatory disorders, Raynaud's disease, NSAID use, multiple sclerosis

fenugreek

Uses: Loss of appetite, inflamed areas of the skin, water retention, cancer, constipation, diarrhea, high cholesterol, high blood glucose, calcium oxalate stones

feverfew

Uses: Migraines, cluster headaches, fever, psoriasis, inflammation

flaxseed

Uses: Constipation, as a source of omega-3 fatty acids

fo-ti

Uses: Tiredness, constipation, elevated cholesterol

garcinia cambogia

Uses: Appetite control, weight loss, high cholesterol

garlic

Uses: Vascular disease, elevated LDL, elevated triglycerides, low HDL, high blood pressure, poor circulation, risk of cancer, inflammatory disorders, childhood ear infection, yeast infection

ginger

Uses: Nausea, motion sickness, indigestion, inflammation

ginkgo

Uses: Poor circulation; age-related decline in cognition, memory; diabetes; vascular disease; cancer; inflammatory disorders; impotence; degenerative nerve conditions

ginseng

Uses: Physical and mental exhaustion, stress, viral infections, diabetes, sluggishness, fatigue, weak immunity, convalescence

goldenseal

Uses: High blood pressure, poor appetite, infections, menstrual problems, minor sciatic pain, muscle spasms, eye washes

gotu kola

Uses: Chronic wounds, psoriasis

grape seed

Uses: Antioxidant, chronic disease prevention, inflammation

green tea

Uses: Cancer prevention, heart disease prevention, hypercholesterolemia, diarrhea

guggul

Uses: High LDL cholesterol, elevated triglycerides, weight loss

gymnema sylvestre

Uses: High blood glucose levels

hawthorn

Uses: Poor circulation, chest pain, irregular heartbeat, high blood fats, high blood pressure

hops

Uses: Mild sedative, diuretic, weak antibiotic, insomnia, hyperactivity, pain, fever, jaundice, improve appetite

horse chestnut

Uses: Fever, fluid retention, frostbite, hemorrhoids, inflammation, lower extremity swelling, phlebitis, varicose veins, wounds

horsetail

Uses: Diuretic, genitourinary astringent, anti-hemorrhagic, Bell's palsy, healing broken bones

kava

Uses: Anxiety, restlessness, sleep disturbances, stress

khat

Uses: Obesity, gastric ulcers, stimulant

kombucha

Uses: Numerous claims for a wide variety of ills; none has been substantiated to date

konjac

Uses: Blood glucose control, constipation, high blood fats, high blood pressure, excessive appetite

kudzu

Uses: Alcohol cravings, menopausal symptoms

lapacho (pau d'arco)

Uses: Cancer, inflammation, infection

lemon balm (melissa)

Uses: Abdominal gas and cramping, cold sores

licorice

Uses: Allergies, arthritis, asthma, constipation, esophagitis, gastritis, hepatitis, inflammatory conditions, peptic ulcers, poor adrenal function, poor appetite

maitake

Uses: Immunostimulant activity, diabetes, hypertension, high cholesterol, obesity

maté

Uses: Diuretic, depurative

melatonin

Uses: Jet lag, insomnia, cancer protection, oral contraceptive

milk thistle

Uses: Protection for alcoholic cirrhosis and hepatitis, antiinflammatory

monascus

Uses: Maintaining acceptable cholesterol levels

morinda

Uses: Headache, digestive, heart and liver conditions, arthritis

nettle

Uses: Diuretic, hay fever

octacosanol

Uses: Herpes, inflammation of the skin, physical endurance

passionflower

Uses: Antifungal, hypertension, sedative, group A hemolytic streptococcus

peppermint

Uses: GI disorders

pygeum

Uses: Benign prostate hypertrophy, antiinflammatory

raspberry leaves

Uses: Facilitation of childbirth, dysmenorrhea, uterine tonic, fever, vomiting

red clover

Uses: Antispasmodic, expectorant, sedative, psoriasis, eczema, amenorrhea

rose hips

Uses: Source of vit C, cold, fever, mild infection

st. john's wort

Uses: Depression, antiviral

sarsaparilla

Uses: Antiinflammatory, antiseptic, syphilis, skin diseases, rheumatism, necrosis, mercury poisoning

sassafras

Uses: Banned in the United States

saw palmetto

Uses: Benign prostatic hypertrophy

schisandra

Uses: GI disorders, liver protection, tonic

skullcap

Uses: Antibacterial, sedative

senna

Uses: Laxative

siberian ginseng (eleuthero)

Uses: Improve appetite, memory loss, hypertension, insomnia, rheumatism, circulation, heart ailments, diabetes, headache

tea tree oil

Uses: Topical use for infections; inhaled for respiratory disorders

uva ursi

Uses: Diuretic, urinary tract infections, contact dermatitis, arthritis

valerian

Uses: Sedative

vitex

Uses: Premenstrual and menstrual disorders, spasms, estrogen gestagen imbalance

yarrow

Uses: To decrease bleeding, Gi disorders, hypertension, thrombi, to improve circulation

yohimbine

Uses: Male organic impotence

Appendix J

FDA Pregnancy Categories

A   No risk demonstrated to the fetus in any trimester
B   No adverse effects in animals, no human studies available
C   Only given after risks to the fetus are considered; animal studies have shown adverse reactions, no human studies available
D   Definite fetal risks, may be given in spite of risks if needed in life-threatening conditions
X   Absolute fetal abnormalities; not to be used anytime during pregnancy

Appendix K

Controlled Substance Chart

DRUGS	UNITED STATES	CANADA
Heroin, LSD, peyote, marijuana, mescaline	Schedule I	Schedule H
Opium (morphine), meperidine, amphetamines, cocaine, short-acting barbiturates (secobarbital)	Schedule II	Schedule G
Glutethimide, paregoric, phendimetrazine	Schedule III	Schedule F
Chloral hydrate, chlordiazepoxide, diazepam, mazindol, meprobamate, phenobarbital (Canada-G)	Schedule IV	Schedule F
Antidiarrheals with opium (Canada-G), antitussives	Schedule V	Schedule F

Appendix L

Commonly Used Abbreviations

abd abdomen
ABG arterial blood gas
ac before meals
ACE angiotensin-converting enzyme
ACT activated clotting time
ADA American Diabetes Association
ADH antidiuretic hormone
ALT alanine aminotransferase
ANA antinuclear antibody
AP anteroposterior
APTT activated partial thromboplastin time
ASA acetylsalicylic acid, aspirin
ASHD arteriosclerotic heart disease
AST aspartate aminotransferase (SGOT)
AV atrioventricular
bid twice a day
BM bowel movement
BMR basal metabolic rate
B/P blood pressure
BPH benign prostatic hypertrophy
BPM beats per minute
BS blood sugar
BUN blood urea nitrogen
C Celsius (centigrade)
Ca cancer
CAD coronary artery disease
cap capsule
Cath catheterization or catheterize
CBC complete blood cell count
CC chief complaint
cc cubic centimeter
CHF congestive heart failure
cm centimeter
CNS central nervous system
CO₂ carbon dioxide
cont continuous
COPD chronic obstructive pulmonary disease
CPAP continuous positive airway pressure

CPK creatinine phosphokinase
CPR cardiopulmonary resuscitation
CCr creatinine clearance
C&S culture and sensitivity
C sect cesarean section
CSF cerebrospinal fluid
CV cardiovascular
CVA cerebrovascular accident
CVP central venous pressure
D&C dilatation and curettage
dir inf direct infusion
dr dram
D₅W 5% glucose in distilled water
ECG electrocardiogram (EKG)
EDTA ethylenediamine tetraacetic acid
EEG electroencephalogram
EENT ear, eye, nose, and throat
EPS extrapyramidal symptoms
ESR erythrocyte sedimentation rate
ext rel extended release
EXTRA STREN extra strength
susp suspension
FBS fasting blood sugar
FHT fetal heart tones
FSH follicle-stimulating hormone
g gram
GABA γ-aminobutyric acid
GI gastrointestinal
gr grain
GTT glucose tolerance test
gtt drops
GU genitourinary
H₂ histamine₂
hCG human chorionic gonadotropin
Hct hematocrit
HDCV human diploid cell rabies vaccine

Hgb hemoglobin
H&H hematocrit and hemoglobin
5-HIAA 5-hydroxyindoleacetic acid
HIV human immunodeficiency
virus (AIDS)
H₂O water

HOB head of bed
HR heart rate
hr hour
hs at bedtime
IgG immunoglobulin G
IM intramuscular
inf infusion
INH inhalation
inj injection
I&O intake and output
IPPB intermittent positive-
pressure breathing
ITP idiopathic thrombocyto-
penic purpura
IUD intrauterine device
IV intravenous
IVP intravenous pyelogram
K potassium
kg kilogram
L liter
lb pound
LDH lactic dehydrogenase
LE lupus erythematosus
LH luteinizing hormone
LLQ left lower quadrant
LMP last menstrual period
LOC level of consciousness
LR lactated Ringer's solution
LUQ left upper quadrant
M meter
m minim
m² square meter
MAOI monoamine oxidase
inhibitor
mcg microgram
mEq milliequivalent
mg milligram
MI myocardial infarction
min minute
ml milliliter
mm millimeter
mo month
Na sodium
neg negative
NPO nothing by mouth (Lat.
nulla per os)
NS normal saline
O₂ oxygen
OBS organic brain syndrome

OD right eye
OR operating room
OS left eye
OTC over-the-counter
OU each eye
oz ounce
p̄ after
P56 plasma-lyte 56
PaCO₂ arterial carbon dioxide
tension (pressure)
PaO₂ arterial oxygen tension
(pressure)
PAT paroxysmal atrial tachycardia
PBI protein-bound iodine
PCWP pulmonary capillary wedge
pressure
PEEP positive end-expiratory
pressure
PERRLA pupils equal, round, react to
light and accommodation
pH hydrogen ion concentration
PO by mouth
postop postoperative
PP postprandial
preop preoperative
prn as required
PT prothrombin time
PTT partial thromboplastin time
PVC premature ventricular
contraction
q every
qAM every morning
qd every day
qh every hour
q2h every 2 hours
q3h every 3 hours
q4h every 4 hours
q6h every 6 hours
q12h every 12 hours
qid four times daily
qod every other day
qPM every night
qs sufficient quantity
qt quart
R right
RAIU radioactive iodine uptake
RBC red blood count or cell
RLQ right lower quadrant
ROM range of motion
RUQ right upper quadrant
SC subcutaneous
SIMV synchronous intermittent
mandatory ventilation
SL sublingual

SLE	systemic lupus erythematosus	**tsp**	teaspoon
SOB	shortness of breath	**TT**	thrombin time
sol	solution	**UA**	urinalysis
ss	one half	**UTI**	urinary tract infection
supp	suppository	**UV**	ultraviolet
sus rel	sustained release	**vag**	vaginal
syr	syrup	**VMA**	vanillylmandelic acid
T&A	tonsillectomy and adenoid-ectomy	**vol**	volume
		VS	vital sign
tab	tablet	**WBC**	white blood cell count
tbsp	tablespoon	**wk**	week
temp	temperature	**wt**	weight
tid	three times daily	**yr**	year
tinc	tincture	**>**	greater than
TPN	total parenteral nutrition	**<**	less than
top	topical	**=**	equal
TRANS	transdermal	**°**	degree
TSH	thyroid-stimulating hormone	**%**	percent
		γ	gamma
		β	beta

- For a list of The Institute for Safe Medicine Practices (ISMP) error prone abbreviations, symbols, and dose designations, please see http://www.ismp.org/PDF/ErrorProne.pdf.
- For frequently asked questions regarding the 2004 National Patient Safety Goals, please visit the Joint Commission on Accreditation of Healthcare Organizations (JCAHO) website at http://www.jcaho.org/accredited+organizations/patient+safety/04+npsg/04_faqs.htm

Appendix M

IV Drug/Solution Compatibility Chart

	D_5	D_{10}	D_5 ½S	D_5 S	NS	R	LR	OTHER
AcetaZOLAMIDE	C	C	C	C	C	C	C	
Acyclovir	C							
Alpha$_1$-proteinase inhibitor								Sterile water for inj
Alprostadil	C	C			C			
Alteplase								Sterile water for inj
Amdinocillin	C	C	C	C	C	C	C	D_5 in R
Amikacin	C				C			
Aminocaproic acid			C	C	C	C		D in distilled water
Ammonium Cl					C			May add KCl to solution
Amphotericin B	C							
Ampicillin	C				C			
Amrinone lactate					C			0.45% saline
Antithrombin III	C				C			Sterile water for inj
Ascorbic acid	C				C	C	C	Sodium lactate
Azlocillin	C		C		C			
Atenolol	C				C			0.45% saline
Aztreonam	C	C			C	C	C	Normosol-R
Bretylium tosylate	C				C			
Cefamandole	C				C			
Cefazolin	C				C			
Cefotetan	C				C			
Cefoxitin	C	C			C	C	C	Aminosol
Ceftrazidime	C		C	C	C	C	C	M/G Sodium lactate
Ceftriaxone	C				C			
Cefuroxime	C		C	C			C	M/G Sodium lactate
Cephalothin	C				C	C	C	M/G Sodium lactate

This chart is not inclusive and is based on manufacturers' recommendations.

Key

C = Compatible
D_5 = Dextrose 5%
D_{10} = Dextrose 10%
D_5½S = Dextrose 5% in saline 0.45%

D_5S = Dextrose 5% in saline 0.9%
NS = Sodium chloride 0.9% (normal saline)
R = Ringer's solution
LR = Lactated Ringer's solution

	D$_5$	D$_{10}$	D$_5$ ½S	D$_5$ S	NS	R	LR	OTHER
Cephapirin	C				C			
Ciprofloxacin	C				C			
CycloSPORINE	C				C			Use only glass containers
DOBUTamine					C			Sodium lactate
DOPamine	C		C	C	C		C	M/G sodium lactate
Doxycycline	C				C			Invert sugar 10%
Edetate Na	C	C						Isotonic saline
Ganciclovir	C				C	C	C	
Gentamicin	C				C			Normosol-R
Heparin Na	C	C			C	C		
Ifosfamide	C				C		C	Sterile water for inj
Isoproterenol	C			C	C	C		Invert sugar 5% & 10%
Kanamycin	C				C			
Metaraminol	C			C	C	C	C	Normosol-R
Methicillin	C			C				
Metoclopramide	C			C		C	C	
Mezlocillin	C	C	C	C	C	C	C	Fructose 5%
Moxalactam	C	C	C	C	C	C	C	M/G sodium lactate
Netilmicin	C	C		C	C	C	C	Normosol-R
Norepinephrine	C	C		C			C	
Nitroglycerin	C	C			C			
Piperacillin	C			C	C		C	
Ritodrine	C							
Ticarcillin	C				C		C	
Tobramycin	C				C			
Vidarabine	C	C			C			

Appendix N

Nomogram for Calculation of Body Surface Area

Place a straight edge from the patient's height in the left column to his or her weight in the right column. The point of intersection on the body surface area column indicates the body surface area (BSA). In Behrman RE, Kliegman RM, Jenson HB: *Nelson textbook of pediatrics*, ed 17, Philadelphia, 2004, WB Saunders; Nomogram modified from data of E. Boyd by CD West.

Alternative (Mosteller's formula):

$$\text{Surface area (m}^2) = \sqrt{\frac{\text{Height (cm)} \times \text{Weight (kg)}}{3600}}$$

Index

Entries can be identified as follows: generic name, Trade Name, DRUG CATEGORY, *Combination Product.*

Entries can be identified as follows: generic name, Trade Name, DRUG CATEGORY, *Combination Product.*

Entries can be identified as follows: generic name, Trade Name, DRUG CATEGORY, *Combination Product.*

Entries can be identified as follows: generic name, Trade Name, DRUG CATEGORY, *Combination Product*.

Entries can be identified as follows: generic name, Trade Name, DRUG CATEGORY, *Combination Product.*

Entries can be identified as follows: generic name, Trade Name, DRUG CATEGORY, *Combination Product.*

Entries can be identified as follows: generic name, Trade Name, DRUG CATEGORY, *Combination Product.*

Entries can be identified as follows: generic name, Trade Name, DRUG CATEGORY, *Combination Product.*

I

Entries can be identified as follows: generic name, Trade Name, DRUG CATEGORY, *Combination Product.*

Entries can be identified as follows: generic name, Trade Name, DRUG CATEGORY, *Combination Product.*

Entries can be identified as follows: generic name, Trade Name, DRUG CATEGORY, *Combination Product.*

Entries can be identified as follows: generic name, Trade Name, DRUG CATEGORY, *Combination Product.*

Entries can be identified as follows: generic name, Trade Name, DRUG CATEGORY, *Combination Product*.

Entries can be identified as follows: generic name, Trade Name, DRUG CATEGORY, *Combination Product.*

Entries can be identified as follows: generic name, Trade Name, DRUG CATEGORY, *Combination Product.*

Entries can be identified as follows: generic name, Trade Name, DRUG CATEGORY, *Combination Product.*

Entries can be identified as follows: generic name, Trade Name, DRUG CATEGORY, *Combination Product.*

Entries can be identified as follows: generic name, Trade Name, DRUG CATEGORY, *Combination Product.*

Entries can be identified as follows: generic name, Trade Name, DRUG CATEGORY, *Combination Product.*

2006 Update to Mosby's Drug Guide for Nurses
Sixth Edition

Following are the monographs for 20 drugs that have received FDA approval since the publication of *Mosby's Drug Guide for Nurses*, 6th edition. These monographs follow the same format as those in the book. They are arranged in alphabetical order by generic name, and trade names are given for all medications in common use. Each monograph contains the same subsections as those listed and described on pages vii through x of the preface to this book.

Drug Monographs in this Update

GENERIC	TRADE
abarelix	Plenaxis
acomprosate	Camprel
apomorphine	Apokyn
azacitidine	Vidaza
bevacizumab	Avastin
cetuximab	Erbitux
cinacalcet	Sensipar
duloxetine	Cymbalta
erlotinib	Tarceva
flavocoxid	Limbrel
lanthanum	Fosrenol
pegaptanib	Macugen
pemetrexed	Alimta
poly-L-lactic Acid	Sculptra
rifaximin	Xifaxan
solifenacin	VESIcare
telithromycin	Ketek
tinidazole	Tindamax
tiotropium	Spiriva
trospium	Sanctura

abarelix (Rx)
(a-ba-rel'iks)
Plenaxis
Func. class.: Gonadotropin-releasing hormone antagonist
Chem. class.: Synthetic decapeptide

Pregnancy category X

Action: Inhibitor of pituitary gonadotropin secretion; inhibits LH, FSH, thereby reducing testosterone

→**Therapeutic Outcome:** Reduction in tumor size

Uses: Palliative treatment of prostate cancer

Dosage and routes
Adult: IM 100 mg in buttock on day 1, 15, 29 (week 4) and every 4 wks, thereafter

Available forms: Powder for inj 113 mg

Adverse effects
(*italic* = common; **bold** = life-threatening)
CNS: *Headache, dizziness, fatigue, sleep disturbance*
ENDO: Breast enlargement, nipple tenderness
GI: *Nausea, constipation, diarrhea*
GU: *Dysuria, frequency, retention, UTI*
INTEG: Pain on inj; local site reactions
MISC: *Pain including back pain, hot flashes*
SYST: **Anaphylaxis, systemic allergic reaction,** decreased bone density (long term treatment)

Contraindications: Pregnancy X, hyper-
P sensitivity, latex allergy, lactation, children

Pharmacokinetics	
Absorption	Unknown
Distribution	Protein binding 96-99%
Metabolism	Unknown
Excretion	Urine
Half-life	Depends on dosage

Pharmacodynamics
Unknown

Interactions: None known

NURSING CONSIDERATIONS
Assessment
• Assess patient for anaphylaxis: swelling of face, throat, eyes, tongue, chest tightness, difficulty breathing; hypotension, fainting, shock; if these occur, usually occur within ½ hr of administration
• Monitor blood studies: ALT, AST, GGT, alk phosphatase

Nursing diagnoses
☑ Injury, risk for (adverse reactions)
☑ Infection, risk for (adverse reactions)
☑ Knowledge, deficient (teaching)

Implementation
• Reconstitute 1 vial with provided diluent (50 mg/ml)
• Prior to reconstitute gently shake vial; hold at 45° angle and tap lightly to break caking; withdraw 2.2 ml of 0.9% NaCl inj using 18g, 1½ inch needle and 3 ml syringe enclosed; discard remaining, unused diluent
• Keeping vial upright, insert needle all the way in the vial and inject diluent quickly; withdraw needle, removing 2.2 ml of air; shake for several seconds; allow vial to stand for 2 min; tap to remove foam, swirl.
• Store between 59-80° F; use within 1 hr of reconstitution

Patient/family education
• Instruct patient to notify prescriber if family members have QTc interval prolongation
• Instruct patient to notify prescriber immediately of chest, throat tightness, flushing, lightheadedness, shortness of breath
◆•• Inform patient that chances of serious or life-threatening allergic reaction may increase with each injection

Evaluation
Positive therapeutic outcome
• Reduction in growth of tumor

acamprosate (Rx)
Camprel
Func. class.: Antialcoholic agent

Dosage and routes
Adult: PO 666 mg tid

Renal dose
Adult: PO 333 mg tid

Uses: For maintenance of abstinence from alcohol in alcohol dependence

Contraindications: Hypersensitivity, severe renal disease, CCr <30 ml/hr

apomorphine (Rx)
(a-poe-mor'feen)
Apokyn
Func. class.: Antiparkinson agent
Chem. class.: Dopamine-receptor agonist, non-ergot

Pregnancy category D

Action: Selective agonist for D_2 subfamily receptors (presynaptic/postsynaptic sites); binding at D_3 receptor may contribute to antiparkinson effects

➡ **Therapeutic Outcome:** Decrease in on/off periods in Parkinsonism

Uses: Parkinsonism: for acute, intermittent treatment of hypomobility (off) episodes in advanced Parkinsonism

Dosage and routes
Adult: SUBCUT 0.2 ml (2 mg) titrate upward, max 0.6 ml (6 mg), administer a test dose of 0.2 ml (2 mg) and closely monitor B/P; to be used concomitantly with antiemetic

Renal dose
Reduce test dose and starting dose to 0.1 ml (1 mg)

Available forms: Inj 10 mg/ml

Adverse effects
(*italic* = common; **bold** = life-threatening)
CNS: *Agitation,* psychosis, hallucination, depression, dizziness, headache, confusion, **sleep attacks,** yawning, dykinesias, drowsiness, somnolence
CV: *Orthostatic hypotension,* edema, syncope, tachycardia
EENT: Blurred vision, rhinorrhea, sweating
GI: *Nausea,* vomiting, *anorexia,* constipation, dysphagia, dry mouth
GU: Impotence, urinary frequency
HEMA: **Hemolytic anemia, leukopenia, agranulocytosis**

Contraindications: Hypersensitivity

Precautions: Pregnancy C, renal, hepatic, cardiac disease, MI with dysrhythmias, affective disorders, psychosis, preexisting dyskinesias, elderly

Pharmacokinetics
Absorption	Unknown
Distribution	Unknown
Metabolism	Minimal
Excretion	Unknown
Half-life	Unknown

Pharmacodynamics
Unknown

Interactions
Individual drugs
◆ Ondansetron, granisetron, dolasetron (5HT3 antagonists): do not give concurrently, profound hypotension may occur
Levodopa, cimetidine, ranitidine, diltiazem, triamterene, verapamil, quinidine: ↑ apomorphine levels
Levodopa: ↑ effect of levodopa
Drug classifications
DOPamine antagonists, phenothiazines, metoclopramide, butyrophenones: ↓ apomorphine levels
⊘ *Herb/drug*
Chaste tree fruit, kava: ↓ effect of apomorphine

NURSING CONSIDERATIONS
Assessment
• Assess B/P supine/standing predose, and 20, 40, 60 min post dose
• Monitor renal, hepatic, cardiac studies baseline
• Assess for involuntary movements in parkinsonism: akinesia, tremors, staggering gait, muscle rigidity, drooling
• Assess mental status: affect, mood, behavioral changes, depression; complete suicide assessment
• Assess for risk of QT prolongation, this drug may increase QT prolongation and possibility of prodysrrthmias

Nursing diagnoses
✓ Mobility, impaired (uses)
✓ Injury, risk for (uses)
✓ Knowledge, deficient (teaching)
✓ Noncompliance (teaching)

Implementation
• Adjust dosage to patient response
◆ • Do not give **IV**
• Use a test dose of 0.2 ml (2 mg), those that tolerate this dose, but achieve no response, give 0.4 ml (4 mg) at the next "off"
• Give antiemetic usually trimethobenzemide 300 mg tid PO 3 day prior to beginning apomorphine and continue for 2 months
• Provide assistance with ambulation during beginning therapy
• Store at 77° F, excursion permitted to 59°-86° F

Patient/family education
• Instruct patient to notify prescriber if pregnancy is planned or suspected

Evaluation

Positive therapeutic outcome
- Decrease in end of dose wearing off and unpredictable on/off episodes

---

⚠ HIGH ALERT

azacitidine (Rx)
(a-za-sie-ti'deen)
Vidaza
Func. class.: Antineoplastic hormone
Chem. class.: DNA demethylation agent

Pregnancy category D

Action: Cytotoxic by producing damage to double-strand DNA during DNA synthesis

⇒ **Therapeutic Outcome:** Improved blood counts in refractor anemia

Uses: Myelodysplastic syndrome (MDS)

Dosage and routes
Adult: SUBCUT 75 mg/m² daily × 7 days, q 4 weeks, premedicate with antiemetic, dose may be increased to 100 mg/m² if no response is seen after 2 treatment cycles, minimum treatment 4 cycles

Available forms: Powdered for inj, lyophilized 100 mg

Adverse effects
(*italic* = common; **bold** = life-threatening)
CNS: Anxiety, depression, dizziness, fatigue, headache
CV: Cardiac murmur, hypotension, tachycardia
GI: **Diarrhea**, nausea, vomiting, anorexia, constipation, abdominal pain, distension, tenderness, hemorrhoids, mouth hemorrhage, tongue ulceration, stomatitis, dyspepsia, **hepatotoxicity, hepatic coma**
GU: **Real failure, renal tubular acidosis**, dysuria, UTI
HEMA: **Leukopenia, anemia, thrombocytopenia, neutropenia**, ecchymosis
INTEG: Irritation at site, rash, sweating, pyrexia
META: Hypokalemia

Contraindications: Pregnancy **D**, hypersensitivity to this drug or mannitol, advanced malignant hepatic tumors

P **Precautions:** Lactation, children, elderly,
G renal and hepatic disease; a man should not father a child while taking this drug

Pharmacokinetics
Absorption	Rapid
Distribution	Unknown
Metabolism	Liver
Excretion	Urine
Half-life	35-49 min

Pharmacodynamics
Onset	Unknown
Peak	½ hr
Duration	Unknown

Interactions: None known

NURSING CONSIDERATIONS
Assessment
- Assess for CNS symptoms: fever, headache, chills, dizziness
- Monitor hematologic response with patients with baseline WBC = to 3 × 10⁹/L, absolute neutrophil count (ANC) = 1.5 × 10⁹/L, and platelets = 75 × 10⁹/L, adjust dose; ANC < 0.5 × 10⁹/L, platelets < 25 × 10⁹/L, give 50% dose next course; ANC 0.5 – 1.5 × 10⁹/L, platelets 25 – 50 × 10⁹/L, give 67% next course
- Assess buccal cavity q8h for dryness, sores, or ulceration, white patches, oral pain, bleeding, dysphagia
- Assess for signs of bone marrow depression: bruising, bleeding, blood in stools, urine, sputum, emesis

Nursing diagnoses
☑ Injury, risk for (adverse reactions)
☑ Body image, disturbed (adverse reactions)
☑ Infection, risk for (adverse reactions)
☑ Knowledge, deficient (teaching)

Implementation
- Administer antiemetics and dexamethasone 10 mg at least ½ hr before antineoplastics
IV **IV route**
- Reconstitute with 4 ml sterile water for inj (25 mg/ml), inject diluent slowly into vial, invert vial 2-3 times and gently rotate, sol will be cloudy, use immediately, divide doses greater than 4 ml into 2 syringes, resuspend the contents 2-3 times and gently roll syringe between the palms for 30 sec immediately prior to administration
- Rotate injection site
- Increase patient's fluid intake to 2-3 L/day to prevent dehydration, unless contraindicated
- Assist patient with rinsing of mouth tid-qid with water, club soda; brushing of teeth bid-tid with soft brush or cotton-tipped applicator for stomatitis; use unwaxed dental floss
- Provide a nutritious diet with iron, vitamin supplement, low fiber, few dairy products

---

☑ Herb/drug   🚫 Do Not Crush   ◆ Alert   ◆π Key Drug   **G** Geriatric   **P** Pediatric

Patient/family education
- Instruct patient to avoid foods with citric acid or hot or rough texture if stomatitis is present; to drink adequate fluids
- Instruct patient to report stomatitis; any bleeding, white spots, ulcerations in mouth; tell patient to examine mouth daily, report symptoms
- Advise patient to use contraception during therapy
- Advise patient not to father a child while receiving this drug

Evaluation
Positive therapeutic outcome
- Improvement in blood counts in refractory anemia, or refractory anemia with excess blasts

---

❗ HIGH ALERT

bevacizumab (Rx)
(beh-va-kiz'you-mab)
Avastin
Func. class.: Miscellaneous antineoplastic
Chem. class.: Monoclonal antibody

Pregnancy category C

Action: DNA-derived monoclonal antibody selectively binds to and inhibits activity of human vascular endothelial growth factor to reduce microvascular growth and inhibition of metastatic disease progression

➡ Therapeutic Outcome: Decreased tumor size

Uses: Metastatic carcinoma of the colon or rectum in combination with 5-FU IV

Investigational uses: Adjunctive in breast, renal cancer

Dosage and routes
Adult: **IV** inf 5 mg/kg q 14 days given over 90 min; if well tolerated, the next infusion may be given over 60 min; if 60 min infusions are well tolerated, subsequent infusions may be given over 30 mins.

Available forms: Inj 25 mg/ml

Adverse effects
(*italic* = common; **bold** = life-threatening)
CNS: Asthenia, dizziness
CV: **Deep vein thrombosis,** hypertension, hypotension, **hypertensive crisis**
GI: Nausea, vomiting, anorexia, diarrhea, constipation, abdominal pain, colitis, stomatitis, **GI hemorrhage**

GU: Proteinuria, urinary frequency/urgency, **nephrotic syndrome**
HEMA: **Leukopenia, neutropenia, thrombocytopenia**
META: Bilirubinemia, hypokalemia
MISC: **Exfoliative dermatitis, hemorrhage**
RESP: Dyspnea, upper respiratory infection

Contraindications: Hypersensitivity

P Precautions: Pregnancy **C**, lactation, **G** children, elderly, CHF, blood dyscrasias, cardiovascular disease, hypertension

---

Pharmacokinetics

Absorption	Unknown
Distribution	Unknown
Metabolism	Unknown
Excretion	Unknown
Half-life	20 days

Pharmacodynamics

Onset	Unknown
Peak	Unknown
Duration	Steady state 100 days

Interactions: None known

NURSING CONSIDERATIONS
Assessment
- Monitor B/P q 3-4 wk
- Assess for symptoms of infection; may be masked by drug
- Monitor CNS reaction: dizziness, confusion
- ◆● Assess for GI perforation, serious bleeding, nephrotic syndrome, hypertensive crisis, drug should be discontinued permanently; proteinuria, or surgery, drug should be discontinued temporarily

Nursing diagnoses
- ✓ Injury, risk for (adverse reactions)
- ✓ Body image, disturbed (adverse reactions)
- ✓ Infection, risk for (adverse reactions)
- ✓ Knowledge, deficient (teaching)

Implementation
IV IV route
- Do not give by **IV** bolus, or **IV** push
- Give as **IV** infusion over 90 min for first dose and 60 min thereafter, if well tolerated

Patient/family education
- Instruct patient to avoid hazardous tasks, since confusion, dizziness may occur
- Instruct patient to report signs of infection: sore throat, fever, diarrhea, vomiting
- Advise patient not to become pregnant while taking this drug, or for several months after discontinuing treatment

- Advise patient to notify prescriber if pregnant or planning a pregnancy

Evaluation
Positive therapeutic outcome
- Decrease in size of tumors

---

cetuximab (Rx)
(se-tux'i-mab)
Erbitux
Func. class.: Misc. antineoplastic, monoclonal antibody
Chem. class.: Epidermal growth factor receptor inhibitor

Pregnancy category C

Action: Not fully understood. Binds to epidermal growth factor receptors (EGFR); inhibits phosphorylation and activation of receptor associated kinase resulting in inhibition of cell growth.

⇒**Therapeutic Outcome:** Decrease in tumor size

Uses: Alone or in combination with irinotecan for EGFR expressing metastatic colorectal carcinoma

Dosage and routes
Adult: **IV** inf 400 mg/m² loading dose given over 120 min, max infusion rate 5 ml/min, weekly maintenance dose (all other infusions) is 250 mg/m² given over 60 min, max infusion rate 5 ml/min. Premedicate with an H₁ antagonist (diphenhydrAMINE 50 mg **IV**); dosage adjustments are made for infusion reactions or dermatologic toxicity

Available forms: Inj 50 ml, single use vial with 100 mg of cetuximab (2 mg/ml)

Adverse effects
(*italic* = common; **bold** = life-threatening)
CNS: *Headache, insomnia, depression*
GI: *Nausea, diarrhea, vomiting, anorexia, mouth ulceration, dehydration, constipation, abdominal pain*
HEMA: **Leukepenia, anemia**
INTEG: *Rash, pruritus, acne, dry skin,* **toxic epidermal neurolysis, angioedema,** *blepharitis, cheilitis, cellulitis, cysts, alopecia, skin/nail disorder*
MISC: *Conjunctivitis, asthema, malaise, fever,* **renal failure**
MS: *Back pain*
RESP: **Interstitial lung disease**, *cough, dyspnea,* **pulmonary embolus,** *peripheral edema*
SYST: **Anaphylaxis, sepsis, infection**

Contraindications: Hypersensitivity to this drug or murine proteins

Precautions: Pregnancy **C**, renal/hepatic ☐ disease, ocular, pulmonary disorders, lacta-☐ tion, children, elderly

Pharmacokinetics	
Absorption	Unknown
Distribution	Unknown
Metabolism	Unknown
Excretion	Unknown
Half-life	114 hrs

Pharmacodynamics	
Onset	Unknown
Peak	168-235 g/ml, trough 41-85 g/ml
Duration	Steady state by 3rd weekly infusion

Interactions: None known

NURSING CONSIDERATIONS
Assessment
◆• Monitor pulmonary changes: lung sounds, cough, dyspnea; interstitial lung disease may occur, my be fatal; discontinue therapy if confirmed
◆• Assess for toxic epidermal necrosis, angioedema, anaphylaxis
- Assess GI symptoms: frequency of stools, dehydration, abdominal pain, stomatitis

Nursing diagnoses
✓ Injury, risk for (adverse reactions)
✓ Body image, disturbed (adverse reactions)
✓ Infection, risk for (adverse reactions)
✓ Knowledge, deficient (teaching)

Implementation
IV **IV infusion**
- Administer by **IV** infusion only, do not give by **IV** push or bolus
- Do not shake or dilute
- Infusion pump: draw up volume of a vial using appropriate syringe/needle (a vented spike or other appropriate transfer device); fill Erbitux into sterile evacuated container/bag, repeat until calculated volume has been put into the container. Use a new needle for each vial; give through in-line filter (low protein binding 0.22-micrometer); affix infusion line and prime before starting infusion, max rate 5 ml/min; flush line at end of infusion with 0.9% NaCl
- Syringe pump: Draw up volume of a vial using appropriate syringe/needle (a vented spike); place syringe into syringe driver of a syringe pump and set rate; use an in-line filter

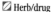

0.22 micrometer (low protein binding); connect infusion line and start infusion after priming; repeat until calculated volume has been given.
• Use a new needle and filter for each vial, max 5 ml/min rate; use 0.9% NaCl to flush line after infusion
• Do not piggyback to patient infusion line
• Observe patient for adverse reactions for 1 hr after infusion
• Infusion reactions: if mild (Grade 1 or 2) reduce all doses by 50%; if severe (Grade 3 or 4) permanently discontinue
• Store refrigerated 36-46° F, discard unused portions

Patient/family education
• Instruct patient to report adverse reactions immediately: SOB, severe abdominal pain, skin eruptions
• Explain reason for treatment, expected results
• Instruct patient to use contraception during treatment, pregnancy **C**
• Advise patient to wear sunscreen and hats to limit sun exposure. Sun exposure can exacerbate any skin reactions

Evaluation
Positive therapeutic outcome
• Decrease growth, spread of EGFR expressing metastatic colorectal carcinoma

---

cinacalcet (Rx)
(sin-a-kal'set)
Sensipar
Func. class.: Calcium receptor agonist
Chem. class.: Polypeptide hormone

Pregnancy category C

Action: Directly lowers PTH levels by increasing sensitivity of calcium sensing receptors to extracellular calcium

Therapeutic Outcome: Decreased symptoms of hypercalcemia

Uses: Hypercalcemia in parathyroid carcinoma, secondary hyperparathyroidism in chronic kidney disease on dialysis

Dosage and routes
Parathyroid carcinoma
Adult: PO 30 mg bid, titrate q 2-4 wks, with sequential doses of 30 mg bid, 60 mg bid, 90 mg bid, 90 mg tid-qid to normalize calcium levels

Secondary hyperparathyroidism
Adult: PO 30 mg daily, titrate no more

frequently than 2-4 wks with sequential doses of 30, 60, 90, 120, 180 mg daily

Available forms: Tabs 30, 60, 90 mg

Adverse effects
(*italic* = common; **bold** = life-threatening)
CNS: Dizziness
CV: Hypertension
GI: Nausea, diarrhea, vomiting, anorexia
MISC: Access infection, noncardiac chest pain, asthenia
MS: Myalgia

Contraindications: Hypersensitivity

P Precautions: Pregnancy **C**, children, lactation, seizure disorders, hepatic disease

Pharmacokinetics
Absorption	93-97% bound to plasma
Distribution	Unknown
Metabolism	Proteins metabolized by CYP3A4, 2D6, 1A2
Excretion	Renal (80% renal, 15% feces)
Half-life	30-40 hrs

Pharmacodynamics
Unknown

Interactions
Individual drugs
Ketoconazole, erythromycin, itraconazole (drugs metabolized by CYP3A4); flecainide, vinBLAStine, thioridazine, tricyclics (drugs metabolized by CYP2D6): adjustments may be necessary
Drug classifications
Tricyclics (metabolized by CYP2D6): adjustments may be necessary
Food/drug
High-fat meal: ↑ action

NURSING CONSIDERATIONS
Assessment
• Assess for hypocalcemia: cramping, seizures, tetany, myalgia, paresthesia
• Monitor calcium, phosphorous within 1 wk and iPTH 1-4 wks after initiation or dosage adjustment when maintenance is established; measure calcium, phosphorus monthly; iPTH q 1-3 mo, target range 150-300 pg/ml for iPTH level
• If calcium < 8.4 mg/dl, do not start therapy

Nursing diagnoses
☑ Injury, risk for (uses)
☑ Knowledge, deficient (teaching)

Implementation
- Can be used alone or in combination with vit D sterols and/or phosphate binders

Secondary hyperthyroidism
- Titrate q 2-4 wks to target iPTH consistent with National Kidney Foundation-Kidney Disease Outcomes Quality Initiative (NKF-/DOQI) for chronic kidney disease patient on dialysis of 150-300 pg/ml; if iPTH drops below 150-300 pg/ml, reduce dose of cinacalcet and/or vit D sterols or discontinue treatment
- Store at <77° F (25° C)

Patient/family education
- Instruct patient to take with food or shortly after a meal
- Instruct patient to take tabs whole, do not divide
- Instruct patient to immediately report cramping, seizures, muscle pain, tingling, tetany

Evaluation
Positive therapeutic outcome
- Calcium levels 9-10 mg/dl, decreasing symptoms of hypercalcemia

---

duloxetine (Rx)
(du-lox'uh-teen)
Cymbalta
Func. class.: Miscellaneous antidepressant
Chem. class: Serotonin, norepinephrine reuptake inhibitor
Pregnancy category C

Action: Unknown, may potentiate serotonergic, nonadrenergic activity in the CNS. In studies duloxetine is a potent inhibitor of neuronal serotonin and norepinephrine reuptake

Therapeutic Outcome: Decreased depression, decreased neuropathic pain

Uses: Major depressive disorder (MDD), neuropathic pain associated with diabetic neuropathy

Dosage and routes
Depression
Adult: PO 20 mg bid, may increase to 30 mg bid if needed
Diabetic neuropathy
Adult: PO 60 mg q day
Available forms: Caps 20, 30, 60 mg

Adverse effects
(*italic* = common; **bold** = life-threatening)
CNS: Insomnia, anxiety, dizziness, tremor, fatigue, decreased appetite, decreased weight
CV: Thrombophlebitis, peripheral edema
EENT: Abnormal vision
GI: Constipation, diarrhea, dysphagia, nausea, vomiting, anorexia, dry mouth, colitis, gastritis
GU: Abnormal ejaculation, urinary hesitation, ejaculation delayed, erectile dysfunction
INTEG: Photosensitivity, bruising, sweating

Contraindications: Hypersensitivity, narrow-angle glaucoma

Precautions: Pregnancy C, mania, lactation, children, elderly, hypertension, cardiac disease, narrow-angle glaucoma, renal disease, hepatic disease, seizures

Pharmacokinetics
Absorption	Well absorbed
Distribution	90% protein binding
Metabolism	Extensively metabolized (CYP 2D6, CYP 1A2) in the liver to an active metabolite
Excretion	70% of drug recovered in urine, 20% in feces
Half-life	12 hr

Pharmacodynamics
Unknown

Interactions
Individual drugs
Alcohol: ↑ ALT, bilirubin
Drug classifications
MAOIs: coadministration is contraindicated or within 14 days of MAOIs use: hyperthermia, rigidity, rapid fluctuations of vital signs, mental status changes, neuroleptic malignant syndrome
Opioids, antihistamines, sedative/hypnotics: ↑ CNS depression
CYP 1A2 inhibitors (fluvoxamine, quinolone antiinfectives); CYP 2D6 (fluoxetine, quinidine, paroxetine): ↑ action of duloxetine
CYP 2D6 extensively metabolized drugs (flecainide, phenothiazines, propafenone, tricyclics, thioridazine): narrow therapeutic index
Herb/drug
Chamomile, hops, kava, lavender, skullcap, valerian: ↑ CNS depression
Corkwood, jimsonweed: ↑ anticholinergic effect
SAM-e, St. John's wort: serotonin syndrome
Yohimbe: ↑ hypertension

⊘ Herb/drug   🚫 Do Not Crush   ◆ Alert   ◆ᴛᴛ Key Drug   🆅 Geriatric   🅿 Pediatric

NURSING CONSIDERATIONS
Assessment
- Assess B/P lying, standing; pulse q/4 h; if systolic B/P drops 20 mm Hg, hold drug, notify prescriber; take VS q4h in patients with cardiovascular disease
- Monitor hepatic studies: AST, ALT, bilirubin
- Monitor weight qwk; weight loss or gain; appetite may increase; peripheral edema may occur
- Offer sugarless gum, hard candy, frequent sips of water for dry mouth
- Assess mental status: mood, sensorium, affect, suicidal tendencies, increase in psychiatric symptoms; depression, panic
- Assess for withdrawal symptoms: headache, nausea, vomiting, muscle pain, weakness; not usual unless drug is discontinued abruptly

Nursing diagnoses
- ✓ Injury, risk for (uses)
- ✓ Knowledge, deficient (teaching)
- ✓ Noncompliance (teaching)

Implementation
- Store in tight container at room temperature; do not freeze
- Provide assistance with ambulation during beginning therapy, since drowsiness, dizziness occur
- Check to see if PO medication was swallowed

Patient/family education
- Advise that drug is dispensed in small amounts because of suicide potential, especially in the beginning of therapy
- Teach patient/family to use caution when driving or other activities requiring alertness because of drowsiness, dizziness, blurred vision
- Advise patient to avoid alcohol ingestion, MAOIs, other CNS depressants
- Advise patient not to discontinue medication quickly after long-term use; may cause nausea, headache, malaise
- Advise patient to wear sunscreen or large hat, since photosensitivity may occur
- 🚫 Teach patient to swallow caps whole; do not crush, chew, or break; do not sprinkle on food or mix with liquid
- Advise patient to notify prescriber if pregnancy is planned or suspected, or if breastfeeding
- Tell patient that improvement may occur in 1-4 wk

Evaluation
Positive therapeutic outcome
- Decreased depression

---

erlotinib (Rx)
(er-loe′tye-nib)
Tarceva
Func. class.: Misc. antineoplastic
Chem. class.: Epidermal growth factor receptor inhibitor

Pregnancy category D

Action: Not fully understood. Inhibits intracellular phosphorylation of cell surface receptors associated with epidermal growth factor receptors.

⇥**Therapeutic Outcome:** Decrease in tumor size

Uses: Nonsmall cell lung cancer (NSCLC)

Dosage and routes
Adult: PO 150 mg daily taken at least 1 hr before or 2 hrs after food
CYP3A4 inducers concurrently (such as rifampin or phenytoin)
Dosage increase is advised
CYP3A4 inhibitors (atazanavir, clarithromycin, indinavir, itraconazole, ketoconazole, telithromycin, ritonavir, saquinavir, troleandomycin, nelfinavir
Dosage reduction may be needed.

Available forms: Tabs 25, 100, 150 mg

Adverse effects
(*italic* = common; **bold** = life-threatening)
GI: Nausea, diarrhea, vomiting, anorexia, mouth ulceration
INTEG: Rash
MISC: Conjunctivitis, eye pain, fatigue, infection
RESP: **Interstitial lung disease,** *cough, dyspnea*

Contraindications: Pregnancy **D**, hypersensitivity

Precautions: Renal, hepatic, ocular, 🅿 pulmonary disorders, lactation, children, 🅖 elderly

Pharmacokinetics
Absorption	Slowly absorbed
Distribution	Unknown
Metabolism	Metabolized by CYP3A4
Excretion	Feces (86%), urine (<4%)
Half-life	36 hrs

Pharmacodynamics
Onset	Unknown
Peak	3-7 hrs
Duration	Unknown

Interactions
Individual drugs
Warfarin, metoprolol: ↑ plasma concentrations

Drug classifications
CYP3A4 inhibitors (atazanavir, clarithromycin, indinavir, itraconazole, ketoconazole, telithromycin, ritonavir, saquinavir, troleandomycin, nelfinavir: ↑ erlotinib concentrations
CYP3A4 inducers (phenytoin, rifampin, carbamazepine, phenobarbital): ↓ erlotinib levels

 Herb/drug
St. John's Wort: ↓ erlotinib levels

NURSING CONSIDERATIONS
Assessment
• Assess for pulmonary changes: lung sounds, cough, dyspnea; interstitial lung disease may occur, may be fatal; discontinue therapy if confirmed
• Assess for ocular changes: eye irritation, corneal erosion/ulcer, aberrant eyelash growth
• Assess for GI symptoms: frequency of stools, if diarrhea is poorly tolerated, therapy may be discontinued for up to 14 days

Nursing diagnoses
☑ Injury, risk for (adverse reactions)
☑ Body image, disturbed (adverse reactions)
☑ Infection, risk for (adverse reactions)
☑ Knowledge, deficient (teaching)

Implementation
• Administer PO, 1 hour before or 2 hours after food

Patient/family education
• Teach patient to report adverse reactions immediately: SOB, severe abdominal pain, persistent diarrhea or vomiting, ocular changes, skin eruptions
• Explain reason for treatment, expected results
• Advise patient to use contraception during treatment, pregnancy **D**

Evaluation
Positive therapeutic outcome
• Decrease non-small cell lung cancer cells

---

flavocoxid (Rx)
(flav-uh-kox'id)
Limbrel
Func. class.: Oral nutritional supplement

Pregnancy category UK

Action: Exhibits anti-inflammatory, analgesic properties, thought to be due to inhibition of prostaglandin synthesis via inhibition of cyclo-oxygenase

➡ **Therapeutic Outcome:** Decreased pain, inflammation in osteoarthritis

Uses: For dietary management of osteoarthritis

Dosage and routes
Adult: PO 250 mg q 12 hrs

Available forms: Cap 250 mg

Adverse effects
(*italic* = common; **bold** = life-threatening)
MISC: Hypertension, increase in varicose veins, psoriasis
MS: Fluid accumulation in the knees

Contraindications: Hypersensitivity

Precautions: Pregnancy **UK**, lactation, children <18 yrs, history of stomach ulcers

Pharmacokinetics	
Absorption	Unknown
Distribution	Unknown
Metabolism	Primarily via glucuronidation and sulfation
Excretion	Unknown
Half-life	Unknown

Pharmacodynamics
Unknown

Interactions: None known

NURSING CONSIDERATIONS
Assessment
• Assess for pain of rheumatoid arthritis, osteoarthritis; check ROM, inflammation of joints, characteristics of pain

Nursing diagnoses
☑ Injury, risk for (uses)
☑ Knowledge, deficient (teaching)

Implementation
PO route
• Administer 1 hr before or after meals

Patient/family education
• Teach patient that drug does not take the place of other drugs including corticosteroids for osteoarthritis
• Advise patient to notify prescriber if pregnancy is planned or suspected

Evaluation
Positive therapeutic outcome
• Decreased pain, inflammation in arthritic conditions

---

lanthanum (Rx)
Fosrenol
Func. class.: Phosphate binder

Dosage and routes
Adult: **PO** 750-1500 mg daily in divided doses with meals. Titrate dose q 2-3 wks until an acceptable phosphate level is reached. Tablets should be chewed completely before swallowing; intact tablets should not be swallowed.

Uses: End stage renal disease

Contraindications: Hypophosphatemia, hypersensitivity

pegaptanib (Rx)
(peg-ap'ta-nib)
Macugen
Func. class: Misc. ophthalmic agent

Pregnancy category B

Action: Binds to vascular endothelial growth factor (VEGF), thereby inhibiting angiogenesis

➡ Therapeutic Outcome: Stabilization of vision in macular degeneration

Uses: Treatment of neovascular (wet) age-related macular degeneration. May be used alone or with photodynamic therapy (PDT).

Dosage and routes
Adult: Intravitreal inj 0.3 mg injected q 6 wks

Available forms: Inj 0.3 mg, single glass syringes

Adverse effects
(*italic* = common; **bold** = life-threatening)
EENT: *Anterior chamber inflammation, blurred vision, conjunctival hemorrhage, corneal edema, cataract, eye discharge, eye pain, increased intraocular pressure, punctuate keratitis, reduced visual acuity, vitreous floaters, vitreous opacities, blepharitis, conjunctivitis, photophobia,* retinal detachment, iatrogenic traumatic cataract

Contraindications: Hypersensitivity, ocular or periocular infections

Precautions: Pregnancy **B**, inflammatory eye disease, ocular hypertension

Pharmacokinetics
Absorption	Unknown
Distribution	Unknown
Metabolism	Unknown
Excretion	Unknown
Half-life	87-100 hrs in vitreous humor of the monkey

Pharmacodynamics
Onset	Unknown
Peak	Unknown
Duration	May remain fully active in the eye for 7-28 days

Interactions: None known

NURSING CONSIDERATIONS
Assessment
- Test visual acuity periodically
- Assess treated eye for increased intraocular pressure, infection, endophthalmitis
- Monitor perfusion of the optic nerve head immediately after injection, tonometry ½ hr after inj, biomicroscopy 2-7 days after inj

Nursing diagnoses
☑ Sensory perception, disturbed: visual (uses)
☑ Knowledge, deficient (teaching)

Implementation
- Administer anesthesia and a broad spectrum anti-infective prior to injection
- The injection should be done under aseptic conditions
- Store at 36°-46° F, do not freeze or shake vigorously

Patient/family education
- Instruct patient to report any inflammation, bleeding, eye discharge, opacities to prescriber.
- Instruct patient to continue with follow up care during treatment

Evaluation
Positive therapeutic outcome
- Macular degeneration stabilized

❗ HIGH ALERT

pemetrexed (Rx)
(pem-ah-trex'ed)
Alimta
Func. class.: Antineoplastic-antimetabolite
Chem. class.: Folic acid antagonist

Pregnancy category D

Action: Inhibits an enzyme that reduces folic acid, which is needed for cell replication

➡ **Therapeutic Outcome:** Decreased spread of mesothelioma, decreased tumor size

Uses: Malignant pleural mesothelioma in combination with cisplatin; non-small cell lung cancer as a single agent

Dosage and routes
Adult: **IV** inf 500 mg/m² given over 10 min on Day 1 of a 21-day cycle with cisplatin 75 mg/m² infused over 2 hrs beginning ½ hr after end of pemetrexed infusion
Nadir ANC < 500/mm³ and platelets = 50,000/mm³ 75% of previous dose

Available forms: Injection, single use vials, 500 mg

Adverse effects
(*italic* = common; **bold** = life-threatening)
CNS: *Fatigue, fever, mood alteration, neuropathy*
CV: **Thrombosis/embolism,** *chest pain*
GI: *Nausea, vomiting, anorexia, diarrhea, ulcerative stomatitis, constipation, dysphagia, dehydration*
GU: **Renal failure,** *creatinine elevation*
HEMA: **Neutropenia, leukopenia, thrombocytopenia, myelosuppression, anemia**
INTEG: *Rash, desquamation*
RESP: *Dyspnea*
SYST: **Infection with/without neutropenia**

Contraindications: Pregnancy **D,** hypersensitivity, ANC <1500 cells/mm³, CCr < 45 ml/min, thrombocytopenia (<100,000/mm³), anemia

Precautions: Renal disease, lactation, **P** children, hepatic disease

Pharmacokinetics	
Absorption	Unknown
Distribution	81% protein binding
Metabolism	Not metabolized
Excretion	Excreted in urine (unchanged 70-90%) Not known if it is excreted in breast milk
Half-life	3.5 hrs

Pharmacodynamics
Unknown

Interactions
Drug classifications
Nephrotoxic drugs (NSAIDs): ↓ pemetrexed clearance

NURSING CONSIDERATIONS
Assessment
◆● Monitor CBC, differential, platelet count, monitor for Nadir and recovery; a new cycle should not begin if ANC < 1500 cells/mm³, platelets are < 100,000 cells/mm³, creatinine clearance < 45 ml/min
• Monitor renal studies: BUN, serum uric acid, urine CCr, electrolytes before, during therapy
• Monitor I&O ratio; report fall in urine output to <30 ml/hr
• Monitor temp q4h; fever may indicate beginning infection; no rectal temps
• Assess bleeding time, coagulation time during treatment; bleeding: hematuria, guaiac, bruising or petechiae, mucosa or orifices q8h
• Assess buccal cavity q8h for dryness, sores, ulceration, white patches, oral pain, bleeding, dysphagia
◆● Assess for symptoms indicating severe allergic reaction: rash, urticaria, itching, flushing

Nursing diagnoses
✓ Injury, risk for (adverse reactions)
✓ Body image, disturbed (adverse reactions)
✓ Infection, risk for (adverse reactions)
✓ Knowledge, deficient (teaching)

Implementation
• Administer vit B₁₂ and low dose folic acid as a prophylactic measure to treat related hematologic, GI toxicity. At least 5 daily doses of folic acid must be taken in the 7 days preceding first dose
• Premedicate with a corticosteroid (dexamethasone) given PO bid the day before, day of, and day after administration of pemetrexed
IV **IV route**
• Use aseptic technique during reconstitution, dilution
• Reconstitute 500 mg vial/20 ml 0.9 % NaCl injection (preservative free) = 25 mg/ml, swirl until dissolved, further dilute with 100 ml 0.9% NaCl injection (preservative free) give as **IV** infusion over 10 mg
• Use only 0.9 % NaCl injection (preservative free) for reconstitution, dilution
• Follow strict medical asepsis and protective isolation if WBC levels are low
• Use a liquid diet: carbonated beverage, Jell-O; dry toast, crackers may be added when patient is not nauseated or vomiting
• Assist patient with rinsing of mouth tid-qid with water, club soda; brushing of teeth bid-tid with soft brush or cotton-tipped applicators for stomatitis; use unwaxed dental floss

- Store at 77° F, excursions permitted 59-86° F, not light sensitive, discard unused portions

Patient/family education

- Instruct patient to report any complaints, side effects to nurse or prescriber: black tarry stools, chills, fever, sore throat, bleeding, bruising, cough, shortness of breath, dark or bloody urine
- Instruct patient to avoid foods with citric acid, hot or rough texture if stomatitis is present
- Instruct patient to report stomatitis: any bleeding, white spots, ulcerations in mouth to prescriber; tell patient to examine mouth daily, report symptoms to nurse, use good oral hygiene
- Advise patient that contraceptive measures are recommended during therapy and for at least 8 wk following cessation of therapy, to discontinue breastfeeding; toxicity to infant may occur
- Advise patient to avoid alcohol, salicylates, live vaccines
- Advise patient to avoid use of razors, commercial mouthwash

Evaluation

Positive therapeutic outcome

- Decreased spread of malignancy

---

poly-L-lactic acid (Rx)

Sculptra
Func. class.: Physical adjuncts

Dosage and routes

Adult: Inj injected deep into dermic or subcut layer to avoid superficial inj using a 26-G sterile needle. The number of inj depends on quantity of fat loss

Uses: Facial fat loss (lipoatrophy) in those with HIV

Contraindications: Hypersensitivity

---

rifaximin (Rx)
(rif-ax'i-min)
Xifaxan
Func. class: Misc. antiinfective
Chem. class: Analog of rifampin

Pregnancy category C

Action: Binds to bacterial DNA dependent RNA polymerase, thereby inhibiting bacterial R synthesis.

➡ **Therapeutic Outcome:** Bacterial action against *E. coli*

Uses: Traveler's diarrhea in those ≥12 yrs old, caused by *E. coli*

Dosage and routes

Adult and child ≥12 yrs.: PO 200 mg tid × 3 days without regard to meals

Available forms: Tabs 200 mg

Adverse effects

(*italic* = common; **bold** = life-threatening)
CNS: Abnormal dreams, dizziness, insomnia
GI: *Abdominal pain, constipation, defecation urgency, flatulence, nausea, rectal tenesmus,* vomiting
MISC: *Headache, pyrexia*

Contraindications: Hypersensitivity

Precautions: Pregnancy **C**, lactation, P children

Pharmacokinetics	
Absorption	Unknown
Distribution	Unknown
Metabolism	Induces P450 3A4 (CYP3A4)
Excretion	Feces
Half-life	6 hrs

Pharmacodynamics
Unknown

Interactions: None known

NURSING CONSIDERATIONS
Assessment

- Assess for GI symptoms: amount character of diarrhea, abdominal pain, nausea, vomiting
◆• Assess for overgrowth of infection and pseudomembranous colitis

Nursing diagnoses

☑ Infection, risk for (uses)
☑ Noncompliance (teaching)
☑ Knowledge, deficient (teaching)

Implementation
- May be administered without regard to food

Patient/family education
- Instruct patient to discontinue rifaximin and notify prescriber if diarrhea persists for more than 24-48 hrs, if diarrhea worsens, or if blood is in stools and fever is present

Evaluation
Positive therapeutic outcome
- Absence of infection

solifenacin (Rx)
(sol-i-fen'a-sin)
VESIcare
Func. class.: Overactive bladder product, anticholinergic
Chem. class.: Muscarinic receptor antagonist

Pregnancy category C

Action: Relaxes smooth muscles in urinary tract by inhibiting acetylcholine at postganglionic sites

➡ Therapeutic Outcome: Decreased dysuria, frequency, nocturia, incontinence

Uses: Overactive bladder (urinary frequency, urgency, incontinence)

Dosage and routes
Adult: PO 5 mg daily, max 10 mg daily

Renal/hepatic dose
Adult: PO CCr <30 ml/min 5 mg daily

Available forms: Tabs 5, 10 mg

Adverse effects
(*italic* = common; **bold** = life-threatening)
CNS: Anxiety, paresthesia, fatigue, *dizziness,* headache
CV: Chest pain, hypertension
EENT: Vision abnormalities, xerophthalmia
GI: Nausea, vomiting, anorexia, abdominal pain, *constipation,* dry mouth, dyspepsia
GU: Dysuria, urinary retention, frequency, UTI
INTEG: Rash, pruritus
RESP: Bronchitis, cough, pharyngitis, URI

Contraindications: Hypersensitivity, uncontrolled narrow-angle glaucoma, urinary retention, gastric retention

Precautions: Pregnancy C, lactation,
P children, renal/hepatic disease, controlled narrow-angle glaucoma

Pharmacokinetics
Absorption	Rapid
Distribution	98% highly protein bound
Metabolism	Extensively metabolized by CYP3A4
Excretion	Excreted in urine/feces
Half-life	Terminal half-life 45-68 hr

Pharmacodynamics
Unknown

Interactions
Drug classifications
CYP3A4 inducers (ketoconazole): ↑ action of solifenacin (dose > 5 mg is not recommended)

NURSING CONSIDERATIONS
Assessment
- Assess urinary patterns: distention, nocturia, frequency, urgency, incontinence
- Assess for allergic reactions: rash; if this occurs, drug should be discontinued

Nursing diagnoses
✓ Urinary patterns, change in (uses)
✓ Knowledge, deficient (teaching)

Patient/family education
- Caution patient to avoid hazardous activities; dizziness may occur
- Advise patient that constipation, blurred vision may occur
- Instruct patient to call prescriber if severe abdominal pain or constipation lasts for 3 or more days
- Advise patient that heat prostration may occur if used in a hot environment

Evaluation
Positive therapeutic outcome
- Urinary status: dysuria, frequency, nocturia, incontinence

telithromycin (Rx)
(teh-lih-throw-my'sin)
Ketek
Func. class.: Antiinfective
Chem. class.: Ketolides

Pregnancy category C

Action: Binds to 50S ribosomal subunits of susceptible bacteria and suppresses protein synthesis

➡ Therapeutic Outcome: Bacterial action against *Streptococcus pneumoniae, Hae-*

mophilus influenzae, Moraxella catarrhalis, Staphylococcus aureus

Uses: Acute bacterial exacerbation of chronic bronchitis caused by *Streptococcus pneumoniae, Haemophilus influenzae, Moraxella catarrhalis*; acute bacterial sinusitis caused by *S. pneumoniae, H. influenzae, M. catarrhalis, Staphylococcus aureus*, community acquired pneumonic

Dosage and routes
Acute bacterial exacerbation of bronchitis
Adult: PO 800 mg daily × 5 days

Acute bacterial sinusitis
Adult: PO 800 mg daily × 5 days

Community-acquired pneumonia
Adult: PO 800 mg daily × 7-10 days

Available forms: Tabs 400 mg

Adverse effects
(*italic* = common; **bold** = life-threatening)
CNS: Dizziness, headache, insomnia, increased sweating
EENT: Blurred vision, diplopia, difficulty focusing
GI: *Nausea, vomiting, diarrhea*, hepatitis, abdominal pain/distension, stomatitis, anorexia
GU: *Vaginitis, moniliasis*
INTEG: Rash, urticaria
MISC: Atrial dysrythmias
MS: Muscle cramps
SYST: **Anaphylaxis**

Contraindications: Hypersensitivity

Precautions: Pregnancy **C**, lactation, children, elderly, myasthenia gravis, ongoing prodysrrhymias, hepatic disease

Pharmacokinetics	
Absorption	Unknown
Distribution	Protein binding 60%-70%
Metabolism	Liver
Excretion	Bile, feces
Half-life	Unknown

Pharmacodynamics	
Onset	Unknown
Peak	1 hr
Duration	Unknown

Interactions
Individual drugs
Atorvastatin, digoxin, ergots, lovastatin, metoprolol, midazolam, simvastatin, theophylline: ↑ action, toxicity

Pimozide: serious dysrhythmias; do not use together
Rifampin, phenytoin, carbamazepine, phenobarbital: ↓ action of telithromycin
Sotalol: ↓ action
Itraconazole, ketoconazole: ↑ telithromycin
Herb/drug
Do not use acidophilus with antiinfectives
Lab test interferences:
↑ AST/ALT

NURSING CONSIDERATIONS
Assessment
• Assess for infection: temp, sputum, WBCs, baseline and periodically
• Assess for oliguria in renal disease
• Monitor hepatic studies: AST, ALT, if patient is on long-term therapy
• Monitor C&S before drug therapy; drug may be given as soon as culture is taken; C&S may be repeated after treatment
• Monitor bowel pattern before, during treatment
• Assess for skin eruptions, itching

Nursing diagnoses
✓ Infection, risk for (uses)

Implementation
• May take without regard to food
• Store at room temperature
• Provide adequate intake of fluids (2 L) during diarrhea episodes

Patient/family education
• Teach patient to report sore throat, fever, fatigue (could indicate superinfection)
• Teach patient to notify nurse of diarrhea stools, dark urine, pale stools, jaundice of eyes or skin, and severe abdominal pain
• Teach patient to report blurred vision, if interfering with daily activities
• Advise patient to avoid driving, hazardous activities if blurred vision occurs
• Instruct patient to take as prescribed, do not double or skip doses
• Instruct patient not to use this drug if using Class 1A or III antidysrythmics
• Advise patient to avoid simvastatin, lovastatin or atorvastatin
• Inform patient that medication may be taken without regard to meals

Evaluation
Positive therapeutic outcome
• Decreased symptoms of infection

Treatment of hypersensitivity:
Withdraw drug; maintain airway; administer epINEPHrine, aminophylline, O_2, **IV** corticosteroids

tinidazole (Rx)
(tye-ni'da-zole)
Tindamax
Func. class.: Antiprotozoal
Chem. class.: Nitroimidazole derivative

Pregnancy category C

Action: Interferes with DNA/RNA synthesis in protozoa

→ **Therapeutic Outcome:** Decrease in infection

Uses: Amebiasis, giardiasis, trichomoniasis

Dosage and routes
Amebiasis
Adult: PO 2 g /day × 3-5 days

P *Child >3 yrs:* PO 50 mg/kg/day × 3-5 days, max 2 g

Giardiasis
Adult: PO 2 g as a single dose

P *Child >3 yrs:* PO 50 mg/kg as a single dose, max 2 g

Trichomoniasis
Adult: PO 2 g as a single dose

Available forms: Tabs 250, 500 mg

Adverse effects
(*italic* = common; **bold** = life-threatening)
CNS: *Dizziness, headache,* **seizures,** *peripheral neuropathy*
GI: *Nausea, vomiting,* anorexia, increased AST and ALT, constipation, abdominal pain
HEMA: **Leukopenia,** neutropenia
INTEG: Pruritus, urticaria, *rash,* oral monilia
SYST: **Angioedema**

Contraindications: Hypersensitivity to this product or nitroimidazole derivative, pregnancy 1st trimester

P **Precautions:** Pregnancy **C,** hepatic disease,
G lactation, children, elderly, CNS depression

Pharmacokinetics	
Absorption	Unknown
Distribution	Crosses blood/brain barrier
Metabolism	Extensively in the liver
Excretion	Unchanged (20-25%) in urine, (12%) feces
Half-life	12-14 hr

Pharmacodynamics
Unknown

Interactions
Individual drugs
Do not use within 2 wks of taking disulfiram
Cyclosporine, tacrolimus, fluorouracil, lithium: ↑ action
Drug classifications
CYP 3A4 inducers (phenobarbital, rifampin, phenytoin); cholestyramine, oxytetracycline: ↓ action of tinidazole
CYP 3A4 inhibitors (cimetidine, ketoconazole): ↑ action of tinidazole
Anticoagulants, hydantoins: ↑ action

NURSING CONSIDERATIONS
Assessment
• Assess for signs of infection, anemia
• Assess bowel pattern before, during treatment

Nursing diagnoses
☑ Infection, risk for (uses)
☑ Knowledge, deficient (teaching)

Implementation
PO route
• Administer to those over 3 yrs old

Patient/family education
• Instruct patient to take with food to increase plasma concentrations, minimize epigastric distress and other GI effects; not to use alcoholic beverages during or for 3 days afterward
• Advise patient that in cases of trichomoniasis, both partners should be treated

Evaluation
Positive therapeutic outcome
• Decreased in infection as evidenced by negative culture

tiotropium (Rx)
(ty-oh'tro-pee-um)
Spiriva
Func. class.: Anticholinergic, bronchodilator
Chem. class.: Synthetic quaternary ammonium compound

Pregnancy category C

Action: Inhibits interaction of acetylcholine at receptor sites on the bronchial smooth muscle, resulting in decreased cGMP and bronchodilation

→ **Therapeutic Outcome:** Improved breathing

Uses: COPD, for long term treatment, once daily maintenance of bronchospasm, associated with COPD including chronic bronchitis and emphysema

 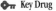

Dosage and routes
Adult: Inh content of 1 cap daily using HandiHaler inhalation device

Available forms: Powder for inhalation 18 mcg in blister packs containing 6 caps with inhaler

Adverse effects
(*italic* = common; **bold** = life-threatening)
CNS: Depression
CV: Chest pain, increased heart rate
EENT: Dry mouth, blurred vision, glaucoma
GI: Vomiting, abdominal pain, constipation, dyspepsia
INTEG: Rash
MISC: Urinary difficulty, urinary retention
RESP: Cough, worsening of symptoms, sinusitis, URI, epistaxis, pharyngitis

Contraindications: Hypersensitivity to this drug, atropine or its derivatives

Precautions: Pregnancy **C**, lactation, children, narrow-angle glaucoma, prostatic hypertrophy, bladder neck obstruction, elderly

Pharmacokinetics
Absorption	Unknown
Distribution	Does not cross blood-brain barrier
Metabolism	Very little metabolized in the liver
Excretion	Excreted in urine
Half-life	5-6 days in animals

Pharmacodynamics
Unknown

Interactions
Drug classifications
Anticholinergics: avoid use with other anticholinergics
Herb/drug
Black catechu: ↑ constipation
Jaborandi tree, pill-bearing spurge: ↓ anticholinergic effect
Butterbur, jimsonweed: ↑ anticholinergic effect
Green tea (large amts), guarana: ↑ bronchodilator effect

NURSING CONSIDERATIONS
Assessment
• For tolerance over long-term therapy; dose may have to be increased or changed

Nursing diagnoses
✓ Breathing pattern, ineffective (uses)
✓ Knowledge, deficient (teaching)

Implementation
• Caps are for INH only; do not swallow
• Immediately prior to administration, peel back foil until cap is visable; until "stop" line, open dust cap of HandiHaler by pulling upwards, then open mouthpiece
• Place cap in center chamber; firmly close mouthpiece until it clicks, leaving dust cap open
• Hold HandiHaler with mouthpiece upwards; press button in once, completely and release; this allows for medication to be released
• Breathe out completely; do not breathe into mouthpiece at any time
• Raise device to mouth and close lips tightly around mouthpiece
• With head upright, breathe in slowly/deeply, but allowing the cap to vibrate; breathe until lungs fill; hold breath and remove mouthpiece; resume normal breathing
• Repeat
• Remove used capsule and dispose; close the mouthpiece and dust cap; store.

Patient/family education
• Teach patient how to use Handihaler
• Teach patient signs of narrow angle glaucoma
• Advise patient that drug is used for long term maintenance, not for immediate relief of breathing problems
• Caution patient to avoid getting the powder in the eyes; may cause blurred vision and pupil dilation

Evaluation
Positive therapeutic outcome
• Ability to breathe easier

---

trospium (Rx)
(trose'pee-um)
Sanctura
Func. class.: Anticholinergic, overactive bladder product
Chem. class.: Muscarinic receptor antagonist

Pregnancy category C

Action: Relaxes smooth muscles in bladder by inhibiting acetylcholine effect on muscarinic receptors

Therapeutic Outcome: Absence of urinary distention, nocturia, frequency, urgency, incontinence

Uses: Overactive bladder (urinary frequency, urgency)

Dosage and routes
Adult: PO 20 mg bid, give 5 ml ≥ 1 hr prior to meals

Renal dose
Adult: PO CCr < 30 ml/min 20 mg daily at bedtime

Elderly ≥ 75 yrs: PO titrate down to 20 mg daily based on response and tolerance

Available forms: Tabs 20 mg

Adverse effects
(*italic* = common; **bold** = life-threatening)
CNS: Fatigue, dizziness, headache
EENT: Dry eyes, vision abnormalities
GI: Flatulence, abdominal pain, *constipation, dry mouth*, dyspepsia

Contraindications: Hypersensitivity, uncontrolled narrow-angle glaucoma, urinary retention, gastric retention

Precautions: Pregnancy **C**, lactation, children, renal/hepatic disease, controlled narrow-angle glaucoma, ulcerative colitis, intestinal atony, myasthenia gravis

Pharmacokinetics
Absorption	Rapidly absorbed (10%)
Distribution	Protein bound (50–85%)
Metabolism	Not fully understood in humans
	Extensively metabolized
Excretion	Urine (6%)/feces (85%)
	Excreted in urine by active tubular secretion
Half-life	Unknown

Pharmacodynamics
Unknown

Interactions
Individual drugs
Alcohol: ↑ drowsiness
Food/drug
High fat meal: ↓ absorption

NURSING CONSIDERATIONS
Assessment
• Assess urinary patterns: distention, nocturia, frequency, urgency, incontinence

Nursing diagnoses
☑ Urinary patterns, change in (uses)
☑ Knowledge, deficient (teaching)

Patient/family education
• Advise patient to avoid hazardous activities; dizziness may occur
• Instruct patient to take 1 hr prior to meals or on empty stomach
• Caution patient that alcohol may increase drowsiness
• Inform patient about anticholinergic effects that may occur

Evaluation
Positive therapeutic outcome
• Correction of urinary status: absence of dysuria, frequency, nocturia, incontinence